Principles and Practice of Particle Therapy

Principles and Practice of Particle Therapy

Edited by

Timothy D. Malouff and Daniel M. Trifiletti

Mayo Clinic
Jacksonville, Florida, USA

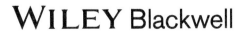

Registered Offices
John Wiley & Sons, Inc., 111 River Street, Hoboken, NJ 07030, USA
John Wiley & Sons Ltd, The Atrium, Southern Gate, Chichester, West Sussex, PO19 8SQ, UK

Editorial Office
9600 Garsington Road, Oxford, OX4 2DQ, UK

For details of our global editorial offices, customer services, and more information about Wiley products visit us at www.wiley.com.

Wiley also publishes its books in a variety of electronic formats and by print-on-demand. Some content that appears in standard print versions of this book may not be available in other formats.

Library of Congress Cataloging-in-Publication Data
Names: Malouff, Timothy D., editor. | Trifiletti, Daniel M., editor.
Title: Principles and practice of particle therapy / edited by Timothy D. Malouff, Daniel M. Trifiletti.
Description: Hoboken, NJ : John Wiley & Sons, 2022. | Includes bibliographical references and index.
Identifiers: LCCN 2021052728 (print) | LCCN 2021052729 (ebook) | ISBN 9781119707516 (hardback) | ISBN 9781119707400 (pdf) |
    ISBN 9781119707523 (epub) | ISBN 9781119707530 (ebook)
Subjects: LCSH: Radiotherapy.
Classification: LCC RM847 .P758 2022 (print) | LCC RM847 (ebook) | DDC 615.8/42--dc23/eng/20211116
LC record available at https://lccn.loc.gov/2021052728
LC ebook record available at https://lccn.loc.gov/2021052729

Cover image: © PopTika/Shutterstock
Cover design by Wiley

Set in 9.5/12.5pt STIXTwoText by Integra Software Services Pvt. Ltd, Pondicherry, India

SKYBAD5BA11-CF9A-4E73-B5CA-D30995F67F32_050522

Contents

Preface

Although radiation has been used therapeutically for over 100 years, we are currently in the midst of a renaissance in our field, especially with the use of particle irradiation. Over the past several years, access to particle therapy, whether it be proton therapy or heavy ion therapy, has increased dramatically. In the United States, more patients are able to benefit from proton therapy than ever before, with the number of centers and indications for proton therapy growing rapidly. Outside of the United States, many centers, including those in Japan and Germany, are gaining expertise as they push the envelope with carbon ion radiotherapy, something that was recently announced in the United States. There is also a renewed interest in using other heavy ions, and even combining radiation treatment modalities to improve oncologic outcomes while minimizing adverse effects.

With the widespread use of proton therapy worldwide, as well as growth of carbon ion therapy throughout Europe, Asia, and soon to be the United States, it became clear that a concise, yet comprehensive, resource was needed for the growing number of radiation oncologists treating with particle therapy. Our inspiration for *Principles and Practice of Particle Therapy* was exactly this – to provide a go-to, clinically oriented resource that can be referenced by both experienced clinicians and those who are just beginning their venture into particle therapy.

To meet this goal, our text is divided into three sections. In the first section, we discuss the most pertinent background information related to particle therapy. The clinically relevant physics, radiobiological, and practical aspects of developing a particle therapy program, including less-commonly discussed topics such as treatment planning software, are included. Our next section is one that focuses on "niche" treatments, many of which are still in their relative infancy, including FLASH, BNCT, and GRID therapy. A special focus is given to how these novel therapeutics can be implemented in the context of particle therapy. Our final section aims to be a clinical reference, organized by disease site, reviewing both the clinical data as well as providing a practical reference for practicing radiation oncologists. Each chapter includes discussions on the simulation process, target volume delineation, and unique treatment planning considerations for each disease site. When applicable, each clinical chapter also includes a discussion on less common ions, such as fast neutrons or helium, which we hope will become more pertinent as our understanding and experience of treating with heavy ions grows. The authors for each chapter were carefully chosen, and represent experts from around the world, and we hope their diversity of experiences in treating with particle therapy helps provide a framework in which to build your own practice.

We recognize that the field of particle therapy is evolving rapidly, and we hope this text will provide a guide map as to the next questions that should be asked in our understanding of the role of particle therapy in patient care. It is our sincere hope that our text will be obsolete in the near future, with well-designed trials and increased expertise in particle therapy answering many of the currently unanswered questions. Until that time, we hope this textbook provides insight and improves your ability to care for your patients, as this is the ultimate goal of our field.

List of Contributors

Armin R. Afshar, MD, MBA, MAS
Assistant Professor,
Department of Ophthalmology,
Wayne & Glady Valley Center for Vision, University of
California San Francisco, San Francisco,
CA, USA

Gregory Alexander, MD
Resident Physician, Department of Radiation Oncology,
University of Maryland School of Medicine,
Baltimore, MD, USA

Aman Anand, PhD
Assistant Professor, Department of Radiation Oncology,
Mayo Clinic, Phoenix, AZ, USA

Justin D. Anderson, MD
Resident Physician, Department of Radiation Oncology,
Mayo Clinic, Phoenix, AZ, USA

Jonathan B. Ashman, MD, PhD,
Assistant Professor, Department of Radiation Oncology,
Mayo Clinic, Phoenix, AZ, USA

Ronik S. Bhangoo, MD
Resident Physician, Department of Radiation Oncology,
Mayo Clinic, Phoenix, AZ, USA

Julie A. Bradley, MD
Associate Professor, Department of Radiation Oncology,
University of Florida College of Medicine,
Jacksonville, FL, USA

Martin Bues, PhD
Associate Professor,
Department of Radiation Oncology, Mayo Clinic,
Phoenix, AZ, USA

Justin Cohen, MD
Resident Physician, Department of Radiation Oncology,
University of Maryland School of Medicine,
Baltimore, MD, USA

Danielle A. Cunningham, MD
Resident Physician, Department of Radiation Oncology,
Mayo Clinic, Rochester, MN, USA

Bertil E. Damato, MD, PhD, FRCOphth
Professor, Oxford Eye Hospital,
University of Oxford, Oxford, UK

Xuanfeng Ding, PhD
Medical Physicist, Department of Radiation Oncology,
Beaumont Health System,
Oakland University William Beaumont School of Medicine,
Royal Oak, MI, USA

J. Michele Dougherty, PhD
Medical Physicist, Department of Radiation Oncology,
Mayo Clinic, Jacksonville, FL, USA

Daniel K. Ebner, MD, MPH
Resident Physician, Hospital of the National Institutes of
Quantum and Radiological Science and Technology (QST
Hospital), Chiba, Japan

Omar El Sherif, PhD
Clinical Medical Physicist, Department of Radiation Oncology,
Mayo Clinic, Rochester, MN, USA

Dr. Piero Fossati
Radiation Oncologist,
MedAustron Ion Therapy Center,
Wiener Neustadt, Austria

Keith M. Furutani, PhD
Associate Professor of Medical Physics, Department of
Radiation Oncology, Mayo Clinic,
Jacksonville, FL, USA

Fantine Giap, MD
Resident Physician, Department of Radiation Oncology,
University of Florida College of Medicine,
Jacksonville, FL, USA

Michael P. Grams, PhD
Assistant Professor of Medical Physics, Department of
Radiation Oncology, Mayo Clinic,
Rochester, MN, USA

Christopher L. Hallemeier, MD
Associate Professor, Department of Radiation Oncology,
Mayo Clinic, Jacksonville, FL, USA

Steven Herchko, DMP, MS
Instructor in Medical Physics,
Department of Radiation Oncology,
Mayo Clinic, Jacksonville, FL, USA

Prof. Dr. Eugen B. Hug
Medical Director, MedAustron Ion Therapy Center,
Wiener Neustadt, Austria

Daniel J. Indelicato, MD
Professor, Department of Radiation Oncology,
University of Florida College of Medicine,
Jacksonville, FL, USA

Elizabeth B. Jeans, MEd, MD
Resident Physician, Department of Radiation Oncology,
Mayo Clinic, Rochester, MN, USA

Krishnan R. Jethwa, MD
Assistant Professor, Department of Therapeutic Radiology,
Yale University School of Medicine,
New Haven, CT, USA

Peyman Kabolizadeh, MD, PhD
Director of Proton Therapy Center, Department of Radiation
Oncology, Beaumont Health System,
Oakland University William Beaumont School of Medicine,
Royal Oak, MI, USA

Andrzej Kacperek, PhD
Emeritus Physics, Clatterbridge Cancer Centre,
Wirral, UK

Rupesh Kotcha, MD
Assistant Professor, Department of Radiation Oncology,
Miami Cancer Institute, Baptist Health South Florida, Miami,
FL, USA and Herbert Wertheim College of Medicine, Florida
International University, Miami, FL, USA

Sunil Krishnan, MBBS, MD
Professor, Department of Radiation Oncology, Mayo Clinic,
Jacksonville, FL, USA

Anna Lee, MD, MPH
Assistant Professor, Department of Radiation Oncology,
University of Texas MD Anderson Cancer Center,
Houston, TX, USA

Nancy Y. Lee, MD, FASTRO
Vice Chair, Department of Radiation Oncology,
Memorial Sloan Kettering Cancer Center,
New York, NY, USA

Xiaoqiang Li, PhD
Medical Physicist, Department of Radiation Oncology,
Beaumont Health System, Oakland University William
Beaumont School of Medicine,
Royal Oak, MI, USA

Xingzhe (Dillion) Li, MD, MPH
Resident Physician, Department of Radiation Oncology,
Memorial Sloan Kettering Cancer Center,
New York, NY, USA

Xiaoying Liang, PhD
Associate Professor, Department of Radiation Oncology,
University of Florida College of Medicine,
Jacksonville, FL, USA

Steven H. Lin, MD, PhD
Associate Professor, Department of Radiation Oncology,
University of Texas MD Anderson Cancer Center,
Houston, TX, USA

Daniel J. Ma, MD
Associate Professor, Department of Radiation Oncology,
Mayo Clinic, Rochester,
MN, USA

Anita Mahajan, MD
Professor, Department of Radiation Oncology,
Mayo Clinic, Rochester, MN, USA

Raymond Mailhot Vega, MD, MPH
Assistant Professor, Department of Radiation Oncology,
University of Florida College of Medicine,
Jacksonville, FL, USA

Timothy D. Malouff, MD
Resident Physician, Department of Radiation Oncology,
Mayo Clinic, Jacksonville, FL, USA

Minesh P. Mehta, MD
Professor, Deputy Director, and Chief of Radiation Oncology,
Department of Radiation Oncology,
Miami Cancer Institute, Baptist Health South Florida,
Miami, FL, USA and Herbert Wertheim College of Medicine,
Florida International University,
Miami, FL, USA

Robert Miller, MD, MBA, FASTRO
Director, Division of Radiation Oncology,
UT Medical Center at the University of Tennessee,
Knoxville, TN, USA

Kavita K. Mishra, MD, MPH
Professor, Director, Ocular Tumor Radiation Therapy
Program, Department of Radiation Oncology,
University of California San Francisco,
San Francisco, CA, USA

Mark V. Mishra, MD
Associate Professor, Department of Radiation Oncology,
University of Maryland School of Medicine,
Baltimore, MD, USA

Osama Mohamad, MD, PhD
Assistant Professor, Department of Radiation Oncology,
University of California San Francisco,
San Francisco, CA, USA

Pranshu Mohindra, MD, MBBS
Associate Professor, Department of Radiation Oncology,
University of Maryland School of Medicine and Maryland
Proton Treatment Center, Baltimore, MD, USA

Sina Mossahebi, PhD
Physicist, Department of Radiation Oncology,
University of Maryland School of Medicine,
Baltimore, MD, USA

Matthew S. Ning, MD, MPH
Assistant Professor, Department of Radiation Oncology,
University of Texas MD Anderson Cancer Center,
Houston, TX, USA

Deanna Pafundi, PhD
Assistant Professor of Medical Physics,
Department of Radiation Oncology, Mayo Clinic,
Jacksonville, FL, USA

Chirayu G. Patel, MD, MPH
Instructor, Department of Radiation Oncology,
Massachusetts General Hospital, Boston, MA, USA

Ariel E. Pollock, MD
Resident Physician, Department of Radiation Oncology,
University of Maryland School of Medicine and
Maryland Proton Treatment Center,
Baltimore, MD, USA

Jill S. Remick, MD
Assistant Professor, Department of Radiation Oncology,
Winship Cancer Institute,
Emory University Hospital, Atlanta, GA, USA

Pouya Sabouri, PhD
Medical Physicist, Department of Radiation Oncology,
Miami Cancer Institute, Baptist Health South Florida,
Miami, FL, USA

Santanu Samanta, MD
Resident Physician, Department of Radiation Oncology,
University of Maryland Medical Center,
Baltimore, MD, USA

Jessica Scholey, MA
Clinical Instructor, Department of Radiation Oncology,
University of California San Francisco,
San Francisco, CA, USA

Danushka Seneviratne, MD, PhD
Resident Physician, Department of Radiation Oncology,
Mayo Clinic, Jacksonville, FL, USA

Christopher Serago, PhD
Associate Professor of Medical Physics, Department of
Radiation Oncology, Mayo Clinic,
Jacksonville, FL, USA

Sherif G. Shaaban, MB ChB
Resident Physician, Department of Radiation Oncology,
University of Minnesota,
Minneapolis, MN, USA

Jiajian (Jason) Shen, PhD
Associate Professor, Department of Radiation Oncology,
Mayo Clinic, Phoenix, AZ, USA

Makoto Shinoto, MD, PhD
Physician, Hospital of the National
Institutes of Quantum and Radiological Science and
Technology (QST Hospital), Chiba, Japan

Matthew Spraker, MD, PhD
Assistant Professor, Department of Radiation Oncology,
Washington University in St. Louis,
St. Louis, MO, USA

Cameron S. Thorpe, MD
Resident Physician, Department of Radiation Oncology,
Mayo Clinic, Phoenix, AZ, USA

Raees Tonse, MBBS
Clinical Research Fellow,
Department of Radiation Oncology,
Miami Cancer Institute, Baptist Health South Florida,
Miami, FL, USA

Daniel M. Trifiletti, MD
Associate Professor, Department of Radiation Oncology,
Mayo Clinic, Jacksonville, FL, USA

Yolanda D. Tseng, MD
Associate Professor, Department of Radiation Oncology,
University of Washington, Seattle, WA, USA

Dr. Slavisa Turbin
Radiation Oncologist, MedAustron Ion Therapy Center,
Wiener Neustadt, Austria

Carlos E. Vargas, MD
Associate Professor, Department of Radiation Oncology,
Mayo Clinic, Phoenix, AZ, USA

Vivek Verma, MD
Radiation Oncologist, Department of Radiation Oncology,
University of Texas MD Anderson Cancer Center,
Houston, TX, USA

Mark R. Waddle, MD
Assistant Professor, Department of Radiation Oncology,
Mayo Clinic, Rochester, MN, USA

Eric Welch, DMP
Clinical Medical Physicist,
Department of Radiation Oncology, Mayo Clinic, Rochester,
MN, USA

Shigeru Yamada, MD, PhD
Director of Department of Charged Particle Therapy
Research, Hospital of the National Institutes of Quantum and
Radiological Science and Technology (QST Hospital),
Chiba, Japan

James E. Younkin, PhD
Assistant Professor, Department of Radiation Oncology,
Mayo Clinic, Phoenix, AZ, USA

Elaine M. Zeman, PhD
Associate Professor, Department of Radiation Oncology,
University of North Carolina School of Medicine,
Chapel Hill, NC, USA

Foreword

Introduction: Improving Precision and Efficacy in Cancer Treatment

Eleanor A. Blakely

Particle radiotherapy for cancer treatment is a rapidly evolving field that has progressed significantly since its clinical origins using newly discovered radioisotopes within university chemistry and physics laboratories in Europe more than twelve decades ago. It is difficult to capture succinctly in a single textbook all of the educational background information available on this topic. *Principles and Practice of Particle Therapy* is intended to summarize the essential updated information one must master to practice the optimization of safely controlling precision non-invasive particle radiation applications to the human body for the purpose of eliminating disease.

The review of this specialty discipline includes the following topics: historical invention and development of accelerator-based radiation physics, creation and importance of patient imaging and immobilization approaches, progressive advancement of spatial- and time-dependent particle delivery options, overview of the discovery of underlying radiobiological principles at the molecular, cellular, tissue, and organismic levels, and understanding of quantitative theoretical modeling codes and treatment planning skills necessary to implement personalized particle therapies. Despite its still limited availability in the United States, the long journey bringing particle therapy to where it is today has been led by notable international giants in the multidisciplinary fields of radiation oncology and biophysics with an ultimate goal to improve precision and efficacy, and to reduce toxicities in cancer treatment.

Principles and Practice of Particle Therapy comprehensively and compactly provides an updated text for clinical education, training and a reference for radiation oncology with particle beams, and introduces a new generation of particle research pioneers. The text is divided into three sections: the first seven chapters review the historical background and status of essential scientific disciplines, followed by five chapters on special topics pertinent to particle therapy, including emerging novel approaches and technical improvements of established targeting therapies, and discussions of the fiscal impacts of particle therapy. Finally, the text concludes with fifteen chapters detailing approaches to treat individual tumor sites for which clinical experiences with the various particle therapy modalities from protons to heavy ions are increasing globally.

Exciting technological progress has been made in quantum imaging detection and mixed radiation field particle track visualization using the miniaturized ADVACAM MinPIX-TimePIX camera at CERN, NASA, and the European Space Agency for various applications, such as particle radiotherapy (see Figures 1 and 2 from Granja et al., Nuclear Inst. and Methods in Physics Research, A 2018, 908 60-71). Recent data measured at the NPI-CAC cyclotron Rez/Prague, and at the medical ion synchrotrons at HIT-Heidelberg/Germany and HIMAC-Chiba/Japan have been reported (see Figures 3 and 4 from Felix-Bautista et al., Med Phys, in Press 2021).

This work demonstrated non-invasive monitoring of pencil beam positions in an anthropomorphic head phantom with an observed *precision* that ranged from 0.61 to 1.49 mm and from 0.27 to 1.39 mm for the vertical and horizontal coordinates, respectively. The *accuracy* ranged from 0.49 to 1.24 mm and from 0.34 mm to 1.20 mm for the vertical and horizontal coordinates, respectively. These investigators indicate that their significant progress in enhancing the quantitation of particle precision demonstrated in passage through the absorbing range modification uncertainties introduced by a human phantom potentially will allow online monitoring in future clinical trials with particle therapy to improve efficacy. This will be a powerful tool for following generations of particle radiation oncologists, including those benefitting from the use of this insightful textbook.

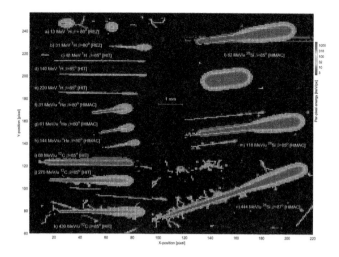

Figure 1   Taken from ADVACAM's public news announcement of their radiation cameras used for particle tracking (ADVACAM, August 31, 2018).

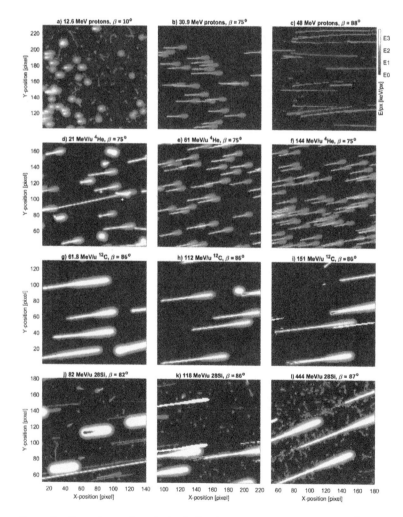

Figure 2   Detection and track simulation for protons (top row) and ions ^{4}He (2nd row), ^{12}C (3rd row), and ^{28}Si (bottom row) at selected energies and incident elevation angles. Equivalent regions of the pixelated sensor are shown (130 pixels x 130 pixels = approximately ¼ of the whole sensor size) for all data. Equal range of per-pixel energy response and area of the pixel matrix displayed for all data. All events registered are shown. Primary beam charged particles are registered as wide tracks of varying thickness and high values of per-pixel energy from protons up to heavy ions. Granja C. et al., (2018)/ Figure 4/with permission of Elsevier.

Ion Track Reconstruction and Back-projection

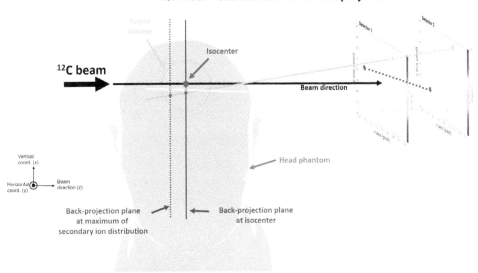

Figure 3 Representation of the ion hits matching (colored clusters of hit pixels), ion track reconstruction (colored dashed lines) and back-projection (colored solid lines) onto different planes perpendicular to the beam axis. The green circle represents the irradiated tumor volume. The figure is not drawn to scale. (Fig. 3 from Feliz-Bautista et al., 2021).

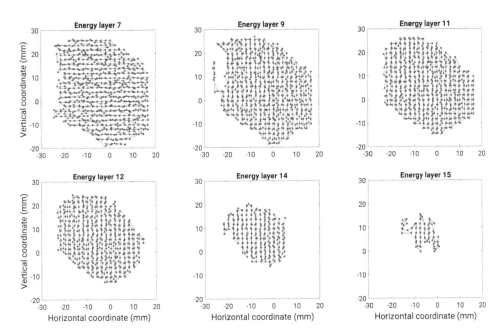

Figure 4 Examples of the reference (red dots) and the measured pencil beam positions (blue triangles) in the plane perpendicular to the carbon beam axis at a depth of 50 mm upstream of the isocenter. The scanning movements of the reference are well reproduced by the measured pencil beam positions. (Fig. 9 from Feliz-Bautista et al., 2021).

Abbreviations

2D:	2-Dimensional	ATP:	Adenosine Triphosphate
3D:	3-Dimensional	ATRT:	Atypical Teratoid Rhabdoid Tumor
3DCRT:	3-Dimensional conformal radiotherapy	AVF:	Azimuthally Varying Field
4D:	4-Dimensional	B:	Boron
4D-BsPTV:	4-Dimensional Beam Specific PTV	BBB:	Blood Brain Barrier
5-FU:	5-Fluorouracil	BCCA:	British Columbia Cancer Agency
6D:	6-Dimensional	BCG:	Bacillus Calmette-Guérin
A:	Atomic Mass	BCLC:	Barcelona Clinic Liver Cancer Staging System
AAPM:	American Association of Physicists in Medicine	BCS:	Breast Conserving Surgery
ABCS:	Active Breathing Controlled Spirometers	BCVA:	Best Corrected Visual Accuity
ABVD:	Adriamycin, Bleomycin, Vinblastine, Dacarbazine	BE:	Beryllium
		BEACOPP:	Bleomycin, Etoposide, Adriamycin, Cyclophosphamide, Oncovin, Procarbazine, Prednisone
ABVE-PC:	Adriamycin, Bleomycin, Vincristine, Etoposide, Prednisone, Cyclophosphamide	BED:	Biologically Effective Dose
ACC:	Adenoid Cystic Carcinoma	BID:	Twice Daily
ACNU:	Nimustine Hydrochloride	BMI:	Body Mass Index
ACR:	American College of Radiology	BNCT:	Boron Neutron Capture Therapy
ACROP:	Advisory Committee on Radiation Oncology Practice	BOPP:	Boronated Porphyrin
		bp:	Base Pair
ADT:	Androgen Deprivation Therapy	BPA:	Boronophenylalanine
AE:	Adverse Event	BS:	Bone Sarcoma
AER:	Absolute Excess Risk	BSH:	Sodium borocaptate
AFP:	Alpha-fetoprotein	BsPTV:	Beam-specific Planning Target Volume
AI:	Anterior Inferior	C:	Carbon
AJCC:	American Joint Commission on Cancer	CAD:	Coronary Artery Disease
ALARA:	As Low as Reasonably Achievable	CAPOX:	Capecitabine and Oxaliplatin
ALBI:	Albumin-Bilirubin Grade	CAR-T:	Chimeric Antigen Receptor T-cells
ALT:	Alanine Aminotransferase	CB:	Ciliary Body
AMU:	Atomic Mass Unit	CBCT:	Cone-beam Computed Tomography
AO:	Anterior Oblique	CDDP:	Cisplatin
AP:	Anteroposterior	CERN:	European Council for Nuclear Research
APC:	Antigen Presenting Cell	CGE:	Cobalt-Gray Equivalent
ART:	Adaptive Radiotherapy	cHL:	Classic Hodgkin Lymphoma
AST:	Aspartate Transaminase	CI:	Confidence Interval
ASTRO:	American Society for Radiation Oncology	CIRT:	Carbon Ion Radiotherapy
		CLSS :	Continuous Line Scanning System

CMMI:	Center for Medicare and Medicaid Innovation
CMS:	Center for Medicare and Medicaid Services
CNAO:	National Centre for Oncological Hadrontherapy
CNS:	Central Nervous System
Co:	Cobalt
COG:	Children's Oncology Group
COMS:	Collaborative Ocular Melanoma Study
CONV RT:	Conventional radiotherapy
COPDAC:	Cyclophosphamide, Oncovin, Prednisone, Dacarbazine
CP:	Child-Pugh Score
CPT:	Charged Particle Therapy
CPT:	Current Procedural Terminology
CRC:	Colorectal Cancer
CSC:	Cancer Stem-like Cells
CSF:	Cerebrospinal Fluid
CSI:	Craniospinal Irradiation
CSS:	Cause-Specific Survival
CT:	Computed Tomography
CTCAE:	Common Terminology Criteria for Adverse Events
CTL:	Cytotoxic T Lymphocytes
CTLA-4:	Cytotoxic T-Lymphocyte Antigen 4
CTV:	Clinical Target Volume
CVD:	Cardiovascular Death
DAMPS:	Danger Associated Molecular Patterns
DC:	Dendritic Cell
DET:	Distal Edge Tracking
DFS:	Disease-free Survival
DIBH:	Deep Inspiration Breath Hold
DICOM:	Digital Imaging and Communications in Medicine
DKFZ:	German Center for Cancer Research
DLBCL:	Diffuse Large B-cell Lymphoma
DLCO:	Diffusing Capacity for Carbon Monoxide
DM:	Distant Metastasis
DMFS:	Distant Metastasis-Free Survival
DNA:	Deoxyribonucleic Acid
DO:	Density-Override
DSB:	Double-strand break
DSS:	Disease Specific Survival
DTC:	Differentiated Thyroid Cancer
DVH:	Dose-Volume Histogram
EBM:	Evidence-Based Medicine
EBRT:	External Beam Radiation Therapy
EBV:	Epstein-Barr Virus
ECOG:	Eastern Cooperative Oncology Group
EFS:	Event-free Survival
EGFR:	Epidermal Growth Factor Receptor
EHCC:	Extrahepatic Cholangiocarcinoma
ELST:	Energy Layer Switching Time
EOR/Gy:	Excessive Odds Ratio Per Gray
EORTC:	European Organisation for Research and Treatment of Cancer
EPIC:	Expanded Prostate Cancer Index Composite
EQD2:	Equivalent Dose in 2 Gray
ERCP:	Endoscopic Retrograde Cholangiopancreatography
ERR:	Excess Relative Risk
ERS:	Extended Range Shifter
ESCC:	Esophageal Squamous Cell Carcinoma
ESFT:	Ewing Sarcoma Family of Tumors
ESMO:	European Society for Medical Oncology
ESR:	Erythrocyte Sedimentation Rate
ESS:	Energy Selection System
ESTRO:	European Society for Radiotherapy and Oncology
EUS:	Endoscopic Ultrasound
eV:	Electronvolts
EVH:	Error Bar Volume Histogram
FACT-P:	Functional Assessment of Cancer Therapy for Prostate Cancer Patients
FDA:	Food and Drug Administration
FDG:	Fluorodeoxyglucose
FFCD:	Fédération Francophone de Cancérologie Digestive
FFDR:	Freedom from Distant Recurrence
FFLP:	Freedom from Local Progression
FFLR:	Freedom from Locoregional Recurrence
FFRR:	Freedom from Regional Recurrence
FISH:	Fluorescent *in-situ* Hybridization
FLAIR:	Fluid Attenuated Inversion Recovery
FLR:	Future Liver Remnant
FLT:	Flourothymidine
FNT:	Fast Neutron Therapy
FOLFIRINOX:	Folinic Acid, Fluorouracil, Irinotecan, Oxaliplatin
FOLFOX:	Folinic acid, Fluorouracil, Oxaliplatin
FRAX:	Fracture Risk Assessment Tool
FSRT:	Fractionated Stereotactic Radiotherapy
FU:	Follow Up
Fx:	Fraction
G:	Grade
GBCA:	Gallbladder Cancer
GBM:	Glioblastoma
GEM:	Genetically Engineered Mouse
GEP:	Gene Expression Profile
GETUG:	Genitourinary Group

gEUD: Generalized Equivalent Uniform Dose
GI: Gastrointestinal
GIST: Gastrointestinal Stroma Tumor
GSI: Gesellschaft für Schwerionenforschung
GTR: Gross Total Resection
GTV: Gross Tumor Volume
GU: Genitourinary
Gy (RBE):   Gray, Relative Biological Effectiveness
Gy: Gray
GyE: Gray Equivalent
H&N: Head and Neck
H: Hydrogen
HBV: Hepatitis B Virus
HCC: Hepatocellular Carcinoma
HCL: Harvard Cyclotron Laboratory
HCP: Heavy Charged Particles
HCV: Hepatitis C Virus
He: Helium
HF: Hypofractionation
HFPV: High-frequency Percussive Ventilation
HFV: High-frequency Ventilation
HGG: High-grade Gliomas
HIF-1α: Hypoxia-inducible Factor 1-alpha
HIMAC: Heavy Ion Medical Accelerator in Chiba
HIT: Heidelberg Ion Beam Therapy Center
HL: Hodgkin Lymphoma
HMA: Homovanillic Acid
HMGB1:   High Mobility Group Protein B1
HNC: Head and Neck Cancer
HNSCC: Head and Neck Squamous Cell Carcinoma
HPV: Human Papillomavirus
HR: Hazard Ratio
HR: Homologous Recombination
HSG: Human Salivary Gland
HT: Helical Therapy
HU: Hounsfield Units
ICD: Immunogenic Cell Death
ICER: Institute for Clinical and Economic Review
ICRU: International Commission on Radiation Units & Measurements
iCTV: Internal Clinical Target Volume
IDH: Isocitrate Dehydrogenase
IFRT: Involved Field Radiation Therapy
IFSO: Individual Field Simultaneous Optimization
IGF: Insulin Growth Factor
IGRT: Image guided radiotherapy
iGTV: Internal Gross Tumor Volume
IHCC: Intrahepatic Cholangiocarcinoma
IL: Interleukin

ILROG: International Lymphoma Radiation Oncology Group
IMPT: Intensity Modulated Proton Therapy
IMPT-PBS: Intensity Modulated Proton Therapy Pencil Beam Scanning
IMRT: Intensity Modulated Radiation Therapy
INRGSS: International Neuroblastoma Risk Group Staging System
INRT: Involved Node Radiation Therapy
INSS: International Neuroblastoma Staging System
IOERT: Intraoperative Electron Radiotherapy
IR: Ionizing Radiation
IRB: Institutional Review Board
IRSG: Intergroup Rhabdomyosarcoma Study Group
IS: Interstitial
ISRT: Involved Site Radiation Therapy
ITV: Internal Target Volume
IV: Intravenous
J-CROS: Japan Carbon-Ion Radiation Oncology Group
JPY: Japanese Yen
keV: Kiloelectronvolts
KPS: Karnofsky Performance Status
kV: Kilovolt
LAD: Left Anterior Descending Artery
LAO: Left Anterior Oblique
LAPC: Locally Advanced Pancreatic Cancer
LAT1:   L-type amino acid transporter
LBNL: Lawrence Berkley National Laboratory
LC: Local Control
LCD: Local Coverage Determination
LDH: Lactate Dehydrogenase
LED: Light-Emitting Diode
LEM: Local Effect Model
LET: Linear Energy Transfer
LET_D: Dose-Averaged Linear Energy Transfer
LGG: Low-grade Glioma
Li: Lithium
LI-RADS: Liver Imaging Reporting and Data System
LMA: Large Mediastinal Adenopathy
LN: Lymph nodes
LOH: Loss of Heterozygosity
LQ: Linear Quadratic
LRC: Locoregional Control
LRF: Locoregional Failure
LRPFS: Locoregional Progression Free Survival
LRR: Locoregional Recurrence
LRRC: Locally Recurrent Rectal Cancer
LRT: Lattice Radiotherapy
LS-SCLC: Limited-Stage Small Cell Lung Cancer

LVSI:	Lymphovascular Space Invasion	NASA:	National Aeronautics and Space Administration
LYL:	Life Years Lost	NASH:	Nonalcoholic Steatohepatitis
MAC:	Medicare Administrative Contractors	NBL:	Neuroblastoma
MALT:	Mucosa-Associated Lymphoid Tissue	NCCN:	National Comprehensive Cancer Network
MAP:	Methotrexate, Adriamycin, Cisplatin	NCD:	National Coverage Determination
MAPKs:	Mitogen Activated Protein Kinase	NCDB:	National Cancer Database
MBRT:	Microbeam Radiotherapy	NCF:	Neurocognitive Function
MC:	Monte Carlo	NCI CTC:	National Cancer Institute Common Toxicity Criteria
MDACC:	MD Anderson Cancer Center		
MDASI:	MD Anderson Symptom Inventory	NCI:	National Cancer Institute
MDM:	Monocyte-derived Macrophages	NCT:	Neutron Capture Therapy
MDSC:	Myeloid-derived Suppressor Cells	N_e:	Electron Density
MEE:	Multiple Energy Extraction	NED:	No Evidence of Disease
MELD:	Model for End-Stage Liver Disease	NF-κB:	Nuclear Factor-κB
MELE:	Multi-energy Layer Extraction	NGGCT:	Non-Germinomatous Germ Cell Tumors
MeV:	Millielectronvolt	NGS:	Next-Generation Sequencing
MFH:	Malignant Fibrous Histiocytosis	NHEJ:	Non-homologous end joining
MFO:	Multi-Field Optimization	NIDCR:	National Institute of Dental and Cranial Research
MG:	Microglia		
MGH:	Massachusetts General Hospital	NIH:	National Institute of Health
MHC:	Major Histocompatibility Complex	NIRS:	National Institute of Radiological Sciences
MHD:	Mean Heart Dose		
MI:	Myocardial Infarction	NK:	Natural Killer Cells
MIBC:	Muscle Invasive Bladder Cancer	NMSC:	Non-melanomatous Skin Cancer
MIBG:	Metaiodobenzylguanidine	NO:	Nitric Oxide
MID:	Minimally Important Difference	NPC:	Nasopharyngeal Cancer
MIP:	Maximal Intensity Projection	NPX:	Nasopharyngeal
MKM:	Microdosimetric Kinetic Model	NR:	Not Reported
MLC:	Multi-leaf Collimator	NRG:	National
MLD:	Mean Liver Dose	ns:	Not Significant
MLIC:	Multi-layer Ionization Chambers	NSABP:	National Surgical Adjuvant Breast and Bowel Project
MLPA:	Multiplex Ligation-dependent Probe Amplification		
MM:	Motion Management	NSC:	Neural Stem Cells
MMP:	Matrix Metalloproteinase	NSCLC:	Non-Small Cell Lung Cancer
Mo:	Month	NSRL:	NASA Space Radiation Laboratory
MPM:	Malignant Pleural Mesothelioma	NTCP:	Normal Tissue Complication Probability
MPNST:	Malignant Peripheral Nerve Sheath Tumor	NVG:	Neovascular Glaucoma
		OAR:	Organ at Risk
MRCP:	Magnetic Resonance Cholangiopancreatography	OCT:	Optical Coherence Tomography
		OEPA:	Oncovin, Etoposide, Prednisolone, Adriamycin
MRI:	Magnetic Resonance Imaging		
MRT:	Microbeam Radiation Therapy	OER:	Oxygen Enhancement Ratio
MSK:	Memorial Sloan Kettering Cancer Center	OM:	Ocular Melanoma
		ON:	Optic Nerve
MU:	Monitor Unit	ONB:	Olfactory Neuroblastoma
MV:	Millivolt	OPC:	Oropharyngeal Cancer
MVA:	Multivariate Analysis	OPSCC:	Oropharyngeal Squamous Cell Carcinoma
MWA:	Microwave Ablation		
N:	Nitrogen	OR:	Odds Ratio
N_A:	Avogadro's Number	ORN:	Osteoradionecrosis
NAFLD:	Nonalcoholic Fatty Liver Disease		

OS: Overall Survival
OTV: Optimization Target Volume
PA: Posteroanterior
PBA: Pencil Beam Analytical
PBI: Partial Breast Irradiation
PBRT: Proton Beam Radiation Therapy
PBS: Pencil Beam Scanning
PBT: Proton Beam Therapy
PCG: Proton Collaborative Group
PCORI: Patient-Centered Outcomes Research Institute
pCR: Pathologic Complete Response
pCT: Proton Computed Tomography
PD-1: Programmed Cell Death Protein 1
PDD: Percent Depth Dose
PDL-1: Programmed Death Ligand 1
PET: Positron Emission Tomography
PFS: Progression Free Survival
PI3K: Phosphatidylinositide 3-kinase
PIDE: Particle Irradiation Data Ensemble
pMBRT: Proton Minibeam Radiation Therapy
PNET: Primitive Neuroectodermal Tumors
PO: Posterior Oblique
POG: Pediatric Oncology Group
PR: Partial Response
PR: Pathological Response
PRAME: Preferentially Expressed Antigen in Melanoma
pRG: Proton Radiography
PRO: Patient Reported Outcomes
PRV: Planning Organ-at-risk Volume
PSA: Prostate-specific Antigen
PSC: Primary Sclerosing Cholangitis
PSI: Paul Scherrer Institute
PSPT: Passive Scatter Proton Therapy
PSQA: Patient Specific Quality Assurance
PT: Particle Therapy
PTCOG: Particle Therapy Co-Operative Group
PTV: Planning Target Volume
QA: Quality Assurance
QACT: Quality Assurance Computed Tomography
QALY: Quality-Adjusted Life-Years
QD: Once Daily
QOL: Quality-of-life
QS: Quad Shot
QST: National Institutes of Quantum and Radiological Science and Technology
QUANTEC: Quantitative Analysis of Normal Tissue Effects
r/r: Relapsed/Refractory
RAI: Radioactive Iodine

RAO: Right Anterior Oblique
RB: Retinoblastoma
RBE: Relative Biological Effectiveness
RC: Regional Control
RCT: Radio(chemo)therapy
RCT: Randomized Controlled Trials
RECIST: Response Evaluation Criteria In Solid Tumours
RF: Radiofrequency
RFA: Radiofrequency Ablation
RFS: Relapse-free Survival
RIBC: Radiation Induced Brain Changes
RIBE: Radiation-induced Bystander Effects
RILD: Radiation-Induced Liver Disease
RION: Radiation Induced Optic Neuropathy
RMS: Rhabdomyosarcoma
RNI: Regional Nodal Irradiation
RO-APM: Radiation Oncology Alternative Payment Model
ROS: Reactive Oxygen Species
RP: Radiation Pneumonitis
RPA: Recursive Partitioning Analysis
RPO: Right Posterior Oblique
RPS: Retroperitoneal Sarcoma
RR: Radiological Response
RR: Relative Risk
RS: Repair Saturation
RSP: Relative Stopping Power
RT: Radiotherapy
RTOG: Radiation Therapy Oncology Group
RT-PCR: Reverse Transcription Polymerase Chain Reaction
RVH: Root Mean Square Deviation Dose Volume Histogram
S: Stopping Power
SABR: Stereotactic Ablative Radiotherapy
SBRT: Stereotactic Body Radiotherapy
SCC: Squamous Cell Carcinoma
SCLC: Small Cell Lung Cancer
SEER: Surveillance, Epidemiology, and End Results Program
SFO: Single-Field Optimization
SFRT: Spatially Fractionated Radiotherapy
SFUD: Single Field Uniform Dose
SGRT: Surface-guided Radiation Therapy
SIB: Simultaneous Integrated Boost
SIOPE: European Society for Paediatric Oncology
SIRT: Selective Internal Radiotherapy
SLD: Sublethal Damage
SOBP: Spread-out Bragg Peak
SPArc: Spot Scanning Proton Arc Therapy
sPBT: Scanning Proton Beam Therapy

SPECT:	Single Photon Emission Computed Tomography	TURBT:	Transurethral Resection of Bladder Tumor
SPHIC:	Shanghai Proton and Heavy Ion Center	TURP:	Transurethral Resection of the Prostate
SPR:	Stopping Power Ratio	UCLBL:	University of California Lawrence Berkeley Laboratory
SRS:	Stereotactic Radiosurgery	UCSF:	University of California San Francisco
SSB:	Single-strand breaks	UFPTI:	University of Florida Proton Therapy Institute
SSD:	Source Surface Distance		
SST:	Spot Scanning Time	UK:	United Kingdom
STING:	Stimulator of Interferon Genes	UM:	Uveal Melanoma
STR:	Subtotal Resection	UNOS:	United Network for Organ Sharing
STS:	Soft-Tissue Sarcoma	UPS:	Undifferentiated Pleomorphic Sarcoma
STV:	Scanning Target Volume	US:	Ultrasound
SUV:	Standardized Uptake Value	US:	United States
SWOG:	Southwest Oncology Group	USD:	United States Dollars
TA:	Tumor Antigens	UT:	University of Texas
TACE:	Transarterial Chemoembolization	UTI:	Urinary Tract Infections
TAE:	Transarterial embolization	UV:	Ultraviolet
TAM:	Tumor-Associated Macrophages	VA:	Visual Acuity
TARE:	Transarterial Radioembolization	VAC:	Vincristine, Actinomycin-D, Cyclophosphamide
TCP:	Tumor Control Probability		
TGF-β:	Tumor Growth Factor- β	VEGF:	Vascular Endothelial Growth Factor
TIL:	Tumor Infiltrating Lymphocytes	VMA:	Vanillylmandelic Acid
TIVA:	Total Intravenous Anesthesia	VMAT:	Volumetric Modulated Arc Therapy
TLN:	Temporal Lobe Necrosis	WBC:	White Blood Cell
TNFα:	Tumor necrosis factor alpha	WEPL:	Water Equivalent Path Length
TPS:	Treatment Planning System	WET:	Water-Equivalent Thickness
TRAIL:	Tumor Necrosis Factor Related Apoptosis-Inducing Ligand	WHO:	World Health Organization
		Y:	Yttrium
Tregs:	Suppressive Regulatory T Cells	Z:	Atomic Number
TTB:	Total Toxicity Burden		

Section I

Background

1

A Brief History of Particle Radiotherapy

Timothy D. Malouff, Christopher Serago, and Daniel M. Trifiletti

Department of Radiation Oncology, Mayo Clinic Florida Address: 4500 San Pablo Road South, Jacksonville, FL, USA 32224

1.1 History of the Clinical Use of Particles

One of the most revolutionary events in the history of medicine was the discovery of X-rays by Wilhelm Röntgen in 1895 [1]. Within 2 months of their discovery, they were used experimentally for diagnostic imaging, as well as the treatment of a multitude of malignant and benign diseases, to varying degrees of success [1,2]. Since that time, the indications for radiation therapy have become better established, with an estimated 60% of cancer patients receiving radiation as part of their treatment course [3]. Corresponding to this increase in usage of radiation therapy over the past century, there have been a multitude of technological advances aimed at improving the "therapeutic window" of radiotherapy, whereby the efficacy of treatment is maximized and the toxicity is minimized, leading to the development of high-energy accelerators and techniques such as intensity-modulated radiation therapy (IMRT). At its heart, the use of particle therapy for therapeutic purposes attempts to maximize the "therapeutic window" and provide highly efficacious therapies with a greater degree of safety.

Occurring at approximately the same time as Röntgen's experiments with X-ray irradiation, Ernest Rutherford made a discovery that would revolutionize our understanding of chemistry and physics: the proton. Hans Wilhelm Geiger and Sir Ernest Marsden, while working in Rutherford's lab, conducted experiments with alpha particles shot into a sheet of metal foil. Based on the reflected angles of the alpha particles,

Rutherford hypothesized that the alpha particles, and therefore atoms, contained a positively charged central structure of large size that was surrounded by negatively charged particles [1]. Rutherford continued his work after World War I, when he irradiated nitrogen gas with alpha particles, creating oxygen and dense hydrogen nuclei. Based on this reaction, he concluded that nitrogen must contain hydrogen nuclei, which he named "proton," based on the Greek word for "first." [1,4].

Though the existence of neutrons was hypothesized by Rutherford in 1923, it was not until later that the idea of the neutron was formalized. Walther Wilhelm Georg Franz Both and Herbert Becker created a radiation beam that was more penetrating than gamma rays by using alpha particles shot at boron and beryllium, and the subsequent work by Joliot-Curies and Sir James Chadwick formally identified the neutron [1].

The physical advantages of proton and heavy ion radiation for therapeutic purposes began to be understood in 1904, when Sir William Henry Bragg reported on the characteristic energy deposition for charged particles in a given medium in which a small amount of energy is deposited entering the tissue, with a large amount deposited at the distal portion of the path. This "Bragg-peak" remains one of the defining physical and dosimetric advantages when using particle therapy [1,2,5].

Clinically, charged particles have been used for over 60 years. With the discovery of a method to accelerate particles

Principles and Practice of Particle Therapy, First Edition. Edited by Timothy D. Malouff and Daniel M. Trifiletti.
© 2022 John Wiley & Sons Ltd. Published 2022 by John Wiley & Sons Ltd.

without the use of high voltage, Earnest O. Lawrence helped develop the first cyclotron in 1929. Interestingly, the first model of the cyclotron was only 4 in. in diameter and was featured on a cover of *Time*. Larger cyclotrons were eventually constructed at the University of California Berkeley, and, in 1938, 24 patients were treated with a single fraction of fast neutron therapy using a 37-in. cyclotron. The early successes of these treatments led to a total of 226 patients treated with fast neutrons from 1938 to 1943 [2], although the toxicities were later judged to be too severe to continue treatment [6]. Although the concerns of fast neutron therapy led to the decrease in use in the US, Gerald Kruger, in 1938, hypothesized that tumors can be treated with alpha particles emitted from boron when irradiated with neutrons [2]. This technique, which is now known as "boron neutron capture therapy," is gaining interest and is discussed extensively in subsequent sections of this text.

Fast-neutron therapy enjoyed a reemergence in the late 1960s, with the development of the cyclotron at the Hammersmith Hospital in London. Based on this, the US National Cancer Institute began funding research at the University of Washington in Seattle, Washington, in 1971. Initially, five cyclotrons were to be used in clinical trials, mostly based out of physics laboratories. In 1984, the University of Washington was brought into service, although development of clinical equipment at the other sites was hampered due to financial problems [7]. Today, the University of Washington is the only site in the US treating with fast neutron therapy, most commonly for locally advanced and unresectable salivary gland tumors.

1.2 History of Proton Therapy

In his innovative paper published in 1946, Dr. Robert R. Wilson proposed the use of accelerated protons, and heavy ions, for oncologic treatment in humans [2,8]. Given the high energy needed to accelerate heavy ions, a 184-in. synchrocyclotron was developed at Berkley in 1947, which was subsequently used by Cornelius Tobias and John Lawrence in animal models with some success [2,4,9].

This preclinical work led to the first patients treated with proton therapy in Berkley in 1954. The first patient treated with proton therapy was a patient with widely metastatic breast cancer who underwent pituitary irradiation, mirroring earlier experiments with pituitary irradiation in a dog model [2,4]. The pituitary provided an ideal location to treat, as it could be located readily using orthogonal X-ray films and rigid immobilization [4]. Although she initially responded well to therapy, she unfortunately died several months after treatment [2,10]. Furthermore, approximately 700 patients with acromegaly were treated with proton therapy [11]. In 1957, the use of proton therapy at Berkley was discontinued and the

accelerator began to be used as a source of helium ions and other heavy charged particles until the particle treatment program was discontinue in 1992 [12]. In total, approximately 2,000 patients were treated at Berkley with protons, helium, and other heavy charged particles [13].

Given these early successes, another particle beam facility was developed in Uppsala, Sweden (now the Svedberg Laboratory), at the Gustaf Werner Institute where Sture Falkmer, Bertil Fors, Borje Larsson, and colleagues treated their first patient with proton therapy in 1957 [14]. Borje Larson, Lars Leksel, and colleagues described some of their first proton irradiation experiments of animals in their impactful manuscript in *Nature* in 1958 [15]. The early work at Uppsala used a 195-MeV synchrocyclotron beam, and the early, if not first, range modulator or "ridge-filter" described by Wilson was used to spread out the Bragg peak to produce a large uniform dose [16].

Subsequently, approximately 9,000 patients were treated at the Harvard Cyclotron Laboratory (HCL) in collaboration with Massachusetts General Hospital (MGH) from its opening in 1961 until closing in 2002. The Harvard cyclotron was built in 1949 under the leadership of Robert Wilson following the publication of his seminal paper in 1946 [8]. The Harvard cyclotron produced a fixed-beam 90-MeV proton beam which increased to 160 MeV in 1956 and was used for physics research until 1961 when it was modified for clinical use [17]. Raymond Kjellberg and William Sweet, two MGH neurosurgeons, began the clinical use of HCL proton beam for single fraction treatment of small intracranial tumors, arteriovenous malformations, and other neurological indications [18–20]. In late 1973 and early 1974, Herman Suit, Michael Goitein, and colleagues from the MGH Department of Radiation Oncology initiated treatment of large fields using fractionated therapy [21,22]. Their proton treatments included innovations such as a 6D couch (Figure 1.1), vertical CT scanner for

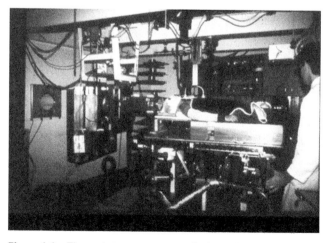

Figure 1.1 The early treatment room for large field treatments at the Harvard Cyclotron Laboratory.

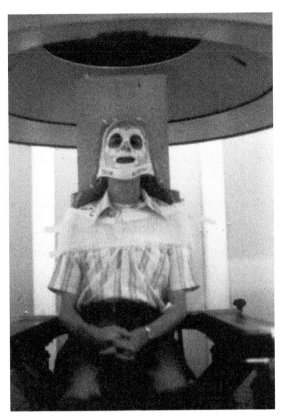

Figure 1.2 A vertical CT scanner for patients treated in the seated position. Treatment in the seated position allows for more comfortable treatment positions, as well as reproducibility, when using a fixed beam for treatment. This technique became largely obsolete following the development of rotating gantries, although there has been renewed support for treating patients in the seated position with the increasing use of fixed-beam heavy ions.

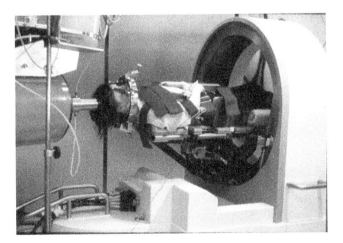

Figure 1.3 An early patient treated for an intracranial malignancy with protons at the Harvard Cyclotron Laboratory with the STereotactic Alignment Radiosurgery (STAR) isocenter patient immobilization and positioning device. The "fixed beam" required the patients to be rotated to allow multiple beam angles. Subsequent developments led to rotating gantries, rendering these current setups obsolete for proton therapy.

treatment in the seated position (Figure 1.2), daily bi-planer radiographs, three-dimensional treatment planning with heterogeneity, beams eye view, dose volume histogram, and calculation of dose uncertainty. Techniques for flattening the proton beam and modulating the range of the beam were developed by Andreas Koehler [23,24]. Advances to the intracranial proton radiosurgery program, such as the novel patient alignment system (Figure 1.3), were made when Paul Chapman and colleagues in neurosurgery at MGH began collaborating with their colleagues in radiation oncology in the early 1990s. Another significant HCL/MGH clinical program was the treatment of uveal melanoma under the guidance of the Massachusetts Eye and Ear Infirmary ophthalmologist Evangelos Gragoudas [25]. The HCL ceased treating patients when the hospital-based proton facility, the Francis H. Burr Proton Therapy Center, at MGH commenced operations in late 2001.

In Russia, the Institute for Theoretical and Experimental Physics opened in Moscow in 1967 [4]. Multiple other centers throughout the world were developed in the following years, and, as of June 2020, over 90 centers worldwide had proton treating capabilities [26] (Figure 1.4).

The world's first hospital based-proton facility was developed by Dr. James Slater at the Loma Linda University Medical Center in 1990 [27]. The proton facility at Loma Linda was the first to use a variable energy 250 MeV synchrotron designed and built by Fermi National Laboratory that was dedicated to medical research and clinical use and included four treatment rooms with three rotating gantries and one fixed-beam line. The fixed-beam line was primarily used for treatment of the eye. To date, more than 21,000 patients have been treated with proton therapy at Loma Linda [2,4].

Perhaps one of the most influential events in the history of particle therapy in the US is the development of proton-specific procedure codes from the American Medical Association, as it indirectly allowed for the expansion of this technology in the US. Prior to the late 1990s, treatment with proton irradiation was considered "experimental" by Medicare and other US insurance carriers, limiting reimbursement. With the approval of proton-specific procedure codes, an effort spearheaded by Loma Linda and Massachusetts General Hospital, the reimbursement rates for patients receiving proton therapy were set by Medicare. With the adoption of the Medicare reimbursement model, proton therapy was no longer considered an experimental therapy, and many private and academic hospitals in the US invested in the technology given the financial incentives [4].

With the concurrent development of protocols involving proton therapy, as well as technological advancements in both treatment planning software and advanced delivery techniques, proton therapy has become a standard option in many centers.

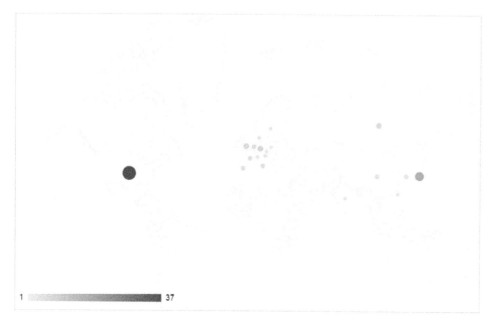

Figure 1.4 Location of Proton Therapy Centers Currently Treating as of June 2020. The reader is referred to the Particle Therapy Co-Operative Group (https://www.ptcog.ch/index.php/facilities-in-operation) for the most up-to-date listing of current and planned centers. Based on [26].

1.3 History of Carbon Ion Therapy

Following the success of his early manuscript, Wilson would later hypothesize that carbon ion radiotherapy was superior to proton radiotherapy [2]. This concept was tested in 1977, when the first patients were treated with carbon ion radiotherapy as part of phase I trials at the Lawrence Berkley National Laboratory (LBNL) [12,28,29]. Although the majority of patients treated at LBNL were with helium and neon ions, the encouraging results from the carbon-ion studies inspired researchers in Japan to further investigate carbon ion therapy. The first heavy ion accelerator in the world, called the Heavy Ion Medical Accelerator in Chiba (HIMAC), was developed at the National Institute of Radiological Sciences in Chiba, Japan, and began treating patients in 1994 [30]. As of June 2012, approximately 6,500 patients were treated with carbon ion therapy in Chiba, and approximately 91% of patients treated with carbon ion radiotherapy occurred in Japan [2]. In Germany, the Gesellschaft für Schwerionenforschung (GSI) began treating patients with carbon ion radiotherapy in 1997 [31]. Haberer et al. developed the active beam scanning method at GSI, allowing for more precise treatment of tumors [31]. In all, approximately 450 patients were treated using active beam scanning at GSI before the center was succeeded by the development of the Heidelberg Ion-Beam Therapy Center (HIT) in 2009 [2,31–34].

Currently, there are 12 centers in 5 countries treating carbon ion radiotherapy in the following countries: Austria, China, Germany, Italy, and Japan. Although currently limited to Europe and Asia, there are eight centers in various stages of development, including in China, France, Japan, South Korea, Taiwan, and the US [26,35,36] (Figure 1.5). Despite no centers currently treating with carbon ion radiotherapy in the US, there is renewed interest in the potential benefit of therapy. In recent years, the University of Texas Southwestern recently opened a phase III trial randomizing patients to carbon radiotherapy (NCT03536182), and Albert Einstein College of Medicine, in collaboration with the Shanghai Proton and Heavy Ion Center, recently completed accrual for a phase I trial investigating carbon radiotherapy (NCT03403049).

1.4 History of Other Heavy Particles

At LBNL, interest in other heavy ions led to the development of the Bevatron, a synchrotron-based facility in 1954, which was designed to test carbon, oxygen, and neon particles. They then modified their 84-in. synchrocyclotron to accelerate helium nuclei in 1957, and again to accommodate neon-ion radiation in 1975. In 1974, the Bevatron was linked to the SuperHILAC linear accelerator, creating the Bevelac. Throughout the 1970s and 1980s, Bevalac was an important component of the research program at LBNL [2].

Approximately 2,000 patients were treated with helium therapy at LBNL, although mainly with passive scattering [37]. Early results were favorable in a variety of disease sites, including unresectable meningiomas, uveal melanoma, and unresectable pancreas cancer [38–40]. Helium was even

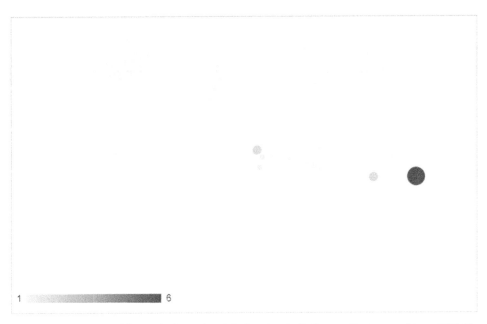

Figure 1.5 Location of Currently Operational Carbon Ion Radiotherapy Centers as of June 2020. The reader is referred to the Particle Therapy Co-Operative Group (https://www.ptcog.ch/index.php/facilities-in-operation) for the most up-to-date listing of current and planned centers.

considered to be used for stereotactic radiosurgery following invention of the Bevelac [41]. Despite strong early clinical results, interest in helium declined with the close of LBNL, as well as the focus on developing facilities with active beam delivery and the ability to provide multiple ion species [37].

By the end of 1988, 433 patients were treated with neon therapy, with 239 patients receiving a minimum dose of 10 Gy. Early results with neon therapy were favorable compared to historical controls for a variety of disease sites, including advanced or recurrent salivary gland tumors, paranasal sinus tumors, sarcomas, and biliary tract carcinomas. Despite the generally favorable results in those disease sites, malignant gliomas, lung cancers, recurrent head, and neck cancers, and many gastrointestinal cancers showed no benefit with neon therapy [28,39].

Unfortunately, LBNL terminated all clinical research programs in 1992 given budget constraints and aging technology. They treated more than 2,000 patients with particle therapy, most of which were treated with helium and neon therapy [2].

1.5 History of Boron Neutron Capture Therapy

The neutron was discovered by James Chadwick in 1932 [1,42]. Shortly after, Goldhaber and Taylor described the reaction underlying boron neutron capture therapy (BNCT), where boron is irradiated with a neutron and produces an alpha particle and lithium ion [43]. The idea to use neutron capture reactions was first proposed by Locher in 1936 [42,44],

and Gerald Kruger first published on his experiments using BNCT in mice in 1940 [45].

The first clinical applications for BNCT were in the treatment of malignant glioma at the Brookhaven Graphite Research Reactor from February 1951 to January 1953 in the United States [42,46–49]. Although promising, all patients eventually died of progressive disease and there was some toxicity due to the large amount of borax. The reactor was subsequently modified, with multiple other boron compounds developed that were less toxic than borax. Despite these advances, the early results were disappointing, leading to the discontinuation of BNCT in the United States in 1961 [42].

Although BNCT was discontinued in the US, in 1968, Hiroshi Hatanaka introduced a new boron compound, BSH, for use in Japan. Additionally, during this time, researchers in Japan made several innovations in the treatment of BNCT, including the use of heavy water to obtain better dose distribution and using BNCT in brain tumors in the pediatric population [42,50,51]. Further, in 1987, Mishima and colleagues began using another boron compound, *p*-boronophenylalanine, which is commonly used today [42].

Clinical research with BNCT was met with renewed interest in the US and Europe in the 1990s, when epithermal neutron sources were developed to treat more deeply seated tumors. Prospective trials were started at Brookhaven and Cambridge in the US, followed by the development of centers in Finland, Sweden, the Czech Republic, Argentina, and Taiwan. Unfortunately, most of these centers closed due to political or economic reasons [42]. As the clinical evidence from these centers was promising, there continues to be interest in developing BNCT facilities, with new centers in development in Europe and Asia.

1.6 Conclusions

Over the past century, the primary goal of radiation therapy has been to maximize clinical effectiveness with minimizing toxicity to normal organs. Treatment with both light and heavy particles hopes to achieve this goal by taking advantage of the physical and radiobiological properties of particles. Over time, it is clear that research and development surrounding in particle therapy have led to the development of technology and applications that have impacted multiple modalities and disciplines and helped to form the basis of radiation therapy today.

References

1 Halperin, E., Wazer, D., Perez, C., Brady, L. (2019). *Perez & Brady's Principles and Practice of Radiation Oncology*, Seventh ed. Wolters Kluwer.

2 Tsujii, H., Kamada, T., Noda, K. et al. (2014). *Carbon-ion Radiotherapy: Principles, Practices, and Treatment Planning.* Japan: Springer.

3 Jimenez-Jimenez, E., Mateos, P., Ortiz, I. et al. (2018). Do patients feel well informed in a radiation oncology service? *Journal of Cancer Education: The Official Journal of the American Association for Cancer Education* Apr 33: 346–351.

4 Giap, H. and Giap, B. (2012). Historical perspective and evolution of charged particle beam therapy. *Translational Cancer Research* 1: 127–136.

5 Bragg, W.R.K. (1904). On the ionization curves of radium. *Philosophical Magazine* 8: 726–738.

6 Stone, R.S. (1948). Neutron therapy and specific ionization. *The American Journal of Roentgenology and Radium Therapy* Jun 59: 771–785.

7 Halperin, E.C. (2006). Particle therapy and treatment of cancer. *The Lancet Oncology* Aug 7: 676–685.

8 Wilson, R.R. (1946). Radiological use of fast protons. *Radiology* Nov 47: 487–491.

9 Tobias, C.A., Anger, H.O., and Lawrence, J.H. (1952). Radiological use of high energy deuterons and alpha particles. *The American Journal of Roentgenology, Radium Therapy, and Nuclear Medicine* Jan 67: 1–27.

10 Lawrence, J.H., Tobias, C.A., Born, J.L. et al. (1958). Pituitary irradiation with high-energy proton beams: A preliminary report. *Cancer Research* Feb 18: 121–134.

11 Lawrence, J.H., Tobias, C.A., Linfoot, J.A. et al. (1976). Heavy-particle therapy in acromegaly and Cushing disease. *JAMA* May 24 235: 2307–2310.

12 Chen, G.T., Castro, J.R., and Quivey, J.M. (1981). Heavy charged particle radiotherapy. *Annual Review of Biophysics and Bioengineering* 10: 499–529.

13 Miller, D.W. (1995). A review of proton beam radiation therapy. *Medical Physics* Nov 22: 1943–1954.

14 Falkmer, S., Fors, B., Larsson, B. et al. (1962). Pilot study on proton irradiation of human carcinoma. *Acta Radiologica* Feb 58: 33–51.

15 Larsson, B., Leksell, L., Rexed, B. et al. (1958). The high-energy proton beam as a neurosurgical tool. *Nature* Nov 1 182: 1222–1223.

16 Larsson, B. (1967). Radiological properties of beams of high-energy protons. *Radiation Research. Supplement* 7: 304–311.

17 Suit, H.D. and Loeffler, J.S. (2011). *Evolution of Radiation Oncology at Massachusetts General Hospital.* New York: Springer.

18 Kjellberg, R.N., Hanamura, T., Davis, K.R. et al. (1983). Bragg-peak proton-beam therapy for arteriovenous malformations of the brain. *The New England Journal of Medicine* Aug 4 309: 269–274.

19 Kjellberg, R.N., Shintani, A., Frantz, A.G. et al. (1968). Proton-beam therapy in acromegaly. *The New England Journal of Medicine* Mar 28 278: 689–695.

20 Kjellberg, R.N., Sweet, W.H., Preston, W.M. et al. (1962). The Bragg peak of a proton beam in intracranial therapy of tumors. *Transactions of the American Neurological Association* 87: 216–218.

21 Goitein, M., Suit, H.D., Gragoudas, E. et al. (1985). Potential for low-LET charged-particle radiation therapy in cancer. *Radiation Research. Supplement* 8: S297–309.

22 Suit, H., Goitein, M., Munzenrider, J. et al. (1982). Evaluation of the clinical applicability of proton beams in definitive fractionated radiation therapy. *International Journal of Radiation Oncology, Biology, Physics* Dec 8: 2199–2205.

23 Koehler, A.M., Schneider, R.J., and Sisterson, J.M. (1977). Flattening of proton dose distributions for large-field radiotherapy. *Medical Physics* Jul-Aug 4: 297–301.

24 Koehler, A.M., Schneider, R.J., and Sisterson, J.M. (1975). Range modulators for protons and heavy ions. In: *Nuclear Instruments and Methods* Volume 131, 3: 437–440. ISSN 0029-554X, https://doi.org/10.1016/0029-554X(75)90430-9. (https://www.sciencedirect.com/science/article/pii/0029554X75904309)

25 Gragoudas, E.S., Goitein, M., Koehler, A.M. et al. (1977). Proton irradiation of small choroidal malignant melanomas. *American Journal of Ophthalmology* May 83: 665–673.

26 Particle therapy facilities in clinical operation (2020). https://www.ptcog.ch/index.php/facilities-in-operation. Accessed June 2020.

27 Slater, J.M., Archambeau, J.O., Miller, D.W. et al. (1992). The proton treatment center at Loma Linda University Medical Center: Rationale for and description of its development. *International Journal of Radiation Oncology, Biology, Physics* 22: 383–389.

28 Castro, J.R., Quivey, J.M., Lyman, J.T. et al. (1980). Radiotherapy with heavy charged particles at Lawrence Berkeley Laboratory. *Journal of the Canadian Association of Radiologists* Mar 31: 30–34.

29 Chatterjee, A., Alpen, E.L., Tobias, C.A. et al. (1981). High energy beams of radioactive nuclei and their biomedical applications. *International Journal of Radiation Oncology, Biology, Physics* Apr 7: 503–507.

30 Tsujii, H., Mizoe, J.E., Kamada, T. et al. (2004). Overview of clinical experiences on carbon ion radiotherapy at NIRS. *Radiotherapy and Oncology: Journal of the European Society for Therapeutic Radiology and Oncology* Dec 73 (Suppl 2): S41–49.

31 Kraft, G. (2000). Tumor therapy with heavy charged particles. *Progress in Particle and Nuclear Physics* 2001 (45): S473–S544.

32 Haberer, T., Becher, W., Schardt, D. et al. (1993). Magnetic scanning system for heavy ion therapy. *Nuclear Instruments & Methods in Physics Research. Section A, Accelerators, Spectrometers, Detectors and Associated Equipment* 10 June 1993 330: 296–305.

33 Combs, S.E., Ellerbrock, M., Haberer, T. et al. (2010). Heidelberg Ion Therapy Center (HIT): Initial clinical experience in the first 80 patients. *Acta Oncologica* Oct 49: 1132–1140.

34 Combs, S.E., Kessel, K.A., Herfarth, K. et al. (2012). Treatment of pediatric patients and young adults with particle therapy at the Heidelberg Ion Therapy Center (HIT): Establishment of workflow and initial clinical data. *Radiation Oncology* Oct 17 7: 170.

35 Particle therapy facilities under construction (2020). https://www.ptcog.ch/index.php/facilities-under-construction. Accessed June 2020.

36 Particle therapy facilities in a planning stage (2020). https://www.ptcog.ch/index.php/facilities-in-planning-stage. Accessed June 2020.

37 Kramer, M., Scifoni, E., Schuy, C. et al. (2016). Helium ions for radiotherapy? Physical and biological verifications of a novel treatment modality. *Medical Physics* Apr 43: 1995.

38 Wang, Z., Nabhan, M., Schild, S.E. et al. (2013). Charged particle radiation therapy for uveal melanoma: A systematic review and meta-analysis. *International Journal of Radiation Oncology, Biology, Physics* May 1 86: 18–26.

39 Linstadt, D., Quivey, J.M., Castro, J.R. et al. (1988). Comparison of helium-ion radiation therapy and split-course megavoltage irradiation for unresectable adenocarcinoma of the pancreas. Final report of a Northern California Oncology Group randomized prospective clinical trial. *Radiology* Jul 168: 261–264.

40 Kaplan, I.D., Castro, J.R., and Phillips, T.L. (1994). Helium charged particle radiotherapy for meningioma: Experience at UCLBL. University of California Lawrence Berkeley Laboratory. *International Journal of Radiation Oncology, Biology, Physics* Jan 1 28: 257–261.

41 Ludewigt, B.A., Chu, W.T., Phillips, M.H. et al. (1991). Accelerated helium-ion beams for radiotherapy and stereotactic radiosurgery. *Medical Physics* Jan-Feb 18: 36–42.

42 Sauerwein, W., Wittig, A., Moss, R. et al. (2012). *Neutron Capture Therapy: Principles and Applications*. Heidelberg New York Dordrecht London: Springer.

43 Taylor, H.J. and Goldhaber, M. (1935). Detection of nuclear disintegration in a photographic emulsion. In: *Nature (London)* 135: 341–348. https://doi.org/10.1038/135341a0

44 Locher, G.L. (1936). Biological effects and therapeutic possibilities of neutrons. *The American Journal of Roentgenology and Radium Therapy* 36: 1–13.

45 Kruger, P.G. (1940). Some biological effects of nuclear disintegration products on neoplastic tissue. *Proceedings of the National Academy of Sciences of the United States of America* Mar 15 26: 181–192.

46 Farr, L.E., Robertson, J.S., and Stickley, E. (1954). Physics and physiology of neutron-capture therapy. *Proceedings of the National Academy of Sciences of the United States of America* Nov 40: 1087–1093.

47 Farr, L.E., Sweet, W.H., Locksley, H.B. et al. (1954). Neutron capture therapy of gliomas using boron. *Transactions of the American Neurological Association* 13: 110–113.

48 Farr, L.E., Sweet, W.H., Robertson, J.S. et al. (1954). Neutron capture therapy with boron in the treatment of glioblastoma multiforme. *The American Journal of Roentgenology, Radium Therapy, and Nuclear Medicine* Feb 71: 279–293.

49 Goodwin, J.T., Farr, L.E., Sweet, W.H. et al. (1955). Pathological study of eight patients with glioblastoma multiforme treated by neutron-capture therapy using boron 10. *Cancer* May-Jun 8: 601–615.

50 Nakagawa, Y., Hatanaka, H., Moritani, M. et al. (1994). Partial deuteration and blood-brain barrier (BBB) permeability. *Acta Neurochirurgica Supplement (Wien)* 60: 410–412.

51 Nakagawa, Y., Kageji, T., Mizobuchi, Y. et al. (2009). Clinical results of BNCT for malignant brain tumors in children. *Applied Radiation and Isotopes: Including Data, Instrumentation and Methods for Use in Agriculture, Industry and Medicine* Jul 67: S27–30.

2

The Physics of Particle Therapy

Steve Herchko, DMP[1], Omar El Sherif, Ph.D.[2], and Eric Welch, DMP[2]

[1] Department of Radiation Oncology, Mayo Clinic Florida, 4500 San Pablo Road, Jacksonville, FL 32224
[2] Department of Radiation Oncology, Mayo Clinic, 200 First St. SW. Rochester, MN 55905

2.1 Introduction

While the fundamental physical principles that provide the basis for particle therapy are well established, the practical use of these principles is continually evolving as the use of particle therapy continues to grow. Once a novelty, particle therapy is now widely available in many parts of the world. Proton therapy is now a routine option for many patients, and multiple facilities in different countries are treating patients with carbon ion therapy as data is gathered to determine the best clinical use of this technology. Pharmaceutical improvements have also revitalized neutron beam therapy when used for boron neutron capture therapy (BNCT), joining several fast neutron therapy (FNT) centers around the world. Compared to traditional photon and electron radiation therapy, heavier particles have some desirable physical characteristics that allow for safer and more effective treatments in certain scenarios. Heavier particles such as neutrons, protons, and carbon ions offer increased linear energy transfer (LET) and relative biological effectiveness (RBE). Heavier charged particles have beneficial dosimetric advantages such as decreased distal, lateral, and integral dose, and neutron beams can be used to generate targeted therapeutic secondary particles.

2.2 Photon and Electron Therapy Physics

The physics of conventional radiation therapy is governed by the interaction of photons and electrons in matter. In the therapeutic energy range, photons primarily interact via the photoelectric, Compton, or pair production process. The photoelectric process dominates at low energies (<0.25 MeV) and involves a low energy photon being fully absorbed by the target atom. This results in the emission of a photoelectron with energy equal to the energy of the incident photon minus the binding energy of the ejected electron. Pair production dominates at high energies (>25 MeV) and occurs when an incident photon with threshold energy greater than 1.02 MeV interacts with a target atom nucleus creating a positive and negative electron pair. The Compton effect dominates at energies in between the photoelectric and pair production processes throughout most of the therapeutic energy range. In a Compton event an incident photon interacts with an orbital electron, transferring some of the energy to the electron. This results in the ejection of the orbital electron and scattering of the incident photon with reduced energy. Photons behave as indirectly ionizing particles, undergoing relatively few interactions in matter that pass on their energy to secondary charge particles which then deposit energy within the medium via additional interactions.

In the therapeutic energy range, electrons primarily interact in matter via inelastic collisions with atomic electrons or inelastic collisions with atomic nuclei. Inelastic collisions with atomic electrons occur when the incident electron passes near the outer edge of the electron orbits, resulting in ionization and excitation events and the creation of additional secondary electrons that can then deposit further energy. Excitation refers to an orbital electron receiving energy that raises the orbital electron to a higher energy state where it then relaxes back to the stable state, while ionization refers to an orbital electron receiving energy in excess of its binding energy and being ejected from the atom. Inelastic collisions with atomic nuclei occur when an incident electron passes near and interacts with the nucleus of an atom. These interactions result in the incident electron being deflected from its original trajectory and transferring energy in the form of an emitted bremsstrahlung photon. The likelihood of bremsstrahlung production increases with both increasing electron energy and atomic number (Z) of the medium. Electrons and other charge particles interact in a fundamentally different manner than uncharged particles due to the Coulomb field associated with the charge particle. This Coulomb field of an incident charged particle interacts with the electrons and nuclei of the atoms it passes, transferring energy along the way. As a result, electrons undergo many interactions compared to photons and follow very tortuous paths as they dissipate their energy.

For an in-depth description of photon and electron interactions in matter, the reader is referred to the works by Attix [1] and Khan [2].

2.3 Neutron Therapy Physics

Neutrons are subatomic particles with neutral charge and mass approximately equal to their positive counterpart, the proton. These two particles together make up the nucleus of atoms. The discovery of neutrons is credited to Chadwick in Ref. [3], building on work by Bothe and Becker, where he proposed a highly energetic neutral particle was produced when Beryllium was irradiated with alpha particles emanating from Polonium, $^9\text{Be}(\alpha,n)^{12}\text{C}$. Following this discovery, scientists further explored the novel particle and its unique properties.

In Ref. [4], Locher hypothesized the potential for neutrons to be absorbed by atoms, namely Boron (^{10}B), consequently releasing energy. This was the advent of neutron capture therapy (NCT) and more specifically BNCT. In the same year, Lawrence described the potential to create neutrons using a cyclotron. Two years later, in Ref. [5], the first FNT study was conducted by Stone et al.

Starting in the 1930s, clinical trials and treatments have been conducted for FNT. BNCT followed in later decades. BNCT and FNT are therapeutics using primary neutrons incident on the patient. These therapies rely on different particle interactions to release energy in tissue damaging cancer cells. The interactions are dependent on the energy of the incident neutron and the material on which the beam is incident.

The following neutron sections will discuss primary neutrons, including energy, interactions, and dose deposition. Accompanying this discussion will be other neutron considerations including secondary neutron production from other therapeutic modalities and rationale behind the use of primary neutrons as therapeutic beams.

2.3.1 Primary Neutrons

The two primary neutron therapies, FNT and BNCT, both use neutron sources as the primary beam. However, the way in which the primary beams are exploited to create damage differs.

Neutrons are analogous to photons in the way that they deposit dose. Neutrons are uncharged particles that interact to create secondary charged particles, which in turn ionize matter and create biologic damage. However, neutrons predominantly interact with the atomic nucleus instead of orbital electrons. FNT has been investigated and utilized due to the higher radiobiological effectiveness and lesser dependence on cell cycle to treat radioresistant tumors. Due to the neutral charge of the particle, manipulation and control of neutron beams is not precise and relies on bulky absorbers and collimators. This lack of control can lead to large normal tissue volumes receiving high dose levels. This delivery strategy relies on normal tissue repair being greater than cancerous tissue to be effective.

If lower energy beams are used, efficiency of neutron interaction, specifically neutron absorption, can be increased. Neutron absorption releases high energy particles (gamma rays, protons, alpha particles, etc.) in the immediate vicinity of the reaction, creating localized damage. This efficiency can be further increased with the addition of elements with high thermal neutron cross-sections, such as boron. The goal of BNCT is to use boron-tagged pharmaceuticals to preferentially damage targets that have taken up the pharmaceuticals, while delivering lower radiation doses to healthy tissue.

Both types of primary neutron therapies require the production of neutron beams. Neutrons can be produced by several different methods, including nuclear reactors, neutron generators, cyclotrons, or radioactive sources. Nuclear reactors and cyclotrons have both been used for therapeutic purposes. These neutron sources are typically in the MeV energy range, usable for FNT. To be used for NCT, the neutron beams need to be moderated to thermal and epithermal energies. This moderation allows for the capture therapy to be effective while sparing normal tissue from fast neutrons.

2.3.2 Secondary Neutrons

Secondary neutrons are not the focus of this work as they are not used for therapeutic purposes but are a consequence of using therapeutic beams. However, because of their impact in radiation doses and selection of radiation modality, they should be addressed. Secondary neutrons are produced from all external beam modalities with different threshold energy and magnitude.

Neutrons are produced from high energy photons striking components in a linear accelerator head as well as the patient. These neutrons are generally referred to as photoneutrons. Photoneutrons have a threshold energy of production corresponding to the binding energy of the nucleons of the material which the therapy beam is incident on. Nucleons are the protons and neutrons within atoms. Nucleons have nuclear-binding energies on the order of 7–8 MeV for most materials. Because of this threshold, low energy photon beams cannot create photoneutrons. Moderate energy photon beams (~10 MeV) produce a low number due to the low percentage of photon energies above the binding energy due to the photon energy spectrum. High-energy photon beams (15–22 MeV) have the potential to create a large number of photoneutrons.

Heavy charged particle (HCP) beams (protons, helium, carbon, and neon) create secondary neutrons through nuclear interactions. HCP can interact with the nuclei of nozzle components of treatment delivery systems, beam modifiers such as range shifters and apertures, and the patient to produce secondary neutrons and other species. Further information on these nuclear interactions will be discussed in later sections of this chapter.

Secondary neutrons will have the same interactions as primary neutrons but will have different energies depending on the mode of production and energy of the primary beam.

2.3.3 Neutron Energy

Neutrons tend to interact differently depending on the energy of the particle. This leads to a natural classification of neutrons by their energy. Neutrons are typically classified as fast neutrons, intermediate neutrons, epithermal neutrons, or thermal neutrons. Table 2.1 shows neutron energy regions associated with neutron therapy beams.

It is important to mention that different sources classify neutron energies differently. These classifications can be highly granular (focusing on major interaction thresholds) or very broad (generalizing interaction types). Most classification systems will include thermal, intermediate, and fast neutrons; however, for therapeutic purposes, epithermal neutrons should be addressed. Table 2.1 is one classification system based on major interaction types. Above 10 keV, elastic scattering is the predominant interaction for human tissue and is the driving force behind FNT. Below 10 keV, neutron capture reactions make up a majority of the dose deposition, which is the driving force behind BNCT.

This interaction preference on energy leads itself to different needs for neutron production. BNCT requires low energy beams to be used to take advantage of interaction probabilities in the thermal and epithermal range. Fast and intermediate energy neutrons should be a small component of the BNCT incident neutron flux so that the neutron capture reaction is the predominant interaction depositing energy locally, sparing normal tissues from the less targeted fast neutrons.

2.3.4 Interactions

As previously mentioned, unlike charged particles and photons, neutrons predominantly interact with the atomic nucleus

Table 2.1 Neutron energy regions associated with neutron therapy beams.

Fast	$E > 1$ MeV
Intermediate	10 keV $< E \leq 1$ MeV
Epithermal	0.025 eV $< E \leq 10$ keV
Thermal	≤ 0.025 eV

rather than the orbital electrons. Neutrons interact by three major methods: elastic scattering with atomic nuclei, inelastic scattering with atomic nuclei, and capture reactions.

Neutrons can interact with nuclei in scattering reactions where kinetic energy is conserved between the neutron and recoil nuclei. This type of reaction is referred to as an elastic scattering reaction. The incident neutron scatters off a nucleus, giving up some fraction of its energy to the nucleus. The energy is split between the neutron and nucleus depending on the angle of scatter and size of nucleus. Equations 2.1 and 2.2 approximate the maximum and average energy that a neutron can transfer to a nucleus in an elastic collision, respectively. E_0 corresponds to the incident neutron energy, M corresponds to the mass of the recoil nucleus, and m corresponds to the mass of the incident neutron.

$$E_{max} = \frac{4MmE_0}{(M+m)^2} \tag{2.1}$$

$$\bar{E} = E_0 \frac{2Mm}{(M+m)^2} \tag{2.2}$$

Neutrons can also interact with nuclei where kinetic energy is not conserved but part of the incident energy is transferred to the atomic nucleus, sending it into an excited state. This type of reaction is referred to as an inelastic scattering reaction. The incident neutron interacts with the nucleus and is briefly held. This results in the brief formation of a compound nucleus. The neutron is ejected from the compound nucleus with a lower kinetic energy and the nucleus is left in an excited state. The excited nucleus then de-excites through the emission of a gamma ray.

Finally, neutrons can also be absorbed by an atomic nucleus, forming a new species. This type of reaction leaves the new nucleus in an excited state. This results in the nucleus needing to remove the excess energy, which can be accomplished in a variety of different particle emissions and fission. Human tissue is predominantly composed of hydrogen, nitrogen, oxygen, and carbon. For epithermal and thermal energies, hydrogen [^{1}H(n,γ)^{2}H] and nitrogen [^{14}N(n,p)^{14}C] capture reactions contribute a majority of the neutron dose. Cross-sections [units: barn = 10^{-24} cm^2] are interaction probabilities. Each element has individual cross-sections for total reaction probabilities and for each reaction. These probabilities are energy and material dependent. Figures 2.1 and 2.2 are plots of the neutron capture cross-section for the major dose deposition reactions of nitrogen and hydrogen, respectively.

Neutron absorption can occur at all neutron energies; however, as the energy of the neutron reaches thermal and epithermal energies, the probability of interaction (cross-section) increases by orders of magnitude. Thermal cross-sections for hydrogen and nitrogen neutron capture are on the order of 0.3–1.4 barns. Boron-10 has a thermal capture cross-section of 3,844 barns. Clinically, boron can be added to pharmaceuticals that can target cancer cells, leading to preferential interaction probabilities in areas of interest creating localized damage from the resultant alpha particle and lithium ion (Figure 2.3). Figure 2.4 shows boron-10 neutron capture cross-section as a function of energy.

The higher probability of interaction and the localized damage that results from the heavy, high-LET particles that come from the interaction are what make BNCT a desirable therapy. Figure 2.5 shows the cross-sections of ^{10}B, ^{14}N, and ^{1}H.

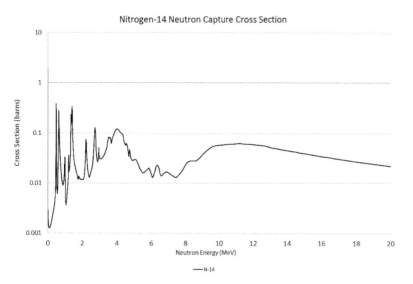

Figure 2.1 Nitrogen-14 neutron capture cross-section ^{14}N(n,p)^{14}C as a function of incident neutron energy (based on D.A. Brown, ENDF 2018 [6]).

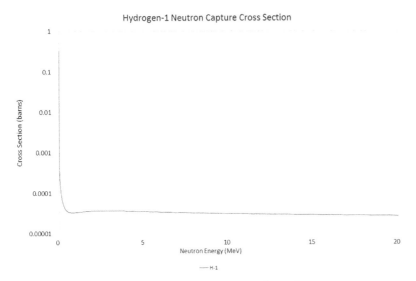

Figure 2.2   Hydrogen neutron capture cross-section $^1H(n,\gamma)^2H$ as a function of neutron energy (based on D.A. Brown, ENDF 2018 [6]).

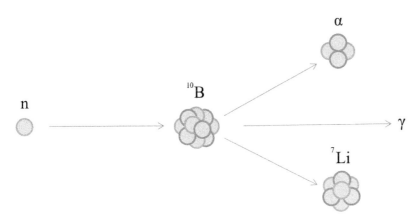

Figure 2.3   Visual representation of $^{10}B(n,\gamma)^7Li$ reaction.

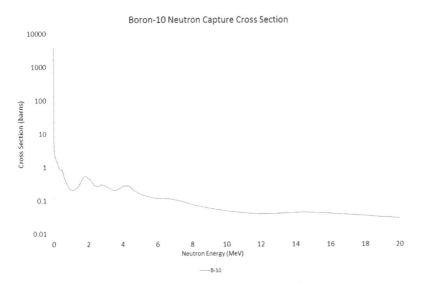

Figure 2.4   Boron-10 neutron captures cross-section $^{10}B(n,\gamma)^7Li$ as a function of incident neutron energy (based on D.A. Brown, ENDF 2018 [6]).

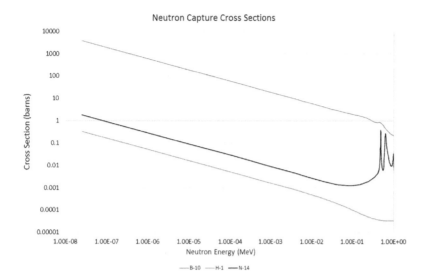

Figure 2.5 Major neutron capture cross-sections for human tissue (based on D.A. Brown, ENDF 2018 [6]).

Boron-10's capture cross-section magnitudes above the other major elements that compose human tissue.

2.3.5 Dose Deposition

Neutrons, like gamma rays and X-rays, are an indirectly ionizing radiation. Fast neutrons predominantly lose energy through elastic scattering interactions with hydrogen nuclei. In this interaction, the neutron can remove the proton from the hydrogen atom which then ionizes the local tissue and deposits dose. Alpha particles and other heavier nuclear fragments can also be produced through interactions with tissue components. Protons, alphas, and other heavy nuclear fragments are all HCPs. In contrast with electrons, HCP produces dense ionization tracks. This dense ionization increases the biologic effectiveness of FNT. FNT dose distributions are similar to a 6–8 MV photon beam with depth of maximum dose equal to ~1.2–1.7 cm [7]. This limits the depth of targets that can be effectively treated with FNT without undesirable normal tissue toxicity.

Thermal neutrons in tissue deposit dose primarily through two interactions with ^{1}H and ^{14}N. Hydrogen absorbs thermal and epithermal neutrons, forming ^{2}H and emitting a 2-MeV gamma ray [8]. This gamma ray then goes on to produce ionizing particles and deposit dose. Nitrogen absorbs thermal and epithermal neutrons, ejecting a proton and forming ^{14}C. The ejected proton and recoil carbon nucleus deposit energy locally. To increase localized damage to tissue, boron can be added to tissues of interest. Boron-10 preferentially absorbs the neutrons compared to the other prominent interactions (3,844 barns vs. 0.3–1.4 barns), leading to high LET dose deposition in those targets.

Compared to photons, neutron radiation has an increased biological effect. The quality factor is often used as a surrogate for biologic effectiveness. Figure 2.6 is a plot of average quality factors per energy for neutrons. Quality factors can be broken into two major regions, corresponding to thermal/epithermal and intermediate/fast neutrons, corresponding to energies listed in Table 2.1. Increased quality factor above 10 keV is attributed to recoil HCP (protons, alphas, and nuclear fragments) formed by intermediate and fast neutrons in elastic scattering reactions. Below 10 keV, quality factors are mostly driven by gamma rays formed from hydrogen neutron capture reactions [8]. This does not include ^{10}B interactions for BNCT. Boron produces high-LET, heavy secondaries that produce damage in the vicinity of the interaction. The alpha particle has an approximate LET of 150 keV/μm. The lithium fragment has an approximate LET of 175 keV/μm [9].

2.4 Proton Therapy Physics

Protons, electrons, and all charged particles are surrounded by an electric field. When protons travel through matter, their electric field interacts with the electric field of the surrounding medium. In general, the result of these interactions can be of the form of energy loss, scattering of the primary particle, and/or fragmentation of secondary particles emerging from the nucleus of the medium. These interactions and their dependencies provide the underpinnings for the radiation dosimetry found within our radiation treatment planning systems. Although these interactions are the same for all the charged particles used in clinical radiotherapy, the differences in their respective mass can significantly alter the observed clinical dose distributions. Take for example the percent depth dose (PDD) observed for a clinical proton versus a clinical electron beam (Figure 2.7); although the two particles have the same magnitude of charge and are undergoing the same types of

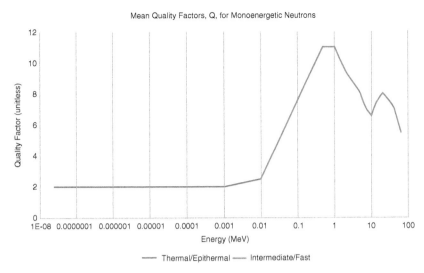

Figure 2.6   Neutron quality factors per energy (based on 10 CFR 20.1004).

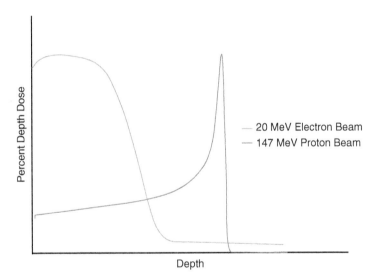

Figure 2.7   Comparison of a clinical proton (red) and electron (blue) measured percent depth dose distributions in water.

interactions, the difference in their masses results in two very contrasting pictures. Due to the increased mass of protons, their interactions differ from electrons by:

- loses only a small fraction of the energy with each interaction
- experiences insignificant energy losses through bremsstrahlung radiation
- predominately moves along its initial path with comparatively smaller scattering angles

These factors lead to the greater depth of penetration and lack of a "buildup" of dose at the beam entrance for protons compared to electrons.

The characteristic shape of the proton depth dose provides a distinct advantage over photon therapy when treating sites such as pediatric CNS and cranial lesions adjacent to critical

organs. For example, the sharp fall-off in dose at the distal edge of the Bragg peak allows proton treatments to treat a spinal column uniformly for craniospinal irradiation, while sparring many of the organs at risk situated beyond the spine. Dosimetric comparison studies have shown reduced integral dose outside the target volume [10,11]. This characteristic can potentially reduce normal tissue complication probabilities and the likelihood of secondary malignancies. Another potential physical advantage of protons is the increased RBE distal to the Bragg peak. The increased RBE is a consequence of the higher density of energy deposition in comparison to photons and may allow for safer dose escalation in radio-resistant cancers.

The above advantages are not without corresponding shortcomings. The sharp dose fall-off increases the uncertainties in the ability to calculate and localize dose during treatment planning compared to photon radiotherapy. Uncertainty in estimating water equivalent path lengths from CT simulation scans exists in both photon and proton planning. With photons a 1-cm error in the path length results in approximately a 2–3% difference in the dose for clinical energies. However, in proton therapy, a 1-cm error in the path length will correspond to a 1-cm shift in the position of the Bragg peak. Such a shift can lead to significantly reduced target coverage and/or delivering the prescription dose to critical organs distal or proximal to the target. This known drawback can be addressed in proton therapy by

- ensuring high-quality simulation scans with little to no artifacts in the vicinity of target or beam entrances
- identifying the composition and accurate water equivalent thicknesses of tissues and medical implants
- regularly monitoring changes in patient anatomy over the course treatment and re-planning when necessary
- implementing motion management strategies for moving targets and other anatomy that may intersect the beam path

2.4.1 Proton Interactions with Matter

2.4.1.1 Stopping Power

The coulombic interaction between the electric field surrounding incident protons and the orbital electrons within the atoms that make up the patient's tissue is the predominant source of energy loss. The amount of energy lost in these interactions will depend on several characteristics of the incident protons and the absorbing material. Knowing these dependencies allows us to estimate the amount of energy lost by the proton per unit length of tissue, referred to as the stopping power (S). The dose of radiation delivered to a patient is related to the stopping power and the number of incident protons traversing the area (referred to as fluence) through Equation 2.3 or 2.4.

$$\text{Dose} = \text{fluence} \times \frac{\text{stopping power}}{\text{density}} \qquad (2.3)$$

$$D = \left(\frac{dN}{dA}\right)\left(\frac{S}{\rho}\right) \qquad (2.4)$$

Table 2.2 lists the stopping power dependencies on the incident particle and absorbing tissue characteristics.

2.4.1.2 Dependence on Mass

The mass of the incident charged particle will dictate if a particle will lose a significant amount of energy when interacting with the orbital electrons of the medium. For particles with masses much greater than an electron (i.e., protons and carbon ions), the energy loss per event is small. Additionally, the mass of the particle impacts the amount of energy transferred

Table 2.2 Stopping power dependencies.

Incident charged particle	Absorbing tissue
Mass[1]	Electron density
Velocity	Mean ionization energy
Charge	Polarization/mass density

[1] For heavy charged particles (>>mass of electron), stopping power is independent of mass.

due to potential radiative losses (bremsstrahlung radiation). For electrons, the amount of energy lost due to bremsstrahlung radiation is significant (can be up to 100% of the kinetic energy); however, this process is insignificant for protons and other HCPs. Bremsstrahlung radiation is inversely proportional to the mass of incident particle. Since HCPs undergo insignificant radiative losses and are much heavier than the orbital electrons, we can consider their stopping power to be independent of the particles' mass.

2.4.1.3 Dependence on Velocity and Kinetic Energy

The amount of energy lost by an incident charged particle will vary depending on the particle's kinetic energy. This relationship is illustrated in Figure 2.8, which can be subdivided into three regions:

1. Low kinetic energy
2. Intermediate kinetic energy
3. Relativistic kinetic energy

When charged particles have low kinetic energy, their stopping power increases with increasing velocity. As the kinetic energy of the particle continues to increase into the intermediate region, this relationship reverses and we begin to observe a decrease in stopping power proportional to the square of the velocity. Once the charged particle begins to move at relativistic speeds, the relationship reverses again leading to an increase in stopping power with increasing kinetic energy. The inverse relationship between velocity and stopping power at the intermediate energy range (Region 2 in Figure 2.8) is partly responsible for the Bragg peak observed at the end of the HCP's range.

2.4.1.4 Dependence on Particle Charge

The amount of energy lost by an incident particle interacting with the electric field of the orbital electrons of the absorber is proportional to the square of the particle's charge (Z^2). Thus when comparing a carbon ion ($Z = 6^+$) to a proton ($Z = 1^+$) of the same velocity, the stopping power of the carbon ion will be 36 times that of the proton and thus lose more energy when interacting with the medium. Particles with increased charge will result in reduced depth of penetration for a given energy compared to particles with less charge.

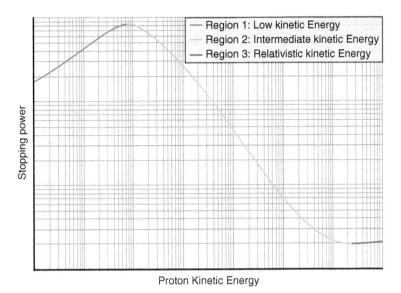

Figure 2.8 The relationship of stopping power with increasing proton kinetic energy. Data obtained from physics.nist.gov.

2.4.1.5 Dependence on Electron Density

The density of the electrons in the tissue also impacts the amount of energy lost by the charged particle as it traverses the medium. The greater the electron density of the absorber, the greater the stopping power. Electron density can be calculated using Equation 2.5.

$$N_e = \frac{N_A Z}{A} \tag{2.5}$$

where N_e, N_A, Z, and A represent the electron density, Avogadro's number, atomic number, and atomic mass, respectively. A list of the electron densities for various tissues can be obtained from ICRU report 46 [12].

2.4.1.6 Dependence on Mean Ionization Energy

When a proton or any charged particle interacts with the electric field of an orbital electron, the minimum amount of energy that can be transferred to the atom has an impact on the stopping power. This energy is referred to as the mean ionization (or excitation) energy. The stopping power of a HCP decreases slightly as the mean ionization energy of the tissue increases. The mean ionization energy typically increases with increasing atomic number (Z). Mean ionization energies for various soft tissues obtained from ICRU report 37 [13] are listed in Table 2.3.

2.4.1.7 Dependence on Mass Density and Polarization

The physical state (i.e., gas, liquid, or solid) of the tissue has an impact on the stopping power. Generally, the stopping power for an absorber in its compressed solid state is decreased in comparison to its gaseous form. This dependency is negligible for HCPs in the low-to-intermediate energy ranges seen in radiotherapy but is significant at the relativistic range.

Table 2.3 Mean ionization energies for soft tissues.

Soft tissue	Mean ionization/Excitation energy (eV)
Muscle	75.3
Compact bone	91.9
Fat	96.2
Lung	75.3
Water	75.0

Modified from ICRU report 37 (1984).

2.4.1.8 Estimating Stopping Powers

The dependencies discussed above can be used to estimate the stopping power of a HCP through Bethe–Bloch Equation (2.6).

$$S = 0.3071 z^2 \frac{Z}{A\beta^2}\left[\ln\frac{2m_e c^2}{I} + \ln\frac{\beta^2}{1-\beta^2} - \beta^2\right] \tag{2.6}$$

where z, Z, A, β, m_e, c, and I represent the incident particle charge, atomic number of absorber, atomic mass of absorber, the ratio of the incident particle's velocity-to-the speed of light, mass of an electron, speed of light, and the absorber's mean ionization/excitation energy, respectively.

Proton stopping power tables for different compounds and tissues can be found in ICRU report 49 [14]. The stopping power can also be related to the range that a given particle will travel within a medium through Equation 2.7.

$$R = \frac{1}{\rho}\int_{T_{initial}}^{T_{final}} \frac{1}{[S/\rho](T)}\,dT \tag{2.7}$$

where R, ρ, and T represent the particle's range in the medium, the mass density of the medium, and the energy of the incident particle, respectively.

2.4.1.9 Multiple Coulomb Scattering

The second interaction to be discussed occurs between the electric field of the incident charged particle and the electric field surrounding the nucleus of the atoms within the tissue (may also occur with electrons of low-z absorbers). This interaction occurs multiple times as the particle travels through tissue and is responsible for the scattering of the incident particles. This process is referred to as multiple coulomb scattering. The lateral spread of the incident charged particle follows a Gaussian distribution with a standard deviation that can be calculated as a function of the water equivalent depth of penetration, the incident particles charge, momentum, and velocity using the Highland formula [15] or the Fermi–Eyges theory [16]. The theory shows that:

- the greater the momentum of the incident particle, the smaller the angular spread
- the angular spread increases with increasing depth and charge

Therefore, higher energy and/or heavier particles have sharper penumbras. This sharper penumbra can lead to better dose conformity around target structures.

2.4.1.10 Nuclear Interactions

The last interaction to be discussed occurs between the incident charged particles and the constituents of the nuclei, this is referred to as nuclear interactions. Nuclear interactions are relatively infrequent compared to the previous interactions discussed above. However, they result in the ejection of particles and/or smaller nuclei that fragment from the atom to deposit additional dose in the form of a "halo" and an "aura" along the path of the incident particle. For heavier particles, these fragments can also deposit non-negligible amounts of dose beyond the Bragg peak, this is often referred to as a fragmentation tail.

2.4.2 Percent Depth Doses and Lateral Profiles

The PDDs for protons of different energy in water are shown in Figure 2.9. Three distinguishing characteristics of a proton PDD are the

1. low entrance dose compared to photons and electrons
2. Bragg peak
3. sharp fall-off distal to the Bragg peak

You will notice in Figure 2.9 that there is increasing longitudinal "spread" in Bragg peak for the particles with increased range (higher energy). The increased distal penumbra seen in Figure 2.9 (referred to as range straggling) is a result of the accumulation of many interactions with differing energy losses by the incident protons as they travel through tissue. The clinical implications of this for spot-scanning systems are that shallow targets require more discrete energy layers to treat an equally sized target volume compared to a deep target. The sharper Bragg peaks and resulting increased number of energy layers may lead to longer field delivery times, increased density of regions with higher relative biologic effectiveness, and potentially greater susceptibility to organ motion.

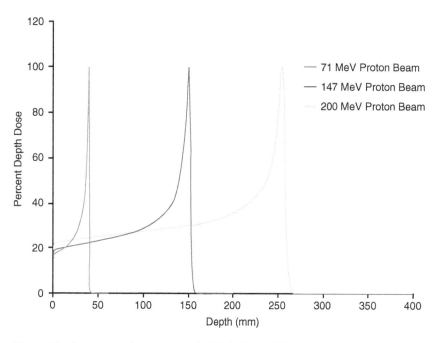

Figure 2.9 Percent depth dose curves for 71, 147, and 200 MeV protons in water. The increased distal penumbra is a result of range straggling and it becomes more pronounced at higher energies.

Similar to photons but to a greater extent, the lateral penumbra of protons increases with increasing depth. The lateral penumbra is typically sharper for protons compared to photons at shallow depths. This can provide improved conformality for shallow targets but equal or sometimes less conformal dose distributions for deep targets such as in some prostate cancer patients [17]. Although the distal penumbra is much sharper than the lateral penumbra, distal target margins created during treatment planning are not made to be more conformal due to proton range uncertainties.

2.4.3 Relative Biological Effectiveness

The mechanism for cell killing by radiation is through single and double strand breaks within the structure of the cell's DNA. It is believed that double strand breaks are more lethal and difficult to repair than single-strand breaks. The likelihood of obtaining a double strand break depends on how densely packed the sites of energy deposition are to each other. The density of energy deposition along the path of a charged particle can be described and estimated in units of keV/μm, referred to as the LET. The LET of a charged particle will vary as it traverses through tissue (see Figure 2.10). The LET increases as we approach the Bragg peak, reaching a maximum value distal to the peak. It is theorized that particles with higher LET will produce more double strand breaks and lead to an increased RBE compared to photon radiotherapy [18]. Using the dose per fraction, LET, and the α/β ratio of tissue, the RBE can be estimated along the beam path and potentially used to treat radio-resistant tumors and/or spare organs at risk [19]. Although the LET is known to vary along the path of an incident proton, it is common clinical practice and the current recommendation by the ICRU to use a single RBE factor of 1.1 regardless of depth when comparing proton and photon doses [20].

This purpose of this chapter was to provide a brief summary for clinicians of the different proton interactions in matter and highlight some of the differences between protons and more conventional radiotherapy modalities such as photons and electron therapy. If the reader is interested in more details on these topics, we direct them to some of the previously published literature from Paganetti [21], Podgorsak [22], and Attix [1].

2.4.4 Helium Ion Therapy

Helium ions (^{4}He) have been used in radiotherapy to treat patients at Lawrence Berkeley National Laboratory (Saunders 1985). [23]. The helium ion has $a + 2$ charge, is ~4 times the mass of a proton, and may theoretically have some clinical advantages over protons [24,25]. The increased mass of ^{4}He results in reduced range straggling, lateral broadening, and generally increased RBE in comparison to protons. Grun *et al.* have shown that the ratio of the RBE at the Bragg peak relative to the entrance is increased for ^{4}He versus protons. However, the ratio of the physical dose at the Bragg peak relative to the entrance is slightly reduced for ^{4}He versus protons. This difference may theoretically lead to reduced RBE-weighted dose to surrounding organs at risk when using ^{4}He. One caveat, when comparing the RBE across different ions, is that this effect will vary depending on tissue type (i.e., α/β ratio), prescription dose, and beam configurations [26], thus making RBE generalizations error prone when comparing ions without situational details.

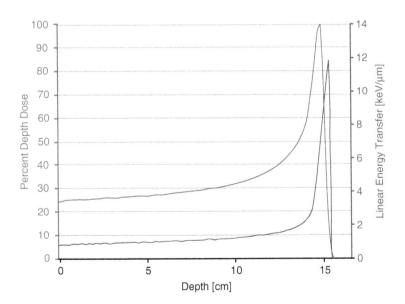

Figure 2.10   The percent depth dose (red) and linear energy transfer (blue) as a function of depth for a 132-MeV proton beam in water.

2.5 Carbon Ion Therapy Physics

The physics of carbon ion and heavy ion therapy differs from proton beam therapy due to the significantly greater charge and mass of heavy ions compared to protons. These physical differences affect the way heavy ions interact and deposit energy in matter. Heavy ion beams offer a greater LET and RBE along with sharper lateral penumbras compared to other therapeutic beams of lesser charge and mass. Like a proton, the large mass of a carbon ion allows the particle to travel a relatively straight course and deposit a substantial portion of its energy at the end of its path. Thus, these beams are well suited for hypoxic radioresistant tumors and tumors adjacent to nearby critical structures. Conversely, heavy ion beams have a greater distal dose compared to proton beams due to the fragmentation tail seen at the end of the beam's path.

2.5.1 Carbon Basics

Carbon represents the sixth-most common element in the universe and the second-most plentiful element in the human body. Carbon-12 atoms contain 6 protons, 6 neutrons, and 6 electrons for a total of 12 nucleons. ^{12}C has an atomic mass of 12 atomic mass units (AMU) by definition. Compared to the other particles previously discussed, the significantly larger mass and charge affect the way a carbon ion beam behaves in matter and will be discussed below. To generate a carbon ion beam used for radiation therapy, the six electrons of the carbon atom are removed leaving a beam of C^{6+} ions which will enter the patient. The creation and acceleration of carbon ions for therapeutic use is an evolving field and will be discussed later in Chapter 4.

2.5.2 Interactions with Matter

Heavy ions such as carbon are governed by the same Coulomb interactions and multiple Coulomb scattering that determine how other charged particles such as electrons and protons interact in matter. Interactions can occur with both atomic electrons and atomic nuclei as the carbon ions travel through a material. The most common interactions occur as inelastic collisions with atomic electrons, which result in ionization and excitation events along with the continuous energy loss of the incident carbon ions. These interactions occur when the incident carbon ion passes near a target atom and primarily interacts with a single atomic electron. Ionization events result in secondary electrons, or delta rays, which can create their own track and undergo additional interactions as previously discussed. Due to the large difference in mass (a carbon ion is roughly 22,000 times heavier than an electron), the energy loss of a carbon ion due to a single interaction with an

orbital electron is quite small, but these interactions are numerous and gradually decrease the velocity of the incident carbon ion as it travels throughout the target material. The number and frequency of these interactions are dependent on the velocity of the projectile and the density of the medium through which the beam is traveling as discussed previously for proton beams. The significant mass difference between the two particles also results in minimal deflection of carbon ions from their original trajectory and contributes to the small lateral penumbra seen with heavier charged particle beams. Compared to an electron which continually changes directions along its path, a carbon ion will maintain a much straighter course. Range straggling is also minimal due to the limited energy loss variation along the path of the incident beam between different particles. Heavy ions deposit their energy in many small steps while lighter charged particles, such as electrons, undergo fewer large interactions with greater variability. Thus, the range of a carbon ion beam's primary particles is well defined.

In addition to Coulomb interactions with atomic electrons, carbon ions undergo nuclear collisions with atomic nuclei. These nuclear interactions may result in the incident particle shattering into many pieces and depositing energy locally at the site of interaction, or more frequently the incident particle will fragment into a few high energy fragments that travel a significant distance from the fragmentation site and cause additional interactions along their path (Figure 2.11). The energy and trajectory of these fragments are similar to that of the incident particle, but the fragments will have a greater range due to their decreased mass. The angular distribution of the fragments is related to the mass of the fragment, with heavier fragments being more forward peaked and lighter fragments scattering with a wider angular distribution [27]. The relative contribution of dose deposition from fragments compared to the contribution from the primary beam increases with increasing depth as more fragments are created and

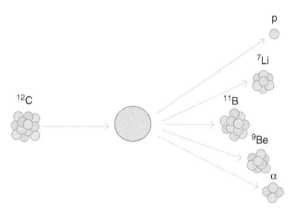

Figure 2.11 Diagram of carbon fragmentation with possible fragments. Note that the lighter fragments travel further and are scattered at greater angles.

deposit their energy downstream. The creation of these fragments results in the fragmentation tail discussed below as the fragments travel beyond the range of the incident particles. Possible fragments of ^{12}C include protons (p), alpha particles (α), Lithium (Li), Beryllium (Be), and Boron (B) [28]. Additionally, a target nucleus may fragment into additional particles with a short range. These target fragments are of minimal concern due to their low energy and short range of travel in tissue [29]. Carbon ion beams also undergo nuclear fusion interactions as ^{12}C fuses with the elements available in human tissue. Radioactive isotopes of fluorine and sodium are potentially created, resulting in future radioactive decay [30]. All of the nuclear interactions discussed above result in the attenuation of the primary beam as incident ions are removed from the beam due to these interactions.

Unlike electrons which undergo radiative losses in the form of bremsstrahlung photons, HCPs do not experience the same deflection in their path as they pass near an atomic nucleus due to their large mass. Thus, radiative losses for HCPs are not a concern and can generally be ignored.

2.5.3 Stopping Power

As discussed previously for proton beam therapy, the rate of energy loss of a particle per unit path length, or stopping power, of a charged particle is dependent on many factors and can be described by the Bethe–Bloch formula (Equation 2.6). As carbon ions are slowed down due to numerous ionization and excitation interactions with atomic electrons, the energy loss gradually increases with depth until a sharp increase is seen near the end of the range. This behavior is due to the inverse dependence on the square of the velocity as previously discussed and results in the characteristic Bragg peak similar to that seen for a proton beam. The stopping power is also dependent on the charge (z) of the particle, and the energy loss will increase as the charge increases. Thus, a carbon ion with the same initial energy as a proton will penetrate a shorter distance within the same material due to increased energy loss per unit path length.

2.5.4 Depth Dose

The depth dose curve of a carbon ion beam exhibits many of the same characteristics previously discussed for proton beams (Figure 2.12). A low entrance dose is observed and the characteristic Bragg peak is seen at the distal end of the beam's path due to the strong dependence of energy loss on the velocity of the particle as described by Bethe–Bloch equation. The width of the Bragg peak is typically a few millimeters, and the depth and width of the Bragg peak both increase as the beam energy increases. Thus, spread-out Bragg peaks (SOBPs) are also employed in carbon ion therapy in order to generate a Bragg peak wide enough to cover clinical target volumes, and the dose proximal to the target increases as the width of the Bragg peak increases. The methods used to generate SOBPs for carbon ion beams will be discussed in Chapter 4.

Beyond the Bragg peak, fragmentation tails are present due to fragments of the ^{12}C beam with lower atomic numbers penetrating further than the primary ^{12}C ions. The dose in

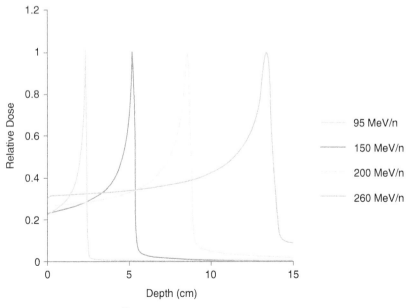

Figure 2.12 Simulated ^{12}C depth dose curves in water for various energies. Note that the relative surface dose, Bragg peak depth, Bragg peak width, and fragmentation tail contribution all increase with increasing energy. Data courtesy of Anissa Bey, Ph.D. and Jiasen Ma, Ph.D.

this region is due to secondary particles generated by fragmentation events as the primary particles cannot penetrate beyond their well-defined range. The dose contribution of the fragmentation tail must be appropriately accounted for in the treatment planning system to avoid unintended regions of high dose beyond the target volume. Correctly accounting for the dose in the fragmentation tail is especially crucial since the dose in this region can be significant and the desire is often to treat targets near critical structures with ^{12}C beams.

2.5.5 Penumbra

The penumbra of a radiation field is dependent on the collimation system and particle in question. Carbon ions provide a lateral penumbra advantage over proton beams as heavier charged particles travel in straighter lines and are less likely to be deflected from their original path due to multiple Coulomb scattering. This advantage is more pronounced with depth as the penumbra of a carbon ion beam is relatively constant with depth compared to the increasing penumbra with depth seen for proton therapy beams [31,32]. Thus, carbon ion beams are well suited to treat deep-seated targets that are adjacent to critical healthy tissues.

2.5.6 LET and RBE

Similar to proton beams, the LET of a carbon ion beam will vary with depth in tissue following the shape of Figure 2.10, but the LET of ^{12}C beams is greater than that of protons such that ^{12}C beams are classified as "high LET" [33]. High LET within the target region is beneficial as the RBE increases with increasing LET, while low LET is desirable proximal to the target to spare more healthy tissue. Unlike proton therapy which has been able to adopt a universal RBE value of 1.1, the RBE of a carbon ion beam is dependent on depth and varies significantly along the beam's path [34]. Thus, a universal RBE value for carbon and other heavy ions has not been adopted and is an active area of ongoing research.

The radiobiological principles of LET and RBE are further discussed in Chapter 3.

2.5.7 Neon and Heavier Charged Particles

The physical principles discussed in this section hold true for heavier charged particles (such as Neon) with the following notable differences:

- Greater mass results in straighter paths with even smaller lateral penumbra
- Greater mass decreases range straggling resulting in sharper Bragg peaks
- Greater charge results in increased energy loss per unit path length and shallower depths of penetration

- Fragmentation tails become more prominent and complex as the particle mass increases and more fragmentation possibilities are available
- Heavier ions provide less sparing to structures within the buildup region and beyond the Bragg peak in the fragmentation tail

2.6 Summary

2.6.1 Neutrons

- Neutrons interact differently depending on the energy of the incident neutrons
- Intermediate and fast neutrons predominantly lose energy through elastic and inelastic collisions
- Elastic scattering with hydrogen in tissue is the primary dose deposition reaction for FNT
- Thermal and epithermal neutrons predominantly interact through neutron capture interactions with hydrogen and nitrogen
- Boron-tagged pharmaceuticals can be introduced to tissues to increase the probability of neutron capture in targets of interest

2.6.2 Protons

- Protons undergo three main interactions with matter:
  1 Coulombic interactions with orbital electrons are the predominant source of energy loss:
     - The amount of energy lost per interaction is inversely proportional to the square of the proton's velocity
     - The amount of energy lost per interaction increases with electron density and decreases with increasing ionization energy of the medium
  2 Multiple coulombic interactions with the nucleus result in scattering of the primary beam
  3 Nuclear interactions result in fragmentation of the nucleus, leading to some additional dose deposition lateral to the primary beam path
- The distal and lateral penumbras increase with depth
- The density of energy deposition and RBE increase with depth to a maximum value distal to the Bragg peak
- The current recommendation by the ICRU is to use a single RBE factor of 1.1 regardless of depth when comparing proton and photon doses

2.6.3 Carbon and Heavy Ions

- Primarily interact with atomic electrons with minimal loss of energy or change in trajectory
- Nuclear interactions result in fragmentation of the incident HCP

- Exhibit a sharp Bragg peak at the end of their range with a characteristic fragmentation tail
  - Fragmentation tail becomes more pronounced for heavier ions
- Small lateral penumbra due to large mass and minimal deflection

Acknowledgments

The authors would like to acknowledge Anissa Bey, Ph.D., and Jiasen Ma, Ph.D., for providing the carbon ion data used in Figure 2.12.

References and Suggested Reading

1 Attix, F.H. (2008). *Introduction to Radiological Physics and Radiation Dosimetry*. John Wiley & Sons.

2 Khan, F.M. and Gibbons, J.P. (2010). *Khan's the Physics of Radiation Therapy*. Philadelphia, PA: Lippincott Williams & Wilkins/Wolters Kluwer.

3 Chadwick, J. (1932). The existence of a neutron. Proceedings of the Royal Society of London. Series A, Containing Papers of a Mathematical and Physical Character, 136, 692–708.

4 Locher, G. (1936). Biological effects and therapeutic possibilities of neutrons. *American Journal of Roentgenology* 36: 1–13.

5 Stone, R.S. and Larkin, J.C., Jr (1942). The treatment of cancer with fast neutrons. *Radiology* 39: 608–620.

6 Brown, D.A., Chadwick, M.B., Capote, R., Kahler, A.C., Trkov, A., Herman, M.W., Sonzogni, A.A., Danon, Y., Carlson, A.D., Dunn, M., Smith, D.L., Hale, G.M., Arbanas, G., Arcilla, R., Bates, C.R., Beck, B., Becker, B., Brown, F., Casperson, R.J., Conlin, J., Cullen, D.E., Descalle, M.A., Firestone, R., Gaines, T., Guber, K.H., Hawari, A.I., Holmes, J., Johnson, T.D., Kawano, T., Kiedrowski, B.C., Koning, A.J., Kopecky, S., Leal, L., Lestone, J.P., Lubitz, C., Márquez Damián, J.I., Mattoon, C.M., Mccutchan, E.A., Mughabghab, S., Navratil, P., Neudecker, D., Nobre, G.P.A., Noguere, G., Paris, M., Pigni, M.T., Plompen, A.J., Pritychenko, B., Pronyaev, V.G., Roubtsov, D., Rochman, D., Romano, P., Schillebeeckx, P., Simakov, S., Sin, M., Sirakov, I., Sleaford, B., Sobes, V., Soukhovitskii, E.S., Stetcu, I., Talou, P., Thompson, I., Van Der Marck, S., Welser-Sherrill, L., Wiarda, D., White, M., Wormald, J.L., Wright, R.Q., Zerkle, M., Žerovnik, G., and Zhu, Y. (2018). ENDF/B-VIII.0: The 8th major release of the nuclear reaction data library with CIELO-project cross sections, new standards and thermal scattering data. *Nuclear Data Sheets* 148: 1–142.

7 Jones, D., Schreuder, A., and Symons, J. (1995). Particle therapy at NAC: Physical aspects. Proceedings of the 14th International Conference on Cyclotrons and their Applications (World Scientific, Singapore 1996), 491.

8 Turner, J.E. (2007). *Atoms, Radiation, and Radiation Protection*. Weinheim: Wiley-VCH.

9 Moss, R.L. (2014). Critical review, with an optimistic outlook, on Boron Neutron Capture Therapy (BNCT). *Applied Radiation and Isotopes: Including Data, Instrumentation and Methods for Use in Agriculture, Industry and Medicine* 88: 2–11.

10 Liu, C., Bhangoo, R.S., Sio, T.T., Yu, N.Y., Shan, J., Chiang, J.S., Ding, J.X., Rule, W.G., Korte, S., Lara, P., Ding, X., Bues, M., Hu, Y., Dewees, T., Ashman, J.B., and Liu, W. (2019). Dosimetric comparison of distal esophageal carcinoma plans for patients treated with small-spot intensity-modulated proton versus volumetric-modulated arc therapies. *Journal Of Applied Clinical Medical Physics / American College of Medical Physics* 20: 15–27.

11 Stromberger, C., Cozzi, L., Budach, V., Fogliata, A., Ghadjar, P., Wlodarczyk, W., Jamil, B., Raguse, J.D., Böttcher, A., and Marnitz, S. (2016). Unilateral and bilateral neck SIB for head and neck cancer patients: Intensity-modulated proton therapy, tomotherapy, and RapidArc. *Strahlentherapie und Onkologie: Organ der Deutschen Rontgengesellschaft. [et al]* 192: 232–239.

12 White, D.R., Griffith, R.V., and Wilson, I.J. (2016). Report 46. Journal of the International Commission on Radiation Units and Measurements.

13 Berger, M., Inokuti, M., Anderson, H., Bichsel, H., and Dennis, J. (1984). ICRU report 37: Stopping powers for electrons and positrons. *Journal of the International Commission on Radiation Units and Measurements* 19.

14 Deasy, J. (1994). ICRU report 49, stopping powers and ranges for protons and alpha particles. *Medical Physics* 21: 709–710.

15 Highland, V.L. (1975). Some practical remarks on multiple scattering. *Nuclear Instruments and Methods* 129: 497–499.

16 Eyges, L. (1948). Multiple scattering with energy loss. *Physical Review* 74: 1534.

17 Underwood, T., Giantsoudi, D., Moteabbed, M., Zietman, A., Efstathiou, J., Paganetti, H., and Lu, H.-M. (2016). Can we advance proton therapy for prostate? Considering alternative beam angles and relative biological effectiveness variations when comparing against intensity modulated radiation therapy. *International Journal of Radiation Oncology, Biology, Physics* 95: 454–464.

18 Mcnamara, A.L., Schuemann, J., and Paganetti, H. (2015). A phenomenological relative biological effectiveness (RBE) model for proton therapy based on all published in vitro cell survival data. *Physics in Medicine and Biology* 60: 8399–8416.

19 Wan Chan Tseung, H.S., Ma, J., Kreofsky, C.R., Ma, D.J., and Beltran, C. (2016). Clinically applicable Monte Carlo-based biological dose optimization for the treatment of head and neck cancers with spot-scanning proton therapy.

International Journal of Radiation Oncology, Biology, Physics 95: 1535–1543.

20 Deluca, P., Wambersie, A., and Whitmore, G. (2007). Prescribing, recording, and reporting proton-beam therapy. *Journal of the ICRU* 7.

21 Paganetti, H. (2019). *Proton Therapy Physics*. Boca Raton, Florida: CRC Press.

22 PodgoršAk, E.B. (2006). *Radiation Physics for Medical Physicists*. Berlin; New York: Springer.

23 Saunders, William, et al. (1985). "Helium-Ion Radiation Therapy at the Lawrence Berkeley Laboratory: Recent Results of a Northern California Oncology Group Clinical Trial."*Radiation Research*, vol. 104, no. 2, Radiation Research Society, pp. S227–34, https://doi.org/10.2307/3576652

24 Grün, R., Friedrich, T., Krämer, M., Zink, K., Durante, M., Engenhart-Cabillic, R., and Scholz, M. (2015). Assessment of potential advantages of relevant ions for particle therapy: A model based study. *Medical Physics* 42: 1037–1047.

25 Krämer, M., Scifoni, E., Schuy, C., Rovituso, M., Tinganelli, W., Maier, A., Kaderka, R., Kraft-Weyrather, W., Brons, S., Tessonnier, T., Parodi, K., and Durante, M. (2016). Helium ions for radiotherapy? Physical and biological verifications of a novel treatment modality. *Medical Physics* 43: 1995.

26 Remmes, N.B., Herman, M.G., and Kruse, J.J. (2012). Optimizing normal tissue sparing in ion therapy using calculated isoeffective dose for ion selection. *International Journal of Radiation Oncology, Biology, Physics* 83: 756–762.

27 Haettner, E., Iwase, H., and Schardt, D. (2006). Experimental fragmentation studies with 12C therapy beams. *Radiation Protection Dosimetry* 122: 485–487.

28 Endo, S., Takada, M., Onizuka, Y., Tanaka, K., Maeda, N., Ishikawa, M., Miyahara, N., Hayabuchi, N., Shizuma, K., and Hoshi, M. (2007). Microsimetric evaluation of secondary particles in a phantom produced by Carbon 290 MeV/nucleon Ions at HIMAC. *Journal of Radiation Research* 48: 397–406.

29 Jäkel, O. (2009). Medical physics aspects of particle therapy. *Radiation Protection Dosimetry* 137: 156–166.

30 Park, S.H. and Kang, J.O. (2011). Basics of particle therapy I: Physics. *Radiation Oncology Journal* 29: 135–146.

31 Suit, H., Delaney, T., Goldberg, S., Paganetti, H., Clasie, B., Gerweck, L., Niemierko, A., Hall, E., Flanz, J., Hallman, J., and Trofimov, A. (2010). Proton vs carbon ion beams in the definitive radiation treatment of cancer patients. *Radiotherapy and Oncology* 95: 3–22.

32 Weber, U. and Kraft, G. (2009). Comparison of carbon ions versus protons. *The Cancer Journal* 15: 325–332.

33 Ohno, T. (2013). Particle radiotherapy with carbon ion beams. *The EPMA Journal* 4: 9-9.

34 Lomax, A.J. (2009). Charged particle therapy: The physics of interaction. *The Cancer Journal* 15: 285–291.

3

The Radiobiology of Particle Therapy

P. Fossati, S. Tubin, and E.B. Hug

MedAustron Ion Therapy Center, Wiener Neustadt, Austria, EBG MedAustron GmbH, Marie Curie-Strasse 5, 2700 Wiener Neustadt, Austria e-mail: piero.fossati@medaustron.at

In this chapter we will highlight the most relevant radiobiological characteristics of particle irradiation, trying to focus on the differences between low and high Linear Energy Transfer (LET).

3.1 Relationship between LET and Complexity of DNA Damage

Several different radiation-induced DNA-damage types have been identified so far [1–3]. The kind of DNA-damage induced by ionizing radiation (IR) plays an essential role in determining its effect. Double-strand breaks (DSBs) are the most common kind of lethal DNA damage [4,5]. The mechanisms behind the radiation-induced DNA-damage and potential DNA (un)repair have important clinical implications for radiation treatment.

DNA injuries can be simple, isolated, and repairable, resulting in cell survival; or more complex, clustered and unrepairable leading to cell death. The most common DNA lesions induced by IR are represented by the isolated single-strand breaks (SSBs) or single base damages, which usually are efficiently addressed by base-excision repair [6]. Being reparable, these lesions don't have much impact on therapeutic efficacy.

Also, DSB can be repaired and the cellular response to non-complex DSBs encompasses non-homologous end-joining (NHEJ) and homologous recombination (HR) [7,8]. However, non-DSBs and DSBs clustered injuries represent a big challenge for cellular repair mechanisms and usually result in cell death.

The radiation quality that is most relevant to determine the kind of DNA damage is the mean distance between two ionization events. A physical parameter closely correlated to the mean distance between ionizations is the energy lost per unit of length or Linear Energy Transfer (LET), which is typically measured in KeV/μm. If the mean distance between two ionizations is much larger than the DNA double helix diameter it is unlikely that a single particle or quantum of energy will result in a DSB or in a complex DNA damage. In this case the radiation is described as low-LET. If, on the contrary, ionization events are denser than the DNA diameter, the radiation is described as high-LET.

High-LET radiation can induce clustered, "dirty" DNA injuries including very complex combinations of SSBs and DSBs that are lethal because they are irreparable.

X-rays, γ-rays, and electrons have low-LET, and fast neutrons have high-LET. Positively charged particles have a variable LET. The LET of charged particles increases as their

Principles and Practice of Particle Therapy, First Edition. Edited by Timothy D. Malouff and Daniel M. Trifiletti.
© 2022 John Wiley & Sons Ltd. Published 2022 by John Wiley & Sons Ltd.

energy decreases. LET in the entrance plateau is lower than in the Bragg peak. Protons can, as a first approximation, be considered low-LET particles because their LET becomes large enough to result in clustered DNA damage only in the very last portion of their Bragg peak, where the dose is extremely low.

Heavy charged particles, such as carbon, oxygen, or nitrogen-ions, produce sparse ionization in the entrance plateau and dense ionization only "in" (carbon) or "a few centimeters before and in" (oxygen) the Bragg peak. This makes them ideal tools for radiotherapy as the high-LET component can be focused in the target while the surrounding healthy tissue will be exposed only to low-LET radiation.

The complex DNA-injuries produced by high-LET radiation are typically clustered within 10–20 bp corresponding to approximately 1–2 helical turns of the DNA [9]. Such an effective induction of irreparable DNA-damages consequent to dense ionization is what makes high-LET radiation biologically highly effective in comparison with low-LET radiation (relative biological effectiveness [RBE] of high-LET carbon-ions is ~ 3–5 folds higher than with low-LET radiation) [10–12]. The relationship between LET and RBE is complex nonlinear and non-monotonous and will be discussed in detail later in this chapter; it can however be assumed that the higher the LET is, the more complex the DNA damage will be [13–16].

The concept of radiation-induced clustered DNA damage has been introduced in 1988 [17]. The dominant role of LET in inducing complex lethal lesions is undisputed. It has been estimated that the amount of complex DNA damage produced by low-LET radiation is two orders of magnitude smaller than that of a similar dose of high-LET radiation [16,18]. Less than 20% of direct DNA damage induced by low-LET radiation is complex enough to be potentially lethal [15,16,19]. Several simulation models have been used to calculate the track structures of a variety of ionizing radiation qualities and have consistently shown that the complexity of DNA lesions increases with LET. For high-LET radiation at least 70% of all DSBs are of complex type [20–26].

The amount of potentially lethal direct DNA damage produced by low-LET radiation is not enough to explain the observed cell death rate. As is well known from classical radiobiology, about two-thirds of the cell killing effect of low-LET radiation is due to indirect DNA damage mediated by free radicals.

3.2 Experimental Methods to Investigate Particle-Induced DNA Damage

Different experimental methods allow investigating the number and spatial distribution of complex DNA damage [27–35]. Currently, the phosphorylated form of histone variant H2AX

(γ-H2AX) is the most used biomarker of DNA damage induced by IR specifically at sites of DNA DSBs [34,35]. The principle is that at each nascent DSB site, H2AX molecules become rapidly phosphorylated as the γ-H2AX foci in the chromatin which can be visualized in situ with the appropriate antibody. For example Mirsch et al. performed in 2015 a quantification of the spatial distribution of DNA lesions following charged particles irradiation by using the γ-H2AX foci technology in biologically relevant material [36]. Using a mouse model tissue, they found that high-LET charged particles damage tissue non-homogenously, confirming their greater biological effectiveness being a function of highly dense ionization events along their path. Pang et al. described the correlation between the killing efficacy and the sizes of DNA fragments following radiation exposure, defining the short DNA fragments as a hallmark of greater RBE of heavy charged particle irradiation [37,38]. They have investigated DNA DSBs following exposure of plasmid DNA to low-LET Co-60 gamma photon and electron irradiation and to high-LET Beryllium and Argon ions with atomic force microscopy. In respect to low-LET irradiation, heavy-charged particles induced a significantly greater proportion of short DNA fragments in irradiated DNA molecules, which was attributed to enhanced biological effectiveness of high-LET irradiations reflecting dense and clustered DNA damage. The same results were previously obtained by neutron irradiated plasmid DNA[39].

Recently the complexity of high-LET radiation-induced DNA damage has been demonstrated in vivo as shown in Figure 3.1 [40].

The lower part of the figure shows distribution of foci diameter for carbon ion (in red) or X-rays (in blue).

This figure has been modified from Oike et al. [40].

Finally, an increasing number of in vitro studies confirmed the essential role of clustered DNA damage in determining improved tumor cells killing after exposure to high-LET charged particles including carbon ions, calcium ions, iron ions, uranium ions, lead ions, tin ions, etc. [41–43].

3.3 Chromosomal Effects of Particle Irradiation

From the above considerations we would expect that few cells are able to repair high-LET-induced DNA damage and that the result of such repair would be unpredictable. We would therefore expect that, in comparison to low-LET, high-LET irradiation would produce fewer but more complex chromosomal aberrations.

Using the technique of premature chromosome condensation, the group from GSI (Gesellschaft fur SchwerIonen Forschung) in Germany, investigated chromosomes fragmentation in non-cycling cells after exposure to different kind of radiation [44]. Analogously to what was demonstrated in the

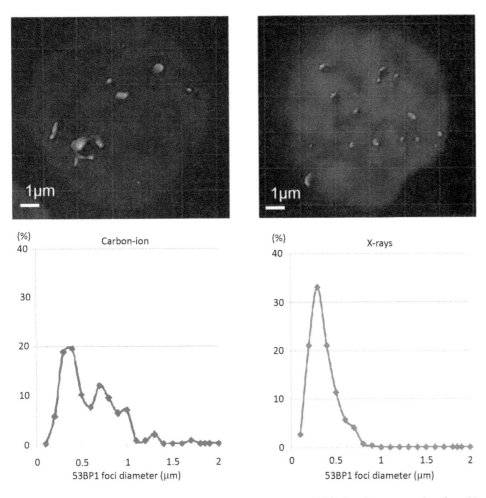

Figure 3.1 DSB are visualized with an antibody against p53 (53BP1). Specimens are taken from biopsies obtained from irradiated patients (biopsy taken 30 min after RT). The figure shows 53BP1 foci in tissue obtained from patients irradiated with carbon ions (upper left side) or X-rays (upper right side) [40].

simpler plasmid model, they could show that heavy particles produce and over-dispersion in the length of chromosome fragments which can be interpreted as the effect of clustered damages produced by a single ion.

The group from National Institute of Radiological Sciences (NIRS) in Japan, confirmed that early rejoining of damaged chromosomes is significantly rarer after high-LET irradiation [45].

Consistent results were obtained examining chromosomal aberrations in peripheral blood of patients treated with photons IMRT or with carbon ion RT, with patients treated with carbon displaying fewer but more complex aberrations [46].

However in vitro data have shown that high-LET radiation produces not only more complex but also more frequent chromosome aberrations than low-LET irradiation [47]. Interestingly most of the excess aberrant rejoining of high LET occurs early (10 hours) after irradiation [48]. The low yield of aberrations in patients can be explained by the reduced volume of circulating blood treated with particles, but the in vitro data suggest that the simplistic idea of almost completely non-repairable damage induced by high LET has to be revised.

3.4 In Vitro Cell Survival

The radiation dose necessary to exert the same tumor cell killing effect is lower for high-LET than for low-LET radiation[49]. This increase in killing efficiency with LET has been clearly proven by several in vitro studies over the years, starting in early eighties. Data of cell survival after irradiation with ions or photons for more than 1100 cell lines have been collected and are freely available online within the PIDE (Particle Irradiation Data Ensemble) project sponsored by GSI [50]. In very general terms dose survival curves of high-LET radiation are steeper and less curved than those of low-LET radiation.

Moreover it is known since the historical experiments performed in the seventies at Berkeley heavy-ion linear accelerator that response to high LET depends only minimally on the cell cycle phase [51].

Recently Ando et al. have reviewed the dose survival curves of 45 cell lines irradiated with X-rays or carbon ions [52]. These curves have been fitted with the linear quadratic (LQ) models, and the α- and β parameter have been extracted. The α parameter did, as expected, show a strong dependence on LET confirming that high LET is more effective in killing cells. The increase of α with LET well agrees with the idea that a single track of high-LET radiation can produce lethal damage. However, rather surprisingly, the β parameter of all cell lines displayed minimal dependence on LET. This finding is also confirmed by in vivo data based on mouse intestinal crypt survival [53]. The square component in the LQ model should represent cell killing due to damage produced by two radiation tracks and therefore also β should increase with LET. The authors of this interesting study suggested an alternative model based on a modified version of the repair saturation model (RS) initially proposed by Goodhead in 1985 [54]. The underlying hypothesis behind this model is that DNA damages are repaired by an existing pool of enzymes whose capacity can be saturated.

High-LET cell killing is therefore mediated by both reparable and non-reparable DNA damages. The increased killing efficacy is due to both an increase of non-repairable damages and a saturation of repair mechanism. Mathematically many alternative models can achieve a good fit of cell survival data; the most interesting aspect of the RS model is that its theoretical background agrees with the data on chromosome aberrations. Further confirmation of the potential reparability even of high-LET-induced DNA damage comes from the work of Suzuki et al. [55] who compared single and fractionated irradiation with X-ray and carbon ions of different LET of different cancer and normal tissues cell lines.

These authors compared the surviving fraction of cells plated immediately after irradiation and of cells incubated in favorable conditions for 24 hours after irradiation and before plating. They could demonstrate higher survival of the incubated cells for X-ray and also for carbon ion at all LET values and attributed this finding to repair of potentially lethal damage. In the same paper the authors investigated the effect of fractionated irradiation. Interestingly, the surviving fraction after X-ray irradiation increased from the third fraction onward (or in other words the radiosensitivty decreased) whereas the effect of carbon ion remained constant at all fractions.

3.5   Oxygen Effect

Regardless if potentially reparable or not, most of the damage induced by high-LET radiation is due to the direct interaction between particles and DNA. The role of free radicals mediated damage is almost negligible. Oxygen stabilizes free radicals and therefore enhances the effect of low-LET radiation, but it is expected to play a minor role in determining the response to high LET. Blakely et al. examined the biological effects of high energy (e.g., 308–670 MeV/u) heavy-ion charged particle beams on variety of in vitro cellular systems showing that the Bragg peak of carbon, neon, and argon ion beams effectively reduced the radioresistance of tumor cells due to hypoxia and intercellular factors within multicellular spheroids [56]. The oxygen enhancement ratio (OER) represents the ratio of the radiation dose required to produce a specific radiobiological effect, like killing tumor cells, in the absence of oxygen to the dose required for the same effect in its presence [57]. The above-mentioned experiments allowed estimating OER for high LET in comparison to OER for X-rays or γ-rays. The oxygen effect is greater for low-LET than for high-LET radiation. OER varies with level of effect but can be 2.5–3-fold for low-LET radiations which means that up to 3 times higher radiation dose of photons is required to kill hypoxic tumor cells in respect to normoxic cells [58]. Experimental data consistently show that OER starts to reduce with LET above 100 keV/μm, reaching unity at high dose averaged LET-values of ~ 500 keV/μm [59–62]. Because of this property high-LET radiation is usually used in the treatment of hypoxic tumors.

3.6   Mechanisms of Cell Death Induced by High-LET Irradiation

Accumulating evidence shows that the different kind of DNA damage induced by high-LET radiations result in a different cascade of intra- and intercellular signaling. *Fournier et al.* investigated the accumulation of the cell cycle regulators TP53 and CDKN1A comparing the effects of X-rays and carbon-ions, xenon, bismuth, and uranium-ions in normal human fibroblasts [63]. Accumulation of TP53 protein and increase in CDKN1A levels were both dose- and LET-dependent. Jakob et al. explored, in the same cell line, the immunocytochemical response to DNA damage induced by bismuth and carbon ions (LETs ranging from about 300 to 13,600 keV/μm) describing very similar arrangements of protein clusters for H2AX, PCNA, p21, and MRE11B [64]. These experiments suggested that factors like compaction or confined movement of chromatin may play a role in the observed clustering of proteins. Additionally, it has been suggested also by *Chang et al.* that LET effects probably play a role in the misregulation of gene function in normal cultured differentiating human lens epithelial cells exposed to high-energy accelerated iron-ions, protons, and X-rays [65]. These authors showed that transcription and translation of CDKN1A were both temporally regulated after a single 4 Gy radiation dose. It is indeed clear that not only does high-LET radiation produce more and more complex lethal DNA damage but that it does also result in different gene activation and signaling and ultimately in different mechanism of death. For example, *Iwadate et al.* investigated in vitro the mechanisms behind the radiation-induced apoptosis by comparing the cytotoxic effects of high-LET carbon versus low-LET X-ray radiation. Considering that a mutation in the *p53 gene* plays an essential role in the radioresistance of many cancer cell lines, they used either knock-out or wild-type p53 glioma cell lines. Apoptosis was detected by colony-forming assay and flow cytometric. Their results showed higher cytotoxic effectiveness of high-LET charged particle radiation against glioma cells in respect to X-rays. Interestingly this paper also showed that cell death other than p53-dependent apoptosis may participate in the cytotoxicity of heavy-charged particles[66]. Those results were confirmed by *Tsuboi et al.* who compared the cytotoxicity of high-LET carbon-ions and y-rays by irradiating human glioblastoma cell lines and fibroblasts, with or without p53-mutation[67]. Cell inactivation was assessed by colony formation assay, morphological detection of apoptosis, and flow-cytometry, while the expression of p53 and p21 were analyzed by immunoblotting. Carbon-ions induced an effective anti-proliferative effect in all glioma cells in a LET-dependent manner regardless of p53 status whereas y-ray radiosensitivities differed substantially according to p53 status. Their findings suggested that high-LET radiation might specifically increase the radiosensitivity of glioblastoma cells by molecular targeting focused on the modulation of G2/M check point.

Hamada et al. demonstrated the potential role of high-LET radiation in treatment of radioresistant tumor cells, like those, for example, characterized by an overexpression of Bcl-2 antiapoptotic protein determining radioresistance [68]. In their study, Bcl-2 overexpressing "HeLa" cells and neomycin-resistant gene-expressing "HeLa" cells were exposed to y-rays or high-LET helium, and carbon- and neon-ions, and assessed for the clonogenic survival, apoptosis, and cell cycle distribution. The findings showed that high-LET heavy ions overwhelmed Bcl-2-related tumor radioresistance, which may be caused by the enhanced apoptotic response and prolonged G2/M arrest.

Miszczyk et al. explored the types of cell-killing induced by protons and X-rays in an ex vivo human peripheral blood lymphocyte model [69]. The cells were irradiated with 60 MeV proton beam or 250-kV X-rays in the dose range of 0.3–4.0 Gy. Interestingly, they found that x-rays and protons induce cell-killing by different modes where protons caused relatively higher yields of cell death that appears to be necrosis compared to X-rays. Similarly, *Maalouf et al.* performed the experiment exploring the types of cell-killing induced by carbon-ions and X-rays in head and neck squamous cell carcinoma cell lines [70]. Their findings indicated that different types of cell death were induced by carbon ions (33.6 and 184 keV/μm) and X-rays, respectively. High-LET radiation induced clonogenic cell death for both radiosensitive (SCC61) and radioresistant (SQ20B) cells and was more effective compared with X-rays.

Additional studies assessed and compared the effects of high-LET versus low-LET radiation on changes in expression of genes associated with cell death and cell cycle in human oral tumor squamous cell lines, and what they all had in common is gene up-regulation being dose-responsive to carbon- and neon-ions, but to a much lesser extent to X-rays [71–73]. Five specific genes: *E2F transcription factor 3, Cyclin D1* (both related to cell cycle), *E3 ubiquitin ligase, TGF-β receptor 2, and bone morphogenic protein 7* (all linked to TGF-β signaling pathway) were assessed by quantitative PCR validation showing that gene expression was specific to carbon- and neon-ions but not affected by X-rays. Finally, *Matsumoto et al.* studied the molecular changes in human melanoma cells after exposure to 2 Gy carbon-ions and X-rays using single-color microarrays identifying 22 genes that were exclusively reactive to carbon-ions [74]. All these were related to cell death, cell cycle progression, cell communication, and cell proliferation.

In conclusion, in vitro data consistently confirm that high LET has greater efficacy in killing cells, that the effect is less dependent on hypoxia and viability of apoptotic pathways and that the mechanism of cell death differs from that of low-LET irradiation.

3.7 Relative Biological Effectiveness (RBE)

From what has been discussed above we can highlight three fundamental properties of high LET positively charged particle irradiation: (i) the same physical dose results in more cell killing as compared to low-LET irradiation, or in other words they have an increased effectiveness, (ii) this increased effectiveness depends on LET, (iii) the results are relatively independent from many factors that influence the results of low-LET irradiation (such as oxygenation and viability of apoptotic pathways).

The increase in cell killing efficacy is typically described in terms of Relative Biological Effectiveness (RBE).

RBE is the ratio between the physical absorbed dose of a reference radiation and of a test radiation that produce the same effect.

$$RBE = \frac{D_{ref}}{D_{test}}$$

Obviously RBE depends on the radiation quality and on the selected endpoint; if the dose response curve (for either the test or the reference radiation) is non-linear, RBE will also depend on dose.

Let us consider for example cell survival of the melanoma cell line C32TG for X-ray and carbon ion with LET of 77 KeV/μm or of 55 KeV/μm [52] . All dose response curves can be fitted with the linear quadratic model.

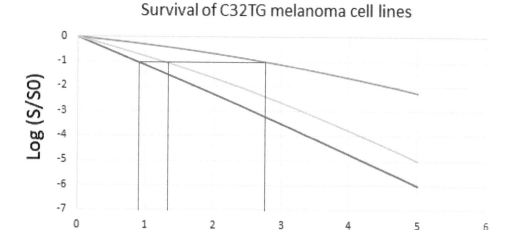

Figure 3.2   Survival of melanoma cell line, based on [52].

As can be seen in Figure 3.2, carbon curves are steeper and less curved than the X-ray curve, and the higher LET carbon curve is steeper and straighter than the middle LET one.

The dose of X-ray that produces 10% survival (1 log kill) is approximately 2.8 Gy whereas the same survival is achieved with carbon ion at 1.3 Gy (55 KeV/µm) or at 0.9 Gy (77 KeV/µm).

If we aim at 1% survival (2 log kills) we need 4.7 Gy with X-ray, 2.35 Gy with carbon (55 KeV/µm), and 1.75 Gy with carbon (77 KeV/µm).

Quantitatively different results would be obtained with other cell lines; however, even after clearly selecting the biological model we cannot possibly describe the increase in killing efficacy of high-LET particles with a constant number. From the example above we can readily see that the RBE can vary significantly, in this example ranging between 2 (1% survival of mid LET carbon vs. X-ray) and 3.11 (10% survival of high-LET carbon vs. X-ray) as summarized in Table 3.1.

Cellular experiments are carried out in conditions that differ from those of clinical treatments. Most importantly the irradiation setup is typically designed in such a way that the cells are exposed to an almost uniform radiation quality. As

known, positively charged particles deposit their energy in multiple ionization events. As they penetrate matter they lose energy and therefore they modify their probability of further interaction. On the macroscopic scale this results in the well-known shape of the depth dose profile called Bragg peak and described by the Bethe Block equation. On the microscopic scale this results in an increase of LET along each particle track. In an experimental set up a thin layer of cells can be irradiated by any portion of the Bragg peak by simply interposing a variable amount of material in front of the sample to be irradiated. We can therefore measure the properties of each particle at different LET values in uniform and controlled conditions. In the clinical setting the patient and tumor anatomy is on the contrary fixed and each portion of the tumor and of the surrounding healthy tissue is exposed to a complex mixed field of primary particles with different distribution of LET (different LET spectra). Moreover, due to inelastic nuclear interactions, not only primary particles but also several fragments will contribute to the complexity of the mixed field of irradiation. Mathematical models are needed to extrapolate the RBE derived from simple experimental data to such a complex scenario. Two different approaches have been

Table 3.1   Changes in RBE with LET and dose.

	55 KeV/µm Carbon ions	77 KeV/µm Carbon ions
10% Survival	RBE = 2.15	RBE = 3.11
	(2.8 Gy X-ray/1.3 Gy carbon)	(2.8 Gy X-ray/0.9 Gy carbon)
1% Survival	RBE = 2.15	RBE = 2.69
	(4.7 Gy X-ray/2.35 Gy carbon)	(4.7 Gy X-ray/1.75 Gy carbon)

used in clinical practice. The first one is based on the local effect model (LEM). This model, developed at GSI, is based on the assumption that dense ionization can still be described in terms of absorbed physical dose if this is modeled in the nanometer scale. Low LET has a uniform dose distribution so the mean dose in a voxel of 1 mm does not differ from the dose in each subvoxel of 1 μm or even of 1 nm. On the contrary with high LET the same dose to a voxel of 1 mm derives from subvoxels with very high dose (around the single particle tracks) and subvoxel with little or no dose. The higher the LET the more inhomogeneous the dose distribution on the nanometer scale.

Moreover, according to the LEM model the probability of inducing a lethal event depends only on physical dose in the nanometer scale. The last main assumption of this model is that we can derive the microscopic probability of lethal events from the global cell killing measurable in low LET. Four different version of the LEM model have been described in detail [75–84]. The LEM model has excellent agreement with experimental data on survival of different cell lines. It can be used to describe any mixed field of particles and is therefore well suited to active scanning particle therapy. The LEM model can correctly predict the change of RBE with dose per fraction. This model has been originally created to be used with carbon ions but can be used also with other particles including protons, helium, etc. The underlying hypothesis of the LEM model has been, to some extent, confirmed by an elegant experiment that could show how focusing low-LET protons to the sub-micrometric scale could increase RBE [85].

The LEM model is used in clinical routine by European and Chinese facilities. Among the free parameters that have to be provided as input to the model there are the α and β values of the photons dose response curve for the endpoint under investigation. Interestingly four version have been developed but only the first version has ever been used in the clinics.

The second strategy has been developed at NIRS in Japan [86,87]. With an empiric and pragmatic approach, NIRS researchers selected a single cell line (derived from normal human salivary glands) and measured survival curves in several positions along the Bragg peak. They confirmed a linear quadratic dose response curve and measured the relative α and β values at different depths. They designed a passive irradiation system in which a spread out Bragg peak was created with a ridge filter. The ridge filter was designed to produce a tapered physical dose profile with the distal portion receiving a lower dose in order to achieve a constant HSG survival at the 10% survival level.

Assuming a mixed field of particle with each component contributing a dose d_i to a total dose D, and having a dose survival curve described by α_i and β_i, the overall dose survival curve was described by mixed α_{mix} and β_{mix} estimated with the Zaider Rossi formula.

$$\alpha_{mix} = \sum \alpha_i \frac{d_i}{D}$$

$$\sqrt{\beta}_{mix} = \sum \sqrt{\beta}_i \frac{d_i}{D}$$

This approach was theoretically valid only for the dose corresponding to 10% survival of HSG (i.e. 1.83 Gy of X-ray); however, the NIRS group considered that the underlying uncertainties of the clinical scenario were substantial and mandated an even further empirical approach. They introduced a scaling factor between the measurable in vitro endpoint (HSG cell survival) and the non-measurable clinically relevant endpoints (such as severe skin toxicity or mucositis). According to past experience with neutrons and in vivo experiments of pig skin reddening, they set this value at (about) 1.5. Therefore, the non-uniform carbon ion SOBP, which was biologically equivalent to 1.83 Gy of X-ray, was deemed to be clinically equivalent to 2.7 Gy of X-ray. Finally, in NIRS clinical practice, dose escalation trials were conducted and the prescription dose was scaled disregarding the known change of RBE with dose per fraction. This had to do with practical difficulties in manufacturing a new ridge filter for each new dose level. When going from the initial dose, supposed to be clinically equivalent to 2.7 Gy of X-ray, to the final prescription dose that was found to be necessary, e.g,. in osteosarcoma, they simply increased the absorbed physical dose 1.63 times and described this as clinically equivalent to 4.4 Gy of photons (2.7 Gy x 1.63). Ultimately prescription dose and dose constraints for organs at risk were determined within clinical dose escalation trials.

This RBE model, usually called the Kanai semi-empirical model, was not suitable for active scanning, could not predict the survival curve of different cell lines, and could not be used for different ions. Despite these potential drawbacks, initial clinical results at NIRS were excellent and comparable with initial results obtained at GSI with the more refined LEM model [88–90].

The Kanai semi-empirical model was used by all Japanese facilities. When spot scanning was introduced in Japan a new RBE model had to be employed and a modified version of the microdosimetric kinetic model (MKM) was developed [91,92]. The MKM model, initially created by Hawkins [93], despite a different mathematical formalism, is based on assumptions similar to those of the LEM model. In LEM, the absorbed dose is modeled in very small sub-micrometric voxels.

The discrete nature of ionization events produced by a single particle is disregarded mediating over many scenarios and the amorphous track structure is considered. With this spatial resolution dose is supposed to be homogeneous in each voxel. In MKM, the scale is limited to domains of typically 5 μm. In these larger domains the inhomogeneity of the dose cannot be disregarded and a quality factor is introduced to account for the denser or sparser ionization events. The peculiarity of the MKM model is that this quality factor is related to a quantity (the lineal energy) that can be directly measured with a physical device (the micro-dosimeter, and hence the model name).

In order to keep consistency with the wealth of data accumulated during dose escalation trials performed with the Kanai semi-empirical model, the modified MKM model used in Japan is no longer considering X-ray as the reference irradiation (this would hardly have been possible considering that dose escalation was performed formally disregarding RBE dependence on dose per fraction). The reference radiation is the carbon ion optimized with the Kanai model considered in the center of the SOBP [91]. Considering that the Kanai model had X-ray as reference radiation, the modified MKM is still referring to X-ray but in an indirect way.

Considering the major unaccounted for sources of uncertainty related to the clinical setting, the practical Japanese approach was widely regarded as justified. Interestingly and somewhat surprisingly, a recent evaluation of different RBE models performed by the German group in Heidelberg has shown that the modified MKM may not only be as good as, but even superior, to any version of the LEM model in fitting patients data [94].

From the clinical point of view, the difference between the two models has important implications. Dose prescription and dose constraints derived from clinical experience obtained with one RBE model cannot be used at nominal value in the other model and require a dedicated effort to convert the numbers [95–103]. Moreover, special care has to be exerted in designing multi-centric prospective trail involving institutions using different RBE models [104].

In the recent ICRU Report 93 on carbon ions [105] it is recommended to prescribe, record, and report RBE weighted dose. The selection of the RBE model (as well as that of the model free parameters if any) is left to the treating institution. RBE models are a validated tool, widely used in clinical practice and recommended by ICRU. It is however worthwhile to briefly review their intrinsic limitations.

As previously mentioned, the effect of the high-LET component of carbon ion irradiation is relatively independent from many factors that influence the response to low-LET. Using low-LET as reference irradiation can therefore lead to artificial changes in RBE. From a purely radiobiological point of view the ideal reference radiation should be as stable as possible: heavy-charged particles are not ideal because their properties change along their penetration path (variable LET); X-rays are not good candidates because their properties change with any change of the irradiated system such as hypoxia and mutations (low-LET). Fast neutrons, having a fixed and high-LET would be the ideal reference radiation. For historical reasons it is not possible

to abandon X-rays as reference, because the overwhelming majority of available clinical data has been obtained with this modality. Despite having been used for more than 100 years and despite millions of patients treated, the basic dose response curve of X-rays is still not known for several clinically relevant endpoints (e.g., risk of renal failure for homogenous kidney RT). No model can predict the RBE relative to an unknown dose response curve; it is however possible to optimistically believe that the status of our knowledge will improve in the future. Notwithstanding that, there are other more fundamental theoretical issues. The RBE concept is based on the assumptions that both the reference and the test radiation dose response curve are measurable. This is of course true for low-LET such as X-ray or high-LET such as fast neutrons. For charged particles there is not a single dose response curve but rather many curves according to the LET or to the position in the Bragg peak. For cell survival we can have the dose response curve of carbon at 55 or at 77 KeV/μm (see Figure 3.1). For clinically relevant endpoints, for example xerostomia induced by parotid irradiation, it is impossible to measure a carbon dose response curve. It is in fact impossible to irradiate a target whose dimension is in the order of magnitude of several centimeters with carbon ions of uniform quality. The same absorbed physical dose may have a two- to threefold difference in effect according to the mix of high and low LET. What is implicitly assumed is that, if we already have a voxel by voxel RBE model, and if we apply a non-uniform absorbed physical dose of carbon ion in such a way that the resulting RBE weighted dose is uniform, and if the macroscopic observable endpoint is identical to that obtained with a uniform dose of X-ray, then our voxel by voxel RBE model was correct. It is immediately evident that this way of reasoning is flawed as there are many (potentially infinite) different non-uniform X-ray dose distributions that would result in the identical macroscopic endpoint. As a confirmation of this statement we could consider how infinite dose distributions result in the same generalized equivalent uniform dose (gEUD) used in one of the most classic NTCP model [106].

When only a single data point is available from clinical data (such as in the case of xerostomia, renal insufficiency, malabsorption, dysphagia, dyspnea, neurocognitive impairment, and radiation-induced liver disease) it is even theoretically impossible to test RBE models against clinical data. There is not enough information in the spatially global measurable endpoint to validate the voxel by voxel RBE.

A similar situation applies regarding to time. In basically all clinical scenarios we can only measure the endpoint at the end (and often a long time after the end) of a fractionated irradiation. In all RBE models used in the clinic we are assuming (typically without even stating it explicitly) that the effect of each fraction of low-LET would be identical and that the effect of each fraction of particle therapy is identical and therefore that the RBE is constant over the treatment. We have already highlighted that this approximation does not even correspond to measurable data from fractionated cell lines irradiation [55]. In the much more complex clinical scenario all the adaptive changes of the tumor and healthy tissue during (and in large part due to) irradiation have a major impact on outcome and are completely neglected by current RBE models.

Some authors believe that better and more complex RBE models will be able to cope with all these issues; we are on the contrary convinced that the proliferation of new RBE models would be detrimental. In our opinion it would fail to improve clinical results and would complicate exchange of information. A more practical approach would be to use the existing and clinically validated model being aware of their limits and trying to optimize additional parameters beside the RBE-weighted dose.

3.8 Fractionated Carbon Irradiation in the Animal Model

Despite all the complexities highlighted in the previous paragraph there have been several attempts to investigate the effect of fractionated carbon ion radiotherapy in vivo.

In particular, the issue of inhomogeneity in absorbed physical dose has been elegantly tackled by the group of the German Center for Cancer Research (DKFZ) focusing on a small organ: the rat spinal cord, in which the physical dose inhomogeneity of a clinically optimized carbon plan can be considered negligible as a first approximation [107–110].

As expected, the results of single fraction experiments differed from those of fractionated exposure. RBE models prediction (namely different versions of LEM) showed reasonable agreement with observed data. These experiences however confirm that cell lines data cannot be used to predict in vivo response to fractionated carbon ion RT without being validated by specific in vivo/ clinical data.

The same group investigated the response of different prostate tumors in rats. As expected the tumor heterogeneity had minimal impact on tumor response with both single exposure and fractionated carbon ions RT [111–113]. These results are to be commended as one of the first attempt to measure in experimental condition phenomena that are of paramount importance for clinical result and elude any in vitro modeling.

Finally, the group from DKFZ explored the effect of carbon ions on microvasculature in comparison to photons. They studied dynamic contrast enhancement MRI of rats treated for prostate tumors [114,115]. These authors could demonstrate a faster and bigger increase in permeability after carbon ion irradiation in comparison to photons for poorly differentiated tumors but not for moderately differentiated ones. These results can be considered the first attempts to measure, if not to model, the increased efficacy of carbon ion in inducing a faster and better re-oxygenation.

3.9 Intracellular Signaling, Invasiveness, Motility

Metastases represent the main cause of cancer death [116, 117]. The hallmarks of cancer progression to an invasive and metastatic stage are loss of cell polarity and adhesion [118] and enhanced motility and invasiveness. Thus, the metastatic process requires transition of primarily differentiated and organized cancer cells, to cells with a migratory and invasive phenotype. The metastatic process is beyond the scope of this paragraph and more details on its mechanisms can be found elsewhere [119].

However, since at least half of the oncological patients will be treated with radiation therapy [120], it is extremely relevant to study the role of RT, and specifically of high-LET RT on tumor cells intracellular signaling, invasiveness, and motility.

Interestingly, it has been shown that radiation has that potential of modulating the behavior of tumor cells in terms of their aggressiveness [121]. Depending on radiation and cell type, radiation can promote or reduce the invasiveness of the irradiated cancer cells [119]. For example, several preclinical studies showed that photon irradiation promotes the metastatic spread of tumor cells. *Fujita et al.* investigated the effects of X-rays and y-rays on motility and invasiveness of two human *pancreatic cancer cell lines* who exhibit a different mode of movement: mesenchymal or amoeboid, respectively [122]. The cells were irradiated with 0.2 and 4 Gy. X-ray irradiation enhanced the migration and promoted the invasion of both cell lines. The same conclusions were met by *Qian et al.* who performed the similar in vitro experiments using three different cell lines from *human pancreatic cancer* [123]. Additionally, *Wild-Bode et al.* established that X-rays can enhance the migration and invasiveness of human malignant glioma cells [124]. In their experiments, sublethal irradiation of rat 9 L glioma cells resulted in the formation of a greater number of tumor satellites in the rat brain in vivo suggesting that the pharmacological inhibition of migration and invasion during radiotherapy may represent a new therapeutic approach to improve the therapeutic efficacy of radiotherapy for malignant glioma. Additionally, several other in vitro and in vivo studies brought to light the comparable findings in sarcoma, lung, colon, cervical, head and neck, liver, or prostate cancer cell lines [125–132].

Metastatic spread is a very complex process consisting of multiple steps in which large number of molecules are involved, especially the *integrins*, *GTPases* gene family, or *matrix metalloproteinases* (MMPs) [133–135]. *Integrins* are involved in almost all steps of carcinogenesis including cell proliferation, survival, adhesion, motility, angiogenesis, tumor growth, and finally metastatic process [136]. Thus, integrins constitute as very attractive anti-tumor targets and are currently under clinical evaluation for drug development. The *GTPases* RAC1 and Ras homolog gene family are considered to be of critical importance for cell motility and metastatic process [137]. RAC1 and RHOA signaling pathways play an essential role in the plasticity of cell migration regulating cellular architecture. *Proteases* are proteolytic enzymes which, being involved in the remodeling of the extracellular matrix, increase the migratory capacity allowing cancer cells to penetrate the extracellular matrix [138–141]. Most in vitro and in vivo studies that showed an increase in metastatic potential following photon irradiation focused on the expression of integrins, GTPases, and proteases [129,142–145]. In addition to it, *Park et al.* observed that photon irradiation of glioma cells induces epidermal growth factor receptor (EGFR) activation, which promotes MMP-2 expression resulting in an amplified irradiation-induced invasive potential of these cancer cells [146]. Migration of follicular (FTC133) and anaplastic (8505 c) thyroid carcinoma cells following X-ray irradiation with up to 6 Gy was evaluated by *Burrows et al.* focusing on phosphatidylinositide 3-kinase (PI3K) and associated pathways. Interestingly, the irradiated cells showed increased migration upon irradiation, which were associated with increased hypoxic inducible factor 1-α (HIF-α) activity [147].

Significantly different results were obtained with particles.

Ogata et al. compared the effects that photons, protons, and carbon-ions exert on motility and invasiveness of highly aggressive HT1080 human fibrosarcoma cells and LM8 in the syngeneic mice osteosarcoma [148]. That study assessed the metastatic process in terms of cell adhesion to extracellular matrix, integrins expression, cell migration, cell invasive capability, and matrix metalloproteinase-2 activity. X-ray irradiation promoted cell migration and invasion concomitant with up-regulation of the α Vβ3 integrin. On the other hand, both proton and carbon ion irradiation decreased cell migration and invasion in a dose-dependent manner by strongly inhibiting matrix metalloproteinase-2 activity. They concluded that radiation with charged particles unlike conventional photon beam therapy has the potential to prevent metastases development in irradiated malignant tumor cells. Interestingly, also protons behaved in this regard as high-LET irradiation. Several other studies confirmed the role of charged particles in reducing cancer cell migration and invasiveness in glioma, non-small cell lung, pancreatic, and colon cancer cell lines [142,149–153].

Rieken et al. showed that carbon-ion irradiation inhibits glioma cell migration through downregulation of integrin expression [142]. In another study, Badiga et al. showed that carbon-ion irradiation of glioma cells resulted in decreased integrin and MMP expression negatively affecting their invasive potential [143]. Interestingly and surprisingly, it has been shown that carbon-ion and photon irradiation might exert their migratory-modulating effects "targeting" different molecular pathways: photon irradiation of U87 EGFR++ glioblastoma cells increased EGFR/AKT/ERK1/2 pathway activation resulting in improved cancer cells migratory capacity [154]. In the same experiment, carbon-ions decreased cells migratory capacity in an EGFR-independent manner.

Finally, to get a deeper understanding on the signaling pathways involved in radiation-modulating invasion effect, Fujita et al. analyzed the effects of 2 Gy carbon-ions irradiation in 31 different tumor cell lines [155]. In many of those, the invasive- and migratory-potential of cancer cells was significantly reduced which was not the case with those irradiated with X-rays. However, in two cell lines (the pancreatic cancer cell line PARC-1 and the glioblastoma cell line SF126) also irradiation with carbon-ions induced an increase of invasiveness. The enhanced invasiveness of PANC-1 seemed to be related to serine protease activation following carbon-ion irradiation.

The preclinical evidence suggests that particle irradiation might be able of suppressing metastatic potential of cancer cells in experimental conditions, while photon irradiation exerts promotion of cell migration and invasiveness. Thus, limited to the in vitro studies, it might be considered that ion beam radiotherapy displays preventive anti-metastatic potential in most even if not in all investigated cell lines. The generalizability of these results and ultimate clinical relevance still need to be clarified. Integrins, GTPases gene family, and matrix metalloproteinases, due to their important role in carcinogenesis and metastatic process, represent potentially novel attractive targets for modulation and prevention of metastases in an eventual setting of concurrent therapy with carbon-ion radiotherapy, and thus merit future investigation.

3.10 Bystander Effect

The bystander effect is a biological effect on non-irradiated cells induced by signaling from irradiated cells. The signaling can be either direct (detectable co-culturing irradiated and non-irradiated cells) or medium mediated (detectable culturing non-irradiated cells with the medium of irradiated cells). The bystander effect was first described in the 1990s [156]. Since then several effects have been demonstrated in non-irradiated cells, including micronuclei formation [157,158], increased plating efficacy [157, 158], chromosome aberrations [156,159], mutations [159,160], and apoptotic death [159–161].

The bystander effect has been linked to either intercellular communication through gap junctions [161–163] or to production of nitric oxide (NO) [157,158,164].

The role of gap junctions appears to be more relevant for high-LET than for low-LET radiation [163,165]. Also, the pathways mediated by NO and other ROS differ according to LET. In particular, p53 mutated cells do not efficiently induce NO mediated bystander effect in response to low-LET whereas high-LET irradiation results in NO production through mitochondrial damage and therefore, ultimately the bystander effect is independent from the p53 status [166].

Very interestingly the bystander effect has also been shown to impact the cytokine production of non-irradiated, immune-relevant cells [167–169].

Despite being known for a long time and despite an in-depth understanding of its mechanism, the role of the bystander effect in the clinical setting is still poorly understood for both low and high-LET irradiation and it remains a topic in need of further investigation.

3.11 Future Perspectives

Particle therapy is becoming more and more clinically available. At present protons and carbon ions are used in the clinical setting and helium and oxygen ions are being intensively investigated for clinical use. A better understanding of particle radiobiology may potentially contribute to an improvement of clinical results. One of the future challenges is how to exploit the efficacy of particle therapy against hypoxic tumors in the best way.

Several researchers are investigating the possibility to optimize clinical treatment with heavy particle by increasing the amount of high-LET radiation delivered to hypoxic tumor sub-volumes. As an example Bassler et al. developed "LET-painting" targeting high LET to the hypoxic tumor segments [170,171]. Similarly, Scifoni et al. integrated tumor oxygen status in treatment planning for carbon-ions [172].

Figure 3.3 shows a potential approach with multi ions plan optimized against hypoxia.

Antonovic et al. have studied "*in silico*" the complex role of hypoxia and re-oxygenation together with a clinical carbon ion treatment (combining a low-LET and a high-LET component) [174]. This analysis showed that hypoxia and fractionation (which may be negligible in the very-high-LET part of a carbon Bragg peak) retain their relevant role in a realistic clinical scenario. Besides being interesting in themselves these approaches are also an example of a more general desirable future development: namely the attempt to abandon the RBE weighted dose as the single relevant parameter acknowledging the need to optimize LET distribution also in consideration of additional, unknown/uncertain parameters.

Another very interesting possible area of future development is the interaction between high-LET irradiation, immune response, and immune-modulating drugs.

Radiation-induced immunogenic cell death represents a specific pattern of tumor cell death that has a high chance of initiating immune response [71]. Following irradiation, cancer cells expose on their surface and release several "immunogenic" molecules known as damage-associated molecular patterns (DAMPs) which interact with immune cells, like dendritic cells (DCs) resulting in "*anticancer vaccine effect*" leading to immunogenic cell death [175]. For example, immunogenic dead cells translocate calreticulin from the endoplasmic reticulum to the cellular periphery and subsequently to the cell surface, providing an "eat me" signal resulting in cancer cell phagocytosis by DCs [176]. This protein represents the hallmark of immunogenic cell death playing the main role in activating anti-tumor immunity. Huang et al. assessed the effects of X-rays, protons, and carbon-ions radiation on calreticulin exposure. Human A549 (lung adenocarcinoma), U251MG (glioma), Tca8113 (tongue squamous carcinoma), and CNE-2 (nasopharyngeal carcinoma) cancer cell lines were irradiated with 2, 4 and 10 Gy (physical dose). They found that

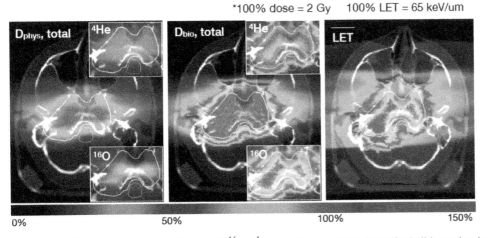

Figure 3.3 "Biologically optimized four-field $^{16}O + ^4He$ plan for a partially hypoxic skull base chordoma). (a-left) Total physical dose, insets correspond to the partial contributions from ^{16}O and ^4He fields. (b-middle) Total biological (RBE-OER-weighted) dose, insets correspond to the partial contributions from ^{16}O and ^4He fields. (c- right) Dose-averaged LET distribution, insets correspond to the partial contributions from ^{16}O and ^4He fields. For (a) and (b) the color scale represents the relative dose compared to the dose of 2 Gy, for (c) the relative LET compared to the LET of 60 keV μm − 1 ." Reproduced from Sokol et al. [173].

proton and photon irradiation showed a similar effectiveness increasing calreticulin exposure with dose escalation inducing the highest value at 10 Gy, while carbon-ion increased most calreticulin exposure at 4 Gy having significantly stronger effects than proton and photon [177].

In addition to calreticulin two more DCs activators are needed in order to process tumor-derived antigens and induce cross-priming of CD8 lymphocytes: High-Mobility-Group-Protein B1 (HMGB1) and ATP [178]. Ideally, this DCs-associated cross-priming of CD8 and cytotoxic T lymphocytes might lead to induction of a systemic anti-tumor immune response known as the abscopal effect [179]. *Radiation-induced abscopal effect* represents a non-targeted immune-mediated regression in tumor lesions outside of the irradiated field. These still rare phenomena, initially observed following X-rays irradiation in 1950s [180], were described also after particle therapy [181,182]. An anecdotal case of dramatic abscopal effect has been described in a patient affected by Merkel cells carcinoma receiving anti PD1 drugs and treated with fast neutrons for palliation[183]. In vitro data suggest that high LET could be more effective in inducing surrogates of immunogenic cell death such as CRT[184] and HMGB1 [185], even though this last effect may be similar to that of low LET after correcting for cell killing RBE [186]. In vivo data have shown initial promising responses by combining carbon ions RT and immunomodulating drugs in an osteosarcoma mouse model [187,188]. The rational combination of high-LET and immuno-modulating drugs demands extensive preclinical radiobiological research. This is once more an example of a broader, interesting category: i.e., exploring the combination of high-LET and targeted systemic treatment focused on the specific cellular response to high LET.

References

1 Friedberg, E.C., Walker, G.C., Siede, W., Wood, R.D., Schultz, R.A., and Ellenberger, T. (2005). *DNA Repair and Mutagenesis*, 2nd ed. Washington, DC, USA: ASM Press. 10.1128/9781555816704.

2 Compe, E. and Egly, J.-M. (2016). Nucleotide excision repair and transcriptional regulation: TFIIH and beyond. *Annual Review of Biochemistry* 85: 265–290. 10.1146/annurev-biochem-060815-014857.

3 Wallace, S.S. (2014). Base excision repair: A critical player in many games. *DNA Repair* 19: 14–26. 10.1016/j.dnarep.2014.03.030.

4 Curtis, S.B. (1986). Lethal and potentially lethal lesions induced by radiation – A unified repair model. *Radiation Research* 106 (2): 252. 10.2307/3576798.

5 Frankenberg, D., Frankenberg-Schwager, M., Blöcher, D., Harbich, R., and Blocher, D. (1981). Evidence for DNA double-strand breaks as the critical lesions in yeast cells irradiated with sparsely or densely ionizing radiation under oxic or anoxic conditions. *Radiation Research* 88 (3): 524. 10.2307/3575641.

6 Mullins, E.A., Rodriguez, A.A., Bradley, N.P., and Eichman, B.F. (2019). Emerging roles of DNA glycosylases and the base excision repair pathway. *Trends in Biochemical Sciences* 44 (9): 765–781. 10.1016/j.tibs.2019.04.006.

7 Scully, R., Panday, A., Elango, R., and Willis, N.A. (2019). DNA double-strand break repair-pathway choice in somatic mammalian cells. *Nature Reviews. Molecular Cell Biology* 20 (11): 698–714. 10.1038/s41580-019-0152-0.

8 Shrivastav, M., De Haro, L.P., and Nickoloff, J.A. (2008). Regulation of DNA double-strand break repair pathway choice. *Cell Research* 18 (1): 134–147. 10.1038/cr.2007.111.

9 Nickoloff, J.A., Sharma, N., and Clustered, T.L. (2020). DNA double-strand breaks: Biological effects and relevance to cancer radiotherapy. *Genes (Basel)* 11 (1): 99. 10.3390/genes11010099.

10 Schardt, D., Elsässer, T., and Schulz-Ertner, D. (2010). Heavy-ion tumor therapy: Physical and radiobiological benefits. *Reviews of Modern Physics* 82 (1): 383–425. 10.1103/RevModPhys.82.383.

11 Tommasino, F. and Durante, M. (2015). Proton radiobiology. *Cancers (Basel)* 7 (1): 353–381. 10.3390/cancers7010353.

12 Krämer, M. (2001). Treatment planning for heavy-ion radiotherapy: Biological optimization of multiple beam ports. *Journal of Radiation Research* 42 (1): 39–46. 10.1269/jrr.42.39.

13 Sørensen, B.S., Overgaard, J., and Bassler, N. (2011). In vitro RBE-LET dependence for multiple particle types. *Acta Oncologica* 50 (6): 757–762. 10.3109/0284186X.2011.582518.

14 Allen, C., Borak, T.B., Tsujii, H., and Nickoloff, J.A. (2011). Heavy charged particle radiobiology: Using enhanced biological effectiveness and improved beam focusing to advance cancer therapy. *Mutation Research* 711 (1-2): 150–157. 10.1016/j.mrfmmm.2011.02.012.

15 Lomax, M.E., Folkes, L.K., and O'Neill, P. (2013). Biological consequences of radiation-induced DNA damage: Relevance to radiotherapy. *College of Radiologists Clinical Oncology* 25 (10): 578–585. 10.1016/j.clon.2013.06.007.

16 Ward, J.F. (2000). Complexity of damage produced by ionizing radiation. *Cold Spring Harbor Symposia on Quantitative Biology* 65: 377–382. 10.1101/sqb.2000.65.377.

17 Ward, J.F. (1988). DNA damage produced by ionizing radiation in mammalian cells: Identities, mechanisms of formation, and reparability. In 95–125. doi:10.1016/S0079-6603(08)60611-X

18 Georgakilas, A.G., O'Neill, P., and Stewart, R.D. (2013). Induction and repair of clustered DNA lesions: What do we know so far? *Radiation Research* 180 (1): 100–109. 10.1667/RR3041.1.

19 Eccles, L.J., O'Neill, P., and Lomax, M.E. (2011). Delayed repair of radiation induced clustered DNA damage: Friend or foe? *Mutation Research/Fundamental and Molecular Mechanisms of Mutagenesis* 711 (1-2): 134–141. 10.1016/j.mrfmmm.2010.11.003.

20 Nikjoo, H., O'Neill, P., Terrissol, M., and Goodhead, D.T. (1999). Quantitative modelling of DNA damage using Monte Carlo track structure method. *Radiation and Environmental Biophysics* 38 (1): 31–38. 10.1007/s004110050135.

21 Goodhead, D.T. (2006). Energy deposition stochastics and track structure: What about the target? *Radiation Protection Dosimetry* 122 (1-4): 3–15. 10.1093/rpd/ncl498.

22 McMahon, S.J. and Prise, K.M. (2019). Mechanistic modelling of radiation responses. *Cancers (Basel)* 11 (2): 205. 10.3390/cancers11020205.

23 Nikjoo, H., Uehara, S., Wilson, W.E., Hoshi, M., and Goodhead, D.T. (1998). Track structure in radiation biology: Theory and applications. *International Journal of Radiation Biology* 73 (4): 355–364. 10.1080/095530098142176.

24 Friedland, W., Schmitt, E., Kundrát, P. et al. (2017). Comprehensive track-structure based evaluation of DNA damage by light ions from radiotherapy-relevant energies down to stopping. *Scientific Reports* 7 (1): 45161. 10.1038/srep45161.

25 Friedland, W., Dingfelder, M., Kundrát, P., and Jacob, P. (2011). Track structures, DNA targets and radiation effects in the biophysical Monte Carlo simulation code PARTRAC. *Mutation Research/Fundamental and Molecular Mechanisms of Mutagenesis* 711 (1-2): 28–40. 10.1016/j.mrfmmm.2011.01.003.

26 Semenenko, V.A. and Stewart, R.D. (2006). Fast Monte Carlo simulation of DNA damage formed by electrons and light ions. *Physics in Medicine and Biology* 51 (7): 1693–1706. 10.1088/0031-9155/51/7/004.

27 Martin, R.G. and Ames, B.N. (1961). A method for determining the sedimentation behavior of enzymes: Application to protein mixtures. *The Journal of Biological Chemistry* 236: 1372–1379. http://www.ncbi.nlm.nih.gov/pubmed/13767412.

28 Bradley, M.O. and Kohn, K.W. (1979). X-ray induced DNA double strand break production and repair in mammalian cells as measured by neutral filter elution. *Nucleic Acids Research* 7 (3): 793–804. 10.1093/nar/7.3.793.

29 Schwartz, D.C. and Cantor, C.R. (1984). Separation of yeast chromosome-sized DNAs by pulsed field gradient gel electrophoresis. *Cell* 37 (1): 67–75. 10.1016/0092-8674(84)90301-5.

30 Olive, P.L., Wlodek, D., and Banáth, J.P. (1991). DNA double-strand breaks measured in individual cells subjected to gel electrophoresis. *Cancer Research* 51 (17): 4671–4676. http://www.ncbi.nlm.nih.gov/pubmed/1873812.

31 Smith, C.L. and Klco, S.R.C.C. (1988). Pulsed-field gel electrophoresis and the technology of large DNA molecules. In: *Genome Analysis: A Practical Approach* (editor K. Davies), 41–72. Oxford, England: IRL Press.

32 Fairbairn, D.W., Olive, P.L., and O'Neill, K.L. (1995). The comet assay: A comprehensive review. *Mutation Research* 339 (1): 37–59. 10.1016/0165-1110(94)00013-3.

33 Collins, A.R. (2004). The comet assay for DNA damage and repair: Principles, applications, and limitations. *Molecular Biotechnology* 26 (3): 249–261. 10.1385/MB:26:3:249.

34 Pilch, D.R., Sedelnikova, O.A., Redon, C., Celeste, A., Nussenzweig, A., and Bonner, W.M. (2003). Characteristics of γ-H2AX foci at DNA double-strand breaks sites. *Biochemistry and Cell Biology* 81 (3): 123–129. 10.1139/o03-042.

35 Sedelnikova, O.A., Rogakou, E.P., and Panyutin, I.G.B.W. (2002). Quantitative detection of 125IdU-induced DNA double-strand breaks with γ-H2AX antibody. *Radiation Research* 158 (4): 486–492.

36 Mirsch, J., Tommasino, F., Frohns, A. et al. (2015). Direct measurement of the 3-dimensional DNA lesion distribution induced by energetic charged particles in a mouse model tissue. *Proceedings of the National Academy of Sciences of the United States of America* 112 (40): 12396–12401. 10.1073/pnas.1508702112.

37 Pang, D., Chasovskikh, S., Rodgers, J.E., and Short, D.A. (2016). DNA fragments are a hallmark of heavy charged-particle irradiation and may underlie their greater therapeutic efficacy. *Frontiers in Oncology* 6: 10.3389/fonc.2016.00130.

38 Pang, D., Rodgers, J.E., Berman, B.L., Chasovskikh, S., and Dritschilo, A. (2005). Spatial distribution of radiation-induced double-strand breaks in plasmid DNA as resolved by atomic force microscopy. *Radiation Research* 164 (6): 755–765. 10.1667/rr3425.1.

39 Pang, D., Berman, B.L., Chasovskikh, S., Rodgers, J.E., and Dritschilo, A. (1998). Investigation of neutron-induced damage in DNA by atomic force microscopy: Experimental evidence of clustered DNA lesions. *Radiation Research* 150 (6): 612. 10.2307/3579883.

40 Oike, T., Niimi, A., Okonogi, N., Murata, K., Matsumura, A., Noda, S.E., Kobayashi, D., Iwanaga, M., Tsuchida, K., Kanai, T., Ohno, T., Shibata, A., and Nakano, T. (2016, Mar 1). Visualization of complex DNA double-strand breaks in a tumor treated with carbon ion radiotherapy. *Scientific Reports* 6: 22275. 10.1038/srep22275. Springer Nature / CC BY 4.0.

41 Timm, S., Lorat, Y., Jakob, B., Taucher-Scholz, G., and Rübe, C.E. (2018). Clustered DNA damage concentrated in particle trajectories causes persistent large-scale

rearrangements in chromatin architecture. *Radiotherapy and Oncology : Journal of the European Society for Therapeutic Radiology and Oncology* 129 (3): 600–610. 10.1016/j.radonc.2018.07.003.

42 Zhang, X., Ye, C., Sun, F., Wei, W., Hu, B., and Wang, J. (2016). Both complexity and location of DNA damage contribute to cellular senescence induced by ionizing radiation. *PLoS One* 11 (5): e0155725. 10.1371/journal.pone.0155725.

43 Averbeck, N.B., Ringel, O., Herrlitz, M., Jakob, B., Durante, M., and Taucher-Scholz, G. (2014). DNA end resection is needed for the repair of complex lesions in G1-phase human cells. *Cell Cycle* 13 (16): 2509–2516. 10.4161/15384101.2015.941743.

44 Gudowska-Nowak, E., Nasonova, E., Ritter, S., and Scholz, M. (2004). Chromosome fragmentation after irradiation with C ions. *Radiotherapy and Oncology : Journal of the European Society for Therapeutic Radiology and Oncology* 73 (Suppl 2): S123–6. 10.1016/s0167-8140(04)80032-x.

45 Sekine, E., Okada, M., Matsufuji, N., Yu, D., Furusawa, Y., and Okayasu, R. (2008). High LET heavy ion radiation induces lower numbers of initial chromosome breaks with minimal repair than low LET radiation in normal human cells. *Mutation Research* 652 (1): 95–101. 10.1016/j.mrgentox.2008.01.003.

46 Hartel, C., Nikoghosyan, A., Durante, M. et al. (2010). Chromosomal aberrations in peripheral blood lymphocytes of prostate cancer patients treated with IMRT and carbon ions. *Radiotherapy and Oncology : Journal of the European Society for Therapeutic Radiology and Oncology* 95 (1): 73–78. 10.1016/j.radonc.2009.08.031.

47 Virsik-Köpp, P. and Hofman-Huether, H. (2004). Chromosome aberrations induced by high-LET carbon ions in radiosensitive and radioresistant tumour cells. *Cytogenetic and Genome Research* 104 (1-4): 221–226. 10.1159/000077493.

48 Durante, M., Furusawa, Y., George, K. et al. (1998). Rejoining and misrejoining of radiation-induced chromatin breaks. IV. charged particles. *Radiation Research* 149 (5): 446. 10.2307/3579784.

49 Krämer, M., Weyrather, W.K., and Scholz, M. (2003). The increased biological effectiveness of heavy charged particles: From radiobiology to treatment planning. *Technology in Cancer Research & Treatment* 2 (5): 427–436. 10.1177/153303460300200507.

50 Friedrich, T., Scholz, U., Elsässer, T., Durante, M., and Scholz, M. (2013). Systematic analysis of RBE and related quantities using a database of cell survival experiments with ion beam irradiation. *Journal of Radiation Research* 54 (3): 494–514. 10.1093/jrr/rrs114.

51 Bird, R.P. and Burki, H.J. (1975). Survival of synchronized Chinese hamster cells exposed to radiation of different linear-energy transfer. *International Journal of Radiation Biology and Related Studies in Physics, Chemistry, and Medicine* 27 (2): 105–120. 10.1080/09553007514550121.

52 Ando, K. and Goodhead, D.T. (2016). Dependence and independence of survival parameters on linear energy transfer in cells and tissues. *Journal of Radiation Research* 57 (6): 596–606. 10.1093/jrr/rrw058.

53 Fukutsu, K., Kanai, T., Furusawa, Y., and Ando, K. (1997). Response of mouse intestine after single and fractionated irradiation with accelerated carbon ions with a spread-out Bragg peak. *Radiation Research* 148 (2): 168–174. http://www.ncbi.nlm.nih.gov/pubmed/9254736.

54 Goodhead, D.T. (1985). Saturable repair models of radiation action in mammalian cells. *Radiation Research* 104 (2): S58. 10.2307/3576633.

55 Suzuki, M., Kase, Y., Kanai, T., and Ando, K. (2000). Change in radiosensitivity with fractionated-dose irradiation of carbon-ion beams in five different human cell lines. *International Journal of Radiation Oncology, Biology, Physics* 48 (1): 251–258. 10.1016/s0360-3016(00)00606-4.

56 Blakely, E.A., Ngo, F.Q.H., Curtis, S.B., and Tobias, C.A. (1984). Heavy-ion radiobiology: Cellular studies. In 295–389. 10.1016/B978-0-12-035411-5.50013-7.

57 Gray, LK. (1961). Radiobiologic basis of oxygen as a modifying factor in radiation therapy. *The American Journal of Roentgenology, Radium Therapy, and Nuclear Medicine* 85: 803–815. http://www.ncbi.nlm.nih.gov/pubmed/13708070.

58 Hall, E. and Giaccia, A. (2006). *Radiobiology for the Radiologist*, 6th Ed. Philadelphia: Lippincott Williams & Wilkins.

59 Furusawa, Y., Fukutsu, K., Aoki, M. et al. (2000). Inactivation of aerobic and hypoxic cells from three different cell lines by accelerated (3)He-, (12)C- and (20)Ne-ionbeams. *Radiation Research* 154 (5): 485–496. 10.1667/0033-7587(2000)154[0485:ioaahc]2.0.co;2.

60 Tobias, C.A., Blakely, E.A., Alpen, E.L. et al. (1982). Molecular and cellular radiobiology of heavy ions. *International Journal of Radiation Oncology* 8 (12): 2109–2120. 10.1016/0360-3016(82)90554-5.

61 Barendsen, G.W., Koot, C.J., van Kersen, G.R., Bewley, D.K., Field, S.B., and Parnell, C.J. (1966). The effect of oxygen on impairment of the proliferative capacity of human cells in culture by ionizing radiations of different LET. *International Journal of Radiation Biology and Related Studies in Physics, Chemistry, and Medicine* 10 (4): 317–327. 10.1080/09553006614550421.

62 Brahme, A. (2011). Accurate description of the cell survival and biological effect at low and high doses and

LET's. *Journal of Radiation Research* 52 (4): 389–407. 10.1269/jrr.10129.

63 Fournier, C., Wiese, C., and Taucher-Scholz, G. (2004). Accumulation of the cell cycle regulators TP53 and CDKN1A (p21) in human fibroblasts after exposure to low- and high-LET radiation. *Radiation Research* 161 (6): 675–684. 10.1667/RR3182.

64 Jakob, B., Scholz, M., and Taucher-Scholz, G. (2003). Biological imaging of heavy charged-particle tracks. *Radiation Research* 159 (5): 676–684. 10.1667/0033-7587(2003)159[0676:biohct]2.0.co;2.

65 Chang, P.Y., Bjornstad, K.A., Rosen, C.J. et al. (2005). Effects of iron ions, protons and X rays on human lens cell differentiation. *Radiation Research* 164 (4 Pt 2): 531–539. 10.1667/rr3368.1.

66 Iwadate, Y., Mizoe, J.-E., Osaka, Y., Yamaura, A., and Tsujii, H. (2001). High linear energy transfer carbon radiation effectively kills cultured glioma cells with either mutant or wild-type p53. *International Journal of Radiation Oncology* 50 (3): 803–808. 10.1016/S0360-3016(01)01514-0.

67 Tsuboi, K., Moritake, T., Tsuchida, Y., Tokuuye, K., Matsumura, A., and Ando, K. (2007). Cell cycle checkpoint and apoptosis induction in glioblastoma cells and fibroblasts irradiated with carbon beam. *Journal of Radiation Research* 48 (4): 317–325. 10.1269/jrr.06081.

68 Hamada, N., Hara, T., Omura-Minamisawa, M. et al. (2008). Energetic heavy ions overcome tumor radioresistance caused by overexpression of Bcl-2. *Radiotherapy and Oncology : Journal of the European Society for Therapeutic Radiology and Oncology* 89 (2): 231–236. 10.1016/j.radonc.2008.02.013.

69 Miszczyk, J., Rawojć, K., Panek, A. et al. (2018). Do protons and X-rays induce cell-killing in human peripheral blood lymphocytes by different mechanisms? *Clinical and Translational Radiation Oncology* 9: 23–29. 10.1016/j.ctro.2018.01.004.

70 Maalouf, M., Alphonse, G., Colliaux, A. et al. (2009). Different mechanisms of cell death in radiosensitive and radioresistant p53 mutated head and neck squamous cell carcinoma cell lines exposed to carbon ions and x-rays. *International Journal of Radiation Oncology, Biology, Physics* 74 (1): 200–209. 10.1016/j.ijrobp.2009.01.012.

71 Zhou, J., Wang, G., Chen, Y., Wang, H., Hua, Y., and Cai, Z. (2019). Immunogenic cell death in cancer therapy: Present and emerging inducers. *Journal of Cellular and Molecular Medicine* 23 (8): 4854–4865. 10.1111/jcmm.14356.

72 Higo, M., Uzawa, K., Kawata, T. et al. (2006). Enhancement of SPHK1 in vitro by carbon ion irradiation in oral squamous cell carcinoma. *International Journal of Radiation Oncology* 65 (3): 867–875. 10.1016/j.ijrobp.2006.02.048.

73 Fushimi, K., Uzawa, K., Ishigami, T. et al. (2008). Susceptible genes and molecular pathways related to heavy ion irradiation in oral squamous cell carcinoma cells. *Radiotherapy and Oncology : Journal of the European Society for Therapeutic Radiology and Oncology* 89 (2): 237–244. 10.1016/j.radonc.2008.04.015.

74 Matsumoto, Y., Iwakawa, M., Furusawa, Y. et al. (2008). Gene expression analysis in human malignant melanoma cell lines exposed to carbon beams. *International Journal of Radiation Biology* 84 (4): 299–314. 10.1080/09553000801953334.

75 Friedrich, T., Scholz, U., Elsässer, T., Durante, M., and Scholz, M. (2012). Calculation of the biological effects of ion beams based on the microscopic spatial damage distribution pattern. *International Journal of Radiation Biology* 88 (1-2): 103–107. 10.3109/09553002.2011.611213.

76 Elsässer, T., Krämer, M., and Scholz, M. (2008). Accuracy of the local effect model for the prediction of biologic effects of carbon ion beams in vitro and in vivo. *International Journal of Radiation Oncology, Biology, Physics* 71 (3): 866–872. 10.1016/j.ijrobp.2008.02.037.

77 Elsässer, T. and Scholz, M. (2006). Improvement of the local effect model (LEM)–implications of clustered DNA damage. *Radiation Protection Dosimetry* 122 (1-4): 475–477. 10.1093/rpd/ncl521.

78 Scholz, M. and Kraft, G. (2004). The physical and radiobiological basis of the local effect model: A response to the commentary by R. Katz. *Radiation Research* 161 (5): 612–620. 10.1667/rr3174.

79 Krämer, M. and Scholz, M. (2000). Treatment planning for heavy-ion radiotherapy: Calculation and optimization of biologically effective dose. *Physics in Medicine and Biology* 45 (11): 3319–3330. 10.1088/0031-9155/45/11/314.

80 Kraft, G., Scholz, M., and Bechthold, U. (1999). Tumor therapy and track structure. *Radiation and Environmental Biophysics* 38 (4): 229–237. 10.1007/s004110050163.

81 Kraft, G., Krämer, M., and Scholz, M. (1992). LET, track structure and models. A review. *Radiation and Environmental Biophysics* 31 (3): 161–180. 10.1007/BF01214825.

82 Jäkel, O., Debus, J., Krämer, M., Scholz, M., and Kraft, G. (1999). Treatment planning for light ions: How to take into account relative biological effectiveness (RBE). *Strahlentherapie Und Onkologie : Organ Der Deutschen Rontgengesellschaft ... [Et Al]* 175 (Suppl): 12–14. 10.1007/BF03038877.

83 Krämer, M., Weyrather, W.K., and Scholz, M. (2003). The increased biological effectiveness of heavy charged particles: From radiobiology to treatment planning. *Technology in Cancer Research & Treatment* 2 (5): 427–436. 10.1177/153303460300200507.

84 Krämer, M., Jäkel, O., Haberer, T. et al. (2004). Treatment planning for scanned ion beams. *Radiotherapy and Oncology : Journal of the European Society for Therapeutic Radiology and Oncology* 73 (Suppl 2): S80–5. 10.1016/s0167-8140(04)80021-5.

85 Schmid, T.E., Greubel, C., Hable, V. et al. (2012). Low LET protons focused to submicrometer shows enhanced radiobiological effectiveness. *Physics in Medicine and Biology* 57 (19): 5889–5907. 10.1088/0031-9155/57/19/5889.

86 Kanai, T., Endo, M., and Minohara, S. et al. (1999). Biophysical characteristics of HIMAC clinical irradiation system for heavy-ion radiation therapy. *International Journal of Radiation Oncology, Biology, Physics* 44 (1): 201–210. 10.1016/s0360-3016(98)00544-6.

87 Kanai, T., Matsufuji, N., Miyamoto, T. et al. (2006). Examination of GyE system for HIMAC carbon therapy. *International Journal of Radiation Oncology, Biology, Physics* 64 (2): 650–656. 10.1016/j.ijrobp.2005.09.043.

88 Tsujii, H., Mizoe, J.-E., Kamada, T. et al. (2004). Overview of clinical experiences on carbon ion radiotherapy at NIRS. *Radiotherapy and Oncology : Journal of the European Society for Therapeutic Radiology and Oncology* 73 (Suppl 2): S41–9. 10.1016/s0167-8140(04)80012-4.

89 Kamada, T., Tsujii, H., Blakely, E.A. et al. (2015). Carbon ion radiotherapy in Japan: An assessment of 20 years of clinical experience. *The Lancet Oncology* 16 (2): e93–e100. 10.1016/S1470-2045(14)70412-7.

90 Schulz-Ertner, D., Nikoghosyan, A., Thilmann, C. et al. (2004). Results of carbon ion radiotherapy in 152 patients. *International Journal of Radiation Oncology, Biology, Physics* 58 (2): 631–640. 10.1016/j.ijrobp.2003.09.041.

91 Inaniwa, T., Furukawa, T., Kase, Y. et al. (2010). Treatment planning for a scanned carbon beam with a modified microdosimetric kinetic model. *Physics in Medicine and Biology* 55 (22): 6721–6737. 10.1088/0031-9155/55/22/008.

92 Inaniwa, T., Kanematsu, N., Matsufuji, N. et al. (2015). Reformulation of a clinical-dose system for carbon-ion radiotherapy treatment planning at the National Institute of Radiological Sciences, Japan. *Physics in Medicine and Biology* 60 (8): 3271–3286. 10.1088/0031-9155/60/8/3271.

93 Hawkins, R.B. (1998). A microdosimetric-kinetic theory of the dependence of the RBE for cell death on LET. *Medical Physics* 25 (7 Pt 1): 1157–1170. 10.1118/1.598307.

94 Mein, S., Klein, C., Kopp, B. et al. (2020). Assessment of RBE-weighted dose models for carbon ion therapy toward modernization of clinical practice at HIT: In vitro, in vivo, and in patients. *International Journal of Radiation Oncology, Biology, Physics* 108 (3): 779–791. 10.1016/j.ijrobp.2020.05.041.

95 Dale, J.E., Molinelli, S., Vischioni, B. et al. (2020). Brainstem NTCP and Dose Constraints for Carbon Ion RT-Application and Translation From Japanese to European RBE-Weighted Dose. *Frontiers in Oncology* 10: 531344. 10.3389/fonc.2020.531344.

96 Zhang, L., Wang, W., Hu, J., Lu, J., and Kong, L. (2020). RBE-weighted dose conversions for patients with recurrent nasopharyngeal carcinoma receiving carbon-ion radiotherapy from the local effect model to the microdosimetric kinetic model. *Radiation Therapy* 15 (1): 277. 10.1186/s13014-020-01723-z.

97 Choi, K., Molinelli, S., Russo, S. et al. (2019). Rectum dose constraints for carbon ion therapy: Relative biological effectiveness model dependence in relation to clinical outcomes. *Cancers (Basel)* 12: 1. 10.3390/cancers12010046.

98 Wang, W., Huang, Z., Sheng, Y. et al. (2020). RBE-weighted dose conversions for carbon ionradiotherapy between microdosimetric kinetic model and local effect model for the targets and organs at risk in prostate carcinoma. *Radiotherapy and Oncology : Journal of the European Society for Therapeutic Radiology and Oncology* 144: 30–36. 10.1016/j.radonc.2019.10.005.

99 Molinelli, S., Bonora, M., Magro, G. et al. (2019). RBE-weighted dose in carbon ion therapy for ACC patients: Impact of the RBE model translation on treatment outcomes. *Radiotherapy and Oncology : Journal of the European Society for Therapeutic Radiology and Oncology* 141: 227–233. 10.1016/j.radonc.2019.08.022.

100 Dale, J.E., Molinelli, S., Vitolo, V. et al. (2019). Optic nerve constraints for carbon ion RT at CNAO – Reporting and relating outcome to European and Japanese RBE. *Radiotherapy and Oncology : Journal of the European Society for Therapeutic Radiology and Oncology* 140: 175–181. 10.1016/j.radonc.2019.06.028.

101 Molinelli, S., Magro, G., Mairani, A. et al. (2016). Dose prescription in carbon ion radiotherapy: How to compare two different RBE-weighted dose calculation systems. *Radiotherapy and Oncology : Journal of the European Society for Therapeutic Radiology and Oncology* 120 (2): 307–312. 10.1016/j.radonc.2016.05.031.

102 Fossati, P., Molinelli, S., Matsufuji, N. et al. (2012). Dose prescription in carbon ion radiotherapy: A planning study to compare NIRS and LEM approaches with a clinically-oriented strategy. *Physics in Medicine and Biology* 57 (22): 7543–7554. 10.1088/0031-9155/57/22/7543.

103 Steinsträter, O., Scholz, U., Friedrich, T. et al. (2015). Integration of a model-independent interface for RBE predictions in a treatment planning system for active particle beam scanning. *Physics in Medicine and Biology* 60 (17): 6811–6831. 10.1088/0031-9155/60/17/6811.

104 Fossati, P., Matsufuji, N., Kamada, T., and Karger, C.P. (2018). Radiobiological issues in prospective carbon ion therapy trials. *Medical Physics* 45 (11): e1096–e1110. 10.1002/mp.12506.

105 *ICRU Report 93* (2016). https://academic.oup.com/jicru/issue/16/1-2.

106 Marks, L.B., Yorke, E.D., Jackson, A. et al. (2010). Use of normal tissue complication probability models in the clinic. *International Journal of Radiation Oncology, Biology, Physics* 76 (3 Suppl): S10–9. 10.1016/j.ijrobp.2009.07.1754.

107 Saager, M., Glowa, C., Peschke, P. et al. (2014). Carbon ion irradiation of the rat spinal cord: Dependence of the relative biological effectiveness on linear energy transfer. *International Journal of Radiation Oncology, Biology, Physics* 90 (1): 63–70. 10.1016/j.ijrobp.2014.05.008.

108 Saager, M., Glowa, C., Peschke, P. et al. (2015). Split dose carbon ion irradiation of the rat spinal cord: Dependence of the relative biological effectiveness on dose and linear energy transfer. *Radiotherapy and Oncology : Journal of the European Society for Therapeutic Radiology and Oncology* 117 (2): 358–363. 10.1016/j.radonc.2015.07.006.

109 Saager, M., Glowa, C., Peschke, P. et al. (2016). The relative biological effectiveness of carbon ion irradiations of the rat spinal cord increases linearly with LET up to 99 keV/μm. *Acta Oncologica* 55 (12): 1512–1515. 10.1080/0284186X.2016.1250947.

110 Saager, M., Glowa, C., Peschke, P. et al. (2020). Fractionated carbon ion irradiations of the rat spinal cord: Comparison of the relative biological effectiveness with predictions of the local effect model. *Radiation Therapy* 15 (1): 6. 10.1186/s13014-019-1439-1.

111 Glowa, C., Karger, C.P., Brons, S. et al. (2016). Carbon ion radiotherapy decreases the impact of tumor heterogeneity on radiation response in experimental prostate tumors. *Cancer Letters* 378 (2): 97–103. 10.1016/j.canlet.2016.05.013.

112 Glowa, C., Peschke, P., Brons, S. et al. (2017). Carbon ion radiotherapy: Impact of tumor differentiation on local control in experimental prostate carcinomas. *Radiation Therapy* 12 (1): 174. 10.1186/s13014-017-0914-9.

113 Glowa, C., Peschke, P., Brons, S., Debus, J., and Karger, C.P. (February, 2021). Effectiveness of fractionated carbon ion treatments in three rat prostate tumors differing in growth rate, differentiation and hypoxia. *Radiotherapy and Oncology : Journal of the European Society for Therapeutic Radiology and Oncology* 10.1016/j.radonc.2021.01.038.

114 Bendinger, A.L., Seyler, L., Saager, M. et al. (2020). Impact of single dose photons and carbon ions on perfusion and vascular permeability: A dynamic contrast-enhanced MRI pilot study in the anaplastic rat prostate tumor R3327-AT1. *Radiation Research* 193 (1): 34–45. 10.1667/RR15459.1.

115 Bendinger, A.L., Peschke, P., Peter, J., Debus, J., Karger, C.P., and Glowa, C. (2020). High doses of photons and carbon ions comparably increase vascular permeability in R3327-HI prostate tumors: A dynamic contrast-enhanced MRI study. *Radiation Research* 194 (5): 465–475. 10.1667/RADE-20-00112.1.

116 Hanahan, D. and Weinberg, R.A. (2011). Hallmarks of cancer: The next generation. *Cell* 144 (5): 646–674. 10.1016/j.cell.2011.02.013.

117 Mehlen, P. and Puisieux, A. (2006). Metastasis: A question of life or death. *Nature Reviews. Cancer* 6 (6): 449–458. 10.1038/nrc1886.

118 Gandalovičová, A., Vomastek, T., Rosel, D., and Brábek, J. (2016). Cell polarity signaling in the plasticity of cancer cell invasiveness. *Oncotarget* 7 (18): 25022–25049. 10.18632/oncotarget.7214.

119 Fujita, M., Yamada, S., and Imai, T. (2015). Irradiation induces diverse changes in invasive potential in cancer cell lines. *Seminars in Cancer Biology* 35: 45–52. 10.1016/j.semcancer.2015.09.003.

120 Delaney, G., Jacob, S., Featherstone, C., and Barton, M. (2005). The role of radiotherapy in cancer treatment: Estimating optimal utilization from a review of evidence-based clinical guidelines. *Cancer* 104 (6): 1129–1137. 10.1002/cncr.21324.

121 Moncharmont, C., Levy, A., Guy, J.-B. et al. (2014). Radiation-enhanced cell migration/invasion process: A review. *Critical Reviews in Oncology/hematology* 92 (2): 133–142. 10.1016/j.critrevonc.2014.05.006.

122 Fujita, M., Otsuka, Y., Yamada, S., Iwakawa, M., and Imai, T. (2011). X-ray irradiation and Rho-kinase inhibitor additively induce invasiveness of the cells of the pancreatic cancer line, MIAPaCa-2, which exhibits mesenchymal and amoeboid motility. *Cancer Science* 102 (4): 792–798. 10.1111/j.1349-7006.2011.01852.x.

123 Qian, L.-W., Mizumoto, K., Urashima, T. (2002). et al. Radiation-induced increase in invasive potential of human pancreatic cancer cells and its blockade by a matrix metalloproteinase inhibitor, CGS27023. *Clinical Cancer Research : An Official Journal of the American Association for Cancer Research* 8 (4): 1223–1227. http://www.ncbi.nlm.nih.gov/pubmed/11948136.

124 Wild-Bode, C., Weller, M., Rimner, A., Dichgans, J., and Wick, W. (2001). Sublethal irradiation promotes migration and invasiveness of glioma cells: Implications for radiotherapy of human glioblastoma. *Cancer Research* 61 (6): 2744–2750. http://www.ncbi.nlm.nih.gov/pubmed/11289157.

125 Furmanova-Hollenstein, P., Broggini-Tenzer, A., Eggel, M., and Millard A-L, P.M. (2013). The microtubule stabilizer patupilone counteracts ionizing radiation-induced matrix metalloproteinase activity and tumor

cell invasion. *Radiation Therapy* 8 (1): 105. 10.1186/1748-717X-8-105.

126 Ghosh, S., Kumar, A., Tripathi, R.P., and Chandna, S. (2014). Connexin-43 regulates p38-mediated cell migration and invasion induced selectively in tumour cells by low doses of γ-radiation in an ERK-1/2-independent manner. *Carcinogenesis* 35 (2): 383–395. 10.1093/carcin/bgt303.

127 Kawamoto, A., Yokoe, T., Tanaka, K. et al. (2012). Radiation induces epithelial-mesenchymal transition in colorectal cancer cells. *Oncology Reports* 27 (1): 51–57. 10.3892/or.2011.1485.

128 Su, W.-H., Chuang, P.-C., Huang, E.-Y., and Yang, K.D. (2012). Radiation-induced increase in cell migration and metastatic potential of cervical cancer cells operates via the K-ras pathway. *The American Journal of Pathology* 180 (2): 862–871. 10.1016/j.ajpath.2011.10.018.

129 Yan, S., Wang, Y., Yang, Q. et al. (2013). Low-dose radiation-induced epithelial-mesenchymal transition through NF-κB in cervical cancer cells. *International Journal of Oncology* 42 (5): 1801–1806. 10.3892/ijo.2013.1852.

130 Pickhard, A.C., Margraf, J., Knopf, A. et al. (2011). Inhibition of radiation induced migration of human head and neck squamous cell carcinoma cells by blocking of EGF receptor pathways. *BMC Cancer* 11: 388. 10.1186/1471-2407-11-388.

131 Cheng, J.C.-H., Chou, C.H., Kuo, M.L., and Hsieh, C.-Y. (2006). Radiation-enhanced hepatocellular carcinoma cell invasion with MMP-9 expression through PI3K/Akt/NF-kappaB signal transduction pathway. *Oncogene* 25 (53): 7009–7018. 10.1038/sj.onc.1209706.

132 Chang, L., Graham, P.H., Hao, J. et al. (2013). Acquisition of epithelial-mesenchymal transition and cancer stem cell phenotypes is associated with activation of the PI3K/Akt/mTOR pathway in prostate cancer radioresistance. *Cell Death & Disease* 4: e875. 10.1038/cddis.2013.407.

133 Ganguly, K.K., Pal, S., Moulik, S., and Chatterjee, A. (2013 May-Jun). Integrins and metastasis. *Cell Adhesion & Migration* 7 (3): 251–261. 10.4161/cam.23840 Epub 2013 Apr 5. PMID: 23563505; PMCID: PMC3711990.

134 Cook, D.R., Rossman, K.L., and Der, C.J. (2014). Rho guanine nucleotide exchange factors: Regulators of Rho GTPase activity in development and disease. *Oncogene* 33 (31): 4021–4035. 10.1038/onc.2013.362.

135 Chaudhary, A.K., Pandya, S., Ghosh, K., and Nadkarni, A. (2013 Jul-Sep). Matrix metalloproteinase and its drug targets therapy in solid and hematological malignancies: An overview. *Mutation Research* 753 (1): 7–23. 10.1016/j.mrrev.2013.01.002. Epub 2013 Jan 28. PMID: 23370482.

136 Stupack, D.G. (2007). The biology of integrins. *Oncology (Williston Park)* 21 (9Suppl 3): 6–12. http://www.ncbi.nlm.nih.gov/pubmed/17927025.

137 Sadok, A. and Marshall, C.J. (2014). Rho GTPases: Masters of cell migration. *Small GTPases* 5: e29710. 10.4161/sgtp.29710.

138 Mason, S.D. and Joyce, J.A. (2011). Proteolytic networks in cancer. *Trends in Cell Biology* 21 (4): 228–237. 10.1016/j.tcb.2010.12.002.

139 Jacob, A. and Prekeris, R. (2015). The regulation of MMP targeting to invadopodia during cancer metastasis. *Frontiers in Cell and Developmental Biology* 3: 4. 10.3389/fcell.2015.00004.

140 Ossowski, L. and Aguirre-Ghiso, J.A. (2000). Urokinase receptor and integrin partnership: Coordination of signaling for cell adhesion, migration and growth. *Current Opinion in Cell Biology* 12 (5): 613–620. 10.1016/s0955-0674(00)00140-x.

141 Yadav, L., Puri, N., Rastogi, V., Satpute, P., Ahmad, R., and Kaur, G. (2014). Matrix metalloproteinases and cancer – Roles in threat and therapy. *Asian Pacific Journal of Cancer Prevention : APJCP* 15 (3): 1085–1091. 10.7314/apjcp.2014.15.3.1085.

142 Rieken, S., Habermehl, D., Wuerth, L. et al. (2012). Carbon ion irradiation inhibits glioma cell migration through downregulation of integrin expression. *International Journal of Radiation Oncology, Biology, Physics* 83 (1): 394–399. 10.1016/j.ijrobp.2011.06.2004.

143 Badiga, A.V., Chetty, C., Kesanakurti, D. et al. (2011). MMP-2 siRNA inhibits radiation-enhanced invasiveness in glioma cells. Lesniak MS, ed. *PLoS One* 6 (6): e20614. 10.1371/journal.pone.0020614.

144 Furmanova-Hollenstein, P., Broggini-Tenzer, A., Eggel, M., and Millard A-L, P.M. (2013). The microtubule stabilizer patupilone counteracts ionizing radiation-induced matrix metalloproteinase activity and tumor cell invasion. *Radiation Therapy* 8: 105. 10.1186/1748-717X-8-105.

145 Nalla, A.K., Asuthkar, S., Bhoopathi, P., Gujrati, M., Dinh, D.H., and Rao, J.S. (2010). Suppression of uPAR retards radiation-induced invasion and migration mediated by integrin β1/FAK signaling in medulloblastoma. *PLoS One* 5 (9): e13006. 10.1371/journal.pone.0013006.

146 Park, C.-M., Park, M.-J., Kwak, H.-J. et al. (2006). Ionizing radiation enhances matrix metalloproteinase-2 secretion and invasion of glioma cells through Src/epidermal growth factor receptor-mediated p38/Akt and phosphatidylinositol 3-kinase/Akt signaling pathways. *Cancer Research* 66 (17): 8511–8519. 10.1158/0008-5472.CAN-05-4340.

147 Burrows, N., Telfer, B., Brabant, G., and Williams, K.J. (2013). Inhibiting the phosphatidylinositide 3-kinase pathway blocks radiation-induced metastasis associated with Rho-GTPase and Hypoxia-inducible factor-1 activity. *Radiotherapy & Oncology* 108 (3): 548–553. 10.1016/j.radonc.2013.06.027.

148 Ogata, T., Teshima, T., Kagawa, K. (2005). et al. Particle irradiation suppresses metastatic potential of cancer cells. *Cancer Research* 65 (1): 113–120. http://www.ncbi.nlm.nih.gov/pubmed/15665286.

149 Fujita, M., Imadome, K., Endo, S., Shoji, Y., Yamada, S., and Imai, T. (2014). Nitric oxide increases the invasion of pancreatic cancer cells via activation of the PI3K-AKT and RhoA pathways after carbon ion irradiation. *FEBS Letters* 588 (17): 3240–3250. 10.1016/j.febslet.2014.07.006.

150 Gonzalez, E. and McGraw, T.E. (2009). Insulin-modulated Akt subcellular localization determines Akt isoform-specific signaling. *Proceedings of the National Academy of Sciences of the United States of America* 106 (17): 7004–7009. 10.1073/pnas.0901933106.

151 Akino, Y., Teshima, T., Kihara, A. et al. (2009). Carbon-ion beam irradiation effectively suppresses migration and invasion of human non-small-cell lung cancer cells. *International Journal of Radiation Oncology, Biology, Physics* 75 (2): 475–481. 10.1016/j.ijrobp.2008.12.090.

152 Goetze, K., Scholz, M., Taucher-Scholz, G., and Mueller-Klieser, W. (2010). Tumor cell migration is not influenced by p21 in colon carcinoma cell lines after irradiation with X-ray or (12)C heavy ions. *Radiation and Environmental Biophysics* 49 (3): 427–435. 10.1007/s00411-010-0297-x.

153 Goetze, K., Scholz, M., Taucher-Scholz, G., and Mueller-Klieser, W. (2007 Nov-Dec). The impact of conventional and heavy ion irradiation on tumor cell migration in vitro. *International Journal of Radiation Biology* 83 (11-12): 889–896. 10.1080/09553000701753826. PMID: 18058372.

154 Stahler, C., Roth, J., Cordes, N., Taucher-Scholz, G., and Mueller-Klieser, W. (2013). Impact of carbon ion irradiation on epidermal growth factor receptor signaling and glioma cell migration in comparison to conventional photon irradiation. *International Journal of Radiation Biology* 89 (6): 454–461. 10.3109/09553002.2013.766769.

155 Fujita, M., Otsuka, Y., Imadome, K., Endo, S., Yamada, S., and Imai, T. (2012). Carbon-ion radiation enhances migration ability and invasiveness of the pancreatic cancer cell, PANC-1, in vitro. *Cancer Science* 103 (4): 677–683. 10.1111/j.1349-7006.2011.02190.x.

156 Nagasawa, H. and Little, J.B. (1992). Induction of sister chromatid exchanges by extremely low doses of alpha-particles. *Cancer Research* 52 (22): 6394–6396. http://www.ncbi.nlm.nih.gov/pubmed/1423287.

157 Shao, C., Aoki, M., and Furusawa, Y. (2001). Medium-mediated bystander effects on HSG cells co-cultivated with cells irradiated by X-rays or a 290 MeV/u carbon beam. *Journal of Radiation Research* 42 (3): 305–316. 10.1269/jrr.42.305.

158 Shao, C., Furusawa, Y., Aoki, M., Matsumoto, H., and Ando, K. (2002). Nitric oxide-mediated bystander effect induced by heavy-ions in human salivary gland tumour cells. *International Journal of Radiation Biology* 78 (9): 837–844. 10.1080/09553000210149786.

159 Hamada, N., Ni, M., Funayama, T., Sakashita, T., and Kobayashi, Y. (2008). Temporally distinct response of irradiated normal human fibroblasts and their bystander cells to energetic heavy ions. *Mutation Research* 639 (1-2): 35–44. 10.1016/j.mrfmmm.2007.11.001.

160 Suzuki, M., Yasuda, N., and Kitamura, H. (2020). Lethal and mutagenic bystander effects in human fibroblast cell cultures subjected to low-energy-carbon ions. *International Journal of Radiation Biology* 96 (2): 179–186. 10.1080/09553002.2020.1683637.

161 Harada, K., Nonaka, T., Hamada, N. et al. (2009). Heavy-ion-induced bystander killing of human lung cancer cells: Role of gap junctional intercellular communication. *Cancer Science* 100 (4): 684–688. 10.1111/j.1349-7006.2009.01093.x.

162 Shao, C., Furusawa, Y., Aoki, M., and Ando, K. (2003). Role of gap junctional intercellular communication in radiation-induced bystander effects in human fibroblasts. *Radiation Research* 160 (3): 318–323. 10.1667/rr3044.

163 Autsavapromporn, N., Suzuki, M., Funayama, T. et al. (2013). Gap junction communication and the propagation of bystander effects induced by microbeam irradiation in human fibroblast cultures: The impact of radiation quality. *Radiation Research* 180 (4): 367–375. 10.1667/RR3111.1.

164 Shao, C., Aoki, M., and Furusawa, Y. (2004). Bystander effect in lymphoma cells vicinal to irradiated neoplastic epithelial cells: Nitric oxide is involved. *Journal of Radiation Research* 45 (1): 97–103. 10.1269/jrr.45.97.

165 Autsavapromporn, N., Plante, I., Liu, C. et al. (2015). Genetic changes in progeny of bystander human fibroblasts after microbeam irradiation with X-rays, protons or carbon ions: The relevance to cancer risk. *International Journal of Radiation Biology* 91 (1): 62–70. 10.3109/09553002.2014.950715.

166 He, M., Dong, C., Konishi, T. et al. (2014). Differential effects of p53 on bystander phenotypes induced by gamma ray and high LET heavy ion radiation. *Life Sciences in Space Research* 1: 53–59. 10.1016/j.lssr.2014.02.003.

167 Mutou-Yoshihara, Y., Funayama, T., Yokota, Y., and Kobayashi, Y. (2012). Involvement of bystander effect in suppression of the cytokine production induced by heavy-ion broad beams. *International Journal of Radiation Biology* 88 (3): 258–266. 10.3109/09553002.2012.636138.

168 Dong, C., He, M., Tu, W. et al. (2015). The differential role of human macrophage in triggering secondary bystander effects after either gamma-ray or carbon beam irradiation. *Cancer Letters* 363 (1): 92–100. 10.1016/j.canlet.2015.04.013.

169 Diegeler, S. and Hellweg, C.E. (2017). Intercellular communication of tumor cells and immune cells after exposure to different ionizing radiation qualities. *Frontiers in Immunology* 8: 664. 10.3389/fimmu.2017.00664.

170 Bassler, N., Jäkel, O., Søndergaard, C.S., and Petersen, J.B. (2010). Dose- and LET-painting with particle therapy. *Acta Oncologica* 49 (7): 1170–1176. 10.3109/0284186X.2010.510640.

171 Bassler, N., Toftegaard, J., Lühr, A. et al. (2014). LET-painting increases tumour control probability in hypoxic tumours. *Acta Oncologica* 53 (1): 25–32. 10.3109/0284186X.2013.832835.

172 Scifoni, E., Tinganelli, W., Weyrather, W.K., Durante, M., Maier, A., and Krämer, M. (2013). Including oxygen enhancement ratio in ion beam treatment planning: Model implementation and experimental verification. *Physics in Medicine and Biology* 58 (11): 3871–3895. 10.1088/0031-9155/58/11/3871.

173 Sokol, O., Krämer, M., Hild, S., Durante, M., and Scifoni, E. (2019, Feb 8). Kill painting of hypoxic tumors with multiple ion beams. *Physics in Medicine and Biology* 64 (4): 045008. 10.1088/1361-6560/aafe40.

174 Antonovic, L., Lindblom, E., Dasu, A., Bassler, N., Furusawa, Y., and Toma-Dasu, I. (2014). Clinical oxygen enhancement ratio of tumors in carbon ion radiotherapy: The influence of local oxygenation changes. *Journal of Radiation Research* 55 (5): 902–911. 10.1093/jrr/rru020.

175 Formenti, S.C. and Demaria, S. (2012). Radiation therapy to convert the tumor into an in situ vaccine. *International Journal of Radiation Oncology* 84 (4): 879–880. 10.1016/j.ijrobp.2012.06.020.

176 Menger, L., Vacchelli, E., Adjemian, S. et al. (2012). Cardiac glycosides exert anticancer effects by inducing immunogenic cell death. *Science Translational Medicine* 4 (143): 143ra99. 10.1126/scitranslmed.3003807.

177 Huang, Y., Dong, Y., Zhao, J., Zhang, L., Kong, L., and Lu, J.J. (2019). Comparison of the effects of photon, proton and carbon-ion radiation on the ecto-calreticulin exposure in various tumor cell lines. *The Annals of Translational Medicine's* 7 (20): 542. 10.21037/atm.2019.09.128.

178 Ma, Y., Kepp, O., Ghiringhelli, F. et al. (2010). Chemotherapy and radiotherapy: Cryptic anticancer vaccines. *Seminars in Immunology* 22 (3): 113–124. 10.1016/j.smim.2010.03.001.

179 Demaria, S. and Formenti, S.C. (2020). The abscopal effect 67 years later: From a side story to center stage. *The British Journal of Radiology* 93 (1109): 20200042. 10.1259/bjr.20200042.

180 Mole, R.H. (1953). Whole body irradiation; radiobiology or medicine? *The British Journal of Radiology* 26 (305): 234–241. 10.1259/0007-1285-26-305-234.

181 Brenneman, R.J., Sharifai, N., Fischer-Valuck, B. et al. (2019). Abscopal effect following proton beam radiotherapy in a patient with inoperable metastatic retroperitoneal sarcoma. *Frontiers in Oncology* 9: 10.3389/fonc.2019.00922.

182 Ebner, D.K., Kamada, T., and Yamada, S. (2017). Abscopal effect in recurrent colorectal cancer treated with carbon-ion radiation therapy: 2 case reports. *Advances in Radiation Oncology* 2 (3): 333–338. 10.1016/j.adro.2017.06.001.

183 Schaub, S.K., Stewart, R.D., Sandison, G.A. et al. (2018). Does neutron radiation therapy potentiate an immune response to merkel cell carcinoma? *International Journal of Therapy and Rehabilitation* 5 (1): 183–195. 10.14338/IJPT-18-00012.1.

184 Huang, Y., Huang, Q., Zhao, J. et al. (2020). The Impacts of Different Types of Radiation on the CRT and PDL1 Expression in Tumor Cells Under Normoxia and Hypoxia. *Frontiers in Oncology* 10: 1610. 10.3389/fonc.2020.01610.

185 Onishi, M., Okonogi, N., Oike, T. et al. (2018). High linear energy transfer carbon-ion irradiation increases the release of the immune mediator high mobility group box 1 from human cancer cells. *Journal of Radiation Research* 59 (5): 541–546. 10.1093/jrr/rry049.

186 Yoshimoto, Y., Oike, T., Okonogi, N. et al. (2015). Carbon-ion beams induce production of an immune mediator protein, high mobility group box 1, at levels comparable with X-ray irradiation. *Journal of Radiation Research* 56 (3): 509–514. 10.1093/jrr/rrv007.

187 Takahashi, Y., Yasui, T., Minami, K. et al. (2019). Carbon ion irradiation enhances the antitumor efficacy of dual immune checkpoint blockade therapy both for local and distant sites in murine osteosarcoma. *Oncotarget* 10 (6): 633–646. 10.18632/oncotarget.26551.

188 Helm, A., Tinganelli, W., Simoniello, P. et al. (2021). Reduction of lung metastases in a mouse osteosarcoma model treated with carbon ions and immune checkpoint inhibitors. *International Journal of Radiation Oncology, Biology, Physics* 109 (2): 594–602. 10.1016/j.ijrobp.2020.09.041.

4

Practical Aspects of Particle Therapy Accelerators

J. Michele Dougherty, Ph.D. and Keith M. Furutani, Ph.D.

Department of Radiation Oncology, Mayo Clinic Florida 4500 San Pablo Road, Mayo 1 North, Jacksonville, Florida, USA, 32224

4.1   Introduction

Particle accelerators were invented in the 1930s as research instruments to probe the structure of matter and to unveil fundamental physics principles. The first cyclotron constructed by Lawrence and Livingston was only 11.4 cm in diameter and accelerated the hydrogen ions to 80 keV. Today, there are more than 30,000 particle accelerators in operation around the world. The largest particle accelerator (Large Hadron Collider at CERN) can produce particle energy in the tera-electron volt range, which is 10^9 times what the first cyclotron could produce.

Some smaller accelerators are built for more practical purposes. For instance, the accelerators designed for particle therapy need to be more compact in size to be built around existing medical facilities or urban surroundings. Larger equipment design not only requires more building material but also more concrete for shielding radiation produced from the particle therapy system. The cost of construction is more expensive with larger facilities. For protons, the therapeutic energy range is less than 300 MeV, which is achievable with commercially manufactured accelerators of the following type: isochronous cyclotron, synchrocyclotron, and synchrotron. The choice of accelerator impacts the dose rate for proton therapy treatment. It also leads to important considerations for the total treat-

ment delivery time and patient throughput. In addition, particle accelerators and the transport beamline are made of various electromagnetic equipment that require high-voltage power supplies. The energy consumption of this equipment is another practical consideration from a cost perspective.

The purpose of this chapter is to provide a brief overview of the three main types of accelerators that are commercially available for proton therapy today. We will also explore the basic physics principles of accelerator operation.

4.2   Accelerators

4.2.1   Basic Cyclotron Equations

To understand how a particle accelerator works, one must first know these two principles:

- A charged particle moving through a magnetic field will turn in a circular path.
- A charged particle is accelerated by an electric field.

In a linear accelerator, a series of electric fields accelerates particles in a straight path; however, it cannot accelerate particles to high enough energies for particle therapy within a practical

Principles and Practice of Particle Therapy, First Edition. Edited by Timothy D. Malouff and Daniel M. Trifiletti.
© 2022 John Wiley & Sons Ltd. Published 2022 by John Wiley & Sons Ltd.

distance. The cyclotron was invented as a solution to accelerate particles to high energies within a small area. A cyclotron accelerates particles in a spiral pattern through a constant magnetic field. Electric fields are applied as the particle rotates to add energy during each revolution.

Despite the design differences between medical particle accelerators, some fundamental physics equations are presented here to help us understand their basic operational principles. A positively charged particle, like a hydrogen nucleus, moving through a magnetic field in a perpendicular direction will follow a circular path due to the centripetal force provided by the magnetic field acting on the particle. This directional vector quantity is called the Lorentz force. This force is a result of the magnetic field acting on a particle traveling in a perpendicular direction to the magnetic field. The vector directions of the magnetic field, Lorentz force, and the particle velocity can be visualized using the right-hand rule. As depicted in Figure 4.1, a charged particle with mass m moves in a circular path with a constant velocity v, when it is placed in a uniform magnetic field B. For a particle traveling much slower than the speed of light (non-relativistic), the centripetal force F_c is

$$F_c = \frac{mv^2}{r} \tag{4.1}$$

where m is the mass of the proton, v is the velocity, and r is the radius of the circular path. Because the centripetal force is equal to the Lorentz force of the magnetic field B, the Lorentz force is

$$F_L = qvB \tag{4.2}$$

where q is the charge of the particle. Equating these two forces, we get

$$\frac{mv^2}{r} = qvB \tag{4.3}$$

We can then obtain the rotational frequency or the angular frequency of the charged particle by moving parameters around

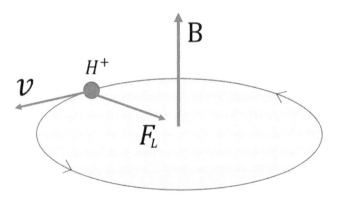

Figure 4.1 A proton moves in circular path with a constant velocity when it is placed in a uniform magnetic field.

$$\omega = \frac{v}{r} = \frac{qB}{m} \tag{4.4}$$

From this equation, we can state that the rotational frequency of the particle ω is a constant under the influence of a constant magnetic field. It is also independent on its traveling radius, velocity, and energy.

Figure 4.2 illustrates the principles of a classical cyclotron where the particles travel with a velocity much slower than the speed of light. At the center of the cyclotron, two semicircular disks are located perpendicularly to the magnetic field. These copper disks are called the dees. A gap is left in between the two dees, which are connected to a sinusoidal RF generator. The frequency of the RF generator is equal to the rotational frequency of the particles. The particles are then accelerated as they pass through the electric field in the gap. Because the RF generator creates an alternating electric field, the protons are accelerated twice per revolution, each time they pass through the gap. Because of the increase in particle speed and energy, the radius of the particle trajectory is incrementally increased and results in an enlarging spiral path. The particles reach their maximum energy at the outer most trajectory and then exit the cyclotron.

4.2.2 Isochronous Cyclotron

The classical cyclotron created by Ernest O. Lawrence at University of California Berkeley [1] only has a beam energy range of 10–20 MeV. The energy is limited due to relativistic effects. As the particle velocity reaches a fraction of the speed of light, the mass of the particle increases as well. The resting mass of a particle m needs to be corrected by a factor γ, given by

$$\gamma = \frac{1}{\sqrt{1 - (v^2/c^2)}} \tag{4.5}$$

where c is the speed of light. As the speed of a particle approaches the speed of light, the γ term gets larger and larger, along with the mass of the particle. A 20-MeV proton is traveling at 20% of the speed of light and has a γ factor equal to 1.02. However, a 230-MeV proton travels at roughly 60% of the speed of light; this proton has a resulting mass increase of 1.25 times its resting mass. Because of the increase in particle mass, the rotational frequency of the particle decreases, and it is no longer in resonance with the RF generator frequency. The particle will no longer be accelerated by the dee voltage. To overcome this limit, an isochronous cyclotron will increase its magnetic field strength with radius to maintain the isochronism condition, defined by

$$\omega_c = \omega_{\mathrm{RF}} = \frac{qB\gamma}{m\gamma} \tag{4.6}$$

Classic Cyclotron Design

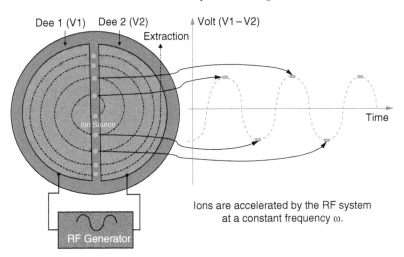

Ions are accelerated by the RF system
at a constant frequency ω.

Figure 4.2   The classic cyclotron design where particles can be accelerated with an electric field oscillating at constant frequency.

where ω_c is the rotational frequency of the particles in the cyclotron, and ω_{RF} is the frequency of the RF generator. The isochronism condition requires the cyclotron magnetic field to increase also by the γ factor to compensate for the relativistic particle mass increase. With the increase in magnetic field, the particle's trajectory will deviate from the mid-plane of the cyclotron and eventually become lost by colliding with the cyclotron interior vacuum walls. To keep the particle beams mid-plane, a focusing magnetic field with the opposite direction is required to refocus the particles by decreasing the magnetic field. It is practically impossible to both increase the magnetic field and decrease the magnetic field at the same time, since the need of maintaining isochronism and the need of refocusing the particles within the cyclotron at mid-plane are contradicting actions against each other.

In 1938, Llewellyn H. Thomas from Ohio State University [2] introduced a clever solution to the problem by designing an azimuthally varying field (AVF) cyclotron. In order to keep the revolution frequency of the particle in a constant, the average magnetic field of an isochronous cyclotron at mid-plane has to be shaped accordingly as a function of radius. By modulating the magnetic field also in the azimuthal direction, the particles experience a strong net vertical focusing effect to keep them captured in their spiral accelerating path. Figure 4.3 shows the magnetic field distribution on the hills and valleys of an AVF cyclotron. The magnetic field strength is higher in the hill sectors and lower at the valley sectors. When a particle travels through the junction between a valley and a hill, the particle will experience a net vertical focusing force large enough to overcome the vertical defocusing force due to the radially increasing average magnetic field. In addition, the alternating

magnetic field created by the sectors of hills and valleys will distort the circular path. In 1954, Donald W. Kerst realized that the symmetrical straight sectors can be replaced with spirally shaped sectors [3], which will further enhance the strong vertical focusing effect. The magnitude of the focusing force from the spiral sectors depends on the field strength difference between the hills and the valleys, as well as the pitch of the spiral. The majority of proton therapy facilities today use this type of isochronous cyclotron design.

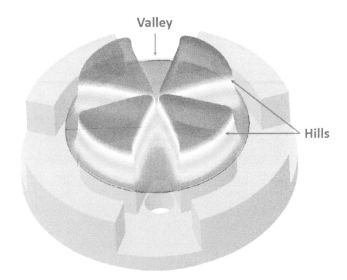

Figure 4.3   Magnetic field modulation with valley and hill sectors inside of an AVF cyclotron (adapted from Simon Zaremba and Wiel Kleeven from Ion Beam Application (IBA), Cyclotrons: Magnetic Design and Beam Dynamics, CERN Document Server, and https://cds.cern.ch/record/2315180?ln=en).

4.2.3 Synchrocyclotron

A typical average magnetic field strength from a commercial isochronous cyclotron for proton ions is around 2.3 T with a diameter of 4–5 m across and a height of approximately 2.5 m (Figure 4.5). Naturally, a smaller accelerator corresponds to a smaller building footprint; hence, it is more suitable for operation at a hospital facility. To shrink the accelerator size or the particle bending radius, one can increase the average magnetic field to be greater than 4 T with a superconducting magnet. Most of the commercially available isochronous cyclotron and synchrocyclotrons for particle therapy nowadays are made of superconducting magnet.

The theoretical concept of the synchrocyclotron was independently reported by Edward M. McMillan at UC Berkeley [4] in 1945 and by a Soviet experimental physicist, Vladimir I. Veksler [5] in 1944. In a synchrocyclotron accelerator, the RF generator changes its frequency to match the particle rotational frequency. As the particle-traveling speed approaches a significant fraction of the speed of light, the relativistic effects will increase the particle mass. Instead of keeping the RF generator at a constant frequency, the synchrocyclotron varies the frequency applied to the electrodes to match the sagging particle revolution frequency. By doing so, the particle experiences a continuous acceleration during each revolution. Furthermore, the magnetic field within the synchrocyclotron decreases radially so that a weak focusing is obtained. The weak focusing effect provides the particles with orbital stability and prevents them from deviating from the mid-plane trajectory. Because the RF supply varies cyclically in frequency, only a short burst of the particles can be captured and accelerated up to the max radius. The frequency at which the parti-

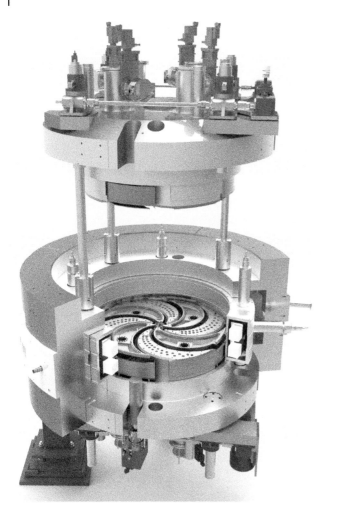

Figure 4.4 A Varian ProBeam superconducting isochronous cyclotron has high efficiency beam production and low energy consumption (image courtesy of Varian Medical Systems, Inc. All rights reserved).

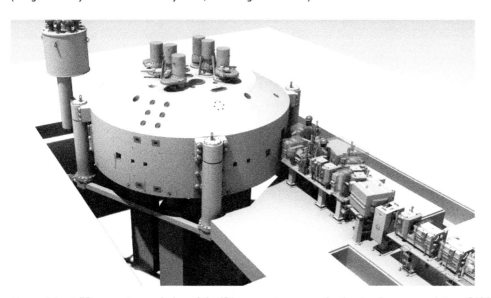

Figure 4.5 A 3D computer rendering of the IBA compact superconducting isochronous cyclotron C400 designed to accelerate proton, helium, and carbon ions. The C400 has an outer diameter of 6.6 m and a height of 3.4 m. The total weight of the magnet system is 700 t. The max field strength is 4.5 T at the hill sectors. The final extraction energy of the ions is 265 MeV/amu for protons and 400 MeV/amu for carbon (image courtesy of IBA. All rights reserved).

cles are pulsed from the accelerator equals the duration of each RF frequency sweep. Hence, the beam production duty cycle from a synchrocyclotron is much lower than the continuous beam current produced with an isochronous cyclotron.

In a synchrocyclotron, a particle starts with small orbits at the center of the accelerator; it crosses the gap between the large hollow dee and a grounded electrode twice per revolution. Because the electric potential difference needed for particle acceleration is much smaller, only one hollow dee is needed (Figure 4.6). The magnitude of the RF energy applied is much lower in a synchrocyclotron, so it will take a particle tens of thousands of revolutions before it can reach its desired clinical range. In comparison, the number of revolutions is much lower (around a thousand) in the isochronous cyclotron. As mentioned earlier, the cyclotron needs to maintain a state of isochronism to accelerate relativistic particles. Similarly, the synchrocyclotron varies its RF frequency to preserve synchronism. In an ideal condition, there exists a synchronous particle who orbits in the accelerator with the same frequency as the RF frequency and it is perfectly synchronous with the RF field by having the exact same phase. However, in reality, a group of particles captured in the synchrocyclotron accelerator will not have identical orbital position, energy, frequency, or phase as the idealized synchronous particle. The physical parameters of these particles (energy and phase) will actually oscillate around the synchronous particle. These particles will remain stable for acceleration as long as their longitudinal phase space stay within a stability zone (or a bucket). The particles which have an initial phase offset that is within the

bucket will slowly oscillate in phase around the synchronous phase. If the particles have an initial phase offset that is not within the bucket, the particle will eventually lose their energy and be lost in the accelerator (Figure 4.7). The bucket width is controlled by the dee voltage, the RF system, and the magnetic field. The concept of the particle phase stability zone or the bucket is illustrated in Figure 4.4.

4.2.4 Synchrotron

The synchrotron accelerator was invented around the same time as the synchrocyclotron. Vladimir I. Veksler first published the principles of synchrotron in 1944 [5]. A year later, Edwin McMillan constructed the first synchrotron for electron beam [6]. Sir Marcus Oliphant designed and built the first proton beam synchrotron in 1952. The primary drawback of the cyclotron or the synchrocyclotron is its limitation in max particle energy with a given magnet size. Larger magnets are more expensive to construct and maintain. As a result, a fixed radius synchrotron concept was developed to maximize particle energy. For a relativistic particle, the orbital radius is defined, as

$$r = \frac{E}{qcB} \tag{4.7}$$

where E is the energy of the charged particle, B is the magnetic field strength, c is the speed of light, and q is the charge of the

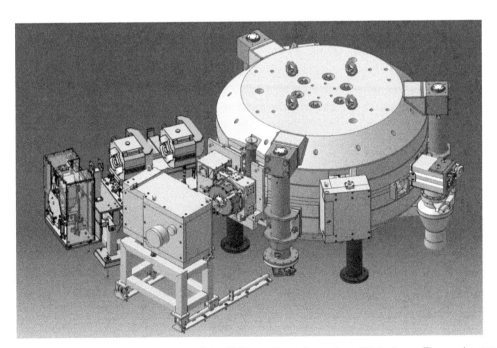

Figure 4.6 A 3D computer rendering of the S2C2 synchrocyclotron from IBA is shown. The accelerator has a yoke radius of 1.25 m with cryogenic cooling for the superconducting magnet system. The max magnetic field strength is 5.7 T (image courtesy of IBA.

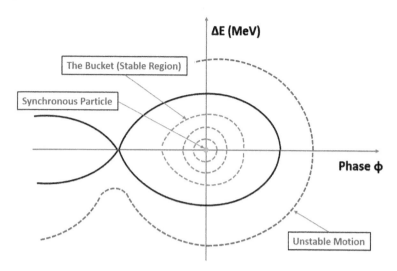

Figure 4.7 The phase space stable region where particles oscillate in the synchronous phase. Particles with unstable motion will be lost in the accelerator.

particle. From this equation, we can deduce that since r is a constant, then the ratio of the particle energy and magnetic field E/B must be a constant. Hence, the magnetic field must synchronously increase with the energy of the particles. In general, the synchrotron accelerator is characterized by two conditions:

- The magnetic field varies synchronously with the particle energy
- The electric field (RF) varies synchronously with the particle orbital frequency, which depends on the particle energy and the magnetic field

In order to modulate the electric field and the magnetic field in synchronism with the particle energy, the beam current is pulsed for a synchrotron.

A synchrotron is not capable of accelerating a particle with zero initial velocity. It requires pre-accelerated particles to be injected into the system. Generally, a linear accelerator is used to provide protons with an initial energy in the range of several MeV. The particles can be either injected all at once or gradually into the synchrotron ring. In order to reduce treatment delivery time, it is critical to fill the ring with as many protons as possible to prolong the extraction time. Higher initial injection energy enables more protons to be stored in the ring due to the reduced coulomb repulsion forces. Also, the injection of the particles needs to be synchronized with respect to the RF frequency of the ring. During each acceleration cycle or spill, 2–10 billion protons are injected into the synchrotron ring. It takes less than 1–2 s to accelerate the protons to the desired energy (typically 70–250 MeV). Then, the protons are slowly extracted during the extraction phase, which lasts from 4 to 7 s. Once the extraction is complete, the unused protons are decelerated and dumped at low energy. This operation cycle is repeated until all

the doses are delivered to a treatment volume. Typically, it takes a couple minutes to deliver 2 Gy to a 1-l volume. The motion of the protons inside of the synchrotron ring, under the influence of both electric and magnetic field, is like that of a harmonic oscillator. Similar to the synchrocyclotron, as long as the protons phase space stays within the stability zone, they will be safe from loss. Alternatively, a RF "kicker" signal can be introduced with the goal of perturbing the phase space of the circulating protons for extraction. Once the protons are kicked out of the stability zone, they will deviate from the acceleration orbit and move into the extraction septum (Figure 4.8).

Since the protons circulate in the synchrotron ring, many thousands of times before the extraction process, it is unavoidable for them to deviate from the ideal path. It is necessary to use focusing magnets to guide them back to the correct path. There are three types of magnets to achieve the goal of bending and focusing the protons. They are categorized by the number of poles. The dipole magnet bends the particles to a desired angle. The quadruple magnets provide strong focusing effect to the beam, but it might introduce more energy spread in the beam. The sextupole ensures particles with all energy offset (dispersed by the quadrupole) are focused back to the same point. The arrangement of the bending and focusing magnets in a synchrotron system is called the focusing lattice. These different magnetic elements in the focusing lattice work together to ensure optimal beam quality and treatment delivery time.

To further shrink the synchrotron size, Hitachi introduced a compact synchrotron design in 2013 [7] (Figure 4.9). The traditional Hitachi focusing lattice consists of 16 magnet elements. The compact system has only a total of eight elements by combining the coupling functions of the quadruple magnets to the ends of the bending magnet. The orbital diameter is reduced

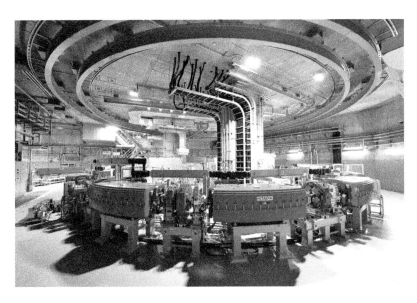

Figure 4.8   A carbon ion synchrotron accelerator system by Hitachi has a circumference of 58 m and 18 m in diameter (in the courtesy of Osaka Heavy Ion Therapy Center. All rights reserved).

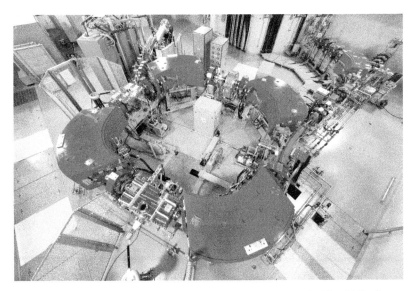

Figure 4.9   A compact proton synchrotron accelerator system by Hitachi (in the courtesy of Hokkaido University Proton Beam Therapy Center. All rights reserved).

from 7.8 m to 5.1 m. The reduction in accelerator size means less shielding materials during a facility construction.

Since the total treatment delivery time is a crucial factor in the selection of a proton therapy system, it is advantageous to increase the synchrotron extraction time by recycling unused protons instead of disposing them. The Hitachi ProBeat V PBS system employs incremental beam deceleration during the extraction phase to deliver multiple energy layers per spill. This process is called the multiple energy extraction (MEE) technique. Instead of reaccelerating a spill of protons to the requested discrete energy layer, multiple energy layers (2–4) are extracted from a single spill of protons. The MEE delivery technique was reported to reduce

the total beam delivery time by 35% on average in comparison with the single energy extraction technique [8].

4.2.5   Energy Selection

Generally, a range of energy layers is needed to cover a target volume robustly in three-dimensional space. A single energy layer is consisting of tens of thousands of ion spots of the same energy. For protons and other heavy ion particles, a particle accelerator system needs to generate the required energy levels according to a DICOM treatment plan. An energy selection process is necessary on a layer-by-layer basis. The energy selection system will vary depending on the type of accelerator used. Both cyclotrons and synchro-cyclotrons deliver a mono-energetic beam that requires external devices to select the beam energy to be delivered. Many cyclotrons and synchrocyclotrons today deliver a 230-MeV proton beam that would reach the equivalent range of about 33 cm of depth in water or 33 g/cm². The typical treatment energies for proton are between 70 MeV and 230 MeV or 4 g/cm² and 33 g/cm². To deliver to the shallower ranges, the beam must pass through a material, such as carbon, to degrade the beam to lower energies. Then, a series of dipole magnets is used to filter the energies of the beam to ensure a single energy is delivered to the patient per spot. To deliver proton energy lower than 70 MeV, an external range pull-back device is placed immediately up stream of the treatment surface to modify the location of the Bragg peaks. Hence, the proton spots can deposit their dose at shallower surface of a breast tissue as opposed to a deep-seated tumor in the prostate. A synchrotron does not require an energy selection system because it selects the particle energy based on the number of revolutions in the synchrotron. The typical treatment energies are between 70 MeV and 230 MeV for proton and 120 MeV/amu and 430 MeV/amu for carbon ions. During a typical commissioning process of synchrotron particle therapy system, the energy levels are discretely chosen to meet the clinical needs. In contrast, for a cyclotron or a synchrocyclotron system, a range of energy levels are defined instead.

4.2.6 Proton Linear Accelerator

Recently, a new commercial proton linear accelerator system was introduced to the particle therapy world [9]. As we have mentioned briefly at the beginning of this chapter, particles can also be accelerated in a linear beamline by an alternating electric field. This type of particle accelerating system is called a linear accelerator. The concept of a linear accelerator was first invented in 1924 by a Swedish physicist Gustav Ising [10]. Nearly 100 years later, under collaboration with CERN, the LIGHT proton linear accelerator system is developed by combining three different

linac sections into one accelerator beamline. The LIGHT accelerator has a total linear length of 25 m, with an energy range of 37.5–230 MeV. It produces a pulsed beam that can be modulated in both the beam intensity and energy. Unlike the circular accelerators (cyclotron, synchrocyclotron, and synchrotron), the energy selection in a LIGHT accelerator can be achieved from a pulse to pulse basis, making it extremely ideal for pencil beam scanning delivery. Because of the extremely small energy switching time, the delivery of the proton spots can be modulated in the energy or range dimension to correct for range differences. With the circular accelerators, the spots in the deepest energy layer are generally delivered first, then the second deepest energy layer is delivered next. This type of de-escalation delivery scheme is no longer needed with the LIGHT accelerator due to the extremely fast energy switching time. Furthermore, because a beam degrader is no longer needed to create low energy proton spots, there is almost no beam loss with the LIGHT accelerator. Minimal beam loss also means fewer shielding materials needed during the construction of a facility with a LIGHT accelerator. All these unique features of the LIGHT proton linear accelerator make it a promising new accelerator technology for spot scanning proton therapy soon.

4.3 Summary

The AVF isochronous cyclotron with spiral pole sectors, the compact superconducting synchrocyclotron with pulsed beam current, and the synchrotron are the three main types of accelerator systems employed for particle therapy around the world. As the need for proton and ion beam therapy increases in the next coming decades, construction footprint, dose rate, total treatment delivery time, and cost will remain the primary considerations when choosing a particle therapy system. It is important to understand basic accelerator physics and operation principles to make informed decisions.

References

1 Lawrence, E.O. and Livingston, M.S. (1932). The production of high speed light ions without the use of high voltages. *Physical Review* 40 (1): 19–35.

2 Thomas, L.H. (1938). The paths of ions in the cyclotron I. Orbits in the magnetic field. *Physical Review* 54 (8): 580–588.

3 Kerst, D.W. (1955). Constant Frequency Cyclotrons with Spiral Ridged Poles, 64. Midwestern Universities Research Association: University of Illinois.

4 McMillan, E.M. (Inventor). (1947). Synchro-cyclotron.

5 Veksler, V.I. (1944). A new method of accelerating relativistic particles. The Proceedings of USSR Academy of Sciences 43 (8): 3.

6 McMillan, E.M. (1945). The synchrotron—A proposed high energy particle accelerator. Physical Review 68 (5-6): 143–144.

7 Umezawa, M., Fujimoto, R., Umekawa, T., et al. (2013). Development of the compact proton beam therapy system dedicated to spot scanning with real-time tumor-tracking technology. AIP Conference Proceedings 1525 (1): 360–363.

8 Younkin, J.E., Bues, M., Sio, T.T., et al. (2018). Multiple energy extraction reduces beam delivery time for a synchrotron-based proton spot-scanning system. Advances in Radiation Oncology 3 (3): 412–420.

9 Degiovanni AS, P. and Ungaro, D. Light: A linear accelerator for proton therapy. Paper presented at: NAPAC2016. Chicago, IL, USA.

10 Ising, G. (1924). Principle of a method for producing high-voltage canal beams. *Arkiv för Matematik, Astronomi och Fysik* 18 (30): 4.

5

Treatment Planning for Scanning Beam Proton Therapy

Aman Anand and Martin Bues

Department of Radiation Oncology, Mayo Clinic, Phoenix, AZ – 85050

This chapter is dedicated to our patients treated with proton therapy whose disease continues to serve as a tutor for all of us to learn this art of treatment planning.

5.1 Introduction

Since the foundational work by Robert Wilson (Wilson, 1946) describing the advantages of using proton beams for clinical use, proton therapy has undergone fundamental change and this change has been accelerated in the last two decades. Passive scattering proton beam therapy and uniform scanning proton beam therapy have been superseded by active scanning proton beam delivery. Hence, our chapter will focus entirely on discussing the techniques that are relevant to scanning beam proton therapy (sPBT). While the first patient was treated with sPBT in 1954 (Tobias et al., 1958), it wasn't until

Principles and Practice of Particle Therapy, First Edition. Edited by Timothy D. Malouff and Daniel M. Trifiletti.

late 1996 when PSI incorporated works of Jäkel et al. to develop and treat patients with narrow scanning pencil beams (Pedroni et al., 1999; Jäkel et al., 2001; Karger et al., 2010). Please refer to the work by Judy Adams for information regarding planning for the older forms of proton beam therapy (Bussière and Adams, 2003).

Our text will cover the characterization, optimization, and planning nuances relevant to scanning proton beam therapy as it applies to the treatment planning for various disease sites. While treatment planning is a procedure that considers both machine and patient specific information, the rules of planning and delivery remain very specific to the site of treatment. Ultimately treatment planning is a vehicle to make the physician's vision of how the patient's condition should improve a reality. Unlike most conventional treatment planning texts, we also provide key notes on the "Do's and Do-not's" of sPBT planning. We also provide some exercises which will allow the novice sPBT planner to gain some hands-on experience with some of the concepts presented here.

5.2 Basics of sPBT Planning

5.2.1 Spot Characteristics

Proton treatment planning, or any radiation treatment planning for that matter, requires prior knowledge of the physical characteristics of the treatment beam. In sPBT, obtaining this knowledge is comparatively simple. Since in sPBT any clinical dose distribution is created as a superposition of individual quasi-monoenergetic pencil beams, it is sufficient to characterize these individual pencil beams that make up the fundamental blocks for treatment planning. Modern day proton therapy is best delivered either by utilizing a synchrotron-based or a cyclotron-based accelerator system (Smith et al., 2009). We will not be discussing hardware specific details of sPBT, but one can familiarize through these references (Pedroni et al., 1999; Smith et al., 2009; Gillin et al., 2010). In each case, a sPBT is delivered by super positioning multiple pencil beams that get carefully weighted and optimized for delivering therapeutic doses to the target volumes by actively painting doses across the target volumes (Smith et al., 2009). Such mechanisms require very large number of pencil beams that get arranged across the target and hence it is extremely important that each pencil beamlet, as described below, gets characterized accurately for commissioning of treatment planning systems. In this chapter, we will highlight some of the necessary and important characteristics of pencil beams that a planner should familiarize themselves with in order to be able to make judicious choices while selecting: beam angles, spacing between the pencil beamlets, and effective treatment planning margins in order to generate robust treatment plans.

Developing an understanding of spot profiles, planar integral doses, and characteristics of spot profiles as a function of energy would make planning of any complicated tumors less burdensome and reduce the multiple-iterative optimization as the planner will have a better know-how of preparing for margins and beam angles. We provide in the following subsection an overview of spot profile and the depth doses in sPBT.

5.2.1.1 Spot Profile

In sPBT, a spot can be understood as a Gaussian distribution (as seen in Figure 5.1) of radiation spreading perpendicular to the direction of travel of the beams (Trofimov and Bortfeld, 2003; Safai et al., 2008). Whenever a magnetically scanned proton beam traverses through a medium, the dose distribution from each beam can then be described by the incident lateral fluence profile combined with the planar integral spot dose along the depths of travel in the medium (Anand et al., 2012 "A Procedure to Determine the Planar Integral Spot Dose Values of Proton Pencil Beam Spots"; Sawakuchi et al., 2010). For a typical proton beam traversing through water, both primary and secondary particles due to elastic and inelastic interactions will start contributing dose lateral to their depths of travel (Figure 5.2a and b).

Such doses are often characterized by their full widths at half maximum (known as spot size) which continues to vary with depths and energies. Each particle accelerator has a unique mechanism of accelerating protons; however, irrespective of their delivery mechanisms, scanning beam systems end up generating a low-dose envelope off the lateral axis from each pencil beam as they continue to travel through a homogeneous phantom.

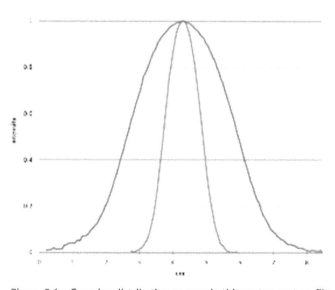

Figure 5.1 Gaussian distribution as seen in this proton spot profile.

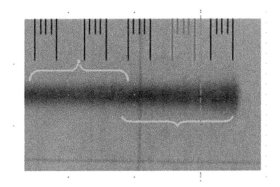

Figure 5.2a A radiographic image of proton beam traveling through medium showing dose deposition lateral to the direction of travel.

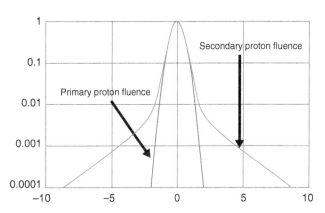

Figure 5.2b Proton beam generating primary and secondary particles as they continue to travel along the medium.

To generate a broad beam dose distribution to cover the target, treatment planning systems, whether analytical or Monte Carlo, end up creating broad field dose distribution by accounting dose from each individual pencil beam. Since these individual pencil beams are now the building blocks for broad beam distributions, it is thus very important to understand lateral characteristics of these beams and the analytical treatment of their Gaussian profiles to be able to create a better lateral fall-off while generating a clinical treatment plan.

For a given shape and geometry of a tumor, sPBT can be delivered volumetrically by constructing what is known as spread-out Bragg peak (SOBP) (Jette and Chen, 2011). Essentially, for each beam necessary to cover the target, multiple pencil beams are delivered with the most distal Bragg peak to the target getting weighted heavily, while the subsequently superpositioned Bragg peaks of lower energies get reduced weighting thereby leading to the creation of a homogenous dose distribution within the target.

5.2.1.2 Depth Dose

Much of the dosimetric advantage of proton beam therapy stems from its depth dose characteristics, often referred to as the Bragg peak. It is important that the Bragg, as shown in Figure 5.3, is that of a narrow pencil beam and that the depth dose curve of an SOBP beam would look quite different due to the super-positioning of individual pencil beams.

We typically treat targets with many pencil beams so that there is always lateral equilibrium present to cover the volumetric shape of the tumor with adequate dose. Due to diminished exit doses, there are some distinct advantages that charged particle therapy offers (Lomax, 2009). Protons tend to lose their energy gradually as they travel through the medium and ultimately exhaust themselves toward the end of range. The inverse relationship between the rate of energy being deposited and the kinetic energy of these particles as they travel in the medium shows that the maximum amount of dose gets deposited toward the end of their travel, thereby leading to this characteristic depth dose curve known as the Bragg peak.

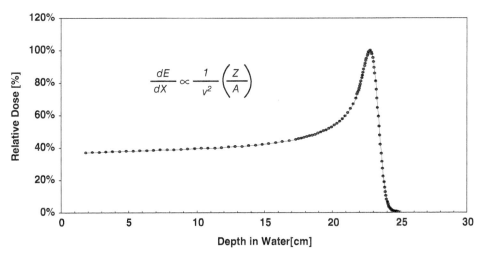

$$\frac{dE}{dX} \propto \frac{1}{v^2}\left(\frac{Z}{A}\right)$$

Figure 5.3 Depth dose distribution of a single monoenergetic proton beam traveling in water.

5.2.2 Dosimetric Advantages of Proton over X-ray Therapy

When embarking on learning proton beam therapy planning, it is important to appreciate how the dose deposition characteristics of protons can offer advantages over other forms of radiotherapy (Patyal, 2007). What we describe in the section later is a water-phantom-based in-silico experiment which highlights some differences between photon and proton-based dosimetric profile both in lateral as well as in the depth-dose directions. It is also advised for users to generate similar dosimetric profiles for their own particle beam line at their facility to establish some working knowledge about the lateral and distal penumbrae of their proton beams. To aid, we provide a simple workbook example toward the end of this section for anyone to practice this dosimetry for their own clinic. The details and step-by-step guide of these exercises have been provided in the Appendix.

As seen in Figure 5.4, we have a spherical target with a radius of 2.5 cm created whose center is at a depth of 10 cm in a water phantom. With dosimetric beamline calculation to cover this target with 60 Gy in 30 fractions, we created three distinct plans: (a) a four-field box with a 6-MV X-ray beam; (b) a two-field rapid arc plan for a 6-MV volumetric modulated arc therapy (VMAT) delivery, and (c) a single-field scanning beam proton plan with a range of 14 cm in water within our treatment planning system (Eclipse V. 15.6). For similar clinical target volume (CTV) coverages (D95 maintained at 95% for all three plans), we then performed dosimetric profile comparisons to highlight differences between these three separate modes of radiotherapy delivery. In Figure 5.5, dosimetric comparison along the lateral profile and along the depth doses between a VMAT and a proton plan is shown.

One can clearly appreciate that for a homogeneous medium the lateral profiles show increased low doses distributed far from the target with X-rays, while protons show reduction in the lateral penumbra due to the properties of the Bragg peak and the reduced need for multiple beam angles. Lateral dose distribution in single-field distribution of protons versus multiple-field distributions of photons will always be superior but the conformality of a rapid arc-based delivery may be superior over the proton-based delivery in some clinical cases. This is due to higher degrees of freedom in delivering radiotherapy doses as an arc compared to only a few discrete angles that are utilized in delivering dose using protons.

Figure 5.5 demonstrates that the entrance dose for protons is higher than for photons. This is due to the summation of plateau doses of the Bragg peaks of different energies. The larger the target in beam direction, the more pronounced this summation effect becomes. In extreme cases, it is sometimes possible to treat the proximal target without placing Bragg peaks in the proximal region of the target. Also notice that protons do not afford the skin sparing effect of high-energy X-rays (see exercise later to learn more). We see the benefits of protons on the distal end of the curve (red). At the end of the SOBP, proton therapy offers sharper dose fall-offs compared to the photon-based delivery and as a result proton-based therapy spares larger volumes of healthy tissues and organs at risk that sit distal to the end of the Bragg peak. We illustrate these basic features of proton dose distributions for didactical purposes only. The actual clinical advantage or disadvantages of protons relative to X-rays will depend on the specifications of the proton beam delivery system and can only be understood through comparative treatment planning. We provide the enthusiastic reader with a few initiating exercises that could help them better appreciate dosimetric characteristics of proton pencil beams as they interact with the medium.

5.2.3 Exercises

5.2.3.1 Exercise 1: Understand Lateral Penumbra

a) As a function of discrete energy
b) As a function of depth in medium for a specific energy

5.2.3.2 Exercise 2: Compare Widths of Bragg Peaks between Low, Medium, and High Energies

Compare widths of various Bragg peaks between low, medium, and high energies to appreciate the amount of distal end fall-offs necessary.

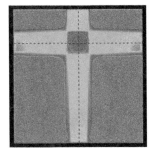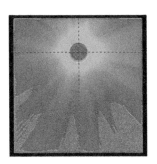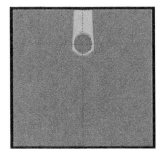

Figure 5.4 Comparing dose distribution from a four-field box X ray, rapid arc X ray, and a single sPBT beam.

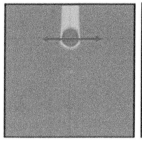
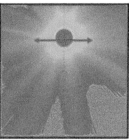
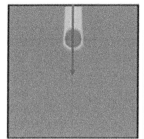
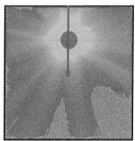

Lateral profile comparison between Protons (left) and X-rays (Right)

Depth-Dose profile comparison between Protons (left) and X-rays

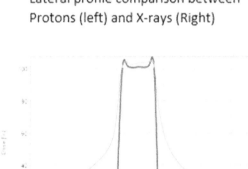
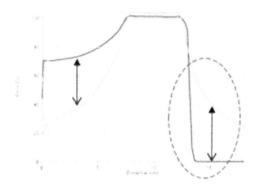

Figure 5.5   Comparing lateral profiles and depth-dose profiles between sPBT and 6-MV rapid arc X-ray beam.

5.2.3.3   Exercise 3: Understanding Skin Dose in sPBT

Understanding the skin sparing effects, or lack of thereof in a single-field plan for various tumor thicknesses and depths.

Since most beam arrangements in clinical situation often go through either oblique incidences and/or heterogeneous mediums (such as air, tissues, and bones), consequently, Bragg peaks at the anterior and posterior margins of the target would have varying penetration depths thereby leading to what is also known as distal end degradation of the SOBPs (Urie et al., 1986). It is thus very important for each clinic to develop basic rules for selecting beam angles as often there will be necessary compromises that will be required for generating safe treatment plans.

5.2.4   Challenges of Proton Beam Radiotherapy

While proton beam therapy is associated with advancement delivering conformal radiotherapy, this technology continues to remain extremely challenging, with higher capital costs (Goitein and Jermann, 2003; Lundkvist et al., 2005; Lievens and Pijls-Johannesma, 2013). Dosimetrically, protons present unique challenges. Charged particle therapy in general remains extremely sensitive to any anatomical changes in

their path lengths as well as the dose distribution can be significantly disturbed due to organ motion (Liu and Chang, 2011), thereby making it extremely difficult for treatment planners to design and deliver a highly conformal radiotherapy plans under such circumstances (Jäkel et al., 2001; Antony J. Lomax, 2009; Karger et al., 2010). Most of the cancer patients requiring radiotherapy undergo tumor resection, which thereby leads to introduction of metal prosthesis and other reconstructive procedures. High atomic number metallic objects are often a deterrent in charged particle therapy and the cases with such metallic implants (Verburg and Seco, 2013) require high precision, labor-intensive contouring for overriding of the element, or in certain situations lead to disqualifying patient completely from receiving proton-based radiotherapy. In spite of many challenges, protons in clinical settings offer hope for improved radiotherapy outcomes in large cohorts of cancer patients.

5.2.5   Margins and Understanding Uncertainties

With reference to spot characterization and dosimetric characteristics of a typical spot scanning-based radiotherapy, we will now switch our focus toward margins necessary to adequately generate a safe deliverable proton treatment plan (Thomas, 2006; Albertini et al., 2011; Schuemann et al., 2014). These margins, in all practical purposes, are a way to define placement of spots as a way of restricting the search space for the optimizer. The problem of spot position optimization is entirely intractable given today's computational resources. Hence, conventionally, generating radiotherapy plans requires creation of planning target volumes (PTVs), which essentially encapsulates the CTVs. These planning structures are generated by isotropic expansion and in some cases anisotropic expansions to address various uncertainties that can originate during delivery of these radiotherapy treatments. The extent/magnitude of uncertainties in beam alignment, patient setup, anatomical organ deformations, motion of the tumor, and/or neighboring organs will govern the margins necessary for expanding these planning volumes (Albertini et al., 2011). In an X-ray treatment, these margins are a simple geometric expansion based on the CTVs and are referred to as PTVs.

Proton therapy is also based on the use of such PTV to provide adequate dose distributions in the presence of geometrical uncertainties; however, in the presence of range uncertainties, proton-based plans yield dose inhomogeneities not only on the edges of the target but also within the target, thereby leaving the overall distribution of dose extremely sensitive to any external or internal perturbations.

There are several confounding factors (Albertini et al., 2011; Paganetti, 2012) that contribute toward the range uncertainties, summarized in Figure 5.6.

There are now several methods that explicitly govern construction of the PTVs to overcome these systematic range uncertainties originating from the source of scanning of these patients. Methods such as beam-specific margins (Park et al., 2012), split target-based optimization volumes (Anand et al., 2019 "Individual Field Simultaneous Optimization (Ifso) in Spot Scanning Proton Therapy of Head and Neck Cancers"), and optimization of plans with robust optimization routines inbuilt in the cost functions (Chen et al., 2012) are some of the most widely used approaches. There is enough literature available to familiarize with these methods, and we describe below some of the routine methods followed in our clinical practice to generate such planning margins (Chen et al., 2012; Bai et al.,

2019; Liu et al., 2012a "Influence of Robust Optimization in Intensity-Modulated Proton Therapy with Different Dose Delivery Techniques"; Liu et al., 2012b "Robust Optimization of Intensity Modulated Proton Therapy").

Depending upon the depths of the target scanning, proton pencil beams will have spot sizes that can range anywhere between 3 mm and 1.2 cm sigma. Generating PTVs will require an adequate understanding of such spot sizes to provide enough margins to envelope the entire spot. Shown in the next section is a typical expansion scheme that we follow within our practice.

5.2.5.1 Clinical Considerations for Generating Margins

ICRU 50 and ICRU 62 form the basis of generating PTVs (Purdy, 2004) that account for patient setup and delivery-related uncertainties. However, in particle therapy, creation of such planning margins is not so straightforward and there are only a few clinical sites where a pre-established protocol for margins exist. Often, the margins are system specific and require adequate background of various immobilization and imaging solutions, and calibration of the CT scanner (Yang et al., 2012; Ainsley and Yeager, 2014); they all play an important role in defining rules for the overall expansion of margins from the CTVs. However, particle therapy, being unique in the sense that such margins also require incorporating values, associated with range uncertainties that exist due to the inherent physics of calibrating CT scanners in particle therapy. We are not going to discuss how in radiotherapy these margins get generated. Readers can find ample literature resources that can discuss the construction of such margins. Instead, we share below a clinical scenario in which a treatment planner within our institution accomplishes the creation of specific margins under extremely tight-spot placement conditions.

In situations where the tumor gets expressed all the way to the surface, there remains a struggle on how to find adequate tissue margins that could allow enough volume for spot placements such that adequate fluence gets built up for delivering therapeutic doses. For such situations, we share below a typical workflow that we follow within our own proton practice.

Step A: Establish an understanding of the available tissue margins for expanding any PTVs. In Figure 5.7a, we notice

Range Calculation Errors by Treatment Planning Systems				Planning and Delivery Errors
CT based errors				• Contouring
HU/Relative Stopping Power calculation	Beam Energy and HU dependence	Binning and reconstruction errors	Heterogeneities and metal artifacts	• Anatomical Changes • Heterogeneities and path length changes • Setup errors • Tumor motion related errors (Interplay and Inter-Field)

Figure 5.6 All major contributors to the range uncertainty in sPBT.

there is an extremely small sliver of tissue available between the red CTV and the external BODY contour marked in orange. For such a scenario, care must be taken to not place any spots that would extend outside the patient's body surface.

Step B: We accomplish this by modifying the available tissue space for optimization target volume (OTV). Seen in Figure 5.7b is a shaded region between the CTV and the patient's external BODY that will require generation of planning margins to place proton spots. Now since the PTV is a geometrical construct to account for setup uncertainties, care must be taken that in proton therapies there is also need for an additional margin to account for range uncertainties. Hence, a plain geometrical construct like that of a PTV may not suffice.

Step C: In situations where there is limited availability of tissue to contain these spots, one of the approaches that works with an **en face beam** is to create a subvolume shrunk by a small amount (2–3 mm), again this value depends upon each institution's Bragg peak widths, and such croppings should be made only in the direction of the beam travel. In all other directions, such a margin is an expansion and gets utilized as the OTV shown in Figure 5.7c. This inward reduction should

happen only in the direction of beam propagation and rest of the volume should be a geometric expansion as one would expect to make with PTVs. As we can see in Figure 5.7c, the red-dotted line depicts such a construct of an OTV volume. This structure then gets heavily utilized during the routine optimization. For our clinic, we choose anywhere between 2 and 3 mm of reduction of this OTV from the body in the direction of the beam travel (arrow lines depicting lateral and anterior and posterior obliques as plausible beam directions). In other possible directions, this OTV continues to remain a geometric expansion in both lateral as well as distal direction.

Step D: Once an OTV gets generated, it is then necessary to define the limits for placement of all the spots in order to meet the lateral penumbral dose falls for these spots. Knowing that the proton spot dosimetry is Gaussian (Sawakuchi et al., 2010), therefore, a margin with at least one full sigma should be added in addition to the existing OTV margins. At our practice, we call such margins the scanning target volumes (STV). STV can be considered as the virtual collimation and is essentially an expansion from the OTV all the way to the external BODY in such cases as seen in Figure 5.7d.

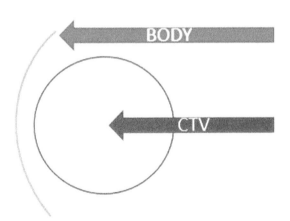

Figure 5.7a   Constructing planning margins by assessing spacing between BODY and the CTV.

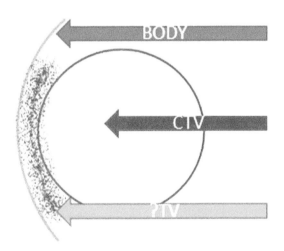

Figure 5.7b   Identifying shaded region to place proton spots.

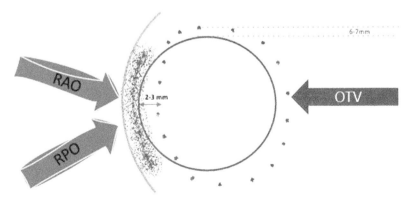

Figure 5.7c   Constructing an optimization target volume.

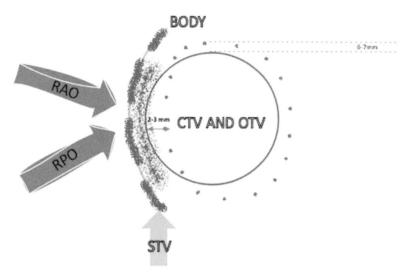

Figure 5.7d Constructing a scanning target volume.

5.2.5.1.1 *To Summarize*

A spot scanning beam line system will require beam-specific and machine-specific information to generate optimal planning and optimization volumes. With scanning volumes being the outmost layer of spot positioning boundaries, margins for the STVs rely mostly on the beam directions and account for the range uncertainties. Such volumes can then also be cropped from any neighboring/abutting OARs in order to limit the placement of Bragg peaks within the OAR themselves as can be seen in Figure 5.8.

A word of caution: Since in actual clinical practice, these Bragg peaks are arranged in a three-dimensional space around the target volumes, when initiating a new site, it is recommended that each patient's plan preparation be reviewed slice by slice to ascertain adequate positioning of these Bragg peaks and ensure no beams:

(a) Traverse critical organs,
(b) heterogeneity, or

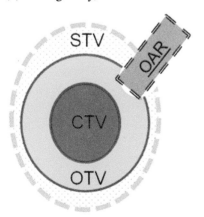

Figure 5.8 Selective cropping of the STV margins from any abutting organs at risk.

(c) get accidentally placed outside the deliverable capabilities (i.e., field size) of an individual machine.

5.2.6 Optimization

Once these margins are generated and Bragg peaks get placed for each individual beamlet, the next part of treatment planning involves beam weight optimization. There are some routinely used techniques in spot scanning which have been listed below. Essentially, all treatment planning systems condition model pencil beams incident on patient to fall parallel to each other along the direction of their travel, upon which the optimization algorithm can then either deliver doses like single-field uniform dose (also known as single-field optimized dose) or a multifield optimized dose (MFO). While there are a number of kinds of optimization algorithms that are currently available, such as worst case (Liu et al., 2012b "Robust Optimization of Intensity Modulated Proton Therapy"; Pflugfelder et al., 2008) and least squares (Pflugfelder et al., 2008), simulated annealing (Joanne H. Kang et al., 2007), minimization (Van Der Voort et al., 2016), etc.; the focus of this chapter remains to highlight the strengths and weaknesses between a single-field optimization (SFO) versus MFO in relation to some disease sites that get treated with sPBT. In general, techniques of optimization (worst case, min–max, etc.) used for a conventional photon plan can also be integrated within proton-based beam weight optimization. It is just that the photon optimization involves two-dimensional modulation of fluence that is generally perpendicular to the plane of beam direction, whereas in protons, there is another additional degree of freedom in which the dose localization can be achieved by modulating beamlets both in perpendicular to travel direction as well as in the direction of depth doses.

To best understand the differences between the single and the MFO, we will utilize example from four different disease sites. We elaborate in next few sections the strengths, weaknesses, and opportunities that are presented with spot sPBT while treating tumors of the

- Head and neck
- Breast
- Gynecological
- Ano-rectal malignances

5.3 Treatment Planning for Four Distinct Disease Sites

Based on our experience of treating head and neck, breast, and tumors of the pelvis with sPBT, we elected to use these disease sites to highlight the must-know details for proton therapy of these tumor sites. While each site utilizes the MFO, the head and neck example will be discussed in more details to also highlight some of the limitations of SFO and why those methods do not allow planning complicated tumors of the oral cavity. We hope that this section will bring out the practical aspects of treating major critical sites with sPBT.

5.3.1 sPBT Treatment Planning of Head and Neck Tumors

5.3.1.1 Introduction

Malignancies of the head and neck demand critical planning techniques as there are several serial and parallel structures that abut and/or overlap with the target volumes that can be of high, intermediate, and low-risk grade types. Sparing midline structures (Anand et al., 2019 "Individual Field Simultaneous Optimization (Ifso) in Spot Scanning Proton Therapy of Head and Neck Cancers") while treating tumors either in the base of skull, oral cavity, or nasal cavity requires that the arrangement of beams be selectively chosen to avoid: heterogeneities, beams passing through organs at risks and at the same time be able to modulate doses to multiple-dose levels. As shown in Figure 5.9, we can clearly appreciate the dose bath that gets deposited in the midline structures (right) when compared with split target-based sPBT (left). With tumors expressed all the way to the surface, there is also need for arranging beams to deposit Bragg peaks all the way up to the surface for adequate tumor coverages. Also, with the help of this site-specific example, we will discuss the best optimization methods along with requirements for other ancillary devices and other necessary details to kept in mind for the planners to design a safe and a robust proton-based treatment plan.

5.3.1.2 Immobilization

Head and neck treatments require both high levels of precision and accuracy. It is thus appropriate to first give credit to our industries who have evolved very quickly to keep up with the growing needs of particle therapy clinics. One of such industries being the immobilization industry. It is very important to bring solutions that are rigid and that allow large reproducibility. A high-quality solution will aid in reducing the burden of replans for proton practice. Head and neck tumors

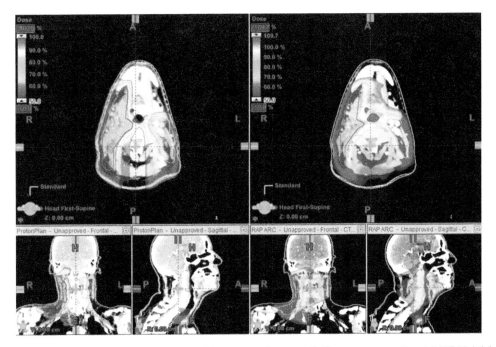

Figure 5.9 Midline dose bath compared between split-target (left) versus conventional IMPT (right)-based sPBT.

otherwise can be notoriously time consuming for dosimetry as it can continuously keep them busy with adaptive replanning. At our practice, we use these Qfix®-based solutions, not only that they are rigid and less deformable. Such patient support device as seen in Figure 5.10 with rigid mask and a head rest with no protruding support material as can be seen in this image brings higher degrees of freedom when choosing beam arrangements to treat these tumors.

5.3.1.3 Challenges with Shallow Tumors

Proton treatment planning requires understanding the size, shape, and location of tumors as these factors govern what type of beam arrangements and placement of Bragg peaks is necessary. Almost every case in head and neck tumors requires that the Bragg peaks are placed all the way to the surface of the patients. Modern delivery systems have their limitations as to how shallow can these Bragg peaks be deposited. For example, in synchrotron-based accelerator systems with discrete energies available, the lowest possible energy available remains 4.0 g/cm^2 in water. Anytime a shallower Bragg peak is needed, as we see in a typical H&N CT scan shown in Figure 5.11, there is then need for external devices to pull back the Bragg peaks and bring them all the way to the surface to adequately cover the proximal margins of CTV. There are various methods by which these energies can be pulled back (Both et al., 2014).

At our practice, we employ two distinct methods to pull back the Bragg peak. These Bragg peaks can be pulled back by either utilizing a device that can be placed directly within the nozzle of the delivery system seen in Figure 5.12 (left), known

as the extended range shifter (ERS), or by utilizing a device that can be placed near the patient's setup, known as bolus helmet as seen in Figure 5.12 (right). Each method offers its own unique advantages. More importantly, due to the airgaps between the ERS and the patient's surface, the physics of ERSs leads to creation of larger spot sizes impinging on the patient's surface, thereby leading to larger penumbral dose. For cases such as nasopharyngeal carcinomas infiltrating the optical apparatus, there is always need for strict penumbral fall-offs. In such situations, those cases are planned with range-shifting materials that are placed next to the patient's habitus.

Use of proper hardware and immobilization solution can setup a good starting point for planning of these head and neck cases. A more critical and important step in the process remains understanding the optimization algorithms that should be employed for the case. While there are several kinds of algorithms that are now widely discussed in literature, we will highlight the two most widely used and referred to methods in planning with sPBT.

5.3.1.4 Flavors of Optimization

5.3.1.4.1 Single-field optimization and Multifield Optimization

Treatment planning for sPBT involves inverse methods of optimizing spot fluence based on individualized patient's anatomical information. By controlling position, energy, and optimizing the weight distribution of proton Bragg peaks within tumor boundaries, one can achieve adequate target coverage while maximizing on the sparing of the healthy tissues (AJ Lomax et al., 2001, 2004; AJ Lomax, 2008, 2009; Schwarz, 2011; McGowan et al., 2013).

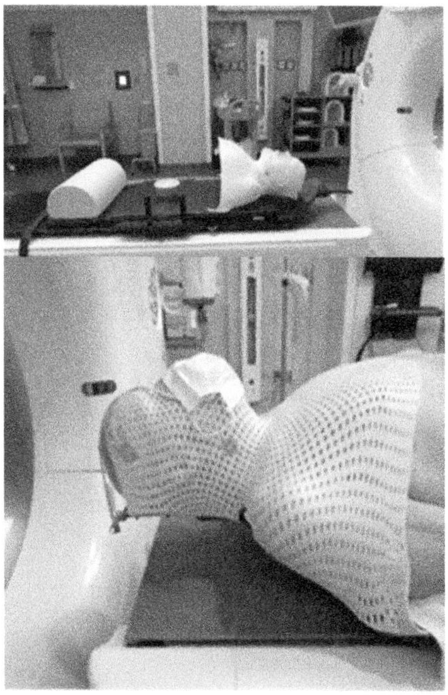

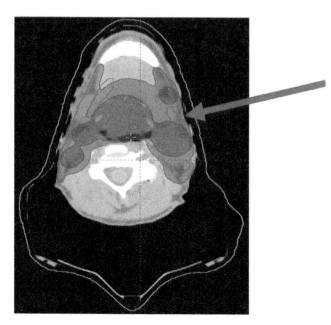

Figure 5.10 Rigid patient support device used to treat head and neck tumors with sPBT.

Figure 5.11 H&N CT scan of a patient showing target margins expressed all the way up to skinline.

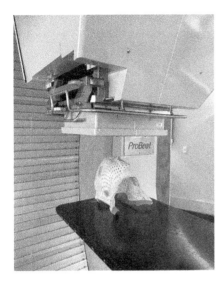

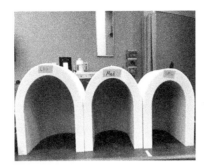

Courtesy Image: Dr. Dan Mundy

Figure 5.12 (Left) Extended range shifter in the nozzle of the gantry. (Right) Bolus helmet brought closer to the patient's surface to reduce the air gap (Image Credits: Dr. Daniel Mundy).

Treating tumors of the head and neck involves several radiosensitive visceral risk organs requiring strict preparations of planning structures and establishing complex mathematical optimization routines to deliver efficacious therapy with reduced side effects (Quan et al., 2013; Frank et al., 2014). While the methods of treatment planning in proton therapy continue to be evolutionary in nature, to date there are two distinct optimization routines that are being used globally in scanning beam proton treatment clinics: SFO and MFO (Quan et al., 2013).

SFO methods optimize by distributing weights from each field individually, as seen in Figure 5.13, and thereby reduce the degree of modulation of spot-weight laterally across the targets. Such a method reduces the gradients generated between multiple fields and results in a nearly uniform dose across the target. SFO-based plans are generally robust, thus remaining less sensitive to setup and range errors. However, since the SFO method does not allow modulation of the spot-weight across the widths of the targets, this method happens to remain less effective in sparing any organs at risks that wraps/abuts around the targets.

Instead, another method, widely known as MFO (Lomax et al., 2001), has gained significant traction in radiotherapy clinics utilizing sPBT. In an MFO-based plan, one can fully modulate proton spots weight distribution across the lateral margins of the target. MFO fields remain quite heterogeneous, as each beam delivers in-homogenous doses to avoid shooting through any radiosensitive organs in proximity to the target as seen in Figure 5.14; however, spots from all beams reaching target from different directions are optimized together to achieve adequate target coverages. Due to the high modulation nature of optimization, MFO-based methods remain sensitive to minor perturbations in both patient setup and range-based errors.

5.3.1.5 Individual Field Simultaneous Optimization

At our practice, we have introduced an approach borrowed from passive scattered 3D planning with split target-based optimization to mitigate these effects of MFO-based treatment plans as depicted in Figure 5.15. Our technique, known as individual field simultaneous optimization (IFSO) (Anand et al., 2019 "Individual Field Simultaneous Optimization (Ifso) in Spot Scanning Proton Therapy of Head and Neck Cancers"), can be quite instrumental in producing robust treatment plans as they avoid beams traversing through heterogeneous medium and thereby reduces the degree of modulation necessary to eliminate doses in unwanted regions, plus due to beam specific optimization, these plans receive doses as they would have in an SFO-based optimized planning. It is beyond the scope of this chapter to discuss the details of IFSO but further resources can be found in the references. Essentially, by splitting the target such that each subtarget receives its own independent beams allows us to achieve superior dosimetry as the

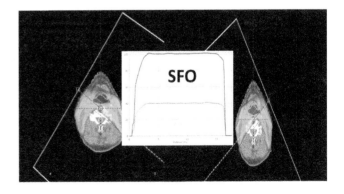

Figure 5.13 Uniform dose distribution from two fields in a single-field-optimized plan.

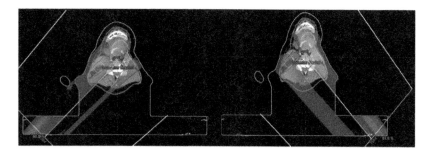

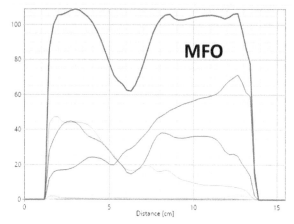

Figure 5.14   Sharp dose gradients and heterogenous dose distribution from each field in a multifield optimization plan.

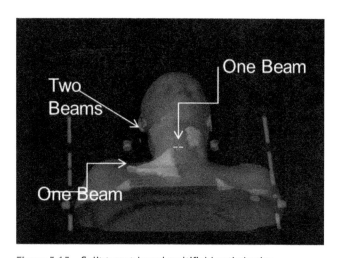

Figure 5.15   Split target-based multifield optimization.

fluence from each beam is nearly uniform in distribution and thus delivering dose that reflects more of SFO plans.

Since the technique of match line-based optimization relies on the integrity of match lines, it is very important to make sure the nominal plan will offer smooth-dose profile gradients along the junction line in order to mitigate any intrafraction errors due to interfield misalignments (Anand et al.).

5.3.1.6   Hardware Issues in Head and Neck Tumors

Patients with head and neck tumors inevitably present with the challenge of metallic hardware implants (Beddok et al.,

2020). These can be either dental or from surgical procedures requiring stomal intubations or regrafting of the tumor cavity with a metal implant as depicted in Figure 5.16. In such situations, a few things need to be kept in mind:

(a) Utilize metal artifact reduction tools (Meyer et al., 2010; Wang et al., 1996; Huang et al., 2015) at the time of simulations to reduce the scatter artifacts. This can improve with contouring and delineations.

(b) Try avoiding beams to traverse through this hardware with high atomic numbers.

(c) Obtain accurate atomic composition of how this hardware was constructed. Such information can then be used to derive appropriate relative stopping power ratios (Fippel

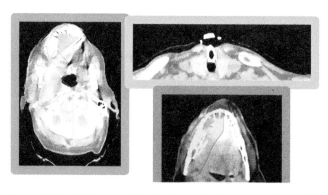

Figure 5.16   Various metallic hardware implants in patients with head and neck cancers.

and Soukup, 2004) and hence more accurate Hounsfield units can then be assigned to the material, should traveling of the beam through this hardware remain unavoidable.

(d) Lastly, but also equally important, should traveling through the beam be unavoidable, care should be taken to select a beam angle that would travel through the shortest possible path length of this metal in order to reduce the effects of range uncertainties. One of the compounded steps of this process also requires that the range uncertainty margins being folded in the planning structure volumes should account for approximately 5% of absolute path length errors that could exist in such beams.

Evaluation of plans: Head and neck planning with proton treatments is labor intensive yet a rewarding task. Once the plan gets completed, a careful slice-by-slice evaluation of dose distribution followed by evaluation of the robustness of these plans should be done for each single case. A slice-by-slice evaluation as seen in Figure 5.17 has a potential to highlight any dose break-ups within the target leading to a cold spot or can yield information regarding any potential hot spots that could be present either within the target or outside the target and thereby risking radiotoxicities within these patients. At our practice, a routine evaluation entails checking for dose distributions around the target as well as the DVH analysis under modeled uncertainties as seen in Figure 5.18. We maintain a metric of modeling setup errors in the order of 3 mm along with range uncertainties compounded to 3%. For these uncertainties, we then estimate that under all possible scenarios the worst-case coverage D95 to remain 95% for all prescribed target doses, and at the same time all OARs remain under their tolerances.

Each case is then also evaluated for their biological effectiveness, but computing a dose averaged linear energy transfer (LET) distribution. Modeling a 6-keV/μm dose wash from LET remains a conservative approach to make sure no critical

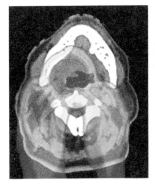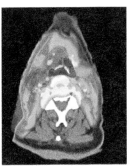

Figure 5.17 Dose colorwash showing an individual slice with dose distribution for plan evaluation.

structures receive such LET doses in areas with high proton fluence. In situations where our LET tests fail, these plans then go back for re-optimization with modified beam arrangements that would allow LET wash-offs (Unkelbach et al., 2016).

Last but not the least, when planning proton treatments for tumors of the nasopharynx, care must be taken to ensure no direct beams anterior to the target point directly at any critical structure. Studies show that there are expected significant changes in the tissue–air ratios during treatments, thereby leading to significant range uncertainties which could then lead into serial structures as can be understood from Figure 5.19 (Fukumitsu et al., 2014; Shusharina et al., 2019).

At our institution, we have had greater than 5 years of experience treating both definitive and postop cases of head and neck tumor with proton beam therapy. At the time of this writing, there are many reports and clinical trials that are being prepared discussing patient-related outcomes from our clinical practice of treating these tumor types with sPBT. Readers are encouraged to watch out for newer publications as they continue to percolate soon.

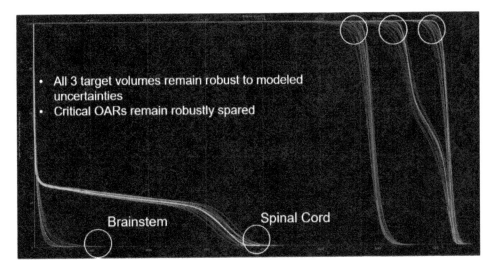

- All 3 target volumes remain robust to modeled uncertainties
- Critical OARs remain robustly spared

Brainstem   Spinal Cord

Figure 5.18 Robustness evaluation of a sPBT plan comparing target coverage versus OAR sparings.

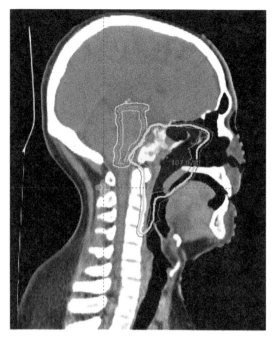

Figure 5.19 Heterogenous anatomy posing significant challenges for treating nasopharynx tumors with sPBT.

5.3.2 sPBT Treatment Planning of Breast Tumors

Introduction: While the treatment with photons for breast malignancies is widely practiced, there are now very large studies demonstrating the radiation-induced late toxicities related to photon irradiation. Out of the many late toxicities, the risk of radiation-induced secondary malignancies in the lungs, sarcomas, and esophagus and/or cardiac toxicities leading to fatalistic outcomes remain major concerns with patients and in radiotherapy clinics (Schneider, 2011). A very large risk-assessment study with a meta-analysis from a systematic review of 762,468 patients indicates significant risks of second nonbreast cancer after radiotherapy for breast cancer (Grantzau and Overgaard, 2015). Such long-term outcome indicators have naturally influenced many clinics to consider radiotherapy techniques that can reduce the exposure of healthy tissue to these carcinogenic ionizing radiations. Proton therapy, due to its characteristics of reducing volumes of low-dose baths, becomes highly attractive in terms of developing solutions for treating comprehensive breast cancers. As can be seen in Figure 5.20, protons yield promising dosimetry in sparing of both lungs, the heart, and especially the left anterior descending arteries (LAD), compared to conventional X-ray therapy with tangents for both right-sided and left-sided tumors.

Immobilization, contouring, and planning preparation: Immobilization of the intact breasts remains a subject of

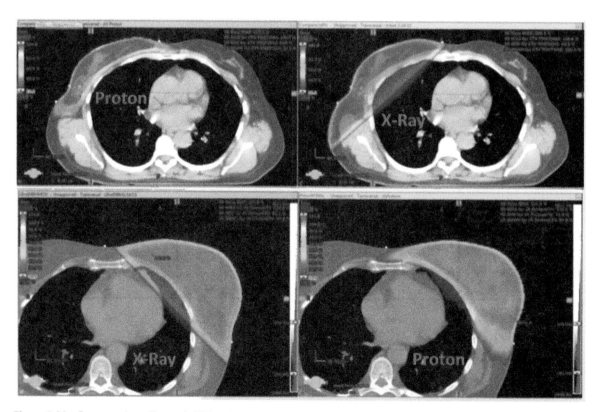

Figure 5.20 Dose-sparing effects of sPBT to the lungs and heart muscle compared against X-ray therapy.

academic interest and there are a variety of solutions available, including thoracic and breast masks. At our practice, we have been using Orfit-based thoracic/breast masks to immobilize patients, and there are developmental efforts underway to incorporate surface-guided imaging system to facilitate easier and efficient setups.

Designing a robust treatment plan for the breast starts with good contouring practice and clear understanding of beam arrangements that would be necessary to cover all levels of the nodal chains and the breast gland. Unlike X-ray-based radiotherapy where a pair of opposite tangent beams with collimation is used for treatments, proton radiotherapy is best designed with nearly en face beams. Arrangements like tangent beams for proton therapy can yield unwanted effects due to breathing-related excursion of the breast gland which can leave the target undercovered due to interplay between the motion and the beam delivery. Instead, en face beams, or nearly en face beams, help mitigate such issues from the breathing motion (Mutter et al., 2021). It is worthwhile mentioning that, unlike photon radiotherapy, the source to surface distance in proton therapy is not relevant; hence, it renders advantages in choosing beams in the direction of breathing motion. When planning with multiple beams, it will be necessary to maintain good hinge angles between beams contributing toward same target areas. These hinge angles can vary depending upon the spot dosimetry. In general practice, an angle of 30° between two complimentary beams will avoid creating hot spots on the surface of the skin.

Also, the target size and contouring of skin folds play an important role in determining the number of beam arrangements to adequately cover the entire length of the target with nearly uniform dose. Often there exists sharp subcutaneous skin folds at the site of the breast gland. Such regions end up receiving grazing and oblique incidences of Bragg peaks and thereby generating large hot spots. This can be avoided by taking care of patient positioning at the time of the simulation to expose as much surface area as possible to the en face beams. It is thus considered good practice to have a representative from the planning team to be in constant communication with the team responsible for creating patient simulations.

While skin sparing is not a strength of proton radiotherapy, there will be clinical requests to provide skin sparings for individual cases in the practice. While it is beyond the scope to list all possible techniques for generating plans for skin sparing, here are a few "rules of thumb" listed below that may help with managing clinical objectives:

(a) Avoid an angle that will go through deep and longer targets. Such an approach will end up generating larger SOBPs and thus leading to larger skin doses.
(b) Use multiple beams where possible to spread out the dose around the skin.

(c) When explicitly required to optimize to skin structure, it should be made sure that the skin contours are drawn accurately by adjusting the CT window thresholds to delineate skin outlines.
(d) It is also encouraged to work with the physician in communicating the potential surface doses so that clinical care with topical creams could be provided to patients early in their treatment schedules.
(e) There are certain occasions where there will be need for sparing the ribs of the chest wall. Since most of our beam arrangements will end up pointing/ranging into chest wall, there will be a needed discussion with the physician to determine the degree of compromise between target coverage and CW sparing for a given case. In such situations, carve out the STVs from the chest wall to avoid placing any Bragg peaks into the bony anatomy of the chest.

Proton-based radiotherapy plans for breast are usually optimized utilizing SFO, where beam weighting gets adjusted depending upon the preferential usefulness of beams involved in planning. Beams more oblique in incidence or going through larger lung volumes can be adjusted to have lower weights for minimizing their contribution to the target dose and hence also reduce dose to the OARs. An example of a SFO plan is shown below, where the dose distributions reveal a uniform dose across the target, as seen by drawing a line profile through the target. With little to no modulation, such plans are safe and robust to deliver and should be favored over IMPT as much as possible.

There are anecdotal opinions of considering deep inspiration breath hold-based treatments for left-sided breast cancers to reduce any extraneous dose to the heart. We have not yet evaluated any potential advantages of such motion management techniques in our proton breast clinic.

Flavors of optimization: Depending upon the extent of the disease, most breast plans can be planned utilizing SFO technique with either two or three beams. Most cases receive equally weighted beams to deliver the dose across the target. However, in cases with large comprehensive nodal chains, there may be the need for utilizing either the split target technique, such as previously discussed IFSO-based methods, or use of SFO with unequal weight distributions between the beams.

Challenges: Treatment planning for breast cancers can be complicated, especially for patients with either larger or reconstructed breasts with expanders/implants. Readers are alerted to literature that discuss the challenges of treating patients with implanted devices (Howarth et al., 2017; Yixiu Kang et al., 2018). Often these devices consist of metallic ports that are used to fill these expanders with the necessary medium. In the process of inflating these devices, there are air bubbles that get introduced in inflating these devices. Careful evaluation of the

CT dataset before initiating a treatment plan is useful strategy to treat these devices. Also, since the expanders will have high Z elements in them, the physics team is encouraged to do a careful relative stopping power assessments of these materials, as well as generate a model in Monte Carlo to compute the effects of elastic and inelastic scatterings of protons in and around these devices.

Evaluation of plans: Evaluation of sPBT plans for breast cancer is no different than the methods discussed earlier for head and neck plans. The dose distributions are evaluated on a slice-by-slice basis, and care is maintained to assess the dose spilling into structures like chest wall, lungs, and heart. When treating comprehensive nodal chain, it is also prudent to take care of dose to the contralateral side. Even though the understanding of radiobiological effectiveness of protons for various disease sites is still a topic of scientific debate, at the time of this work, evaluation of LET doses for breast cases remains identical as that discussed earlier for head and neck sites.

5.3.3 sPBT Treatment Planning of Gynecological Tumors

Introduction: Gynecological tumors, such as endometrial cancer, have thus far been treated with brachytherapy and external beam radiotherapy. With either modality, there are several organs at risk, such as bone marrow, bladder, rectum, femoral heads, small bowel, and large bowel, that end up receiving large dose baths which can be avoided with use of proton-based radiotherapy. However, since charged particle therapy remains very sensitive to minor anatomical changes, this site continues to challenge efficacy in delivering therapeutic doses with radiation. Consequently, there are still several clinics who feel less comfortable incorporating proton radiotherapy within their gynecologic radiation oncology (GYN) practice. At our facility, we have been treating these patients with sPBT and we share below some of our own experiences and issues that are faced commonly. Discussed below are the rationale and challenges when treating pelvis malignancies with protons.

In the early days, it was discovered that, due to significant large volumes of bone marrow producing structures in the pelvis (Levine et al., 1994), these patients exhibited various forms of toxicities, such as hematological (Klopp et al., 2013), insufficiency fractures (Ikushima et al., 2006), incontinence (Dunberger et al., 2010), and vaginal stenosis (Brand et al., 2006; Morris et al., 2017). For us, the objective of designing treatment plans with protons involves sparing of the bone marrow, femoral heads, and rectum.

It is known that the low-dose bath (V10, V20) to the bone marrow leads to neutropenia and leukopenias in patients undergoing systemic treatments (Mell et al., 2006 "Dosimetric Predictors of Acute Hematologic Toxicity in Cervical Cancer Patients Treated with Concurrent Cisplatin and Intensity-Modulated Pelvic Radiotherapy"). By utilizing split target-based MFO, there lies tremendous opportunities to mitigate such issues.

Flavors of optimization: Various proton clinics choose to treat these malignancies using either convention methods of intensity-modulated proton beam therapy or can elect to treat the site with split target-based methods, such as the one discussed using IFSO methods. At our center, we use the split-target technique of IFSO to treat the tumor around the vaginal site, and splitting the beams to treat the prophylactic targets such as the iliac nodes with their own individual beams as further discussed in the sections that follow.

Challenges: Since treatment of GYN tumors involves prophylactic treatment of lymphatic chains, there is significant involvement of anatomy that remains fluidic. Figure 5.21 on the right is used to highlight four key areas of challenges posed during the sPBT of GYN tumors.

Location 1: Bladder. Being fluidic in nature, bladder volumes are extremely hard to reproduce. Consequentially due to variability in filling of bladder volumes, extreme excursions in the vaginal target are noticed. It is thus best to avoid using beams as far as possible traveling through bladder.

Location 2: Vaginal target. Especially with the apex of vagina that can both collapse and displace, treating this volume has always been a challenge that gets discussed in scientific community at large.

Location 3: Rectum: Both distensibility of the rectal walls and content fillings of the rectum can again lead to displace the vaginal target seen in Figure 5.22 as well as lead to any range errors in case of use of any beams traveling through rectum.

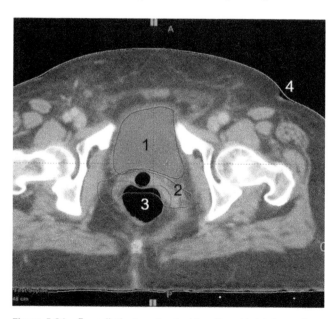

Figure 5.21 Four distinct anatomical locations that bring unique challenges of treating vaginal targets with sPBT.

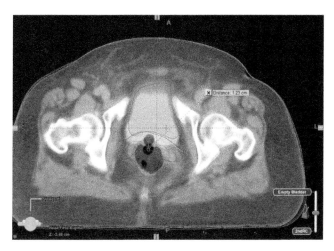

Figure 5.22 Showing vaginal excursion due to nonreproducible bladder filling.

Location 4: Certain large patients can also present with challenging pannus that can fall into the beam and altering the range of those beams significantly.

So, some of the recommended strategies to help mitigate these issues are discussed below.

To avoid exposing large volumes of bone marrow to low doses, and avoiding traversing through heterogeneous anatomies such as large and small bowel, bladder, and rectum, it becomes necessary to consider splitting of the target and treat each subtarget site with its respective beams.

In Figure 5.23, one can evaluate different ways of splitting the target such that the common iliac nodes and if involved para-aortic nodes get their own beam arrangements preferably a posterior beam whereas the vaginal target gets treated by a pair of near-opposed laterals. Also, to mitigate any possible vaginal excursions, we utilize the aid of endorectal balloons to arrest any distensibility of rectum and sim these patients with empty bladder to bring more reproducibility.

The dosimetry achieved is comprehensive and significantly sparing in nature. A color wash of a typical dose distribution seen in Figure 5.24 shows significant sparing of bony structures, thereby reducing risks of any hematologic side effects or injuries due to insufficiency bone fractures.

Evaluation of plans: Robustness evaluations of each of our GYN plans are modeled to 5 mm of setup and 3% of range errors, with 95% of the target covered by at least 95% of prescription doses. In addition, there is a verification simulation scan suggested during the 3rd week of radiotherapy course to ensure safer treatments in progress. Each individual clinic will be developing their own custom verification schedule based on physician preference. However, we feel that a verification scan toward the middle of second week of treatment allows ample opportunity to adapt to improve any insufficiencies that may start appearing on certain challenging cases.

5.3.4 sPBT Treatment Planning of Anorectal Cancers

Introduction: Just as we discussed in the treatment of GYN malignancies, cancers of the rectum and anus are also potential sites that can be treated with protons. Due to the significant sparing of the bone marrow that is achievable with protons, there are now studies that discuss the advantages of utilizing proton beams to treat anorectal tumors. RTOG 0529 (Kachnic et al., 2013) is a useful resource understanding the dose prescriptions and the delineation of these targets. Diseases of the anus/rectum often involve treating areas involving anal verge, rectum, and inguinal nodes.

Flavors of optimization: Due to the proximity of the target to several OARs such as bladder, femoral heads, bone marrow structures, bowel bag, and genitalia (Figure 5.25), the treatment planning involves MFO for dose-carving and shaving off extraneous doses from all these OARs. Again, since the target involves heterogeneous paths for these beamlines to traverse, it is important to choose angles that would avoid traversing heterogeneous and fluidic anatomies such as the bladder and bowel bag. For example, in this cross-sectional view, we identify that in treating the tumor of the anus with prophylactic treatments of inguinal nodes there is a large volume of involvement of the bladder. Hence, the ideal

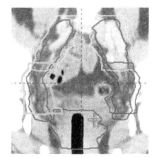
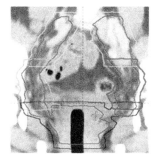
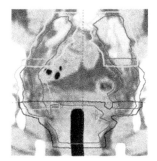
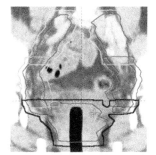

Figure 5.23 A representative slide showing various ways of splitting a postop endometrial target with lymphatic nodes.

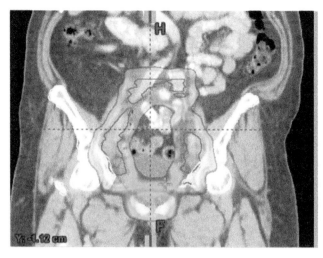

Figure 5.24 A dose color wash showing significant sparing of bony anatomy while treating GYN target with sPBT and.

beam arrangement for such a situation requires that the targets be split between the anterior and the posterior portions for being able to treat them with beams coming in direction of closest approach and avoid crossing bladder and other OARs. At our practice, we utilize an IFSO-based split target optimization approach and the advantages of utilizing such a technique compared over the conventional rapid arc methods can be seen in the image of the dose color wash on the right. With utilizing one to two posterior beams to treat the anal/rectal target and anterior/anterior oblique beams for inguinal nodes happen to be the most probable choices to treat these targets. Sections where the gross disease margins start coming closer to the anterior portions of the inguinal nodes, a gradient-based overlap between the anterior and posterior margins ensures mitigating over and underranging effects in the junction planes. There is a very large and significant reduction in the intergral dose bath to the healthy tissues when treating with protons compared to photons. There are studies/guidelines that recommend reduction in

the low-dose volumes of bone marrow in patients undergoing concurrent chemoradiotherapy for cancers of the anus and rectum, as that reduces risks of hematologic toxicity (Albuquerque et al., 2011; Anand et al., 2015 "Scanning Proton Beam Therapy Reduces Normal Tissue Exposure in Pelvic Radiotherapy for Anal Cancer"; Mell et al., 2006 "Dosimetric Predictors of Acute Hematologic Toxicity in Cervical Cancer Patients Treated with Concurrent Cisplatin and Intensity-Modulated Pelvic Radiotherapy"; Mell et al., 2008 "Dosimetric Comparison of Bone Marrow-Sparing Intensity-Modulated Radiotherapy Versus Conventional Techniques for Treatment of Cervical Cancer").

Challenges: While there are large advantages of using charged particle therapy to treat such targets, like gynecological malignancies, there are many areas of concerns that should be kept in mind while treating this site with protons.

(a) The issue or rectal filling and distensibility, as seen in Figure 5.26.
(b) Bleeding of dose into genitalia and bladder. A typical slice seen in Figure 5.27 showing potential of distal end dose bleeding into the genitalia due to variation in rectal content.
(c) Patient setup and immobilization and reproducibility of the gluteal muscles.

In all other pelvic sites with intact rectum, there is value of utilizing an endorectal balloons as those devices continue to arrest any anatomical excursions in the pelvis, but in the case of anal tumors, use of endorectal balloons is not permissible. Due to large variations in both the rectal filling as well as the distension of the walls of the rectal tube, there is a possibility of over and underranging of the target and thereby can increase both the dose and the LET within OARs such as the bladder and/or genitalia as discussed.

Compared to male anatomy, there is less margin of sparing that exists between the anus and the genitalia thereby increas-

Usual Prescription based on RTOG 0529

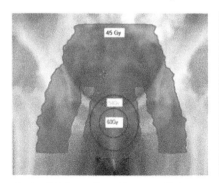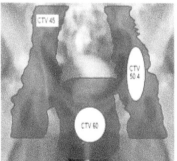

OARs: **Bi-Hips** **Bone Marrow** **Bladder** **Small Bowel** **Large Bowel** **Genitalia**

Figure 5.25 Various OARs while treating anorectal tumors with sPBT.

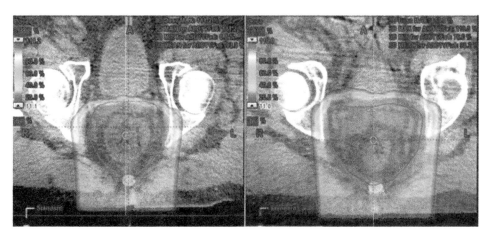

Figure 5.26 Rectal filling and distensibility affecting the overall dose distribution between two setup conditions (left and right).

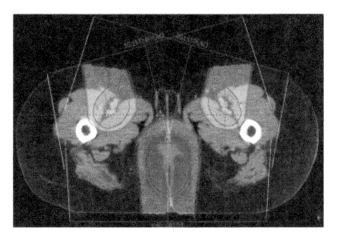

Figure 5.27 A representative slice indicating potential of sPBT ranging into the genitalia due to variation in the rectal content.

ing the risks of beam overranging into the OAR. It is thus being suggested that a frequent verification scans, that is, at least twice during treatments, be considered for select cases that are presented with large content and flatulence at the time of their treatment scans.

Immobilization: Immobilization of this site is also very important due to the nature of beam arrangements. The majority of the clinics treating anorectal cancers with protons utilize some arrangements of posterior beams. These can be either a straight posterior beam or a pair of posterior oblique to treat anal verge and the underlying gross disease. For supine setups, there remains a possibility of gluteal muscles not reproducing and having interfractional setup issues, and thus lead to large dose-perturbations. Especially the folding of gluteal fat into the gluteal cleft can significantly pull back the range of the protons thereby leading to underdosing of the target. At our practice, we have implemented an approach of prone setups (Figure 5.28, left) along with a pelvis mask that gets wedged in the separation of the gluteal muscles thereby avoiding such an issue from happening.

Often an aid of a belly board when positioning patients prone as seen in Figure 5.28 can come in handy as it allows to both for the belly as well as bowel bag to fall out of the beam's path. There are other contingencies situations requiring switching from protons to X-ray therapy. In such cases, these patients will require to be resimulated with a super-flab-based bolus to treat the superficial skin level target in the anal region. Seen in the image on the right, a small super-flab positioned in the gluteal cleft under the mask allows to treat these cases in a prone setup. Again, just like in the case of gynecological tumors, tumors of the anus/rectum are surrounded by fluidic anatomy hence guidelines for obtaining verification scans during treatments can ensure safe treatments of this site with protons.

Plan evaluation: We suggest the guidelines to evaluate plans computed for ano-rectal and gynecological disease site follow the same recipe as discussed for other disease sites. Slice-by-slice evaluation of target coverage, followed by robustness checks utilizing 5% of the range and 3 mm of setup errors to ensure safe and superior quality of plans for treating this site. There are no other unique indications for assessing LET distributions either, hence this site remains subject of same dosimetric assessments as other sites. Organ-specific details for plan evaluation have purposefully been omitted from our discussions. Readers are encouraged to follow their individual clinical guidelines to make sure the quality of prescription is upheld for their practice.

5.4 Future of Treatment Planning in Proton Therapy

sPBT was introduced in the United States around 2008 (Gillin et al., 2010), with limited choice of algorithms and treatment planning systems available at the time. Since then tremendous amounts of developments have been made to

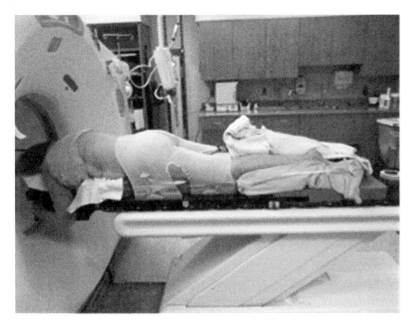

Figure 5.28 Prone setup with a belly board and a pelvis mask.

advance the field of treatment delivery. It is not possible to discuss the entire evolution of treatment planning, but the most important remains the recent introductions of 4D robust optimization utilizing Monte Carlo Systems (Liu et al., 2016 "Exploratory Study of 4d Versus 3d Robust Optimization in Intensity Modulated Proton Therapy for Lung Cancer"), biological dose optimization by incorporating density corrected LET-based evaluations and optimizations (Unkelbach et al., 2016; Unkelbach and Paganetti, 2018), and real-time adaptive radiotherapy based on deep machine learning models (Brock, 2019). At our center, we have developed in-house software that allows us to assess our plans for their dose averaged LET distributions and efforts are underway to develop much more advanced software that will allow incorporating some of the aforementioned wish list.

We hope to have covered some major treatment planning nuances within this chapter, we have left out the discussions of treatment planning for motion-related tumors as it is a completely unique and different topic that has been discussed independently in a separate chapter.

5.5 A Typical List of Do's and Don'ts for Treatment Planners

We list below some of major do's and don'ts along with some rationale for designing proton-based treatment plans.

(a) Establish beam angles that achieves nearly enface incidence for majority of the target volumes. Such an approach can avoid dose grazing and extraneous hot spots due to insufficiency in tissue areas for adequate spot placements.

(b) Avoid going through sharp edges of materials that could affect the path lengths of the calculated beams. Scenarios such as edge of patient positioning devices, immobilization devices with sharp cut-outs, and any hardware to support patient happen to be the most predominant situations.

(c) Must be familiar of the machine's field size and relevant output factors for deciding margins.

(d) Careful choices should be made while selecting angle of attack for each beam. There are often compromises necessary between going through a long versus short lengths of the tumor. Longer dimension would construct larger SOBPs thereby increasing skin doses, whereas shorter dimensions sometimes could be situated at deeper depths thereby increasing the penumbral doses as well as range uncertainties.

(e) Avoid treating through high-density materials both external and/or internal to patient's anatomy.

(f) Avoid treating through critical organs with multiple beams. On similar subject avoid using beam angles with multiple beams that point directly at the critical structures.

(g) Avoid going through areas of high heterogeneities.

(h) When trying to achieve organ sparings through distal end margins, use of shortest beam range will allow generating smaller margins to account for range uncertainties.

(i) When possible select beam angles that generate smaller SOBPs.

(j) Use multiple beam arrangements that traverse away from each other to effectively wash away the effects of linear energy transfers.

(k) Avoid angles prone to collisions with beam delivery systems.

(l) Select beam arrangements with larger hinge angles. Depending upon the spot dosimetry, a separation of hinge angle greater than 30° will be helpful.

(m) Contouring for patients with metal artifacts should be performed on datasets processed through any commercial software for metal artifact reductions.

While the list above (which by the way is not exhaustive) sheds some light on criteria to keep in mind, planners are also encouraged to pay attention to nondosimetric details that can affect quality of treatment. For example, individual site, patient's habitus, prior health history, machine's imaging capabilities, immobilization solutions available for the site, general agreements in clinical practice group for verification of Tx, and dose-calculation capabilities of treatment planning systems are some of the important considerations to be kept in mind. While it is beyond the scope of this chapter to discuss each item in detail, readers are encouraged to refer to some previously published work on these individual items.

5.6 Conclusion

Proton therapy, although arduous and sensitive to a whole lot of anatomical issues, the advantages offered by this modality continues to inspire us develop techniques in this field for safer and efficacious treatments. With decades worth of experience utilizing sPBT in treating majority of various cancers, we have started to realize that the field offers rich opportunity to learn the art of treatment planning.

Acknowledgments

We remain grateful to our institution that has invested significant amount of resources in making this technology available to our patients. The authors would like to thank Mr. Richard Amos, Dr. Chris Beltran, Dr. Wei Liu, Dr. Jiajian Shen, Dr. Xiaoning Ding and Dr. Dan Mundy for sharing their knowledge and experiences with us. We also thank the dosimetry team at both Mayo Clinic's proton centers (Rochester, MN and Phoenix, AZ) for developing state-of-the-art treatment planning routines that we now use in our clinics. Last but not the least, special word of thanks to our radiation oncologists and the care giving team for making our practice safe and superior.

Appendix and Glossary

Nomenclature and terms used

sPBT: scanning proton beam therapy
SFO: single-field optimization
MFO: multifield optimization
IFSO: individual-field optimization
IMPT: intensity-modulated proton therapy
CTV: clinical target volume
PTV: planning target volume
OTV: optimization target volume
STV: scanning target volume

Exercise details

Step-by-step instructions

Exercise 1: Understand lateral penumbra

Preparation: Create or scan a water phantom block with dimensions 40 cm-by-40 cm-by-40 cm cube

- Create three spherical CTVs: CTV1, CTV2, CTV3 with same diameter but their centers placed at depths of 5 cm, 10cm, and 15 cm.
- Expand for each CTV a planning target/optimization target volume with an additional 5 mm margin.
- Generate separate sPBT plans for each target described above using any treatment planning software by utilizing a single field in an anterior–posterior direction to deliver 60 Gy in 30 fx.
- Optimization criteria should be maintained identical for all three separate plans.
- Once the dose distribution is achieved, normalize all three plans to D95 coefficient receiving 95% of the prescription doses.
  (a) Understanding lateral penumbra as a function of energy.
- Compare the dose profiles across the center of the target by drawing a dose profile perpendicular to the direction of travel of beam in each of those three plans.
- From each of those three profiles, compare the value of full-width half maximum and plot it as a function of the nominal energy of the beam.
  (b) Understanding lateral penumbra as a function of depth.

- Pick any of the plan from the exercise above and draw dose profiles for that beam along a few different depths.
- For each profile, compute the full-width half maximum.
- Plot the values of full-width half maximum as a function of depth for the given energy.

Exercise 2: Compare widths of Bragg peaks between low, medium, and high energies

- Use water phantom, targets, and the plan from Exercise 1.
- Draw a dose profile along the direction of depth dose for each of those plans.
- Plot width for the proximal and distal R50, proximal and distal R80 on the Bragg peaks for each of those three beams.
- Compare the Bragg peak widths as a function of energy and observe the widening of the Bragg peaks for higher energies.

Exercise 3: Understanding skin dose in sPBT

- Use the water phantom from Exercise 1.
- Draw two rectangular targets one that is 10 cm long and 2 cm wide, and the other that is 2 cm long and 10 cm wide.

- Both targets should be placed at the same depths such that each target should begin at a depth of 5 cm from the surface of the phantom.
- Expand for each CTV a planning target/optimization target volume with an additional 5-mm margin.
- Also draw a skin line, which is a 3-mm rind drawn from the external body contour.
- Place an anterior–posterior beam for each of those targets and deliver 60 Gy in 30 fractions.
- Optimize these plans using single-field uniform dose optimization, and make sure that the 100% isodose line covers the target in each plan. Essentially, optimization criteria should be maintained identical for each of those plans.
- No other optimization to skin line is necessary.
- Compare the dose–volume histograms for skin structure in each of those plans and at the same time also estimate the number of energy layers being used for each of those plans.
- Side note: Should there be an ambitious desire to compare this skin dose with X-ray therapy, same targets can be optimized utilizing static or rapid arc-based X-rays. Plot an intercomparison dose to the skin OAR between the X-ray and proton plans for each target type.

References

Ainsley, C.G. and Yeager, C.M. (2014). Practical considerations in the calibration of Ct scanners for proton therapy. *Journal of Applied Clinical Medical Physics* 15 (3): 202–220.

Albertini, F. et al. (2011). Is it necessary to plan with safety margins for actively scanned proton therapy? *Physics in Medicine and Biology* 56 (14): 4399.

Albuquerque, K. et al. (2011). Radiation-related predictors of hematologic toxicity after concurrent chemoradiation for cervical cancer and implications for bone marrow–sparing pelvic IMRT. *International Journal of Radiation Oncology, Biology, Physics* 79 (4): 1043–1047.

Anand, A. et al. (2012). A procedure to determine the planar integral spot dose values of proton pencil beam spots. *Medical Physics* 39 (2): 891–900.

Anand, A. et al. (2015). Scanning proton beam therapy reduces normal tissue exposure in pelvic radiotherapy for anal cancer. *Radiotherapy and Oncology* 117 (3): 505–508.

Anand, A. et al. (2019). Individual Field Simultaneous Optimization (IFSO) in spot scanning proton therapy of head and neck cancers. *Medical Dosimetry* 44 (4): 375–378.

Bai, X. et al. (2019). Robust optimization to reduce the impact of biological effect variation from physical uncertainties in intensity-modulated proton therapy. *Physics in Medicine and Biology* 64 (2): 025004.

Beddok, A. et al. (2020, Jun). Proton therapy for head and neck squamous cell carcinomas: A review of the physical and clinical challenges. *Radiotherapy and Oncology* 147: 30–39. doi: 10.1016/j.radonc.2020.03.006. Epub 2020 Mar 27. PMID: 32224315.

Both, S. et al. (2014). Development and clinical implementation of a universal bolus to maintain spot size during delivery of base of skull pencil beam scanning proton therapy. *International Journal of Radiation Oncology, Biology, Physics* 90 (1): 79–84.

Brand, A.H. et al. (2006, Jan-Feb). Vaginal stenosis in patients treated with radiotherapy for carcinoma of the cervix. *International Journal of Gynecologic Cancer* 16 (1): 288–93. doi: 10.1111/j.1525-1438.2006.00348.x. PMID: 16445647.

Brock, K.K. (2019, Jul). Adaptive radiotherapy: Moving into the future. *Seminars in Radiation Oncology* 29 (3): 181–184 NIH Public Access, . doi: 10.1016/j.semradonc.2019.02.011. PMID: 31027635; PMCID: PMC7219982.

Bussière, M.R. and Adams, J.A. (2003). Treatment planning for conformal proton radiation therapy. *Technology in Cancer Research & Treatment* 2 (5): 389–399.

Chen, W. et al. (2012). Including robustness in multi-criteria optimization for intensity-modulated proton therapy. *Physics in Medicine and Biology* 57 (3): 591.

Dunberger, G. et al. (2010, Apr). Fecal incontinence affecting quality of life and social functioning among long-term gynecological cancer survivors. *International Journal of Gynecologic Cancer* 20 (3): 449–460. doi: 10.1111/IGC.0b013e3181d373bf. PMID: 20375813.

Fippel, M. and Soukup, M. (2004). A Monte Carlo dose calculation algorithm for proton therapy. *Medical Physics* 31 (8): 2263–2273.

Frank, S.J. et al. (2014). Multifield optimization intensity modulated proton therapy for head and neck tumors: A translation to practice. *International Journal of Radiation Oncology, Biology, Physics* 89 (4): 846–853.

Fukumitsu, N. et al. (2014). Dose distribution resulting from changes in aeration of nasal cavity or paranasal sinus cancer in the proton therapy. *Radiotherapy and Oncology* 113 (1): 72–76.

Gillin, M.T. et al. (2010). Commissioning of the discrete spot scanning proton beam delivery system at the University of Texas MD Anderson Cancer Center, Proton Therapy Center, Houston. *Medical Physics* 37 (1): 154–163.

Goitein, M. and Jermann, M. (2003). The relative costs of proton and X-Ray radiation therapy. *Clinical Oncology* 15 (1): S37–S50.

Grantzau, T. and Overgaard, J. (2015). Risk of second non-breast cancer after radiotherapy for breast cancer: A systematic review and meta-analysis of 762,468 patients. *Radiotherapy and Oncology* 114 (1): 56–65.

Howarth, A.L. et al. (2017. Jun 23). Tissue expanders and proton beam radiotherapy: What you need to know. *Plastic and Reconstructive Surgery Global Open* 5 (6): e1390. doi: 10.1097/GOX.0000000000001390. PMID: 28740794; PMCID: PMC5505855.

Huang, J.Y. et al. (2015). An evaluation of three commercially available metal artifact reduction methods for CT imaging. *Physics in Medicine and Biology* 60 (3): 1047.

Ikushima, H. et al. (2006). Pelvic bone complications following radiation therapy of gynecologic malignancies: Clinical evaluation of radiation-induced pelvic insufficiency fractures. *Gynecologic Oncology* 103 (3): 1100–1104.

Jäkel, O. et al. (2001). Treatment planning for heavy ion radiotherapy: Clinical implementation and application. *Physics in Medicine and Biology* 46 (4): 1101.

Jette, D. and Chen, W. (2011). Creating a spread-out Bragg peak in proton beams. *Physics in Medicine and Biology* 56 (11): N131.

Kachnic, L.A. et al. (2013). Rtog 0529: A phase 2 evaluation of dose-painted intensity modulated radiation therapy in combination with 5-fluorouracil and mitomycin-c for the reduction of acute morbidity in carcinoma of the anal canal. *International Journal of Radiation Oncology, Biology, Physics* 86 (1): 27–33.

Kang, J.H. et al. (2007). Demonstration of scan path optimization in proton therapy. *Medical Physics* 34 (9): 3457–3464.

Kang, Y. et al. (2018). Evaluating proton pencil beam scanning treatment for breast cancer patients with breast tissue expander. *Medical Physics* 45: WILEY 111 RIVER ST, HOBOKEN 07030-5774, NJ USA, E126–E126. https://doi.org/10.26226/morressier.5cb72190a e0a090015830845

Karger, C.P. et al. (2010). Dosimetry for ion beam radiotherapy. *Physics in Medicine and Biology* 55 (21): R193.

Klopp, A.H. et al. (2013). Hematologic toxicity in Rtog 0418: A phase 2 study of postoperative IMRT for gynecologic cancer. *International Journal of Radiation Oncology, Biology, Physics* 86 (1): 83–90.

Levine, C.D. et al. (1994). Pelvic marrow in adults. *Skeletal Radiology* 23 (5): 343–347.

Lievens, Y. and Pijls-Johannesma, M. (2013, Apr). Health economic controversy and cost-effectiveness of proton therapy. *Seminars in Radiation Oncology* 23(2): Elsevier, 134–141. doi: 10.1016/j.semradonc.2012.11.005. PMID: 23473691.

Liu, H. and Chang, J.Y. (2011). Proton therapy in clinical practice. *Chinese Journal of Cancer* 30 (5): 315.

Liu, W. et al. (2012a). Influence of robust optimization in intensity-modulated proton therapy with different dose delivery techniques. *Medical Physics* 39 (6): Part1, 3089–3101.

Liu, W. et al. (2012b). Robust optimization of intensity modulated proton therapy. *Medical Physics* 39 (2): 1079–1091.

Liu, W. et al. (2016). Exploratory study of 4d versus 3d robust optimization in intensity modulated proton therapy for lung cancer. *International Journal of Radiation Oncology, Biology, Physics* 95 (1): 523–533.

Lomax, A.J. et al. (2001). Intensity modulated proton therapy: A clinical example. *Medical Physics* 28 (3): 317–324.

Lomax, A.J. (2008). Intensity modulated proton therapy and its sensitivity to treatment uncertainties 2: The potential effects of inter-fraction and inter-field motions. *Physics in Medicine and Biology* 53 (4): 1043.

Lomax, A.J. et al. (2004). The clinical potential of intensity modulated proton therapy. *Zeitschrift Für Medizinische Physik* 14 (3): 147–152.

Lomax, A.J. (2009). Charged particle therapy: The physics of interaction. *The Cancer Journal* 15 (4): 285–291.

Lundkvist, J. et al. (2005). Proton therapy of cancer: Potential clinical advantages and cost-effectiveness. *Acta Oncologica* 44 (8): 850–861.

McGowan, S.E. et al. (2013). Treatment planning optimisation in proton therapy. *The British Journal of Radiology* 86 (1021): 20120288-20120288.

Mell, L.K. et al. (2006). Dosimetric predictors of acute hematologic toxicity in cervical cancer patients treated with concurrent cisplatin and intensity-modulated pelvic radiotherapy. *International Journal of Radiation Oncology, Biology, Physics* 66 (5): 1356–1365.

Mell, L.K. et al. (2008). Dosimetric comparison of bone marrow-sparing intensity-modulated radiotherapy versus conventional techniques for treatment of cervical cancer. *International Journal of Radiation Oncology, Biology, Physics* 71 (5): 1504–1510.

Meyer, E. et al. (2010). Normalized Metal Artifact Reduction (NMAR) in computed tomography. *Medical Physics* 37 (10): 5482–5493.

Morris, L. et al. (2017, May 2). Radiation-induced vaginal stenosis: Current perspectives. *International Journal of Women's Health* 9: 273–279. doi: 10.2147/IJWH.S106796. PMID: 28496367; PMCID: PMC5422455.

Mutter, R.W. et al. (2021, Oct 1). Proton therapy for breast cancer: A consensus statement from the Particle Therapy Cooperative Group (PTCOG) breast cancer subcommittee. *International Journal of Radiation Oncology, Biology, Physics* 111(2): 337–359. doi: 10.1016/j.ijrobp.2021.05.110. Epub 2021 May 25. PMID: 34048815; PMCID: PMC8416711.

Paganetti, H. (2012). Range uncertainties in proton therapy and the role of Monte Carlo simulations. *Physics in Medicine and Biology* 57 (11): R99.

Park, P.C. et al. (2012). A beam-specific Planning Target Volume (PTV) design for proton therapy to account for setup and range uncertainties. *International Journal of Radiation Oncology, Biology, Physics* 82 (2): e329–e336.

Patyal, B. (2007). Dosimetry aspects of proton therapy. *Technology in Cancer Research & Treatment* 6 (4_suppl): 17–23.

Pedroni, E. et al. (1999). Initial experience of using an active beam delivery technique at psi. *Strahlentherapie Und Onkologie* 175 (2): 18–20.

Pflugfelder, D. et al. (2008). Worst case optimization: A method to account for uncertainties in the optimization of intensity modulated proton therapy. *Physics in Medicine and Biology* 53 (6): 1689.

Purdy, J.A. (2004, Jan). Current ICRU definitions of volumes: Limitations and future directions. *Seminars in Radiation Oncology* 14: Elsevier, 27–40. doi: 10.1053/j.semradonc.2003.12.002. PMID: 14752731.

Quan, E.M. et al. (2013). Preliminary evaluation of multifield and single-field optimization for the treatment planning of spot-scanning proton therapy of head and neck cancer. *Medical Physics* 40 (8): 081709.

Safai, S. et al. (2008). Comparison between the lateral penumbra of a collimated double-scattered beam and uncollimated scanning beam in proton radiotherapy. *Physics in Medicine and Biology* 53 (6): 1729.

Sawakuchi, G.O. et al. (2010). Experimental characterization of the low-dose envelope of spot scanning proton beams. *Physics in Medicine and Biology* 55 (12): 3467.

Schneider, U. (2011). Modeling the risk of secondary malignancies after radiotherapy. *Genes* 2 (4): 1033–1049.

Schuemann, J. et al. (2014). Site-specific range uncertainties caused by dose calculation algorithms for proton therapy. *Physics in Medicine and Biology* 59 (15): 4007.

Schwarz, M. (2011). Treatment planning in proton therapy. *The European Physical Journal Plus* 126 (7): 1–10.

Shusharina, N. et al. (2019). Impact of aeration change and beam arrangement on the robustness of proton plans. *Journal of Applied Clinical Medical Physics* 20 (3): 14–21.

Smith, A. et al. (2009). The MD Anderson Proton Therapy System. *Medical Physics* 36 (9): Part1, 4068–4083.

Thomas, S.J. (2006). Margins for treatment planning of proton therapy. *Physics in Medicine and Biology* 51 (6): 1491.

Tobias, C.A. et al. (1958). Pituitary irradiation with high-energy proton beams a preliminary report. *Cancer Research* 18 (2): 121–134.

Trofimov, A. and Bortfeld, T. (2003). Optimization of beam parameters and treatment planning for intensity modulated proton therapy. *Technology in Cancer Research & Treatment* 2 (5): 437–444.

Unkelbach, J. et al. (2016). Reoptimization of intensity modulated proton therapy plans based on linear energy transfer. *International Journal of Radiation Oncology, Biology, Physics* 96 (5): 1097–1106.

Unkelbach, J. and Paganetti, H. (2018, Apr). Robust proton treatment planning: Physical and biological optimization. *Seminars in Radiation Oncology* 28: Elsevier, 88–96. doi: 10.1016/j.semradonc.2017.11.005. PMID: 29735195; PMCID: PMC5942229.

Urie, M. et al. (1986). Degradation of the Bragg peak due to inhomogeneities. *Physics in Medicine and Biology* 31 (1): 1.

Van Der Voort, S. et al. (2016). Robustness recipes for minimax robust optimization in intensity modulated proton therapy for oropharyngeal cancer patients. *International Journal of Radiation Oncology, Biology, Physics* 95 (1): 163–170.

Verburg, J.M. and Seco, J. (2013). Dosimetric accuracy of proton therapy for chordoma patients with titanium implants. *Medical Physics* 40 (7): 071727.

Wang, G. et al. (1996). Iterative deblurring for CT metal artifact reduction. *IEEE Transactions on Medical Imaging* 15 (5): 657–664.

Wilson, R.R. (1946). Radiological use of fast protons. *Radiology* 47 (5): 487–491.

Yang, M. et al. (2012). Comprehensive analysis of proton range uncertainties related to patient stopping-power-ratio estimation using the stoichiometric calibration. *Physics in Medicine and Biology* 57 (13): 4095.

6

Image-Guided Particle Therapy and Motion Management

James E. Younkin Ph.D., Martin Bues Ph.D., and Aman Anand Ph.D.

Corresponding Author Details: anand.aman@mayo.edu Tel: 480-342-0231
Department of Radiation Oncology, Mayo Clinic, Phoenix, AZ – 85050

TABLE OF CONTENTS

6.1 Introduction

Image-guided radiotherapy (IGRT) and motion management (MM) are distinct yet related subjects in particle therapy. This chapter will focus primarily on the challenges in image guidance and MM as they are related to particle therapy, with an emphasis on techniques unique to particle therapy. Proton beam therapy (PBT) will be used as a model for heavy charged particle therapy; however, the techniques can readily be extended to other particles. Image guidance has a long history in PBT. Notably 3D volumetric imaging for the purpose of 3D treatment planning was first introduced at the Massachusetts

Principles and Practice of Particle Therapy, First Edition. Edited by Timothy D. Malouff and Daniel M. Trifiletti.
© 2022 John Wiley & Sons Ltd. Published 2022 by John Wiley & Sons Ltd.

General Hospital in Boston shortly after the invention of the CT scanner with the intent to better estimate the range of proton beam with the help of 3D voxelized Hounsfield unit (HU) information [1,2]. Due to the difference in transport properties between photons and protons, detailed knowledge of the distribution of HUs within the patients is far more important in the case of PBT than in photons. This is evidenced by the fact that for many years after invention of the CT-based treatment planning photon-based codes assumed all patient tissues to be water [3,4].

MM in PBT is by comparison a newer phenomenon. Much of the early work in PBT was focused on intracranial malignancies where MM, once the patient is immobilized, is not an issue. Some of the early lung cancer trials were conducted at Loma Linda PBT center [5]. These trials were carried out in the context of passive scattering PBT. The relatively higher importance of MM in protons derives from the fact that in PBT organ motion may deform the dose cloud and lead to geographic target misses even if the target does not move relative to isocenter. In other words, the static dose cloud approximation, while reasonable in conventional radiotherapy, fails in the case of PBT.

In this chapter, we will describe the principles and practice of IGRT and MM in PBT. We will pay special attention to those IGRT procedures and MM strategies in our own proton practice at Mayo Clinic in Arizona. The chapter will be organized along the chain of radiation therapy beginning with simulation and ending with daily treatment. We will also discuss the important topic of verification imaging, which is more important in protons due to reasons discussed earlier in this volume.

The sections of this chapter are as follows: In the section following this introduction, we will discuss imaging procedures and MM during pretreatment imaging including CT simulation. We will also discuss patient immobilization equipment and ancillary devices used in IGRT and MM in this phase of the treatment process, including a decision tree used at our institution that describes how patient treatment is adapted to motion detected at this point in the radiotherapy workflow. The section after that will focus on MM during treatment planning. We will describe how the various motion-related images enter into the plan optimization and plan evaluation process. The planning scenarios will include planning based on 4D CT with and without gating and deep inspiration breath hold (DIBH). The following section will address IGRT and MM during treatment. We will discuss various imaging protocols and MM techniques currently in use in PBT and the decisions therapists make during treatment in interpreting images and how to apply MM techniques. The penultimate section will discuss imaging for treatment verification which is carried out with and without MM. We will discuss the decision process regarding whether a patient requires replanning or not. In the final

section, we will briefly touch upon advanced approaches to IGRT and MM, which are under development at various centers, and which have not yet made their way into clinical use or are only used in very few centers.

6.2 Pretreatment Imaging

6.2.1 Immobilization for Moving Targets Treated with Particle Radiotherapy

For moving tumors undergoing conformal radiotherapy treatments (whether conventional or charged particle-based), it is important that the immobilization solutions allow high-precision dose delivery [6–8]. Taking advantage of the precision dose delivery of particle-based therapies requires maintaining even tighter tolerances on interfractional setup uncertainties compared to conventional conformal modalities (e.g., IMRT). Patient setup for treatment of moving tumors in the lungs, pancreas, and liver will also require managing any variability in patient breathing characteristics in addition to daily setup uncertainties. In this section, we discuss choices of immobilization devices that result in improved patient setup with reduction in inter- and intra-fractional variability. The ideal immobilization device for a conformal radiotherapy treatment would combine robust positioning with reproducible indexing of the patient. Immobilization devices that assist in comfortable patient positioning, e.g., of the arms through features such as hand poles and arm incline supports (shown in Figure 6.1), are also desirable since they allow patients to better tolerate long radiotherapy sessions.

Proton therapy centers should invest effort into designing and carefully testing immobilization solutions for each treatment site. For example, daily translational and rotational setup uncertainties are reduced by using appropriately sized thoracic masks for lung lesions or pelvic masks for abdominal or gastrointestinal malignancies. At the time of this writing, particle therapy clinics typically assume a 2–3-mm daily setup error for thoracic sites and 3–4-mm daily setup error for pelvic sites to model the robustness of treatment plans [9]. Hence, it is necessary to ensure that before every treatment, the customized or commercial immobilization devices are capable of positioning these patients within these tolerances. Either a body fix bag and/or expanded foam in conjunction with a T-bar or a pole as shown in Figure 6.1 has proven to be effective in reducing daily setup errors to less than 3 mm in each of the cardinal directions [10]. When designing these immobilization solutions, it is important to ensure that no components with high Z elemental composition (such as BBs or scar wires) will be positioned in the path of the proton beam during treatment. There are also special cases in which the radiotherapy treatments of the extra-cranial tumors such as those in the

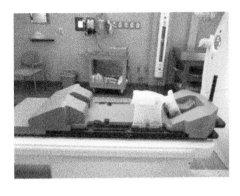
(a)

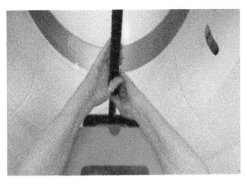
(b)

Figure 6.1   A typical thoracic immobilization device to support patient's arms, elbows, and immobilizing the body with a thoracic mask.

lungs, liver, and pancreatic tumors can be delivered in less number of fractions as compared to conventional fractionations. Such hypofractionated treatments as defined by the American Society of Radiation Oncology and American College of Radiology are a method to deliver very precisely high dose radiation to a small target within the body [11,12]. When preparing patients for such radiotherapy procedures, there have to be available resources that can limit the excursions of tumor due to respiratory motion and in addition provide extreme patient reproducibility to minimize the interfractional setup errors. For selected sites and clinical indications, methods such as abdominal compressions, active breathing controls, breath holds, beam gating, real-time tumor tracking, and near rigid body fix bags have been developed to mitigate the effects of motion for safer deliveries of these special procedures. While fiducial markers used to track localization of tumors with respect to the neighboring anatomy are used in the same way that they are typically employed in conventional radiotherapy, the type of fiducial marker should be chosen with great care. The fiducial markers should be as small as possible yet still visible on the radiographs used for image guidance. The composition of fiducial markers and their relative stopping power should be determined prior to treatment so that they can be contoured and overridden to appropriate HU values on the patient CT. It should be kept in mind that novel markers may have an elemental composition that does not correspond to any value available on the CT calibration curves in the treatment planning system (TPS), thereby leading to additional uncertainties in the range of the particle therapy beams.

In our clinical practice, we take great care in implementing radiotherapy markers that would allow better target localization, avoid artifacts that otherwise could perturb the proton-based treatments, and provide superior imaging during the IGRT procedures. The use of VISICOIL™ (Visicoil; RadioMed, Barlett, TN) has proven to be quite effective within our practice.

In addition to the VISICOIL-based surrogates, we also employ use of carbon-based markers where possible. When performing special MM procedures such as DIBH (discussed later), the use of fiducial markers for daily IGRT is a must within our practice, unless there happens to be clearly visible anatomical demarcation to utilize for setups. In special circumstances when fiducial markers are clinically not indicated, we can utilize in-room CT on rails within one of our gantries as depicted in Figure 6.2 to perform volumetric-based patients' setup. The use of CT on rails is fraught with uncertainties due to the fact that the CT on rails isocenter is different from treatment isocenter. We always verify through portal imaging using 2D–3D match at the treatment isocenter to validate the CT on rails setup.

6.2.2   CT Simulation and Motion Quantification

6.2.2.1   CT Simulation of Moving Target Anatomy

Using a 3D CT to image a moving target (e.g., in the thorax or abdomen) can result in severe motion artifacts [13]. In conventional radiotherapy, these artifacts are a source of uncertainty in the lateral target margins; however, in particle therapy, it becomes impossible to plan treatments using a 3D CT of a moving target because the resulting artifacts cause severe miscalculation of charged particle range in the patient geometry. The range miscalculation due to CT artifacts could result in reduced coverage, geometric miss, and overshoot, possibly into critical normal tissues. Therefore, a 4D CT simulation that can capture patient anatomy at many fixed points over the respiratory cycle is required for any particle therapy involving any target volume that has significant motion (e.g., lung, esophagus, or liver).

6.2.2.2   4D CT Simulation

The purpose of 4D CT simulation is to construct multiple 3D CTs of stationary anatomical states representative of anatomical

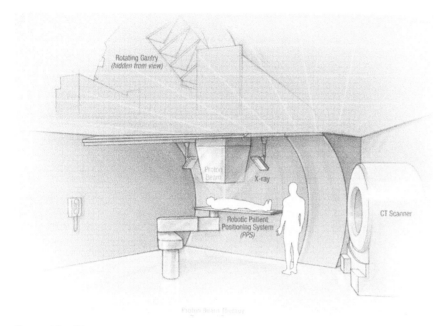

Figure 6.2 CT on rails within gantry for volumetric imaging and treatment setup verifications.

motion during the patient respiratory cycle [13–15]. These 3D CTs are known as *breathing phases*, and the *4D CT dataset* is a collection of breathing phases that covers the entire respiratory cycle. CT projection data are collected under free breathing conditions and used to reconstruct CT images at each position (*slices*), which are combined to form breathing phases. Slices are reconstructed using either *prospective gating* (data acquisition starts at preselected respiratory states) or *retrospective gating* (slices are reconstructed post-scan based on measurements of patient respiration) [16]. This chapter will only be concerned with retrospective gating. CT projection data may be acquired in either helical [13] or ciné [15] (axial) modes. On modern CT simulators, helical scans are typically used to reduce scanning time [16].

6.2.2.3   Sorting CT Images into Breathing Phases

An *external respiratory signal* (also known as the *surrogate signal*) is a high-frequency measurement of some physical property whose amplitude is used to characterize the respiratory state as a function of time. The external respiratory signal is synchronized with the start of the scan, which allows matching CT projection data to an external respiratory signal amplitude by time values. Examples of external respiratory signals used for 4D CT include surrogate motion tracking [13] and spirometry [15] whose amplitudes are the superior–inferior position of an object attached to the patient surface and the volume of air measured by a spirometer, respectively. *Sorting* is the process of dividing the external respiratory signal into bins (in time) that are associated with breathing phases and then binning the CT projection data. The binned CT projection data can then be reconstructed into slices for each breath-

ing phase. In general, slice reconstruction can use *phase-based sorting* [13,14,17] or *amplitude-based sorting* [15,17–19], which are different methods of locating bin midpoints within the external respiratory signal. Both methods start by dividing the external respiratory signal into respiratory cycles at time values that correspond to either peaks or troughs.

Phase-based sorting divides respiratory cycles into equal-time parts; the boundaries between these parts become the midpoints of bins [18]. Amplitude-based sorting first divides each respiratory cycle into inhalation and exhalation according to whether the external respiratory signal amplitude is rising or falling. In some procedures, amplitude-based sorting has not distinguished inspiration from exhalation [15] but this may not be advisable since, for example, lung tumor motion is known to exhibit hysteresis [20]. Bin midpoints are located at the time points when the external respiratory signal crosses preselected amplitude levels. There are two types of amplitude-based sorting. *Global amplitude-based sorting* uses identical amplitude levels over all respiratory cycles [15,18,21]. For example, amplitude levels may be a percentage of the difference between the average peak amplitude and the average trough amplitude across all respiratory cycles [21]. In *local amplitude-based sorting*, amplitude levels are a percentage of the amplitude of each single inspiration or exhalation and thus may vary in absolute magnitude between respiratory cycles [19]. While global amplitude-based sorting generates slices corresponding to consistent external respiratory signal amplitudes [18], local amplitude-based sorting ensures that breathing phases will not be missing slices if the external respiratory signal amplitude does not cross a global amplitude threshold in some respiratory cycles [19,21]. These three methods of sorting projection data into breathing phases are shown in Figure 6.3.

The external respiratory signal was generated using a sin [4] model with a constant baseline shift of 0.21 units per second. (a) Phase-based sorting selects bin midpoints (red Xs) by dividing the time between consecutive peaks into even parts. Boundaries of projection data bins are vertical gray lines, and labels showing the corresponding breathing phases of 10 example bins are printed to the right of the vertical line marking the start of the

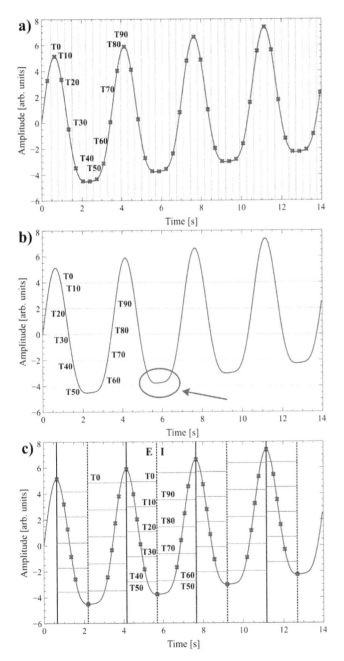

bin. (b) Global amplitude-based sorting uses average peak and trough amplitudes (here defined by zero baseline shift) to define bin midpoints that are evenly spaced in amplitude. Bin boundaries are marked by horizontal gray lines, and the corresponding breathing phases of 10 example bins are labeled. Due to the sudden baseline shift, the external respiratory signal does not reach the T50 bin for several respiratory cycles (red circle and arrow), which can result in missing slices in the T50 breathing phase. (c) In contrast, local amplitude-based sorting considers the peak-to-trough amplitude of each exhalation (E) and inhalation (I) portion of each respiratory cycle (peak inhalation is marked by solid black vertical lines and maximum exhalation is marked by dotted black vertical lines). Bin midpoints (red Xs) are evenly spaced in amplitude between each peak and trough, and the boundaries are marked by short gray horizontal lines between solid and dotted vertical lines. The breathing phases corresponding to ten example bins are labeled.

Generally speaking, 4D CT datasets are obtained using helical scans and multislice CT scanners [22]. The critical parameters of the scan are the pitch and the gantry rotation speed [14]. The gantry must rotate with sufficient speed so that slices are acquired during a sufficiently small fraction of the respiratory cycle; the anatomy must be relatively fixed for the duration of each image acquisition. A data sufficiency condition determines the maximum pitch given the need to obtain images at each position over the entire breathing cycle [16]. Modern CT simulators generally have built-in 4D CT scan parameter presets that control gantry rotation speed and pitch. Parameter presets are selected based on the patient respiratory period, as discussed in greater detail below.

6.2.2.4 Irregular Respiratory Motion and Image Artifacts

Slice reconstruction can become problematic in the presence of significantly irregular respiratory motion. Hypothetically, if CT scans were performed in ciné mode, then slices affected by irregular respiratory motion could be re-scanned, but this is not possible for helical scans [16,17]. Irregular respiratory motion can lead to image artifacts in breathing phases of a variety of types that have been well documented in the literature [23]. However, it should be noted that even in the absence of visually recognizable artifacts, irregular respiratory motion can result in breathing phases that are not an accurate representation of a realistic anatomical state. For example, with local amplitude-based sorting baseline drift might result in adjacent slices that are only slightly inconsistent with one another, but two slices from the beginning and the end of a scan might correspond to very different anatomical positions [17].

6.2.2.5 Limitations of 4D CT Techniques

The 4D CT is a representation of the patient anatomy constructed from the particular respiratory cycles that occurred

Figure 6.3 Defining projection data bins for reconstructing breathing phases of a 10-phase 4D CT dataset using (a) phase-based (based on [18]), (b) global amplitude-based [15,18,21], and (c) local amplitude-based sorting (based on [19]).

during simulation. It is impossible to extrapolate beyond the respiratory amplitude recorded during 4D CT simulation. If the patient respiratory amplitude exceeds this range during treatment, then the normal tissues or the tumor may be in a position relative to the beam that was not anticipated during treatment planning. The 4D CT uses an external respiratory signal under the assumption that the respiratory motion, including the tumor position, is completely characterized by the signal amplitude. However, the relationship between the signal amplitude and tumor motion is more complex, and there is no perfect correlation between surrogate motion and tumor position [24].

6.2.2.6 CT Simulation with Deep Inspiration Breath Hold

DIBH is a MM technique developed by researchers at Memorial Sloan Kettering [25–27]. The DIBH technique is particularly useful in scanning proton beam therapy (sPBT) since respiratory motion is arrested during the breath hold, which prevents the deleterious effects of relative motion between the scanned beam and a moving target. Preparing patients for DIBH treatment requires a more time-consuming initial CT simulation procedure that often involves several CT scans [28]. Similar to 4D CT or respiratory gating, DIBH requires an external respiratory signal to monitor the respiratory state (e.g., surrogate motion tracking [13] or spirometry [15]) and in particular the reproducibility of the breath hold. CT simulation for DIBH is performed in the breath hold position.

6.2.2.7 4D CT Simulation Workflow

At our institution, initial simulation for the lung, esophagus, liver, and pancreas treatment sites follows a 4D CT-based workflow. After patient setup, a small plastic block with infrared reflectors is reproducibly attached to the anterior surface of the patient as a motion surrogate. An infrared camera measures the motion surrogate amplitude in the superior–inferior direction by tracking infrared reflectors on the plastic block. This platform can provide the motion surrogate amplitude as a function of time elapsed since the start of the CT scan as an external respiratory signal for 4D CTs. Prior to the scan, the respiratory signal is monitored for several respiratory cycles to determine the respiratory period. The respiratory period is used to select from built-in 4D CT scan parameter presets, which are listed in Table 6.1.

Table 6.1 4D CT scan parameter presets are selected based on patient respiratory period. These scan techniques are built in to our institution's CT simulators.

Respiratory period	4D CT scan technique
Less than 5 s	Trigger 12
5–6.5 s	Trigger 9
More than 6.5 s	Trigger 6

After the scan, the maximum exhalation peaks in the trace of the external respiratory signal are identified by a qualified medical physicist or medical physicist assistant, and then 10 breathing phases are reconstructed using phase-based sorting. An animation of breathing phases is examined for any artifacts near the treatment site that would require a repeat scan. After verifying the scan, the tumor motion is measured in the superior–inferior, anterior–posterior, and left–right directions using a software tool. If the motion amplitude is less than 10 mm, then average intensity projection and the maximum intensity projection of the 10 phases are calculated (minimum intensity projection is also calculated for the liver site). Then, these projections and the breathing phases are exported for treatment planning.

If the motion is greater than 10 mm, then the patient may be treated using the DIBH technique. This requires coaching the patient on how to perform the breath hold; they are instructed to hold their breath at a comfortable level for approximately 20 s. Patients are given audiovisual cues for the breath hold and when to resume normal breathing. The patient performs two initial breath holds, which are used to set an amplitude gating window. This gating window is used to verify the reproducibility of breath holds; the CT scan and beam delivery are manually controlled by therapists. A standard (non-4D) helical CT scan is performed during breath hold, and the resulting 3D CT image is exported to the TPS.

6.3 Treatment Planning of Tumors with Motion and Heterogeneities

6.3.1 Overview of Proton Treatment Planning in the Presence of Motion

The development of sPBT is a remarkable milestone as it offers effective and efficient ways of delivering conformal proton therapy with much less hardware. Readers are encouraged to familiarize themselves with the mechanisms of sPBT [29,30] and the ways to deliver intensity modulated proton therapy [31]. There are several safety considerations that should be considered when delivering this form of radiation to targets that vary drastically in size, shape, homogeneity, and inter- and intra-fractional localizations. The interaction between charged particles and the medium is sensitive to the physical characteristics of the medium as well as any tumor specific motions that could perturb proton range and dose homogeneities within the target. Potential dose uncertainties, especially those due to any movement of the tumor, can quickly become a major impediment when treating tumors of the lungs, pancreas, liver, and prostate.

In addition, to the challenges of beam delivery for moving targets, one also needs to be fully aware of the clinical details such as capabilities of TPS in use with respect to dose calculations in heterogeneous medium, availability of various immobilization solutions in their practice, and the forms of image guidance tools available for daily setups when treating moving targets. In dosimetry when preparing a treatment plan for moving targets, it will be important that a preplanning consultation be made with the physician and physics in order to establish the planning goals of target coverage and prescription describing the constraints for organs at risk. Planning volumes being generated should be based on the 4D CT-based motion assessment of the tumor and all margins should follow guidelines as suggested by ICRU 50 and 62 [32]. Tumors prone to respiratory-based internal motions warrant use of beam angles that would get least perturbed and maintain their range accuracies required to cover the target. Those should also be consulted with physician and physics group when in doubt. Maintaining sufficient awareness of these design principles remains fundamental to any particle therapy-based clinics that wish to treat moving tumors as targets. In the next few subsections, we will discuss the essentials of treatment planning and the necessary treatment planning preparation strategies for the safe delivery of particle-based treatments. In these subsections, we highlight challenges involving dose calculation algorithms, discrepancies between planned and delivered doses caused by motion, and modeling target volumes in the presence of motion. We also discuss various strategies that are presently available along with highlighting promising future technologies that can further mitigate the effects of motion-related uncertainty in particle-based treatment plans. Any unique anatomy-specific details will be discussed within the context of these aforementioned sections wherever necessary.

6.3.2 Proton Treatment Planning for Moving Targets

6.3.2.1 Proton Dose Calculation Algorithms

The fundamental objective of ionization beam therapies is to achieve maximum tumor kill while preserving significant amounts of healthy tissues. Any associated uncertainties with dose calculations will have a direct and a strong impact on the overall success of the treatments. Hence, accuracy in dose calculations remains of paramount importance in this field. When computing treatment plans to treat cancers especially in lung tumors, dose calculation algorithms have their own special limitations. Even though such limitations are not precisely correlated with motion, however, motion when compounded with heterogeneities can have a significant impact on the overall treatments of these patients. Particle therapy practice currently relies on either a pencil beam and analytical algorithm [33] or the Monte Carlo algorithm [34,35]. The PBA-based dose calculations rely on ray tracing of individual beams through the medium, whereas the Monte Carlo method tracks individual particles through the medium, thereby offering a

higher accuracy summation of dose through any kind of medium.

Especially in heterogeneous medium such as in the case of lungs, PBA models the medium to be homogeneous on either sides of central axis, whereas in actual clinical situations that assumption is not necessarily accurate, thereby limiting the overall accuracy of doses. Now compounding the issue of lateral heterogeneities along with the motion of the overall target, studies show that pencil-beam-based dose calculations could be off by approximately 30% along the tissue/air interfaces [36,37]. Hence, care must be taken in selecting TPS which can provide a comparison of these doses against a full MC system. In clinics that are not equipped to support a MC-based treatment system, it is extremely important to have at least another independent TPS to perform secondary checks on the doses computed by the primary TPS used for these treatments. The issue of MC versus analytical dose calculations tends to reduce with increase in homogeneities of the target such as in the case of liver-based treatments. However due to the motion of these tumor types, there remains a possibility for these particle beams to traverse through different medium that could result in variations of their path lengths.

At the time of this work within our practice, we have commissioned three completely independent TPSs to perform various checks as required on a case-by-case basis. While the primary treatment planning is routinely performed using a commercial TPS that calculates plans on analytical algorithms, we also have an independent dose-engine system developed in-house that can compute doses using both analytical as well as full MC algorithms.

6.3.2.2 Dose Uncertainties Caused by Target Motion and the Interplay Effect

Target volume expansion can compensate for motion uncertainties in conventional external beam therapy. However, treatment modalities that use dynamic beam delivery must contend with an additional motion effect that cannot be corrected by margins. Dynamically delivered beams, e.g., using IMRT or sPBT, deliver time-dependent nonuniform doses. When delivered to a static target, the sum of doses delivered by these dynamic beams creates a homogeneous dose distribution. But if there is significant motion during dynamic beam delivery, then the target volume will have a different geometric configuration and anatomical position at each time point that the nonuniform doses are delivered, and the sum of these doses will no longer result in a homogenous dose distribution within the target volume. The target-dose inhomogeneity created by relative motion between dynamically delivered beams and a moving target volume is known as the interplay effect [38]. The interplay effect can be recognized by characteristic hot and cold spots throughout the target volume that have no substantial effect on mean target dose compared to the nominal

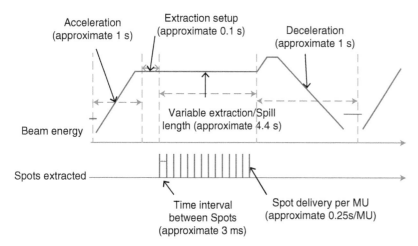

Figure 6.4 Accelerator cycle for discrete scanning beam particle therapy system showing some parameters that influence interplay effects*.
*Figure reprinted with permission from Elsevier (# 4892750953318).

plan dose [39,40]. If not corrected, target-dose inhomogeneity caused by the interplay effect could have serious consequences for local tumor control [41].

Fractionation is generally sufficient to manage interplay effects for photon-based dynamic beam modalities such as IMRT [38]. Randomization of the relative motion between the dynamic beams and the target volume for each fraction averages out the dose inhomogeneity. However, for sPBT the interplay effect causes more severe-dose degradation [42]. This is particularly true for tumors that exhibit large amplitude motion [43] and fractionation alone may not be sufficient to remove dose inhomogeneity caused by the interplay effect [44]. Therefore, additional strategies are used to either increase the amount of averaging (e.g., by rescanning [42,44–46]) or reduce the target motion (e.g., delivering during DIBH [25–27]). Robust optimization of treatment plans has also been shown to mitigate the effects of target motion, including the interplay effect [47]. Regardless of the strategies used to reduce the effects of interplay, the Particle Therapy Co-Operative Group (PTCOG) recommends performing a motion analysis prior to treating thoracic sites with sPBT to determine the severity of dose degradation caused by motion [48].

The relative motion between the scanned proton beam and the target depends on the beam characteristics of both the proton delivery system including spot size, scanning speed, energy switching time, etc. as also seen in Figure 6.4 and patient respiration (including motion amplitude, respiratory period, and irregularity of patient respiratory motion) [39,44]. In addition, the relative phase between the patient respiratory motion and the spot delivery sequence, which is randomly determined at the start of beam delivery, has a non-trivial effect on the amount of dose inhomogeneity [39]. Therefore, it is not currently possible to predict the interplay effect *a priori* even with perfect knowledge of patient respiratory motion and the proton therapy system.

For these reasons, pretreatment motion analysis requires a *4D dynamic dose distribution* that incorporates patient respiratory

motion [49]. The 4D dynamic dose (also known as 4D dynamically accumulated dose) is calculated on the 4D dataset acquired during 4D CT simulation. The first step in the 4D dynamic dose calculation is assigning each proton spot to a particular breathing phase. Delivery times for each spot measured from the start of the spot delivery sequence can be obtained from a beam delivery model [50,51] or from machine log files [52]. Based on data from the external respiratory signal, spots are assigned to one of the breathing phases based on their time values. Importantly, the initial phase must be randomized for each fraction (i.e., the first spot has an equal chance to be registered to any of the breathing phases). Then, a dose calculation algorithm is used to compute the dose to each breathing phase from all spots registered to that phase. One of the breathing phases (typically the phase corresponding to maximum exhalation) is selected as the *reference phase* onto which the 4D dynamic dose is accumulated. A deformable image registration algorithm registers all other breathing phases to the reference phase. The resulting deformation vector fields make it possible to transform the dose to each breathing phase into the resulting dose on the reference phase, and the sum of the breathing phase doses on the reference phase is the 4D dynamic dose.

Unfortunately, commercial TPSs do not yet offer the capability to calculate 4D dynamic dose (although with some scripting 4D dose calculations can be performed in RayStation™ (Raysearch Laboratories, Sweden) [53]). Therefore, proton treatment centers treating thoracic malignancies that are affected by respiratory motion (e.g., in the lung) must rely on in-house developed software to calculate 4D dynamic dose distributions. At our institution, we have developed and commissioned a dose engine [54] as part of a TPS that has the capability to perform deformable image registration of breathing phases, and this software is used to perform motion analysis on all lung and esophagus treatment plans. We follow the recommendations of PTCOG and calculate 4D dynamic dose on two breathing phases (maximum inhalation and maximum exhalation) to get a worst-case estimate of the interplay effect [48]. A custom export filter is used to send the DICOM files corresponding to the proton treatment plan, the structure files, the nominal plan dose, and the CT images corresponding to these two breathing phases to a remote workstation. A web interface is provided through which users can run 4D dynamic dose calculations on this workstation. One of the input parameters is the patient respiratory period. The initial phase is determined by choosing a random time between zero and the respiratory period, corresponding to the start of the maximum inhalation phase and the end of the exhalation phase, respectively. Spots are assigned to one of the two phases starting from this initial time, alternating between the two phases every one-half breathing period. While this method does not consider the irregularity of respiratory motion as measured by the external respiratory signal, irregular respiratory motion contributes to averaging out dose inhomogeneity caused by the interplay effect [44] (similar to fractionation or rescanning), and so this method is consistent with our intent to perform a worst-case motion analysis. After the calculation, a copy of the dose DICOM containing the calculated 4D dynamic dose distribution is re-imported to the TPS. The DVH calculated from dose in the GTV is used for motion analysis. Our clinical requirement is that GTV dose coverage ($D_{95\%}$) in the 4D dynamic dose distribution should be greater than 95% of the prescription dose.

6.3.2.3 Modeling Patient Geometries in Moving Targets

Every particle therapy treatment plan essentially begins with a computed tomography scan of a patient. With the CT scan of a patient becomes available a spatial and density information specific to that patient requiring a treatment plan. The overall accuracy of their treatments relies strongly upon the integrity of these scanned data. Now for tumors that involve internal motions such as lungs, liver, and pancreas particularly the organ motion can lead to large uncertainties in representing both the spatial and density information. Particularly since the CT algorithms that reconstruct anatomical information works best for static datasets, utilizing those methods to compute plans for moving targets could be highly detrimental. Hence, it is extremely important to introduce mathematical solutions that allow reconstructing patient specific information which will account for breathing motion related displacements in the spatial localization of tumors as well as provide better information on the differences in the water equivalent thicknesses due to displacements of the tissues caused by respiratory motions. In order to overcome such difficulties, there are now commercial solutions such as 4D CT which allows to represent the internal anatomical changes that occur over the entire breathing cycle of these patients. The methods of reconstructing 4D CT can be found in an earlier section (CT simulation and motion quantification) and further details can be found in the literature [18]. However, it is important to men-

tion that challenges that still persist with these techniques. 4D CT-based imaging remains prone to misrepresentation of tumor volumes due to high respiratory breathing amplitudes and frequencies. Since this technique reconstructs patient data based on the specific time intervals and amplitudes, there are often cases where the two parameters remain irregular and erratic. Both the spatial representation of the tumor location as well as the extent of motion of the tumor can be misrepresented, which will then have an impact on the planning of the treatment margins. Such degradations will have a direct consequence on the temporal accuracy of dose calculations and thereby on the overall prognosis of the treatments. It is therefore quite necessary to validate the breathing cycles and reproducibility of motion-related patterns for these patients before selecting a given dataset to generate their treatment plans.

6.3.3 Mitigating Motion-related Uncertainties

There are three major strategies across the majority of particle therapy facilities that have been utilized to mitigate motion related uncertainties, which are summarized in a schema as seen in Figure 6.5. All these strategies discussed within the schematics have been discussed in sections that follow.

6.3.3.1 Generating Robust Plans

Generating robust treatment plan happens to be one of the foremost steps when it comes to managing the motion-related uncertainties in particle therapy-based treatments. Known to us the two most important ways to generate robust treatment plans are:

1 By selecting optimal beam angles and margins for preparing planning structures
2 By utilizing robust plan optimization capabilities of TPSs

Discussed below are some pertinent studies that describe various ways of generating robust plans in particle therapy for managing motion-related uncertainties.

6.3.3.1.1 *Optimal Beam Angle Selection and Margins for Preparing Planning Structures*

Whether generating a particle therapy treatment plan for a site with static tumors or for any moving tumors, the foremost rule of planning employs careful arrangements of beam angles and structure preparations for optimization. Originally suggested by Rietzel and Bert [55], the idea of selecting planning target volume margins specific to the orientation of the beam opened up several possibilities of generating plans with nearly uniform dose in the spread out Bragg peak regions. The concept of beam-specific PTVs was found to be extremely helpful in creating margins to compensate for range uncertainties along the

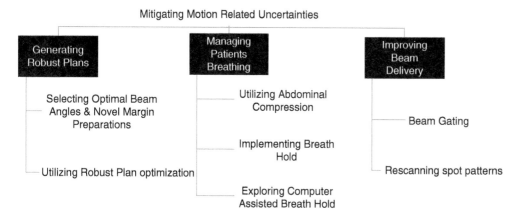

Figure 6.5   Schema showing various possible methods to mitigate motion related uncertainties in radiotherapy practice for particle therapy.

direction of the beams. The similar concept of beam-specific PTVs was then further extended to compensate for tissue misalignments due to tumor motion.

Particle therapy beams are extremely sensitive to tissue heterogeneities, objects that can cause variations in the path lengths of the particles, and hence when expanding the margins from the CTV to form a planning target volume margins, it is necessary to account for these factors that can influence the overall variations in the range of the particle beams. By selecting beam-specific margins which are estimated on the beam angle in use, one is able to generate planning target volumes that helps generating a nearly uniform dose within these moving tumors [56].

This methodology [56] was then further extended to the 4D CT dataset which allows to then incorporate phase-specific path length variations that can happen for a given beam angle. By using this information, one is then able to generate beam-specific planning volumes which will account for the motion-specific variations in the path lengths of the particles in that particular direction. Essentially such margins are four-dimensional beam-specific PTV (4D-bsPTV). At our own institution, we follow a specific procedure in how we generate all the planning volumes within our practice. Shown in Figure 6.6 is a typical workflow for lung-based proton treatment planning practiced at our own.

6.3.3.1.2   Robust Plan Optimization

Intensity-modulated proton therapy plans modulate the fluence from each beam in order to limit the dose to critical organs abutting the target volume. However, the cumulative doses from all the beams lead to a homogeneous dose to the entire targets. Due to such high modulation of individual beams, intensity-modulated particle therapy plans are highly susceptible to minute perturbations in the medium along the path of travel of these beams. There has now been much progress in the development of robust optimization in which the optimizer takes into account all possible scenarios of uncertainties

that could disturb the dose homogeneities within the target. There are now several algorithms that describe various ways of implementing 3D robust optimization [57]. The tools of robust optimization essentially incorporate setup and range-specific errors per beam, thereby accounting for all possible scenarios that could yield worst cases of either target coverages and/or sparing of the OARs. While it is beyond the scope of this current work, readers are encouraged to review separate literature that discusses methods such as minimax optimization [58] and voxel-wise robust optimization [57] and object-wise robust optimization [59,60]. When performed on a 3D CT dataset, any of these methods prove valuable and effective in generating robust treatment plans. However, all of these algorithms in their nascent state would fail to account for accurate delivery time structures of the beams, phase-based displacements of the target due to internal motion, and consequently calculate incorrect path lengths of particle beams due to periodical deformation of the anatomy due to internal breathing-related tumor motions. As discussed earlier, unless incorporated within the optimizer, it is nearly impossible to predict the phase-specific interplay effects which can lead to serious local under or over dosages to the target and nearby structures.

Keeping these factors in mind, there has now been advancements made in the field of 4D robust optimization [61] where the optimizer explicitly takes into account from all breathing phases the excursion of the tumor as well as any shape changes of the anatomy due to breathing. We believe readers and potential new users planning to adopt novel techniques such as 4D-based robust optimization should familiarize themselves with various methods of performing robust optimizations for moving targets as they have been shown to be better than 3D robust optimization. Liu et al. [61] have demonstrated that their methods of deforming of all 10 phases of doses with respect to their reference phases and by incorporating within the optimization the time structure of their beam delivery system allow to better optimize their spot pattern to correct phase and therefore providing more robust and homogeneous doses

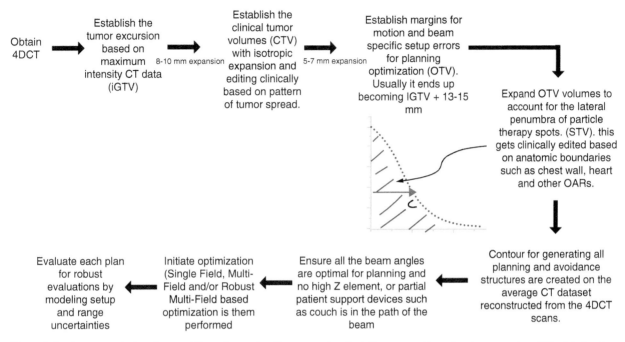

Figure 6.6 A treatment planning workflow at a proton therapy center depicting generation of various margins utilized in treatment planning of a lung tumor.

to the target. Similarly, Furukawa et al. [62] have shown online phase controlled rescanning of the carbon ion beams yields much better particle numbers per spot that get matched to correct delivery phases of their beams. Due to both the interplay effect and motion associated setup uncertainties, treatment of moving tumors with particle beam requires extremely sophisticated treatment planning platforms that can support verification of interplay effects and allow the planners to use powerful methods of motion-specific robust optimization of these plans. While we are on this subject of robust optimization, as discussed earlier, the algorithms for dose calculations also play an important role in establishing the overall accuracy of the treatment delivery. Hence, we would be amiss to not mention the ongoing developmental work in this field which is looking at incorporating motion-specific robust optimization of these moving targets using the Monte Carlo dose computational platform. It is believed that 4D-RO for heterogeneous targets when performed on a MC-based platform will yield utmost accurate and robust treatment plans for particle-based therapy.

6.3.3.1.3 *Treatment Planning for Moving Targets in Our Practice*

Irrespective of choice of MM, we utilize an in-house designed algorithm that suggests the option of either planning with either 3D robust optimization with free breathing techniques or utilizing DIBH in cases where the motion of the target exceeds 10 mm in either directions. There are also efforts underway developing tools that in the future would allow us to use the power of or using the 4D robust optimization methods [61]. Essentially depending upon the respiratory motion

amplitudes and the tumor volume a reasonable choice can be made to select what type of optimization routine would yield the most robust plan. The original plan irrespective of the type of algorithms are calculated on the average CT dataset and in addition two verification plans generated on breathing phase T0 and breathing phase T50 of the 4D CT dataset is also computed to make sure the plans are inherently robust to motion. The criterion for assessment of planning robustness is asking for 95% of the tumor coverage under all of the worst case scenarios. Usually two to three beams with margins suited for individual beams (discussed in Figure 6.6) is common practice in our clinic for planning lung and liver treatments.

6.3.3.2 Managing Patient Breathing

Besides utilizing tools made available through TPSs, there have been wide-spread studies and discussions over how patients' breathing could be managed through an aid of either mechanical support or computer and audio–video-assisted breath holds. Devices assisting with abdominal compressions and techniques of deep inspirational breath holds have been subject of ongoing clinical research and development. The usage and their limitations have been discussed in sections below.

6.3.3.2.1 *Abdominal Compression for Motion Management*

Mechanically compressing patient's abdominal region has shown to reduce the diaphragmatic motion, which then aids in reducing the amplitude of lung motions [35,63]. Although the abdominal compression techniques as studied and reported [64] show efficacies in reducing tumor motions that are closer to the diaphragm, there have also been some controversial findings related to these methods. One study analyzing the immobilization of the GTV with their daily CBCT showed that the interfractional variations in the localization of tumor were larger in cases with abdominal compression than those without, which made this technique less favorable for its widespread use [65]. Also, when utilizing any such methods that employ compression devices such as abdominal belt, there remains the risk of perturbing the particle beams if they end up being in the path of the beam angles necessary for treating the lesion. Hence, special care must be taken in order to avoid any high density objects that could perturb the overall range of these charged particles.

6.3.3.2.2 *Implementing Deep Inspiration Breath Hold*

One of the most widely accepted and robust methods to mitigate motion in the patients is by using breath hold or DIBH techniques using either an **audiovisual feedback** or by **computer-assisted breath control devices** which control the breath by temporarily blocking the airways. The managing of these breath hold scans has now been made easier through the use of audiovisual feedback mechanism in which a block of reflective marker is placed on the patient's abdominal area (closest) around the site of treatment or where as stable as possible (shown in Figure 6.7).

The infrared enabled monitoring system, seen in Figure 6.8a, then maps in real time the complete cycle of inhalation and exhalation during the time of simulation and allows the clinical team members to establish a zone of comfortable position with upper and lower threshold of breathing window, as depicted in Figure 6.8b, in which the patient is then coached to hold their breath. Typically, the most popular and widely used mechanism of this technique being inspirational phase for the breath hold [26].

Such a method proves advantageous in not only immobilization of the moving target(s) but also allow in creating radiological separation between the tumor site and the lung/heart volumes and thereby reducing the amount of volumes for

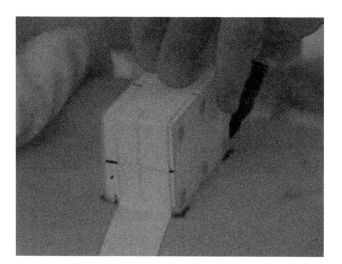

Figure 6.7 A block of reflective marker used for infrared enable monitoring patients' active breathing.

these OARs receiving high doses [66]. When utilizing these tools in the clinic, it is advisable to perform a few consecutive scans (three or more) in order to establish confidence in the breathing trends for these patients and also be able to confirm the reproducibility of the setup, as well as breath holding patterns. Patients who are able to voluntarily practice DIBH have shown substantial reduction in target motion [25,35,67]. Even though there remains residual motion between breathing phases, with the aid of robust optimization and when holding breath in a moderate and comfortable position, one can achieve superior dosimetry as well as overall treatment qualities [68]. Such a technique can be usefully applied to sites such as lungs, liver, and pancreatic tumors. There are also commercially available products such as active breathing controlled spirometers (ABCS) which is a computer controlled device that can temporarily immobilizes the patient's breathing pathways and thereby arresting the tumor motion [69,70].

6.3.3.3 Improved Beam Delivery

For patients who struggle to cooperate with the aforementioned methods such as breath holds, deep inspirational breath holds, and computer-assisted breathing there are some also advanced and alternate strategies of managing treatments for moving targets. Briefly discussed in this section are two main currently available techniques of *beam gating* and *rescanning spot patterns*.

6.3.3.3.1 *Beam Gating*

Beam gating is a motion mitigation technique in which beam delivery is limited to a fraction of the patient respiratory cycle [71,72]. Theoretically, this limits tumor motion to the subset of breathing phases during which beam is delivered. The most reproducible breathing phase(s) that remains stable for a duration of time is selected for a given patient at the time of CT simulation. From these scans, one is then able to extract an upper and a lower threshold which end up defining the window for management of beam delivery. Treatment delivery units for protons/carbon can then be coined through a transistor to a transistor logic circuit in order to gate the delivery of particle beams while the excursion of the tumor remains to be within the breathing cycle window. Constant monitoring of either through techniques like fluoroscopy [73] or through the infrared reflective marker tracking will be essential in order to make sure there are no drifts or irregularities in the breathing pattern for that patient on any given day of their treatments. Patient-specific challenges and machine characteristics such as the overall beam delivery times can affect the overall quality of the treatments. Beam gating is considered to be the most wide-spread method of mitigating motion related uncertainties when treating such tumors as in the case of lungs and liver. Since a large beam delivery time due to the machine characteristics or increased number of energy layers due to finer placements of spots during the treatment planning of these tumors will require prolonged treatments, utmost care

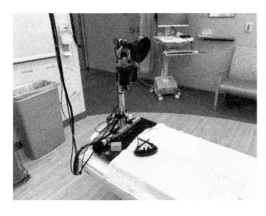
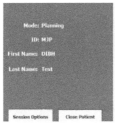
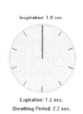
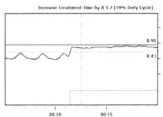

(a)   (b)

Figure 6.8 Example of an infrared-based monitoring system (left) used for monitoring patients' breathing cycles and a gating window (right) with thresholds to coach patients hold their breaths within the upper and lower thresholds based on each patient's comfort level.

must be taken when establishing treatment planning methods within each center. Readers are referred to the literature in order to advance their knowledge in understanding the intricate relationships between accelerator types, pulsed versus continuous beams, variable flat-top phase operations [35,74,75], and multiple-gated irradiation [74] to understand how could one further improve the gated treatments and further reduction of residual errors in gated treatments which are also subject to interplay effects (discussed earlier).

6.3.3.3.2 Rescanning Spot Patterns

Rescanning refers to any delivery technique that divides a treatment field into parts in such a way that the beam is scanned over portions of the target volume more than once. While beam delivery time is increased, the dose is delivered more evenly throughout the respiratory cycle and thereby reduces target-dose inhomogeneity caused by the interplay effect. Rescanning is commonly used with both proton [42] and carbon-ion [76] therapy systems. It has been reported that such scanning methods in conjunction with 4D robust optimization can significantly reduce the fluctuations in local doses due to interplay effects [77]. There are two distinct methods in which these patterns of particle beams could be delivered. Either these can delivered as a layer-by-layer rescans in which partial "packets" of dose are delivered at a fixed spot per energy layer before moving onto the next energy layer (isolayer rescanning). Or one can also execute rescanning as a volumetric repainting of the dose in which the entire volume of the target gets painted by a fraction of a dose per scan and repeated until the entire dose for the fraction is delivered (volumetric rescanning). Both methods are known to have their own clinical merits [35]. Volumetric rescanning may lead to increased delivery times depending upon the energy switching times. Managing large tumors with breath hold and isolayer rescanning have been widely used in particle therapy centers including our own at the time of this work.

At our institution, all patient treatments are delivered using an isolayer rescanning technique since, given the duration of our synchrotron's energy switching time (2 s), volumetric rescanning would greatly increase beam delivery time. We use the "cut and append" rescanning method provided by our TPS, which sets a maximum number of monitor units (MU) for each spot. When the tumor motion amplitude is less than 5 mm, the maximum is set to 0.04 MU, and when the tumor motion amplitude is greater than 5 mm, the maximum is set to 0.01 MU. Any spot above this limit is divided into several spots, each less than the maximum MU limit. These additional spots are appended to the end of the energy layer's spot delivery sequence for rescanning.

6.4 Treatment Delivery and Verification

6.4.1 Treatment Delivery

It is difficult to summarize treatment delivery and verification of treatments in particle therapy since there significant variations in procedures between different treatment sites. Owing to large differences in the particle therapy delivery solutions that are present across various institutions, it is beyond the scope of this work to discuss in detail the diverse aspects of treatment delivery with particles; however, we provide below a brief description of our own practice that we follow in delivering proton-based radiotherapy for tumors susceptible to motions.

Each day prior to the delivery of their treatments, the patients are immobilized using the devices that were prepared for them at the time of CT simulation. In our practice, we have benefitted from the use of CIVCO™ (Civco Radiotherapy, Orange City, IA, USA)-based wing boards along with BodyFix bags. Additional details of the immobilization have been discussed in earlier sections of this chapter and can also be seen in Figure 6.1. The patients are immobilized initially using the three point marks on the patient's skin and with the aid of in-room laser systems the tumor isocenter is localized prior to any X-ray-based image guidance. At our site, we utilize a customized solution for the camera system that utilizes infrared-based detection of the marker block which is placed on the patient's belly when performing DIBH-based treatments. DIBH patients are often coached before the respiratory position monitoring is enabled. Once comfortable depending upon the MM strategy needed, visual feedback is enabled to provide breathing window/gating information to the patient. At the onset of image guidance, the necessary screens showing patients' their breathing instructions are turned on and based on each patient's compliance the therapists then establish their IGRT-based corrections. For computing setup error margins during each session, we utilize a pair of flat panel-based X-ray detectors which have been synchronously coined to generate 3D anatomical information using a pair of 2D X-ray units recessed in floor (see Figure 6.9). The method is useful as it allows interlacing with low energy X rays for soft tissue visualizations and is capable of being operated in fluoroscopic modes when needed to image real-time soft tissue movements. Also, housed within one of the gantry units is a CT on rails system which allows for volumetric imaging of tumors involving soft tissues (liver/pancreas). Such a system proves to be very useful in certain clinical situations when the patients are presented in the clinic without any implanted surrogate markers in and around the tumor/tumor bed. Under those circumstances, a 3D (volumetric) imaging using CT on rails proves to be immensely helpful. There are other commercial solutions that are also available (such as cone beam CTs); however, due to the half-gantry rotation solution of our proton equipment, implementation of CBCTs was not possible.

Each solution available in our practice (2D–3D image guidance or CT on rails) is integrated with our MM equipment used for either breathing monitoring or for performing DIBH. Also, the process of image guidance needs to be carefully chosen as often times there are situations where patients are not able to reproduce their breathing patterns as established at the time of their simulations. Under such circumstances, there are risks of geometric misses. In our practice, we maintain necessary physics support to assist "re-establishing" of their breathing baselines (Figure 6.7) during the time of the treatment by adjusting the breathing specific gating window levels in situations where patients are not able to reproduce their breathing patterns established at the time of their simulation scans. Such a technique always requires re-imaging of the bony anatomy and also making sure proper localization of the tumor as per the instructions of the treatment planners who always mention the setup tolerances based on the beam and setup margins selected at the time of the planning. Once an IGRT is complete, the particle beams are turned on and where necessary they continue to remain gated with the breathing monitoring signals for robust

delivery of the treatment plans. A typical thoracic and lower GI malignancies can take anywhere between 45 min to an hour each day for the treatment setup and delivery of their radiotherapy plans. Hence, care must be taken in order to make sure appropriate checks are in place to make these patients feel comfortable throughout the course of delivery of their treatments.

6.4.2 Treatment Verification

For a majority of thoracic and liver lesions, our clinic has policies in place that mandate weekly CT scans to verify the robustness of treatment plans. Each 4D CT dataset collected in verification simulations is registered to the original 4D CT dataset and then a forward calculation of the treatment plan is computed on the verification 4D CT dataset in which the necessary targets and OAR contours get propagated from the original dataset and then verified by the physician group for their accurate projections. Each verification plan is then evaluated to ensure adequate target coverage and organ sparing is achieved. At our facility we like to maintain 95% of CTV coverage with at least 95% of the prescription dose as our basic evaluation metric to confirm adequate treatment delivery. Under circumstances where the verification plans fail to meet the tolerances of target coverage and/or OAR sparing, then per the physician's requests planners are required to regenerate a new plan in order to adapt and improve the cumulative doses for the delivery of their treatments. The process of replanning receives complete clinical support similar to that in the case of preparing an original treatment plans. Adaptive replanning for motion managed tumors is of paramount interests in the particle therapy community.

6.4.3 Patient-specific Quality Assurance for DIBH Treatments

At our institution, a measurement-based patient-specific quality assurance (PSQA) procedure is used to verify the delivery of every proton plan before patient treatment [78]. For DIBH treatments, this procedure includes manually testing beam gating during field delivery to verify the related plan settings in the TPS. During treatment field measurement for PSQA, a pause signal is sent through the gating system to ensure interruption of beam delivery. This is sufficient to ensure proper operation of the gating system during the patient's DIBH treatment.

6.5 Future Technologies

In the penultimate section of this chapter we touch upon four promising technologies related to IGRT and MM that are currently under development in a few centers and have not yet

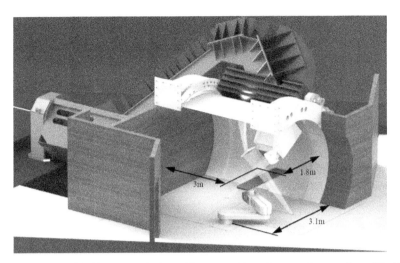

Figure 6.9 A half gantry solution with recessed imaging panels to perform 2D–3D image registrations at the treatment isocenter.

found their way into the mainstream of PBT. The list of topics presented here is far from exhaustive and reflects the interests of the authors.

6.5.1 Real-Time Tumor Tracking

The idea of imaging the actual excursion of tumors in all three dimensions with an aid of fluoroscopic imaging has been a subject of greater interest in the research frontiers of this topic. It is considered that the real-time volumetric imaging with precise tumor movements can allow for advanced treatment deliveries in which the radiological path length changes and spatiotemporal movements of the internal anatomy could be imaged in real time and adapted for improved sequencing of Bragg peaks for their accurate and precise deliveries. Although this subject is still in its infancy and will require ultrafast computing, significantly increased scanning speed, and a treatment delivery system to perform fast range adaptation, there has been significant effort put into development of this technology [79–82].

6.5.2 Proton Radiography and Proton CT

An imaging technique that has attracted significant interest in recent years is proton radiography, and proton CT in particular. The main attraction of this technique lies in mapping the stopping power directly, either in a single projection in the case of proton radiography or in three dimensions in the case of proton CT. In the 3D case, a direct mapping of the stopping power eliminates the need of converting HUs to proton stopping power, which is a source of range uncertainty. Few centers have accelerators powerful enough to generate beam energies high enough to penetrate every part of the patient's anatomy. Therefor, research efforts currently focus on the

brain, head and neck, and the lung. The types of detectors used in proton radiography are diverse and included Multi-layer Ionization Chambers (MLICs) [83] silicon pixel detectors [84] and calorimeters in conjunction with particle trackers [85].

6.5.3 High-frequency Percussive Ventilation

High-frequency ventilation (HFV) can be applied in radiotherapy to reduce respiratory motion to negligible levels during treatment [86,87]. HFV would be particularly beneficial for scanned particle therapy of thoracic treatment sites as it has the potential to virtually eliminate the interplay effect without appreciable increase in beam delivery time. The latest technology, high-frequency percussive ventilation (HFPV), uses high-frequency but low-pressure bursts of air that can be adapted to create an apnea-like state at full inspiration without causing barotrauma [88]. The patient interface is noninvasive and HFPV does not require general anesthesia [89,90]. Healthy volunteers have been able to achieve breath holds of up to 20 min, achieved motion amplitude variation as small as 1 mm, and were able to tolerate several successive breath holds [88–91]. In one study, four out of five patients (including lung cancer patients) were able to tolerate HFPV and achieve breath holds for 5–10 min, allowing treatment in an apnea-like state [88]. In addition to its therapy applications, HFPV has also been used to reduce motion blurring to improve lung tumor delineation in PET/CT [92] and increase spatial resolution in chest MRI [93].

6.5.4 Prompt Gamma and PET Activation Imaging for Proton Range Verification

PBT is plagued by range uncertainty and there is a clinical need for verifying proton range *in vivo*. Two imaging techniques have emerged to achieve this goal. One is positron emission tomography (PET) [94–96], and the other is prompt gamma ray detection [97]. Both methods rely on the detection of gamma rays. In the case of PET, high-energy photons are generated in the destruction of a positron with an electron in a matter–antimatter interaction. The positron activity is generated in nuclear interaction of the protons with the patient's tissues. The positron activity persists for a few minutes, until the positron emitters have decayed to undetectable levels of have been washed out by the patients' natural blood flow. In the case of prompt gamma imaging high-energy photons (gamma rays) are generated in nuclear interactions between protons and nuclei in the patient's tissue. The nuclei are lifted into an excited state and subsequently emit their excess energy quasi instantaneously in the form of gamma rays.

In both approaches, the spatial distribution of photon emitters is imaged in highly sensitive gamma detectors, which in the case of PET may take the form of a commercially available PET CT. The distribution of photon emitters in the patient is then correlated to the range of the protons through Monte Carlo modeling. Neither approaches have found wide application in clinical practice yet. In the case of prompt gamma this failure may be traced to the relatively low prompt gamma signal which is at the edge of what can to date be reliably detected with today's detector technology. In addition, the measurement is confounded by the presence of neutrons. In the case of PET, biologic washout presents a significant barrier to widespread adoption.

6.6 Conclusions

IGRT and MM for PBT are far from fully developed, and much work remains to be done to fully address the significant challenges in appropriately addressing the heightened requirements for IGRT and MM in PBT compared to the corresponding requirements in external beam therapy with photons. As pointed out in the introduction section of this chapter, there once was a time when PBT was far ahead in image guidance relative to photons. However, these days have long passed. PBT equipment vendors have only recently introduced 3D volumetric imaging and are beginning to offer 4D volumetric imaging at the isocenter of the treatment room, thereby catching up with what has been the standard in photon beam therapy for approximately a decade. MM tools in commercially available PBT treatment planning software are often still in rudimentary state and PBT centers must rely on in-house developed software to address the challenges associated with planning PBT for moving targets.

In this chapter, we have aimed to give an overview of the tools and techniques that are available for IGRT and MM in PBT with a heavy emphasis on what we are doing in this regard at the Mayo Clinic in Arizona. A consensus is forming in the PBT community concerning what tools are needed and how to address these issues. The Report of AAPM Task Group 290: Respiratory Motion Management for Particle Therapy should be helpful in solidifying this consensus.

Acknowledgments

We are grateful to the other physicists who have developed the MM and IGRT workflows used in our department. We would like to specifically thank Dr. Wei Liu, Dr. Yanle Hu, Dr. Xiaoning Ding, and Dr. Chris Beltran for useful discussions that helped us prepare this literature. Providing high-quality proton radiotherapy procedures is necessarily a community effort, and we wish to express our appreciation to all of the physicians, physicists and physicist assistants, dosimetrists, therapists, and administrators at Mayo Clinic Arizona whose collective efforts ensure that our patients receive the best possible care. We also wish to acknowledge Mayo Clinic Scientific Publications for their assistance with our literature research.

References

1 Goitein, M., Abrams, M., Rowell, D., Pollari, H., and Wiles, J. (1983). Multi-dimensional treatment planning: II. Beam's eye-view, back projection, and projection through CT sections. *International Journal of Radiation Oncology, Biology, Physics* 9 (6): 789–797.

2 Suit, H., Chen, G., Bortfeld, T. et al. (2017). Michael Goitein, 1939-2016: A giant of modern medical physics. *International Journal of Radiation Oncology, Biology, Physics* 97 (4): 654–658.

3 Day, M.J. (1950). A note on the calculation of dose in X-ray fields. *The British Journal of Radiology* 23 (270): 368–369.

4 Das, I.J., Cheng, C.-W., Cao, M., and Johnstone, P.A.S. (2016). Computed tomography imaging parameters for inhomogeneity correction in radiation treatment planning. *Journal Of Medical Physics / Association of Medical Physicists of India* 41 (1): 3–11.

5 Bush, D.A., Slater, J.D., Shin, B.B., Cheek, G., Miller, D.W., and Slater, J.M. (2004). Hypofractionated proton beam radiotherapy for stage I lung cancer. *Chest* 126 (4): 1198–1203.

6 Fiorino, C., Reni, M., Bolognesi, A., Bonini, A., Cattaneo, G.M., and Calandrino, R. (1998). Set-up error in supine-positioned patients immobilized with two different modalities during conformal radiotherapy of prostate cancer.

Radiotherapy and Oncology: Journal of the European Society for Therapeutic Radiology and Oncology 49 (2): 133–141.

7 Herfarth, K., Debus, J., Lohr, F. et al. (2000). Extracranial stereotactic radiation therapy: Set-up accuracy of patients treated for liver metastases. *International Journal of Radiation Oncology, Biology, Physics* 46 (2): 329–335.

8 Negoro, Y., Nagata, Y., Aoki, T. et al. (2001). The effectiveness of an immobilization device in conformal radiotherapy for lung tumor: Reduction of respiratory tumor movement and evaluation of the daily setup accuracy. *International Journal of Radiation Oncology, Biology, Physics* 50 (4): 889–898.

9 van der Merwe, D., Van Dyk, J., Healy, B. et al. (2017). Accuracy requirements and uncertainties in radiotherapy: A report of the international atomic energy agency. *Acta Oncologica* 56 (1): 1–6.

10 Halperin, R., Roa, W., Field, M., Hanson, J., and Murray, B. (1999). Setup reproducibility in radiation therapy for lung cancer: A comparison between T-bar and expanded foam immobilization devices. *International Journal of Radiation Oncology, Biology, Physics* 43 (1): 211–216.

11 Potters, L., Kavanagh, B., Galvin, J.M. et al. (2010). American Society for Therapeutic Radiology and Oncology (ASTRO) and American College of Radiology (ACR) practice guideline for the performance of stereotactic body radiation therapy. *International Journal of Radiation Oncology*Biology*Physics* 76 (2): 326–332.

12 Sahgal, A., Roberge, D., Schellenberg, D. et al. (2012). The Canadian Association of Radiation Oncology scope of practice guidelines for lung, liver and spine stereotactic body radiotherapy. *Clinical Oncology* 24 (9): 629–639.

13 Vedam, S., Keall, P., Kini, V., Mostafavi, H., Shukla, H., and Mohan, R. (2002). Acquiring a four-dimensional computed tomography dataset using an external respiratory signal. *Physics in Medicine and Biology* 48 (1): 45.

14 Ford, E.C., Mageras, G.S., Yorke, E., and Ling, C.C. (2003). Respiration-correlated spiral CT: A method of measuring respiratory-induced anatomic motion for radiation treatment planning. *Medical Physics* 30 (1): 88–97.

15 Low, D.A., Nystrom, M., Kalinin, E. et al. (2003). A method for the reconstruction of four-dimensional synchronized CT scans acquired during free breathing. *Medical Physics* 30 (6): 1254–1263.

16 Pan, T. (2005). Comparison of helical and cine acquisitions for 4D-CT imaging with multislice CT. *Medical Physics* 32 (2): 627–634.

17 Rietzel, E., Pan, T., and Chen, G.T.Y. (2005). Four-dimensional computed tomography: Image formation and clinical protocol. *Medical Physics* 32 (4): 874–889.

18 Wink, N.M., Panknin, C., and Solberg, T.D. (2006). Phase versus amplitude sorting of 4D-CT data. *Journal Of Applied Clinical Medical Physics / American College of Medical Physics* 7 (1): 77–85.

19 Vásquez, A., Runz, A., Echner, G., Sroka-Perez, G., and Karger, C. (2012). Comparison of two respiration monitoring systems for 4D imaging with a Siemens CT using a new dynamic breathing phantom. *Physics in Medicine and Biology* 57 (9): N131.

20 Seppenwoolde, Y., Shirato, H., Kitamura, K. et al. (2002). Precise and real-time measurement of 3D tumor motion in lung due to breathing and heartbeat, measured during radiotherapy. *International Journal of Radiation Oncology • Biology • Physics* 53 (4): 822–834.

21 Li, H., Noel, C., Garcia-Ramirez, J. et al. (2012). Clinical evaluations of an amplitude-based binning algorithm for 4DCT reconstruction in radiation therapy. *Medical Physics* 39 (2): 922–932.

22 Keall, P., Starkschall, G., Shukla, H. et al. (2004). Acquiring 4D thoracic CT scans using a multislice helical method. *Physics in Medicine and Biology* 49 (10): 2053.

23 Yamamoto, T., Langner, U., Loo, B.W., Jr, Shen, J., and Keall, P.J. (2008). Retrospective analysis of artifacts in four-dimensional CT images of 50 abdominal and thoracic radiotherapy patients. *International Journal of Radiation Oncology, Biology, Physics* 72 (4): 1250–1258.

24 Feng, M., Balter, J.M., Normolle, D. et al. (2009). Characterization of pancreatic tumor motion using cine MRI: surrogates for tumor position should be used with caution. *International Journal of Radiation Oncology, Biology, Physics* 74 (3): 884–891.

25 Hanley, J., Debois, M.M., Mah, D. et al. (1999). Deep inspiration breath-hold technique for lung tumors: The potential value of target immobilization and reduced lung density in dose escalation. *International Journal of Radiation Oncology*Biology*Physics* 45 (3): 603–611.

26 Rosenzweig, K.E., Hanley, J., Mah, D. et al. (2000). The deep inspiration breath-hold technique in the treatment of inoperable non–small-cell lung cancer. *International Journal of Radiation Oncology*Biology*Physics* 48 (1): 81–87.

27 Mah, D., Hanley, J., Rosenzweig, K.E. et al. (2000). Technical aspects of the deep inspiration breath-hold technique in the treatment of thoracic cancer. *International Journal of Radiation Oncology*Biology*Physics* 48 (4): 1175–1185.

28 Mageras, G.S. and Yorke, E. (2004). Deep inspiration breath hold and respiratory gating strategies for reducing organ motion in radiation treatment. *Seminars in Radiation Oncology* 14 (1): 65–75.

29 Pedroni, E., Bacher, R., Blattmann, H. et al. (1995). The 200-MeV proton therapy project at the Paul Scherrer Institute: Conceptual design and practical realization. *Medical Physics* 22 (1): 37–53.

30 Gillin, M.T., Sahoo, N., Bues, M. et al. (2010). Commissioning of the discrete spot scanning proton beam delivery system at the University of Texas M.D. Anderson Cancer Center, Proton Therapy Center, Houston. *Medical Physics* 37 (1): 154–163.

31 Lomax, A., Boehringer, T., Coray, A. et al. (2001). Intensity modulated proton therapy: A clinical example. *Medical Physics* 28 (3): 317–324.

32 Stroom, J.C. and Heijmen, B.J.M. (2002). Geometrical uncertainties, radiotherapy planning margins, and the ICRU-62 report. *Radiotherapy and Oncology: Journal of the European Society for Therapeutic Radiology and Oncology* 64 (1): 75–83.

33 Hong, L., Goitein, M., Bucciolini, M. et al. (1996). A pencil beam algorithm for proton dose calculations. *Physics in Medicine and Biology* 41 (8): 1305.

34 Grassberger, C., Daartz, J., Dowdell, S., Ruggieri, T., Sharp, G., and Paganetti, H. (2014). Quantification of proton dose calculation accuracy in the lung. *International Journal of Radiation Oncology, Biology, Physics* 89 (2): 424–430.

35 Han, Y. (2019). Current status of proton therapy techniques for lung cancer. *Radiation Oncology Journal* 37 (4): 232–248.

36 Widesott, L., Lorentini, S., Fracchiolla, F., Farace, P., and Schwarz, M. (2018). Improvements in pencil beam scanning proton therapy dose calculation accuracy in brain tumor cases with a commercial Monte Carlo algorithm. *Physics in Medicine and Biology* 63 (14): 145016.

37 Saini, J., Traneus, E., Maes, D. et al. (2018). Advanced proton beam dosimetry Part I: Review and performance evaluation of dose calculation algorithms. *Translational Lung Cancer Research* 7 (2): 171–179.

38 Bortfeld, T., Jokivarsi, K., Goitein, M., Kung, J., and Jiang, S.B. (2002). Effects of intra-fraction motion on IMRT dose delivery: Statistical analysis and simulation. *Physics in Medicine and Biology* 47 (13): 2203.

39 Dowdell, S., Grassberger, C., Sharp, G.C., and Paganetti, H. (2013). Interplay effects in proton scanning for lung: a 4D Monte Carlo study assessing the impact of tumor and beam delivery parameters. *Physics in Medicine and Biology* 58 (12): 4137–4156.

40 Bert, C., Grozinger, S.O., and Rietzel, E. (2008). Quantification of interplay effects of scanned particle beams and moving targets. *Physics in Medicine and Biology* 53 (9): 2253–2265.

41 Grassberger, C., Dowdell, S., Lomax, A. et al. (2013). Motion interplay as a function of patient parameters and spot size in spot scanning proton therapy for lung cancer. *International Journal of Radiation Oncology, Biology, Physics* 86 (2): 380–386.

42 Phillips, M.H., Pedroni, E., Blattmann, H., Boehringer, T., Coray, A., and Scheib, S. (1992). Effects of respiratory motion on dose uniformity with a charged particle scanning method. *Physics in Medicine and Biology* 37 (1): 223.

43 Lambert, J., Suchowerska, N., McKenzie, D., and Jackson, M. (2005). Intrafractional motion during proton beam scanning. *Physics in Medicine and Biology* 50 (20): 4853.

44 Kraus, K., Heath, E., and Oelfke, U. (2011). Dosimetric consequences of tumour motion due to respiration for a scanned proton beam. *Physics in Medicine and Biology* 56 (20): 6563.

45 Knopf, A.-C., Hong, T.S., and Lomax, A. (2011). Scanned proton radiotherapy for mobile targets – The effectiveness of re-scanning in the context of different treatment planning approaches and for different motion characteristics. *Physics in Medicine and Biology* 56 (22): 7257.

46 Engwall, E., Glimelius, L., and Hynning, E. (2018). Effectiveness of different rescanning techniques for scanned proton radiotherapy in lung cancer patients. *Physics in Medicine and Biology* 63 (9): 095006.

47 Liu, W., Liao, Z., Schild, S.E. et al. (2015). Impact of respiratory motion on worst-case scenario optimized intensity modulated proton therapy for lung cancers. *Practical Radiation Oncology* 5 (2): e77–e86.

48 Chang, J.Y., Zhang, X., Knopf, A. et al. (2017). Consensus guidelines for implementing pencil-beam scanning proton therapy for thoracic malignancies on behalf of the PTCOG thoracic and lymphoma subcommittee. *International Journal of Radiation Oncology • Biology • Physics* 99 (1): 41–50.

49 Paganetti, H., Jiang, H., and Trofimov, A. (2005). 4D Monte Carlo simulation of proton beam scanning: Modelling of variations in time and space to study the interplay between scanning pattern and time-dependent patient geometry. *Physics in Medicine and Biology* 50 (5): 983.

50 Shen, J., Tryggestad, E., Younkin, J.E. et al. (2017). Technical Note: Using experimentally determined proton spot scanning timing parameters to accurately model beam delivery time. *Medical Physics* 44 (10): 5081–5088.

51 Younkin, J.E., Bues, M., Sio, T.T. et al. (2018). Multiple energy extraction reduces beam delivery time for a synchrotron-based proton spot-scanning system. *Advances in Radiation Oncology* 3 (3): 412–420.

52 Johnson, J.E., Beltran, C.Chan, W., and Tseung, H. et al. (2019). Highly efficient and sensitive patient-specific quality assurance for spot-scanned proton therapy. *PLoS One* 14 (2): e0212412.

53 Pfeiler, T., Bäumer, C., Engwall, E., Geismar, D., Spaan, B., and Timmermann, B. (2018). Experimental validation of a 4D dose calculation routine for pencil beam scanning proton therapy. *Zeitschrift Für Medizinische Physik* 28 (2): 121–133.

54 Younkin, J.E., Morales, D.H., Shen, J. et al. (2019). Clinical validation of a ray-casting analytical dose engine for spot scanning proton delivery systems. *Technology in Cancer Research & Treatment* 18: 1533033819887182.

55 Rietzel, E. and Bert, C. (2010). Respiratory motion management in particle therapy. *Medical Physics* 37 (2): 449–460.

56 Park, P.C., Zhu, X.R., Lee, A.K. et al. (2012). A beam-specific planning target volume (PTV) design for proton therapy to account for setup and range uncertainties. *International Journal of Radiation Oncology, Biology, Physics* 82 (2): e329-e336.

57 Unkelbach, J., Chan, T.C., and Bortfeld, T. (2007). Accounting for range uncertainties in the optimization of intensity modulated proton therapy. *Physics in Medicine and Biology* 52 (10): 2755.

58 Fredriksson, A., Forsgren, A., and Hårdemark, B. (2011). Minimax optimization for handling range and setup uncertainties in proton therapy. *Medical Physics* 38 (3): 1672–1684.

59 Chen, W., Unkelbach, J., Trofimov, A. et al. (2012). Including robustness in multi-criteria optimization for intensity-modulated proton therapy. *Physics in Medicine and Biology* 57 (3): 591.

60 Liu, W., Li, Y., Li, X., Cao, W., and Zhang, X. (2012). Influence of robust optimization in intensity-modulated proton therapy with different dose delivery techniques. *Medical Physics* 39 (6Part1): 3089–3101.

61 Liu, W., Schild, S.E., Chang, J.Y., Liao, Z., Y-h, C., and Wen, Z. (2016 May 1). Exploratory study of 4D versus 3D robust optimization in intensity modulated proton therapy for lung Cancer. *International Journal of Radiation Oncology, Biology, Physics* 95 (1):523–533. doi: 10.1016/j.ijrobp.2015.11.002. Epub 2015 Nov 10. PMID: 26725727; PMCID: PMC4834263.

62 Furukawa, T., Inaniwa, T., Sato, S. et al. (2010). Moving target irradiation with fast rescanning and gating in particle therapy. *Medical Physics* 37 (9): 4874–4879.

63 Rasheed, A., Jabbour, S.K., Rosenberg, S. et al. (2016). Motion and volumetric change as demonstrated by 4DCT: The effects of abdominal compression on the GTV, lungs, and heart in lung cancer patients. *Practical Radiation Oncology* 6 (5): 352–359.

64 Han, C., Sampath, S., Schultheisss, T.E., and Wong, J.Y. (2017). Variations of target volume definition and daily target volume localization in stereotactic body radiotherapy for early-stage non–small cell lung cancer patients under abdominal compression. *Medical Dosimetry: Official Journal of the American Association of Medical Dosimetrists* 42 (2): 116–121.

65 Mampuya, W.A., Nakamura, M., Matsuo, Y. et al. (2013). Interfraction variation in lung tumor position with abdominal compression during stereotactic body radiotherapy. *Medical Physics* 40 (9): 091718.

66 Remouchamps, V.M., Vicini, F.A., Sharpe, M.B., Kestin, L.L., Martinez, A.A., and Wong, J.W. (2003). Significant reductions in heart and lung doses using deep inspiration breath hold with active breathing control and intensity-modulated radiation therapy for patients treated with locoregional breast irradiation. *International Journal of Radiation Oncology, Biology, Physics* 55 (2): 392–406.

67 Rydhög, J.S., De Blanck, S.R., Josipovic, M. et al. (2017). Target position uncertainty during visually guided deep-inspiration breath-hold radiotherapy in locally advanced lung cancer. *Radiotherapy and Oncology: Journal of the European Society for Therapeutic Radiology and Oncology* 123 (1): 78–84.

68 Lee, D., Greer, P.B., Lapuz, C. et al. (2017). Audiovisual biofeedback guided breath-hold improves lung tumor position reproducibility and volume consistency. *Advances in Radiation Oncology* 2 (3): 354–362.

69 Burnett, S.S., Sixel, K.E., Cheung, P.C., and Hoisak, J.D. (2008). A study of tumor motion management in the conformal radiotherapy of lung cancer. *Radiotherapy and Oncology: Journal of the European Society for Therapeutic Radiology and Oncology* 86 (1): 77–85.

70 Cheung, P.C., Sixel, K.E., Tirona, R., and Ung, Y.C. (2003). Reproducibility of lung tumor position and reduction of lung mass within the planning target volume using active breathing control (ABC). *International Journal of Radiation Oncology, Biology, Physics* 57 (5): 1437–1442.

71 Minohara, S., Kanai, T., Endo, M., Noda, K., and Kanazawa, M. (2000). Respiratory gated irradiation system for heavy-ion radiotherapy. *International Journal of Radiation Oncology*Biology*Physics* 47 (4): 1097–1103.

72 Lu, H.-M., Brett, R., Sharp, G. et al. (2007). A respiratory-gated treatment system for proton therapy. *Medical Physics* 34 (8): 3273–3278.

73 Matsuura, T., Miyamoto, N., Shimizu, S. et al. (2013). Integration of a real-time tumor monitoring system into gated proton spot-scanning beam therapy: An initial phantom study using patient tumor trajectory data. *Medical Physics* 40: 7.

74 Yamada, T., Miyamoto, N., Matsuura, T. et al. (2016). Optimization and evaluation of multiple gating beam delivery in a synchrotron-based proton beam scanning system using a real-time imaging technique. *Physics in Medicine \& Biology* 32 (7): 932–937.

75 Ciocca, M., Mirandola, A., Molinelli, S. et al. (2016). Commissioning of the 4-D treatment delivery system for organ motion management in synchrotron-based scanning ion beams. *Physics in Medicine \& Biology* 32 (12): 1667–1671.

76 Furukawa, T., Inaniwa, T., Sato, S. et al. (2007). Design study of a raster scanning system for moving target irradiation in heavy-ion radiotherapy. *Medical Physics* 34 (3): 1085–1097.

77 Schätti, A., Meer, D., and Lomax, A.J. (2014). First experimental results of motion mitigation by continuous line scanning of protons. *Physics in Medicine and Biology* 59 (19): 5707.

78 Hernandez Morales, D., Shan, J., Liu, W. et al. (2019). Automation of routine elements for spot-scanning proton patient-specific quality assurance. *Medical Physics* 46 (1): 5–14.

79 Grözinger, S.O., Rietzel, E., Li, Q., Bert, C., Haberer, T., and Kraft, G. (2006). Simulations to design an online motion compensation system for scanned particle beams. *Physics in Medicine and Biology* 51 (14): 3517.

80 Lüchtenborg, R., Saito, N., Durante, M., and Bert, C. (2011). Experimental verification of a real-time compensation functionality for dose changes due to target motion in scanned particle therapy. *Medical Physics* 38 (10): 5448–5458.

81 Eley, J.G., Newhauser, W.D., Lüchtenborg, R., Graeff, C., and Bert, C. (2014). 4D optimization of scanned ion beam tracking therapy for moving tumors. *Physics in Medicine and Biology* 59 (13): 3431.

82 Zhang, Y., Knopf, A., Tanner, C., and Lomax, A. (2014). Online image guided tumour tracking with scanned proton beams: A comprehensive simulation study. *Physics in Medicine and Biology* 59 (24): 7793.

83 Hammi, A., König, S., Weber, D.C., Poppe, B., and Lomax, A.J. (2018). Patient positioning verification for proton therapy using proton radiography. *Physics in Medicine and Biology* 63 (24): 245009.

84 Gehrke, T., Gallas, R., Jäkel, O., and Martišíková, M. (2018). Proof of principle of helium-beam radiography using silicon pixel detectors for energy deposition measurement, identification, and tracking of single ions. *Medical Physics* 45 (2): 817–829.

85 Plautz, T., Bashkirov, V., Feng, V. et al. (2014). 200 MeV proton radiography studies with a hand phantom using a prototype proton CT scanner. *IEEE Transactions on Medical Imaging* 33 (4): 875–881.

86 Chang, H.K. and Harf, A. (1984). High-frequency ventilation: A review. *Respiration Physiology* 57 (2): 135–152.

87 Bert, C. and Durante, M. (2011). Motion in radiotherapy: Particle therapy. *Physics in Medicine and Biology* 56 (16): R113.

88 Péguret, N., Ozsahin, M., Zeverino, M. et al. (2016). Apnea-like suppression of respiratory motion: First evaluation in radiotherapy. *Radiotherapy and Oncology: Journal of the European Society for Therapeutic Radiology and Oncology* 118 (2): 220–226.

89 Ogna, A., Bernasconi, M., Belmondo, B. et al. (2017). Prolonged apnea supported by high-frequency noninvasive ventilation: A pilot study. *American Journal of Respiratory and Critical Care Medicine* 195 (7): 958–960.

90 Sala, I.M., Nair, G.B., Maurer, B., and Guerrero, T.M. (2019). High frequency percussive ventilation for respiratory immobilization in radiotherapy. *Technical Innovations & Patient Support in Radiation Oncology* 9: 8–12.

91 Audag, N., Van Ooteghem, G., Liistro, G., Salini, A., Geets, X., and Reychler, G. (2019). Intrapulmonary percussive ventilation leading to 20-minutes breath-hold potentially useful for radiation treatments. *Radiotherapy and Oncology: Journal of the European Society for Therapeutic Radiology and Oncology* 141: 292–295.

92 Prior, J.O., Peguret, N., Pomoni, A. et al. (2016). Reduction of respiratory motion during PET/CT by pulsatile-flow ventilation: a first clinical evaluation. *Journal of Nuclear Medicine: Official Publication, Society of Nuclear Medicine* 57 (3): 416–419.

93 Beigelman-Aubry, C., Peguret, N., Stuber, M. et al. (2017). Chest-MRI under pulsatile flow ventilation: A new promising technique. *PLoS One* 12 (6): e0178807.

94 Handrack, J., Tessonnier, T., Chen, W. et al. (2017). Sensitivity of post treatment positron emission tomography/ computed tomography to detect inter-fractional range variations in scanned ion beam therapy. *Acta Oncologica* 56 (11): 1451–1458.

95 Bauer, J., Chen, W., Nischwitz, S. et al. (2018). Improving the modelling of irradiation-induced brain activation for in vivo PET verification of proton therapy. *Radiotherapy and Oncology: Journal of the European Society for Therapeutic Radiology and Oncology* 128 (1): 101–108.

96 Helmbrecht, S., Enghardt, W., Parodi, K. et al. (2013). Analysis of metabolic washout of positron emitters produced during carbon ion head and neck radiotherapy. *Medical Physics* 40 (9): 091918.

97 Verburg, J.M., Riley, K., Bortfeld, T., and Seco, J. (2013). Energy-and time-resolved detection of prompt gamma-rays for proton range verification. *Physics in Medicine and Biology* 58 (20): L37.

7

Advanced Particle Therapy Delivery

A Review of Advanced Techniques for Particle Therapy Delivery

Peyman Kabolizadeh M.D., PhD., Xuanfeng Ding Ph.D., and Xiaoqiang Li Ph.D.

Department of Radiation Oncology, Beaumont Health System, Oakland University William Beaumont School of Medicine.
*Corresponding Author: Peyman Kabolizadeh MD/PhD

TABLE OF CONTENTS

7.1 Introduction

7.1.1 Advanced Proton Therapy Delivery

In 1946, Robert Wilson first proposed the use of accelerated protons and heavier ions in radiation treatment for human cancers. His hypothesis relied upon the Bragg peak characteristic of particle therapy in which the deposited dose increases quite sharply and yields a distinct, localized high-dose region that could potentially be used to concentrate a conformal dose to the tumor. Delivery of proton therapy matured over recent years from single scattering and double scattering into intensity-modulated proton therapy pencil beam scanning (IMPT-PBS), which has been used in clinics more often. IMPT-PBS is a more efficient and more conformal way of delivering proton therapy to patients as there is no need to use brass aperture, range compensators, or range modulators. In order to enhance efficiency, conformity, and clinical use, more concepts have been introduced such as line scanning, proton arc therapy, flash therapy (reviewed in a separate chapter), linear energy transfer (LET)/RBE optimization, proton imaging, and prompt gamma. We will cover IMPT and arc therapy in detail follow by discussing other new concepts briefly.

7.2 Intensity-Modulated Proton Therapy

Given the finite penetration range of proton particles and limited scatter, proton therapy delivers superior dose distributions including dose conformity, homogeneity, and sparing of

---

the adjacent healthy tissues. In recent years, another feature of proton particle that helped molding its future of clinical use was its positive charge which enables magnetic scanning of narrow pencil beams. Using pencil beam scanning technology, a narrow beam of protons enters the patient from different sites and magnetic scanning angles them via deflecting the beams (Figure 7.1).

Historically, the first case of proton pencil beam scanning was reported from Japan using a low energy 70-MeV proton beam which was not adequate to be used in clinical setting. Subsequently, significant development was made in PBS technology with pion therapy program at the Paul Scherrer Institute (PSI, formerly SIN) which resulted in treating about 500 patients between 1981 and 1992 [1]. The study reported treating patients using dynamic beam delivery using 60 converging pion beams by moving the patients in three dimensions using water bolus and CT-based inverse planning system [2,3]. This helped to develop this technique further for clinical treatment at PSI which started in 1990s for treatment of deep seeded tumors. Proton beam scanning is a precise efficient method to deliver treatment as no field specific hardware is needed and all fields are being delivered without any entry into the treatment room. However, the disadvantage of beam scanning is its higher sensitivity to organ motion and having a less sharp penumbra. Further improvements in proton therapy include motion management and development of proton arc therapy.

7.2.1 Brief Physics of IMPT-PBS

Pencil beam scanning technology delivers the dose to the target via multiple small physical proton beamlets with the help of a magnetic field in 3D conformal dose distribution. This technology does not need patient-specific hardware, which reduces the manpower, cost, storage, and mounting of hardware such as collimators and compensators. This results in increase of treatment efficiency, decreased treatment time, and therefore increasing patient throughput. The region of 100% dose can be strictly confined to the target via PBS which is in contrast to modulation of a spread-out Bragg peak (SOBP)

in passive scattering system which results in spillage of unwanted dose. Hence, this is an important concept especially in treating targets with complex shapes and geometry (Figure 7.1). Another advantage of PBS is reduction of proton interaction with field-specific devices which ultimately results in minimizing the neutron dose to the patient. This can be an important property, especially in treating pediatrics to reduce the risk of secondary malignancies. Moreover, given the simultaneous optimization of spot intensities, IMPT encompasses more degrees of freedom in predicting more conformal treatment planning. Therefore, the advantages of IMPT consist of designing the dose distribution to targets with convexities and complex 3D structure while sparing adjacent critical normal organs.

7.2.2 Limitations of IMPT Use in Clinical Practice

7.2.2.1 Target Motion

It is important to note that pencil beam scanning is sensitive to organ motion during delivery which reduces the homogeneity of the dose to the target volume. Consequently, initially only well-immobilized tumors were treated with IMPT. Several approaches have been developed to address this issue. One solution is to repaint dose multiple times over a period of organ motion to reach an averaging of the dose. Additional number of times to repaint would cause more averaging of the dose and therefore a better tumor motion control, however, with the caveat of prolonging of the treatment time. Other solutions include reducing the organ motion through management of breathing cycle or via synchronizing the beam delivery with the motion or phases of breathing cycle.

Furthermore, there are two modes that pencil beam scanning can be calculated. The first is called single field uniform dose (SFUD) planning in which the fluences are calculated and optimized for each field individually while achieving a homogeneous dose covering the whole target volume from each individual field. IMPT, on the other hand, consists of number of individually inhomogeneous fields calculated in a

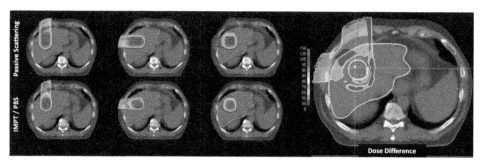

Figure 7.1 Example of comparison between pencil beam scanning (IMPT) versus passive beam scattering.

way that, when combined, results in a homogenous and conformal dose to the target volume. Hence, in full IMPT, not every beam covers the whole target volume; therefore, the effect of motion in delivering dose is less evident when using SFUD [4].

While delivering dose using pencil beam technology in tumors with motions, every effort should be made to decrease the target motion along with concept of repainting while using SFUD. If full IMPT planning is used, the risk of undercovering the target with hot and cold spots should be taken into account with its associated clinical consequences.

7.2.2.2 Robustness

As it was mentioned above, proton particles lose their energy as they penetrate into the matter, exhibiting Bragg peaks with low entrance dose and negligible dose beyond the range. However, proton particles are sensitive to tissue density variations in the beam path. The planned dose distribution with steep gradient could easily get deteriorated by different types of uncertainties and ultimately diminish its effectiveness. These uncertainties consist of systematic and random uncertainties associated with patient immobilization, patient daily setup, proton range, intra- and inter-fractional motion, physiological changes, and machine delivery systems.

Compared with traditional passive scatter proton therapy (PSPT), spot-scanning beam intensity-modulated proton therapy (IMPT) not only eliminates the use of range modulation wheel, beam-specific block and compensator, but also has the advantages to produce a more conformal dose distribution. In spot-scanning proton therapy, thousands of mono-energetic spots from different beam angles are optimized simultaneously and magnetically scanned to superpose a desired dose distribution. Although this active scanning delivery system provides the greatest flexibility to shape to the target volume, the dose distributions from individual beam could be very heterogeneous. Therefore, due to the different beam paths of each beam, such uncertainties could have more significant impact in spot-scanning proton beam therapy.

Traditionally adding margins around the clinical target volume (CTV) to form a planning target volume (PTV) has been used to compensate setup uncertainties. It is important to note that in conventional photon therapy, the planned dose distributions are not significantly affected by the rigid body shifts; therefore, using PTV could assure the CTV's coverage under setup uncertainties. However, such traditional margin approach is not applicable to proton therapy, where the dose distributions could be strongly affected, by the heterogeneities in each beam path. Therefore, Park et al. [5] proposed the concept to create a beam-specific PTV for planning, where each beam has a specific margin to account for its setup and range uncertainties. Unfortunately, such method works only for

PSPT or single-field optimization (SFO) and has limitations to be applied to full IMPT.

In IMPT, in order to achieve a highly conformal dose to the target while sparing the adjacent critical structures, the dose contribution from individual beam could be inhomogeneous or even highly heterogeneous. In case of any errors, the planned dose could result not only in degradation of the target edges, but more severely in hot and cold spots throughout the target volume. However, it should be noted that in some circumstances, the added margin approach could be possibly used to account for the setup and range uncertainties for IMPT. Albertini et al. [6] demonstrated proper margins could improve the plan robustness for IMPT plans with low gradient, but not for high gradient IMPT plans. Therefore, during IMPT treatment planning, the planner has to be very careful to choose the proper margin and to control the gradient of the IMPT plan.

More importantly, the planner needs to quantitatively evaluate the robustness of the plan. Several common methods used are perturbed dose-volume histogram (DVH) approach, error bar volume histogram (EVH), and root mean square deviation (RMSD) dose-volume histograms (RVH). At our institution, evaluation of IMPT plan is done under a multidisciplinary manner involving dosimetry and physics and physicians where we have used the perturbed dose approach to evaluate the robustness. The planned dose is re-recalculated with isocenter shifts in the anterior–posterior, superior–inferior, and right–left directions under the nominal proton beam range, with proton beam range uncertainties, corresponding to a total of 26 dose distribution scenarios. The perturbed doses and DVHs are analyzed to evaluate the robustness of the plan.

Moreover, the most effective way to account for setup and range uncertainties in IMPT treatment planning is robust optimization. In general, there are two types of robust optimizations, probabilistic optimization and worst-case scenario robust optimization. Due to degeneracy of the IMPT planning, both concepts have tried to include a robust solution by incorporating the setup and range uncertainties into the planning. More specifically, those algorithms consider the target coverage and normal tissue sparing under associated uncertainties by simulating all or a portion of the uncertainties scenarios. The planner could also modify the objective function to balance the plan quality and robustness. The probabilistic optimization minimizes the expected value of the objective function among the scenarios while the worst-case robust optimization minimizes the objective function from the worst-case scenario at each iteration. The robust optimization has been incorporated into commercial treatment planning system and has shown significant advantages to improve the robustness of IMPT plans and even the plan quality compared to margin approach.

7.3 Spot-scanning Proton Arc Therapy

7.3.1 Introduction

Compared to photon radiotherapy and passive-scattering proton therapy, IMPT-PBS provides superior tumor coverage and conformity while delivering less body integral dose. However, the robustness and dosimetric quality of a proton plan still rely heavily on the number of fields as well as beam angle selections. Unfortunately, the total number of beam angles that IMPT-PBS can deliver to each patient per faction is limited by current available planning and beam delivery techniques as well as the limited proton machine efficiency [7,8]. To improve the quality of proton beam therapy, the concept of arc delivery remains of interest since Sandison et al. in 1997 [9] investigated the benefits of normal lung integral dose reduction using passive-scattering proton arc therapy. As mentioned above, with the development of spot-scanning technique [10,11], a range modulation wheel and beam-specific compensator were no longer required. As a result, clinical operation and workflow became less complicated and more efficient [12]. Compared to the passive-scattering technique, spot-scanning proton therapy produces a more conformal dose distribution to the target volume while reducing the dose to the adjacent critical normal structures [13,14]. There is, however, still room to further increase the conformity and dosimetric quality of the proton beam treatments. Thus, proton arc therapy using a spot-scanning technique is of great interest to researchers and clinicians. Seco et al. [15] explored the potential advantage of proton arc therapy to minimize the range uncertainties for treatment of non-small cell lung cancer. Meanwhile, Sanchez-Parcerisa and Carabe-Fernandez [16] presented a radiobiological optimized treatment planning approach based on a mono-energetic proton arc therapy. Subsequently, a concept of distal edge tracking (DET) was introduced in recent years to reduce the energy layers and to improve delivery efficiency with 12–24 static proton beams [17,18]. However, DET is a forward planning approach based on the target volume contour which does not take into account the robustness in sparing of the organ-at-risks (OARs). Furthermore, previous attempts of proton arc therapy failed to demonstrate clinical feasibility, as an extensive amount of computation was required to calculate and deliver a robust proton arc plan with continuous sampling frequency. Therefore, currently, the major limitations in the implementation of proton spot-scanning arc therapy into routine clinical practice are the treatment delivery efficiency and having a robust proton plan quality [19]. None of the previous studies have been able to address such obstacles. Here in this section, we present a novel proton arc therapy optimization algorithm and platform based on the current clinical PBS proton therapy machine and gantry.

This algorithm can generate a robust and delivery-efficient proton spot-scanning plan for potential continuous and dynamic arc treatment delivery.

7.3.2 Basic Physics of Proton Arc Therapy

As the current clinical proton beam therapy still relies on the limited number of beam angles, the potential to provide superior treatment to cancer patients in terms of dosimetric quality, treatment robustness, and delivery efficiency has reached a plateau. Our group at Beaumont developed and tested the first robust and delivery-efficient spot-scanning proton arc therapy (SPArc) therapy concept and algorithm [20]. SPArc algorithm is based on an iterative inverse optimization approach integrated with (a) control point re-sampling, (b) control point energy layer re-distribution, (c) energy layer filtration, and (d) energy layer re-sampling. This is the first critical step toward clinical implementation of proton arc therapy (Figure 7.2) [21]. Further improvement of initial algorithm with SPArc_seq optimization algorithm was made to improve the beam delivery time. An iterative energy layer sorting and redistribution mechanism following the direction of the gantry rotation was implemented into the original SPArc algorithm [22]. Subsequently, the Beaumont team reported the first prototype of dynamic proton arc delivery on a clinical proton therapy system successfully delivered. The measurements and simulations demonstrated the feasibility of SPArc treatment within the clinical requirements. The planar iso-dose lines' comparisons for the calculated and measured SPArc with 2 cm solid water buildup and the gamma index map calculated with 3% and 3 mm between the two doses were both reported. The gamma index reached 98.6%, which indicates the good agreement between the calculated and measured doses [23].

7.3.3 Clinical Implications of Proton Arc Therapy

The preliminary results of SPArc plan analysis demonstrated potential clinical benefits by providing not only a better conformal robust plan but also an efficient treatment delivery system. Examples of different treatment body sites and its potential benefits are detailed in the following section.

Lung Cancer

Lung cancer remains the leading cause of cancer deaths in the United States [24], and for patients with locally advanced lung cancer, radiotherapy has been part of the standard of care. Although spot scanning proton therapy has the greatest flexibility to shape to the target volume, one of the major challenges with spot scanning beam in treatment of lung cancer is the interplay effect between the patient-specific

Figure A

Figure B

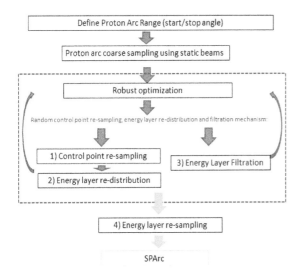

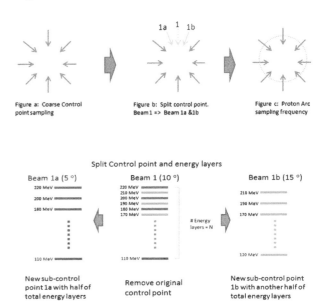

Figure 7.2   A. Scanning proton arc (SPArc) algorithm and workflow. B. Control point re-sampling and energy layer re-distribution mechanism in SPArc. (a) SPArc starts with static coarse control point sampling. (b) The original control was split into a pair of adjacent sub-control points. (c) New control points are added randomly and in an interactive way to reach a desired arc-sampling frequency. (d) Energy layer re-distribution mechanism. A pair of sub-control points (±5°) was generated adjacent to the original control points via splitting mechanism. The new sub-control point carries over half of the original energy layers, spot position, and MU weighting [21].

respiratory motion and the spot scanning delivering sequence. Such interplay effect could lead to severe dose distortion, especially in cases of large tumor motion [25,26]. Using Arc therapy not only improved the conformality and dosimetric results but also decreased the interplay effect. The degree of dose alteration is significantly less via SPArc as shown in Figure 7.3 [27]. Such improvement could be explained by the washout effect of SPArc's hundreds of beamlets.

Moreover, further studies on effectiveness of motion interplay effect mitigation using SPArc in stereotactic body radiotherapy of lung tumors showed that SPArc is capable of effectively mitigating the interplay effect and therefore has potential to deliver SBRT treatment while keeping delivery efficient without undergoing any number of repaintings. The study reported that the effectiveness of such motion mitigation using SPArc was about 5–7 times of IMPT without any repainting. Although repainting would help diminishing the interplay effect of IMPT, it will cause the delivery time to increase by approximately 40% [28].

Head and Neck Cancer

Treating head and neck cancer with proton therapy is challenging as treating higher cervical lymph nodes would lead to the inability to spare the parotid glands as the beams enter through the parotid glands on the affected side. Conversely,

SPArc would provide the means for better conformity and sparing of OARs in head and neck cancer patient while keeping the delivery efficiency the same. As it was presented by the Beaumont team, proton arc could ultimately spare the parotid, optic nerves, chiasm, and brain stem in any head and neck cancer patients including base of skull malignancies [29,30]. Future studies are undergoing.

Breast Cancer

The initial role of SPArc is recently published which showed SPArc technique can spare OARs including heart and lung, thus reducing the probability of normal tissue complications in patients with left-sided breast cancer (Figure 7.4) [31]. The RVH analysis showed SPArc provided a significantly better plan robustness in OARs sparing while the average estimated treatment delivery was comparable to vertical intensity-modulated proton therapy (vIMPT) plans in modern proton therapy centers with the ELST of about 0.5 s [32].

Brain Malignancy

The role and benefit of proton arc therapy in treatment of patients with brain malignancies is vast. One area of interest is hippocampal and cochlear sparing that drawn significant interest in order to minimize the neurocognitive toxicity and the risks of hearing loss. In a dosimetric study done by Ding et al., SPArc plans showed significant dosimetric improve-

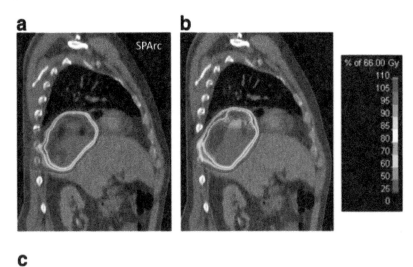

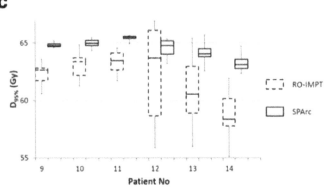

Figure 7.3 Single-fraction 4D dynamic dose distributions without considering rescanning on exhale phase for (a) SPArc and (b) RO-IMPT plan and the boxplot of the doses encompassing 95% ($D_{95\%}$) ITV on exhalation phase based on single-fraction 4D dynamic dose simulated with different starting breathing phase (c) [27].

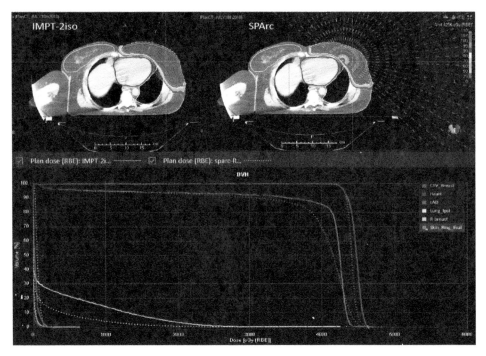

Figure 7.4 A representative of the radiation treatment plan. The comparison of (a) patient dose distribution, beam angle, and (b) dose volume histograms (DVHs) (solid and dash lines for vIMPT and SPArc) [31].

ments in multiple dosimetric parameters including the mean dose to the hippocampus, D100% to the hippocampus, mean and max dose to the cochlea. The mean dose to the cochlea was reduced to 6.2 Gy via SPArc in comparison to 10.89 and 9.38 in VMAT and RO-IMPT, respectively [33].

Gastrointestinal Malignancy

The role of SPArc in treating GI malignancy is still being investigated. Initial studies in treating large liver tumors are showing that SPArc could significantly improve dosimetric profile in patients that would require dose escalation which was otherwise unachievable with standard RO-IMPT. This ultimately could result in better clinical outcome.

SRS/SBRT

Given the range uncertainties, large lateral penumbra, and motion uncertainties, the role of spot scanning proton therapy is limited. Therefore, it would be challenging to treat target volumes with concepts of radiosurgery or stereotactic body radiotherapy. Initial studies presented at multiple conferences showed that SPArc therapy provides dosimetric advantages over IMPT with superior sparing of adjacent critical normal structures while offering improved conformity index and delivery efficiency. Moreover, it was shown that proton arc therapy was more tolerating toward target motion than IMPT and could offer equivalent or better dosimetry parameters compared to repainting technique (PTCOG 2019) [34–37].

7.3.4 Linear Energy Transfer and Relative Biological Effectiveness

Clinically, most centers use a presumed constant relative biological effectiveness (RBE) value of 1.1 regardless of the dose, LET, physiological and biological factors, or clinical end point [38]. Historically, the RBE value was chosen based on the *in vitro and in vivo* data at the center of SOBP [39]. However, recent data have shown that RBE value may increase toward the distal dose fall-off of SOBP as the LET increases to the magnitude of 1.7 [40]. Hence, more than expected rate of clinical toxicities could be seen if the distal end of the Bragg peaks terminates in the adjacent critical normal organs [41]. Hence, having the ability to control the location of high LET would be beneficial to further improve clinical outcomes.

Unfortunately, in the era of passive-scattering proton therapy, the high LET region is inevitably located at the distal end of each beam and is impossible to change its distribution. To avoid any overlapping high LET regions with the adjacent critical organs, it is common to use the beam angles without aiming directly toward the critical organs. The emergence of intensity-modulated proton therapy based on PBS technique not only improved the clinical workflow and the plan conformity but also enabled us to potentially modify the LET distribution by incorporating the LET optimization into the planning process. However, the obstacle is that the ability of IMPT to spatially place the LET value is limited by the number of beam angles used [42], Nevertheless, SPArc can provide the means to overcome such obstacle since it delivers hundreds of beam angles selected from a smart energy and spot selection algorithm discussed above. This results in greater optimization and therefore further improves the LET distribution while still maintaining the delivery efficiency. As shown in Figure 7.5, SPArc has the ability to concentrate and maximize the LET distribution in the target volume wherever is desired and therefore averts the high LET away from the adjacent normal organs at risk. Moreover, this can also be used as a technique for dose escalation inside the target volume by concentrating the high LET points and ultimately respective higher RBE. Further work regarding this area is in work for publication in a very close future [43].

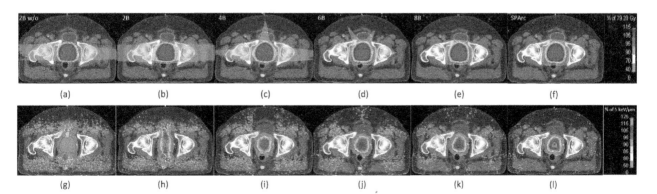

Figure 7.5 The dose (upper row) and the LET$_d$ (lower row) distributions for two beams without LET$_d$-based optimization (2Bw/o, a, g), and with LET$_d$-based optimization for 2 (2B, b, h), 4 (4B, c, i), 6 (6B, d, j), 8 (8B, e, k) beams and SPArc (f, l) for a prostate clinical case [43].

7.4 Other Future Directions on Proton Therapy Delivery

7.4.1 Treatment Delivery Efficiency

In comparison with the passive-scattering technique, which delivers a uniform proton beam across the target volume using SOBP, the new treatment technique, IMPT, is based on the pencil beam scanning technique, which actively scans the target volume spot by spot and energy layer by energy layer [12,44–46]. Although IMPT is able to further spare the adjacent OARs and reduce the total integral dose compared to the passive-scattering technique, there are questions regarding its feasibility, robustness, and reliability in the clinical setting given the prolonged treatment delivery time and complicated radiation intensity modulation [47–49]. However, as the PBS system hardware related to the energy layer selection system and spot scanning controller become more advanced, IMPT has been gradually replacing passive-scattering technique as the main treatment technique in the particle therapy [8,50,51]. As of today, the majority of the new particle therapy centers under construction are equipped with PBS technique alone.

Generally, an IMPT plan contains hundreds of the energy layers and thousands of spots which results in at least several minutes for treatments to be delivered for each individual field. Thus, there are two main challenges that need to be addressed for more efficient treatment delivery: energy layer switching time (ELST) [8] and spot scanning time (SST) [52]. ELST depends on the different types of the accelerators. It generally takes couple of seconds to change from one proton energy layer to another in a synchrotron-based proton therapy system due to the acceleration cycling [53]. For a cyclotron-based accelerator proton therapy system, the recent improvement of the mechanical energy layer selection system and the degrader could shorten the ELST from 5 s to about 1 s [52]. For an IMPT plan with hundreds of energy layers, it would cost about a couple of minutes just to switch between all the energy layers. In order to further reduce the total ELST, several techniques were recently proposed such as multi-energy layer extraction method (MELE) for HITACHI ProBeat synchrotron system [54] and energy layer reduction algorithm [7]. The recent study reports that the MELE method could result in an efficient IMPT delivery in synchrotron accelerator proton therapy system platform [54]. On the other hand, the energy layer reduction method proposed by Cao et al. was able to maintain the plan quality while significantly reducing the treatment delivery time. It's important to know that such method would play a significant role in proton centers with ELST longer than 1 s [7]. However, the improvement by reducing energy layers would be negligible when the ELST continue to improve to less than 0.2 s [7].

The second main challenge is to reduce the SST, although current scanning time with the same energy can be as fast as 10–20 ms^{-1}. When considering an IMPT plan with tens of thousands of spots, it takes more than a couple of minutes just to allow the magnet switching the spots one by one [53]. Moreover, in order to reduce the dosimetric impact from interplay, the repainting technique is now widely adopted in the routine clinical practice in treating targets with motions [55–57]. Hence, an IMPT plan with three volumetric repainting would triple the total SST result; however, this would lead into more uncertainties involving patient's intra-fraction motion and setup [58]. In 2015, National Cancer Center Hospital East, Chiba, Japan in collaboration with Sumitomo Heavy Industries, Ltd. reported the development of a prototype called continuous line scanning system (CLSS) for treatment of prostate cancer [59]. In contrast to discrete spot scanning technique that has been widely implemented in the clinical settings, the CLSS controls beam position and scanning velocity with a pair of scanning magnets to maintain constant beam intensity while scanning the proton beams in the x and y directions. The maximum and minimum scanning speeds of this system were reported to be 7 mm/ms and 0.1 mm/ms, respectively, at the isocenter plane [59]. Recently, PSI reported new developments with the Gantry 2 where a spherical target of 0.5 l was irradiated with 0.1 Gy in pure line scanning mode in 6 s using 18 different proton energies delivered in sequence [60]. These new developments indicated that such technique may have the potential to further improve treatment delivery efficiency.

7.4.2 Novel Imaging Techniques and Their Applications in Proton Therapy

Imaging techniques play a critical role in the improvement of the radiation treatment delivery accuracy. One of the examples is the development of CBCT, where it was first commercially available for dentomaxillofacial imaging in 2001 [61]. Such new concepts led to the development of the Imaging Guided Radiotherapy (IGRT) technique for linear accelerators, where it could provide 3D view of the patient setup in the treatment position and monitor patient position changes during treatments [62]. This new IGRT technique introduced by Jaffary et al. in 2002 was able to directly reduce the treatment setup margin and therefore would ultimately result in lower dose around the target to adjacent critical organs. Moreover, in combination of Intensity Modulated Radiation Therapy, dose escalation to the target also became possible [63]. IGRT represents a new paradigm in the delivery of highly precise radiation therapy [24]. Moreover, CBCT could verify the patient geometric variation during the treatment course. With such 3D imaging information, adaptive radiotherapy (ART) was introduced to re-optimize the plan during the treatment course [64–66]. Due to the complexity of the particle therapy system, the first CBCT on gantry wasn't developed until 2014 [67]. Using a fast range-corrected dose distribution virtual CT scan based on daily CBCTs, a clinical decision could be made based on the offline recalculated proton dose on the vCT scan [67].

Besides the setup uncertainties and geometry changes, the range uncertainty has been another topic on interest in proton beam therapy. Several imaging techniques have been proposed to reduce the range uncertainty such as prompt gamma camera [68], acoustic emissions [69], dual-energy CT scan [70], and proton imaging [71]. One of the imaging techniques that has been implemented in the clinical setting is the prompt gamma camera, where Xie et al. reported the first *in vivo* range verification for proton therapy in treating a brain cancer patient in 2017 [72]. A stand-alone, trolley-mounted, prototype prompt gamma system utilizing a knife-edge slit collimator design was developed. A submillimeter accuracy of the spot positions has been measured during the six treatment fractions over 3 weeks [72]. More recently, a full-scale clinical prototype prompt gamma-ray spectroscopy system was developed in Massachusetts General Hospital (MGH) [73] where the system was mounted on a rotating frame which made it easier to rotate with different gantry angle. In addition, a new algorithm has been developed for the measurement of energy- and time-resolved gamma-ray spectra during proton irradiation at a clinical dose rate [74].

Another imaging technique that has the potential to be implemented in the clinical setting in the near future is proton radiography (pRG) and tomography (pCT). Although it has been over 50 years since the introduction of such concept [75], this technique has been slow to reach clinical practice due to the technical challenges as well as the costs [71]. Multiple scattering effects remain the fundamental obstacles as proton particles do not move through a medium in straight lines. Most-likely-path was introduced [76] to solve the problem which make it one step closer into the clinical product. The above issues have limited the proton image quality in comparison to X-rays. The reason that proton transmission imaging is still of great interest is because this technique could show the reality behind the proton range *in vivo*. Recent development of proton imaging into the rotational gantry and PBS technique could allow such concept to be integrated into the clinical workflow just like the CBCT [52,77]. In order to reconstruct the proton imaging from each individual proton spot, a spot decomposition method was introduced to increase efficiency of pCT using PBS technique demonstrating the feasibility of using PBS gantry for pCT [77]. Furthermore, with the modulation capability of PBS technique, a fluence field modulation pCT was introduced by Dedes et al. in 2017. These new technique developments further pushed the field forward toward the clinical implementation of pCT on a proton beam rotating gantry [78].

7.4.3 Heavy Charged Particle Radiotherapy

In the current era of cancer therapy, the questions are always raised on how much local control and overall survival benefit is important while decreasing treatment toxicities. Charges particles, including proton and heavier ions, could provide better dose distribution and, in case of heavier ions, better and larger RBE. This could result in improved local control while reducing the associated morbidity given smaller volumes of adjacent critical structures are being irradiated. It is known that conventional photon beams and neutron beams are characterized for their absorption of dose with depth while protons and other heavier ions such as carbons provide a high dose region known as Bragg peak in the medium. The energy spread and range straggling of the particles are smaller for carbon ions than protons. In addition, the penumbra of the ion beam becomes smaller as the mass of particle increases. Moreover, carbon ion undergoes unclear interactions with fragmentation of the primary beam into lower atomic number particles producing a fragmentation tail after the distal end of the Bragg peak. Note the biological effect of such tail is small as it only contains low atomic number fragments. Therefore, carbon ion dose distribution, the lateral fall-off around the target volume, is more rapid with carbon ions than protons.

The world first heavy ion accelerator facility devoted to medical use is the HIMAC in Chiba. This large facility consists of one story above the ground and three stories below the ground spanning about approximately 100 m × 50 m × 30 m in size.

Although the RBE of carbon ion beams is larger than that of proton, the interest lies in the differential effect noted between the tumor and normal tissue which can increase the therapeutic gain. Because of carbon unique physical and biological properties, it is possible to use hypo-fractionated carbon therapy to increase the therapeutic gain. It is reported that increasing the fraction size tends to lower RBE for both tumor and normal tissue; however, the RBE for the tumor would not decrease as rapidly as the RBE for normal tissue increases. Hence, the therapeutic ratio increases rather than decreases with carbon ion hypo-fractionation.

Presently, carbon ion beam scanning is used only in limited number of centers but it has the advantage of low maintenance costs and the potential of intensity-modulated particle therapy to deliver a better conformal plan. Moreover, recent research development is showing the advantage of a concept called spot scanning hadron arc (SHArc) therapy with heavy ion gantry. Such small study showed potential treatment benefits including normal tissue sparing and its ability to mitigate tumor hypoxia-induced loss of efficacy [79].

7.4.3.1 Multi-Ion Particle Therapy

Given that proton therapy and carbon ion therapy each have different properties, multi-ion particle therapy is gaining momentum. Neither proton therapy nor carbon ion therapy is considered perfect. Proton therapy has a narrow range of RBE, therefore reduced uncertainty in biological response and ultimately decreased risk of late tissue effect. On the other hand, it exhibits larger lateral penumbra and range straggling which can affect treatment when precision is critical. However, carbon ion therapy shows significant RBE variations due to its higher LET and therefore potential for greater tumor control. Combining two ions in a single filed treatment resulted in more robust biological and more conformal dose distribution compared to conventional particle therapy. Further studies have been designed to validate combined ion-beam therapy for improved treatment efficacy, robustness, and normal tissue sparing [80].

References

1 Von Essen, C. et al. (1985). The positron II: methods and initial results of dynamic pion therapy in phase II studies. *International Journal of Radiation Oncology, Biology, Physics* 11: 217–226.

2 Pedroni, E. et al. (1979). Development of the therapy planning programs for the 60 beams SIN-pion therapy facility. *Radiation and Environment Biophysics* 16: 211–217.

3 Pedroni, E. et al. (1981). Therapy planning system for the SIN pion therapy facility. In: *Treatment Planning for External Beam Therapy with Neutrons* (ed. G. Burger and J.J. Broerse), 60–69. Munich: Urban & Schwarzenberg.

4 Delaney, T.F. and Kooy, H.M. (2008). *Proton and Charged Particle Radiotherapy*. Philadelphia, PA: Lippincott Williams & Wilkins.

5 Park, P.C. et al. (2012). A beam-specific planning target volume (PTV) design for proton therapy to account for setup and range uncertainties. *International Journal of Radiation Oncology, Biology, Physics* 82 (2): e329–36.

6 Albertini, F., Hug, E.B., and Lomax, A.J. (2011). Is it necessary to plan with safety margins for actively scanned proton therapy? *Physics in Medicine & Biology* 56: 4399–4413.

7 Cao, W., Lim, G., Liao, L.*et al.* (2014). Proton energy optimization and reduction for intensity-modulated proton therapy. *Physics in Medicine & Biology*59: 6341–6354.

8 vande Water, S., Kooy, H.M., Heijmen, B.J.M.*et al.* (2015). Shortening delivery times of intensity modulated proton therapy by reducing proton energy layers during treatment plan optimization. *International Journal of Radiation Oncology, Biology, Physics*92: 460–468.

9 Sandison, G.A., Papiez, E., Bloch, C. *et al.* (1997). Phantom assessment of lung dose from proton arc therapy. *International Journal of Radiation Oncology, Biology, Physics* 38: 891–897.

10 Pedroni, E., Bacher, R., Blattmann, H. *et al.* (1995). The 200-MeV proton therapy project at the Paul Scherrer Institute: Conceptual design and practical realization. *Medical Physics* 22: 37–53.

11 Pedroni, E., Scheib, S., Böhringer, T. *et al.* (2005). Experimental characterization and physical modelling of the dose distribution of scanned proton pencil beams. *Physics in Medicine & Biology* 50: 541.

12 Lomax, A.J., Boehringer, T., Coray, A.*et al.* (2001). Intensity modulated proton therapy: a clinical example. *Medical Physics*28: 317–324.

13 Ding, X., Dionisi, F., Tang, S. *et al.* (2014). A comprehensive dosimetric study of pancreatic cancer treatment using three-dimensional conformal radiation therapy (3DCRT), intensity-modulated radiation therapy (IMRT), volumetric-modulated radiation therapy (VMAT), and passive-scattering and modulated-scanning proton therapy (PT). *Medical Dosimetry Official Journal* of the American Association of Medical Dosimetrists 39: 139–145.

14 Zhang, X., Li, Y., Pan, X. *et al.* (2010). Intensity-modulated proton therapy reduces the dose to normal tissue compared with intensity-modulated radiation therapy or passive scattering proton therapy and enables individualized radical radiotherapy for extensive stage IIIB non-small-cell lung cancer: A virtual clinical study. *International Journal of Radiation Oncology, Biology, Physics* 77: 357–366.

15 Seco, J., Gu, G., Marcelos, T. *et al.* (2013). Proton arc reduces range uncertainty effects and improves conformality compared with photon volumetric modulated arc therapy in stereotactic body radiation therapy for non-small cell lung cancer. *International Journal of Radiation Oncology, Biology, Physics* 87: 188–194.

16 Carabe-Fernandez, A., Kirk, M., Sanchez-Parcerisa, D. *et al.* (2015). SU-E-T-640: proton modulated arc therapy using scanned pencil beams. *Medical Physics* 42: 3483–3483.

17 Zhang, M., Flynn, R.T., Mo, X. *et al.* (2012). The energy margin strategy for reducing dose variation due to setup uncertainty in intensity modulated proton therapy (IMPT) delivered with distal edge tracking (DET). *Journal of Applied Clinical Medical Physics American College of Medical Physics* 13: 3863.

18 Flynn, R.T., Barbee, D.L., Mackie, T.R. *et al.* (2007). Comparison of intensity modulated x-ray therapy and intensity modulated proton therapy for selective subvolume boosting: a phantom study. *Physics in Medicine & Biology* 52: 6073–6091.

19 Berman, A.T., James, S.S., and Rengan, R. (2015). Proton beam therapy for non-small cell lung cancer: Current clinical evidence and future directions. *Cancers* 7: 1178–1190.

20 Ding, X., Li, X., Jm, Z. *et al.* (2016). Spot-Scanning Proton Arc (SPArc) therapy: The first robust and delivery-efficient Spot-Scanning Proton Arc Therapy. *International Journal of Radiation Oncology, Biology, Physics* 96: 1107–1116.

21 Reprinted from Int J Radiat Oncol Biol Phys, 96/5, Xuanfeng Ding, X., Li, J., Zhang, M., Kabolizadeh, P., Stevens, C., and Yan, D. (2016). Spot-Scanning Proton Arc (SPArc) therapy: The first obust and delivery efficient Spot-Scanning Proton Arc therapy, Figure 1-2, Copyright. with permission from Elsevier.

22 Liu, G., Li, X., Zhao, L., Zheng, W., Qin, A., Zhang, S., Stevens, C., Yan, D., and Kabolizadeh, P. (2020). Ding X A novel energy sequence optimization algorithm for efficient spot-scanning proton arc (SPArc) treatment delivery. *Acta Oncologica* 59 (10): 1178–1185.

23 Li, X., Liu, G., Janssens, G., De Wilde, O., Bossier, V., Lerot, X., Pouppez, A., Yan, D., Stevens, C., Kabolizadeh, P., and Ding, X. (2019). Radiotherapy oncology. 137: 130–136.

24 Siegel, R.L., Miller, K.D., and Jemal, A. Cancer statistics. (2016). *CA: A Cancer Journal for Clinicians* 2016 66: 7–30.

25 Li, Y., Kardar, L., Li, X. et al. (2014). On the interplay effects with proton scanning beams in stage iii lung cancer. *Medical Physics* 41: 021721.

26 Kardar, L., Li, Y., Li, X. et al. (2014). Evaluation and mitigation of the interplay effects of intensity modulated proton therapy for lung cancer in a clinical setting. *Practical Radiation Oncology* 4: e259–68.

27 Reprinted from Radiation Oncology, 13/35 Li, X., Kabolizadeh, P., Yan, D., Qin, A., Zhou, J., Hong, Y., Guerrero, T., Grills, I., Stevens, C., and Ding, X. (2018). Improve dosimetric outcome in stage III non-small cell lung cancer treatment using spot-scanning proton arc (SPArc) therapy, Figure 4, Copyright. with permission from Springer Nature.

28 Liu, G., Li, X., Yan, D., Stevens, C., Grills, I., Kabolizadeh, P., and Ding, X. (2020). Lung stereotactic body radiotherpay (SBRT) using spot scanning proton arc (SPArc) therapy: A feasibility study, PTCOG58. *International Journal of Particle Therapy* 6: 45–491.

29 Liu, G., Li, X., Qin, A., Zheng, W., Yan, D., Zhang, S., Stevens, C., Kabolizadeh, P., and Ding, X. (2020). Improve the dosimetric outcome in bilateral head and neck cancer (HNC) treatment using spot-scanning proton arc (SPArc) therapy: A feasibility study. *Radiation Oncology* 15 (1): 21.

30 Hyde, C., Liu, G., Li, X., Chen, P.Y., Yan, D., Stevens, C., Kabolizadeh, P., Deraniyagala, R., and Ding, X. (2020). Spot scanning proton arc therapy (SPArc) versus intensity modulated proton therapy (IMPT) for parotid sparing in unilateral tonsil cancer, PTCOG58. *International Journal of Particle Therapy* 6: 45–49.

31 Reprinted from Radiation Oncology, 15/232 Chang, S., Liu, G., Zhao, L., Dilworth, J.T., Zheng, W., Jawad, S., Yan, D., Chan, P., Stevens, C., Kabolizadeh, P., Li, X., and Ding, X., (2020). Feasibility study: Spot scanning proton arc therapy (SPArc) for left sided whole breast radiotherapy, Figure 4, Copyright. with permission from Springer Nature.

32 Chang, S., Liu, G., Zhao, L., Dilworth, J., Zheng, Q., Jawad, S., Yan, D., Chen, P., Stevens, C., Kabolizadeh, P., Li, X., and Ding, X. (2020). Feasibility study: Spot scanning proton arc therapy (SPArc) for left-sided whole breast radiotherapy. *Radiation Oncology* 15: 232.

33 Ding, X., Zhou, J., Li, X., Blas, K., Liu, G., Wang, Y., Qin, A., Chinnaiyan, P., Yan, D., Stevens, C., Grills, I., and Kabolizadeh, P. (2019). Improving dosimetric outcome of hippocampus and cochlea sparing whole brain radiotherapy using spot-scanning proton arc therapy. *Acta Oncologica* 58 (4): 483–490.

34 Zhou, J., Kabolizadeh, P., Grills, I., Li, X., Wang, Y., Yan, D., and Ding, X. (2017). Fiest feasibility study: Spot scanning proton arc stereotactic radiosurgery (SRS) for localized spine metastasis. *International Journal of Radiation Oncology, Biology, Physics* 99:: E747.

35 Sura, K., Grills, I., Kabolizadeh, P., Zhou, J., Li, X., Yan, D., Krauss, D., Chinnaiyan, P., and Ding, X. (2017). Feasibility of spot scanning proton arc fractionated radiosurgery to the post operative cavity for brain metastasis. *International Journal of Radiation Oncology, Biology, Physics* 99: E725.

36 Thompson, A., Ding, X., Abbott, V., Ja, P., Palermino, J., Frankenfield, A., Kabolizadeh, P., and Dj, K. (2019). Proton Stereotactic Body Radiotherapy as a Nephron-Sparing Approach for Patients with Localized Renal Cell Carcinoma: A Dosimetric Analysis. *International Journal of Radiation Oncology, Biology, Physics* 1051: E713.

37 Ding, X., Li, X., Zhou, J., Stevens, C., Sura, K., Chinnaiyan, P., Grills, I., Di, Y., and Kabolizadeh, P. (2018). *Radiotherapy and Oncology* 127: S491–492.

38 Newhauser, W. (2009). International commission on radiation units and measurements report 78: Prescribing. *Recording and Reporting Proton-beam Therapy. Radiation Protection Dosimetry* 133 (1): 60–62.

39 Paganetti, H. et al. (2002). Relative biological effectiveness (RBE) values for proton beam therapy. *Int J Radiat Oncol Biol Phys* 53 (2): 407–421.

40 Paganetti, H. (2014). Relative biological effectiveness (RBE) values for proton beam therapy. Variations as a function of biological endpoint, dose, and linear energy transfer. *Physics in Medicine & Biology* 59 (22): R419–72. Figure 02, p 03 / Frontiers Media S.A. / CC BY 4.0.

41 Harrabi, S. et al. (2017). OC-0514: Radiation necrosis after proton beam therapy – when and where does it happen? *Radiotherapy and Oncology* 123: S271.

42 Toussaint, L. et al. (2019). Towards proton arc therapy: Physical and biologically equivalent doses with increasing number of beams in pediatric brain irradiation. *Acta Oncologica* 58 (10): 1451–1456.

43 Li, X. et al., (2019, Jul). Linear energy transfer incorporated spot scanning proton Arc therapy (SPArc) optimization, AAPM. 14–18.

44 Lomax, A. (1999). Intensity modulation methods for proton radiotherapy. *Physics in Medicine & Biology* 44: 185.

45 Lomax, A.J. (2008). Intensity modulated proton therapy and its sensitivity to treatment uncertainties 2: The potential effects of inter-fraction and inter-field motions. *Physics in Medicine & Biology* 53: 1043–1056.

46 Lomax, A.J., Pedroni, E., Rutz, H. et al. (2004). The clinical potential of intensity modulated proton therapy. *Z. Medical Physics* 14: 147–152.

47 Chen, W., Unkelbach, J., Trofimov, A. et al. (2012). Including robustness in multi-criteria optimization for intensity-modulated proton therapy. *Physics in Medicine & Biology* 57: 591–608.

48 Li, Y., Zhang, X., and Mohan, R. (2011). An efficient dose calculation strategy for intensity modulated proton therapy. *Physics in Medicine & Biology* 56: N71.

49 Hyer, D.E., Hill, P.M., Wang, D. et al. (2014). A dynamic collimation system for penumbra reduction in spot-scanning proton therapy: Proof of concept. *Medical Physics* 41: 091701.

50 Thorwarth, D., Soukup, M., and Alber, M. (2008). Dose painting with IMPT, helical tomotherapy and IMXT: A dosimetric comparison. *Radiotherapy & Oncology* 86: 30–34.

51 Both, S., Shen, J., Kirk, M. et al. (2014). Development and clinical implementation of a universal bolus to maintain spot size during delivery of base of skull pencil beam scanning proton therapy. *International Journal of Radiation Oncology, Biology, Physics* 90: 79–84.

52 Ding, X., Li, X., Zhang, J.M. et al. (2016). Spot-Scanning Proton Arc (SPArc) therapy: The first robust and delivery-efficient spot-scanning proton arc therapy. *International Journal of Radiation Oncology, Biology, Physics* 96: 1107–1116.

53 Shen, J., Tryggestad, E., Younkin, J.E. et al. (2017). Technical note: Using experimentally determined proton spot scanning timing parameters to accurately model beam delivery time. *Medical Physics* 44: 5081–5088.

54 Younkin, J.E., Bues, M., Sio, T.T. et al. (2018). Multiple energy extraction reduces beam delivery time for a synchrotron-based proton spot-scanning system. *Advance in Radiation Oncology* 3: 412–420.

55 Bert, C., Grözinger, S.O., and Rietzel, E. (2008). Quantification of interplay effects of scanned particle beams and moving targets. *Physics in Medicine & Biology* 53: 2253–2265.

56 Dowdell, S., Grassberger, C., Sharp, G.C. et al. (2013). Interplay effects in proton scanning for lung: A 4D Monte Carlo study assessing the impact of tumor and beam delivery parameters. *Physics in Medicine & Biology* 58: 4137–4156.

57 Grassberger, C., Dowdell, S., Lomax, A. et al. (2013). Motion interplay as a function of patient parameters and spot size in spot scanning proton therapy for lung cancer. *International Journal of Radiation Oncology, Biology, Physics* 86: 380–386.

58 Suzuki, K., Gillin, M.T., Sahoo, N. et al. (2011). Quantitative analysis of beam delivery parameters and treatment process time for proton beam therapy. *Medical Physics* 38: 4329–4337.

59 Kohno, R., Hotta, K., Dohmae, T. et al. (2017). Development of continuous line scanning system prototype for proton beam therapy. *International Journal of Particle. Therapy* 3: 429–438.

60 Safai, S., Bula, C., Meer, D. et al. (2012). Improving the precision and performance of proton pencil beam scanning. *Translational. Cancer Research* 1: 196-206–206.

61 Miracle, A.C. and Mukherji, S.K. (2009). Conebeam CT of the head and neck, part 2: clinical applications. *AJNR American Journal of Neuroradiology* 30: 1285–1292.

62 Jaffray, D.A., Siewerdsen, J.H., Wong, J.W. et al. (2002). Flat-panel cone-beam computed tomography for image-guided radiation therapy. *International Journal of Radiation Oncology, Biology, Physics* 53: 1337–1349.

63 Dawson, L.A. and Jaffray, D.A. (2007). Advances in image-guided radiation therapy. *Journal of Clinical Oncology Off. Journal of American Society of Clinical Oncology* 25: 938–946.

64 Yan, D., Vicini, F., Wong, J. et al. (1997). Adaptive radiation therapy. *Physics in Medicine & Biology* 42: 123–132.

65 Foroudi, F., Wong, J., Kron, T. et al. (2011). Online adaptive radiotherapy for muscle-invasive bladder cancer: results of a pilot study. *International Journal of Radiation Oncology, Biology, Physics* 81: 765–771.

66 Nijkamp, J., Pos, F.J., Nuver, T.T. et al. (2008). Adaptive radiotherapy for prostate cancer using kilovoltage cone-beam computed tomography: first clinical results. *International Journal of Radiation Oncology, Biology, Physics* 70: 75–82.

67 Veiga, C., Janssens, G., Teng, C.-L. et al. (2016). First clinical investigation of CBCT and deformable registration for adaptive proton therapy of lung cancer. *International journal of radiation oncology, biology, physics* 0.

68 Smeets, J., Roellinghoff, F., Prieels, D. et al. (2012). Prompt gamma imaging with a slit camera for real-time range control in proton therapy. *Physics in Medicine & Biology* 57: 3371–3405.

69 Jones, K.C., Stappen, F.V., Bawiec, C.R. et al. (2015). Experimental observation of acoustic emissions generated by a pulsed proton beam from a hospital-based clinical cyclotron. *Medical Physics* 42: 7090–7097.

70 Bär, E., Lalonde, A., Royle, G. *et al.* (2017). The potential of dual-energy CT to reduce proton beam range uncertainties. *Medical Physics* 44: 2332–2344.

71 Schneider, U., Besserer, J., Pemler, P. *et al.* (2004). First proton radiography of an animal patient. *Medical Physics* 31: 1046–1051.

72 Xie, Y., Bentefour, E.H., Janssens, G. *et al.* (2017). Prompt gamma imaging for in vivo range verification of pencil beam scanning proton therapy. *International Journal of Radiation Oncology, Biology, Physics* 99: 210–218.

73 Hueso-González, F., Rabe, M., Ruggieri, T.A. *et al.* (2018). A full-scale clinical prototype for proton range verification using prompt gamma-ray spectroscopy. *Physics in Medicine & Biology* 63: 185019.

74 Verburg, J.M., Riley, K., Bortfeld, T. *et al.* (2013). Energy- and time-resolved detection of prompt gamma-rays for proton range verification. *Physics in Medicine & Biology* 58: L37–49.

75 Cormack, A.M. (1963). Representation of a function by its line integrals, with some radiological applications. *Journal of Applied Physics* 34: 2722–2727.

76 Williams, D.C. (2004). The most likely path of an energetic charged particle through a uniform medium. *Physics in Medicine & Biology* 49: 2899.

77 Zhou, J., Li, X., Kabolizadeh, P., *et al.* (2019). Spot decomposition in a novel pencil beam scanning proton computed tomography. In: *Medical Imaging*.

78 Dedes, G., De Angelis, L., Rit, S. *et al.* (2017). Application of fluence field modulation to proton computed tomography for proton therapy imaging. *Physics in Medicine & Biology* 62: 6026–6043.

79 Mein, S., Tessonnier, T., Kopp, B. *et al.* (2021). Spot-Scanning Hadron Arc (SHArc) therapy: A study with light and heavy ions. *Advances in Radiation Oncology* 6: 100661.

80 Kopp, B., Mein, S., Dokic, I. *et al.* (2020). Development and validation of single field multi-ion particle therapy treatment. *International Journal of Radiation Oncology Biology Physics* 106: 194–205. Figure 04, p 06 / Springer Nature / CC BY 4.0.

8

FLASH Radiotherapy

Santanu Samanta MD[1], Sina Mossahebi PhD[2], and Robert C Miller MD MBA FASTRO[3]

[1] University of Maryland Medical Center
[2] University of Maryland, School of Medicine
[3] University of Tennessee Medical Center

Corresponding author: Robert C Miller, MD MBA FASTRO (corresponding author), Director, Radiation Oncology, University of Tennessee Medical Center, 1926 Alcoa Highway, Building F, Suite #130 Knoxville, Tennessee, 37920

TABLE OF CONTENTS

8.1   Background

Ionizing radiation with ultrahigh dose rates (>40 Gy/s), known as FLASH radiotherapy, has been recently shown to markedly reduce radiation toxicity to normal healthy tissues while inhibiting tumor growth with similar efficacy as compared to conventional dose-rate radiation. Results from preclinical models and limited clinical data had stirred up mixed response of great hope and skepticism regarding the future of FLASH therapy in radiation oncology.

The phenomenon of the increased therapeutic index of FLASH compared to conventional dose-rate irradiation, or the "FLASH effect," has now been reported in multiple preclinical models. Normal tissue sparing by FLASH of multiple organ systems including lung, brain, intestinal tract, and skin has been demonstrated in multiple animal models, while demonstrating a similar tumoricidal effect relative to conventional dose-rate delivery in multiple *in vivo* tumor models. Though results have been encouraging, mechanistic understanding of FLASH effect is very speculative. Some early experiments found reduced damage of tissue at high dose rates and this was attributed to oxygen depletion. At very high dose rate, high total dose depletes oxygen too quickly for diffusion to maintain re-oxygenation. This mimics hypoxia and increases radio-resistance of normal tissue, while a tumor tissue which is naturally hypoxic is minimally impacted, thus widening the TCP-NTCP (tumor control probability-normal tissue control probability) and producing FLASH effect.

8.2 Rationale and Theoretical Benefits of FLASH

The two major hypotheses to explain FLASH include the oxygen depletion hypothesis and the immune hypothesis.

The oxygen depletion hypothesis is believed to be the most important factor behind the FLASH effect that was also seen by relative low yields of ROS (reactive oxygen species) induced by FLASH-RT and reversal of FLASH effects after carbogen breathing [1]. Although the exact mechanism is still speculative, most authors believe that the super-fast delivery of single dose of FLASH-RT depletes oxygen in normal tissues and prevents normal tissue from reoxygenation, thereby increasing their resistance to ionizing radiation. In tumors having abnormal blood vessels, oxygen depletion by FLASH poses negligible impact on the tumor tissues as compared to the normal tissues, thus generating the differential response [2].

There are possible intrinsic differences in immunological responses between normal and tumor tissues in response to ionizing radiation, although the exact mechanism is unknown. Ionizing radiation delivered by either conventional RT (CONV-RT) or FLASH-RT may directly or indirectly change the expression of immune factors, pro-inflammation and anti-inflammation markers, and bring about changes in the microenvironment of the exposed tissue. TGF-β is considered as an important regulator of radiation induced antitumor response. It is also an important component of the inflammatory signals secreted by dead and senescent cells [3]. It is interesting that fibrosis and activation of TGF beta-pathway are not observed in FLASH-RT but seen in CONV-RT. In the experiments, CONV-RT of 17 Gy significantly induced TGF-β signaling; and this signaling was reduced in mice that had been subjected to FLASH-RT [4]. Once again, a greater dose of 30 Gy delivered by FLASH-RT was required to induce TGF-β signaling to the equivalent extent as seen following irradiation with CONV-RT [5]. Limited TGF-β signaling following FLASH-RT has also been shown in vitro and this study demonstrated that even 24 h post-irradiation, CONV-RT induced threefold greater TGF-β signaling compared to FLASH-RT. There are other hypotheses that FLASH-RT may include sparing of stem cells including epidermal, neural, and intestinal stem cells that may lead to paring of normal tissues [6].

8.3 FLASH Experiments

Preclinical data that laid the foundation for the clinical translation of FLASH has been studied in several animal models like mice, zebrafish, cats, and pig by Bourhis et al. and demonstrated consistent normal tissue protection among species and excellent antitumor effects [7].

Favaudon et al. [4] presented the first lung fibrosis model in mice where he delivered single dose of 30 Gy either with FLASH (40 Gy/s) or conventional dose rates (0.03 Gy/s). The FLASH-RT doses were generated by electron linear accelerator (linac) and compared against conventional radiation with electron beams. Significant reduction in normal tissue damage was found with FLASH-RT while the overall treatment efficacy remains unchanged at similar doses between the two treatment methods [3]. While pulmonary fibrosis was found for 100% of the animals treated with conventional methods, no pneumonitis and late lung fibrosis were observed with FLASH-RT. This study showed that treatment delivery time largely influences normal tissue toxicity while maintaining its antitumor effectiveness [1].

Healthy tissue protection effects were also observed by radiation of the abdomen in mice. This study compared the treatment with conventional dose rate (0.05 Gy/s) and FLASH dose rate (210 Gy/s) at similar doses between 10 and 22 Gy for this study. For treatment, 20 MeV electrons were used as opposed to the lower energy electrons as high-energy electrons are believed to have advantage of smaller dose variation with depth. The results demonstrated significant increase in survival for FLASH radiation where 90% of the FLASH-radiated mice survived 20 days compared to 29% of the conventional radiated mice, at the same time period, confirming advantages of FLASH-RT effect.

With this background evidences, further studies were conducted by Montay-Gruel et al. [8] to demonstrate the long-term cognitive benefits of FLASH radiation. The brain response to FLASH-RT was chosen for investigation as it is an established radiobiology model, where cognitive impairments are the most frequently described functional defects. Dismal neurocognitive outcomes are observed following cranial radiation in both children and adults, due to complex neuropathology that includes reduction of microvascular density, reduced myelination and synapse density, and increased neuro inflammation. Using healthy mouse models, the authors were able to compare between FLASH-RT and conventional radiation and found that FLASH-RT-treated animals did not exhibit neurocognitive decline with spared-associated pathologies. Increasing the dose rate 1,000 times showed a significant increase in the preservation of memory. The authors further demonstrated that by doubling the oxygen content though carbogen breathing, the neurocognitive benefits of FLASH-RT found after normoxic exposure were eliminated, thereby pointing to a fundamental and physicochemical mechanism for neuro protection in FLASH-RT treatment.

Similar studies were conducted by Simmons et al. that showed reduced cognitive impairment and associated neurodegeneration using FLASH-RT, compared to conventional delivery irradiation, potentially through decreased induction of neuroinflammation. In this study, 30 Gy to whole brain of the mice was administered in sub-second (FLASH-RT) versus 240 s conventional delivery time keeping all other parameters constant, using a custom configured clinical linac. At 10 weeks post-irradiation, compared to unirradiated controls, conventional delivery time irradiation significantly impaired novel object location and recognition tasks in mice that was not seen with FLASH-RT animals. A similar study was conducted by Schuler et al. to demonstrate feasibility of using clinical linac to obtain dose rates exceeding 200 Gy/s with excellent dosimetric properties for small animal experiments [9].

Clinical translation of FLASH-RT effect on higher mammals was studied by Vozenin et al. [10] by developing squamous cell carcinoma in cats followed by treatment with FLASH therapy. In this study, a single dose escalation from 25 to 41 Gy was delivered to the squamous cell carcinoma (SCC) of the nasal planum to determine the maximum tolerated dose and progression-free survival of single dose of FLASH-RT. Follow-up at 6 months post-treatment, all the cats achieved complete remission, and three of them were still disease-free after 18 months. Because of the enhanced tolerance of healthy tissue with FLASH therapy, dose escalation was possible that translated to improved outcomes. The cats were found to have permanent depilation at the site of treatment with no other permanent toxicities. A second study to facilitate transfer of FLASH-RT to the clinic involved the irradiation of a pig skin, which was used to mimic the reactions of a human skin to the different dose-rate irradiations (FLASH-RT at 300 Gy/s vs. CONV-RT at 0.08 Gy/s). Transient acute toxicity was found 3 weeks after irradiation but lasted only 4 weeks for doses smaller than 31 Gy. Hair follicles were preserved, whereas in conventional radiotherapy, they were found to be permanently destroyed. No other acute toxicity was observed for the FLASH-RT, whereas skin fibro necrosis was observed in the low dose-rate irradiated skin patches. A dose-protective factor increases of FLASH-RT of at least 20% as compared to CONV-RT was estimated, and together with the results in cats provided rationale for further clinical studies on humans.

8.4 FLASH on Human Patient Study

Bourhis et al. conducted the first human patient study to demonstrate feasibility and safety with favorable outcomes using FLASH-RT therapy [11]. In this study, a 75-year-old man with CD30-positive T-cell diffusely disseminated cutaneous lymphoma was treated using 5.6 MeV linac specifically designed for FLASH-RT, with a prescription dose of 15 Gy in 90 ms to one of the most resistant and progressive skin lesions. There was a rapid, complete, and durable treatment response with minimal skin reaction not exceeding grade 1 at 3 week follow-

up. While no definite conclusions can be drawn based on only one patient, the study has shown that the high FLASH dose could be administered safely, with complete, durable, and rapid tumor response in the follow-up period of 6 months, supporting further implementation of FLASH therapy in the clinic.

8.5 Physics of FLASH

FLASH-RT involves dose delivery at ultrahigh dose rates generally several thousand times higher than the ones currently used in routine clinical practice. While FLASH-RT, as compared to CONV-RT, has been differentiated by dose rate (>40 Gy/s for FLASH-RT vs. 0.03–0.05 Gy/s for conventional RT), its full definition also includes other physical parameters like repetition rate, pulses, and duration of exposure. In the most recent studies, FLASH-RT effect was found to be reproducible with 1–10 pulses per 1.8–2 μs, overall time of less than 200 ms, and a dose rate within the pulse above 1.8×10^5 Gy/s. It is also important to point out that in all these studies, the total RT dose was delivered in single fraction.

8.5.1 Proton FLASH

Patriarca et al. [12] published the first attempt for proton FLASH-RT utilizing clinical cyclotron to deliver proton spread-out Bragg peak (SOBP) with FLASH beam for thorax radiation of mice. Beyreuther et al. [13] developed proton FLASH delivery utilizing horizontal fixed beam. The setup allowed for delivery of 224 MeV proton either by continuous beam at conventional dose rate (5 Gy/min) or by proton FLASH (100 Gy/s). Methods were implemented to reduce the proton fluence on central beam axes for the delivery of the conventional dose rate and homogenize the dose distribution over the sample area. A homogeneous dose distribution was achieved by placing scatterer with minimum reduction in proton fluence for proton FLASH. Homogeneity over the radiation field was monitored with scintillator detector and films at target position revealing maximum dose inhomogeneities of ±3%. The dose homogeneity along the proton depth dose curve was verified by multilayer ionization chamber detector.

8.5.2 Electron FLASH

In proton therapy, the FLASH dose rate (up to 200 Gy/s) within a Bragg peak is readily available. In order to use electron beam at FLASH dose rate, typically one (or more) electron energy of linac is converted to deliver at FLASH-RT dose rates by adjusting the beam magnet current and tuning the radiofrequency driver to increase the dose rate.

8.5.3 Technical Requirements of FLASH

FLASH radiotherapy needs ultrahigh dose rates (typically >40 Gy/s) [14]. Currently, FLASH irradiation has been produced using X-rays generated in a synchrotron facility, electrons generated by linear accelerators when it's running at the highest beam current, and high-energy proton beam (>200 MeV) using isochronous cyclotron and synchrocyclotron. The isochronous cyclotron gives quasi-continuous radiation, while the output radiation from a synchrocyclotron is pulsed. The maximum (or output) energy of the protons in a cyclotron is fixed and an energy selection system (ESS) or range degraders are used to reduce the energy and range of the protons. Synchrocyclotron system can provide high instantaneous dose rate instead of high average dose rate as it provides pulsed output. There is still an open question if the average dose rate or instantaneous dose rate should be considered for FLASH radiotherapy.

Regarding treatment planning system for FLASH radiotherapy, currently there is no commercial treatment planning system available. Some research groups have developed in-house programs to provide dose and dose-rate distribution of treatment plans.

8.5.4 Beam Configuration with FLASH

The current beam configuration uses the transition mode (plateau region) of proton beam for FLASH irradiation. This is dictated by the limitation of the current proton therapy systems in delivering FLASH dose rate over clinically sufficient beam range span. The major factor that limits achieving the FLASH delivery using any proton beam energy is the limited beam current density available at the treatment room isocenter and difficult to steer spots fast enough to produce conformal irradiation using SOBP. Although the extraction of the beam current from the accelerators (cyclotron) can be significantly increased with appropriate technology changes, the limits on the available beam current at the treatment room isocenter are strongly governed by the proton machine beamline efficiency or ESS. This efficiency commonly varies between a maximum of 10% at the very higher energy limit, with double wedge of ESS minimally in place, down to 0.05% at the lowest energy limit. Therefore, very high-energy proton beam can produce the high dose rate (FLASH) and most of proton FLASH therapy preclinical research are done in the transmission mode (plateau region) using the highest available proton energy where the Bragg peaks reside outside the patient.

Most clinical tumor targets are deeply located inside the patient. Usually linacs have 20 MeV as the highest electron energy. The practical range of 20 MeV electron beam is about 10 cm but normally R80 and R90 (range of 80% and 90%) are considered as the reasonable range to provide high and uniform dose. These ranges for 20 MeV electron beam are less than 7 cm which still considered as shallow depth for radiation treatment. Additional to the special characteristics of proton beam (Bragg peak, higher RBE), very high-energy proton beam (>200 MeV) can be easily produced by the commercially available accelerating systems. The range of these high-energy proton beams can be more than 30 cm, which are suitable for radiation therapy. Therefore, FLASH radiotherapy clinical trials on deep-seated tumors can only be performed with high-energy proton beams.

8.5.5 Modification Needed to Deliver FLASH with Protons

Generally, there is no need to modify the cyclotron as long as the high beam current can be produced from the cyclotron and the beamline transmission is acceptable to deliver to the nozzle in the treatment room. For nonefficient systems, FLASH capabilities and dose rate can be improved by (1) increasing the cyclotron beam current output, (2) improving the efficiency of beamline ESS, and (3) modify the beam quality at the nozzle exit. In the cyclotron systems, the efficiency can be also improved by fully retract the double wedge at the ESS and reach to the maximum achievable dose rate (transmission efficiency ≈ 100%). For other beam energies, the dose-rate value strongly depends on the beamline transmission efficiency, which varies in average between 10% and 0.05%. For synchrocyclotron, some modifications in pulse width are needed to deliver ultrahigh dose rates.

8.5.6 Modification Needed to Deliver FLASH with ELECTRONS

There are a couple of ways to convert a linac to FLASH dose rate. One method involves using electron mode with the scattering foil in place and does not involve removing the photon target. Therefore, there is no need to touch the target or modify the carousel. In this method, the modulator is tweaked to run with the highest beam current. This requires boosting the RF generation and electron gun current which can boost the dose rate about 100 times (from 0.1–0.4 Gy/s to about 10–35 Gy/s). Dose rate of 35 Gy/s can be still low for FLASH therapy. The rest of the dose-rate increase can be obtained by reducing SSD and applying inverse square law. By reducing SSD, the dose rate can be increased from 35 Gy/s at isocenter to about 110 Gy/s at the faceplate and about 375 Gy/s at the jaw level (Figure 8.1). The downside of lower SSD is the smaller field size. Therefore, there is a trade-off between dose rate and field size. Generally, the faceplate level is the most convenient and a good compromise between dose rate (~100 Gy/s) and field size ($14 \times 14 \text{ cm}^2$).

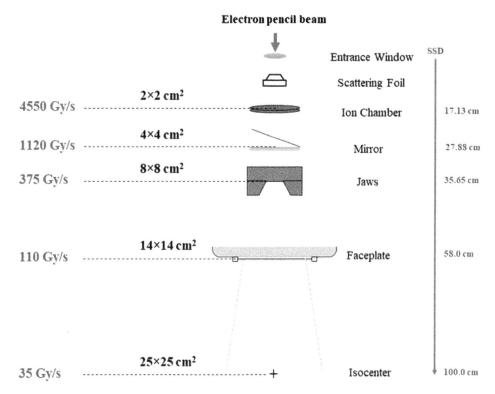

Figure 8.1 The effect of SSD on dose rate for the linac that is tweaked to deliver 35 Gy/s at isocenter. The conventional dose rate at isocenter is typically less than 0.4 Gy/s.

Another way that requires more physical modification of linac is using the photon mode and high beam current by withdrawing the target and scattering foil to deliver high dose-rate electron beam while the linac is running in X-ray mode. Similarly, the smaller SSD is still needed to provide ultrahigh dose rate (>100 Gy/s).

In both methods, monitor chambers and dynamic beam steering system are not functional as the monitor chambers are being completely saturated due to high dose rate. Therefore, the corresponding dosimetric interlocks, dose servos, and symmetry check should be deactivated. Time interlock can be used to control the beam but due to high increment (0.01 min for C-series), the dose delivery can't be reproducible. Therefore, a gating circuit board or auxiliary beam stopper needed to count pulses and assert interlock.

There shouldn't be any significant difference between FLASH and non-FLASH beam parameters. From the physics aspect (not radiobiologically), electrons behave similarly in both scenarios. Unfortunately, the current and commonly used detection systems (ion chamber, film) are not designed to function in very high dose rate or they have inherent uncertainties.

Researchers have used a range of electron beam energies. The low-energy electron beam (4–10 MeV) has sharper dose fall-off which can reduce dose (mainly non-FLASH) to the distal part of the target. The disadvantage of low-energy electron beam is less homogenous beam profile and small practical range.

The high-energy electron beam (16–20 MeV) has larger practical range and provides more homogenous beam profile as its more forwarded peak and scattered less compared to low-energy electron beam. The downside is the slower dose fall-off which can be not suitable for normal tissue sparing.

8.6 Challenges in Developing FLASH Program

The mechanism of FLASH radiotherapy is still unknown. Researchers are still debating the effect of oxygenation and hypoxia, travel of free radicals, and immunology. Additionally, there are many unresolved physics/radiobiology questions regarding FLASH therapy such as single fraction versus fractionation, and effect of dose per pulse versus average dose rate. Moreover, the availability of FLASH beam can be a challenge as it can be usually produced by very high dose-rate electron beam which is not commercially available and needs some modification in the current linacs or high-energy proton beam which currently can be used only in the transmission mode.

Another challenge is defining treatment margin and control intra-fractional motion as the FLASH beam is delivered in a fraction of second.

8.7 Future Directions

The clinical translation of FLASH-RT has been substantiated by multiple experiments that confirm the differential effect between the tumors and the normal tissue, as compared to conventional dose-rate radiation. Recent clinical studies further validate the potential benefits of FLASH-RT. However, studies utilizing proton therapy to deliver FLASH-RT effect have not been very promising and further research will be required to determine if FLASH effect can be reproducible in photon and proton therapy. While there are only very few systems available of delivering low-energy electron beams at those rates required for FLASH-RT, the development of X-ray, proton, and possible heavy ion FLASH will pose technical challenge requiring advanced accelerators. The other major challenges for FLASH effect include dose-rate conformity, hypoxia induction, and narrow therapeutic index.

While the current evidence of FLASH effect seems to be very promising, there are several issues that need to be explored. It is of paramount importance to understand the threshold dose, dose rate, and adequate length of exposure. Also, not all tumors may respond in the same way and response based on histology would be pertinent. Even normal tissue response may be different at different sites of the body. Multiple pre-clinical tumor models to measure differential tissue effects to establish normal tissue toxicity constraints for lung and pancreas trials are awaited. It is also important to know the oxygen tension impact as well as role of hyperthermia coupled with FLASH-RT effect. Also, it is of paramount importance to understand the effect of FLASH dose on a radiation induced antitumor immunity.

References

1 Montay-gruel, P. et al. (2020). Erratum: Long-term neurocognitive benefits of FLASH radiotherapy driven by reduced reactive oxygen species. (Proceedings of the National Academy of Sciences of the United States of America (2019) 116 (10943-10951) DOI: 10.1073/pnas.1901777116). *Proceedings of the National Academy of Sciences of the United States of America* 117: 25946–25947.

2 Zhou, G. (2020). Mechanisms underlying FLASH radiotherapy, a novel way to enlarge the differential responses to ionizing radiation between normal and tumor tissues. *Radiation Medicine and Protection* 1: 35–40.

3 Yilmaz, M.T., Hurmuz, P., and Yazici, G. (2020). FLASH-radiotherapy: A new perspective in immunotherapy era? *Radiotherapy and Oncology : Journal of the European Society for Therapeutic Radiology and Oncology* 145 137.

4 Favaudon, V. et al. (2019). Erratum: Ultrahigh dose-rate FLASH irradiation increases the differential response between normal and tumor tissue in mice. (Science Translational Medicine DOI: 10.1126/scitranslmed.3008973). *Science Translational Medicine* 11: 1–10.

5 Arina, A. et al. (2019 Sep 2). Tumor-reprogrammed resident T cells resist radiation to control tumors. *Nature Communications* 10(1): 3959. DOI: 10.1038/s41467-019-11906-2. PMID: 31477729; PMCID: PMC6718618.

6 Loo, B.W. et al. (2017). (P003) Delivery of ultra-rapid flash radiation therapy and demonstration of normal tissue sparing after abdominal irradiation of mice. *International Journal of Radiation Oncology, Biology, Physics* 98: E16

7 Bourhis, J. et al. (2019). Clinical translation of FLASH radiotherapy: Why and how? *Radiotherapy and Oncology: Journal of the European Society for Therapeutic Radiology and Oncology* 139: 11–17.

8 Montay-gruel, P., Acharya, M.M., Petersson, K., Alikhani, L., and Yakkala, C. (2019). Long-term neurocognitive benefits of FLASH radiotherapy driven by reduced reactive oxygen species. 116.

9 Schüler, E. et al. (2017). Experimental platform for ultra-high dose rate FLASH irradiation of small animals using a clinical linear accelerator. *International Journal of Radiation Oncology, Biology, Physics* 97: 195–203.

10 Vozenin, M.C. et al. (2019). The advantage of FLASH radiotherapy confirmed in mini-pig and cat-cancer patients. *Clinical Cancer Research : An Official Journal of the American Association for Cancer Research* 25: 35–42.

11 Bourhis, J. et al. (2019). Treatment of a first patient with FLASH-radiotherapy. *Radiotherapy and Oncology : Journal of the European Society for Therapeutic Radiology and Oncology* 139: 18–22.

12 Patriarca, A. et al. (2018). Experimental set-up for FLASH proton irradiation of small animals using a clinical system. *International Journal of Radiation Oncology, Biology, Physics* 102: 619–626.

13 Beyreuther, E. et al. (2019). Feasibility of proton FLASH effect tested by zebrafish embryo irradiation. *Radiotherapy and Oncology : Journal of the European Society for Therapeutic Radiology and Oncology* 139: 46–50.

14 Durante, M., Bräuer-krisch, E., and Hill, M. (2018). Faster and safer? FLASH ultra-high dose rate in radiotherapy. *British Journal of Radiology* 91: 6–9.

9

Boron Neutron Capture Therapy

Danushka Seneviratne, Timothy Malouff, Deanna Pafundi, Daniel Trifiletti, and Sunil Krishnan

Department of Radiation Oncology, Mayo Clinic Florida 4500 San Pablo Road, Jacksonville, FL 32224

TABLE OF CONTENTS

9.1   General Principles

Boron neutron capture theory (BNCT) is an innovative method of treating tumors by selectively irradiating cancer cells that have accumulated boron compounds. The advantage of BNCT lies in its ability to localize lethal damage to malignant cells while limiting injury to normal surrounding tissues. In order to achieve this goal, BNCT involves a bimodal approach. The first component involves the delivery of boron-containing compounds into the tumor cells in a higher concentration than the surrounding normal tissues. This is achieved through the use of various methods including antibody-mediated boron locali-

zation, boron porphyrins, liposomes, etc. This aspect of BNCT is discussed in detail below.

The second component of BNCT involves exposing the boron-containing tumor cells to low-energy thermal neutrons or high-energy epithermal neutrons that become thermalized as they penetrate tissues. This interaction between the boronated cells harboring a non-radioactive isotope of boron, Boron-10 (^{10}B), and the thermal neutrons (<0.025 eV) results in a nuclear capture and fission reaction. The reaction leads to the production of high linear energy transfer (LET) α particles and recoiling lithium-7 nuclei (^{10}B + n$_{th}$ → [^{11}B] → ^{4}He (α) + ^{7}Li + 2.38 MeV γ). The high LET α particles of

Principles and Practice of Particle Therapy, First Edition. Edited by Timothy D. Malouff and Daniel M. Trifiletti.
© 2022 John Wiley & Sons Ltd. Published 2022 by John Wiley & Sons Ltd.

approximately 150 keV/μm and ^{7}Li-nucleus of approximately 175 keV/μm have path ranges in water and tissue in the range of 4.5–10 μm, leading to energy deposition within the diameter of a single cell. This highly limited path range theoretically allows for the selective irradiation of tumor cells that have taken up boron while sparing normal tissues. Once the neutrons penetrate the tumor at the reference neutron velocity of 2,200 m/s, neutron absorption occurs due to the fact that Boron-10 has an absorption cross-section of 3,837 barns (Nedunchezhian et al., 2016a).

General principles of the BNCT reaction are shown in Figure 9.1.

Boron (generally delivered as BPA or BSH intravenously) largely accumulates in the tumor while sparing normal tissue. When cells harboring the non-radioactive isotope, Boron-10, are exposed to neutrons that become thermalized as they penetrate tissues, a nuclear capture and fission reaction occurs producing high LET α particles and recoiling lithium-7 nuclei. The resulting localized dose deposition allows for selective irradiation of tumor cells.

9.2 Boron Pharmacokinetics

9.2.1 Delivery of Boron and the Differential Accumulation in Tissues

In order for BNCT to be effective, studies have indicated that 20 μg/g of ^{10}B per weight of tumor is required. As alpha particles have a path length range of 5–9 μm, their impact is limited to boron-containing cells. Therefore, the impact of BNCT is theoretically limited to boron-containing tumor cells and spares normal tissues.

The general requirements for boron delivery agents include low *in-vivo* toxicity, high tumor uptake, low normal tissue uptake, and ability to achieve rapid clearance following completion of treatment (Barth, Mi, and Yang, 2018). Delivery of BNCT has primarily been performed with two boron compounds, sodium undecahydro-mercapto*closo*-dodecaborate ($Na_2B_{12}H_{11}SH$, also referred to as sodium borocaptate or BSH), and 4-dihydroxyborylphenylalanine (boronophenylalanine or BPA). Studies have shown that BPA is robustly taken up by a variety of cell types, including glioma and gliosarcoma cells, which overexpress the L-type amino acid transporter (LAT1) membrane protein that preferentially transports neutral branched-chain and aromatic amino acids. Clinical trials in the United States, Japan, and Sweden have indicated that BPA, particularly when complexed to fructose to form BPA-F, had a higher therapeutic effectiveness in comparison to BSH (Yoshino et al., 1989).

In BNCT, the absorbed dose depends on the concentration of boron and the distribution of the compound in the volume of irradiated tissue. Ideally, boron accumulation should be high in tumor and low in normal tissues. Witting et al. performed a study using a mouse model to assess the uptake of boron delivered using BPA or BSH. The investigators noted that after BPA delivery, the boron concentration was high in the kidneys and the spleen and was low in the brain. Following BSH injection, boron levels were high in the kidneys and low in brain and muscle tissues. Combined injection of BPA and BSH led to an additive effect of the two compounds within the organs. They concluded that boron uptake differed signifi-

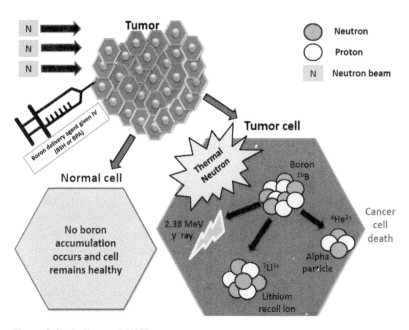

Figure 9.1 Delivery of BNCT.

cantly between different tissues and the biodistribution of boron largely depended on the boron delivery agent utilized (Wittig et al., 2009). In a similar study of biodistribution and pharmacokinetics of boron in dogs following administration of boronated porphyrin (BOPP), boron was found to primarily accumulate in the liver, lymph nodes, adrenal, and kidney tissues with very low level accumulation in the brain (Tibbitts et al., 2000).

9.2.2 Boron Accumulation Heterogeneity within Tumors

For BNCT to achieve optimal tumor control, there must be relatively high and homogenous buildup of boron throughout the tumor with minimal accumulation in normal tissues. The heterogeneity of boron delivery that allows for high concentrations in tumor tissues is advantageous for increasing tumor cell killing while sparing normal tissues. However, this tendency of boron to accumulate in a heterogeneous manner can also lead to inconsistent buildup within the tumor itself. Prior investigations have demonstrated that biodistribution of boron can differ widely between different parts of the tumor. Goodman et al. investigated tumor and normal brain tissue biodistribution of BSH in 25 patients with glioblastoma or anaplastic astrocytoma who were candidates for debulking surgery. These patients were administered BSH intravenously and at varying doses ranging from 15 to 50 mg/kg of body weight and multiple samples of brain tissues were obtained at either 3–7 or 13–15 h following infusion. The boron content of the tissue samples was then assessed using atomic emission spectroscopy. The authors found that the mean tumor boron concentrations were 17.1 µg/g ± 5.8 for glioblastoma multiformes (GBMs), while normal tissue concentrations were 4.6 µg/g ± 5.1. The large standard deviation values reflected the heterogeneity in boron uptake in tumor and normal tissues (Goodman et al., 2000). Another study of 98 patients treated with BPA-F in Finland also showed that there is significant heterogeneity in BPA levels in tumor and the normal brain tissues (Haapaniemi et al., 2016).

Animal studies have further confirmed this boron uptake heterogeneity as noted by the boron concentration variability in tissues in the F98 rat glioma model and the nude rat model of neuron capture therapy for intracerebral melanoma (Barth et al., 1994). As significant boron accumulation in tissues is necessary for the production of alpha particles, it is discernable that higher boron concentrations in tumors are likely associated with increased tumor response to BNCT therapy. This concept was demonstrated initially in rat glioma models in which the rats receiving higher doses of BPA experienced increasing survival times without evidence of increased toxicity. Further highlighting the importance of tissue boron concentration on therapeutic efficacy of BNCT, a study by Barth et al. showed that intracarotid injection of BSH or BPA followed by radiation led to superior survival in F98 glioma rats in comparison to intravenous injection. The highest tumor concentrations of boron were achieved via the intracarotid injection, and the survival increase noted with intracarotid injection was further enhanced by disruption of the blood–brain barrier with mannitol. Analysis of normal brain tissues 1 year following boron administration showed minimal radiation-related changes and no clear histopathological differences between the radiated and non-radiated controls or those who received intravenous or intracarotid boron (Barth et al., 1997, 2000).

Given that microlocalization of boron compounds within the tumor is crucial to the success of BNCT, the combined administration of different boronated compounds with various properties and uptake mechanisms have been investigated as a method to allow for more homogenous tumor delivery. A comparison of the properties of BSH and BPA is illustrated in Table 9.1. BPA is transported across the cell membrane by the L-amino acid transport system and therefore BPA uptake depends largely on the cell viability and metabolic status. In contrast, BSH appears to have lower selectivity due to their lack of a cell-specific transport system. BSH is also only capable of entering the brain when the blood–brain barrier has been disrupted. However, in comparison to BPA, BSH has 12 times more ^{10}B per molecule and therefore can lead to a higher accumulation of boron within the tumor (Futamura et al., 2017). Using a combination of these BPA and BSH or developing novel boronated compounds for delivery are potential options to overcome tumor heterogeneity while preserving the selectivity of boron accumulation between tumor and normal tissues. For instance, an institution in Osaka, Japan, has published on the use of ACBC (1-amino-3-fluorocyclobutane-1-carboxylic acid) conjugated to BSH as a potential boron delivery agent. The authors of this work demonstrate that ACBC is an unnatural amino acid which is actively taken up by cells with LAT1s and can be conjugated to BSH to derive ACBC-BSH. This conjugated derivative was found to selectively accumulate in the tumor cells of F98 cell line bearing xenografted rats at higher concentrations in comparison to BPA and led to significantly increased survival among the cohort treated with the conjugate (Futamura et al., 2017).

Based on the above-noted findings and evident shortcomings of currently utilized boronated compounds, further investigations are certainly warranted to determine optimal type and the method of delivery of boron for BNCT treatments.

9.3 Neutron Sources

9.3.1 Neutron Producing Reactions for Accelerator-based BNCT

Although nuclear reactors have been used with success for the production of neutrons, low-energy particle accelerators appear

Table 9.1 Comparison of the properties of the most common BNCT delivery agents (adapted from Porcari, P.C., Silvia; Saverio Pastore, Francesco, 2011)

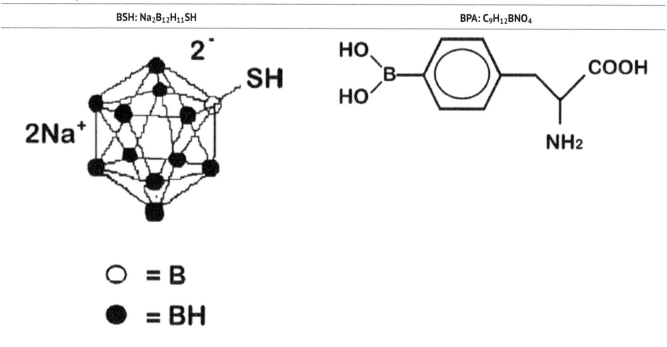

BSH: $Na_2B_{12}H_{11}SH$	BPA: $C_9H_{12}BNO_4$
No specific cell-membrane transporter	Transported across cell membrane by L-amino acid transport system
Uptake is generally independent of cell cycle phase or metabolic status	Uptake depends on cell viability and metabolic status BPA accumulation increases during S phase of cell cycle
Has 12× more ^{10}B per molecule compared to BPA	Lower ^{10}B content in BPA can theoretically limit BNCT effectiveness
Is soluble in aqueous solutions/hydrophilic	Has low solubility in aqueous solutions and therefore must be administered in complex with fructose
Enters brain only when blood–brain barrier is disrupted	Can enter brain without disruption of blood–brain barrier

to be the most promising method of BNCT delivery within standard hospital environments. Accelerator-based BNCT has several advantages over reactor-based BNCT, including the ability to be turned off when the neutron field is no longer required, lower cost of installation and maintenance, and the softer neutron energy spectrum generated which allows for an ideal epithermal neutron spectrum. The nuclear fission of ^{235}U induced by thermal neutrons occurs within nuclear reactors and yields high-energy fragments with an average energy of 2 MeV. These neutrons need to be moderated to thermal energies to treat superficial lesions or epithermal energies to treat deep-seated tumors. Another form of generating neutrons is through the use of charged particles. In this process, a certain projectile is accelerated to a high energy to overcome the Coulombic forces and attacks the target nucleus leading to the production of a residual nucleus and a neutron. These reactions can be termed exothermic if they do not require a minimum kinetic energy of the projectile (Kreiner et al., 2014; Suzuki, 2020).

9.3.2 Neutron Beam Design and Dose Monitoring

The main objective of beam design for neutron capture therapy is to produce a uniform distribution of low-energy neutrons in the targeted treatment volume. Given that tumor dose conformity is achieved primarily by the selective capture of thermal neutrons within the tumor during irradiation, there is limited need for intricate modulation of the beam spatial profile. However, neutron beams should be collimated to help reduce irradiation of organs and peripheral normal tissues that may have absorbed some of the boron. Studies have shown that a variety of neutron beam energies are advantageous for external beam neutron capture therapy. The optimal energy for a particular tumor type appears to depend on tumor location, tumor size, the constraints of normal tissues, and boron uptake. Given that BNCT-absorbed dose is derived from neutron interactions within cells, monitoring the absorbed dose accurately presents a challenge. Uranium-lined fission counters, helium, and boron-filled gas-filled detectors have been used previously in some clinical centers. Additionally, neutron fluence can also be monitored *in situ* with the use of foils or wires inserted into the cavity following surgical resection of the tumor (Perks et al., 1988; Zaidi et al., 2018).

9.3.3 Endothermic Reaction of Neutron Production

$^{7}Li(p,n)^{7}Be$ reaction is the most frequently studied endothermic reaction that serves as a neutron source for BNCT. This is often displayed as $^{7}Li + p \rightarrow {}^{7}Be + n$. Given that this is an endothermic reaction, the Q value is in the negative range and measures –1.644 MeV. The emitted neutron energy can be modulated with the bombarding proton energy and depends largely upon the emerging proton angle. With decrease in neutron energy, moderation of the neutrons is more easily accomplished; however, it must be noted that as energy decreases, the neutron yield also decreases proportionally. The ideal neutron energy involves achieving a balance between neutron moderation and yield. This endothermic reaction works near its threshold of 1.88 MeV. In comparison to other neutron production reactions that yield higher energies, this reaction yields maximum energies of about 100 keV and thus is more useful for obtaining energies that can be successfully utilized in BNCT (Kreiner et al., 2014; Minsky and Kreiner, 2015).

9.4 Dosimetry and Treatment Planning in BNCT

The main advantage of BNCT lies in the fact that its therapeutic benefits occur primarily locally at the cellular level. In order to obtain an accurate dose calculation for BNCT, nuclear interactions of neutrons with different tissue elements must be performed along with patient geometry modelling. Generally, patient models are created using CT and MRI images and imaging information from different modalities are combined to help create accurate models for dose calculations. Given that BNCT is an uncommon treatment modality, there are no widely accepted consensus guidelines regarding beam dosimetry. The work toward developing coherent dosimetry guidelines was started in 1998. There are several methods of assessing BNCT dosimetry. When epithermal neutrons are used, reasonable dosimetric accuracy has been achieved via ionization chambers. The use of dual ionization chambers is recommended for dose measurements and is often used to determine photon and fast neutron dose when mixed beams are utilized. The use of miniature proportional counters is also popular in BNCT treatments as they reduce the issue of dose pile-up at high intensities. Silicon diode-based microdosime-

ters can be used to measure the total neutron and photon dose easily with a small detector. Additional methods of assessing photon and neutron dosimetry for BNCT include the use of thermoluminescent dosimeters, gel dosimeters, and alanine detectors. Given that there is no definite consensus regarding the optimal method of performing BNCT dosimetry, novel techniques continue to evolve (Burmeister, Kota, and Maughan, 1999; Kumada et al., 2004).

There are several Monte-Carlo-based treatment planning methods for BNCT developed over the last several decades. NCTPLAN was one of the earliest planning systems involving Monte Carlo based calculations that was developed in the late 1990s with the support of the Massachusetts Institute of Technology BNCT program. NCTPLAN uses CT image data to create a mathematical model of relevant anatomic parts. It was initially validated via experiments involving mixed field dosimetry utilizing cranial parallel-opposed epithermal neutron beam irradiation of a human subject with glioblastoma (Zamenhof et al., 1996). Nievaart et al. presented a relatively comprehensive review of Monte-Carlo-based treatment planning systems for BNCT used in the Netherlands. This publication discussed the successful use of the BNCT_rtpe system for treatment planning in glioblastoma and the use of NCTPLAN for treatment planning of melanoma. Additionally, they also noted that, more recently, another *ad-hoc* PET-based treatment planning system known as BDTPS has also been implemented in order to integrate real macroscopic boron distribution data obtained from PET scanning. The authors noted that in general, a well-designed BNCT treatment planning system should have a pre-processing phase with CT/MRI scans to create a geometric solid model, the ability to perform calculations of 3D radiation transport and estimate neutron and gamma fluences, as well as a post processing phase (Nievaart, Daquino, and Moss, 2007).

9.5 Clinical Applications

To date, BNCT has been studied clinically in several disease sites, including GBM, meningioma, head and neck cancers, lung cancers, breast cancers, hepatocellular carcinoma, sarcomas, cutaneous malignancies, extra-mammary Paget's disease, recurrent cancers, pediatric cancers, and metastatic disease.

Below is an attempt to provide a comprehensive review of the clinical studies for each of these disease sites, as well as a review on the challenges limiting the widespread adoption of BNCT. Data pertaining to select disease sites are outlined in Table 9.2.

9.5.1 Glioblastoma Multiforme

GBM is a primary brain malignancy with a dismal prognosis, despite multimodality therapy consisting of maximum resection,

Table 9.2 Studies of select disease sites and outcomes with the use of BNCT

Study	Number of patients	Boron carrier	Outcomes
Henriksson et al. (2008)	30	BPA-F	Median OS: 14.2 months Median time to progression: 5.8 months
Chanana et al. (1999)	38	BPA-F	Median OS: 13 months Median time to progression: 31.6 weeks
Miyatake et al. (2016)	167	BPA-F	Median survival: 9.6 months
Shiba et al. (2018)	7	Combination BPA with bevacizumab	Median OS: 15.1 months Median time to progression: 5.4 months

Head and neck

Study	Number of patients	Boron carrier	Outcomes
Head and neck (definitive)			
Kankaanranta et al. (2012)	30	BPA-F	Response rate: 76% Median PFS: 7.5 months 2-year OS: 30%
Head and neck (recurrent)			
Suzuki et al. (2014)	62	BPA alone or BPA and BSH	Median survival: 10.1 months Response rate: 58% 2-year OS: 24.2%
Koivunoro et al. (2019)	79	BPA-F	Complete response rate: 36% 2-year LRPFS 38% 2-year OS 21%
Wang et al. (2014, 2018)	23	BPA-F	2-year locoregional control: 28% 2-year OS: 47%

Melanoma

Study	Number of patients	Boron carrier	Outcomes
Menendez et al. (2009)	7	BPA-F	Overall response rate: 69% Grade 3 toxicity rate: 30%

Meningioma

Study	Number of patients	Boron carrier	Outcomes
Takeuchi et al. (2018)	31	BPA-F	Median OS: 24.6 months

radiation, and adjuvant chemotherapy (Stupp et al., 2005). Due to this, BNCT has been theorized as a potentially beneficial treatment option in the upfront and recurrent settings to achieve localized dose escalation within the tumor. BNCT is believed to be very feasible in the treatment of difficult to treat CNS malignancies given that boron has been shown to possess direct tumoricidal activity and many boronated compounds can cross the blood–brain barrier (Altinoz, Topcu, and Elmaci, 2019). A report by Miyatake et al. documented the treatment of 167 cases of malignant brain tumors and high-grade meningiomas with BNCT from 2002 to 2014. BPA was used at the boron delivery agent in these cases. The median survival time following BNCT administration for GBM was 9.6 months (Miyatake et al., 2016). In another report, 30 patients with glioblastoma in Sweden were treated between 2001 and 2003 with BNCT. BPA-F at a high dose of 900 mg/kg was used as the boron carrier and irradiation with neutrons was performed 2 h after the infusion. In this patient cohort, the median OS was 14.2 months and the time to progression was 5.8 months following treatment. Toxicity assessment revealed seizures in seven patients, thromboembolic events in five patients, and grades 1–3 skin toxicity in eight patients. Unfortunately, patient quality of life was found to have considerably deteriorated following BNCT treatment due to toxicities and/or disease progression (Henriksson et al., 2008). There is limited North American data regarding the use of BNCT in GBM treatment. A study that is often quoted as being exemplary of a US study is a phase I/II trial assessing the feasibility of single fraction BNCT in the treatment GBM performed at Brookhaven National Laboratory during the 1990s. BPA fructose was used as the delivery agent and a total of 38 patients were treated as part of a Phase I/II dose escalation study. The median time to tumor progression following treatment was 31.6 weeks, with a median survival of 13.0 months. There were no reported grade 3 or 4 toxicity (Chanana et al., 1999).

Given that there are very limited options for the treatment of recurrent high-grade gliomas, BNCT was also tested in a phase I study for recurrent disease. L-BPA-fructose was used as the boron delivery agent, and increasing doses of boron ranging from 290 mg/kg to 450 mg/kg were administered to patients with high-grade gliomas. Following treatment, the median survival was 7 months and the maximum tolerated dose of L-BPA-fructose was found to be 450 mg/kg. The authors concluded that BNCT therapy with L-BPA-fructose administration at a dose of 400 mg/kg as a 2-h infusion is a reasonable option for the treatment of recurrent gliomas (Kankaanranta et al., 2011b).

One of the concerns of BNCT in the setting of malignant gliomas is the high rates of symptomatic pseudoprogression and radionecrosis that is observed following treatment (Miyatake et al., 2018). In one series, at 3 months following BNCT, 11 out of 52 malignant gliomas and 3 out of 13 malignant meningioma patients developed worsening edema (Miyatake et al., 2009). In an attempt to reduce the rate of radionecrosis following BNCT, a pilot study involving the use of BNCT in combination with bevacizumab was performed in Japan. Bevacizumab was started 2–6 weeks after BNCT and was given at biweekly doses of 10 mg/kg. From 2013 to 2014, seven patients were treated with BNCT and bevacizumab. Median overall survival (OS) and progression-free survival (PFS) were 15.1 months and 5.4 months, respectively. No radionecrosis was seen through December 2017, and the authors concluded that bevacizumab treatments appeared to limit radionecrosis and lead to prolonged OS and acceptable toxicity levels (Shiba et al., 2018). Additionally, bevacizumab at a dose of 5 mg/kg was shown to improve symptomatic pseudoprogression in two patients treated with BNCT for recurrent gliomas. In support of these findings, Miyatake et al. reported on four patients with recurrent malignant gliomas treated in Osaka, Japan with BNCT and bevacizumab. Three RPA class 4 patients had survival times of 14, 16.5 and over 23 months following BNCT. The authors concluded that BNCT with bevacizumab improved symptoms of symptomatic pseudoprogression or radionecrosis and prolonged survival (Miyatake et al., 2014).

In a histopathological study of patients treated with BNCT for GBM performed at the time of salvage surgery or autopsy, residual tumor cells were noted in 4/8 patients. The authors concluded that at least a dose of 68 Gy to the GTV and 44 Gy to the CTV was needed to achieve a histopathologic cure (Kageji et al., 2014). In one interesting case, a patient with gliosarcoma who was previously treated with BNCT, only the sarcomatous component was found to recur 6 months following-BNCT (Miyatake et al., 2006). Radiographic analysis of a portion of patients treated with BNCT as part of the EORTC 11961 trial revealed that approximately 50% of patients had cerebral changes within the first year following treatment with atrophy affecting 42% of patients (Vos et al., 2005).

Currently, there are several accruing or completed clinical trials investigating the use of BNCT in high-grade gliomas in Japan. The Tsukuba BNCT trial is a phase II study evaluating photon irradiation with concurrent temozolomide combined with BNCT using 250 mg/kg BPA as the boron delivery agent (Yamamoto et al., 2011).

Although there is limited data available to date supporting the use of BNCT in high-grade gliomas, the existing studies paint an encouraging picture, particularly as a possible treatment option for multiply recurrent disease with limited local and systemic therapy options.

9.5.2 Meningioma

Miyatake et al. described the treatment of seven cases of malignant meningiomas with BNCT, including three anaplastic meningiomas, two papillary meningiomas, one atypical meningioma, and one sarcoma that had transformed from an initial diagnosis of a meningioma. Following treatment, two of the three anaplastic meningiomas showed a complete response, with all patients showing radiographic improvement (Miyatake et al., 2007). Stenstam et al. described two patients with recurrent meningeal tumors treated with BNCT following surgery, radiation, or salvage surgery. The authors concluded that BNCT is a potentially effective treatment modality for recurrent malignant intracranial meningeal tumors (Stenstam et al., 2007).

A retrospective review from the Osaka Medical College Hospital and the Kyoto University Research Reactor Institute investigated 31 patients treated with recurrent high-grade meningiomas. PET scans revealed that boron accumulation was much higher in the meningiomas compared to normal brain. Following treatment, all lesions showed a decrease in size. Median survival was 24.6 months following BNCT (Takeuchi et al., 2018).

In an interesting case report by Tamura et al., a 25-year-old patient with a recurrent malignant meningioma was treated with BNCT following two failed resections and three courses of Gamma Knife radiosurgery. Following treatment, she regained the ability to ambulate within one week after the first treatment of BNCT and radiographic decrease in tumor size was seen at 26 weeks post-treatment (Tamura et al., 2006).

Histopathological data following BNCT treatment of meningiomas remains limited. Autopsy studies of a 70-year-old male who died from systemic metastasis from an anaplastic meningioma indicated that the meningioma recurrences treated with BNCT showed significantly lower proliferative activity compared to untreated metastatic liver lesions (Kawaji et al., 2015). Additional pathology studies have showed that despite the positive treatment impact of BNCT, high doses of BNCT to the neural parenchyma can lead to radiation-induced focal venular fibrinoid necrosis and multifocal demyelination (Aziz et al., 2000).

9.5.3 Definitive Head and Neck Cancers

Although the majority of clinical trials investigated the use of BNCT in the recurrent head and neck setting, BNCT has also been used for definitive therapy in select cases. Kankaanranta et al. reported on a 53-year-old patient who was successfully treated with BNCT for a large 7.4-cm intranasal mass in the definitive setting. Patient was initially administered 400 mg/kg L-BPA-fructose, which was followed by IMRT with a dose of 44 Gy with concurrent IV cetuximab and cisplatin. The patient experienced grade 3 mucositis, alopecia, fatigue, and xerophthalmia. Following treatment, the patient achieved a complete response and had no evidence of disease at 6 month follow-up (Kankaanranta et al., 2011a). The authors concluded that BNCT is reasonable with moderate toxicity in the setting of first line therapy for head and neck cancers. Another case report documented the successful utilization of single fraction BNCT using BPA-F at a dose of 400 mg/kg for the treatment of unresectable, undifferentiated sinonasal carcinoma. The patient recurred after 6 months. As per the report, following BNCT treatment, quality of life was improved, and mucositis was the main toxicity experienced by the patient (Kouri et al., 2004). Kimura et al. reported on a 78-year-old patient with a papillary cystadenocarcinoma of the upper lip that was treated with BNCT in two fractions, using 500 mg/kg BPA as the boron carrier. At a follow up of 5 months, the tumor size decreased by 86% (Kimura et al., 2009).

In a prospective phase I/II trial (NCT00114790) of 30 patients treated for inoperable, locally advanced head and neck cancer with BNCT between December 2003 and September 2008 in Finland showed promising results. Patients were treated with surgery and radiation therapy to a median dose of 60 Gy, with 33% of patients receiving concurrent chemotherapy. BNCT was administered in two fractions with 400 mg/kg L-BPA-fructose. A response rate of 76% was noted among the evaluable patients. The median PFS was 7.5 months, and the 2-year OS and PFS were 30% and 20%, respectively.

Acute toxicities primarily included grade 3 mucositis and oral pain which were observed in 54% of patients. Long-term toxicities included osteoradionecrosis in three patients, soft tissue necrosis in one patient, and grade 3 xerostomia in six patients (Kankaanranta et al., 2012).

One of the main concerns regarding BNCT in the treatment of head and neck cancers includes the risk of fatal carotid blowout. A recent study reported that carotid blowout syndrome occurred in 2 out of 33 patients treated with BNCT and occurred between 1 and 3 months after BNCT (Aihara et al., 2015). Although there is limited data regarding the use of BNCT in the definitive treatment of head and neck cancers, early data indicates that it is a promising modality for certain aggressive pathologies.

9.5.4 Recurrent Head and Neck Cancers

Given the poor prognosis of recurrent head and neck cancer, there have been several investigations into BNCT as a possible treatment modality for this patient population. Kato et al. reported on the first six patients treated with BNCT for recurrent head and neck cancers, using a combination of BPA and BSH as the boron delivery agent. Following treatment, there was considerable reduction in tumor volume in five patients and patient reported improvement in quality of life (Kato et al., 2004). In a report of 62 recurrent head and neck patients treated with BNCT at Kyoto University with BPA alone or BPA/BSH combination, a median survival of 10.1 months and an overall response rate of 58% were observed at 6 months. The 2-year OS was 24.2%. The most common acute grade 3+ toxicity was hyperamylasemia and the second most common toxicity was grade 3+ mucositis. Following treatment, two patients experienced fatal carotid blowout, and one patient died due to anorexia (Suzuki et al., 2014). A retrospective study of seventy-nine patients with unresectable, recurrent squamous cell carcinoma of the head and neck region that were treated with BNCT in Finland was recently reported. It showed a 68% response rate, with 38% of patients achieving a complete response. Patients who were treated with BNCT twice showed increased response rates. The median follow-up was 7.8 years, the 2-year locoregional progression-free survival was 38%, and 2-year OS was 21%. Statistical analysis revealed that a minimum GTV dose of 18 Gy was associated with increased survival (Koivunoro et al., 2019). In a report from Osaka, Japan, twenty-six patients with recurrent head and neck cancer were treated with BNCT, the authors reported an 85% response rate with a median survival of 13.6 months. Transient mucositis and alopecia were the most common side effects, with three patient developing osteomyelitis (Kato et al., 2009). Another study from Japan reported on 12 patients with unresectable, recurrent, locally advanced head and neck cancers who were treated with BNCT. Ten patients received BNCT twice, and two patients were treated once. Following treatment, 83% of patients showed some response. Two patients had grade 3+ toxicity consisting of xerostomia or dysphagia (Kankaanranta et al., 2007).

BNCT has shown some promise particularly in difficult to treat recurrent tumors such as recurrent salivary gland tumors. In a report by Aihara et al. a 48-year-old patient with recurrent submandibular gland malignancy showed complete regression after therapy (Aihara et al., 2006). The same authors also reported on two patients with recurrent salivary gland cancer and three patients with newly diagnosed T4 salivary gland cancers treated with BNCT between 2003 and 2007. All of these patients achieved a complete response within 6 months. The median survival was 32 months, with two patients eventually developing distant metastatic disease. There were no grade 3+ toxicities (Aihara et al., 2014). BNCT has also been used successfully in treating nodal recurrences in head and neck cancer. In a report of four patients undergoing treatment with BNCT for regional nodal recurrences following definitive treatment for oral cavity cancer, all patients showed some response (Ariyoshi et al., 2007).

Given the promising results from case reports and case series regarding the use of BNCT in recurrent head and neck malignancies, a phase I/II trial was opened at the National Tsing-Hua University. This trial enrolled 17 patients with recurrent head and neck cancer between 2010 and 2013. A fructose complex of L-boronophenylalanine was used as the boronated compound. Patients were then treated to a prescription dose of 20 Gy in two fractions using a single field with a 28-day interval between the fractions. With a median follow up of 19.9 months, 15 patients received both fractions, and 6 had a complete response. Low-grade oral mucositis, radiation dermatitis, and alopecia were the most common acute toxicities. The reported severe long-term toxicities included grade 4 acute laryngeal edema, carotid hemorrhage, and grade 3 cranial neuropathy. The authors reported a 2-year OS of 47% (Wang et al., 2014, 2016, 2018). The locoregional control rate was 28%. Based on the results from this trial, a second clinical trial using image-guided IMRT for radiation delivery was opened with the aim of further improving local control. In the second protocol, radiation treatment was initiated 28 days following administration of BNCT. A total of seven patients were treated on this protocol; complete response was seen in three patients with a calculated median OS of 56% (Wang et al., 2018).

9.5.5 Lung Cancers

BNCT has been proposed in the treatment of diffuse, nonresectable lung tumors (Trivillin et al., 2014), as well as for inoperable malignant pleural mesothelioma; however, the data remain limited (Suzuki et al., 2006, 2007b, 2008). A report of two patients with diffuse pleural tumors treated with BNCT with BPA-fructose as the boron carrier indicated promising results. The tumors remained stable or regressed by the 6-month follow-up without evidence of grade 3+ toxicity (Suzuki et al., 2008). Another study by Farias et al. indicated that BNCT may be appropriate in the treatment of shallow lung tumors; however, there are no studies to date investigating the use of BNCT in deeper tumors (Farias et al., 2014).

9.5.6 Breast Cancers

There are very limited data regarding the use of BNCT in breast cancer. Promising preclinical data have indicated that BNCT may be an option in at least HER2 overexpressing breast malignancies. In preclinical studies, immunoliposomes, such as those labeled with trastuzumab, have been used as boron carriers to selectively target HER2 overexpressing cells (Gadan et al., 2015). Further clinical work needs to be performed to determine whether BNCT is a viable option in the treatment of aggressive breast malignancies.

9.5.7 Hepatocellular Carcinoma

A case report from Japan of a patient with hepatocellular carcinoma with Child–Pugh grade B cirrhosis who underwent irradiation of the right lobe with BNCT demonstrated stable tumor at 1 month following treatment. The patient however had disease progression 3.5 months following treatment (Suzuki et al., 2007a). Yanagie et al. performed a pilot study using selective intra-arterial infusion to deliver a BSH containing emulsion to a left liver lobe lesion in a 63-year-old man with hepatocellular carcinoma. The patient was considered to have stable disease on initial imaging following treatment; however, he eventually developed multiple lung and additional liver nodules (Yanagie et al., 2014). The data regarding treatment of hepatocellular carcinoma with BNCT are sparse, and further research is needed prior to adopting it as a possible treatment option.

9.5.8 Sarcoma

Osteosarcoma has been shown to be effectively and safely treated with BNCT. A report of a temporomandibular joint osteosarcoma treated with BNCT showed no evidence of disease recurrence after 2 years (Uchiyama et al., 2014). In a report by Futamura et al., a 54-year-old female was treated with BNCT for a recurrent radiation-induced osteosarcoma in the left occipital skull. BPA was used as the boron delivery agent. Although she was unable to ambulate at diagnosis, she regained the ability to ambulate without aid approximately 3 weeks following BNCT. The treatment was well tolerated, with the patient experiencing alopecia as the only reported toxicity (Futamura et al., 2014).

9.5.9 Melanoma

Patients diagnosed with melanoma often have poor prognoses despite optimal treatments. Gonzalez et al. reported on a case of 54-year-old woman treated with BNCT for cutaneous melanoma as part of a 30-patient cohort. Of the 25 skin nodules on these patients, 21 showed complete response approximately 8 weeks following treatment with grade 1 acute skin reaction as the primary toxicity (Gonzalez et al., 2004). Menendez et al. reported on seven patients treated with BNCT for cutaneous melanoma with multiple skin metastases treated with BNCT in Argentina between 2003 and 2007. All patients received 14 mg/m^2 of BPA. The overall response rate was 69%. Grade 3 toxicity rate was 30% with the primary adverse effect being ulceration (Menendez et al., 2009).

Most recently, the Third Xiangya Hospital of Central South University in Changsha China developed a protocol for treating malignant melanoma using BNCT in 30 patients (NCT02759536). In this study, a BPA-F complex was used as the boron delivery agent, with 350 mg/kg infused into the patient over 90 min. The estimated dose was determined using the Monte Carlo N Particle Transport Code 6 program. The authors reported on the first patient treated on this trial in 2014. The patient only experienced mild dandruff 1 week following irradiation, although this progressed to grade 2 dermatitis by 4 weeks. Biopsy performed at 9 months post-BNCT and PET scan 24 months post-BNCT showed no evidence of disease (Yong et al., 2016).

9.5.10 Extra-mammary Paget's Disease

Due to the morbidity associated with wide local excision of extra-mammary Paget's disease of the genitals, there has been increased interest in alterative treatment options. Hiratsuka et al. treated four patients with extra-mammary Paget's disease between 2005 and 2014 with BNCT. ^{10}B-enriched L-BPA was used as the boron delivery agent. All four patients had a complete response in 6 months. With regard to toxicity, two patients developed grade 2 erosions and one patient developed grade 1 mucositis (Hiratsuka et al., 2018).

Makino et al. reported on the first two cases of extra-mammary Paget's disease of the genitals treated with BNCT. Approximately 12 months post-treatment, both patients had complete response with no evidence of recurrence or metastatic disease (Makino et al., 2012; Nedunchezhian et al., 2016b).

9.5.11 Metastatic Disease

Although BNCT has sparingly been used in the treatment of primary tumors as noted above, given that there are limited data and a plethora of other viable options when treating in the definitive setting, BNCT may be a better option in the recurrent or metastatic disease settings. The EORTC 11001 protocol is a translational phase I trial with the goal to measure the uptake of two boronated compounds in tissues and the blood in patients treated with BNCT for metastatic liver disease. BSH and BPA were administered prior to surgical resection of hepatic metastasis. The trial has completed accrual. In an initial report of the trial results, the authors noted that there was no toxicity associated with the delivery of the boronated compounds. They also noted that BSH may not be a suitable carrier, as the concentration of the compound in the liver was higher than in the metastatic lesions. The authors concluded that BPA may be used for extracorporeal irradiation of the liver with BNCT (Wittig et al., 2008).

Clinically, BNCT has been shown to lead to suppression of tumor growth in a 72-year-old patient with recurrent gastric cancer and a left cervical node lesion (Yanagie et al., 2012; Nedunchezhian et al., 2016a).

Interestingly, a proof of principle study using rats treated with BNCT showed that BNCT is capable of inducing the abscopal effect in rats inoculated with colon cancer cells (Trivillin et al., 2017). Given the limited studies and the available promising results, further studies are warranted to assess the efficacy and feasibility of BNCT in the metastatic setting.

9.5.12 Pediatrics

BNCT has been shown to be safe and efficacious in the treatment of pediatric malignant brain lesions. A case series of 23 patients under the age of 15 with malignant brain tumors including glioblastoma, astrocytoma, PNET, pontine glioma, and anaplastic ependymoma showed encouraging results with 4/6 anaplastic astrocytomas and a single patient with anaplastic ependymoma showing no evidence of disease recurrence following treatment completion. The authors concluded that BNCT may be used in select pediatric brain malignancies (Nakagawa et al., 2009a).

Zhang et al. assessed the secondary malignancy risk in pediatric patients treated with BNCT for brain tumors in China. When comparing neutron beam geometries, the authors concluded that the lifetime attributable risk of secondary malignancy was lower with posterior-to-anterior arrangement of beams compared to right-lateral and top-to-bottom beam arrangements. Younger age and female gender significantly associated with increased risk of secondary malignancy (Zhang et al., 2019). In Japan, only 1 out of 180 patients treated for malignant brain tumors since 1968 developed multiple radiation-induced meningiomas in the treatment field (Kageji et al., 2015).

9.5.13 Discussion

Although there are currently limited data, BNCT is a promising treatment modality that appears to be safe and efficacious in the treatment of patients with advanced tumors. The above-noted studies however exhibit a high degree of heterogeneity with regard to the inclusion criteria, the type of boronated compounds used, times for infusion, and neutron radiation dose. This leads to some difficulty when assessing the results of the studies. Coupled with this heterogeneity of clinical features of patients on trials, tumor heterogeneity results in variable uptake of boronated compounds by tumors of the same type in different patients. Lack of routine use of ^{18}F-BPA PET to account for this variability and for treatment planning also probably contributes to inconsistencies in outcomes reported across studies. Given these concerns, there is certainly a need for phase II/III trials to further assess the role of BNCT in the treatment of primary and recurrence malignancies. It is important to note that the available data to date suggests that despite good responses particularly in difficult to treat tumors, toxicity rates remain relatively high. Whether this is due to intermixing of fast neutrons, persistent boronated compounds in normal tissues (and vasculature) during irradiation, limited beam orientations used to reduce dose to upstream normal tissues in the beam path, and/or lack of fractionation remains unclear. Nevertheless, further research to develop more selective boronated compounds that may improve the therapeutic ratio will certainly improve treatment outcomes and increase the acceptability of BNCT as a routine oncologic therapy. A considerable barrier to the adoption of BNCT is the high cost of developing and maintaining a BNCT treatment center. Currently, Nakagawa et al. estimated that a BNCT facility in Japan costs approximately 1,200 million Yen (approximately $11.4 million) to construct with an annual personnel cost of 113 million Yen (approximately $1 million) (Nakagawa et al., 2009b). If further studies indicate that BNCT is safe and efficacious, the costly investment of developing a *de novo* BNCT center in the United States may be considered a worthy goal.

Boron neutron capture therapy represents an emerging targeted therapy with promising results and acceptable toxicity in early clinical studies. Further prospective research is necessary to define the role of BNCT in clinical practice.

References

1 Aihara, T., Hiratsuka, J., Ishikawa, H., Kumada, H., Ohnishi, K., Kamitani, N., Suzuki, M., Sakurai, H., and Harada, T. (2015). Fatal carotid blowout syndrome after BNCT for head and neck cancers. *Applied Radiation and Isotopes: Including Data, Instrumentation and Methods for Use in Agriculture, Industry and Medicine* 106: 202–206.

2 Aihara, T., Hiratsuka, J., Morita, N., Uno, M., Sakurai, Y., Maruhashi, A., Ono, K., and Harada, T. (2006). First clinical case of boron neutron capture therapy for head and neck malignancies using 18F-BPA PET. *Head & Neck* 28: 850–855.

3 Aihara, T., Morita, N., Kamitani, N., Kumada, H., Ono, K., Hiratsuka, J., and Harada, T. (2014). Boron neutron capture therapy for advanced salivary gland carcinoma in head and neck. *International Journal of Clinical Oncology* 19: 437–444.

4 Altinoz, M.A., Topcu, G., and Elmaci, I. (2019). Boron's neurophysiological effects and tumoricidal activity on glioblastoma cells with implications for clinical treatment. *The International Journal of Neuroscience* 129: 963–977.

5 Ariyoshi, Y., Miyatake, S., Kimura, Y., Shimahara, T., Kawabata, S., Nagata, K., Suzuki, M., Maruhashi, A., Ono, K., and Shimahara, M. (2007). Boron neuron capture therapy using epithermal neutrons for recurrent cancer in the oral cavity and cervical lymph node metastasis. *Oncology Reports* 18: 861–866.

6 Aziz, T., Peress, N.S., Diaz, A., Capala, J., and Chanana, A. (2000). Postmortem neuropathological features secondary to boron neutron capture therapy for glioblastoma multiforme. *Journal of Neuropathology and Experimental Neurology* 59: 62–73.

7 Barth, R.F., Matalka, K.Z., Bailey, M.Q., Staubus, A.E., Soloway, A.H., Moeschberger, M.L., Coderre, J.A., and Rofstad, E.K. (1994). A nude rat model for neutron capture therapy of human intracerebral melanoma. *International Journal of Radiation Oncology, Biology, Physics* 28: 1079–1088.

8 Barth, R.F., Mi, P., and Yang, W.L. (2018). Boron delivery agents for neutron capture therapy of cancer. *Cancer Communications* 38.

9 Barth, R.F., Yang, W., Rotaru, J.H., Moeschberger, M.L., Boesel, C.P., Soloway, A.H., Joel, D.D., Nawrocky, M.M., Ono, K., and Goodman, J.H. (2000). Boron neutron capture therapy of brain tumors: Enhanced survival and cure following blood-brain barrier disruption and intracarotid injection of sodium borocaptate and boronophenylalanine. *International Journal of Radiation Oncology, Biology, Physics* 47: 209–218.

10 Barth, R.F., Yang, W., Rotaru, J.H., Moeschberger, M.L., Joel, D.D., Nawrocky, M.M., Goodman, J.H., and Soloway, A.H. (1997). Boron neutron capture therapy of brain tumors: Enhanced survival following intracarotid injection of either sodium borocaptate or boronophenylalanine with or without blood-brain barrier disruption. *Cancer Research* 57: 1129–1136.

11 Burmeister, J., Kota, C., and Maughan, R.L. (1999). Dosimetry of the boron neutron capture reaction for BNCT and BNCEFNT. *Strahlentherapie Und Onkologie: Organ Der Deutschen Rontgengesellschaft. [Et Al]* 175 (Suppl 2): 115–118.

12 Chanana, A.D., Capala, J., Chadha, M., Coderre, J.A., Diaz, A.Z., Elowitz, E.H., Iwai, J., Joel, D.D., Liu, H.B., Ma, R., *et al.*

(1999). Boron neutron capture therapy for glioblastoma multiforme: Interim results from the phase I/II dose-escalation studies. *Neurosurgery* 44: 1182–1192. discussion 1192-1183.

13 Farias, R.O., Bortolussi, S., Menendez, P.R., and Gonzalez, S.J. (2014). Exploring Boron Neutron Capture Therapy for non-small cell lung cancer. *Medical Physics* 30: 888–897.

14 Futamura, G., Kawabata, S., Nonoguchi, N., Hiramatsu, R., Toho, T., Tanaka, H., Masunaga, S.I., Hattori, Y., Kirihata, M., Ono, K., *et al.* (2017). Evaluation of a novel sodium borocaptate-containing unnatural amino acid as a boron delivery agent for neutron capture therapy of the F98 rat glioma. *Radiation Oncology* 12: 26.

15 Futamura, G., Kawabata, S., Siba, H., Kuroiwa, T., Suzuki, M., Kondo, N., Ono, K., Sakurai, Y., Tanaka, M., Todo, T., *et al.* (2014). A case of radiation-induced osteosarcoma treated effectively by boron neutron capture therapy. *Radiation Oncology* 9: 237.

16 Gadan, M.A., Gonzalez, S.J., Batalla, M., Olivera, M.S., Policastro, L., and Sztejnberg, M.L. (2015). Application of BNCT to the treatment of HER2+ breast cancer recurrences: Research and developments in Argentina. *Applied Radiation and Isotopes: Including Data, Instrumentation and Methods for Use in Agriculture, Industry and Medicine* 104: 155–159.

17 Gonzalez, S.J., Bonomi, M.R., Santa Cruz, G.A., Blaumann, H.R., Calzetta Larrieu, O.A., Menendez, P., Jimenez Rebagliati, R., Longhino, J., Feld, D.B., Dagrosa, M.A., *et al.* (2004). First BNCT treatment of a skin melanoma in Argentina: Dosimetric analysis and clinical outcome. *Applied Radiation and Isotopes: Including Data, Instrumentation and Methods for Use in Agriculture, Industry and Medicine* 61: 1101–1105.

18 Goodman, J.H., Yang, W., Barth, R.F., Gao, Z., Boesel, C.P., Staubus, A.E., Gupta, N., Gahbauer, R.A., Adams, D.M., Gibson, C.R., *et al.* (2000). Boron neutron capture therapy of brain tumors: Biodistribution, pharmacokinetics, and radiation dosimetry sodium borocaptate in patients with gliomas. *Neurosurgery* 47: 608–621. discussion 621-602.

19 Haapaniemi, A., Kankaanranta, L., Saat, R., Koivunoro, H., Saarilahti, K., Makitie, A., Atula, T., and Joensuu, H. (2016). Boron Neutron Capture Therapy in the treatment of recurrent laryngeal cancer. *International Journal of Radiation Oncology, Biology, Physics* 95: 404–410.

20 Henriksson, R., Capala, J., Michanek, A., Lindahl, S.A., Salford, L.G., Franzen, L., Blomquist, E., Westlin, J.E., and Bergenheim, A.T., and Swedish Brain Tumour Study, G.. (2008). Boron neutron capture therapy (BNCT) for glioblastoma multiforme: A phase II study evaluating a prolonged high-dose of boronophenylalanine (BPA). *Radiotherapy and Oncology: Journal of the European Society for Therapeutic Radiology and Oncology* 88: 183–191.

21 Hiratsuka, J., Kamitani, N., Tanaka, R., Yoden, E., Tokiya, R., Suzuki, M., Barth, R.F., and Ono, K. (2018). Boron neutron capture therapy for vulvar melanoma and genital extramammary Paget's disease with curative responses. *Cancer Commun (Lond)* 38: 38.

22 Kageji, T., Mizobuchi, Y., Nagahiro, S., Nakagawa, Y., and Kumada, H. (2014). Correlation between radiation dose and histopathological findings in patients with glioblastoma treated with boron neutron capture therapy (BNCT). *Applied Radiation and Isotopes: Including Data, Instrumentation and Methods for Use in Agriculture, Industry and Medicine* 88: 20–22.

23 Kageji, T., Sogabe, S., Mizobichi, Y., Nakajima, K., Shinji, N., and Nakagawa, Y. (2015). Radiation-induced meningiomas after BNCT in patients with malignant glioma. *Applied Radiation and Isotopes: Including Data, Instrumentation and Methods for Use in Agriculture, Industry and Medicine* 106: 256–259.

24 Kankaanranta, L., Saarilahti, K., Makitie, A., Valimaki, P., Tenhunen, M., and Joensuu, H. (2011a). Boron neutron capture therapy (BNCT) followed by intensity modulated chemoradiotherapy as primary treatment of large head and neck cancer with intracranial involvement. *Radiotherapy and Oncology: Journal of the European Society for Therapeutic Radiology and Oncology* 99: 98–99.

25 Kankaanranta, L., Seppala, T., Koivunoro, H., Saarilahti, K., Atula, T., Collan, J., Salli, E., Kortesniemi, M., Uusi-Simola, J., Makitie, A., *et al.* (2007). Boron neutron capture therapy in the treatment of locally recurred head and neck cancer. *International Journal of Radiation Oncology, Biology, Physics* 69: 475–482.

26 Kankaanranta, L., Seppala, T., Koivunoro, H., Saarilahti, K., Atula, T., Collan, J., Salli, E., Kortesniemi, M., Uusi-Simola, J., Valimaki, P., *et al.* (2012). Boron neutron capture therapy in the treatment of locally recurred head-and-neck cancer: Final analysis of a phase I/II trial. *International Journal of Radiation Oncology, Biology, Physics* 82: e67–75.

27 Kankaanranta, L., Seppala, T., Koivunoro, H., Valimaki, P., Beule, A., Collan, J., Kortesniemi, M., Uusi-Simola, J., Kotiluoto, P., Auterinen, I., *et al.* (2011b). L-boronophenylalanine-mediated boron neutron capture therapy for malignant glioma progressing after external beam radiation therapy: A Phase I study. *International Journal of Radiation Oncology, Biology, Physics* 80: 369–376.

28 Kato, I., Fujita, Y., Maruhashi, A., Kumada, H., Ohmae, M., Kirihata, M., Imahori, Y., Suzuki, M., Sakrai, Y., Sumi, T., *et al.* (2009). Effectiveness of boron neutron capture therapy for recurrent head and neck malignancies. *Applied Radiation and Isotopes: Including Data, Instrumentation and Methods for Use in Agriculture, Industry and Medicine* 67: S37–42.

29 Kato, I., Ono, K., Sakurai, Y., Ohmae, M., Maruhashi, A., Imahori, Y., Kirihata, M., Nakazawa, M., and Yura, Y. (2004). Effectiveness of BNCT for recurrent head and neck malignancies. *Applied Radiation and Isotopes: Including Data, Instrumentation and Methods for Use in Agriculture, Industry and Medicine* 61: 1069–1073.

30 Kawaji, H., Miyatake, S., Shinmura, K., Kawabata, S., Tokuyama, T., and Namba, H. (2015). Effect of boron neutron capture therapy for recurrent anaplastic meningioma: An autopsy case report. *Brain Tumor Pathology* 32: 61–65.

31 Kimura, Y., Ariyoshi, Y., Miyatake, S., Shimahara, M., Kawabata, S., and Ono, K. (2009). Boron neutron capture therapy for papillary cystadenocarcinoma in the upper lip: A case report. *International Journal of Oral and Maxillofacial Surgery* 38: 293–295.

32 Koivunoro, H., Kankaanranta, L., Seppala, T., Haapaniemi, A., Makitie, A., and Joensuu, H. (2019). Boron neutron capture therapy for locally recurrent head and neck squamous cell carcinoma: An analysis of dose response and survival. *Radiotherapy and Oncology: Journal of the European Society for Therapeutic Radiology and Oncology* 137: 153–158.

33 Kouri, M., Kankaanranta, L., Seppala, T., Tervo, L., Rasilainen, M., Minn, H., Eskola, O., Vahatalo, J., Paetau, A., Savolainen, S., et al. (2004). Undifferentiated sinonasal carcinoma may respond to single-fraction boron neutron capture therapy. *Radiotherapy and Oncology: Journal of the European Society for Therapeutic Radiology and Oncology* 72: 83–85.

34 Kreiner, A.J., Baldo, M., Bergueiro, J.R., Cartelli, D., Castell, W., Thatar Vento, V., Gomez Asoia, J., Mercuri, D., Padulo, J., Suarez Sandin, J.C., et al. (2014). Accelerator-based BNCT. *Applied Radiation and Isotopes: Including Data, Instrumentation and Methods for Use in Agriculture, Industry and Medicine* 88: 185–189.

35 Kumada, H., Yamamoto, K., Yamamoto, T., Nakai, K., Nakagawa, Y., Kageji, T., and Matsumura, A. (2004). Improvement of dose calculation accuracy for BNCT dosimetry by the multi-voxel method in JCDS. *Applied Radiation and Isotopes: Including Data, Instrumentation and Methods for Use in Agriculture, Industry and Medicine* 61: 1045–1050.

36 Makino, E., Sasaoka, S., Aihara, T., Sakurai, Y., Maruhashi, A., Ono, K., Fujimoto, W., and Hiratsuka, J. (2012). 1013 the first clinical trial of boron neutron capture therapy using 10B-para-boronophenylalanine for treating extramammary paget's disease. *European Journal of Cancer* 48: S244–S245.

37 Menendez, P.R., Roth, B.M., Pereira, M.D., Casal, M.R., Gonzalez, S.J., Feld, D.B., Santa Cruz, G.A., Kessler, J., Longhino, J., Blaumann, H., et al. (2009). BNCT for skin melanoma in extremities: Updated Argentine clinical results. *Applied Radiation and Isotopes: Including Data, Instrumentation and Methods for Use in Agriculture, Industry and Medicine* 67: S50–53.

38 Minsky, D.M. and Kreiner, A.J. (2015). Near threshold (7) Li(p,n) (7)Be reaction as neutron source for BNCT. *Applied Radiation and Isotopes: Including Data, Instrumentation and Methods for Use in Agriculture, Industry and Medicine* 106: 68–71.

39 Miyatake, S., Kawabata, S., Hiramatsu, R., Furuse, M., Kuroiwa, T., and Suzuki, M. (2014). Boron neutron capture therapy with bevacizumab may prolong the survival of recurrent malignant glioma patients: Four cases. *Radiation Oncology* 9: 6.

40 Miyatake, S., Kawabata, S., Hiramatsu, R., Kuroiwa, T., Suzuki, M., Kondo, N., and Ono, K. (2016). Boron Neutron Capture Therapy for Malignant Brain Tumors. *Neurologia Medico-chirurgica* 56: 361–371.

41 Miyatake, S., Kawabata, S., Nonoguchi, N., Yokoyama, K., Kuroiwa, T., Matsui, H., and Ono, K. (2009). Pseudoprogression in boron neutron capture therapy for malignant gliomas and meningiomas. *Neuro-Oncology* 11: 430–436.

42 Miyatake, S., Kuwabara, H., Kajimoto, Y., Kawabata, S., Yokoyama, K., Doi, A., Tsuji, M., Mori, H., Ono, K., and Kuroiwa, T. (2006). Preferential recurrence of a sarcomatous component of a gliosarcoma after boron neutron capture therapy: Case report. *Journal of Neuro-oncology* 76: 143–147.

43 Miyatake, S., Tamura, Y., Kawabata, S., Iida, K., Kuroiwa, T., and Ono, K. (2007). Boron neutron capture therapy for malignant tumors related to meningiomas. *Neurosurgery* 61: 82–90. discussion 90-81.

44 Miyatake, S.I., Kawabata, S., Hiramatsu, R., Kuroiwa, T., Suzuki, M., and Ono, K. (2018). Boron Neutron Capture Therapy of malignant gliomas. *Progress in Neurological Surgery* 32: 48–56.

45 Nakagawa, Y., Kageji, T., Mizobuchi, Y., Kumada, H., and Nakagawa, Y. (2009a). clinical results of bnct for malignant brain tumors in children. *Applied Radiation and Isotopes: Including Data, Instrumentation and Methods for Use in Agriculture, Industry and Medicine* 67: S27–30.

46 Nakagawa, Y., Yoshihara, H., Kageji, T., Matsuoka, R., and Nakagawa, Y. (2009b). Cost analysis of radiotherapy, carbon ion therapy, proton therapy and BNCT in Japan. *Applied Radiation and Isotopes: Including Data, Instrumentation and Methods for Use in Agriculture, Industry and Medicine* 67: S80–83.

47 Nedunchezhian, K., Aswath, N., Thiruppathy, M., and Thirugnanamurthy, S. (2016a). Boron Neutron Capture Therapy - a literature review. *Journal of Clinical and Diagnostic Research: JCDR* 10: Ze01–ze04.

48 Nedunchezhian, K., Aswath, N., Thiruppathy, M., and Thirugnanamurthy, S. (2016b). Boron Neutron Capture Therapy - a literature review. *Journal of Clinical and Diagnostic Research: JCDR* 10: ZE01–04.

49 Nievaart, V.A., Daquino, G.G., and Moss, R.L. (2007). Monte Carlo based treatment planning systems for Boron Neutron Capture Therapy in Petten, The Netherlands. *Journal of Physics. Conference Series* 74.

50 Perks, C.A., Mill, A.J., Constantine, G., Harrison, K.G., and Gibson, J.A. (1988). A review of boron neutron capture therapy (BNCT) and the design and dosimetry of a high-intensity, 24 keV, neutron beam for BNCT research. *The British Journal of Radiology* 61: 1115–1126.

51 Porcari, P.C., Silvia; Saverio Pastore, Francesco (2011). Novel pharmacological and magnetic resonance strategies to enhance Boron Neutron Capture Therapy (BNCT) efficacy in the clinical treatment of malignant glioma, Management of CNS Tumors. In Management of CNS Tumors (Semmelweis University, Hungary: IntechOpen).

52 Shiba, H., Takeuchi, K., Hiramatsu, R., Furuse, M., Nonoguchi, N., Kawabata, S., Kuroiwa, T., Kondo, N., Sakurai, Y., Suzuki, M., *et al.* (2018). Boron Neutron Capture Therapy combined with early successive bevacizumab treatments for recurrent malignant gliomas - a pilot study. *Neurologia Medico-chirurgica* 58: 487–494.

53 Stenstam, B.H., Pellettieri, L., Sorteberg, W., Rezaei, A., and Skold, K. (2007). BNCT for recurrent intracranial meningeal tumours - case reports. *Acta Neurologica Scandinavica* 115: 243–247.

54 Stupp, R., Mason, W.P., Van Den Bent, M.J., Weller, M., Fisher, B., Taphoorn, M.J., Belanger, K., Brandes, A.A., Marosi, C., Bogdahn, U., *et al.* (2005). Radiotherapy plus concomitant and adjuvant temozolomide for glioblastoma. *The New England Journal of Medicine* 352: 987–996.

55 Suzuki, M. (2020). Boron neutron capture therapy (BNCT): A unique role in radiotherapy with a view to entering the accelerator-based BNCT era. *International Journal of Clinical Oncology* 25: 43–50.

56 Suzuki, M., Endo, K., Satoh, H., Sakurai, Y., Kumada, H., Kimura, H., Masunaga, S., Kinashi, Y., Nagata, K., Maruhashi, A., *et al.* (2008). A novel concept of treatment of diffuse or multiple pleural tumors by boron neutron capture therapy (BNCT). *Radiotherapy and Oncology: Journal of the European Society for Therapeutic Radiology and Oncology* 88: 192–195.

57 Suzuki, M., Kato, I., Aihara, T., Hiratsuka, J., Yoshimura, K., Niimi, M., Kimura, Y., Ariyoshi, Y., Haginomori, S., Sakurai, Y., *et al.* (2014). Boron neutron capture therapy outcomes for advanced or recurrent head and neck cancer. *Journal of Radiation Research* 55: 146–153.

58 Suzuki, M., Sakurai, Y., Hagiwara, S., Masunaga, S., Kinashi, Y., Nagata, K., Maruhashi, A., Kudo, M., and Ono, K. (2007a). First attempt of boron neutron capture therapy (BNCT) for hepatocellular carcinoma. *Japanese Journal of Clinical Oncology* 37: 376–381.

59 Suzuki, M., Sakurai, Y., Masunaga, S., Kinashi, Y., Nagata, K., Maruhashi, A., and Ono, K. (2006). Feasibility of boron neutron capture therapy (BNCT) for malignant pleural mesothelioma from a viewpoint of dose distribution analysis. *International Journal of Radiation Oncology, Biology, Physics* 66: 1584–1589.

60 Suzuki, M., Sakurai, Y., Masunaga, S., Kinashi, Y., Nagata, K., Maruhashi, A., and Ono, K. (2007b). A preliminary experimental study of boron neutron capture therapy for malignant tumors spreading in thoracic cavity. *Japanese Journal of Clinical Oncology* 37: 245–249.

61 Takeuchi, K., Kawabata, S., Hiramatsu, R., Matsushita, Y., Tanaka, H., Sakurai, Y., Suzuki, M., Ono, K., Miyatake, S.I., and Kuroiwa, T. (2018). Boron Neutron Capture Therapy for high-grade skull-base meningioma. *Journal of Neurological Surgery. Part B, Skull Base* 79: S322–s327.

62 Tamura, Y., Miyatake, S., Nonoguchi, N., Miyata, S., Yokoyama, K., Doi, A., Kuroiwa, T., Asada, M., Tanabe, H., and Ono, K. (2006). Boron neutron capture therapy for recurrent malignant meningioma. *Case Report: Journal of Neurosurgery* 105: 898–903.

63 Tibbitts, J., Sambol, N.C., Fike, J.R., Bauer, W.F., and Kahl, S.B. (2000). Plasma pharmacokinetics and tissue biodistribution of boron following administration of a boronated porphyrin in dogs. *Journal of Pharmaceutical Sciences* 89: 469–477.

64 Trivillin, V.A., Garabalino, M.A., Colombo, L.L., Gonzalez, S.J., Farias, R.O., Monti Hughes, A., Pozzi, E.C., Bortolussi, S., Altieri, S., Itoiz, M.E., *et al.* (2014). Biodistribution of the boron carriers boronophenylalanine (BPA) and/or decahydrodecaborate (GB-10) for Boron Neutron Capture Therapy (BNCT) in an experimental model of lung metastases. *Applied Radiation and Isotopes: Including Data, Instrumentation and Methods for Use in Agriculture, Industry and Medicine* 88: 94–98.

65 Trivillin, V.A., Pozzi, E.C.C., Colombo, L.L., Thorp, S.I., Garabalino, M.A., Monti Hughes, A., Gonzalez, S.J., Farias, R.O., Curotto, P., Santa Cruz, G.A., *et al.* (2017). Abscopal effect of boron neutron capture therapy (BNCT): Proof of principle in an experimental model of colon cancer. *Radiation and Environmental Biophysics* 56: 365–375.

66 Uchiyama, Y., Matsumoto, K., Murakami, S., Kanesaki, T., Matsumoto, A., Kishino, M., and Furukawa, S. (2014). MRI in a case of osteosarcoma in the temporomandibular joint. *Dento Maxillo Facial Radiology* 43: 20130280.

67 Vos, M.J., Turowski, B., Zanella, F.E., Paquis, P., Siefert, A., Hideghety, K., Haselsberger, K., Grochulla, F., Postma, T.J., Wittig, A., *et al.* (2005). Radiologic findings in patients treated with boron neutron capture therapy for glioblastoma multiforme within EORTC trial 11961. *International Journal of Radiation Oncology, Biology, Physics* 61: 392–399.

68 Wang, L.W., Chen, Y.W., Ho, C.Y., Hsueh Liu, Y.W., Chou, F.I., Liu, Y.H., Liu, H.M., Peir, J.J., Jiang, S.H., Chang, C.W., *et al.* (2014). Fractionated BNCT for locally recurrent head and neck cancer: Experience from a phase I/II clinical trial at Tsing Hua Open-Pool Reactor. *Applied Radiation and Isotopes: Including Data, Instrumentation and Methods for Use in Agriculture, Industry and Medicine* 88: 23–27.

69 Wang, L.W., Chen, Y.W., Ho, C.Y., Hsueh Liu, Y.W., Chou, F.I., Liu, Y.H., Liu, H.M., Peir, J.J., Jiang, S.H., Chang, C.W., *et al.* (2016). Fractionated Boron Neutron Capture Therapy in locally recurrent head and neck cancer: A prospective Phase I/II trial. *International Journal of Radiation Oncology, Biology, Physics* 95: 396–403.

70 Wang, L.W., Liu, Y.H., Chou, F.I., and Jiang, S.H. (2018). Clinical trials for treating recurrent head and neck cancer with boron neutron capture therapy using the Tsing-Hua Open Pool Reactor. *Cancer Commun (Lond)* 38: 37.

71 Wittig, A., Collette, L., Appelman, K., Buhrmann, S., Jackel, M.C., Jockel, K.H., Schmid, K.W., Ortmann, U., Moss, R., and Sauerwein, W.A. (2009). EORTC trial 11001: Distribution of two 10B-compounds in patients with squamous cell carcinoma of head and neck, a translational research/phase 1 trial. *Journal of Cellular and Molecular Medicine* 13: 1653–1665.

72 Wittig, A., Malago, M., Collette, L., Huiskamp, R., Buhrmann, S., Nievaart, V., Kaiser, G.M., Jockel, K.H., Schmid, K.W., Ortmann, U., *et al.* (2008). Uptake of two 10B-compounds in liver metastases of colorectal adenocarcinoma for extracorporeal irradiation with boron neutron capture therapy (EORTC Trial 11001). *International Journal of Cancer. Journal International Du Cancer* 122: 1164–1171.

73 Yamamoto, T., Nakai, K., Nariai, T., Kumada, H., Okumura, T., Mizumoto, M., Tsuboi, K., Zaboronok, A., Ishikawa, E., Aiyama, H., *et al.* (2011). The status of Tsukuba BNCT trial: BPA-based boron neutron capture therapy combined with X-ray irradiation. *Applied Radiation and Isotopes: Including Data, Instrumentation and Methods for Use in Agriculture, Industry and Medicine* 69: 1817–1818.

74 Yanagie, H., Higashi, S., Seguchi, K., Ikushima, I., Fujihara, M., Nonaka, Y., Oyama, K., Maruyama, S., Hatae, R., Suzuki, M., *et al.* (2014). Pilot clinical study of boron neutron capture therapy for recurrent hepatic cancer involving the intra-arterial injection of a (10) BSH-containing WOW emulsion. *Applied Radiation and Isotopes: Including Data, Instrumentation and Methods for Use in Agriculture, Industry and Medicine* 88: 32–37.

75 Yanagie, H., Higashi, S., Seguchi, K., Ikushima, I., Oyama, K., Nonaka, Y., Maruyama, S., Hatae, R., Sairennji, T., and Takahashi, S. (2012). Pilot clinical study of boron neutron capture therapy for recurrent hepatic cancer and gastric cancer. Paper presented at: the international congress on neutron capture therapy, Tsukuba, Japan.

76 Yong, Z., Song, Z., Zhou, Y., Liu, T., Zhang, Z., Zhao, Y., Chen, Y., Jin, C., Chen, X., Lu, J., *et al.* (2016). Boron neutron capture therapy for malignant melanoma: First clinical case report in China. *Chinese Journal of Cancer Research* 28: 634–640.

77 Yoshino, K., Suzuki, A., Mori, Y., Kakihana, H., Honda, C., Mishima, Y., Kobayashi, T., and Kanda, K. (1989). Improvement of solubility of p-boronophenylalanine by complex formation with monosaccharides. *Strahlentherapie Und Onkologie: Organ Der Deutschen Rontgengesellschaft . [Et Al]* 165: 127–129.

78 Zaidi, L., Belgaid, M., Taskaev, S., and Khelifi, R. (2018). Beam shaping assembly design of (7)Li(p,n)(7)Be neutron source for boron neutron capture therapy of deep-seated tumor. *Applied Radiation and Isotopes: Including Data, Instrumentation and Methods for Use in Agriculture, Industry and Medicine* 139: 316–324.

79 Zamenhof, R., Redmond, E., 2nd, Solares, G., Katz, D., Riley, K., Kiger, S., and Harling, O. (1996). Monte Carlo-based treatment planning for boron neutron capture therapy using custom designed models automatically generated from CT data. *International Journal of Radiation Oncology, Biology, Physics* 35: 383–397.

80 Zhang, X., Geng, C., Tang, X., Bortolussi, S., Shu, D., Gong, C., Han, Y., and Wu, S. (2019). Assessment of long-term risks of secondary cancer in paediatric patients with brain tumours after boron neutron capture therapy. *Journal of Radiological Protection* 39: 838–853.

10

Grid Therapy

Elizabeth B. Jeans MEd, MD*, Michael P. Grams PhD*, Matthew B. Spraker MD, PhD^, Elaine M. Zeman PhD†, and Daniel J. Ma MD*

* *Department of Radiation Oncology, Mayo Clinic, 200 2nd Street SW, Rochester, MN 55901*

^ *Department of Radiation Oncology, Washington University in St. Louis, 660 S. Euclid Avenue, St. Louis, MO 63110*

† *Department of Radiation Oncology, University of North Carolina School of Medicine, 101 Manning Drive, Chapel Hill, NC 27514*

Corresponding author: Daniel J. Ma, MD, 200 First Street SW, Rochester, MN 55905

TABLE OF CONTENTS

10.1 Introduction

Grid therapy, the first implementation of spatially fractionated radiotherapy (SFRT), is a technique of radiotherapy (RT) delivery that results in a heterogeneous dose distribution to a target volume. From its historical to modern day use, this technique allows for delivery of evenly spaced high-dose "hotspots" interspersed with low-dose "valleys" of dose distributed within a designated target volume. Historically, this technique was implemented to reduce skin toxicity, which limited effective orthovoltage therapy for the treatment of deeply seated tumors. Orthovoltage units were gradually replaced by megavoltage linear accelerators, which could treat with improved skin toxicity, so spatial fractionation remained niche. In the 1990s, there was a resurgence of this technique, and physicians reported treating large, bulky tumors with excellent effect while adequately sparing dose-limiting organs at risk.

Notably, this technique contrasts with the general modern conventional radiotherapeutic practice of complete, homogeneous dose coverage to a target volume. Further reappearance of and support for this technique has been rooted in the advancement in knowledge of stereotactic body radiotherapy (SBRT), which demonstrated favorable outcomes by heterogeneous dose delivery to a target, allowing for dose escalation and potentiation of the immune system. In the modern era, the advancements in planning techniques and incorporation of particle therapy into routine practice have brought about further use of grid therapy as a possible radiotherapeutic strategy. Additional evidence into the possible radiobiologic and immunologic effects from this technique has led to multiple clinical trials aimed at utilizing this technique to further optimize oncologic control of tumors with poor prognosis.

This chapter will provide a historical perspective of the early use of grid therapy, its re-emergence in the 1990s, its modern day use including proposed radiobiologic effects and open accruing clinical trials, and next steps in this technique.

10.2 Early Days of Grid

The first report of grid therapy was in 1909 by the German radiologist, Alban Köhler. He delivered spatially fractionated kilovoltage X-rays to deeply seated tumors using a handmade 1 mm^2 hole grid crafted from iron wire [1]. This device was secured to the skin prior to treatment and then flushed with the X-ray tube's lead shield [1]. He aimed to treat deep and bulky tumors by overcoming the dose-limiting toxicity of skin erythema and necrosis. Several patients underwent treatment with this technique, successfully delivering doses of up to 60 Gy with improved healing in skin toxicities as compared to prior attempts without the utilization of a grid. Further research in the decade to follow by Dr. Liberson of the New York City US Marine Hospital [2] included further optimization of geometries for multiperforated grids [2]. These two pioneering physicians, as well as the work by further researchers noted that delivery of higher doses of RT, 20 times greater than normal, were deliverable through these multiperforated grids [1–4]. As they observed that small volumes of skin tissue could tolerate higher doses of RT, this technique allowed for better deep target coverage while sparing patients of unpleasant and sometimes devastating skin toxicity.

The use of such techniques ultimately fell out of favor as megavoltage linear accelerators were developed. The first linear accelerator used for medical purposes was developed in London and treated its first patient in 1953 [5]. In the 1990s, several clinicians, including Mohiuddin et al. [6,7], brought the concept of grid therapy back into clinical practice as they aimed to treat patients with bulky or recurrent tumors, for which traditional megavoltage photon planning would be toxic.

10.3 Re-emergence of Grid in 1990s

In 1990, Mohiuddin utilized grid therapy in 22 patients with large or recurrent tumors across a variety of histologies [6]. All patients were noted to have exhausted other options for palliation and were symptomatic [6]. A 50% open and 50% blocked Cerrobend block was placed into a linear accelerator to deliver a single field of 6 MV or 25 MV photons to a dose of 10–15 Gy [6]. Ninety-one percent had a response to treatment with a reasonable side-effect profile [6] (Table 10.1). In two follow-up studies, the use of grid therapy again continued to show a high rate of response with reasonable toxicity profiles [7,8] (Table 10.1). In addition to control rates, additional studies demonstrated further improvement in control with grid doses of greater than or equal to 15 Gy and also when utilized in conjunction with consolidative external beam RT of at least 40 Gy [7,9]. Studies over

the past century have continued to analyze the use of grid in both the definitive and palliative settings in a variety of histologies showing robust control rates and manageable toxicities (Table 10.1) [10–15]. Although retrospective in nature with a highly heterogeneous patient population, treatment indications, and spatially fractionated strategies, these studies demonstrated proof of concept paving the way for modern day trials.

10.4 Proposed Radiobiologic Principles of Grid

The biology of SFRT, of which grid is one type, is poorly understood, multifactorial, and especially difficult to study, because each model system—cells in culture, preclinical animal models, and clinical studies in patients—employs different types and configurations of grid systems, different radiation doses, dose rates and types, and different end points. Further complicating matters is that the historical knowledge base concerning the radiation responses of normal tissues and tumors (i.e., foundational or "classical" radiobiology) is predicated on the fact that the tissues are uniformly irradiated and typically with small, repeated dose fractions over extended periods of time. Not only does grid therapy by its very nature not involve uniform tissue irradiation, but also it typically is hypofractionated, that is, one or only a few large radiation doses delivered in short overall treatment times.

The fundamental paradox of grid and other forms of SFRT is that, simultaneously, the normal tissue in the field is protected, allowing higher doses than usual to be delivered, yet the tumor is radiosensitized. Multiple mechanisms could be responsible for this postulate. Most of the research to date suggests that molecular, cellular, and tissue-level differences in the tumor's microenvironment compared to normal tissues may be responsible.

10.4.1 The Role of Tumor Vasculature

It has long been appreciated that vascular injury is responsible, at least in part, for radiation-induced complications in some normal tissues [19]. The role vascular injury plays in tumors is less well understood; however, the ability of radiation to destroy tumor blood vessels has considerable allure because the loss of a single microvessel has the potential to kill hundreds, if not thousands, of tumor cells [20].

Garcia-Barros et al. and Fuks and Kolesnick [21,22] have suggested that the clinical response of tumors to RT is mediated by the apoptotic death of vascular endothelial cells and that this could be enhanced by the larger doses per fraction characteristic of grid therapy [23]. Their proposed mechanism for this was that radiation activated the acid sphingomyelinase pathway, which is enriched in vascular endothelial cells, lead-

Table 10.1 Summary of Early Clinical Grid Trials (from Billena et al. [16] with permission).

Authors	Treated sites (*n*)	Follow-up, median (range) (month)	Histology	GRID dose, median (range) (Gy)	Prior RT	GRID only	Control rates	Side effects
Mohiuddin et al. [6]	22	NR (1–18)	Diverse	NR (10–15)	27%	36%	Response rate: 91%	1 acute skin erythema, 2 nausea and vomiting, 2 diarrhea, 1 late SBO
Mohiuddin et al. [9]	72	4 (0.5–28)	Diverse	NR (10–25)	24%	44%	Response rate: 91%	No grade 2 or higher acute toxicity
Mohiuddin et al. [7]	87	7 (3–42)	Diverse	15 (10–20)	9%	20%	Response rate: 91%	1 grade 3 acute mucositis, 1 fatal carotid blowout
Kudrimoti et al. [17]	20	NR	Melanoma	15 (12–20)	25%	25%	Response rate: 80%	No grade 3 or higher toxicities
Huhn et al. [11]	27	10 (3–44)	SCC of H&N	15 (15–20)	0%	0%	(1) Neck control rate: 93% (2) neck control rate 92%	(1) acute G 2–3 skin toxicity, 10 late G 2 soft tissue and muscle fibrosis (2) 3 poor postoperative wound healing, 4 fibrosis limiting neck movement
Mohiuddin et al. [18]	44	9 (2–44)	Soft tissue sarcoma	15 (12–20)	NR	9%	Response rate: 76%	2 G 3 acute skin reactions
Penagaricano et al. [15]	14	19.5 (2–38)	SCC of H&N	20	0%	0%	Local control rate: 79%	1 fatal carotid blowout, 11 acute G 2–3 skin reaction, 13 acute G 2–3 mucosal reaction, 4 late G 2–3 skin fibrosis
Neuner et al. [14]	79	2 (0–51.6)	Diverse	15 (10–20)	NR	20%	Pain response rate, block: 95%, pain response rate, MLC: 74%, mass effect response rate, block: 84%, mass effect response rate, MLC: 79%	4 G 3–4 acute skin reactions with block versus 10 G 3–4 acute skin reactions with MLC
Mohiuddin et al. [13]	14	14 (3–43)	Soft tissue sarcoma	18	0%	0%	Local control rate: 100%	1 G 3 acute skin, 2 delayed wound healing
Edwards et al. [10]	53	Mean 34 (1–239)	SCC of H&N	15	NR	0%	Local control rate: 81%	2 late toxicities requiring feeding tubes

ing to the generation of ceramide, a potent mediator of apoptosis. Select preclinical and clinical studies are consistent with this mechanism of action. For example, in genetically engineered animals lacking the acid sphingomyelinase pathway, endothelial cells in tumors were resistant to radiation-induced apoptosis after large single doses, but in animals with this pathway intact, a rapid wave of endothelial cell apoptosis occurred within hours of irradiation, followed 2–3 days later by a second wave of tumor cell death [21]. In select rodent tumors and human tumor xenografts irradiated with single doses of 10 or 20 Gy, Song et al. [24–26] also noted a further

decrease in clonogenic tumor cell survival 2–3 days after irradiation, likewise a time scale consistent with the loss of vascular endothelial cells. In a clinical study by Sathishkumar et al. [23], 11 patients were treated with 15 Gy of SFRT, followed by monitoring of serum ceramide and secretory sphingomyelinase before and at 24, 48, and 72 h after irradiation. Those patients showing a clinical response (67%) had elevated serum secretory sphingomyelinase and ceramide following RT. With the addition of conventional RT following the grid treatment, further sensitization of the tumor occurred, supporting a possible clinical role for this type of combination treatment.

The role of tumor vasculature in radiation response remains controversial, however, in that there are also studies that refute a role for vascular endothelial cell death in overall tumor response. Moding et al. [27] found no influence of the presence or absence of endothelial cell apoptosis on the overall radiation response of primary sarcomas in mice. Further, there are reports in the literature that do not show a further reduction in tumor clonogens in the days immediately following irradiation with a single dose of 20 Gy, e.g., the classic study by Hermens and Barendsen [28] showing a steady *increase* in tumor clonogen numbers after irradiation of a rat rhabdomyosarcoma.

Regardless of an exact mechanism of action, a loss or reduction in tumor vasculature could have opposing consequences. It could act as a radiation sensitizer by causing secondary ischemic death of tumor cells, reducing the tumor's growth rate and/or leading to the phenomenon termed "vascular normalization" [29,30]. Vascular normalization occurs when small, inefficient tumor blood vessels are destroyed, leaving the more mature, larger vessels intact, and potentially facilitating reoxygenation of hypoxic regions of the tumor. On the other hand, loss of small vasculature could also increase tumor hypoxia, causing an increase in radioresistance as well as promoting further tumor progression [31,32]. There is also evidence that radiation can *protect* tumor vasculature by causing the upregulation of proangiogenic factors [33], including following spatially fractionated microbeam irradiation [34].

10.4.2 The Role of the Radiation-Induced Bystander Effect

The radiation-induced bystander effect (RIBE) is defined as the manifestation of radiation injury in cells proximate to irradiated cells, but that were not themselves irradiated, and is mediated by complex signals transmitted directly or indirectly from the nearby irradiated cell(s) [35–39]. The phenomenon was first described by Nagasawa and Little in 1992 [40], who irradiated G1 phase Chinese hamster ovary cells *in vitro* with alpha particles at a low dose and fluence sufficient to only directly irradiate about 1% of the cells. Nevertheless, about 30% of cells showed an increased frequency of sister chromatid exchanges, a type of chromosome aberration indicative of the production and repair of DNA damage. Since that time, the RIBE has been documented both *in vitro* and *in vivo*, for different types of ionizing radiations at different radiation doses and dose rates, for both broad beam and SFRT irradiation arrangements, and for different types of cells and tissues. Although much has been learned since the RIBE was first described *in vitro* [40], its complexity and context dependence leave many aspects of the phenomenon poorly understood. Its general significance *in vivo*, let alone for grid radiation therapy in particular, remains unclear.

The non-targeted effects produced in "bystanders" are quite similar to those of direct irradiation, including, among others, production of various types of DNA damage (e.g., DNA strand breaks and chromosome aberrations [38,40], micronucleus formation [41]), epigenetic changes [42,43], genomic instability [36], mutation induction [39,44], neoplastic transformation [36,38], changes in gene expression [37,45], oxidative stress responses [38,41], and different modes of cell killing, including mitotic catastrophe, apoptosis, and senescence/permanent growth arrest [37–39,46].

The signaling effects leading to the RIBE are facilitated through gap junction intercellular communication between irradiated and bystander cells [47,48] and by the secretion of signaling molecules into the surrounding medium by irradiated cells and macrophage mediators that respond to cellular and tissue damage [48,49]. Many signaling molecules have been proposed as key players in these signaling pathways, including cytokines such as transforming growth factor-β (TGF-β) and interleukin-8 (IL-8), as well as reactive oxygen and nitrogen species [48]. The activation of TGF-β and IL-8 initiates multiple downstream pathways such as the mitogen-activated protein kinase (MAPKs) and nuclear factor-κB (NF-κB) pathways [48,50]. Tumor necrosis factor alpha (TNFα) and tumor necrosis factor-related apoptosis-inducing ligand (TRAIL) have also been implicated in the bystander pathway [51]. Activation of these and other pathways have been linked to increased expression of genes involved in DNA repair, cell cycle arrest, and apoptosis in bystander cells [46,48]. Some of these complex interactions are illustrated in Figure 10.1.

Complex signaling pathways activated as part of the RIBE. Both diffusible substances, some released from tissue-resident macrophages, and direct cell–cell communication through gap junctions transduce signals from irradiated cells to their unirradiated neighbors.

Ultimately, whether the RIBE is considered favorable or detrimental when it comes to grid and other types of SFRT will depend on the exact context. Irradiated *tumor* cells transmitting damage to their nonirradiated counterparts and increasing cell killing, as seems to be the case for grid therapy, is a desirable outcome. Yet, if the same were to occur for cells in the surrounding normal tissue, this would obviously be detrimental. However, it appears that in the case of normal tissues, the opposite is true; normal tissues irradiated with grid are spared, not sensitized to radiation, suggesting something akin to an inverse RIBE in which unirradiated cells communicating with their irradiated neighbors can afford protection from radiation damage. Although less well studied than the traditional RIBE and even less well understood, there is some precedent for this phenomenon, which has been termed the "rescue effect" [52,53]. Both phenomena require further study

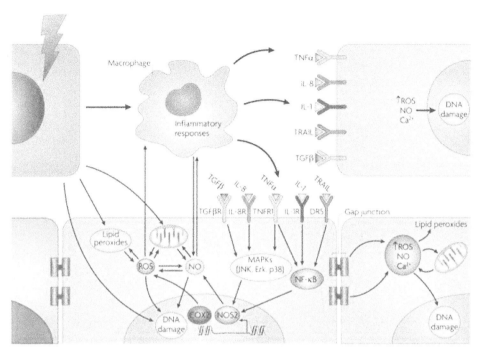

Figure 10.1 Key pathways affecting bystander signals [50].

in order to better understand the biology of grid therapy and, in so doing, better define its clinical utility.

10.4.3 The Role of the Immune System

An emerging paradigm is the use of radiation therapy as a nonspecific immune system stimulant [54–57]. Traditionally, radiation has been considered an immunosuppressant because of, for example, its use to destroy host immunity in advance of a hematopoietic stem-cell transplant due to the exquisite radiosensitivity of lymphocytes. Nevertheless, recognition that radiation also could *elicit* an immune response has long been familiar. First described by Mole in 1953 [58], local radiation therapy to a primary tumor occasionally caused tumor regression at distant, metastatic sites that were not irradiated. A type of bystander effect, albeit operating well outside the radiation field, Mole termed this phenomenon the abscopal effect, from the Latin prefix "ab" meaning "away from" and "scopus" referring to something being targeted, i.e., an off-target effect [59]. Mole postulated that an immune response to fragments of dying tumor cells at the irradiated site was responsible for the abscopal effect at the distant metastatic sites that weren't irradiated [58].

Most human tumors are not particularly immunogenic by nature, presumably because of an immunosuppressive tumor microenvironment that allows them to evade immune system detection [54], one of the hallmarks of cancer [60]. This also likely explains why abscopal effects were so rare historically.

More recently, however, with the introduction of immune checkpoint inhibitors capable of abrogating at least some of this immunosuppression, reports of radiation-induced abscopal effects have become more frequent [61–63], further supporting a role of the immune system in the phenomenon.

If an immune response to fragments of dying tumor cells is indeed the trigger for the abscopal effect, it follows that the more radiation-induced cell death, the better, suggesting that abscopal responses would be more likely for higher doses per fraction than lower ones. This idea has driven considerable research in both animal models [54,64,65] and in the clinic [66–68] on combinations of hypofractionated RT and/or SFRT (with or without immune checkpoint inhibitors) in an attempt to elicit abscopal responses.

At the higher radiation doses used in hypofractionation and SFRT (generally, ≥ 8 Gy per fraction delivered in 1–5 fractions), some of the ways tumor cells die (e.g., mitotic catastrophe, necrosis, and immunogenic cell death) have the potential to liberate large quantities of tumor-associated antigens, release "danger associated molecular patterns" (DAMPS) such as ATP, calreticulin and high mobility group protein B1 (HMGB1), increase MHC 1 expression on tumor cells, and stimulate proinflammatory cytokine and chemokine release [69,70]. Another source of proinflammatory cytokines in lethally irradiated tumor cells is activation of the cGAS/ STING pathway, a cellular defense mechanism triggered by the presence of extranuclear double-stranded DNA, frequently noted in cells that have been infected by viruses, but also in cells that die by radiation-induced mitotic catastrophe [71,72]. Once triggered, this pathway leads to the production and release of type 1 interferons. Together, all of these biological responses enhance antigen presentation and processing by dendritic cells and macrophages, in effect converting the tumor microenvironment into an *in situ* vaccine capable of recruiting and then "educating" CD8+ T lymphocytes to attack tumor cells both locally, and potentially, at distant sites as well [66,68].

In conclusion, the exact biological underpinnings of grid therapy are complex and not fully understood and will require much further research. However, there is compelling evidence from experiments using cells, laboratory animals, and clinical studies in patients for preferential damage to tumor vasculature and the triggering of numerous signaling cascades that instigate bystander and abscopal effects as possible biological factors at play during grid therapy. Yet to be determined from a radiobiologic perspective is whether and why these effects may be greater in tumors than in normal tissues, greater for SFRT like grid than for standard broad beam RT, and greater when grid is combined with molecularly targeted therapies or immune modulating agents. How best to manipulate radiation time, dose, and fractionation patterns in order to maximize these effects is also of considerable importance in further improving grid's therapeutic ratio. Ultimately, the potential of grid for the treatment of otherwise radioresistant tumors, either because of large tumor burden, inherent radioresistance, and/or presence of tumor hypoxia by eliciting off-target effects is especially noteworthy and justifies further exploration of this unique and highly innovative technique.

10.5 Contemporary GRID

Recently, advances in RT planning and delivery have allowed for further investigation into the utilization of grid. In the re-emergence of grid RT in the 1990s, the continued strategy for planning included a physical grid block, which was customized for insertion into the conventional linear accelerator (Figure 10.2). With this grid, two-dimensional plans can be generated using a single field (Figure 10.2).

The use of a physical grid block comes with a few challenges. First, the grid block lacks flexibility in planning as a single field is delivered with a set distance between the holes. It must be utilized in the right clinical scenario, as the dose is distributed more superficially as compared to alternative techniques (Figure 10.2). While it would be feasible to deliver two fields, such as in an AP-PA or two non-opposed fields, in attempting to do so with a brass insert, the peak-to-valley ratio would be decreased, thus diminishing the possible radiobiologic advantages of grid RT. Additionally, the use of a physical block is burdensome on therapists as it often weighs over 30 pounds and requires physical insertion into the gantry head prior to treatment.

Two-dimensional plans can also be delivered with the use of multileaf collimators (MLCs). This technique allows for improved flexibility as the spot size and distance from center to center can be altered, as well as the decision for spot placement within the tumor volume, thus maximizing the delivery of high dose within the tumor and away from the periphery, sparing the surrounding organs at risk. Challenges in the delivery of two-dimensional MLC RT include increased expertise for planning and longer delivery time.

An additional type of grid RT is termed lattice radiotherapy (LRT). This is the delivery of three-dimensional grid. The most

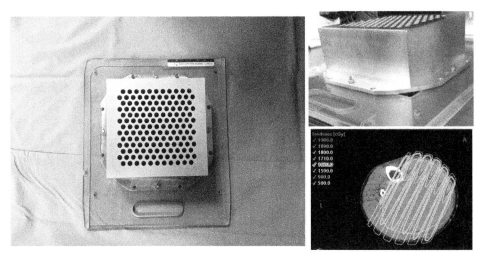

Figure 10.2 Brass grid block for two-dimensional grid delivery (left, top right). Two-dimensional grid plan (bottom right) for a lower extremity sarcoma (blue is ctv1800).

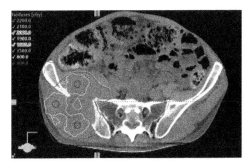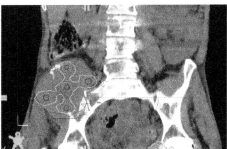

Figure 10.3   Lattice radiotherapy (LRT) utilizing intensity-modulated radiotherapy (IMRT) to treat metastatic sarcoma of the right ilium.

utilized techniques for designing such plans include the use of MLCs, delivered by volumetric arc or intensity-modulated RT (Figure 10.3).

This was initially described by Wu et al. [73] who noted a continued limitation in clinical implementation of grid as inductive therapy was secondary to the volume of normal tissue receiving significant dose. Thus, the concept of a three-dimensional dose lattice was orchestrated, where high doses were concentrated in a lattice arrangement within the tumor volume and lower doses between the vertices, maintaining the peak-to-valley effect seen in two-dimensional grid (Figure 10.4) [73]. This lead to minimal dose being spread outside of the clinical target volume. Notably, this modernized technique continues to have the benefit of other MLC-derived planning, including improved planning flexibility, and improved dose to surrounding organs at risk, in particular skin; however, it comes with challenges of increased expertise and treatment time.

Clinical application of LRT has been shown to be feasible by Amendola et al. [74] who delivered LRT (18 Gy to vertices and 3 Gy to GTV) followed by 45–66 Gy EBRT to 10 patients with advanced stage non-small cell lung cancer. They demonstrated a mean tumor response of 52% and mean overall survival of 22 months [74]. No grade 2 or higher toxicities were seen [74]. Additional other small series have been published [74–76].

Additional RT planning techniques have been explored including the use of tomotherapy-based grid [77,78].

An alternative approach to incorporating the fundamentals of SBRT with SFRT called lattice SBRT is described by Duriseti et al. [79]. In this study, 12 tumors greater than 10 cm were recorded in 11 patients [79]. Lattice SBRT plans were created using a peak–valley dose gradient of 100% to 30%, thereby creating a simultaneous integrated boost of 6,670 cGy to a planned target volume of 2,000 cGy delivered in five fractions utilizing volumetric arc planning [79]. All plans underwent a quality assurance assessment and met prespecified thresholds for approval [79]. This method is now being tested in a prospective study of patients with large tumors needing palliative RT (NCT04133415).

With the increased incorporation of particle therapy into clinical practice, the use of proton grid has been explored.

Protons are particularly attractive due to the rapid dose fall-off past the Bragg peak, as well as their low entrance dose. Thus, there is maximal opportunity to spare surrounding non-targeted structures with proton beam grid. Proton grid was first described by Henry et al. [80] in 2016. In this feasibility study, the authors concluded that utilizing pencil-beam proton scanning and cross-firing millimeter-sized beams allowed for larger separation between beam elements [80]. Comparably, Gao et al. [81] created a SFRT plan using a single pencil beam scanning proton beam, mimicking holes 1 cm in diameter and 2 cm from center to center. This demonstrated a uniform beamlet dose with excellent sparing of organs at risk.

While individual patients have been treated with these techniques [81], no larger clinical series are available for further interpretation. Further investigation into SFRT with particle therapy includes the utilization of carbon ion therapy. Optimal grid planning has been demonstrated with 0.5-mm and 3.0-mm-wide beam elements demonstrating homogeneous dose distribution inside the target volume and low doses in the normal tissues with crossfired, interlaced beams [82].

10.6   Future of SFRT

While SFRT becomes more clinically utilized with advanced planning methods, a few questions remain to be answered, which should be evaluated on prospective studies with specific eligibility criteria and standard measurements of effect (as compared to response rate) and toxicity. The most basic of questions would be which patients will clinically benefit from such a technique. Years of research has shown that delivery of grid in the palliative setting is feasible and demonstrates palliation for patients without unreasonable toxicities. The question of dose escalation in the palliative setting of SFRT remains a question and will further be evaluated by clinical trials.

However, as grid is finessed and refined, the role of this therapy as an inductive measure continues to beg the question: which patients may benefit from this therapy as part of curative-intent treatment. With the development of proton grid and

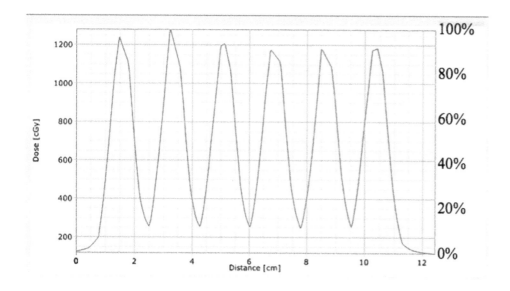

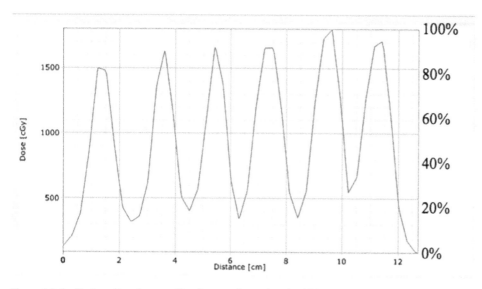

Figure 10.4   Peak–valley dose profiles for two-dimensional grid (top) versus lattice (bottom) [73].

from a radiobiologic standpoint, use of this technique in radioresistant tumors would be of largest benefit; however, there is a lack of clinical trial evidence supporting this case. In a study by Gholami et al. [83], review of retrospective literature demonstrates a clinical total response rate from grid of 50% to 100% across histologic subtype without a clear consensus of who benefits the greatest. Using the linear quadratic and the Hug–Kellerer models, the therapeutic ratio and equivalent uniform dose for different types of tumors were calculated from simulated dose profiles with respect to their radiation sensitivities [83]. From this, the therapeutic ratio values increased with increasing grid doses in radioresistant cells but failed to show more effectiveness in radiosensitive tumors [83]. Therefore, despite true clinical evidence, comparison with clinical

responses of 232 patients from different publications, grid RT appears more effective in radioresistant tumors [83].

A further question that must be answered in subsequent SFRT trials includes standardization of SFRT treatment. This includes a multitude of planning and treatment-related questions regarding the optimal size and spacing of high dose regions, dosing of consolidative external beam RT, sequencing of SFRT to consolidative RT or in relation to subsequent SFRT (multi-fractionated SFRT), as well as quality assurance practices and appropriate dosimetric planning parameters. Additionally, the investigation into the use of concurrent pharmaceutical agents for possible synergistic effects on the tumor microenvironment should be investigated thoroughly in both animal and human models.

Clinical trials standardizing an approach to planning SFRT across disease sites may allow for more information regarding ideal tumor histology as well as further guide optimal planning parameters and SFRT delivery. Clinical trials registered through the National Institute of Health are shown in Table 10.2.

10.7 Microbeam Radiation Therapy and Minibeam Radiation Therapy

Over the past several years, microbeam radiotherapy (MRT) has been further investigated. This utilizes the concept of delivering SFRT using beams that are the width of 25–50 μm and spaced 200–400 μm apart [16]. Spatially distancing entry beams with techniques such as MRT or MBRT (further described below) results in convergence of the beams at the target, resulting in higher radiation doses with improved sparing of healthy tissues. This has been demonstrated as feasible in rodent CNS tumors [84]. Delivery of MRT is characterized by parallel microbeams generated by a high photon fluence at extremely high dose rates to avoid beam smearing due to cardiosynchronous pulsations [85]. Despite preclinical models, MRT has yet to transition into clinical practice due to the need for extremely high dose rates to prevent negating the tissue sparing effect.

Table 10.2   NIH Registered Clinical Trials (As of October 8, 2020).

Title	Status	Study results	Conditions	Interventions	Locations
GRID Therapy as Palliative Radiation for Patients With Advanced and Symptomatic Tumors (NCT02333110)	Recruiting	No results available	• Patients with symptomatic or bulky tumors (more than 8 cm) or with tumors resistant to radiation	• Radiation: spatially fractionated radiation therapy	• Sir Mortimer Jewish General Hospital, Montreal, Quebec, Canada
Randomized MRI-Guided Prostate Boosts Via Initial Lattice Stereotactic versus Daily Moderately Hypofractionated Radiotherapy (NCT02307058)	Recruiting	No results available	• Prostate cancer	• Radiation: LEAD RT	• University of Miami, Miami, Florida, United States
Phase I Clinical Trial of GRID Therapy in Pediatric Osteosarcoma of the Extremity (NCT03139318)	Recruiting	No results available	• Osteosarcoma in children • Radiation toxicity	• Radiation: GRID radiotherapy	• University of Arkansas for Medical Sciences, Little Rock, Arkansas, United States
Neoadjuvant Durvalumab and Tremelimumab Plus Radiation for High Risk Soft-Tissue Sarcoma (NCT03116529)	Recruiting	No results available	• Soft tissue sarcoma	• Combination product: combination radiation, immunotherapy, surgery	• University of Maryland Medical Center, Greenebaum Comprehensive Cancer Center, Baltimore, Maryland, United States
Palliative Lattice Stereotactic Body Radiotherapy (SBRT) (NCT04133415)	Recruiting	No results available	• Cancer • Palliative radiotherapy	• Radiation: lattice stereotactic body Radiation therapy • Procedure: peripheral blood	• Washington University School of Medicine, Saint Louis, Missouri, United States
Palliative Lattice Stereotactic Body Radiotherapy (SBRT) for Patients With Sarcoma, Thoracic, Abdominal, and Pelvic Cancers (NCT04553471)	Recruiting	No results available	• Sarcoma • Thoracic cancer • Abdominal cancer • Pelvic cancer	• Radiation: lattice stereotactic body Radiation therapy • Procedure: peripheral blood	• Washington University School of Medicine, Saint Louis, Missouri, United States
GRID Therapy for Tumors of the Head, Neck, Thorax, Abdomen, Pelvis and Extremitie. (NCT04549246)	Recruiting	No results available	• Radiation therapy Complication • Tumor neck • Tumor abdomen	• Radiation: spatially fractionated radiation (GRID) therapy	• Mayo Clinic in Rochester Rochester, Minnesota, United States
MRI-Guided Lattice Extreme Ablative Dose Radiotherapy For Prostate Cancer (NCT01411319)	Active, not recruiting	Has results	• Prostate cancer	• Radiation: lattice extreme ablative dose radiation therapy	• University of Miami, Miami, Florida, United States

(a) Dose distribution of GRID therapy

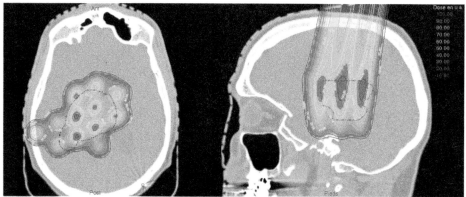

(b) Dose distribution of PMBRT

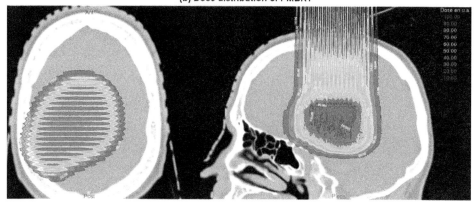

Figure 10.5   Example of planned dose distribution of GRID (a) and pMBRT (b) [90].

Minibeam radiotherapy (MBRT) delivers SFRT at interbeam distances approximately double the width of MRT, 500–700 μm, spaced 1–3 mm apart [77]. The use of MBRT has been demonstrated in preclinical models [86] to be feasible in delivery with increased dose delivery and reduced acute and late toxicities [87]. Furthermore, it is not limited by dose rate and can therefore be clinically implemented. The use of proton minibeam radiation therapy (pMBRT) has been further investigated as it allows for a combination of SFRT with submillimeter field sizes and also would incorporate increased radiobiologic effectiveness and less scattering of dose beyond the target volume [87]. A recent preclinical model delivered 70 Gy peak dose in a single fraction to glioma bearing rats. At 6 months, tumor eradication was seen in 22% of rodents without substantial brain damage [88]. Forefronts to move this preclinical model into patient-centered therapy includes recent dosimetric evaluation in human patients [89], which showed promising results in providing increased target dose with sparing of normal tissues when compared to standard fractionation or traditional SFRT (Figure 10.5) [90]. The potential to utilize pMBRT may be particularly important when considering cases of re-irradiation near critical structures that have already been exposed to ionizing radiation.

Carbon ion minibeams have been investigated at the NASA Space Radiation Laboratory (NSRL) utilizing interlaced beams to ablate a small target in a rabbit brain [91]. CT evaluation at 6 months demonstrated no evidence of damage to the surrounding brain [91]. There are multiple limitations in clinical implementation of carbon ion minibeam therapy, most importantly the lack of carbon ion facilities in the US and lack of experience with planning of carbon ions. However, the clinical implementation of pMBRT is feasible for both pencil beam scanning and passively scattered protons [92]. No phase I or II clinical trials exist for pMBRT.

10.8   Conclusion

SFRT is the modern day term used for grid treatment. This treatment technique allows for delivery of high-dose RT in a single fraction while sparing the non-targeted tissues. Initial studies utilized this technique for mainly palliative indications but demonstrated excellent outcomes with tolerable toxicities. Further understanding of the radiobiologic potential behind this therapy includes RIBEs, activation of the immune system (thus possibly potentiating the abscopal effect), and altering vascular microenvironment resulting in tumor hypoxia. Further insight into grid's potential has resulted in this therapy being utilized as an inductive technique for particularly radioresistant tumors; however, there is a lack of clinical evidence regarding its use in this setting. Proton beam SFRT has the potential to be utilized in the curative-intent setting by further minimizing the dose to nontargeted tissues. Guidance in treatment delivery and planning are needed. The potential to utilize targeted agents and immune modulators with this technique warrants investigation. The possibility to further harness the potential of SFRT with MBRT, in particular pMBRT, has implications in the setting of tumors that continue to have poor prognosis and would benefit from higher radiotherapeutic doses. Clinical trials, in particular phases II and III, are needed to evaluate SFRT to further discern its therapeutic benefit in the upfront setting.

Bibliography

1 Laissue, J.A., Blattmann, H., and Slatkin, D.N. (2012). Alban Köhler (1874-1947): inventor of grid therapy. *Zeitschrift fur Medizinische Physik* 22 (2): 90–99.

2 Liberson, F. (1933). The value of a multi-perforated screen in deep X-ray therapy. *Radiology* 20 (3): 186–195.

3 Marks, H. (1952). Clinical experience with irradiation through a grid. *Radiology* 58 (3): 338–342.

4 Failla, G. (1952). Irradiation through grids. *Radiology* 58 (3): 424–426.

5 Thwaites, D.I. and Tuohy, J.B. (2006). Back to the future: The history and development of the clinical linear accelerator. *Physics in Medicine and Biology* 51 (13): R343–62.

6 Mohiuddin, M., et al. (1990). Palliative treatment of advanced cancer using multiple nonconfluent pencil beam radiation: A pilot study. *Cancer* 66 (1): 114–118.

7 Mohiuddin, M., et al. (1999). High-dose spatially-fractionated radiation (GRID): A new paradigm in the management of advanced cancers. *International Journal of Radiation Oncology, Biology, Physics* 45 (3): 721–727.

8 Mohiuddin, M., Marks, G., and Marks, J. (2002). Long-term results of reirradiation for patients with recurrent rectal carcinoma. *Cancer* 95 (5): 1144–1150.

9 Mohiuddin, M., et al. (1996). Spatially fractionated (GRID) radiation for palliative treatment of advanced cancer. *Radiation Oncology Investigations* 4 (1): 41–47.

10 Edwards, J.M., et al. (2015). Definitive GRID and fractionated radiation in bulky head and neck cancer associated with low rates of distant metastasis. *International Journal of Radiation Oncology*Biology*Physics* 93 (3, Supplement): E334.

11 Huhn, J.L., et al. (2006). Spatially fractionated GRID radiation treatment of advanced neck disease associated with head and neck cancer. *Technology in Cancer Research & Treatment* 5 (6): 607–612.

12 Kudrimoti, M., et al. (2002). Spatially fractionated radiation therapy (SFR) in the palliation of large bulky (>8 cm) melanomas. *International Journal of Radiation Oncology*Biology*Physics* 54 (2, Supplement): 342–343.

13 Mohiuddin, M., et al. (2014). Locally advanced high-grade extremity soft tissue sarcoma: Response with novel approach to neoadjuvant chemoradiation using induction spatially fractionated GRID radiotherapy (SFGRT). *Journal of Clinical Oncology* 32 (15_suppl): 10575–10575.

14 Neuner, G., et al. (2012). High-dose spatially fractionated GRID radiation therapy (SFGRT): A comparison of treatment outcomes with Cerrobend vs. MLC SFGRT. *International Journal of Radiation Oncology, Biology, Physics* 82 (5): 1642–1649.

15 Peñagarícano, J.A., et al. (2010). Evaluation of spatially fractionated radiotherapy (GRID) and definitive chemoradiotherapy with curative intent for locally advanced squamous cell carcinoma of the head and neck: Initial response rates and toxicity. *International Journal of Radiation Oncology*Biology*Physics* 76 (5): 1369–1375.

16 Billena, C. and Khan, A.J. (2019). A current review of spatial fractionation: Back to the future? *International Journal of Radiation Oncology, Biology, Physics* 104 (1): 177–187.

17 Kudrimoti, M. (2002). Spatially fractionated radiation therapy (SFR) in the palliation of large bulky (>8 cm) melanomas. *International Journal of Radiation Oncology, Biology, Physics* 54 (2): 342–343.

18 Mohiuddin, M., et al. (2009). Spatially fractionated grid radiation (SFGRT): A novel approach in the management of recurrent and unresectable soft tissue sarcoma. *International Journal of Radiation Oncology*Biology*Physics* 75 (3, Supplement): S526.

19 Rubin, P. and Casarett, G. (1968). *Clinical Radiation Pathology*. Philadelphia: WB Saunders.

20 Denekamp, J. (1984). Vascular endothelium as the vulnerable element in tumours. *Acta Radiologica. Oncology* 23 (4): 217–225.

21 Garcia-Barros, M., et al. (2003). Tumor response to radiotherapy regulated by endothelial cell apoptosis. *Science* 300 (5622): 1155–1159.

22 Fuks, Z. and Kolesnick, R. (2005). Engaging the vascular component of the tumor response. *Cancer Cell* 8 (2): 89–91.

23 Sathishkumar, S., et al. (2005). Elevated sphingomyelinase activity and ceramide concentration in serum of patients undergoing high dose spatially fractionated radiation treatment: Implications for endothelial apoptosis. *Cancer Biology & Therapy* 4 (9): 979–986.

24 Song, C., et al. (2014). Radiobiological basis of SBRT and SRS. *International Journal of Clinical Oncology* 19 (4): 570–578.

25 Kim, M., et al. (2015). Radiobiological mechanisms of stereotactic body radiation therapy and stereotactic radiation surgery. *Radiation Oncology Journal* 33 (4): 265–275.

26 Song, C.W., et al. (2015). Indirect tumor cell death after high-dose hypofractionated irradiation: Implications for stereotactic body radiation therapy and stereotactic radiation surgery. *International Journal of Radiation Oncology, Biology, Physics* 93 (1): 166–172.

27 Moding, E., et al. (2015). Tumor cells, but not endothelial cells, mediate eradication of primary sarcomas by stereotactic body radiation therapy. *Science Translational Medicine* 7 (278): 278ra34.

28 Hermens, A. and Barendsen, G. (1969). Changes of cell proliferation characteristics in a rat rhabdomyosarcoma before and after X-irradiation. *European Journal of Cancer (Oxford, England: 1990)* 5: 173–189.

29 Goel, S., et al. (2011). Normalization of the vasculature for treatment of cancer and other diseases. *Physiological Reviews* 91 (3): 1071–1121.

30 Lan, J., et al. (2013). Ablative hypofractionated radiotherapy normalizes tumor vasculature in Lewis lung carcinoma mice model. *Radiation Research* 179 (4): 458–464.

31 Semenza, G. (2000). Hypoxia, clonal selection, and the role of HIF-1 in tumor progression. *Critical Reviews in Biochemistry and Molecular Biology* 35 (2): 71–103.

32 Semenza, G. (2010). Defining the role of hypoxia-inducible factor 1 in cancer biology and therapeutics. *Oncogene* 29 (5): 625–634.

33 Moeller, B., et al. (2005). Pleiotropic effects of HIF-1 blockade on tumor radiosensitivity. *Cancer Cell* 8 (2): 99–110.

34 Fontanella, A., et al. (2015). Effects of high-dose microbeam irradiation on tumor microvascular function and angiogenesis. *Radiation Research* 183 (2): 147–158.

35 Mothersill, C. and Seymour, C. (2001). Radiation-induced bystander effects: Past history and future directions. *Radiation Research* 155 (6): 759–767.

36 Heeran, A., Berrigan, H., and O'Sullivan, J. (2019). The radiation-induced bystander effect (RIBE) and its connections with the hallmarks of cancer. *Radiation Research* 192 (6): 668–679.

37 Lyng, F. (2019). Radiation induced bystander signalling. *Radiation Environment and Medicine* 8 (2): 51–58.

38 Mukherjee, S. and Chakraborty, A. (2019). Radiation-induced bystander phenomenon: insight and implications in radiotherapy. *International Journal of Radiation Biology* 95 (3): 243–263.

39 Hu, S. and Shao, C. (2020). Research progress of radiation induced bystander and abscopal effects in normal tissue. *Radiation Medicine and Protection* 1: 69–74.

40 Nagasawa, H. and Little, J. (1981). Induction of chromosome aberrations and sister chromatid exchanges by X-rays in density inhibited cultures of mouse 10T1/2 cells. *Radiation Research* 87: 538–551.

41 Azzam, E., et al. (2002). Oxidative metabolism modulates signal transduction and micronucleus formation in bystander cells from alpha-particle-irradiated normal human fibroblast cultures. *Cancer Research* 62 (19): 5436–5442.

42 Ilnytskyy, Y. and Kovalchuk, O. (2011). Non-targeted radiation effects-an epigenetic connection. *Mutation Research* 714 (1–2): 113–125.

43 Mothersill, C. and Seymour, C. (2012). Are epigenetic mechanisms involved in radiation-induced bystander effects. *Frontiers in Genetics* 3: 74.

44 Mothersill, C., Rusin, A., and Seymour, C. (2019). Relevance of non-targeted effects for radiotherapy and diagnostic radiology; A historical and conceptual analysis of key players. *Cancers (Basel)* 11 (9).

45 Sokolov, M. and Neumann, R. (2018). Changes in gene expression as one of the key mechanisms involved in radiation-induced bystander effect. *Biomedical Reports* 9 (2): 99–111.

46 Tomita, M., et al. (2013). Dose response of soft X-ray-induced bystander cell killing affected by p53 status. *Radiation Research* 179 (2): 200–207.

47 Azzam, E.I., De Toledo, S.M., and Little, J.B. (2001). Direct evidence for the participation of gap junction-mediated intercellular communication in the transmission of damage signals from α-particle irradiated to nonirradiated cells. *Proceedings of the National Academy of Sciences of the United States of America* 98 (2): 473–478.

48 Asur, R., et al. (2015). High dose bystander effects in spatially fractionated radiation therapy. *Cancer Letters* 356 (1): 52–57.

49 Mothersill, C. and Seymour, C. (1998). Cell-cell contact during gamma irradiation is not required to induce a bystander effect in normal human keratinocytes: Evidence for release during irradiation of a signal controlling survival into the medium. *Radiation Research* 149 (3): 256–262.

50 Prise, K. and O'Sullivan, J. (2009). Radiation-induced bystander signalling in cancer therapy. *Nature Reviews. Cancer* 9 (5): 351–360.

51 Yan, W., et al. (2020). Spatially fractionated radiation therapy: History, present and the future. *Clinical and Translational Radiation Oncology* 20: 30–38.

52 Chen, S., et al. (2011). Rescue effects in radiobiology: Unirradiated bystander cells assist irradiated cells through intercellular signal feedback. *Mutation Research* 706 (1–2): 59–64.

53 Yu, K. (2019). Radiation-induced rescue effect. *Journal of Radiation Research* 60 (2): 163–170.

54 Formenti, S. and Demaria, S. (2009). Systemic effects of local radiotherapy. *The Lancet Oncology* 10 (7): 718–726.

55 Demaria, S. and Formenti, S. (2012). Radiation as an immunological adjuvant: Current evidence on dose and fractionation. *Frontiers in Oncology* 2: 153.

56 Demaria, S. and Formenti, S. (2013). Radiotherapy effects on anti-tumor immunity: Implications for cancer treatment. *Frontiers in Oncology* 3: 128.

57 Burnette, B. and Weichselbaum, R. (2015). The immunology of ablative radiation. *Seminars in Radiation Oncology* 25 (1): 40–45.

58 Mole, R. (1953). Whole body irradiation; radiobiology or medicine. *The British Journal of Radiology* 26 (305): 234–241.

59 Siva, S., et al. (2015). Abscopal effects of radiation therapy: A clinical review for the radiobiologist. *Cancer Letters* 356 (1): 82–90.

60 Hanahan, D. and Weinberg, R. (2011). Hallmarks of cancer: The next generation. *Cell* 144 (5): 646–674.

61 Postow, M., et al. (2012). Immunologic correlates of the abscopal effect in a patient with melanoma. *The New England Journal of Medicine* 366 (10): 925–931.

62 Golden, E., et al. (2013). An abscopal response to radiation and ipilimumab in a patient with metastatic non-small cell lung cancer. *Cancer Immunology Research* 1 (6): 365–372.

63 Ngwa, W., et al. (2018). Using immunotherapy to boost the abscopal effect. *Nature Reviews. Cancer* 18 (5): 313–322.

64 Kanagavelu, S., et al. (2014). In vivo effects of lattice radiation therapy on local and distant lung cancer: Potential role of immunomodulation. *Radiation Research* 182 (2): 149–162.

65 Lugade, A., et al. (2005). Local radiation therapy of B16 melanoma tumors increases the generation of tumor antigen-specific effector cells that traffic to the tumor. *Journal of Immunology (Baltimore, Md.: 1950)* 174 (12): 7516–7523.

66 Demaria, S., et al. (2014). The optimal partnership of radiation and immunotherapy: From preclinical studies to clinical translation. *Radiation Research* 182 (2): 170–181.

67 Vatner, R., et al. (2014). Combinations of immunotherapy and radiation in cancer therapy. *Frontiers in Oncology* 4: 325.

68 Ishihara, D., et al. (2017). Rationale and evidence to combine radiation therapy and immunotherapy for cancer treatment. *Cancer Immunology, Immunotherapy: CII* 66 (3): 281–298.

69 Galluzzi, L., et al. (2017). Immunogenic cell death in cancer and infectious disease. *Nature Reviews. Immunology* 17 (2): 97–111.

70 Kalina, J., et al. (2017). Immune modulation by androgen deprivation and radiation therapy: Implications for prostate cancer immunotherapy. *Cancers (Basel)* 9 (2).

71 Rodríguez-Ruiz, M., et al. (2018). Immunological mechanisms responsible for radiation-induced abscopal effect. *Trends in Immunology* 39 (8): 644–655.

72 Wang, Y., et al. (2020). cGAS-STING pathway in cancer biotherapy. *Molecular Cancer* 19 (1): 136.

73 Wu, X., et al. (2010). On modern technical approaches of three-dimensional high-dose lattice radiotherapy (LRT). *Cureus* 2 (3): e9.

74 Amendola, B.E., et al. (2019). Safety and efficacy of lattice radiotherapy in voluminous non-small cell lung cancer. *Cureus* 11 (3): e4263-e4263.

75 Ahmed, A.J.I., Estape, R., and Lambrou, N. (2010). Lattice radiotherapy with RapidArc for treatment of gynecological tumors: Dosimetric and early clinical evaluations.

76 Blanco Suarez, J.M., et al. (2015). The use of lattice radiation therapy (LRT) in the treatment of bulky tumors: A case

report of a large metastatic mixed mullerian ovarian tumor. *Cureus* 7 (11): e389-e389.

77 Yan, W., et al. (2019). Spatially fractionated radiation therapy: History, present and the future. *Clinical and Translational Radiation Oncology* 20: 30–38.

78 Zhang, X., et al. (2016). Spatially fractionated radiotherapy (GRID) using helical tomotherapy. *Journal Of Applied Clinical Medical Physics / American College of Medical Physics* 17 (1): 396–407.

79 Duriseti, S., et al. (2020). Spatially fractionated stereotactic body radiotherapy (Lattice SBRT) for large tumors. medRxiv.

80 Henry, T., et al. (2017). Proton grid therapy: A proof-of-concept study. *Technology in Cancer Research & Treatment* 16 (6): 749–757.

81 Gao, M., et al. (2018). Spatially fractionated (GRID) radiation therapy using proton pencil beam scanning (PBS): Feasibility study and clinical implementation. *Medical Physics* 45 (4): 1645–1653.

82 Tsubouchi, T., et al. (2018). Quantitative evaluation of potential irradiation geometries for carbon-ion beam grid therapy. *Medical Physics* 45 (3): 1210–1221.

83 Gholami, S., et al. (2016). Is grid therapy useful for all tumors and every grid block design? *Journal of Applied Clinical Medical Physics* 17 (2): 206–219.

84 Grotzer, M.A., et al. (2015). Microbeam radiation therapy: Clinical perspectives. *Physica Medica* 31 (6): 564–567.

85 Schültke, E., et al. (2017). Microbeam radiation therapy - grid therapy and beyond: A clinical perspective. *The British Journal of Radiology* 90 (1078): 20170073.

86 Girst, S., et al. (2016). Proton minibeam radiation therapy reduces side effects in an in vivo mouse ear model. *International Journal of Radiation Oncology, Biology, Physics* 95 (1): 234–241.

87 Prezado, Y., et al. (2017). Proton minibeam radiation therapy spares normal rat brain: Long-term clinical, radiological and histopathological analysis. *Scientific Reports* 7 (1): 1–7.

88 Prezado, Y., et al. (2018). Proton minibeam radiation therapy widens the therapeutic index for high-grade gliomas. *Scientific Reports* 8 (1): 16479–16479.

89 Lansonneur, P., et al. (2020). First proton minibeam radiation therapy treatment plan evaluation. *Scientific Reports* 10 (1): 7025–7025.

90 De Marzi, L., et al. (2019). Spatial fractionation of the dose in proton therapy: Proton minibeam radiation therapy. *Cancer Radiotherapie: Journal de la Societe Francaise de Radiotherapie Oncologique* 23 (6–7): 677–681.

91 Dilmanian, F.A., et al. (2012). Interleaved carbon minibeams: An experimental radiosurgery method with clinical potential. *International Journal of Radiation Oncology, Biology, Physics* 84 (2): 514–519.

92 Dilmanian, F.A., et al. (2015). Charged particle therapy with mini-segmented beams. *Frontiers in Oncology* 5: 269–269.

11

Particle Therapy and the Immune System

Sherif G. Shaaban, MB ChB[1], Daniel Ebner, MD, MPH[2], and Osama Mohamad, MD, PhD[3]

[1] Department of Radiation Oncology, University of Minnesota, Minneapolis, MN
[2] Hospital of the National Institutes of Quantum and Radiological Science and Technology (QST Hospital), Chiba, Japan
[3] Department of Radiation Oncology, University of California San Francisco

Corresponding Author: Osama Mohamad, MD, PhD, Department of Radiation Oncology, University of California San Francisco 1825 4th St, Suite L1101 San Francisco, California 94107

11.1 Cancer Immunoediting

The hypothesis of cancer immunosurveillance was first proposed in 1957 by Burnet and Thomas [1] who suggested that thymus-dependent lymphocytes could recognize and eliminate continuously budding transformed cells [1]. Over the years, there has been growing evidence that cancer immunosurveillance plays a crucial role in host protection through inhibition of carcinogenesis and maintenance of cellular homeostasis [2]. Immunosurveillance represents one component of a broader and more complex relationship between the immune system and cancer termed "cancer immunoediting" [3]. Immunoediting is composed of three phases termed the "three Es of immunoediting": elimination, equilibrium, and escape (Figure 11.1).

11.1.1 The Elimination Phase

To better understand the elimination phase, it is essential to recognize the immune cells which protect the host against tumor development and explain the process through which the immune system differentiates between the transformed and the normal host cells [4]. The elimination process involves four main phases [4]:

1 Recognition of tumor by innate immune cells: as the developing tumor acquires blood supply and induces stromal remodeling, proinflammatory cytokine release results in the recruitment of innate immune cells such as natural killer (NK) cells, T cells, macrophages, and dendritic cells (DCs) into the tumor [5,6]

2 Maturation and immigration of DCs and cross-priming of T cells: the recruited immune cells then migrate to nearby tumor-draining lymph nodes, leading to antigen presentation to naive CD4+ T cells and the eventual clonal expansion of cytotoxic T lymphocytes (CTLs) [7]

3 Production of tumor antigen (TA)-specific T cells and release of IL-12 and IFN-γ, which promote cytotoxic mechanisms such as perforin, TRAIL, and reactive oxygen species [8]

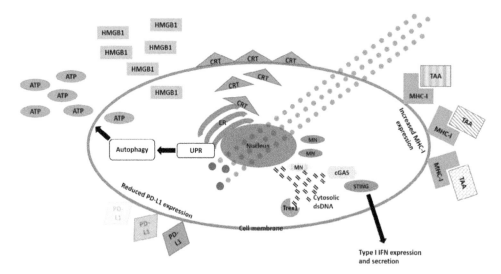

Figure 11.1 Mechanism of immunogenicity of particle radiation. Transformation of normal cells (gray) after exposure to various oncogenic stimuli into tumor cells (red) (top). In the bottom, the three phases of the cancer immunoediting process are illustrated (elimination, equilibrium, and escape). Permission from (Dunn et al., 2004. Cell Press, Elsevier Inc.).

4 Homing of TA-specific T cells to tumor site: TA-specific CD4+ and CD8+ T cells migrate to the tumor, where they eradicate the remaining tumor cells facilitated by the release of IFN-γ [9]. Other T cells differentiate into memory cells that may protect the host from recurrence [10].

11.1.2 The Equilibrium Phase

Although most transformed cells are terminated during the elimination phase, some tumor cells may survive the massive immunosurveillance pressure. While the immune system tries to continuously abolish rapidly mutating cells, the ongoing sculpting of tumor cells, on the other hand, creates cells more resistant to the immune response [2]. This process leads to the selection of tumor cells with reduced immunogenicity and increased capacity for survival in an immunocompetent host [2]. The equilibrium phase is the longest of the three phases of cancer immunoediting and may take place over a period of many years [3].

11.1.3 The Escape Phase

This phase is dominated by tumor cells which have survived the equilibrium phase and overcame the innate and adaptive immune defenses [2]. Malignant cells evade the immune system through various mechanisms. Cancer cells reduce or alter their MHC I expression to evade detection by CD8+ cytotoxic T cells [11] either by directly mutating the MHC I gene or by reducing their sensitivity to IFN-γ which impacts the expression of MHC I [12]. In addition, tumor cells can alter the function of cytotoxic T cells through inhibition of co-stimulatory molecules (CD80 and CD86) [13,14], induction of apoptosis of T lymphocytes (FasL) [15], and expression of PD-L1 which suppresses T-cell function via PD1–PD-L1 interaction [16].

Tumor cells also acquire resistance against NK and cytotoxic CD8+ T cells by overexpressing anti-apoptotic molecules Bcl-2, IAP, or XIAP [17,18]. All these mechanisms are enhanced by the generation of an immunosuppressive tumor microenvironment. Transforming growth factor beta (TGF-β) secreted by tumor cells and myeloid-derived suppressor cells (MDSC) plays an important role in creating an immunosuppressive microenvironment through the conversion of CD4+ T cells into suppressive regulatory T cells (Tregs) [19].

11.2 Ionizing Radiation and Immune Modulation

Radiotherapy (RT) constitutes one of the main pillars in the treatment of cancer. Traditionally, ionizing radiation exerts its cytotoxic effects on tumors directly via DNA strand breakage or indirectly by generating free radicals that result in DNA damage. Additionally, radiation promotes mitochondrial redox imbalances, lipid peroxidation of cell membranes, and a variety of signaling cascades that ultimately result in either permanent radiation-induced cell death or temporary inhibition of cell division to repair the damage [20]. However, the cell killing effect of RT is also modulated via the immune system. Historically, RT has been deemed to be immunosuppressive as localized RT commonly resulted in lymphopenia [21]. These findings were thought to be due to irradiation of the circulating blood pool and the innate radiation sensitivity of immune cells to low doses of radiation [22]. However, there is an established and growing body of evidence that radiation has an immune-stimulatory role and can enhance antitumor immunity [23].

Over the last 20 years, the term "immunogenic cell death" (ICD) has emerged referring to any kind of cell death eliciting an immune response [24]. ICD could be achieved by ATP (adenosine triphosphate) release, cell surface translocation of calreticulin which promotes phagocytosis of tumor cells by DCs, as well as extracellular release of high-mobility group protein B1 (HMGB1) [25,26]. Ionizing radiation induces these molecular proteins and leads to the emission of tumor-specific antigens which in turn steer antigen presenting cells (APCs), primarily DCs, to induce a T-cell-based immune response eventually leading to ICD [27]. RT increases tumor expression of MHC I, enhances production of endogenous peptides for antigen presentation [28], and increases Fas gene expression in tumor cells resulting in enhanced sensitivity to cytotoxic T-cell-mediated killing [29]. By debulking large tumors, RT reduces immune tolerance [30] and destroys the more immune-resistant tumor clones allowing for more effective and robust antitumor immunity [31]. RT thus acts as an "*in-situ* vaccine" [32]. Interestingly, this local immunity could be translated into systemic immunity against distant unirradiated tumor sites, a phenomenon called the "abscopal effect" (discussed later) [31]. That being said, the optimal dose and fractionation required to produce a systemic immunogenic response to RT is still unknown. Indeed, the ability of RT to prime T-cell response is influenced by a number of complex factors including the characteristics of RT delivered, the pre-existing tumor microenvironment, and the impact of RT on immune cells and other elements of the tumor microenvironment [33]. Some preclinical models showed that RT-induced ICD is a dose-dependent process with higher doses producing more immunogenic events [34].

Despite the role of RT in priming the immune response, repeated exposure to moderate doses of radiation may ultimately have a deleterious effect on the immune system, resulting in the elimination of effector cells required for potent antitumor action. The tumor microenvironment exhibits various inhibitory immune cells including tumor-associated macrophages (TAMs), Treg cells, and MDSCs [35]. These cells are effectively modulated by localized RT. TAMs can be evoked by RT to alter expression of chemokines, thus modifying the regulation of T cells [36]. On the other hand, Tregs are CD4+ T cells that secrete inhibitory cytokines, specifically TGF-β and IL-10, which suppress cytotoxic T-lymphocyte (CTL) activation and stimulate MDSCs [37,38]. RT increases the number of Tregs, suggesting that Tregs are more radioresistant than other immune cells or are capable of quicker regeneration [39,40]. RT also recruit MDSCs to irradiated sites, leading to suppression of CTL function [41–43]. Activated antitumor immune cells are exquisitely sensitive to radiation and can be wiped out at much lower doses than required to kill cancer cells [44]. Photon RT plans, especially with intensity modulation, often have significant areas of low-dose bath due to the many overlapping beams used. This exposes large circulating blood volumes to low-dose radiation which eventually compromise the systemic immune response [45]. Several studies have demonstrated that the degree of lymphopenia has a prognostic impact on survival with low nadir lymphopenia shown to be associated with a poor overall

survival across many cancer types [46]. Radiation-induced lymphopenia may also shorten time to progression in patients treated with immunotherapy [47]. Conversely, more advanced radiation techniques are associated with significantly less radiation-induced lymphopenia than conventional RT, including stereotactic body radiotherapy [48] and particle therapy (PT) [49,50].

11.3 Evolution of Immunotherapy

Stimulation of antitumor immunity is a multistep process controlled by several positive and negative signals [51]. Immunotherapy has emerged with drugs targeting one or more steps in this process. The original use of immunotherapy started as early as the 19th century with "Coley's toxin," a bacterial preparation which showed a modest clinical benefit but was an early proof that the immune system can be harnessed to generate an antitumor response. Since then, tremendous progress in immuno-oncology has led to the development of new treatments such as immune checkpoint blockade, monoclonal antibody treatment, adoptive T-cell transfer, cytokine therapy, DC, and peptide vaccines [52]. We will briefly introduce immune checkpoint inhibitors.

Immune checkpoint molecules prevent the over-activation of the immune system and self-recognition by suppressing T-cell activation and effector function, thus sustaining a balance between induction and inhibition of immune functions to prevent autoimmunity [52]. CTL antigen 4 (CTLA-4) is a member of the immunoglobulin superfamily that is overexpressed after T-cell activation and transmits inhibitory signals that suppress T-cell activation and proliferation [53]. CTLA-4 inhibitors work by blocking the inhibitory effect of CTLA-4. On the other hand, PD-1 is an inhibitory cell surface receptor that protects against detrimental autoimmunity by stimulating programmed cell death (apoptosis) of antigen-specific T cells and reducing apoptosis in regulatory suppressive T cells [54,55]. Its ligand, PD-L1, is expressed on several types of cells involving antigen-presentation, epithelial, and endothelial cells. Owing to the extensive research on CTLA-4 and PD-1, an improved understanding of how T-cell pathways could be targeted to induce antitumor T-cell responses subsequently emerged. This has led to the rapid development of antibodies targeting PD-1/PD-L1 and CTLA-4 [56] with widespread success across different tumor types basically changing the landscape of antitumor therapies.

11.4 Photon Radiotherapy and Immune Checkpoint Inhibitor Combinations

In light of the remarkable success of checkpoint inhibitors, there has been a great interest in combining these agents with RT. The biological rationale behind such a strategy is that tumor-antigen release after localized RT will promote specific tumor-targeting by the adaptive immune system, which can be further boosted by systemic immune-stimulating agents [57–59]. On the other hand, immunotherapy augments the action of RT by targeting and modulating different T-cell populations, including both exhausted and newly activated cells [60]. This biological synergism, in addition to spatial and temporal cooperation, provided a strong rationale for this combination. Many *in vitro* and clinical studies have tested this combination to better understand the synergistic action and to help optimize strategies for sequencing and timing of the two modalities to maximize the benefit and reduce treatment-related toxicities [20]. It is noteworthy that most *in vivo* studies suggest that a single or few large fractions of RT synergize with immune checkpoint inhibitors better than multiple small fractions, likely because of depletion of newly recruited activated T cells by repetitive irradiation [61,62]. This is still a subject of intense debate, too. Notably, RT leads to the accumulation of cytosolic DNA which activates a protein called stimulator of interferon genes (STING), ultimately leading to promotion of antitumor immunity in different cancer cells [63,64]. However, higher doses of RT (12–18 Gy) upregulate the DNA exonuclease Trex1 protein [65], which degrades cytosolic DNA and thus reduces immunogenicity.

The preclinical investigation of the combination of RT and immune checkpoint inhibitors have substantially increased over the last few years. Despite the great potential, the best way to utilize this combination remains elusive. Demaria et al. showed that RT followed by CTLA-4 blockade granted superior survival relative to either treatment alone in a 4T1 breast cancer model [66]. Another study utilized murine colon cancer models treated with RT and intratumoral injection of immature DCs and CTLA-4 inhibitor. This combination significantly enhanced antitumor immunity by reducing Treg populations [67]. Likewise, Wu et al. found that RT and CTLA-4 inhibitors significantly boosted the antitumor immunity against mesothelioma cancer cells [68]. Timing of the CTLA-4 blockade with RT was tested in an experiment conducted by Young et al. [69]. The CT26 murine colorectal carcinoma was treated with a single dose of RT (20 Gy) combined with anti-CTLA-4 antibody given either before or after RT. They observed that the best survival results were achieved with administration of CTLA-4 antibody before RT [69]. Similar to CTLA-4, PD1/PDL1 blockade has been tested in combination with RT. Murine intracranial glioma models treated with anti-PD-1 inhibitor plus RT showed superior survival with combined treatment relative to each modality alone, as well as a more robust systemic immunologic memory illustrated by an increased number of CD8+ CTLs and a decreased number of CD4+ Tregs in tumors [70]. Wu et al. treated MB 49 transitional cell bladder cancer models with anti-PDL1 antibody daily on days 0–14 and concurrent RT on days 1 and 14. They found that the combined approach resulted in longer tumor growth delays relative to RT or anti-PDL1 alone [71].

Several retrospective studies have been published reporting on the safety and efficacy of such combinations in different cancer types such as melanoma [72,73], non-small cell lung cancer [74], and others [75,76]. Generally, these studies showed the safety of such combinations but caution is warranted with brain radiosurgery. A few prospective studies have also investigated these combinations with conflicting results of whether such treatments increase efficacy compared to either treatment alone [77–82].

11.4.1 Abscopal Effect

Historically, the RT role was limited to eradication of local disease, maximizing tumor kill while attempting to spare surrounding structures. More recently, RT has been demonstrated to elicit a systemic immune effect, eliminating unirradiated distant tumors [83]. The abscopal effect, hence, refers to the ability of localized RT to provoke systemic antitumor effect, i.e., away from the site of irradiation.

The abscopal effect has been observed in many preclinical and clinical cases. A few observations over decades have suggested that RT alone could induce an abscopal effect. However, these effects remained elusive until Demaria et al. hypothesized that they are immune-moderated [31]. They used the DC growth factor Flt3-L in mice models that were implanted in one flank with mammary 67NR tumor cells alone and in the contralateral flank with both 67NR tumor cells and A20 lymphoma cells. The irradiation of the 67NR tumor cells on one side resulted in significant regression in the contralateral non-irradiated flank 67NR tumors but did not affect the growth of the antigenically unrelated A20 lymphoma [31]. Another study treated Lewis lung carcinoma models with RT reported limitation of growth of non-irradiated T241 fibrosarcoma cells implanted in a second site [84]. The abscopal effect has been also reported with the combined use of RT and immunotherapy. In mouse models of renal cell carcinoma with pulmonary metastases treated with either combined RT and IL-2 or RT alone, the combined modality eliminated more pulmonary metastases compared to localized RT alone [85]. The same combination was used to treat a mouse model of colon adenocarcinoma with liver metastases in another study, again showing that RT with immunotherapy significantly reduced the size of metastatic disease compared to RT alone [86]. Likewise, the combination of RT with CTLA-4 antibodies for treatment of 4T1 mammary carcinoma models led to slowed growth of primary irradiated tumors as well as inhibited development of pulmonary metastases [66]. Zeng et al. also studied the effect of anti-PD-1 antibodies with RT in the treatment of glioblastoma multiforme model. Median survival was greatest with use of combined treatment [70]. The abscopal effect appears to be influenced by many factors including the radiation dose, delivery schedule, dose per fraction, number of fractions, timing of RT, and primary tumor size [87]. Early preclinical reports demonstrated that higher RT dose (20 Gy) is required to provoke an abscopal effect [88]. A recent review suggested that the incidence of abscopal effect in preclinical models corelated with the biologically effective dose (BED) and concluded that probability of observing abscopal effects is more than 50% at BED of 60 Gy [87]. In the clinical setting, the abscopal effect has been reported as well. A study was conducted among patient with different solid tumors and was treated with localized RT 35 Gy in 10 fractions and granulocyte-macrophage colony-stimulating factor. They observed abscopal effect in 26% of the cohort [89]. Postow et al. reported a metastatic melanoma patient who was treated with palliative RT 28.5 Gy in three fractions to a right paraspinal mass plus ipilimumab as maintenance therapy. Four months after RT, irradiated as well as nonirradiated lesions in the right hilar lymph nodes and spleen had decreased in size [90]. The induction of a systemic radiation effect has been rare and inconsistent, however.

11.5 Particle Therapy

PT is a form of external beam RT that uses neutral (such as neutrons) or charged (such as protons, helium, and carbon ions, among others) particles. PT has witnessed a tremendous expansion over the past 20 years particularly using protons. The experience with other heavy particles is limited to a few institutions around the world. The number of patients treated with PT has substantially increased over the past two decades with approximately 250,000 patients treated worldwide; 213,000 with protons, 32,000 with carbon ions, and 3,500 with helium and other ions by end of 2019 [91]. Proton therapy was initially proposed in 1946 by Robert R. Wilson [92] and the first patient was treated at the Lawrence Berkeley National Laboratory in Berkeley, California in 1954. As of April 2020, there were 37 current operating proton centers in the United States with 14 others under construction or in the planning stage [93]. Carbon-ion radiotherapy (CIRT), on the other hand, has increasingly gained attention in treating tumors resistant to other modalities, with multiple operating facilities in Japan, Germany, Italy, China, and Austria.

11.5.1 Particles, Linear Energy Transfer, and Relative Biological Effect

Photon irradiation delivers dose uniformly to target tissue. Particle irradiation, on the other hand, provides for an improved dose distribution, depositing dose relatively selectively within target tissue while minimizing both entrance and exit doses to normal tissues [94] (Figure 11.2). Particles deposit energy at an inverse of their speed: as the particle slows within the body, its energy is gradually released until reaching an

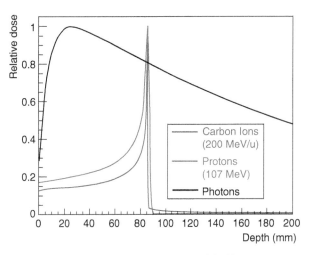

Figure 11.2 Dose deposition of photons (black), protons (blue), and carbon ions (red) as a function of depth in the transverse matter.

asymptotic point—the Bragg peak—where the particle stops and all energy is deposited. Through careful modulation of particle speed and with consideration of intermediary tissues between emitter and target, particles can be used to paint a tumor with dose while functionally limiting irradiation of healthy tissue [95]. These properties allow for more conformal targeting compared to photon RT and potentially have significant biological and immunological implications.

Beyond the physical distribution of these particles, however, are the biological ramifications of particulate irradiation. Heavy-ion beams, such as those made with carbon ions, have a high linear energy transfer (LET), transferring an increased amount of energy per particle per unit distance in comparison with comparatively low LET irradiation, such as photons or even protons. This results in an increased number of ionization events per unit dose deposited [96]. Consequently, high LET radiation generates an enhanced double stranded to single stranded DNA break ratio within irradiated tissue leading to a cell-killing effect relatively independent of cell-cycle and tissue oxygenation [97,98]. These biological differences result in differing biological damage, or kill effect, between identical physical doses of carbon, proton, and photon irradiation. This physical dose to biological effect ratio is termed the relative biological effectiveness (RBE). Though a complex question involving substantial (and evolving) dose-modeling techniques encompassing beam delivery apparatus, as well as tumor target and intermediary tissue types, carbon is generally considered to have an RBE to conventional photon irradiation of ~3 [99], while proton is considered to have an RBE of ~1.1; though these RBEs may notably vary within the beam itself [100]. Owing to this difference in RBE, mounting (pre)clinical evidence with carbon particles has demonstrated particular potential in the treatment of hypoxic and radioresistant disease [97,101,102]. Attention is now directed toward concentrating high LET radiation in radioresistant areas of tumors, as well as to maintain dose uniformity while modifying only LET ("LET painting"); these efforts are ongoing [103–105]. Given these diverging physical and biological properties, PT is thought to have unique downstream biological ramifications, with widely yet unknown local and systemic immune effects.

11.6 Immunogenicity of Particle Therapy

The number of studies investigating the immunogenicity of PT is limited but increasing. Preclinical evidence suggests that higher LET irradiation may be more conducive to generating a systemic immune response and anti-metastatic (abscopal) effect [82,101,102,106,107]. Tumor damage may be enhanced with high-LET beams or by leveraging the advantageous dose distribution of particles for dose escalation. Theoretically, this may increase the rate of cells undergoing ICD, reduce immunosuppression or lymphopenia, or even cause cells to undergo necrosis outright, leading to immune-activation [108]. The improved dose distribution with PT diminishes unnecessary radiation of normal tissues (including nearby draining lymph nodes) that may elicit immunosuppressive responses [45]. High-LET radiation seems to increase the ceramide pathway as well as other pathways that ultimately enhance tumor growth arrest and apoptosis more efficiently than low-LET beams [109]. A preclinical study utilizing a lung carcinoma model reported reduced the levels of IL-6, IL-8, vascular endothelial growth factor (VEGF), and hypoxia-inducible factor 1-alpha (HIF-1α) after treatment with PT resulting in suppression of tumor angiogenesis and growth [110]. A single dose of CIRT to a peripheral tumor, for example, significantly reduced the number of lung metastases when combined with intratumoral DC injection [111]. Resistance to photon therapy is largely attributed to the development of resistant heterogenous clones within the tumor [112,113] along with cancer stem-like cells (CSC) and other quiescent cells promoting further tumor growth and local recurrence. Interestingly, these types of cells were found to be more sensitive to PT and CIRT than photons [114,115]. In addition, multiple *in vivo* studies have demonstrated that carbon ions, relative to photons, increase expression of membrane-associated immunogenic molecules and reduce distant metastasis in different cancer models [116,117]. Taken together, these findings have renewed the interest in the combination of PT with immunotherapy with proposed superior outcomes compared with photon therapy. To what degree this is unique to LET, hypofractionation, or enhanced dose delivery remains under study.

Not all studies, however, showed increased benefit of heavy ions compared to photons. Suetens et al. studied the genomic changes in human prostate cancer cells induced by CIRT. They found that expression of genes involved in cell migration and motility varied in a cancer-type specific and dose- and time-

dependent manner compared with photons [118]. One Japanese study examined the ability of CIRT to induce high mobility group box 1 (HMGB1) release compared to photons. HMGB1 plays a pivotal role in APC activation and promotion of antitumor immune response [119]. They used five human cancer cell lines and reported similar effect between photons and CIRT in stimulation of HMGB1 at different time points after irradiation [120]. Similarly, there was no difference in the incidence or histology of metastatic deposits after irradiation of a primary tumor with CIRT or photons in a murine model [121].

11.7 Particle Therapy and Immunotherapy Combinations

11.7.1 Preclinical Studies

Two Japanese *in vivo* studies examined the immunogenic potential of combining CIRT and DC-based immunotherapy using immunocompetent mice. Matsunaga et al. utilized two models: syngeneic C3H/He mice inoculated with poorly immunogenic squamous cell carcinoma (SCC VII) and mammary carcinoma FM3A cells, whereas Ohkubo et al. used a highly metastatic squamous cell carcinoma (NR-S1)-implanted C3H/HeSlc mouse model. Immunotherapy was administered intratumorally following CIRT. Both experiments showed that this combination resulted in greater induction of antitumor immunity (compared to "no treatment" controls or CIRT only) [111,122]. Matsunaga et al. further showed that the antitumor effect is tumor-specific and acts through CD-8+ T cells. In a recent collaboration between GSI and NIRS, carbon ions were combined for the first time with immune checkpoints inhibitors in a mouse osteosarcoma model. The combination of CIRT and immunotherapy was more effective in controlling the unirradiated contralateral limb tumor and in suppressing lung metastasis compared to photons and immunotherapy [123].

11.7.2 Clinical Studies

In the clinical setting, there are many ongoing clinical trials utilizing PT in treating various types of cancers. Clinical trials combining PT and immunotherapy are still scarce, however. In a phase I safety study, *in situ* tumor vaccination using an immunoadjuvant made of BCG extract bound to hydroxyapatite and micro-particulated tuberculin was combined with proton irradiation in nine patients with hepatocellular carcinoma. The combination was feasible and safe but no further efficacy tests have been reported yet [124]. PT can elicit an abscopal effect either alone or combined with immunotherapy [101]. A few case reports have been published in this setting. A 75-year-old patient with recurrent locally advanced colorectal

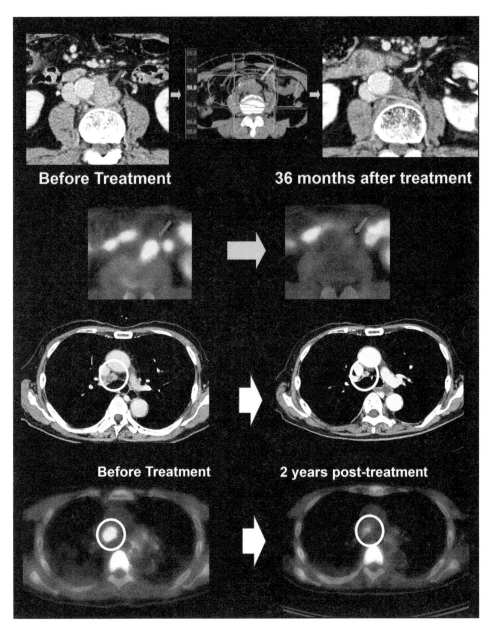

Figure 11.3 An 85-year-old patient received 50.4 GyE in 12 fractions for an ascending colon carcinoma at National Institute of Radiological Sciences, Chiba, Japan (A). At the time of treatment, the patient had mediastinal lymph node metastasis, at computed tomography and methionine positron emission tomography imaging (B). Six months after treatment, resolution of both the irradiated lesion (A) and the metastasis occurred (B).

cancer with multiple hepatic and abdominal metastases received CIRT to a painful recurrence in his left flank. PET CT scan done 1 month after treatment demonstrated notable reduction of both treated and untreated para-iliac artery masses [106]. An 85-year-old patient with recurrent and metastatic colorectal cancer was treated with CIRT to a metastatic aortic lymph node. Posttreatment imaging evaluation after 6 months showed shrinkage of both treated site and untreated right subclavian node [106] (Figure 11.3). Recently, Brenneman et al. reported a case illustrating the abscopal effect following treatment with protons where a 67-year-old patient with metastatic

inoperable retroperitoneal sarcoma received proton irradiation to the primary site. Post-RT surveillance imaging after 5 months showed complete resolution of all metastatic sites [125].

11.8 Conclusion

There is a growing interest to further understand the interplay between particulate irradiation and the immune system. The favorable physical and radiobiological characteristics of PT could be maximally utilized when used synergistically with different immunotherapeutic agents for the induction of efficient and sustained antitumor effects. Future preclinical and clinical work should be directed to PT and immunotherapy combinations to test the safety and efficacy of these treatments and to maximize patient outcomes. This should include deter-mination of the optimal radiation dose, fractionation, dose per fraction, sequencing of radiation with immunotherapy, and the type of immunotherapeutic agents used in each type of cancer.

References

1 Burnet, M. (1957). Cancer: A biological approach. III. Viruses associated with neoplastic conditions. IV. Practical applications. (in eng), *British Medical Journal* 1 (5023): (Apr 13): 841–847.

2 Kim, R., Emi, M., and Tanabe, K. (2007). Cancer immunoediting from immune surveillance to immune escape. (in eng), *Immunology* 121 (1): (May):1–14.

3 Dunn, G.P., Old, L.J., and Schreiber, R.D. (2004). The three Es of cancer immunoediting. (in eng), *Annual Review of Immunology* 22: 329–360. https://www.annualreviews.org/doi/10.1146/annurev.immunol.22.012703.104803

4 Dunn, G.P., Old, L.J., and Schreiber, R.D. (2004). The Immunobiology of Cancer Immunosurveillance and Immunoediting. *Immunity* 21 (2): (2004/08/01/): 137–148. https://www.annualreviews.org/doi/10.1146/annurev.iy.12.040194.005015

5 Matzinger, P. (1994). Tolerance, danger, and the extended family. (in eng), *Annual Review of Immunology* 12: 991–1045. https://10.1146/annurev.iy.12.040194.005015

6 Smyth, M.J., Godfrey, D.I., and Trapani, J.A. (2001). A fresh look at tumor immunosurveillance and immunotherapy. (in eng), *Nature Immunology* 2 (4): (Apr): 293–299. https://www.nature.com/articles/ni0401_293

7 Ikeda, H., Old, L.J., and Schreiber, R.D. (2002). The roles of IFN gamma in protection against tumor development and cancer immunoediting. *Cytokine & Growth Factor Reviews* 13 (2): England, 95–109.

8 Sinha, P., Clements, V.K., Miller, S., and Ostrand-Rosenberg, S. (2005). Tumor immunity: A balancing act between T cell activation, macrophage activation and tumor-induced immune suppression. (in eng), *Cancer Immunology, Immunotherapy : CII* 54 (11): (Nov): 1137–1142. https://link.springer.com/article/10.1007/s00262-005-0703-4

9 Hollenbaugh, J. A., and Dutton, R.W. (2006). IFN-gamma regulates donor CD8 T cell expansion, migration, and leads to apoptosis of cells of a solid tumor. *Immunology*. 177(5): 3004–3011. doi: 10.4049/jimmunol.177.5.3004. PMID: 16920936.https://www.jimmunol.org/content/177/5/3004.long

10 Aguirre-Ghiso, J.A. (2007). Models, mechanisms and clinical evidence for cancer dormancy. (in eng), *Nature Reviews. Cancer* 7 (11): (Nov): 834–846. https://www.nature.com/articles/nrc2256

11 Daniyan, A.F. and Brentjens, R.J. (2017). Immunotherapy: Hiding in plain sight: Immune escape in the era of targeted T-cell-based immunotherapies. (in eng), *Nature Reviews. Clinical Oncology* 14 (6): (Jun): 333–334.

12 Mojic, M., Takeda, K., and Hayakawa, Y. (2017 Dec 28). The dark side of IFN-γ: Its role in promoting cancer immunoevasion. (in eng), *International Journal of Molecular Sciences* 19 (1): 89. doi: 10.3390/ijms19010089. PMID: 29283429; PMCID: PMC5796039.

13 Tirapu, I. et al. (2006). Low surface expression of B7-1 (CD80) is an immunoescape mechanism of colon carcinoma. *Cancer Research* 66 (4): United States, 2442–2450.

14 Pettit, S.J., Ali, S., O'Flaherty, E., Griffiths, T.R., Neal, D.E., and Kirby, J.A. (1999). Bladder cancer immunogenicity: Expression of CD80 and CD86 is insufficient to allow primary CD4+ T cell activation in vitro. (in eng), *Clinical and Experimental Immunology* 116 (1): (Apr): 48–56.

15 Peter, M.E. et al. (2015). The role of CD95 and CD95 ligand in cancer. (in eng), *Cell Death and Differentiation* 22 (4): (Apr): 549–559.

16 Buchbinder, E.I. and Desai, A. (2016). CTLA-4 and PD-1 Pathways: Similarities, Differences, and Implications of Their Inhibition. (in eng), *American Journal of Clinical Oncology* 39 (1): (Feb): 98–106.

17 Frenzel, A., Grespi, F., Chmelewskij, W., and Villunger, A. (2009). Bcl2 family proteins in carcinogenesis and the treatment of cancer. (in eng), *Apoptosis* 14 (4): (Apr): 584–596.

18 Obexer, P. and Ausserlechner, M.J. (2014). X-linked inhibitor of apoptosis protein – A critical death resistance regulator and therapeutic target for personalized cancer therapy. (in eng), *Frontiers in Oncology* 4: 197.

19 Polanczyk, M.J., Walker, E., Haley, D., Guerrouahen, B.S., and Akporiaye, E.T. (2019). Blockade of TGF-β signaling to enhance the antitumor response is accompanied by dysregulation of the functional activity of CD4(+)CD25(+)Foxp3(+) and CD4(+)CD25(-)Foxp3(+) T cells. (in eng), *Journal of Translational Medicine* 17 (1): (Jul 9): 219.

20 Aliru, M.L. et al. (2018). Radiation therapy and immunotherapy: What is the optimal timing or sequencing? in eng), *Immunotherapy* 10 (4): (Feb 1): 299–316.

21 Campian, J.L., Ye, X., Brock, M., and Grossman, S.A. (2013). Treatment-related lymphopenia in patients with stage III non-small-cell lung cancer. (in eng), *Cancer Investigation* 31 (3): (Mar): 183–188. https://www.tandfonline.com/doi/abs/10.3109/07357907.2013.767342

22 Yovino, S., Kleinberg, L., Grossman, S.A., Narayanan, M., and Ford, E. (2013). The etiology of treatment-related lymphopenia in patients with malignant gliomas: Modeling radiation dose to circulating lymphocytes explains clinical observations and suggests methods of modifying the impact of radiation on immune cells. (in eng), *Cancer Investigation* 31 (2): (Feb): (140–144). https://www.tandfonline.com/doi/abs/10.3109/07357907.2012.762780

23 Zeng, J., Harris, T.J., Lim, M., Drake, C.G., and Tran, P.T. (2013). Immune modulation and stereotactic radiation: Improving local and abscopal responses. (in eng), *BioMed Research International* 2013: 658126. 10.1155/2013/658126.

24 Ma, Y. et al. (2010). Chemotherapy and radiotherapy: Cryptic anticancer vaccines. (in eng), *Seminars in Immunology* 22 (3): (Jun): 113–124. https://www.sciencedirect.com/science/article/pii/S1044532310000369

25 Apetoh, L. et al. (2007). Toll-like receptor 4-dependent contribution of the immune system to anticancer chemotherapy and radiotherapy. (in eng), *Nature Medicine* 13 (9): (Sep): 1050–1059. https://www.nature.com/articles/nm1622

26 Ghiringhelli, F. et al. (2009). Activation of the NLRP3 inflammasome in dendritic cells induces IL-1beta-dependent adaptive immunity against tumors. (in eng), *Nature Medicine* 15 (10): (Oct): 1170–1178. https://www.nature.com/articles/s41577-019-0165-0

27 Demaria, S. and Formenti, S.C. (2007). Sensors of ionizing radiation effects on the immunological microenvironment of cancer. (in eng), *International Journal of Radiation Biology* 83 (11-12): (Nov-Dec 2007): 819–825. https://www.tandfonline.com/doi/abs/10.1080/09553000701481816

28 Reits, E.A. et al. (2006). Radiation modulates the peptide repertoire, enhances MHC class I expression, and induces successful antitumor immunotherapy. (in eng), *The Journal of Experimental Medicine* 203 (5): (May): 1259–1271. https://rupress.org/jem/article/203/5/1259/54491/Radiation-modulates-the-peptiderepertoire

29 Garnett, C.T. et al. (2004). Sublethal irradiation of human tumor cells modulates phenotype resulting in enhanced killing by cytotoxic T lymphocytes. (in eng), *Cancer Research* 64 (21): (Nov): 7985–7994. https://cancerres.aacrjournals.org/content/64/21/7985.long

30 Drake, C.G. (2012). Combination immunotherapy approaches. (in eng), *Annals Of Oncology : Official Journal Of The European Society For Medical Oncology / ESMO* 23 (Suppl 8): (Sep): viii41–6. https://www.sciencedirect.com/science/article/pii/S0923753419376902

31 Demaria, S. et al. (2004). Ionizing radiation inhibition of distant untreated tumors (abscopal effect) is immune mediated. *International Journal of Radiation Oncology, Biology, Physics* 58 (3): United States, 862–870.

32 Formenti, S.C. and Demaria, S. (2012). Radiation therapy to convert the tumor into an in situ vaccine. (in eng), *International Journal of Radiation Oncology, Biology, Physics* 84 (4): (Nov): 879–880. https://www.sciencedirect.com/science/article/pii/S0360301612008462

33 Demaria, S. and Formenti, S.C. (2012). Radiation as an immunological adjuvant: Current evidence on dose and fractionation. (in eng), *Frontiers in Oncology* 2: 153. https://www.frontiersin.org/articles/10.3389/fonc.2012.00153/full

34 Filatenkov, A. et al. (2015). Ablative tumor radiation can change the tumor immune cell microenvironment to induce durable complete remissions. (in eng), *Clinical Cancer Research : An Official Journal of the American Association for Cancer Research* 21 (16): (Aug): 3727–3739. https://clincancerres.aacrjournals.org/content/21/16/3727.long

35 Fridman, W.H., Zitvogel, L., Sautès-Fridman, C., and Kroemer, G. (2017). The immune contexture in cancer prognosis and treatment. (in eng), *Nature Reviews. Clinical Oncology* 14 (12): (Dec): 717–734. https://www.nature.com/articles/nrclinonc.2017.101

36 Inoue, T. et al. (2004). CCL22 and CCL17 in rat radiation pneumonitis and in human idiopathic pulmonary fibrosis. (in eng), *The European Respiratory Journal* 24 (1): (Jul): 49–56. https://erj.ersjournals.com/content/24/1/49.long

37 Burnette, B. and Weichselbaum, R.R. (2013). Radiation as an immune modulator. (in eng), *Seminars in Radiation Oncology* 23 (4): (Oct): 273–280. https://www.sciencedirect.com/science/article/pii/S1053429613000507

38 Facciabene, A., Motz, G.T., and Coukos, G. (2012). T-regulatory cells: Key players in tumor immune escape and angiogenesis. (in eng), *Cancer Research* 72 (9): (May): 2162–2171. https://cancerres.aacrjournals.org/content/72/9/2162.long

39 Balogh, A. et al. (2013). The effect of ionizing radiation on the homeostasis and functional integrity of murine splenic regulatory T cells. (in eng), *Inflammation Research : Official Journal of the European Histamine Research Society . [Et Al.]* 62 (2): (Feb): 201–212. https://link.springer.com/article/10.1007/s00011-012-0567-y

40 Persa, E., Balogh, A., Sáfrány, G., and Lumniczky, K. (2015). The effect of ionizing radiation on regulatory T cells in health and disease. (in eng), *Cancer Letters* 368 (2): 252–261. https://www.sciencedirect.com/science/article/pii/S0304383515001706

41 Condamine, T., Ramachandran, I., Youn, J.I., and Gabrilovich, D.I. (2015). Regulation of tumor metastasis by myeloid-derived suppressor cells. (in eng), *Annual Review of Medicine* 66: 97–110. https://www.annualreviews.org/doi/10.1146/annurev-med-051013-052304

42 Crittenden, M.R., Cottam, B., Savage, T., Nguyen, C., Newell, P., and Gough, M.J. (2012). Expression of NF-κB p50 in tumor stroma limits the control of tumors by radiation therapy. (in eng), *PLoS One.* 7 (6): e39295.

43 Xu, J. et al. (2013). CSF1R signaling blockade stanches tumor-infiltrating myeloid cells and improves the efficacy of radiotherapy in prostate cancer. (in eng), *Cancer Research* 73 (9): (May): 2782–2794. https://cancerres.aacrjournals.org/content/73/9/2782.long

44 Trowell, O.A. (1952). The sensitivity of lymphocytes to ionising radiation. (in eng), *The Journal of Pathology and*

Bacteriology 64 (4): (Oct): 687–704. https://pubmed.ncbi.nlm.nih.gov/13000583/

45 Lee, H.J., Zeng, J., and Rengan, R. (2018). Proton beam therapy and immunotherapy: An emerging partnership for immune activation in non-small cell lung cancer. (in eng), *Translational Lung Cancer Research* 7 (2): (Apr): 180–188. https://tlcr.amegroups.com/article/view/20665/16112

46 Tang, C. et al. (2014). Lymphopenia association with gross tumor volume and lung V5 and its effects on non-small cell lung cancer patient outcomes. (in eng), *International Journal of Radiation Oncology, Biology, Physics* 89 (5): (Aug): 1084–1091. https://www.sciencedirect.com/science/article/pii/S0360301614004969

47 Diehl, A., Yarchoan, M., Hopkins, A., Jaffee, E., and Grossman, S.A. (2017). Relationships between lymphocyte counts and treatment-related toxicities and clinical responses in patients with solid tumors treated with PD-1 checkpoint inhibitors. *Oncotarget* 8 (69): (Dec 26): 114268–114280. https://www.oncotarget.com/article/23217/text/

48 Wild, A.T. et al. (2016). Lymphocyte-sparing effect of stereotactic body radiation therapy in patients with unresectable pancreatic cancer. (in eng), *International Journal of Radiation Oncology, Biology, Physics* 94 (3): (Mar): 571–579. https://www.sciencedirect.com/science/article/pii/S0360301615267648

49 Welsh, J. et al. (2011). Intensity-modulated proton therapy further reduces normal tissue exposure during definitive therapy for locally advanced distal esophageal tumors: A dosimetric study. (in eng), *International Journal of Radiation Oncology, Biology, Physics* 81 (5): (Dec): 1336–1342. https://www.sciencedirect.com/science/article/pii/S0360301610031226

50 Davuluri, R. et al. (2017). Lymphocyte nadir and esophageal cancer survival outcomes after chemoradiation therapy. (in eng), *International Journal of Radiation Oncology, Biology, Physics* 99 (1): (09): 128–135. https://www.sciencedirect.com/science/article/pii/S0360301617309756

51 Chen, D.S. and Mellman, I. (2013). Oncology meets immunology: The cancer-immunity cycle. (in eng), *Immunity* 39 (1): (Jul): 1–10. https://www.sciencedirect.com/science/article/pii/S1074761313002963

52 Kang, J., Demaria, S., and Formenti, S. (2016). Current clinical trials testing the combination of immunotherapy with radiotherapy. (in eng), *The Journal for ImmunoTherapy of Cancer* 4: 51. https://www.ncbi.nlm.nih.gov/pmc/articles/PMC5028964/

53 Peggs, K.S., Quezada, S.A., and Allison, J.P. (2008). Cell intrinsic mechanisms of T-cell inhibition and application to cancer therapy. (in eng), *Immunological Reviews.* 224: (Aug): 141–165. https://onlinelibrary.wiley.com/doi/10.1111/j.1600-065X.2008.00649.x

54 Francisco, L.M., Sage, P.T., and Sharpe, A.H. (2010). The PD-1 pathway in tolerance and autoimmunity. (in eng), *Immunological Reviews* 236: (Jul): 219–242.

55 Fife, B.T. and Pauken, K.E. (2011). The role of the PD-1 pathway in autoimmunity and peripheral tolerance. (in eng), *Annals of the New York Academy of Sciences* 1217: (Jan): 45–59. https://nyaspubs.onlinelibrary.wiley.com/doi/10.1111/j.1749-6632.2010.05919.x

56 Brahmer, J.R. et al. (2012). Safety and activity of anti-PD-L1 antibody in patients with advanced cancer. (in eng), *The New England Journal of Medicine* 366 (26): (Jun): 2455–2465. https://www.nejm.org/doi/full/ 10.1056/nejmoa1200694

57 Gupta, A. et al. (2012). Radiotherapy promotes tumor-specific effector CD8+ T cells via dendritic cell activation. (in eng), *Journal of Immunology (Baltimore, Md. : 1950)* 189 (2): (Jul): 558–566. https://www.jimmunol.org/content/189/2/558

58 Parker, J.J., Jones, J.C., Strober, S., and Knox, S.J. (2013). Characterization of direct radiation-induced immune function and molecular signaling changes in an antigen presenting cell line. (in eng), *Clinical Immunology (Orlando, Fla.)* 148 (1): (Jul): 44–55. https://www.sciencedirect.com/science/article/pii/S1521661613000703

59 Tang, C. et al. (2014). Combining radiation and immunotherapy: A new systemic therapy for solid tumors? (in eng), *Cancer Immunol Res* 2 (9): (Sep): 831–838. https://cancerimmunolres.aacrjournals.org/content/2/9/831.long

60 Weichselbaum, R.R., Liang, H., Deng, L., and Fu, Y.X. (2017). Radiotherapy and immunotherapy: A beneficial liaison? (in eng), *Nature Reviews. Clinical Oncology* 14 (6): (Jun); 365–379. https://www.nature.com/articles/nrclinonc.2016.211

61 Dewan, M.Z. et al. (2009). Fractionated but not single-dose radiotherapy induces an immune-mediated abscopal effect when combined with anti-CTLA-4 antibody. (in eng), *Clinical Cancer Research : An Official Journal of the American Association for Cancer Research* 15 (17): (Sep 1): 5379–5388.

62 Bernstein, M.B., Krishnan, S., Hodge, J.W., and Chang, J.Y. (2016). Immunotherapy and stereotactic ablative radiotherapy (ISABR): A curative approach? (in eng), *Nature Reviews. Clinical Oncology* 13 (8): (08): 516–524. https://www.nature.com/articles/nrclinonc.2016.30

63 Woo, S.R. et al. (2014). STING-dependent cytosolic DNA sensing mediates innate immune recognition of immunogenic tumors. (in eng), *Immunity* 41 (5): (Nov): 830–842. https://www.sciencedirect.com/science/article/pii/S1074761314003938

64 Deng, L. et al. (2014). STING-Dependent Cytosolic DNA sensing promotes radiation-induced type i interferon-dependent antitumor immunity in immunogenic tumors. (in eng), *Immunity* 41 (5): (Nov): 843–852. https://www.sciencedirect.com/science/article/pii/S1074761314003951

65 Vanpouille-Box, C. et al. (2017). DNA exonuclease Trex1 regulates radiotherapy-induced tumour immunogenicity. (in eng), *Nature Communications* 8: (06): 15618. https://www.nature.com/articles/ncomms15618

66 Demaria, S. et al. (2005). Immune-mediated inhibition of metastases after treatment with local radiation and CTLA-4

blockade in a mouse model of breast cancer. (in eng), *Clinical Cancer Research : An Official Journal of the American Association for Cancer Research* 11 (2): Pt 1 (Jan):728–734. [Online]. Available: https://clincancerres.aacrjournals.org/content/11/2/728

67 Son, C.H. et al. (2014). CTLA-4 blockade enhances antitumor immunity of intratumoral injection of immature dendritic cells into irradiated tumor in a mouse colon cancer model. (in eng), *Journal of Immunotherapy (Hagerstown, Md. : 1997)* 37 (1): (Jan): 1–7. https://journals.lww.com/immunotherapy-journal/Fulltext/2014/01000/CTLA_4_Blockade_Enhances_Antitumor_Immunity_of.1.aspx

68 Wu, L. et al. (2015). Targeting the inhibitory receptor CTLA-4 on T cells increased abscopal effects in murine mesothelioma model. (in eng), *Oncotarget* 6 (14): (May): 12468–12480. https://www.oncotarget.com/article/3487/text/

69 Young, K.H. et al. (2016). Optimizing timing of immunotherapy improves control of tumors by hypofractionated radiation therapy. (in eng), *PLoS One* 11 (6): e0157164. https://journals.plos.org/plosone/article?id=10.1371/journal.pone.0157164

70 Zeng, J. et al. (2013). Anti-PD-1 blockade and stereotactic radiation produce long-term survival in mice with intracranial gliomas. (in eng), *International Journal of Radiation Oncology, Biology, Physics* 86 (2): (Jun): 343–349. https://www.sciencedirect.com/science/article/pii/S0360301613000047

71 Wu, C.T., Chen, W.C., Chang, Y.H., Lin, W.Y., and Chen, M.F. (2016). The role of PD-L1 in the radiation response and clinical outcome for bladder cancer. (in eng), *Scientific Reports* 6: (Jan): 19740. https://www.nature.com/articles/srep19740

72 Barker, C.A. et al. (2013). Concurrent radiotherapy and ipilimumab immunotherapy for patients with melanoma. *Cancer Immunol Res* 1 (2): (Aug): 92–98. https://cancerimmunolres.aacrjournals.org/content/1/2/92.long

73 Ahmed, K.A. et al. (2016). Clinical outcomes of melanoma brain metastases treated with stereotactic radiation and anti-PD-1 therapy. *Annals of Oncology: Official Journal of the European Society for Medical Oncology/ESMO* 27 (3): (Mar): 434–441. https://www.sciencedirect.com/science/article/pii/S0923753419356121

74 Shaverdian, N. et al. (2017). Previous radiotherapy and the clinical activity and toxicity of pembrolizumab in the treatment of non-small-cell lung cancer: A secondary analysis of the KEYNOTE-001 phase 1 trial. *The Lancet Oncology* 18 (7): (Jul); 895–903. https://www.sciencedirect.com/science/article/pii/S1470204517303807

75 Martin, A.M. et al. (2018). Immunotherapy and symptomatic radiation necrosis in patients with brain metastases treated with stereotactic radiation. *JAMA Oncology* 4 (8): (Aug 1); 1123–1124. https://jamanetwork.com/journals/jamaoncology/fullarticle/2668527

76 Mohamad, O. et al. (2018). Safety and efficacy of concurrent immune checkpoint inhibitors and hypofractionated body

radiotherapy. *Oncoimmunology* 7 (7): e1440168. https://www.tandfonline.com/doi/full/10.1080/2162402X.2018.1440168

77 Kwon, E.D. et al. (2014). Ipilimumab versus placebo after radiotherapy in patients with metastatic castration-resistant prostate cancer that had progressed after docetaxel chemotherapy (CA184-043): A multicentre, randomised, double-blind, phase 3 trial. *The Lancet Oncology* 15 (7): (Jun): 700–712. https://www.sciencedirect.com/science/article/pii/S1470204514701895

78 Tang, C. et al. (2017). Ipilimumab with stereotactic ablative radiation therapy: Phase i results and immunologic correlates from peripheral T Cells. *Clinical Cancer Research : An Official Journal of the American Association for Cancer Research* 23 (6): (Mar 15): 1388–1396. https://clincancerres.aacrjournals.org/content/23/6/1388.long

79 Antonia, S.J. et al. (2017). Durvalumab after chemoradiotherapy in Stage III non-small-cell lung cancer. *The New England Journal of Medicine* 377 (20): (Nov 16): 1919–1929. https://www.nejm.org/doi/10.1056/NEJMoa1709937

80 Formenti, S.C. et al. (2018). Radiotherapy induces responses of lung cancer to CTLA-4 blockade. *Nature Medicine* 24 (12): (Dec): 1845–1851. https://www.nature.com/articles/s41591-018-0232-2

81 McBride, S. et al. (2020 Jan 1). Randomized Phase II trial of nivolumab with stereotactic body radiotherapy versus nivolumab alone in metastatic head and neck squamous cell carcinoma. *Journal of Clinical Oncology : Official Journal of the American Society of Clinical Oncology* (Aug 21), 39(1):30–37. JCO2000290. https://ascopubs.org/doi/10.1200/JCO.20.00290

82 Theelen, W. et al. (2019 Sep 1). Effect of pembrolizumab after stereotactic body radiotherapy vs pembrolizumab alone on tumor response in patients with advanced non-small cell lung cancer: Results of the PEMBRO-RT Phase 2 randomized clinical trial. *JAMA Oncology* (Jul 11): 5(9):1276–1282. 10.1001/jamaoncol.2019.1478 PMID: 31294749; PMCID: PMC6624814.

83 Hu, Z.I., McArthur, H.L., and Ho, A.Y. (2017). The abscopal effect of radiation therapy: What is it and how can we use it in breast cancer? (in eng), *Current Breast Cancer Reports* 9 (1): 45–51. https://www.ncbi.nlm.nih.gov/pmc/articles/PMC5346418/

84 Camphausen, K. et al. (2003). Radiation abscopal antitumor effect is mediated through p53. (in eng), *Cancer Research* 63 (8): (Apr): 1990–1993. [Online]. Available: https://cancerres.aacrjournals.org/content/63/8/1990.long

85 Dybal, E.J., Haas, G.P., Maughan, R.L., Sud, S., Pontes, J.E., and Hillman, G.G. (1992). Synergy of radiation therapy and immunotherapy in murine renal cell carcinoma. (in eng), *The Journal of Urology* 148 (4): (Oct): 1331–1337. https://pubmed.ncbi.nlm.nih.gov/1404669/

86 Yasuda, K., Nirei, T., Tsuno, N.H., Nagawa, H., and Kitayama, J. (2011). Intratumoral injection of interleukin-2 augments the local and abscopal effects of radiotherapy in murine rectal cancer. (in eng), *Cancer Science* 102 (7): (Jul): 1257–1263. https://onlinelibrary. wiley.com/doi/10.1111/j.1349-7006.2011.01940.x

87 Marconi, R., Strolin, S., Bossi, G., and Strigari, L. (2017). A meta-analysis of the abscopal effect in preclinical models: Is the biologically effective dose a relevant physical trigger? (in eng), *PLoS One* 12 (2): e0171559. https://journals.plos.org/ plosone/article?id=10.1371/journal.pone.0171559

88 Strigari, L. et al. (2015). Abscopal effect of radiation therapy: Interplay between radiation dose and p53 status. (in eng), *International Journal of Radiation Biology* 91 (3): (Mar): 294. https://www.tandfonline.com/doi/abs/10.3109/09553002.201 4.874608

89 Golden, E.B. et al. (2015). Local radiotherapy and granulocyte-macrophage colony-stimulating factor to generate abscopal responses in patients with metastatic solid tumours: A proof-of-principle trial. (in eng), *The Lancet Oncology* 16 (7): (Jul): 795–803. https://www.sciencedirect. com/science/article/pii/S1470204515000546

90 Postow, M.A. et al. (2012). Immunologic correlates of the abscopal effect in a patient with melanoma. (in eng), *The New England Journal of Medicine* 366 (10): (Mar): 925–931. https://www.nejm.org/doi/full/10.1056/nejmoa1112824

91 Particle Therapy Co-Operative Group. https://www.ptcog. ch/index.php/patient-statistics

92 Wilson, R.R. (1946). Radiological use of fast protons. (in eng), *Radiology* 47 (5): (Nov): 487–491. https://pubs.rsna.org/ doi/10.1148/47.5.487

93 Ferre, R.D.Proton therapy centers in the United States. https://proton-therapy-centers.com

94 Kamada, T. et al. (2015). Carbon ion radiotherapy in Japan: An assessment of 20 years of clinical experience. *The Lancet Oncology* 16 (2): (Feb): https://www.sciencedirect.com/ science/article/pii/S1470204514704127

95 Mori, S. et al. (2016). Carbon-ion pencil beam scanning treatment with gated markerless tumor tracking: An analysis of positional accuracy. (in eng), *International Journal of Radiation Oncology, Biology, Physics* 95 (1): (May): 258–266. https://www.sciencedirect.com/science/article/pii/ S0360301616000249

96 Sutherland, B.M. et al. (2001). Clustered DNA damages induced by high and low LET radiation, including heavy ions. (in eng), *Physics in Medicine \& Biology* 17 (Suppl 1): 202–204. [Online]. Available: https://pubmed.ncbi.nlm.nih. gov/11776262/

97 Tinganelli, W. et al. (2015). Kill-painting of hypoxic tumours in charged particle therapy. (in eng), *Scientific Reports* 5: (Nov): 17016. https://www.nature.com/articles/ srep17016

98 Thariat, J. et al. (2019). Hadrontherapy interactions in molecular and cellular biology. (in eng), *International Journal of Molecular Sciences* 21 (1): (Dec): https://www. mdpi.com/1422-0067/21/1/133

99 Karger, C.P. and Peschke, P. (2017). RBE and related modeling in carbon-ion therapy. (in eng), *Physics in Medicine and Biology* 63 (1): (12): 01TR02. https:// iopscience.iop.org/article/10.1088/1361-6560/aa9102

100 Ilicic, K., Combs, S.E., and Schmid, T.E. (2018). New insights in the relative radiobiological effectiveness of proton irradiation. (in eng), *Radiation Oncology* 13 (1): (Jan): 6. https://ro-journal.biomedcentral.com/ articles/10.1186/s13014-018-0954-9

101 Shimokawa, T., Ma, L., Ando, K., Sato, K., and Imai, T. (2016). The future of combining carbon-ion radiotherapy with immunotherapy: Evidence and progress in mouse models. (in eng), *International Journal of Particle Therapy* 3 (1): 61–70. https://meridian.allenpress.com/theijpt/ article/3/1/61/203350/The-Future-of-Combining- Carbon-Ion-Radiotherapy

102 Takahashi, Y. et al. (2019). Carbon ion irradiation enhances the antitumor efficacy of dual immune checkpoint blockade therapy both for local and distant sites in murine osteosarcoma. (in eng), *Oncotarget* 10 (6): (Jan): 633–646. https://www.oncotarget.com/article/26551/text/

103 Bassler, N. et al. (2014). LET-painting increases tumour control probability in hypoxic tumours. (in eng), *Acta Oncologica* 53 (1): (Jan): 25–32. https://www.tandfonline. com/doi/full/10.3109/0284186X.2013.832835

104 Malinen, E. and Søvik, Å. (2015). Dose or 'LET' painting– What is optimal in particle therapy of hypoxic tumors?. (in eng), *Acta Oncologica* 54 (9): 1614–1622. https://www. tandfonline.com/doi/full/10.3109/0284186X.2015.1062540

105 Grassberger, C., Trofimov, A., Lomax, A., and Paganetti, H. (2011). Variations in linear energy transfer within clinical proton therapy fields and the potential for biological treatment planning. (in eng), *International Journal of Radiation Oncology, Biology, Physics* 80 (5): (Aug): 1559– 1566. https://www.sciencedirect.com/science/article/pii/ S0360301610034486

106 Ebner, D.K., Kamada, T., and Yamada, S. (2017). Abscopal effect in recurrent colorectal cancer treated with carbon-ion radiation therapy: 2 Case reports. (in eng), *Advances in Radiation Oncology* 2 (3): (Jul-Sep 2017): 333–338. https:// www.advancesradonc.org/article/S2452-1094(17)30101-X/pdf

107 Durante, M., Reppingen, N., and Held, K.D. (2013). Immunologically augmented cancer treatment using modern radiotherapy. (in eng), *Trends in Molecular*

Medicine 19 (9): (Sep): 565–582. https://www.sciencedirect.com/science/article/pii/S1471491413000968

108 Helm, A. et al. (2018). Combining heavy-ion therapy with immunotherapy: An update on recent developments. (in eng), *International Journal of Particle Therapy* 5 (1): 84–93. https://meridian.allenpress.com/theijpt/article/5/1/84/202616/

109 Alphonse, G. et al. (2013). P53-Independent early and late apoptosis is mediated by ceramide after exposure of tumor cells to photon or carbon ion irradiation. (in eng), *BMC Cancer* 13 (Mar 25): 151.

110 Girdhani, S., Sachs, R., and Hlatky, L. (2013). Biological effects of proton radiation: What we know and don't know. (in eng), *Radiation Research* 179 (3): (Mar): 257–272. https://bioone.org/journals/radiationresearch/volume-179/issue-3/RR2839.1

111 Ohkubo, Y. et al. (2010). Combining carbon ion radiotherapy and local injection of α-galactosylceramide-pulsed dendritic cells inhibits lung metastases in an in vivo murine model. *International Journal of Radiation Oncology, Biology, Physics* 78 (5): United States: © 2010 Elsevier Inc, 1524–1531.

112 Greaves, M. and Maley, C.C. (2012). Clonal evolution in cancer. (in eng), *Nature* 481 (7381): (Jan 18): 306–313.

113 Foo, J. and Michor, F. (2014). Evolution of acquired resistance to anti-cancer therapy. (in eng), *Journal of Theoretical Biology* 355: (Aug): 10–20. https://www.sciencedirect.com/science/article/pii/S0022519314001003

114 Zhang, X., Lin, S.H., Fang, B., Gillin, M., Mohan, R., and Chang, J.Y. (2013). Therapy-resistant cancer stem cells have differing sensitivity to photon versus proton beam radiation. (in eng), *Journal of Thoracic Oncology : Official Publication of the International Association for the Study of Lung Cancer*, 8 (12): (Dec,): 1484–1491. https://www.sciencedirect.com/science/article/pii/S1556086415301301

115 Masunaga, S. et al. (2008). The radiosensitivity of total and quiescent cell populations in solid tumors to 290 MeV/u carbon ion beam irradiation in vivo. (in eng), *Acta Oncologica* 47 (6): 1087–1093. https://www.tandfonline.com/doi/full/10.1080/02841860701821999

116 Ogata, T. et al. (2005). Particle irradiation suppresses metastatic potential of cancer cells. (in eng), *Cancer Research* 65 (1): (Jan): 113–120. [Online]. Available: https://cancerres.aacrjournals.org/content/65/1/113.long

117 Imadome, K. et al. (2008). Upregulation of stress-response genes with cell cycle arrest induced by carbon ion irradiation in multiple murine tumors models. (in eng), *Cancer Biology & Therapy* 7 (2): (Feb): 208–217. https://www.tandfonline.com/doi/abs/10.4161/cbt.7.2.5255

118 Suetens, A. et al. (2015). Dose- and time-dependent gene expression alterations in prostate and colon cancer cells after in vitro exposure to carbon ion and X-irradiation. (in eng), *Journal of Radiation Research* 56 (1): (Jan): 11–21. https://academic.oup.com/jrr/article/56/1/11/2580125

119 Schmid, T.E. and Multhoff, G. (2012). Radiation-induced stress proteins – The role of heat shock proteins (HSP) in anti- tumor responses. (in eng), *Current Medicinal Chemistry* 19 (12): 1765–1770. https://www.eurekaselect.com/96390/article

120 Yoshimoto, Y. et al. (2015). Carbon-ion beams induce production of an immune mediator protein, high mobility group box 1, at levels comparable with X-ray irradiation. (in eng), *Journal of Radiation Research* 56 (3): (May): 509–514. https://academic.oup.com/jrr/article/56/3/509/917013

121 Tamaki, T. et al. (2009). Application of carbon-ion beams or gamma-rays on primary tumors does not change the expression profiles of metastatic tumors in an in vivo murine model. *International Journal of Radiation Oncology, Biology, Physics* 74 (1): (May 1): 210–218. https://www.sciencedirect.com/science/article/pii/S0360301609000911

122 Matsunaga, A. et al. (2010). Carbon-ion beam treatment induces systemic antitumor immunity against murine squamous cell carcinoma. (in eng), *Cancer* 116 (15): (Aug): 3740–3748. https://acsjournals.onlinelibrary.wiley.com/doi/10.1002/cncr.25134

123 Helm, A. et al. (2020). Reduction of lung metastases in a mouse osteosarcoma model treated with carbon ions and immune checkpoint inhibitors. *International Journal of Radiation Oncology, Biology, Physics* In press. 109(2): 594–602. doi: 10.1016/j.ijrobp.2020.09.041. Epub 2020 Sep 24. PMID 32980497

124 Abei, M. et al. (2013). A phase I study on combined therapy with proton-beam radiotherapy and in situ tumor vaccination for locally advanced recurrent hepatocellular carcinoma. *Radiation Oncology (London, England)* 8 (Oct 16): 239. https://ro-journal.biomedcentral.com/articles/10.1186/1748-717X-8-239

125 Brenneman, R.J. et al. (2019). Abscopal effect following proton beam radiotherapy in a patient with inoperable metastatic retroperitoneal sarcoma. (in eng), *Frontiers in Oncology* 9: 922. https://www.frontiersin.org/articles/10.3389/fonc.2019.00922/full

12

The Economics of Particle Therapy

Mark Waddle, MD[1] and Robert Miller, MD, MBA, FASTRO[2]

[1] Department of Radiation Oncology, Mayo Clinic, Rochester MN
[2] Division of Radiation Oncology, UT Medical Center at the University of Tennessee, Knoxville TN

Corresponding Author: Mark Waddle, MD, Department of Radiation Oncology, Mayo Clinic, 200 1st St. SW, Rochester, MN 55905

TABLE OF CONTENTS

12.1 Particle Therapy Growth

12.1.1 Adoption of Proton Therapy in the United States

There has been a nearly exponential increase in the number of proton beam radiation facilities in the United States over the past 20 years, rising from 2 centers and 4 gantries in 2000 to approximately 35 centers and 85 operational gantries in 2020 (Figure 12.1) [1,2]. The proliferation of proton therapy centers has been spurred by the promise of superior dose distribution relative to conventional photon treatments and the hope for reduced toxicity of treatments. Several improvements in key components of treatment delivery such as treatment planning and biologic modeling, dose rates, pencil beam scanning, and reduction in beam spot size have occurred that have refined planning and treatment delivery and facilitated the adoption of proton therapy into the routine practice [3]. Additionally, technology improvements have reduced the construction and operating costs significantly. Multi-gantry facilities are estimated to have construction costs ranging from 100 to 300 million USD while single gantry systems are now available for 25–30 million USD, which has made initiating and sustaining proton therapy programs more attainable [4]. Although challenges remain with proton therapy treatments, such as lower throughput [5] and limited image guidance compared to traditional photon treatments [6], advances continue to be made which offer further promise that proton therapy will be able to deliver on improving the therapeutic ratio of radiation therapy treatment at an acceptable increased cost.

However, despite this promise, the high costs of proton therapy coupled with the lagging clinical evidence demonstrating improvements in clinical outcomes compared to photon radiation for many disease sites have led to concerns about the rapid adoption of this technology [7,8]. Staggering rises in health-care costs in a short period of time have garnered scrutiny from national payers such as the Center for Medicare and Medicaid

Principles and Practice of Particle Therapy, First Edition. Edited by Timothy D. Malouff and Daniel M. Trifiletti.

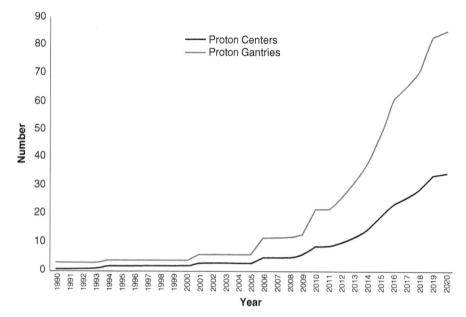

Figure 12.1 Cumulative number of proton centers and gantries in the United States from 1990 to 2020.

Services (CMS) as well as private insurers [9]. Increasing focus on proton facilities by private investors and reduced reimbursement has led to geographic competition among proton therapy facilities and resulted in increased marketing and a reliance on treatment of common cancers, such as prostate cancer, to remain financially solvent. As such, the rise of proton facilities has been compared to other economic "bubbles" [10]. Several proton facilities have faced bankruptcy and required restructuring to remain afloat [11,12]. More recently, the Center for Medicare and Medicaid Innovation (CMMI) has released a mandatory Radiation Oncology Alternative Payment Model (RO-APM) that will result in fixed payments by disease site regardless of treatment modality for those included in the model [13]. This has been estimated to result in 48–71% reductions in reimbursement in an industry already wrought with financial challenges [14].

Despite financial headwinds, proton therapy remains a pinnacle of innovation in radiation therapy. Increasing clinical experience and promising clinical trials have shown that proton therapy represents a valuable treatment option for certain subgroups of patients [15–18]. The key to a sustainable healthcare system moving forward will be identifying and describing these subgroups and ensuring the responsible use and distribution of existing and new proton facilities.

12.1.2 Adoption of Proton Therapy outside of the United States

The adoption of proton beam therapy outside of the United States has taken a slower and more predictable path, likely due to differences in health-care policy and different financial practices and incentives in countries outside the United States, as seen in Table 12.1. Geographic and population distributions likely also contribute to the differences seen in the number and distribution of proton beam facilities, allowing for fewer facilities in certain countries. Several countries, such as Canada, the United Kingdom, and Australia, initially chose to reimburse travel and treatment of select patients at well-regarded proton therapy facilities rather than initiate proton therapy programs in their countries. Other countries, such as the Netherlands, introduced unique systems to choose which patients would have access to a limited supply of proton therapy treatment facilities based on dosimetric advantages seen at the time of radiation planning. Other countries, such as Japan, have fully embraced the promise of particle therapy and now support 24 facilities, the only country in the world rivaling in number the 35 proton therapy facilities present in the United States.

12.2 Finances of Proton Therapy in United States

12.2.1 Capital Requirements and Financing of Proton Therapy

Initial capital costs of proton therapy, as with many new technologies, were staggering. Development costs, the need for testing and validation, and lack of efficient supply chains, among other challenges, all contribute to the financial disadvantages of technology innovations, and proton therapy was

Table 12.1 Number of proton therapy centers per country and the year of first clinically operating facility.

Country	Year first adopted	Number of centers
Austria	2016	2
Belgium	2019	1
China	2004	4
Czech Republic	2012	1
Denmark	2019	1
England*	2018	4
France*	2014	3
Germany	1998	6
India	2019	1
Italy	2002	4
Japan	1998	24
Poland	2011	1
Russia	1999	5
South Korea	2007	2
Spain	2020	2
Sweden	2015	1
Switzerland	1984	1
Taiwan	2015	2
Netherlands	2018	3
United States	1990	35
Total		103

* Excluding fixed beam nonclinical rooms. Based on Particle Therapy Co-Operative Group (PTCOG).

no exception [19]. Construction costs of some of the first multiple gantry systems had costs ranging from $140 to $235 million, which arguably represents the most expensive medical device of all time. Current costs of large proton centers remain high, largely related to the large geographic footprints, massive volumes of shielding, expensive technical equipment such as cyclotrons or synchrotrons, and multi-story gantries to precisely bend the proton beam. The raw numbers for construction of multi-gantry facilities are simply staggering: $200 million, 80,000 square feet, 220-t cyclotrons, 8–12-ft thick concrete shielding, and 30-ft tall gantries. For this reason, these facilities have been pursued only by the largest nonprofit medical centers often with the support of generous benefactors. When compared to the smaller footprint and lower technology costs of photon radiation, which can often be accomplished for costs approaching $5–20 million for facilities capable of treating a similar volume of patients, it is clear that large-scale proton therapy facilities are only feasible for the largest and most profitable medical centers.

More recently, standalone single gantry proton systems have become available at significantly lower costs. In stark contrast to multi-gantry facilities, a single-vault Mevion facil-

ity in Jacksonville, Florida was constructed in an existing radiation facility for only $5 million dollars in infrastructure costs in 2013, bringing the total facility costs to $30 million dollars [20]. This has allowed for investment in this technology by medical centers that were otherwise prohibited by high initial costs. In additional to traditional financing available, private equity has taken note of the possible financial returns available by investing in these facilities. As an example, Proton International is one such investment group backing a total of six proton facilities at the time of writing, three in the United States and three in Europe [21].

Construction costs are only one facet of the financial demands of running a successful proton therapy facility. Operating costs of proton therapy are similarly much larger than those of photon radiation. With a larger facility size comes increased energy requirements and higher fixed operating costs. First year utility costs alone are estimated to be $60,000–$200,000 for smaller facilities and a report by the ECRI Institute found annual electricity costs for a multi-gantry facility to total $1 million dollars per year [4,22]. Similarly, more staff are required to run and maintain proton therapy equipment and specially trained staff, including radiation therapists, physicists, and radiation oncologists, are necessary to ensure appropriate treatment. Finally, due to the complexity of the equipment and long treatment hours, proton therapy demands on-site engineering support typically covered under vendor service contracts in the millions of dollars each year.

High start-up and operating costs have thus required robust financial plans to remain solvent and often demand treatment schedules at full capacity to remain financially viable. Some centers have relied on business plans emulating that of Loma Linda, focused on the least complex and highest throughput cases such as prostate cancer. Other centers have only remained operational through creative financing or by restructuring debts at cents on the dollar.

12.2.2 Insurance Coverage

Proton therapy was first used to treat patient in 1954 and was later approved for treatment in the United States by the United States Food and Drug Administration (FDA) in 1988. For much of the history of proton therapy, reimbursement by national and local payers has been non-uniform and it was unclear which cancer types and indications would be covered. This is largely due to the fact that, despite the longstanding use of proton therapy, Medicare currently does not have a National Coverage Determination (NCD). When NCDs do not exist, Medicare Administrative Contractors (MACs) are tasked with creating local coverage determinations (LCDs) to guide reimbursement for medical procedures by geographic region. MACs work as an intermediary between patients and hospital systems and CMS to facilitate reimbursement for fee-for-service payments. The first Medicare LCDs specific to proton therapy went into effect in 2009 [23,24].

In 2009, in response to local coverage decisions, ASTRO released a Proton Beam Model Policy to help guide insurance coverage and acceptable use of proton therapy. This initial document identified ocular cancer, spinal cord, base of skull, liver, and pediatric patients as medically necessary cases for proton therapy. In 2014, ASTRO updated the published groups deemed medically necessary for proton beam therapy to also include CNS tumors, advanced and/or unresectable head-and-neck cancers, cancers of the paranasal sinuses or accessory sinuses, nonmetastatic retroperitoneal sarcomas, and re-irradiation cases. In 2017, this document now includes hepatocellular carcinoma. ASTRO also clearly indicated the need for improved clinical evidence of proton therapy to guide future coverage decisions and as such suggested that other indications should also be covered under "Coverage with evidence development." Under this system it was suggested that patient enrolled on IRB-approved clinical trials or multi-institutional patient registries meeting Medicare's requirements should also be provided insurance coverage to allow the generation of clinical data to understand the benefits of proton therapy.

Despite local coverage decisions and national specialty guidance, insurance approval, coverage, and reimbursement in the United States remain opaque, burdensome, and frustrating for patients and health-care systems. Although there is the potential for downstream savings with reduced toxicity and improved quality of life, higher initial costs have resulted in intense scrutiny of proton therapy. Because proton radiation offers dosimetric advantages based on the specific location of a tumor relative to organs at risk, it is often an individualized process to identify which patients are most suitable for proton therapy. Insurance companies are not typically designed to apply coverage on a case-by-case basis such as this. As a result, insurance companies will typically send initial denials for all patients of certain cancer types and require an appeal to then initiate an individualized review of the case, followed by a peer-to-peer discussion between the treating physician and insurance representative and the development of photon and proton therapy plans for comparison, and finally a decision.

For private insurance, this has proven particularly impactful on patient care; a study published in 2018 found that 70% of initial head and neck or thoracic cancer proton therapy requests were denied coverage [25]. The subsequent appeal process requires additional staffing, time, and practice resources that are not reimbursed. The denial and appeal process appears to result in delays in treatment – an average delay of 21 days and up to 4 months – which can lead to patient anxiety and the risk of suboptimal cancer outcomes [25,26]. Other studies have found that insurance denials are not logically based on cancer type or ASTRO proton beam model policy guidance, but only based on insurance category [26]. As a result, the prior-authorization process described above has faced intense criticism across specialties as a resource-intensive and time-consuming burden that adversely impacts patient care.

Some centers have collaborated directly with payers on proton therapy coverage pilots and results have been encouraging. One group worked with insurance providers to ensure coverage for a predefined cohort of approximately 200,000 plan enrollees based on evidence supported anatomical sites and clinical trial enrollment. Although the initial modeling predicted increased costs for these patients, no increased costs were identified at three years of follow-up [27]. These findings suggest that appropriate access to proton therapy does not result in overutilization and increased costs, and current efforts are underway by specialty and advocacy groups, as well as CMS to improve the prior-authorization process [28].

In 2018, CMS publicly criticized proton therapy as low-value care due to a rapid proliferation of centers, a 244% increase in spending from 2010 to 2016, and a shift from use primarily for rare adult cancers and pediatric malignancies to more common cancers without high-level evidence of benefit such as prostate cancer [9]. CMS has since targeted radiation oncology for a mandatory RO-APM that would include 40% of Medicare patients and would provide a fixed reimbursement for radiation services regardless of modality [29]. Despite the urging of the radiation oncology community to exclude proton therapy from the RO-APM, CMS confirmed that they believe it is appropriate to include this modality in the model due to the "continued debate around the benefits of proton therapy." Although this program has faced delays and now will be implemented starting in 2022, studies have estimated a staggering reduction in reimbursement for proton therapy of 48–71% for the cancer types included in the model [14]. The result of this model remains to be seen, but changes in reimbursement such as this will likely slow the adoption of proton therapy and threaten the financial stability of existing centers.

12.2.3 Randomized Clinical Trials of Proton Therapy

The United States is undergoing a shift from fee-for-service payments to one of value-based care. Under such a system, it is critical for health-care systems to define the value of any new treatment device or paradigm. Given the high costs and rapid adoption of proton therapy, it is increasingly necessary to show that there are improved cancer outcomes or reduced toxicities that justify the increased costs and to ensure a sustainable health-care system. However, since proton therapy is a substantially equivalent 510(k) FDA-approved medical device, no clinical efficacy superiority trials were necessary prior to introducing this technology into the treatment of patients with cancer. As such, no foundation of clinical evidence existed to compare proton therapy to photon radiation. This is in stark contrast to FDA-approved medications that undergo rigorous clinical evaluations to ensure a measurable benefit over existing medications, trials that are usually funded nearly exclusively by the drug manufacturers.

Clinical trials require massive resource investments and results are not available until years after initiation. Some have argued that randomized clinical trials in proton therapy do not have clinical equipoise and that those resources could be used for other more important clinical questions [30]. These opponents argue that proton therapy has repeatedly been verified to have superior dose distributions when compared with photon radiation treatments and that this evidence is enough. However, the medical community is largely in agreement that randomized evidence is necessary and several clinical trials have been completed with many more currently in progress [31].

Despite widespread agreement that randomized clinical trials are necessary, a review of 219 clinical studies published as of July 2018 found that only 89 studies were prospective, 5 were randomized phase II, and only 3 were randomized phase III [32]. Of the randomized phase III studies, only one was published after 2006 with modern proton therapy equipment

and planning, although this used passive scatter techniques [33]. This study randomized IMRT versus proton therapy in advanced non-small cell lung cancer and failed to find a difference in radiation pneumonitis rates [33]. Since this time, one additional randomized phase IIB study has been published in 2020 which found reduced total toxicity burden of proton therapy as compared with IMRT in locally advanced esophageal cancer, although the symptom burden instrument used in this study is somewhat controversial [15]. It is encouraging that the National Cancer Institute (NCI) and the Patient-Centered Outcomes Research Institute (PCORI) have made large investments into seven randomized clinical trials of proton therapy in breast, lung, prostate, glioblastoma, esophageal, low-grade glioma, and liver cancers.

Other prospective studies have shown certain subgroups of patients which benefit from proton therapy, which is largely reflected in the ASTRO Proton Beam Therapy Model Policy [34]. It is largely agreed that the superior dose distribution and meaningful risks of long-term secondary cancer risks and other long-term effects, such as intellectual abilities and cognitive skills, justify the use of proton therapy in pediatric patients [35]. Choroid melanoma is another site with several studies to justify its use [36,37]. Skull-base lesions and cancers of the paranasal sinus and nasal cavity have been shown to benefit from proton therapy due to close proximity to critical organs such as the brainstem, and in some cases, studies have identified improved disease-free survival and local control [17]. Numerous other studies show benefits of proton therapy in other disease sites as well [38]. However, the gold standard remains randomized controlled trials, and although these studies are in progress, the results will not be available for many years to come.

12.2.4 Cost-Effectiveness of Proton Therapy

Due to lack of randomized controlled trials in proton therapy, it becomes difficult to define the incremental cost-effectiveness of proton therapy versus photon radiation. However, using single arm prospective studies or systematic reviews of retrospective studies, it becomes possible to model these different treatment modalities using a number of assumptions and sensitivity analyses. Although this is considered low quality data, it is a starting point to determine the cost-effectiveness of proton therapy. Studies have identified proton therapy to be cost-effective in certain scenarios for disease sites including pediatric brain tumors, ocular tumors, skull-base tumors, sinonasal cancers, head and neck cancers, esophageal cancer, advanced NSCLC, brain tumors, and breast cancer. Alternatively, studies have largely failed to find cost-effectiveness for prostate cancer. Ultimately, each individual case must be carefully considered for the relative merits of proton therapy in the context of increased costs, and it becomes the physician's responsibility to judiciously use this resource for those who will benefit the most relative to alternative radiation modalities.

In pediatric patients, proton therapy has a substantial chance of reducing long-term side effects due to the sensitivity of the developing body and mind to radiation. As a result of typically high success rates of treatment, high risks of secondary malignancy, and a lifelong reduction in costs associated with managing chronic conditions, proton therapy has been repeatedly found to be cost-effective for children. For medulloblastoma, Markov simulations identified an estimated $23,600 in cost savings and 0.68 quality-adjusted life-years (QALY) gained per patient [39]. Similar findings have been found by other groups using alternative methodologies and different cancer types [40–42]. As a result, proton therapy is the standard radiation modality for all but the most aggressive pediatric malignancies when available.

Several other rare cancers are commonly treated with proton therapy such as ocular, skull base, sinonasal, nasopharyngeal, and hepatocellular cancers due to the ability to dose escalate and/or spare vital organs at risk that have resulted in favorable non-randomized studies using proton therapy. Cost-effectiveness studies have been performed in skull-base tumors [43,44], sinonasal cancer [45], hepatocellular cancers [46], and choroid melanomas [47] and have nearly universally confirmed the cost-effectiveness in these disease sites. As a result, these cancers are routinely treated with proton therapy when available.

Other more common cancers have had mixed results in cost-effectiveness studies, largely related to variation in patient-specific information. For breast cancer, proton therapy has primarily been shown to be cost-effective in young women, those with the most cardiac risk factors, or when a willingness-to-pay threshold of $100,000/QALY was used [48–50]. Other studies have shown proton therapy to be cost effective only with significant differences in dose to organs at risk [50]. Some researches have suggested that proton therapy is cost-effective when one or most cardiac risk factors exist or when the mean heart dose is unable to be kept below 5 Gy [51]. For oropharyngeal cancer, proton therapy was shown to be cost-effective in young patients with the most significant reduction in long-term xerostomia and avoidance of gastrostomy use [52] and found in another study to have a general incremental cost-effectiveness versus IMRT of approximately €60,279 [53]. For advanced lung cancers, one study concluded that proton therapy was "borderline" cost-effective with an incremental cost benefit of $35,309 versus IMRT [54] and another found that proton therapy was only cost-effective for those at the highest risk of toxicity [55]. For esophageal cancer, a study from 2016 found proton therapy to be cost-effectiveness with an ICER of $84,000 per QALY gained.

In contrast, there are certain patient populations that proton therapy generally does not appear to be cost-effective. Although clinical data continue to be acquired, to date there is limited evidence of superior clinical outcomes in prostate cancer. As a result, it appears that conventionally fractionated proton therapy is suboptimally cost-effective for the treatment of prostate cancer, as documented in two older studies [39,56]. Another study published in 2012, which compared IMRT, SBRT, and proton therapy, found SBRT to be the most cost-effective, while proton therapy had a <5% probability of being cost-effective [57]. Despite these findings, significant changes have occurred in the delivery and reimbursement of proton therapy, and contemporary studies comparing photon with proton radiation are in progress. Further, no studies have been completed that have evaluated the cost-effectiveness of proton therapy-based SBRT for prostate cancer. These studies will ultimately aid in concluding if proton therapy is cost-effective for prostate cancer in the modern era.

12.3 Evolving Particle Therapy Treatments

Several other heavy particles have been studied for the treatment of cancer, primarily neutron and carbon ion therapy, and interest in these treatment modalities has increased recently due to technologic advancements. Proton therapy only represents one type of particle therapy, but many of the economic principles of proton therapy apply to other particle therapy treatments. High infrastructure and personnel costs, limited clinical evidence, and uncertain cost–benefit ratios are three important challenges that have limited or need to be overcome for the clinical use of heavy ion treatments.

12.3.1 Neutron Therapy

Fast neutron therapy was first introduced into clinical practice in the late 1930s but was quickly abandoned due to concerns of toxicity [58]. Interest was renewed in the 1960s at Hammersmith Hospital in London, where neutron therapy was again introduced into clinical practice for the treatment of head and neck cancers. Although initial reports showed promising cancer control, results were limited by high rates of severe side effects in early trials [58–60]. Currently, clinically active neutron therapy programs exist in the United States, Russia, Germany, and South Africa [61]. In the United States, a single clinical neutron therapy facility remains at the University of Washington in Seattle, WA. This facility was one of four original neuron therapy centers in the United States funded by a NCI grant and is the only remaining of such facilities. This facility was built for $3 million and the equipment carried a cost of $4 million dollars in 1979 when built (inflation adjusted to $25.9 million in 2021 dollars), and the first patient was treated in 1984. The center has treated over 3000 patients, including 311 in the past 5 years, which have been primarily salivary gland cancers [62]. Other US centers, including those at Fermi National Accelerator Laboratory and Karmanos Cancer Center at Wayne State University, have since decommissioned their clinical practices. Fast neutron therapy will likely remain limited in clinical practice due to the clinical results to-date, high start-up and operating costs, and certain physical properties such as the lack of a Bragg peak. At this time, boron-neutron capture therapy is now being explored to improve the therapeutic ratio of neutron therapy [63].

12.3.2 Carbon Therapy

Carbon ion therapy is another heavy ion which is used in clinical practice and has several unique physical properties including a Bragg peak, high linear energy transfer, and a steep lateral penumbra. This treatment was first introduced clinically in Japan in 1994 at the National Institute of Radiologic Sciences (NIRS) where over 20,000 patients have since been treated [64]. This technology was later adopted in Europe in 2009 at Heidelberg Ion Therapy Center (HIT) [65]. At this time there are currently 12 operational facilities in the world with the majority of centers in Japan (Figure 12.2). Plans now are in place for the first carbon ion therapy facility in North America to be constructed at Mayo Clinic's campus in Jacksonville, FL.

Similar to proton therapy, carbon ion facilities have high construction costs due to the necessary infrastructure, shielding, and accelerators. In addition to increased shielding compared with proton therapy centers, carbon ion gantries must be significantly larger and more costly due to the higher mass of a carbon ion. As a result, most centers in existence treat with a fixed beam and only two centers offer treatment with rotating gantries. It is estimated that a carbon ion facility will cost greater than $200 million and carry costs approximately two to three times those of a similarly sized proton therapy center [66–68].

Although evidence is starting to be collected and reported, there are limited comparative effectiveness studies in carbon ion therapy [64]. As a result, it is difficult to fully define an incremental cost–benefit of carbon ion therapy versus other radiation treatments or surgery. However, despite these limitations, there are a number studies that have suggested a cost-effectiveness of carbon ion therapy for the treatment of skull-base chordomas [69,70], adenoid cystic cancer [71], and locally recurrent rectal cancer [72].

In the United States, there is currently no FDA clearance for carbon ion treatment and no suggested reimbursement, which makes any investment in this technology challenging. FDA clearance will likely follow a similar path to that of proton therapy, with approval as a substantially equivalent 510(k) FDA-approved medical device. Insurance coverage and reimbursement of this technology in the United States have yet to be seen, but this will undoubtedly also follow a similar path as proton therapy ultimately leading to LCDs. This technology will be exempt from alternative payment models until Current Procedural Terminology (CPT) codes are assigned to carbon ion therapy, which will occur 5–10 years after the first patient is treated at the earliest, if at all. In Japan, reimbursement for carbon ion therapy and proton therapy has been established and is covered by national insurance for pediatric cancers, sarcoma, head and neck cancer (excluding oral cavity, larynx, and pharynx), prostate cancer, and ocular melanoma [73]. Reimbursement is a bundled payment, separate from tradi-

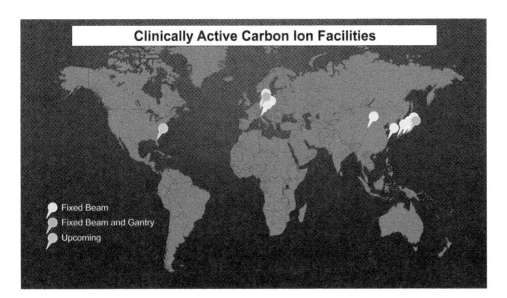

Figure 12.2   Currently active or upcoming clinical carbon ion treatment facilities.

tional fee-for-service payments of photon radiation, and is approximately 2.4 million JPY ($22,923) for sarcoma and head and neck and 1.6 million JPY ($15,282) for prostate cancer [74].

12.4 Closing Thoughts

The clinical use of particle therapy represents one of the most advanced and technologically demanding medical treatments of our time. As a result, extraordinary resources are necessary to initiate and maintain a viable proton therapy or carbon ion treatment center. There are clear indications for the use of this technology and numerous studies to confirm the cost-effectiveness in these cases. However, not all cancers will benefit from this technology, and in the era of value-based medicine in the United States, the path forward for this technology is uncertain. It is increasingly critical to show both clinical benefit as well as incremental cost-effectiveness for these forms of radiation treatment.

Currently, radiation oncology services represent only 1.4% of total Medicare charges and 1.15 billion inflation-adjusted dollars, which can be compared with the estimated 11.6 billion spent in 2014 alone on anticancer medications per Medicare Part-B spending [75,76]. Although national spending on radia-tion therapy, including particle therapy, is dwarfed by other components of oncology care such as systemic therapies, particle therapy has been targeted for reductions in reimbursement [9]. This may in part be due to certain groups across the country that have been incentivized to recoup their investment in this technology quickly by putting through a large volume of patients, especially with prostate cancer, rather than using the technology for those most likely to benefit, such as children [77]. A complex ethical dilemma appears to have emerged that appears to represent two models of proton care; according to Dr. Robert Foote at Mayo Clinic, "one to make money – the other to provide the best care possible for the people who need it" [77].

Therefore, the success of capital-intensive medical treatments such as particle therapy depends on judicious use, clearly defined benefit in clinical trials and cost-effectiveness studies, and a collaboration between patients, radiation oncologists, professional societies, national policy makers, and payers. It is certain that particle therapy has a meaningful role in the treatment – and cure – of cancer. It remains up to all shareholders to approach the development and use of these facilities in an equitable way so that we can maximize the availability and benefit to the patients that need this treatment the most.

References

1 Waddle, M.R., Sio, T.T., Van Houten, H.K. et al. (2017). Photon and proton radiation therapy utilization in a population of more than 100 Million commercially insured patients. *International Journal of Radiation Oncology, Biology, Physics* (In Eng.) 10.1016/j.ijrobp.2017.07.042.

2 PTCOG. (2017). Particle therapy facilities in operation.

3 Mohan, R. and Grosshans, D. (2017). Proton therapy - Present and future. *Advanced Drug Delivery Reviews* 109: 26–44. (In Eng.). 10.1016/j.addr.2016.11.006.

4 Kim, J., Wells, C., Khangura, S., et al. (2017). Proton beam therapy for the treatment of cancer in children and adults: A health technology assessment.

5 Aitkenhead, A.H., Bugg, D., Rowbottom, C.G., Smith, E., and Mackay, R.I. (2012). Modelling the throughput capacity of a single-accelerator multitreatment room proton therapy centre. *The British Journal of Radiology* 85 (1020): e1263–72. (In Eng.). 10.1259/bjr/27428078.

6 Herrmann, H., Seppenwoolde, Y., Georg, D., and Widder, J. (2019). Image guidance: Past and future of radiotherapy. *Radiologe* 59 (Suppl1): 21–27. (In Eng.). 10.1007/s00117-019-0573-y.

7 Hancock, J. (2018). *For Cancer Centers, Proton Therapy's Promise Is Undercut by Lagging Demand.*

8 Zietman, A.L. (2019). Can proton therapy be considered a standard of care in oncology? Lessons from the United States. *British Journal of Cancer* 120 (8): 775–776. (In Eng.). 10.1038/s41416-018-0324-2.

9 Winter, A., Ray, N., and Zarabozo, C. (2018). Medicare coverage policy and use of Low-value care. March 22, 2021 MedPACS. (http://www.medpac.gov/docs/default-source/default-document-library/medicare-coverage-and-use-of-low-value-care_public.pdf?sfvrsn=0)

10 Johnstone, P.A.S. and Kerstiens, J. (2016). Reconciling reimbursement for Proton therapy. *International Journal of Radiation Oncology, Biology, Physics* 95 (1): 9–10. (In Eng.). 10.1016/j.ijrobp.2015.09.037.

11 Lee, J. (2014). As a proton therapy center closes, some see it as a sign. Modern Healthcare.

12 Brickley, P. (2020).Proton therapy centers in Tennessee and Florida file for bankruptcy. *Wall Street Journal.*

13 (2017). (ASTRO) ASfRO. Radiation Oncology Alternative Payment Model (RO-APM).

14 Meeks, S.L., Shah, A.P., Sood, G., et al. (2020). Effect of proposed episode-based payment models on advanced radiotherapy procedures. https://doiorg/101200/OP2000495 (research-article) (In EN). DOI: 10.1200/OP.20.00495.

15 Lin, S.H., Hobbs, B.P., Verma, V. et al. (2020). Randomized phase IIB trial of proton beam therapy versus intensity-modulated radiation therapy for locally advanced esophageal cancer. *Journal of Clinical Oncology: Official Journal of the American Society of Clinical Oncology* 38: 14. 10.1200/JCO.19.02503.

16 Chung, C.S., Yock, T.I., Nelson, K., Xu, Y., Keating, N.L., and Tarbell, N.J. (2013). Incidence of second malignancies among patients treated with proton versus photon radiation. *International Journal of Radiation Oncology, Biology, Physics* 87 (1): 46–52. (In Eng.). 10.1016/j.ijrobp.2013.04.030.

17 Patel, S.H., Wang, Z., Wong, W.W. et al. (2014). Charged particle therapy versus photon therapy for paranasal sinus and nasal cavity malignant diseases: A systematic review and meta-analysis. *The Lancet Oncology* 15 (9): 1027–1038. (In Eng.). 10.1016/S1470-2045(14)70268-2.

18 Shih, H.A., Sherman, J.C., Nachtigall, L.B. et al. (2015). Proton therapy for low-grade gliomas: Results from a prospective trial. *Cancer* 121 (10): 1712–1719. (In Eng.). 10.1002/cncr.29237.

19 Rosenberg, Ka. (1986). *The Positive Sum Strategy: Harnessing Technology for Economic Growth, National Academy Press.* Washington, DC: National Academy Press. 275–304. https://doi.org/10.17226/612.

20 Ackerman, S. (2015). *Building the World's First Private, Physician-Owned Proton Therapy Center.* Scot Ackerman, MD: Applied Radiation Oncology.

21 Proton international. (https://protonintl.com/facilities/) accessed March 22, 2021.

22 (2017). Proton beam radiation therapy systems for cancer Accessed March 22, 2021. https://www.ecri.org/search-results/member-preview/forecast/pages/14187.

23 (2009). Local coverage determination for proton beam therapy. LCD Database ID Number L30314: Highmark Medicare services.

24 (2009). Local coverage determination for proton beam radiotherapy. LCD Database ID Number L29263.: First coast service options, Inc.

25 Ning, M.S., Gomez, D.R., Shah, A.K. et al. (2019). The insurance approval process for proton radiation therapy: A significant barrier to patient care. *International Journal of Radiation Oncology, Biology, Physics* 104 (4): 10.1016/j.ijrobp.2018.12.019.

26 Gupta, A., Khan, A.J., Goyal, S. et al. (2019). Insurance approval for proton beam therapy and its impact on delays in treatment. *International Journal of Radiation Oncology, Biology, Physics* 104 (4): 714–723. (In Eng.). 10.1016/j.ijrobp.2018.12.021.

27 Ning, MS., Palmer, M.B., Shah, A.K. et al. (2020). Three-year results of a prospective statewide insurance coverage pilot for proton therapy: Stakeholder collaboration improves patient access to care. *JCO Oncology Practice* 16 (9): 10.1200/JOP.19.00437.

28 (2021). Medicaid program; Patient protection and affordable care act; reducing provider and patient burden by improving prior authorization processes, and promoting patients' electronic access to health information for Medicaid managed care plans, state Medicaid agencies, chip agencies and chip managed care entities, and issuers of qualified health plans on the federally-facilitated exchanges; health information technology standards and implementation specifications. In: SERVICES DOHAH, ed. Centers for Medicare & Medicaid Services.

29 (2020). Medicare program; Specialty care models to improve quality of care and reduce expenditures. In: (CMS) CfMMS, ed. Federal Register: Centers for Medicare & Medicaid Services (CMS), HHS.

30 Goitein, M. and Cox, J.D. (2016). Should randomized clinical trials be required for proton radiotherapy? https://doiorg/101200/JCO2007144329 (other) (In Eng.). DOI: 10.1200/JCO.2007.14.4329.

31 Glatstein, E., Glick, J., Kaiser, L., and Hahn, S.M. (2016). Should randomized clinical trials be required for proton radiotherapy? An alternative view. https://doiorg/101200/JCO2008171843 (other) (In Eng.). DOI:10.1200/JCO.2008.17.1843.

32 Ofuya, M., McParland, L., Murray, L., Brown, S., Sebag-Montefiore, D., and Hall, E. (2019). Systematic review of methodology used in clinical studies evaluating the benefits of proton beam therapy. *Clinical and Translational Radiation Oncology* 19: 17–26. (In Eng.). 10.1016/j.ctro.2019.07.002.

33 Liao, Z., Lee, J.J., Komaki, R., et al. (2018). Bayesian adaptive randomization trial of passive scattering proton therapy and intensity-modulated photon radiotherapy for locally advanced non–small-cell lung cancer. March 22, 2021 https://doiorg/101200/JCO2017740720 (research-article) (In Eng.). DOI: 10.1200/JCO.2017.74.0720.

34 (2017). ASTRO Model Policy: Proton Beam Therapy. ASTRO.com: American Society of Radiation Oncology (ASTRO). https://www.astro.org/uploadedFiles/_MAIN_SITE/Daily_Practice/Reimbursement/Model_Policies/Content_Pieces/ASTROPBTModelPolicy.pdf

35 Sands, S.A. (2016). Proton beam radiation therapy: The future may prove brighter for pediatric patients with brain tumors. *Journal of Clinical Oncology: Official Journal of the American Society of Clinical Oncology* 34 (10): 1024–1026. (In Eng.). 10.1200/JCO.2015.65.4350.

36 Lane, A.M., Kim, I.K., and Gragoudas, E.S. et al. (2015). Long-term risk of melanoma-related mortality for patients with Uveal Melanoma treated with proton beam therapy. *JAMA Ophthalmology* 133 (7): 10.1001/jamaophthalmol.2015.0887.

37 Verma, V., and Mehta, M.P. (2016). Clinical outcomes of proton radiotherapy for Uveal Melanoma. *Clinical Oncology (Royal College of Radiologists (Great Britain))* 28 (8): 10.1016/j.clon.2016.01.034.

38 Hu, M., Jiang, L., Cui, X., Zhang, J., and Yu, J. (2018). Proton beam therapy for cancer in the era of precision medicine. *Journal of Hematology & Oncology* 11 (1): 136. (In Eng.). 10.1186/s13045-018-0683-4.

39 Lundkvist, J., Ekman, M., Ericsson, S.R., Jönsson, B., Glimelius, B. (2005). Cost-effectiveness of proton radiation in

the treatment of childhood medulloblastoma. *Cancer*103 (4): 10.1002/cncr.20844.

40 Mailhot Vega, R.B., Kim, J., Bussière, M., Hattangadi, J. et al. (2013). Cost effectiveness of proton therapy compared with photon therapy in the management of pediatric medulloblastoma. *Cancer*119: 24. 10.1002/cncr.28322.

41 Hirano, E., Fuji, H., Onoe, T., Kumar, V. et al. (2014). Cost-effectiveness analysis of cochlear dose reduction by proton beam therapy for medulloblastoma in childhood. *Journal of Radiation Research*55 (2): 10.1093/jrr/rrt112.

42 Mailhot Vega, R., Kim, J., Hollander, A. et al. (2015). Cost effectiveness of proton versus photon radiation therapy with respect to the risk of growth hormone deficiency in children. *Cancer*121 (10): 10.1002/cncr.29209.

43 Austin, A.M., Douglass, M.J.J., Nguyen, G.T. et al. (2019). Cost-effectiveness of proton therapy in treating base of skull chordoma. *Australasian Physical & Engineering Sciences in Medicine*42 (4): 10.1007/s13246-019-00810-0.

44 Peeters, A., Grutters, J.P., Pijls-Johannesma, M. et al. (2010). How costly is particle therapy? Cost analysis of external beam radiotherapy with carbon-ions, protons and photons. *Radiotherapy and Oncology: Journal of the European Society for Therapeutic Radiology and Oncology*95 (1): 10.1016/j.radonc.2009.12.002.

45 Li, G., Qiu, B., Huang, Y.X. et al. (2020). Cost-effectiveness analysis of proton beam therapy for treatment decision making in paranasal sinus and nasal cavity cancers in China. *BMC Cancer* 20 (1): 599. (In Eng.). 10.1186/s12885-020-07083-x.

46 Leung, H.W.C. and Chan, A.L.F. (2017). Cost-utility of stereotactic radiation therapy. *Oncotarget* 8 (43): 75568–75576. (In Eng.). 10.18632/oncotarget.17369.

47 Moriarty, J.P., Borah, B.J., Foote, R. L. (2015). Cost-effectiveness of proton beam therapy for intraocular melanoma. *PloS One*10 (5): 10.1371/journal.pone.0127814.

48 Vega, R.M.NYU School of Medicine NY, NY, Formenti SC, NYU School of Medicine NY, NY, MacDonald S, Massachusetts General Hospital B, MA. (2015). Cost-effective analysis of proton therapy for breast irradiation. *International Journal of Radiation Oncology, Biology, Physics* 93 (3): (In English). 10.1016/j.ijrobp.2015.07.218.

49 Xie, Y., Guo, B., Zhang, R. (2020). Cost-effectiveness analysis of advanced radiotherapy techniques for post-mastectomy breast cancer patients. *Cost Effectiveness and Resource Allocation: C/E*18: 10.1186/s12962-020-00222-y.

50 Austin, A.M., Douglass, M.J.J., Nguyen, G.T. et al. (2020). Individualised selection of left-sided breast cancer patients for proton therapy based on cost-effectiveness. *Journal of Medical Radiation Sciences*10.1002/jmrs.416.

51 Mailhot Vega, R.B., Ishaq, O., Raldow, A. et al. (2016). Establishing Cost-effective allocation of proton therapy for breast irradiation. *International Journal of Radiation Oncology, Biology, Physics*95 (1): 10.1016/j.ijrobp.2016.02.031.

52 Sher, D.J., Tishler, R.B., Pham, N.L., Punglia, R.S. (2018). Cost-effectiveness analysis of intensity modulated radiation therapy versus proton therapy for oropharyngeal squamous cell carcinoma. *International Journal of Radiation Oncology, Biology, Physics*101 (4): 10.1016/j.ijrobp.2018.04.018.

53 Ramaekers, B.L., Grutters, J.P., Pijls-Johannesma, M. (2013). Protons in head-and-neck cancer: Bridging the gap of evidence. *International Journal of Radiation Oncology, Biology, Physics*85 (5): 10.1016/j.ijrobp.2012.11.006.

54 Lievens, Y., Verhaeghe, N., DeNeve, W. et al. Proton radiotherapy for locally-advanced non-small cell lung cancer, a cost-effective alternative to photon radiotherapy in Belgium? ISSN: 1556-0864 2013 (info:eu-repo/semantics/publishedVersion) (In Eng.). DOI: http://hdl.handle.net/1854/LU-5777188.

55 Smith, W.P., Richard, P.J., Zeng, J., Apisarnthanarax, S., Rengan, R., and Phillips, M.H. (2018). Decision analytic modeling for the economic analysis of proton radiotherapy for non-small cell lung cancer. *Translational Lung Cancer Research* 7 (2): 122–133. (In Eng.). March 22, 2021 10.21037/tlcr.2018.03.27.

56 Konski, A., Speier, W., Hanlon, A., Beck, J.R., Pollack, A. (2007). Is proton beam therapy cost effective in the treatment of adenocarcinoma of the prostate?*Journal of Clinical Oncology: Official Journal of the American Society of Clinical Oncology*25 (24): 10.1200/JCO.2006.09.0811.

57 Parthan, A., Pruttivarasin, N., Davies, D. et al. (2012). Comparative cost-effectiveness of stereotactic body radiation therapy versus intensity-modulated and proton radiation therapy for localized prostate cancer. *Frontiers in Oncology*210.3389/fonc.2012.00081

58 Svensson, H., Landberg, T. (1994). Neutron therapy–the historical background. *Acta Oncologica (Stockholm, Sweden)*33 (3): 10.3109/02841869409098412.

59 Catterall, M., Sutherland, I., and Bewley, D.K. (1975). First results of a randomized clinical trial of fast neutrons compared with X or gamma rays in treatment of advanced tumours of the head and neck. Report to the Medical Research Council. (In Eng.). DOI: 10.1136/bmj.2.5972.653.

60 Spratt, D.E., Salgado, L.R., Riaz, N., Doran, M.G. et al. (2014). Results of photon radiotherapy for unresectable salivary gland tumors: Is neutron radiotherapy's local control superior?*Radiology and Oncology*48 (1): 10.2478/raon-2013-0046.

61 Neutron therapy centers worldwide March 22, 2021 (http://www.neutrontherapy.com/Worldwidecentres.asp).

62 UWMCF Quick Facts. (2020). In: Washington Uo, ed.

63 Malouff., T, Seneviratne, D., Ebner, D., Stross, W., Waddle, M., Trifiletti, D., and Krishnan, S. (2021). Boron neutron capture therapy: A review of clinical applications |. *Frontiers in Oncology*10.3389/fonc.2021.601820.

64 Lazar, A.A., Schulte, R., Faddegon, B., Blakely, E.A., Roach M 3rd. (2018). Clinical trials involving carbon-ion radiation therapy and the path forward. *Cancer*124 (23): 10.1002/cncr.31662.

65 Combs, S.E., Ellerbrock, M., Haberer, T. et al. (2010). Heidelberg Ion Therapy Center (HIT): Initial clinical experience in the first 80 patients. *Acta Oncologica (Stockholm, Sweden)* 49 (7): 10.3109/0284186X.2010.498432.

66 Pompos, A., Durante, M., and Choy, H. (2016). Heavy ions in cancer therapy. *JAMA Oncol* 2 (12): 1539–1540. (In Eng.). 10.1001/jamaoncol.2016.2646.

67 Durante, M., Orecchia, R., and Loeffler, J.S. (2017). Charged-particle therapy in cancer: Clinical uses and future perspectives. *Nature Reviews. Clinical Oncology* 14 (8): 483–495. (In Eng.). 10.1038/nrclinonc.2017.30.

68 Nakagawa, Y., Yoshihara, H., Kageji, T., and Matsuoka, R. (2009). Cost analysis of radiotherapy, carbon ion therapy, proton therapy and BNCT in Japan. *Applied Radiation and Isotopes: Including Data, Instrumentation and Methods for Use in Agriculture, Industry and Medicine* 67 ((7–8Suppl)): S80–3. (In Eng.). 10.1016/j.apradiso.2009.03.055.

69 Sprave, T., Verma, V., Sterzing, F. et al. (2018). Cost-effectiveness of carbon ion radiation therapy for skull base chordoma utilizing long-term (10-year) outcome data. *Anticancer Research* 38 (8): 4853–4858. (In Eng.). 10.21873/anticanres.12797.

70 Jäkel, O., Land, B., Combs, S.E., Schulz-Ertner, D., and Debus, J. (2007). On the cost-effectiveness of Carbon ion radiation therapy for skull base chordoma. *Radiotherapy and Oncology: Journal of the European Society for Therapeutic Radiology and Oncology* 83 (2): 133–138. (In Eng.). 10.1016/j.radonc.2007.03.010.

71 Jensen, A.D. and Debus, J. (2019). Cost-effectiveness analysis (CEA) of IMRT plus C12 boost vs IMRT only in adenoid cystic carcinoma (ACC) of the head and neck. *Radiat Oncology* 14 (1): 194. (In Eng.). 10.1186/s13014-019-1395-9.

72 Mobaraki, A., Ohno, T., Yamada, S., Sakurai, H., and Nakano, T. (2010). Cost-effectiveness of carbon ion radiation therapy for locally recurrent rectal cancer. *Cancer Science* 101 (8): 1834–1839. (In Eng.). 10.1111/j.1349-7006.2010.01604.x.

73 Huh, S.J., Nishimura, T., Park, W., Onishi, H., Ahn, Y.C., and Nakamura, K. (2020). Current status and comparison of national health insurance systems for advanced radiation technologies in Korea and Japan. *Radiation Oncology Journal* 38 (3): 170–175. (In Eng.). 10.3857/roj.2020.00703.

74 (2020). *The medical fee points list: Radiotherapy*. Tokyo, Japan Igakutushinsya Co. Ltd.

75 Mokhtech, M., Laird, J.H., Maroongroge, S. et al. (2021). Drivers of Medicare spending: A 15 year review of radiation oncology charges allowed by the Medicare physician/supplier fee-for-service program compared to other specialties. *International Journal of Radiation Oncology, Biology, Physics* (In Eng.). 10.1016/j.ijrobp.2020.12.051.

76 (2016). Medicare Part B drug and oncology payment issues. Report to the Congress: Medicare and the healthcare delivery system: MedPac.

77 Epstein, K. (2012). Is spending on proton beam therapy for cancer going too far, too fast? *BMJ* 344: e2488. (In Eng.). 10.1136/bmj.e2488.

Section II

Particle Therapy by Clinical Indication

13

Intracranial Tumors

Principles and Practice of Particle Therapy

Raees Tonse MD[1], Pouya Sabouri PhD[1], Minesh P. Mehta MD[1,2], and Rupesh Kotecha MD[1,2]

[1]Department of Radiation Oncology, Miami Cancer Institute, Baptist Health South Florida, Miami, FL
[2]Herbert Wertheim College of Medicine, Florida International University, Miami, FL
Corresponding author: Rupesh Kotecha, MD, Office 1R203, Department of Radiation Oncology, Miami Cancer Institute, Baptist Health South Florida, Miami, FL 33176

13.1   Introduction

Tumors of the central nervous system (CNS) originate from the brain and spinal cord and encompass a broad range of diseases of differing histopathological and molecular characteristics. The existence of the blood–brain barrier (BBB) acts as a distinction in terms of disease progression patterns; consequently, disease spread through hematogenous or lymphatic routes to other parts of the body is uncommon. Tumors in the CNS may spread to nearby or distant parts of the brain and the spinal cord via white-matter pathways such as the corpus callosum or the leptomeninges.

In adults, meningioma, glioblastoma, and astrocytoma are some of the most common primary brain tumors. The most common malignant primary brain tumor is glioblastoma, while the most common benign intracranial tumor is meningioma. CNS tumors have a 5-year survival rate that has remained reasonably stable over the last 10 years, ranging between 23% and 36% [1].

Since brain tumors have a low tendency for distant metastasis, local control is critical to treating these complex tumors. Radiotherapy (RT) remains an important treatment option for improving local control. Treatment paradigms for various CNS tumors are based on tumor grade and molecular profile; resection or RT is typically used for lower grade primary tumors and triple modality (including systemic therapy) approaches for those of higher grades, although even for some lower grade gliomas, chemotherapy has now become standard.

Particle therapies are used in a dose-escalation setting and also for better dose sparing of organs-at-risk (OARs) for optimal dose conformation [2,3]. In this context, proton therapy (PT) can reduce the incidence and severity of photon therapy-related acute and late toxicity, resulting in a significant increase in the therapeutic ratio of RT [4]. In adult and pediatric patients, PT is used for the treatment of both benign and malignant CNS tumors. The majority of studies looking at the clinical outcomes and side effects of intracranial PT are retrospective in nature; however, prospective studies have recently been published and show promising outcomes. Randomized trials are currently underway, with results anticipated soon.

The basic principles, dosimetric studies, preclinical evidence, and early clinical data supporting the use of particle therapy in patients with CNS tumors will be reviewed in this chapter. A detailed review of the clinical evidence to-date will be provided for the most common primary CNS tumors, meningioma and glioblastoma, but other rare malignancies will also be discussed. Of note, the role of particle therapy for base-of-skull tumors and pediatric CNS malignancies is addressed elsewhere in this book. Critical details important for treatment planning with particle therapy will be reviewed. This chapter provides a comprehensive and evidenced-based approach for those new and experienced with particle therapy for CNS malignancies.

13.2 Basic Science Principles

Neural stem cells (NSCs) are specialized glial cells that reside in neurogenic niches and ultimately differentiate into oligodendrocytes and astrocytes [5]. During the early stages of cell differentiation, the interaction between NSCs and the surrounding vasculature is important within the neurogenic niche [6]. To date, the preclinical evidence indicates that brain tumors originate from or are propelled by cells that mimic the neurogenic niche [7]. Malignant niches with micro-architectural features and signaling properties similar to those found in nonmalignant neurogenic niches have been found to contain stem-like cells [8]. NSCs derived from the parent cells that produce these tumors have been identified in subgroups of brain tumors, suggesting that recurrent mutations in brain tumors can disrupt signaling pathways that control brain development.

From a radiobiological standpoint, particle therapy (protons or carbon ions) may result in differential effects on CNS malignancies, the tumor microenvironment, and surrounding normal tissues. High-LET ions, for example, have unique properties that could help overcome tumor resistance by activating the extrinsic ceramide apoptotic pathway and destroying telomerase-activated cells [9]. Ion-irradiated tumor cells are less susceptible to invasion and mobility, and they adopt a stem-cell-like phenotype, although the cellular mechanism for this differential effect, as well as the ability to selectively target only these subsets of cells, are unclear [10]. Conventional RT with photons has been shown to induce an adaptive response in CNS tumors and their microenvironment, which may promote cellular plasticity and motility, resulting in RT resistance and relapse. Alternatively, high-LET irradiation might be able to mitigate this adaptive tumor response [11]; however, further clinical study is necessary to confirm these radiobiological hypotheses.

Mutational profiling allows for accurate estimation of PFS and OS in subsets of patients with similar brain tumors on histopathological diagnosis. Gliomas that are histologically equivalent are classified as having or not having isocitrate dehydrogenase (IDH) mutations, with histological grade becoming less relevant in recent years. The most important finding is that patients with grade III gliomas who have an IDH mutation have a better prognosis, with subsets of these patients experiencing long-term median survivals [12,13], whereas patients without IDH mutations may experience rapid disease progression [13,14]. For patients with favorable-risk disease, early intervention is important for better outcomes [15]. However, physicians or patients may prefer to postpone photon RT due to concerns about radiation-induced cognitive dysfunction [16]. When compared to advanced photon techniques, the dosimetric advantages of PT lead in superior normal tissue sparing. Patients with more indolent tumors benefit from this in terms of cognitive preservation. The potential benefit of dose-escalated RT for high-grade tumors like glioblastoma may help to overcome the hypoxic microenvironments thought to be responsible for RT's reduced biologic effect and, ultimately, tumor resistance to treatment [17]. Finally, as these patients also receive chemotherapy, either concurrent with RT or in the adjuvant setting, treatment-induced lymphopenia is commonly encountered [18] and has been shown to be related to local control and survival outcomes [19]. Therefore, the use of particle therapy to reduce irradiation of the circulating blood volume remains of key interest.

13.3 Preclinical Data

The biological implications of CNS tumor onset and growth have been studied using a number of animal models [20,21]. Despite the fact that these preclinical models have contributed greatly to our understanding of tumor growth mechanisms, the knowledge gained has only been translated to a limited extent. Several reports show that novel treatment modalities are effective in animal model studies; however, clinical trials in patients have failed [22]. The reason is thought to be multifactorial: rodent tumor models do not adequately or fully match the biological characteristics of human tumors [22]; the pharmacokinetics of the animals used are not the same as in humans [22]; and the cellular and evolutionary heterogeneity of human tumors, especially the interaction with the stromal and immunological milieu, is not reflected in animal models [22].

The use of cell-line-based xenografts in therapeutic trials is the mainstay of preclinical research. The characterization of genomic alterations in gliomas has recently resulted in a better understanding of the genetic mutations and modifications [23]. Using advanced genomic techniques, GEM glioma models based on known genetic changes commonly found in human tumors have been created [24]. These reflect important features of many glioma subtypes and shed light on unique genetic events that contribute to tumor initiation and progression [23].

Preclinical models' inability to accurately demonstrate therapeutic activity for investigational agents in a clinical setting contributes to the lack of progress. Preclinical drug development that allows for accurate prediction of effective drugs is particularly important for CNS malignancies due to the limited number of participants [25,26]. Several factors are currently limiting the development of novel successful therapies for brain tumors. First, rather than more reliable orthotopic, patient-derived xenograft models, legacy models usually use poorly defined *in vitro* systems or subcutaneous tumor xenografts. Second, clinically relevant features such as the BBB, the tumor microenvironment, and the immunological milieu are not characterized. As a result, developing and deploying more accurate preclinical models would necessitate a novel strategy based on a better understanding of brain tumor biology and basic neurobiology leading to more accurate animal models.

At present, there is a paucity of studies using preclinical mouse models to test novel RT techniques such as PT. Historically, two-dimension *in-vitro* tumor cell cultures have been traditionally used to study the cells radiosensitivity [27]. Shai et al. showed that tumor cells grown in cell culture for less than three passages were not representative of the original tumor [28]. *In-vitro* cell cultures often lack cellular complexity because inflammatory and vascular components are not taken into account. Given these limitations, some have proposed that an ectopic xenograft model might be more suitable, as it permits measurement of post-irradiation tumor growth or shrinkage on a frequent basis using minimally invasive techniques such as a caliper or ultrasound. Such flank models, however, do not recapitulate the biology or microenvironment of the unique intracranial setting, and therefore orthotopic xenograft models, especially patient-derived, have been proposed; these require *in-vivo* imaging to evaluate post-treatment tumor growth or regression [29]. Additional research is clearly needed to better understand differences among radiotherapy techniques using advanced preclinical models, as to-date, little "state-of-the-art" radiobiology has been studied in the context of charged or heavy particles. More recently, with the recognition that there is considerable heterogeneity even within each of the histopathologic categories, genetic engineering of tumors in rodents permits elucidation of tumor genome-specific radiation responsiveness. As an example, Akkari et al. recently developed both a p53-deficient and a p53-proficient GBM rodent model to test whether radiation resistance was potentially modulated by a change in tumor-associated macrophages and microglia (MG). Using transgenic mouse glioma models, they demonstrated very elegantly that MG and monocyte-derived macrophages (MDM) display a heterogenous response during RT, but at recurrence, they express a convergent transcriptional signature. When compared to p53-proficient glioblastoma, p53-deficient tumors have a higher MDM-to-MG ratio at baseline, indicating that the underlying cancer cell genetics can sculpt the tumor microenvironment in various ways, including altering the immune milieu. Whether such tumor cell genetics-specific effects are equivalent with all forms of RT remains understudied [30].

13.4 Proton Physics Rationale and Dosimetric Evidence

The dose distribution in PT is characterized by a well-defined maximum range and a clearly defined Bragg peak [31] (see Figure 13.1). When compared to photon therapy, this dose deposition provides better dose conformality and a lower integral dose. This is even more pronounced when using intensity-modulated PT (IMPT) for Pencil Beam Scanning (PBS) systems [32]. CNS tumors are usually found close to a number of essential OARs, making them a relevant indication for PT [33]. RT toxicities have a dose–response relationship, with either volume-based effects or serial-dose constraints. Some examples of this principle include the degree of endocrine dysfunction is related to the mean doses to the hypothalamus and pituitary, mean cochlear dose predicts auditory dysfunction, point doses to the visual apparatus and other cranial nerves predict nerve deficits, and memory effects are related to the volumetric dose to the hippocampus [34,35].

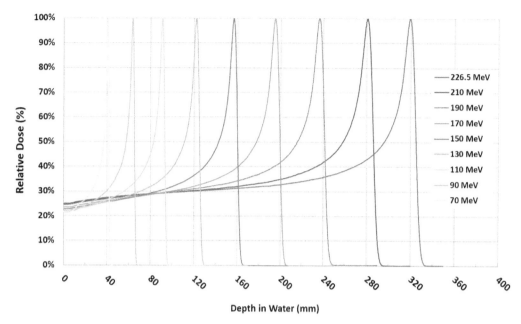

Figure 13.1 The absorbed dose as a function of depth in water from unmodulated (pristine) proton Bragg peaks produced by proton beams of various energies.

Many studies have shown that PT has a dosimetric advantage over photon therapy, but the extent of the clinical gain is less well known. These dosimetric studies have been performed across a variety of CNS tumor subsites. Harrabi et al., for example, found that particle therapy reduced the maximal, mean, and integral dose to essential neurologic structures, areas of neurogenesis, and structures of neurocognitive function in a treatment planning comparison to photon therapy [36]. Moreover, as most primary brain tumors are unilateral in nature, contralateral structures were essentially completely spared with particle therapy. Dosimetric comparisons have also been performed across different types of PT, including passive scatter and IMPT, with demonstrated reductions to dose to important neurocognitive substructures, such as the hippocampus, dentate gyrus, subventricular zone, and uninvolved brain with IMPT [37]. Individual studies have also demonstrated the importance of tumor size and location with regards to differential dose distributions among RT techniques. Adeberg and colleagues assessed the advantage of PT for five different types of brain tumors and concluded that parietal tumors benefitted the most [38]. PT showed better sparing of the circle of Willis, and it has recently been proposed as the key predictor of cerebrovascular events in childhood survivors [39,40]. The dosimetric benefit is also noticeable for large target volumes, such craniospinal irradiation (CSI), where PT can spare the OARs anterior to the vertebrae [41]. Tamura et al. used *in-silico* modeling to predict that PT will result in a significant reduction in the risk of radiation-induced secondary cancers [42]. The dosimetric advantage also translates into a clinical benefit in terms of decreased neurodisability and better quality of life (QOL) [43,44].

PT's superior dose conformity comes at the expense of increased sensitivity to range and setup uncertainties. These dosimetric uncertainties can be mitigated using robust planning and optimization techniques [45,46]. As LET rises, RBE rises as well, and RBE is affected by factors such as total dose, fractionation, biological end point, oxygenation, and cell type [47,48]. Using LET/RBE evaluation and LET optimization of PT plans, high LET areas to critical structures can be avoided [49,50]. Future advances in this area are expected to improve PT's dosimetry, physics, and clinical aspects even further.

13.5 Clinical Indications

To justify the use of PT in the era of evidence-based medicine, high-quality studies are needed. Prospective cohort studies, phase II, and randomized controlled trials have enrolled patients from around the globe. The most common brain tumors included in these trials are meningioma, glioblastoma, and low-grade glioma (LGG). Table 13.1 lists a variety of ongoing CNS tumor prospective trials and tumor registries in the United States and Europe.

13.5.1 Meningioma

Meningiomas are the most common benign neoplasm of the brain [1]. Total resection of the meningioma and its related dural base is the treatment of choice and postoperative risks include neurological deficits, particularly cranial nerve palsies, especially with skull-base locations [51]. Surgery alone is curative in patients with low-grade disease (WHO I) without risk-

Table 13.1 Prospective trials and tumor registries active in the United States and Europe for primary brain tumors treated with particle therapy.

Trial registration no.	Tumor type	Location	Study design	N	Age	Primary end point	Treatment dose/ Fractionation schedule
NCT03267836	Recurrent meningioma (G I–III)	Washington University School of Medicine, USA	Phase Ib	12	≥18 years	Two-year immunogenicity measured by changes of CD8+/CD4+ TILs	20 GyE in 5 fractions with avelumab
NCT02693990	Meningioma (G II/III)	Mass. General/ MD Anderson, USA	Nonrandomized Phase I/II	60	≥18 years	2-year safety and utility of increased dose IMPT: dose-limiting toxicity using NCI CTC 4.0	NA
NCT03180268	Meningioma (G II)	NRG Oncology, USA	Randomized Phase III	148	≥18 years	10-year PFS	59.4 GyE in 33 fractions
NCT02978677	Meningioma (G II/III)	Technische Universität Dresden, Germany	Nonrandomized Phase I/II	90	≥18 years	5-year PFS	68–72 GyE in 34–36 fractions
NCT04278118	Benign brain tumors, meningioma (G I–III)	Emory University, USA	Nonrandomized Phase II	70	≥18 years	3-year LC and AE	NA
NCT03286335	Benign or malignant brain tumor (LGG or grade III anaplastic glioma with either or both IDH1 mutation or 1p/19q co-deletion, and meningioma)	Mass. General Hospital, USA	Observational study	100	≥18 years	2-year LC	NA
NCT01358058	LGG or grade III anaplastic glioma with either or both IDH1 mutation or 1p/19q co-deletion	Mass. General Hospital, USA	Single-arm Phase II	63	≥18 years	7-year efficacy	54–59.4 GyE in 30–33 fractions
NCT02824731	Gliomas (low or high grade), intracerebral meningiomas	University Hospital Carl Gustav Carus, Germany	Nonrandomized Phase II	418	≥18 years	1-year toxicity	54–60 GyE in 27–30 fractions
NCT03180502	IDH mutant Glioma (G II/III)	NRG Oncology, USA	Randomized Phase II	120	≥18 years	10-year cognition	NA
NCT02179086	Glioblastoma	NRG Oncology, USA	Randomized Phase II	606	≥18 years	5-year OS	NA
NCT01854554	Glioblastoma	MD Anderson, USA	Nonrandomized Phase II	90	≥18 years	4-month cognitive failure	NA
NCT02179086	Glioblastoma	NRG Oncology, USA	Randomized Phase II	606	≥18 years	5-year OS	NA

N = Number; G = grade; TILs = tumor infiltrating lymphocytes; GyE = gray equivalent; Mass. = Massachusetts; IMPT = intensity modulated proton therapy; LGG = low-grade glioma; NA = not available; PFS = progression-free survival; LC = local control; AE = adverse event; IDH = isocitrate dehydrogenase; OS = overall survival.

factors for recurrence [52], whereas higher-grade meningiomas (WHO II/III) may benefit from adjuvant RT [53]. Patients with multiple or inoperable meningiomas can be treated with definitive RT [51]. Since meningiomas have a high long-term survival rate, in order to preserve cognition and QOL, there is a greater emphasis on sparing adjacent OARs [54].

PT is effective in the treatment of grade I meningioma as a primary treatment, for those with significant residual tumor following surgery, those at higher risk for disease recurrence, and for those with relapsed disease. Fractionated PT resulted in excellent 5-year local control between 88% and 100% (see Table 13.2). Doses used across the reported studies varied based on institutional preference, tumor grade, and treatment setting (initial vs. recurrent disease) but ranged from 54 to 60 Gy. Hypofractionated stereotactic PT has also been shown to result in local control rates of greater than 90% in 5 years [55,56]. Proton stereotactic radiosurgery (SRS) is normally administered to the 90–95% isodose line, to a dose of 10–15 Gy in 1 fraction [57].

Fractionated PT has been shown to reach high control rates with minimal treatment-related side effects [58]. Toxicity was more significant in patients either with cavernous sinus involvement or if encasing the optic pathway, but it's uncertain if this was due to the treatment or the severity of the disease [58,59]. For example, in the study by Slater and colleagues of the patients who had cavernous sinus involvement at initial diagnosis, 8.3% developed late neurologic symptoms, such as optic neuropathy [59]. None of the patients with non-skull-base tumors experienced high-grade or late complications as a result of PT in the WHO grade I studies. Evidently, even for large tumors, such as those in the Vernimmen et al. series [55], where the majority of the patients had lesions larger than 14 cm^3, the toxicity was low. When compared to SRS, hypofractionated SRT, or fractionated RT, PT, regardless of its mode of administration, produced similar results [60,61]. As a result, PT can be considered a reasonable choice for WHO I meningiomas, especially those in the skull-base, complex geometries, or those that are radiation-induced.

There are fewer PT studies in patients with grade II/III meningiomas in the literature. Hug et al. published the results of grade II/III meningiomas treated with either photon therapy or combination proton-photon RT [62]. PT significantly improved local control as compared to photon RT alone and survival for grade II meningioma patients was significantly higher among those treated with PT to doses >60 Gy. Another research showed that survival was significantly associated with total dose administered when patients were given proton and photon RT [63]. Chan et al. showed patients with grade II/III meningiomas being treated with high doses without any toxicity. Furthermore, there was only one recurrence in this study, in a patient with a grade III meningioma [64]. The ongoing NRG BN003 clinical trial (NCT03180268), in patients with a gross totally resected grade II meningioma randomizes between surveillance and RT, and includes PT. Meningiomas studies using carbon ion irradiation were confined to retrospective data from single institutions. The data of grade II/III meningiomas treated with a combined photon-carbon-ion therapy with a median follow-up of 77 months showed high

Table 13.2 Selected series of particle therapy for meningioma.

Author	Year	Tumor type and grade	No. of patients	Median dose (GyE)	Median FU (months)	Outcome
Halasz et al. [57]	2011	Meningioma G I–II	50	13 (10–15.5)	32	3 y-LC: 94%
Weber et al. [139]	2012	Meningioma G I–III	39	G:I–II 52.2–56, G:III-60.8	55	5 y-LC: G I: 100%, G II/III: 49%
Slater et al. [59]	2012	Meningioma G I–II	72	G:I 50.4–66.6, G:II 54–70.2	74	5 y-LC: 96%
Combs et al. [66]	2013	Meningioma G I–III	107	54 (52.2–57.6)	12	2 y-LC: G I: 100%, G II/III: 33%
McDonald et al. [140]	2015	Meningioma G II	22	63 (54–68.4)	39	5 y-LC: 71.1%
Vlachogiannis et al. [56]	2017	Meningioma G I	170	21.9 (14–46)	84	5 y-PFS: 93%, 10 y-PFS: 85%
Murray et al. [141]	2018	Meningioma G I–III	96	G:I 50.4–64, G:II/III 54–68	57	5 y-LC: 86.4%, 5 y-OS: 88.2%
El Shafie et al. [142]	2018	Meningioma G I–III	110	Protons: 54, carbon: 18	47	5 y-PFS: 96.6%, 5 y-OS: 96.2%

GyE = Gray equivalent; FU = follow-up; y = year; G = grade; LC = local control; PFS = progression-free survival; OS = overall survival.

rates of local tumor control and no high-grade adverse events [65]. In recurrent setting, photon therapy accompanied by a carbon ion boost showed a promising local control (67%), with no high-grade toxicity [66]. The ongoing MARCIE trial (NCT01166321), in which subtotally resected meningioma receives an IMRT base plan followed by carbon ion boost, may address this issue.

Boron neutron capture therapy (BNCT) is based on a nuclear capture reaction in which boron is irradiated with thermal neutrons, generating high-energy short-range particles and recoiling lithium nuclei [67]. This treatment will potentially kill only cancer cells as boron is selectively taken up by them. BNCT was used to treat the first case of recurrent grade III meningioma in 2006 [68]. In recurrent meningioma, Takeuchi et al. found that BNCT therapy showed a mean volume reduction of 64.5% in 2 months [69]. The distinction between tumor recurrence and pseudo-progression with necrosis is difficult to make with BNCT, as it is with conventional RT [70,71]. The 18F-BPA-PET will theoretically differentiate between recurrence and necrosis [72].

Comparisons between particle therapy and photon therapy studies are difficult due to clear differences in patient cohorts [3,73]. Since definitive RT for meningioma is usually reserved for those who are unable to undergo surgery, have incomplete resection, or have high-risk features, each institutional series involves a heterogeneous group of patients [73]. It's also crucial to assess whether particle therapy for high-risk meningiomas actually is superior as compared to photon RT in terms of outcomes. Although particle therapy allows for dose escalation while maintaining low OAR doses [64,74], the importance of dose-escalation should be better established. Ongoing clinical trials evaluating different particle therapy techniques and dose-escalation efforts for meningiomas are summarized in Table 13.3.

Table 13.3 Ongoing particle therapy clinical trials in meningioma.

NCT number	Study name	Study type	Tumor type	Particle therapy	N	Age	Study start	Estimated completion date	Primary outcome	Secondary outcomes
NCT03180268	NA	Phase III	WHO II	NA	148	≥18	06/2017	08/2027	10-year PFS	10-year OS, 5-year OS, DSS, NCF, PRO
NCT02693990	NA	Phase II	WHO II/III	Proton	60	≥18	02/2016	08/2027	2-year safety and utility of increased dose IMPT: dose-limiting toxicity using NCI CTC 4.0	5-year PFS, 2-year OS, 2-year LET
NCT03267836	NA	Phase I	WHO grade I–III	Proton	12	≥18	01/2018	07/2022	2-year immunogenicity measured by changes of CD8+/ CD4+ TILs	6 months safety, 3 months RR and PR, 2-year PFS and OS
NCT02978677	PANAMA	Phase I/II	WHO II/III	Proton	90	≥18	10/2019	12/2028	5-year PFS	5-year late/ acute toxicity, OS, recurrence, QOL
NCT01795300	PINOCCHIO	Phase I/II	WHO I	Proton, carbon ion	80	≥18	05/2020	05/2022	1-year toxicity graded according to CTCAE Version 4.1	3-year OS, PFS, QOL
NCT01166321	MARCIE	Phase II	WHO II	Photons + carbon-ion boost	40	≥18	06/2012	12/2020	3-year PFS	3-year OS

N = Number; NA = not available; WHO = World Health Organization; PFS = progression-free survival; OS = overall survival; DSS = disease-specific survival; NCF = neurocognitive function; PRO = patient-reported outcomes; NCI CTC = National Cancer Institute Common Toxicity Criteria; LET = linear energy transfer; TILs = tumor infiltrating lymphocytes; RR = radiological response; PR = pathological response; QOL = quality of life; CTCAE = Common Terminology Criteria for Adverse Events.

13.5.2 Glioma

Traditionally, LGG includes grade I/II tumors and they account for about 10% of all primary brain tumors [1]. For grade I gliomas, the 10-year recurrence-free survival rate after resection is about 95% [75]. According to the most recent WHO classification, grade II LGGs are characterized by mutations in the IDH1/2 genes and often have 1p/19q co-deletion, indicating a favorable prognosis [76].

Glioblastoma and anaplastic astrocytoma are more commonly IDH wild-type according to the most recent WHO classification [76]. Glioblastoma has a poor prognosis with only about half of patients surviving after 1 year of diagnosis [1]. Patients with promoter methylation of the MGMT gene receiving chemoradiotherapy have a slightly greater survival rate [77] with age, histology, and performance status being important prognostic factors [78]. Anaplastic oligodendroglioma with IDH mutations and 1p/19q co-deletion has a better prognosis, particularly when chemoradiotherapy is used [79].

The dosimetric benefits of particle therapy have shown reduced integral dose to the uninvolved brain, OARs, and the circulating blood pool in the brain, which is correlated with treatment-induced lymphopenia [36,80]. Since these patients are receiving chemoradiotherapy, the reduced adverse effects associated with particle therapy compared to photon therapies, while maintaining comparable survival rates, can translate into the cost-effectiveness of this RT technique [81]. These benefits become particularly significant in a patient population with favorable molecular characteristics and a high probability of long-term survival.

Since LGGs are usually rare, the clinical evidence is limited (see Table 13.4). In a prospective QOL study with LGG with a median follow-up of 5.1 years, there were no declines in multiple neurocognitive QOL parameters [82]. The median PFS of a heterogeneous cohort of LGGs was 4.5 years, with no late toxicities beyond 2 years [83]. Similarly, when patients were treated up to 54 Gy, a retrospective study found no grade 3 toxicities [84]. Dose escalation up to 68.2 Gy for LGG and to 79.7 Gy for anaplastic gliomas has also been performed [85]. The ongoing randomized BN005 trial (NCT03180502) will provide additional evidence for particle therapy in patients with IDH-mutated grade II/III gliomas.

Dose escalation has been evaluated in glioblastoma with PT [86,87]. When compared to standard photon therapy, a retrospective series using 50 Gy photon therapy followed by a 10 Gy proton boost to a reduced target volume showed less acute and chronic toxicity rates [88]. Smaller target volumes were associated with better QOL, neurocognitive, and neurologic function, according to these findings. The majority of recurrences, however, remained in-field, according to patterns-of-failure analysis. Furthermore, at such high doses, 30% of patients developed symptomatic radiation necrosis. The University of Tsukuba reported dose escalation for glioblastoma with an overall median survival of 22 months [86,89].

Table 13.4 Selected series of particle therapy for upfront or recurrent gliomas.

Author	Year	Tumor type and grade	Particle therapy	No. of patients	Median dose (GyE)	Median FU (months)	Outcome
Fitzek et al. [85]	2001	LGG (G II/III)	Proton	20	G II/III: 68.2/79.7	G II/III: 61/55	G II/III: 5 y OS: 71%/23%
Hauswald et al. [127]	2012	LGG (G I/II)	Proton	19	54	NA	NA
Shih et al. [82]	2015	LGG (G II)	Proton	20	54	61	3 y PFS: 85%, 5 y PFS: 40%
Hasegawa et al. [90]	2012	LGG (G II)	Carbon ion	14	50.4/55.2	18/91	5 y OS:43%, 10 y OS: 36%
Fitzek et al. [87]	1999	Glioblastoma	Photon/Proton	23	90	20	2 y OS: 34%, 3 y OS: 18%
Mizoe et al. [91]	2007	HGG	Photon/Carbon ion	48	50 Gy/16.8–24.8 GyE	35	NA
Mizumoto et al. [86]	2010	Glioblastoma	Proton	20	50.4	21.6	2 y LC: 15.5 %, 2 y OS: 45.3%
Mizumoto et al. [89]	2015	Glioblastoma	Photon/Proton	23	50.4 Gy/46.2 GyE	70.9	1 y OS: 78%, 2 y OS: 43%
Adeberg et al. [88]	2017	HGG	Photon/Proton	66	50.0-50.4 Gy/10 GyE	32	2 y OS: 40%

N = Number; GyE = grey equivalent; LGG = low-grade glioma; y = year; G = grade; PFS = progression-free survival; OS = overall survival; LC = local control; NA = not available; HGG = high-grade glioma.

Carbon-ion therapy, either alone or in combination with other treatments, has also been shown to be effective in glioma patients [90,91]. In a study of 48 HGG patients, photon RT was combined with carbon-ion boost and reported no grade ≥3 toxicity [90]. In another study, patients with diffuse grade II astrocytoma were treated to <50.4 Gy, or 55.2 Gy of carbon-ion therapy with no chemotherapy [91]. Patients who received 46.2–50.4 Gy, the median PFS and OS were 18 and 28 months, respectively, with no grade ≥3 late effects in any patients. Similarly, patients with glioblastoma who were treated with BNCT had promising early results, with median survival times ranging from 13 to 27 months [67,92].

Early results from dose-escalation studies of particle therapy have been mixed [93]. Several trials are currently underway to currently evaluate this further (see Table 13.5). The prospective NRG BN001 trial (NCT02179086) randomizes newly diagnosed glioblastoma patients between conventional RT and hypofractionated dose-escalated RT and includes PT in the dose-escalation cohort. The recently completed CLEOPATRA trial (NCT01165671) may also address this question using carbon-ion therapy [94].

In patients undergoing re-treatment, particle therapy has been explored as a means of re-irradiation. In a retrospective review, re-irradiation was assessed in 26 glioma patients, 8 of whom were re-treated with PT [95]. In the PT re-irradiated patients, the median OS was 19.4 months, which was considered favorable in comparison to existing photon literature. The PCG recently published the results with recurrent glioblastoma who were treated with PT and followed up after a median of 20.2 months showing favorable outcomes [96].

Despite the paucity of evidence on particle therapy for glioma, there are a few points worth mentioning. Both LGG and HGG are extremely heterogeneous populations with a broad variety of prognoses that can be stratified using molecular profiling [1]. Toxicity reduction is an important goal, but the occurrence of toxicities is also a function of patient selection [88]. Although many of the aforementioned studies pertain to dose escalation, a clear role for radiation dose-escalation, the correct method of achieving this, in gliomas, has not been established. The role of particle therapy in re-irradiation cannot be overstated; however, various other variables such as tumor volume margins and concurrent chemotherapy must also be considered [95]. The ongoing CINDERELLA study will compare stereotactic photon RT with carbon-ion re-irradiation for recurrent gliomas [97].

13.5.3 Miscellaneous CNS Tumors

Medulloblastoma is a form of primitive neuroectodermal tumor [98]. Adult medulloblastoma varies from pediatric medulloblastoma in terms of clinical outcomes and molecular profile [99,100]. Although CSI is an effective treatment for medulloblastoma with photon therapy, it is usually associated with treatment-related side effects [100–102]. This may have a significant impact on the QOL of the patient [103]. PBT has been suggested to reduce treatment-related morbidity in adults undergoing CSI, and similar results seen in pediatric patients (see corresponding chapter).

Brown et al. compared the efficacy of proton CSI with photon CSI in adult medulloblastoma patients [104]. Proton CSI patients lost less weight than photon CSI patients, had less grade 2 nausea and vomiting, and were less likely to require medical treatment for esophagitis. They also had small reductions in peripheral white blood cell (WBC), hemoglobin, and platelet counts. Similar benefits were observed in a series adult patient of varying histologies treated with vertebral body-sparing proton CSI [105]. These results, along with data on proton CSI in pediatric patients, support the use of particle therapy to treat these extensive target volumes and reduce toxicity.

13.6 Treatment Planning Considerations

13.6.1 Simulation, Target Delineation, and Radiation Dose/Fractionation

CT simulation may be performed with or without intravenous contrast. However, for planning and dose calculation purposes for particle therapy, a non-contrast CT is required [106]. Prior to contrast administration, this CT scan should be reviewed for the extent of any metal artifacts, appropriate chin position, presence of skin folds, reproducibility of the shoulder position, and adequacy of the CT reconstruction technique and resolution. Bite blocks can be used to isolate the tongue and the roof of the mouth in cases with extensive base-of-skull tumors with paranasal sinus involvement or significant inferior extracranial extension [106].

Target volume delineation for the majority of CNS tumors is performed using diagnostic MR imaging to visualize intact tumors or postoperative cavities [107]. Delineation of structures, such as the hippocampus and optic chiasm, may be aided by an MRI [108]. For accurate target volume delineation, the MRI should be registered to the planning CT scan. The dose and fractionation schedule prescribed is determined by the tumor type, grade, and clinical scenario. For particle therapy and photon therapy cases, the expansions of the gross tumor volume (GTV) and clinical target volumes (CTV) are delineated in the similar way [109] (see Table 13.6).

Materials such as implants and metal hardware should be appropriately contoured on the bone window and assigned their proper stopping power ratio (SPR) or mass density before starting the treatment planning process. In cases where the material is unknown, SPR measurements of a sample can be performed using a multi-slit ion chamber. If a sample cannot

Table 13.5 Ongoing particle therapy clinical trials in glioma.

NCT number	Study name	Study type	Tumor type	Particle therapy	N	Age	Study start	Estimated completion date	Primary outcome	Secondary outcomes
NCT02179086	NRG BN001	Phase III	Glioblastoma (initial)	Proton	606	≥18	10/2021	05/2021	5-year OS	PFS, toxicity, neurocognitive function, lymphopenia, imaging features
NCT03180502	NA	Phase II	IDH mutant Grade II or III glioma	Proton	120	≥18	08/2017	01/2030	10-year cognition	10 year QOL, symptoms, cognition, AEs, local control, OS and PFS
NCT02824731	ProtoChoice-Hirn	Phase II	Gliomas (low or high grade), intracerebral meningiomas	Proton	346	≥18	07/2016	07/2026	1-year late toxicity	1- and 2-year LC and OS, 3-month acute toxicity, 2-year late toxicity
NCT01854554	NA	Phase II	Glioblastoma	Proton	90	≥18	05/2013	05/2020	4-month cognitive failure	4-month local control
NCT03286335	NA	Phase II	Benign or malignant brain tumor (LGG or grade III anaplastic glioma with either or both IDH1 mutation or 1p/19q co-deletion, and meningioma)	Proton	100	≥18	09/2018	09/2027	2-year LC	2-year QOL, ototoxicity, vision, neuroendocrine, neurocognition, alopecia and CD4
NCT01358058	NA	Phase II	LGG or grade III anaplastic glioma with either or both IDH1 mutation or 1p/19q co-deletion	Proton	63	≥18	05/2011	08/2022	7-year efficacy	7-year safety, tolerability and OS
NCT04536649	NA	Phase III	Glioblastoma	Proton, Carbon ion	369	≥18	10/2020	09/2025	3-year OS	3-year PFS, 12 month toxicity, recognition function and life quality
NCT01166308	CINDERELLA	Phase I/II	Recurrent glioma	Carbon ion	56	≥18	12/2010	04/2016	1-year OS	1-year PFS

N = Number; OS = overall survival; PFS = progression-free survival; NA = not available; IDH = isocitrate dehydrogenase; QOL = quality of life; AE = adverse events; LC = local control; LGG = low-grade glioma.

Table 13.6 Recommended target volumes and radiation doses for treatment of intracranial tumors

Tumor type	Volume	Definitive	Postoperative	Dose
Meningioma, Grade I	GTV	Tumor delineated including suspicious dural and/or bone involvement by postcontrast T1 MRI	Postoperative cavity, residual enhancing tumor including suspicious dural and/or bone involvement by postcontrast T1 MRI	SRS: 14–16 GyE in 1 fraction FSRT: 20–24 GyE in 4 fraction/25 GyE in 5 fractions Fractionated RT: 52.2–54 GyE at 1.8–2 GyE/fraction
	CTV	0–0.5 cm, reduced around natural anatomic barriers to tumor spread	Anatomically constrained 0–0.5 cm expansion	
	PTV	0–0.3 cm, depending on the radiotherapy technique and daily patient positioning technology 0–1 mm: SRS or HSRT 1–3 mm: fractionated RT	0–0.3 cm, depending on the radiotherapy technique and daily patient positioning technology 0–1 mm: SRS or HSRT 1–3 mm: Fractionated RT	
Meningioma, Grade II	GTV	Tumor delineated including suspicious dural and/or bone involvement by postcontrast T1 MRI	Postoperative cavity, residual enhancing tumor including suspicious dural and/or bone involvement by postcontrast T1 MRI	PTV: 54–59.4 GyE at 1.8 GyE/fraction
	CTV	0.5–1 cm expansion, reduced around natural barriers to tumor spread	0.5–1 cm expansion, reduced around natural barriers to tumor spread	
	PTV	0.3–0.5 cm, depending on daily patient positioning technology	0.3–0.5 cm, depending on daily patient positioning technology	
Meningioma, Grade III	GTV	Tumor delineated including suspicious dural and/or bone involvement by postcontrast T1 MRI	Postoperative cavity, residual enhancing tumor including suspicious dural and/or bone involvement by postcontrast T1 MRI	PTV: 59.4–60 GyE at 1.8–2 GyE/fraction
	CTV	1–1.5 cm expansion, reduced around natural barriers to tumor spread	1–1.5 cm expansion, reduced around natural barriers to tumor spread	
	PTV	0.3–0.5 cm, depending on daily patient positioning technology	0.3–0.5 cm, depending on daily patient positioning technology	
Low-grade glioma (LGG)	GTV	Tumor delineated by the postcontrast, T2 or FLAIR MRI	Postoperative cavity and residual tumor postcontrast, T2 or FLAIR MRI	PTV: 50.4–54 GyE at 1.8–2 GyE/fraction
	CTV	1 cm, reduced around natural barriers to tumor spread	1 cm, reduced around natural barriers to tumor spread	
	PTV	0.3–0.5 cm, depending on daily patient positioning technology	0.3–0.5 cm, depending on daily patient positioning technology	
Anaplastic glioma (enhancing tumor)	GTV	–	GTV1 is defined by the T2 or FLAIR volume, GTV2 is defined by the postoperative cavity and residual tumor by the postcontrast T1 MRI	PTV1: 50.4 GyE at 1.8 Gy/fraction, PTV2: 59.4 GyE at 1.8 Gy/fraction (sequential cone down) PTV1: 54.45 GyE at 1.65 GyE/fraction, PTV2: 59.4 GyE at 1.8 GyE/fraction (simultaneous integrated boost)
	CTV	–	CTV1 is defined by a 1.5-cm expansion, reduced around natural barriers to tumor spread, CTV2 is defined by a 1.0-cm expansion, reduced around natural barriers to tumor spread	
	PTV	–	0.3–0.5 cm, depending on daily patient positioning technology	

(Continued)

Table 13.6 (Continued)

Tumor type	Volume	Definitive	Postoperative	Dose
Anaplastic glioma (non-enhancing tumor) IDH-wild-type diffuse astrocytoma	GTV	–	GTV is defined by the postoperative cavity volume and residual tumor by T2 or FLAIR	PTV: 59.4 GyE at 1.8 GyE/fraction
	CTV	–	1.5 cm expansion, reduced around natural barriers to tumor spread	
	PTV	–	0.3–0.5 cm, depending on daily patient positioning technology	
Glioblastoma	GTV	–	GTV1 is defined by the T2 or FLAIR volume, GTV2 is defined by the postoperative cavity and residual tumor by the postcontrast T1 MRI	PTV1: 46 GyE at 2 GyE/fraction PTV2: 60 GyE at 2 GyE/fraction (sequential cone down) PTV1: 50–51 GyE at 1.67–1.7 GyE/fraction
	CTV	–	CTV1 is defined by a 2-cm expansion, reduced around natural barriers to tumor spread, CTV2 is defined by a 2-cm expansion, reduced around natural barriers to tumor spread	PTV2: 60 GyE at 2 GyE/fraction (simultaneous integrated boost)

GTV = Gross tumor volume; CTV = clinical target volume; PTV = planning target volume; SRS = stereotactic radiosurgery; FSRT = fractionated stereotactic radiotherapy; RT = radiotherapy, GyE = Gray equivalent.

be obtained, an extended scale CT scan can be reconstructed from the simulation scan and may help provide a first estimate for the material composition [110].

13.6.2 Patient Positioning, Immobilization, and Treatment Verification

A three-point mask is generally recommended for simulation; however, a five-point mask can be used for base-of-skull tumors to maintain neck alignment [111]. To check the accuracy of the setup, imaging can be used. Cone-beam CT is recommended to test for possible changes in patient anatomy that could affect the planned dose distribution [111]. In certain situations, such as when tracking cyst growth in an adult craniopharyngioma, weekly MRIs may be recommended [112]. Changes in anatomy that cause clinically relevant perturbations in target coverage or OAR doses identified during verification CTs can necessitate a replan.

13.6.3 Beam Selection

Beam configuration is dictated by anatomical considerations, such as the extent of the healthy brain traversed, proximity of the target volume to nearby OARs, and setup reproducibility [113]. Beam transmission through the paranasal sinuses, postoperative air-cavities, and skin folds should be avoided [114,115]. Additionally, to limit range uncertainties, beams should not traverse through any non-biological implants [116]. Based on the location, extent of disease, and surrounding anatomy, CNS plans have two to four beams, with a typical

dosimetric preference for three. One common configuration is an enface beam, a vertex, and a third beam. For most superficial brain tumors, two-beam arrangements often provide sufficient coverage. When possible, beams should avoid traversing through the contralateral hemisphere or end-ranging in critical OARs. In cases where this latter condition is not possible, an adequate hinge angle between the two beams can minimize distal range overlap toward the OAR.

Due to constraints on the minimum available energy, range shifters are required to treat shallow targets [117]. However, it is important to be cognizant that range shifter use also increases spot size and degrades the spot penumbra. Both of these factors can negatively impact dose conformity and, ultimately, plan quality. Therefore, range shifter use should be avoided when possible. This is typically possible with deeper brain tumors at depths greater than 3 cm.

13.6.4 Passive Scattering and Uniform Scanning

Passive scattering and uniform scanning techniques represent older particle therapy delivery technologies [118,119]. These techniques use a broad field shaped laterally by apertures and distally using beam-specific compensators. A forward planning approach is typically used; first, a rough estimate of the distal range uncertainty is calculated based on the central axis distal range. This factor is modified to account for possible heterogeneity effects and target shape. Subsequently, beam-specific planning target volumes are generated, and a compensator is created to carve the dose's distal end. Due to the uniform nature of the field, there is limited control for shaping the proximal end of the beam. Beams without an adequate hinge angle can generate hot tails proximally, which can be alleviated by widening the hinge angle or introducing additional beams.

13.6.5 Pencil Beam Scanning

The PBS technique delivers a unique pattern of spot positions, and monitor unit (MU) weights that are arranged to generate highly conformal dose distributions [120]. Plans are optimized to be robust with respect to setup and proton range uncertainties [121]. Two ways to accomplish this are by planning to larger beam-specific planning target volumes (beam-specific PTV) or by robustly optimizing to the CTV. In both cases, prescription level dose clouds larger than the CTV are expected. If beam-specific PTVs are used, expansion margins on the distal end must be greater than the proximal and lateral margins to correctly account for range uncertainties.

Due to its higher accuracy, Monte Carlo-based dose optimization and calculation are advised for plans that utilize range shifters, as well as those involving field sizes smaller than 3×3 cm^2 [122]. During the optimization process, a maximum MU/spot threshold can be enforced to avoid heavy MU weighted spots, which could potentially elevate toxicity risks. Two additional parameters that can impact field homogeneity, conformity, and minimum and maximum spot MU are spot energy layer and spatial spacing. The impact of these two parameters on plan quality should be investigated during the optimization process.

The decrease in proton energy in the Bragg peak region is associated with an enhanced RBE. The RBE values in this area are commonly reported to be 1.1 in the entrance region and 1.7 at the distal edge fall off. Reported evidence suggests a sensitivity of the brainstem to PT in situations when the standard RBE-corrected dose exceeds the conventional photon brainstem tolerance [50]. Because of these enhanced effects, good planning practice entails avoidance of heavily weighted spot deposition into critical CNS structures (i.e., brainstem, optic nerve and chiasm, and spinal cord) when possible. Planning strategies include the use of beam-specific optimization structures where regions of overlap with OARs are carved out or the use of beam-specific blocking structures that avoid spot deposition in these specific regions. Additional optimization structures can be used to improve coverage or promote dose drop-off near OARs. Finally, during the optimization process, mean and maximum dose objectives can be provided to a skin rind with a low weight to promote skin sparing in superficial brain tumors.

Multi-field optimization (MFO) and single-field optimization (SFO) are used to create PBS plans. MFO plans are achieved by considering spots from all proton fields together during the optimization process. Individual beams from such plans no longer cover the entirety of the target. The total of all beams in these plans is designed to provide a uniform dose within the target. The beam dose for such plans is highly modulated and contains sharp gradients within and outside the target. Because of these features, MFO plans are extremely vulnerable to setup and range uncertainties [123]. Spots in each proton field are optimized independently from other fields in SFO plans, also known as single field uniform dose (SFUD). As such, the dose contribution from each beam is fairly homogeneous and uniform within the target, with few dose gradient regions within the target. In PBS, the SFO technique is often preferred because it produces the most robust treatment plan; however, there are circumstances where the location and shape of the tumor with respect to surrounding critical OARs require a MFO or a hybrid MFO/SFO approach. In such cases, it is important to limit the extent of modulation per beam. A practical technique is to limit the beam-specific maximum dose contribution to 70% of the prescription (with a secondary goal of 75%). In nearly all cases, this is achievable without compromising the plan quality. Additionally, in cases where an MFO approach is needed, the planner should consider using a hybrid approach where target coverage is MFO while SFO constraints are applied on OARs.

13.6.6 Plan Evaluation

Plan evaluation must include a comprehensive review of several treatment plan quality features with several aspects specific to PT. Key points to consider during the plan evaluation process include spot placement at the most distal layers, and actions taken by the planner to limit placement of such spots in sensitive CNS OARs or air cavities. Additionally, the level of beam modulation in the plan and methodology selected to generate a robust plan should be carefully reviewed. In cases where optimization target structures were used to promote plan robustness, inspection of these structures with respect to their conformity and extent of expansion relative to the original target are highly encouraged. A systematic approach and review with dosimetry and physics is encouraged to ensure adequate and appropriate plan evaluation:

- Plan dose evaluation and clinical goals: The clinician should review the plan dose slice by slice, paying particular attention to target coverage and dose to nearby OARs. OAR planning organ-at-risk volumes (PRVs), which are usually built with 0.3–0.5 cm expansion margins, may be used to assess the effectiveness of dose fall-off.
- Beam-specific dose and spot placement: Each beam should be evaluated to ensure adequate coverage. A good rule of thumb is to limit the beam-specific dose to 110% of the average beam dose. Spot placement for each beam should be reviewed; in general, spots greater than 2 cm water equivalent thickness from target are undesired and can be removed without a loss in plan quality or robustness. It's important to evaluate the level of modulation in each beam in MFO plans. Beam-specific

dose-volume histogram (DVH) for the target should be reviewed to examine the level of modulation and verify that the beam-specific maximum dose is lower than 70% of the prescription. Beam dose should be examined slice by slice to confirm that high-dose regions always lie within the target, and that beam contribution to OAR doses is acceptable.

- Plan robustness: The acceptance threshold for robustness should be institutionally standardized. The 95% isodose line covers at least 95% of the target volume which is a minimum robustness threshold. Target coverage in various scenarios can be examined by viewing the DVH. If robust optimization is used, parameters used for optimization and evaluation should be standardized across the institution. The adherence to and possible reasons for deviations from these values should be discussed during plan evaluation. All critical OARs should be within their dose tolerances when reviewing plan robustness. In general, the maximum dose in the worst scenario should be lower than 120% of the prescription.

In addition to the aforementioned principles, key example cases and teaching points are provided in Figures 13.2–13.4.

13.7 Particle Therapy Toxicities

In dosimetric comparisons, PT for intracranial tumors has demonstrated superior avoidance of critical structures particularly for targets close to critical structures [80, 124]. Although phase III randomized evidence supports stereotactic conformal RT over conventional RT in patients with benign or low-grade primary brain tumors, similar comparisons between IMRT and PT are eagerly awaited [125].

13.7.1 Acute Toxicity

Several studies have reported the acute treatment-related toxicity associated with particle therapy for patients with primary CNS malignancies. Shih et al. in adult LGG patients treated with PT reported fatigue, alopecia, headache, and scalp erythema among the acute toxicities [82]. Combs et al. reported treatment outcomes with PT and carbon-ion therapy. Hair loss was the most common acute toxicity, followed by visual disturbances, fatigue, and headaches [126]. The PCG reported acute adverse effects to be alopecia (81%), dermatitis (78%), fatigue (47%), and

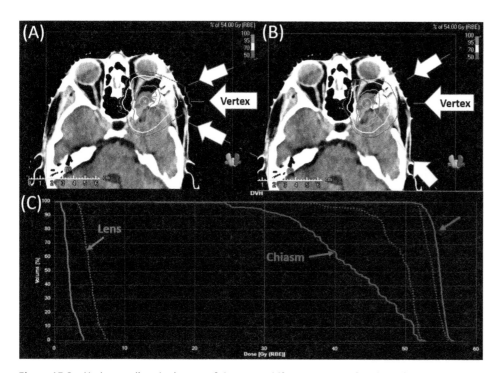

Figure 13.2 Understanding the impact of the range shifter on plan conformity. This figure presents two-beam configurations for an intracranial meningioma adjacent to the left optic nerve. The prescription required 54 Gy in 30 fractions planned robustly to the CTV and prioritized optic nerve sparing over coverage. Both beam arrangements utilized a vertex beam, and two co-planar lateral obliques. The left anterior oblique field in both plans used a 7.5-cm range shifter to cover the target. The left posterior oblique in panel A traversed a depth of ~2.5 cm to arrive at the target and also required a range shifter. Since two beams used the range shifter, the planner included the range shifter on with the vertex beam. In panel B, the left posterior oblique beam was rearranged to traverse a deeper depth and did not utilize a range shifter. The range shifter was also removed from the vertex beam. The impact of the range shifter on plan conformity can be seen from the 54-Gy isodose line (orange) which covers a larger portion of the CTV in panel B while leaving most of the target uncovered in panel A. Despite the improvement in coverage, the plan in panel B had a lower chiasm and lens dose (solid lines in panel C). Finally, an additional concern with the left posterior oblique beam in panel B was that it partially traversed the skin folds of the ear.

headaches (40%) [84]. Hauswald et al. documented in LGG patients who received PT the most common side effects to be alopecia (68%) and fatigue (32%) [127]. Maquilan et al. looked at the short-term side effects of PT with fatigue (67%), anorexia (29%), and headache (20%) being the most common [128].

The studies reported to-date do not demonstrate any increased acute toxicities with particle therapy compared to photon therapy, but prospective standardized reporting with comparative studies along with patient QOL data is encouraged. Treatment-induced lymphopenia has recently been the

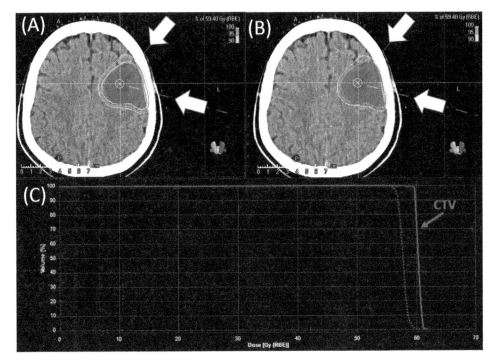

Figure 13.3 Understanding dose calculation. Panel A presents a planar dose sagittal view of an ependymoma of the left frontal gyrus and was prescribed to receive 59.4 Gy in 33 fractions. Due to the shallow nature of the target, two left lateral oblique beams with a 7.5-cm range shifter were used. The plan was optimized and calculated using the pencil beam algorithm which is inadequate for accurately modeling the effects of the range shifter on the proton beam. Upon recomputing the plan dose using the Monte Carlo dose calculation engine, a 5% dose discrepancy in target coverage was observed (B). As observed by the DVH presented in panel C, the loss of coverage is consistent throughout the target.

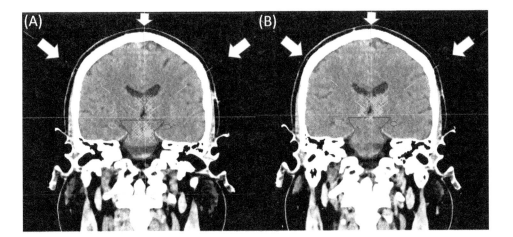

Figure 13.4 Demonstration on the use of blocking structures to avoid spot deposition in OARs. Panel A presents spot contributions from the vertex beam in the treatment of a craniopharyngioma superior to the brainstem. The presented beam configuration consisted of two laterals with couch kicks and a vertex beam. While the lateral obliques efficiently avoid the hippocampi and temporal lobes, there was significant distal range overlap between the vertex beam and the laterals in the brainstem. The plan was reoptimized using a brainstem blocking structure for the vertex beam which resulted in a considerable reduction of spots deposited in the brainstem (B), without a negative impact on coverage or robustness.

topic of increased attention and investigation. A phase II study of photon therapy or PT for newly diagnosed glioblastoma patients found lower rates of grade 3 + lymphopenia (14% vs. 39%, $p = 0.024$) [129]. Additional results from NRG BN001 will help to validate these findings.

13.7.2 Late Toxicity

Long-term outcomes and late toxicities are less reported in the literature for adult CNS patients treated with PT. The most common long-term toxicities with PT for primary brain tumors, according to Shih et al., were headaches, fatigue, and alopecia [82]. Neurocognitive activity, as well as scores for QOL questionnaires, stayed unchanged in this series when compared to baseline values. Neuroendocrine toxicity after treatment should be investigated further, as this study found a 15%, 25%, and 30% risk of developing neuroendocrine dysfunction at 1 year, 3 years, and 5 years, respectively. Sherman et al. looked at the same group of patients for neurocognitive side effects of PT [2]. Patients with left-sided tumors performed poorly on verbal and visual memory, and language tests at the start of the study, on the other hand, patients with right-sided tumors had no impairments. This cohort's output in repeated neuropsychological studies demonstrated no noticeable difference in the cognitive domains studied. In terms of hypofractionated PT, Vlachogiannis et al. used IMPT (4 × 5 Gy or 4 × 6.6 Gy) to treat intracranial meningioma (WHO I) with the majority of the tumors found in the skull base [56]. The presence of a tumor in the anterior cranial fossa was associated to a higher risk of treatment-related complications.

13.8 Future Developments

The field of radiation oncology has been tasked to generate proof that radiotherapy techniques such as PT are superior to modern photon therapy approaches. Nevertheless, the dosimetric advantage of particle therapies as compared to photon therapies is a representation in the advancement of radiotherapy delivery technology. However, unlike different forms of photon therapy delivery, particle therapies require careful evaluation and study in a prospective manner to understand the radiobiologic effects.

There is substantial potential for more technical advances in particle therapy, with treatment planning systems developing and the majority of them offering features like robust optimization [121,130,131]. Combining this with smaller spot sizes has the potential to reduce side scatter and allow for continued efforts and safe dose escalation. In terms of image guidance, PT has traditionally lagged behind in terms of features like CBCT and CT on rails with these features were only recently included in the construction of a new PT facility. Special image-guidance techniques such as in-beam PET may be encouraged [132]. Prognostic molecular data such as IDH mutation status in glioma identify subsets of patients that have a high likelihood of long-term survival and could be treated with PT [133]. It is becoming increasingly recognized that RT combined with immunotherapy can have synergistic effects [134, 135]. The thought that protons could be more immunogenic than photons is still under investigation. There are still many unanswered concerns about PT's efficacy in terms of biological effects [136, 137]. Finally, as discussed elsewhere in this book, the development of FLASH dose rates (>40 Gy/s) with modern PT systems may further unlock the true potential of particle therapy in optimizing tumor control [138].

In conclusion, PT and other particle therapy techniques are still maturing. Although PT has been around for decades, treatment techniques have only recently advanced significantly. These technological advancements have also converged on physicians alongside a deeper understanding of tumor biology. The challenge for practitioners in the modern era is to now integrate particle therapy technology with tumor biology to design appropriate clinical trials.

References

1 Ostrom, Q.T. et al. (2019). CBTRUS statistical report: Primary brain and other central nervous system tumors diagnosed in the United States in 2012–2016. *Neuro Oncology* 21 (Suppl. 5): v1–v100.

2 Sherman, J.C. et al. (2016). Neurocognitive effects of proton radiation therapy in adults with low-grade glioma. *Journal of Neuro-oncology* 126 (1): 157–164.

3 Weber, D.C. et al. (2018). Adjuvant postoperative high-dose radiotherapy for atypical and malignant meningioma: A phase-II parallel non-randomized and observation study (EORTC 22042–26042). *Radiotherapy and Oncology : Journal of the European Society for Therapeutic Radiology and Oncology* 128 (2): 260–265.

4 Weber, D.C. et al. (2020). Proton therapy for brain tumours in the area of evidence-based medicine. *The British Journal of Radiology* 93 (1107): 20190237.

5 Singh, S.K. et al. (2004). Identification of human brain tumour initiating cells. *Nature* 432 (7015): 396–401.

6 Ignatova, T.N. et al. (2002). Human cortical glial tumors contain neural stem-like cells expressing astroglial and neuronal markers in vitro. *Glia* 39 (3): 193–206.

7 Bjornsson, C.S. et al. (2015). It takes a village: Constructing the neurogenic niche. *Developmental Cell* 32 (4): 435–446.

8 Calabrese, C. et al. (2007). A perivascular niche for brain tumor stem cells. *Cancer Cell* 11 (1): 69–82.

9 Li, F. et al. (2016). Radiation induces the generation of cancer stem cells: A novel mechanism for cancer radioresistance. *Oncology Letters* 12 (5): 3059–3065.

10 Atashzar, M.R. et al. (2020). Cancer stem cells: A review from origin to therapeutic implications. *Journal of Cellular Physiology* 235 (2): 790–803.

11 Moncharmont, C. et al. (2014). Radiation-enhanced cell migration/invasion process: A review. *Critical Reviews in Oncology/hematology* 92 (2): 133–142.

12 Olar, A. et al. (2015). IDH mutation status and role of WHO grade and mitotic index in overall survival in grade II-III diffuse gliomas. *Acta Neuropathologica* 129 (4): 585–596.

13 Cancer Genome Atlas Research, N. et al. (2015). Comprehensive, Integrative Genomic Analysis of Diffuse Lower-Grade Gliomas. *The New England Journal of Medicine* 372 (26): 2481–2498.

14 Eckel-Passow, J.E. et al. (2015). *Glioma Groups Based on 1p/19q, IDH, and TERT Promoter Mutations in Tumors. The New England Journal of Medicine* 372 (26): 2499–2508.

15 Buckner, J.C. et al. (2016). Radiation plus Procarbazine, CCNU, and Vincristine in Low-Grade Glioma. *The New England Journal of Medicine* 374 (14): 1344–1355.

16 Laack, N.N., Sarkaria, J.N., and Buckner, J.C. (2015). Radiation Therapy Oncology Group 9802: Controversy or Consensus in the Treatment of Newly Diagnosed Low-Grade Glioma? *Seminars in Radiation Oncology* 25 (3): 197–202.

17 Seidel, S. et al. (2010). A hypoxic niche regulates glioblastoma stem cells through hypoxia inducible factor 2 alpha. *Brain* 133 (Pt 4): 983–995.

18 Hughes, M.A. et al. (2005). Primary brain tumors treated with steroids and radiotherapy: Low CD4 counts and risk of infection. *International Journal of Radiation Oncology, Biology, Physics* 62 (5): 1423–1426.

19 Grossman, S.A. et al. (2011). Immunosuppression in patients with high-grade gliomas treated with radiation and temozolomide. *Clinical Cancer Research : An Official Journal of the American Association for Cancer Research* 17 (16): 5473–5480.

20 Hesselager, G. and Holland, E.C. (2003). Using mice to decipher the molecular genetics of brain tumors. *Neurosurgery* 53 (3): 685–694. discussion 695.

21 Holland, E.C. (2001). Brain tumor animal models: Importance and progress. *Current Opinion in Oncology* 13 (3): 143–147.

22 Kerbel, R.S. (2003). Human tumor xenografts as predictive preclinical models for anticancer drug activity in humans: Better than commonly perceived-but they can be improved. *Cancer Biology & Therapy* 2 (4 Suppl 1): S134–9.

23 Hambardzumyan, D. et al. (2011). Genetic modeling of gliomas in mice: New tools to tackle old problems. *Glia* 59 (8): 1155–1168.

24 Cancer Genome Atlas Research, N. (2008). Comprehensive genomic characterization defines human glioblastoma genes and core pathways. *Nature* 455 (7216): 1061–1068.

25 Northcott, P.A. et al. (2012). Medulloblastomics: The end of the beginning. *Nature Reviews. Cancer* 12 (12): 818–834.

26 Chow, S.C. (2014). Adaptive clinical trial design. *Annual Review of Medicine* 65: 405–415.

27 Franken, N.A. et al. (2006). Clonogenic assay of cells in vitro. *Nature Protocols* 1 (5): 2315–2319.

28 Mehrian Shai, R. et al. (2005). Robustness of gene expression profiling in glioma specimen samplings and derived cell lines. *Brain Research. Molecular Brain Research* 136 (1–2): 99–103.

29 Stangl, S. et al. (2014). Selective in vivo imaging of syngeneic, spontaneous, and xenograft tumors using a novel tumor cell-specific hsp70 peptide-based probe. *Cancer Research* 74 (23): 6903–6912.

30 Pyonteck, S.M. et al. (2013). CSF-1R inhibition alters macrophage polarization and blocks glioma progression. *Nature Medicine* 19 (10): 1264–1272.

31 Lomax, A.J. (2009). Charged particle therapy: The physics of interaction. *The Cancer Journal* 15 (4): 285–291.

32 Lomax, A. (1999). Intensity modulation methods for proton radiotherapy. *Physics in Medicine and Biology* 44 (1): 185–205.

33 Lambrecht, M. et al. (2018). Radiation dose constraints for organs at risk in neuro-oncology; the European particle therapy network consensus. *Radiotherapy and Oncology : Journal of the European Society for Therapeutic Radiology and Oncology* 128 (1): 26–36.

34 Vatner, R.E. et al. (2018). Endocrine deficiency as a function of radiation dose to the hypothalamus and pituitary in pediatric and young adult patients with brain tumors. *Journal of Clinical Oncology : Official Journal of the American Society of Clinical Oncology* 36 (28): 2854–2862.

35 Zureick, A.H. et al. (2018). Left hippocampal dosimetry correlates with visual and verbal memory outcomes in survivors of pediatric brain tumors. *Cancer* 124 (10): 2238–2245.

36 Harrabi, S.B. et al. (2016). Dosimetric advantages of proton therapy over conventional radiotherapy with photons in young patients and adults with low-grade glioma. *Strahlentherapie Und Onkologie : Organ Der Deutschen Rontgengesellschaft . [Et Al]* 192 (11): 759–769.

37 Boehling, N.S. et al. (2012). Dosimetric comparison of three-dimensional conformal proton radiotherapy, intensity-modulated proton therapy, and intensity-modulated radiotherapy for treatment of pediatric craniopharyngiomas. *International Journal of Radiation Oncology, Biology, Physics* 82 (2): 643–652.

38 Adeberg, S. et al. (2018). Dosimetric comparison of proton radiation therapy, volumetric modulated arc therapy, and three-dimensional conformal radiotherapy based on intracranial tumor location. *Cancers (Basel)* 10 (11).

39 Correia, D. et al. (2019). Whole-ventricular irradiation for intracranial germ cell tumors: Dosimetric comparison of pencil beam scanned protons, intensity-modulated radiotherapy and volumetric-modulated arc therapy. *Clinical and Translational Radiation Oncology* 15: 53–61.

40 El-Fayech, C. et al. (2017). Cerebrovascular diseases in childhood cancer survivors: Role of the radiation dose to Willis circle arteries. *International Journal of Radiation Oncology, Biology, Physics* 97 (2): 278–286.

41 Seravalli, E. et al. (2018). Dosimetric comparison of five different techniques for craniospinal irradiation across 15 European centers: Analysis on behalf of the SIOP-E-BTG (radiotherapy working group)(). *Acta Oncology* 57 (9): 1240–1249.

42 Tamura, M. et al. (2017). Lifetime attributable risk of radiation-induced secondary cancer from proton beam therapy compared with that of intensity-modulated X-ray therapy in randomly sampled pediatric cancer patients. *Journal of Radiation Research* 58 (3): 363–371.

43 Kahalley, L.S. et al. (2019). Prospective, longitudinal comparison of neurocognitive change in pediatric brain tumor patients treated with proton radiotherapy versus surgery only. *Neuro Oncology* 21 (6): 809–818.

44 Verma, V., Simone, C.B., 2nd, and Mishra, M.V. (2018). Quality of life and Patient-Reported outcomes following proton radiation therapy: A systematic review. *Journal of the National Cancer Institute* 110 (4).

45 Unkelbach, J. et al. (2018). Robust radiotherapy planning. *Physics in Medicine and Biology* 63 (22): 22TR02.

46 McGowan, S.E. et al. (2015). Defining robustness protocols: A method to include and evaluate robustness in clinical plans. *Physics in Medicine and Biology* 60 (7): 2671–2684.

47 Paganetti, H. (2014). Relative biological effectiveness (RBE) values for proton beam therapy. Variations as a function of biological endpoint, dose, and linear energy transfer. *Physics in Medicine and Biology* 59 (22): R419–72.

48 Luhr, A. et al. (2018). Relative biological effectiveness in proton beam therapy - Current knowledge and future challenges. *Clinical and Translational Radiation Oncology* 9: 35–41.

49 Luhr, A. et al. (2018). "Radiobiology of Proton Therapy": Results of an international expert workshop. *Radiotherapy and Oncology : Journal of the European Society for Therapeutic Radiology and Oncology* 128 (1): 56–67.

50 Haas-Kogan, D. et al. (2018). National Cancer Institute Workshop on Proton therapy for children: Considerations Regarding Brainstem injury. *International Journal of Radiation Oncology, Biology, Physics* 101 (1): 152–168.

51 Buerki, R.A. et al. (2018). An overview of meningiomas. *Future Oncology* 14 (21): 2161–2177.

52 Haddad, A.F. et al. (2020). WHO Grade I Meningioma Recurrence: Identifying High Risk Patients Using Histopathological Features and the MIB-1 Index. *Frontiers in Oncology* 10: 1522.

53 Rogers, C.L. et al. (2020). High-risk Meningioma: Initial outcomes from NRG oncology/RTOG 0539. *International Journal of Radiation Oncology, Biology, Physics* 106 (4): 790–799.

54 Zamanipoor Najafabadi, A.H. et al. (2017). Impaired health-related quality of life in meningioma patients-a systematic review. *Neuro Oncology* 19 (7): 897–907.

55 Vernimmen, F.J. et al. (2001). Stereotactic proton beam therapy of skull base meningiomas. *International Journal of Radiation Oncology, Biology, Physics* 49 (1): 99–105.

56 Vlachogiannis, P. et al. (2017). Hypofractionated high-energy proton-beam irradiation is an alternative treatment for WHO grade I meningiomas. *Acta Neurochir (Wien)* 159 (12): 2391–2400.

57 Halasz, L.M. et al. (2011). Proton stereotactic radiosurgery for the treatment of benign meningiomas. *International Journal of Radiation Oncology, Biology, Physics* 81 (5): 1428–1435.

58 Weber, D.C. et al. (2004). Spot-scanning proton radiation therapy for recurrent, residual or untreated intracranial meningiomas. *Radiotherapy and Oncology : Journal of the European Society for Therapeutic Radiology and Oncology* 71 (3): 251–258.

59 Slater, J.D. et al. (2012). Fractionated proton radiotherapy for benign cavernous sinus meningiomas. *International Journal of Radiation Oncology, Biology, Physics* 83 (5): e633–7.

60 Debus, J. et al. (2001). High efficacy of fractionated stereotactic radiotherapy of large base-of-skull meningiomas: Long-term results. *Journal of Clinical Oncology : Official Journal of the American Society of Clinical Oncology* 19 (15): 3547–3553.

61 Kondziolka, D. et al. (2008). Radiosurgery as definitive management of intracranial meningiomas. *Neurosurgery* 62 (1): 53–58. discussion 58-60.

62 Hug, E.B. et al. (2000). Management of atypical and malignant meningiomas: Role of high-dose, 3D-conformal radiation therapy. *Journal of Neuro-oncology* 48 (2): 151–160.

63 Boskos, C. et al. (2009). Combined proton and photon conformal radiotherapy for intracranial atypical and malignant meningioma. *International Journal of Radiation Oncology, Biology, Physics* 75 (2): 399–406.

64 Chan, A.W. et al. (2012). Dose escalation with proton radiation therapy for high-grade meningiomas. *Technology in Cancer Research & Treatment* 11 (6): 607–614.

65 Combs, S.E. et al. (2010). Carbon ion radiation therapy for high-risk meningiomas. *Radiotherapy and Oncology : Journal* *of the European Society for Therapeutic Radiology and Oncology* 95 (1): 54–59.

66 Combs, S.E. et al. (2013). Prospective evaluation of early treatment outcome in patients with meningiomas treated with particle therapy based on target volume definition with MRI and 68Ga-DOTATOC-PET. *Acta Oncology* 52 (3): 514–520.

67 Barth, R.F., Zhang, Z., and Liu, T. (2018). A realistic appraisal of boron neutron capture therapy as a cancer treatment modality. *Cancer Commun (Lond)* 38 (1): 36.

68 Tamura, Y. et al. (2006). Boron neutron capture therapy for recurrent malignant meningioma. Case report. *Journal of Neurosurgery* 105 (6): 898–903.

69 Takeuchi, K. et al. (2018). Boron Neutron Capture Therapy for High-Grade Skull-Base Meningioma. *Journal of Neurological Surgery. Part B, Skull Base* 79 (Suppl 4): S322–S327.

70 Miyatake, S. et al. (2009). Pseudoprogression in boron neutron capture therapy for malignant gliomas and meningiomas. *Neuro Oncology* 11 (4): 430–436.

71 Kawabata, S. et al. (2013). Boron neutron capture therapy for recurrent high-grade meningiomas. *Journal of Neurosurgery* 119 (4): 837–844.

72 Beshr, R. et al. (2018). Preliminary feasibility study on differential diagnosis between radiation-induced cerebral necrosis and recurrent brain tumor by means of [(18)F] fluoro-borono-phenylalanine PET/CT. *Annals of Nuclear Medicine* 32 (10): 702–708.

73 Wu, A. et al. (2019). Efficacy and toxicity of particle radiotherapy in WHO grade II and grade III meningiomas: A systematic review. *Neurosurgical Focus* 46 (6): E12.

74 Sanford, N.N. et al. (2017). Prospective, randomized study of radiation dose escalation with combined proton-photon therapy for Benign Meningiomas. *International Journal of Radiation Oncology, Biology, Physics* 99 (4): 787–796.

75 Claus, E.B. and Black, P.M. (2006). Survival rates and patterns of care for patients diagnosed with supratentorial low-grade gliomas: Data from the SEER program, 1973-2001. *Cancer* 106 (6): 1358–1363.

76 Louis, D.N. et al. (2016). The 2016 World Health Organization Classification of Tumors of the Central Nervous System: A summary. *Acta Neuropathologica* 131 (6): 803–820.

77 Hegi, M.E. et al. (2005). MGMT gene silencing and benefit from temozolomide in glioblastoma. *The New England Journal of Medicine* 352 (10): 997–1003.

78 Barker, C.A. et al. (2014). Survival of patients treated with radiation therapy for anaplastic astrocytoma. *Radiology and Oncology* 48 (4): 381–386.

79 Abrey, L.E. et al. (2007). Survey of treatment recommendations for anaplastic oligodendroglioma. *Neuro Oncology* 9 (3): 314–318.

80 Dennis, E.R. et al. (2013). A comparison of critical structure dose and toxicity risks in patients with low grade gliomas treated with IMRT versus proton radiation therapy. *Technology in Cancer Research & Treatment* 12 (1): 1–9.

81 Baumann, B.C. et al. (2020). Comparative effectiveness of Proton vs Photon Therapy as part of concurrent Chemoradiotherapy for locally advanced cancer. *JAMA Oncology* 6 (2): 237–246.

82 Shih, H.A. et al. (2015). Proton therapy for low-grade gliomas: Results from a prospective trial. *Cancer* 121 (10): 1712–1719.

83 Tabrizi, S. et al. (2019). Long-term outcomes and late adverse effects of a prospective study on proton radiotherapy for patients with low-grade glioma. *Radiotherapy and Oncology : Journal of the European Society for Therapeutic Radiology and Oncology* 137: 95–101.

84 Wilkinson, B. et al. (2016). low levels of acute toxicity associated with proton therapy for low-grade Glioma: A proton collaborative group study. *International Journal of Radiation Oncology, Biology, Physics* 96 (2S): E135.

85 Fitzek, M.M. et al. (2001). Dose-escalation with proton/photon irradiation for Daumas-Duport lower-grade glioma: Results of an institutional phase I/II trial. *International Journal of Radiation Oncology, Biology, Physics* 51 (1): 131–137.

86 Mizumoto, M. et al. (2010). Phase I/II trial of hyperfractionated concomitant boost proton radiotherapy for supratentorial glioblastoma multiforme. *International Journal of Radiation Oncology, Biology, Physics* 77 (1): 98–105.

87 Fitzek, M.M. et al. (1999). Accelerated fractionated proton/photon irradiation to 90 cobalt gray equivalent for glioblastoma multiforme: Results of a phase II prospective trial. *Journal of Neurosurgery* 91 (2): 251–260.

88 Adeberg, S. et al. (2017). Sequential proton boost after standard chemoradiation for high-grade glioma. *Radiotherapy and Oncology : Journal of the European Society for Therapeutic Radiology and Oncology* 125 (2): 266–272.

89 Mizumoto, M. et al. (2015). Long-term survival after treatment of glioblastoma multiforme with hyperfractionated concomitant boost proton beam therapy. *Practical Radiation Oncology* 5 (1): e9–16.

90 Hasegawa, A. et al. (2012). Experience with carbon ion radiotherapy for WHO Grade 2 diffuse astrocytomas. *International Journal of Radiation Oncology, Biology, Physics* 83 (1): 100–106.

91 Mizoe, J.E. et al. (2007). Phase I/II clinical trial of carbon ion radiotherapy for malignant gliomas: Combined X-ray radiotherapy, chemotherapy, and carbon ion radiotherapy. *International Journal of Radiation Oncology, Biology, Physics* 69 (2): 390–396.

92 Miyatake, S. et al. (2016). Boron neutron capture therapy for Malignant brain tumors. *Neurologia Medico-chirurgica* 56 (7): 361–371.

93 Cardinale, R. et al. (2006). A phase II trial of accelerated radiotherapy using weekly stereotactic conformal boost for supratentorial glioblastoma multiforme: RTOG 0023. *International Journal of Radiation Oncology, Biology, Physics* 65 (5): 1422–1428.

94 Combs, S.E. et al. (2010). Randomized phase II study evaluating a carbon ion boost applied after combined radiochemotherapy with temozolomide versus a proton boost after radiochemotherapy with temozolomide in patients with primary glioblastoma: The CLEOPATRA trial. *BMC Cancer* 10: 478.

95 Mizumoto, M. et al. (2013). Reirradiation for recurrent malignant brain tumor with radiotherapy or proton beam therapy. Technical considerations based on experience at a single institution. *Strahlentherapie Und Onkologie : Organ Der Deutschen Rontgengesellschaft . [Et Al]* 189 (8): 656–663.

96 Saeed, A.M. et al. (2020). Clinical outcomes in patients with recurrent Glioblastoma treated with proton beam therapy Reirradiation: Analysis of the Multi-Institutional Proton Collaborative group registry. *Advances in Radiation Oncology* 5 (5): 978–983.

97 Combs, S.E. et al. (2010). Randomised phase I/II study to evaluate carbon ion radiotherapy versus fractionated stereotactic radiotherapy in patients with recurrent or progressive gliomas: The CINDERELLA trial. *BMC Cancer* 10: 533.

98 Northcott, P.A. et al. (2019). Medulloblastoma. *Nature Reviews Disease Primers* 5 (1): 11.

99 Remke, M. et al. (2011). Adult medulloblastoma comprises three major molecular variants. *Journal of Clinical Oncology : Official Journal of the American Society of Clinical Oncology* 29 (19): 2717–2723.

100 Smoll, N.R. (2012). Relative survival of childhood and adult medulloblastomas and primitive neuroectodermal tumors (PNETs). *Cancer* 118 (5): 1313–1322.

101 Packer, R.J. et al. (2006). Phase III study of craniospinal radiation therapy followed by adjuvant chemotherapy for newly diagnosed average-risk medulloblastoma. *Journal of Clinical Oncology : Official Journal of the American Society of Clinical Oncology* 24 (25): 4202–4208.

102 Merchant, T.E. et al. (1996). Medulloblastoma: Long-term results for patients treated with definitive radiation therapy during the computed tomography era. *International Journal of Radiation Oncology, Biology, Physics* 36 (1): 29–35.

103 Brodin, N.P. et al. (2012). Life years lost–comparing potentially fatal late complications after radiotherapy for pediatric medulloblastoma on a common scale. *Cancer* 118 (21): 5432–5440.

104 Brown, A.P. et al. (2013). Proton beam craniospinal irradiation reduces acute toxicity for adults with medulloblastoma. *International Journal of Radiation Oncology, Biology, Physics* 86 (2): 277–284.

105 Barney, C.L. et al. (2014). Technique, outcomes, and acute toxicities in adults treated with proton beam craniospinal irradiation. *Neuro Oncology* 16 (2): 303–309.

106 Wohlfahrt, P. and Richter, C. (2020). Status and innovations in pre-treatment CT imaging for proton therapy. *The British Journal of Radiology* 93 (1107): 20190590.

107 Farace, P. et al. (2011). Clinical target volume delineation in glioblastomas: Pre-operative versus post-operative/pre-radiotherapy MRI. *The British Journal of Radiology* 84 (999): 271–278.

108 Villanueva-Meyer, J.E., Mabray, M.C., and Cha, S. (2017). Current clinical brain tumor imaging. *Neurosurgery* 81 (3): 397–415.

109 Burnet, N.G. et al. (2004). Defining the tumour and target volumes for radiotherapy. *Cancer Imaging : The Official Publication of the International Cancer Imaging Society* 4 (2): 153–161.

110 Mullins, J.P. et al. (2016). Treatment planning for metals using an extended CT number scale. *Journal Of Applied Clinical Medical Physics / American College of Medical Physics* 17 (6): 179–188.

111 Wroe, A.J. et al. (2015). Clinical immobilization techniques for proton therapy. *Technology in Cancer Research & Treatment* 14 (1): 71–79.

112 Rutenberg, M.S. et al. (2020). Clinical outcomes following proton therapy for adult craniopharyngioma: A single-institution cohort study. *Journal of Neuro-oncology* 147 (2): 387–395.

113 Cao, W. et al. (2012). Uncertainty incorporated beam angle optimization for IMPT treatment planning. *Medical Physics* 39 (8): 5248–5256.

114 Shusharina, N. et al. (2019). Impact of aeration change and beam arrangement on the robustness of proton plans. *Journal Of Applied Clinical Medical Physics / American College of Medical Physics* 20 (3): 14–21.

115 Gu, W. et al. (2019). Robust beam orientation optimization for intensity-modulated proton therapy. *Medical Physics* 46 (8): 3356–3370.

116 Oancea, C. et al. (2018). Perturbations of radiation field caused by titanium dental implants in pencil proton beam therapy. *Physics in Medicine and Biology* 63 (21): 215020.

117 Shen, J. et al. (2015). Impact of range shifter material on proton pencil beam spot characteristics. *Medical Physics* 42 (3): 1335–1340.

118 Liu, H. and Chang, J.Y. (2011). Proton therapy in clinical practice. *Chinese Journal of Cancer* 30 (5): 315–326.

119 DeLaney, T.F. (2011). Proton therapy in the clinic. *Frontiers of Radiation Therapy and Oncology* 43: 465–485.

120 Grosshans, D.R. et al. (2014). Spot scanning proton therapy for malignancies of the base of skull: Treatment planning, acute toxicities, and preliminary clinical outcomes. *International Journal of Radiation Oncology, Biology, Physics* 90 (3): 540–546.

121 Liu, W. et al. (2012). Robust optimization of intensity modulated proton therapy. *Medical Physics* 39 (2): 1079–1091.

122 Ma, J. et al. (2014). A GPU-accelerated and Monte Carlo-based intensity modulated proton therapy optimization system. *Medical Physics* 41 (12): 121707.

123 Quan, E.M. et al. (2013). Preliminary evaluation of multifield and single-field optimization for the treatment planning of spot-scanning proton therapy of head and neck cancer. *Medical Physics* 40 (8): 081709.

124 Jhaveri, J. et al. (2018). Proton vs. Photon Radiation Therapy for Primary Gliomas: An Analysis of the National Cancer Data Base. *Frontiers in Oncology* 8: 440.

125 Jalali, R. et al. (2017). Efficacy of Stereotactic Conformal Radiotherapy vs Conventional Radiotherapy on Benign and Low-Grade Brain Tumors: A Randomized Clinical Trial. *JAMA Oncol* 3 (10): 1368–1376.

126 Combs, S.E. et al. (2013). Proton and carbon ion radiotherapy for primary brain tumors and tumors of the skull base. *Acta Oncology* 52 (7): 1504–1509.

127 Hauswald, H. et al. (2012). First experiences in treatment of low-grade glioma grade I and II with proton therapy. *Radiation Oncology* 7: 189.

128 Maquilan, G. et al. (2014). Acute toxicity profile of patients with low-grade gliomas and meningiomas receiving proton therapy. *American Journal of Clinical Oncology* 37 (5): 438–443.

129 Mohan, R. et al. (2020 Feb 25). Proton therapy reduces the likelihood of high-grade radiation-induced lymphopenia in glioblastoma patients: Phase II Randomized study of Protons vs. Photons. *Neuro Oncology*. 23(2):284–294. doi: 10.1093/neuonc/noaa182. PMID: 32750703; PMCID: PMC7906048.

130 Chen, W. et al. (2012). Including robustness in multi-criteria optimization for intensity-modulated proton therapy. *Physics in Medicine and Biology* 57 (3): 591–608.

131 McGowan, S.E., Burnet, N.G., and Lomax, A.J. (2013). Treatment planning optimisation in proton therapy. *The British Journal of Radiology* 86 (1021): 20120288.

132 Bisogni, M.G. et al. (2017). INSIDE in-beam positron emission tomography system for particle range monitoring in hadrontherapy. *Journal of Medical Imaging (Bellingham)* 4 (1): 011005.

133 Gondim, D.D. et al. (2019). Determining IDH-Mutational status in gliomas using IDH1-R132H antibody and polymerase chain reaction. *Applied Immunohistochemistry & Molecular Morphology : Aimm / official publication of the Society for Applied Immunohistochemistry* 27 (10): 722–725.

134 Wang, Y. et al. (2018). Combining immunotherapy and Radiotherapy for Cancer Treatment: Current challenges and future directions. *Frontiers in Pharmacology* 9: 185.

135 Rajani, K.R. et al. (2018). Harnessing radiation biology to augment immunotherapy for Glioblastoma. *Frontiers in Oncology* 8: 656.

136 Grassberger, C. et al. (2011). Variations in linear energy transfer within clinical proton therapy fields and the potential for biological treatment planning. *International Journal of Radiation Oncology, Biology, Physics* 80 (5): 1559–1566.

137 Mohan, R. et al. (2017). Radiobiological issues in proton therapy. *Acta Oncology* 56 (11): 1367–1373.

138 Montay-Gruel, P. et al. (2020). *Hypo-fractionated FLASH-RT as an Effective Treatment against Glioblastoma that Reduces Neurocognitive Side Effects in Mice*. Clin Cancer Res.

139 Weber, D.C. et al. (2012). Spot scanning-based proton therapy for intracranial meningioma: Long-term results from the Paul Scherrer Institute. *International Journal of Radiation Oncology, Biology, Physics* 83 (3): 865–871.

140 McDonald, M.W. et al. (2015). Proton therapy for atypical meningiomas. *Journal of Neuro-oncology* 123 (1): 123–128.

141 Murray, F.R. et al. (2017). Long-term clinical outcomes of pencil beam scanning proton therapy for Benign and Non-benign Intracranial Meningiomas. *International Journal of Radiation Oncology, Biology, Physics* 99 (5): 1190–1198.

142 El Shafie, R.A. et al. (2018). Clinical outcome after particle therapy for meningiomas of the skull base: Toxicity and local control in patients treated with active rasterscanning. *Radiation Oncology* 13 (1): 54.

143 Parsons, D.W. et al. (2008). An integrated genomic analysis of human glioblastoma multiforme. *Science* 321 (5897): 1807–1812. doi: 10.1126/science.1164382. Epub 2008 Sep 4. PMID: 18772396; PMCID: PMC2820389.

14

Ocular Malignancies

Kavita K. Mishra, MD MPH[1], Armin R. Afshar, MD MBA MAS[2], Scholey Jessica, MA, Andrzej Kacperek, PhD[3], and Bertil E. Damato, MD PhD FRCOphth[4]

1 Director, Ocular Tumor Radiation Therapy Program, Department of Radiation Oncology, University of California San Francisco, San Francisco, CA
2 Ocular Oncology, Department of Ophthalmology, Wayne & Glady Valley Center for Vision, University of California San Francisco, San Francisco, CA
3 Emeritus Physics, Clatterbridge Cancer Centre, Wirral, United Kingdom
4 Ocular Oncology, Oxford Eye Hospital, University of Oxford, United Kingdom
Corresponding author: Kavita K. Mishra, MD MPH Professor, Department of Radiation Oncology Director, Ocular Tumor Radiation Therapy Program University of California San Francisco 1600 Divisadero Street, H-1031San Francisco, CA 94115

TABLE OF CONTENTS

Malignant ocular tumors are rare cancers and can threaten vision, quality of life, and life expectancy. Radiation therapy (RT) with external beam radiation, plaque brachytherapy, stereotactic techniques, and charged particles, including proton (PBRT), helium, and carbon-ion therapy, have been used in treatment. This chapter focuses on the use of particle radiation for treatment of uveal melanomas (UMs), intraocular metastases, and other diseases of the eye and orbit. Ocular particle beam radiotherapy, most commonly proton therapy, for UM is associated with excellent local tumor control and eye preservation compared with other eye-conserving forms of primary treatment. Proton beam is also utilized for other malignant and benign tumors, including conjunctival melanomas, choroidal metastases, circumscribed and diffuse hemangiomas, angiomas, and retinoblastomas, as primary, salvage, or adjuvant treatment with combined modality therapy.

In total, approximately 47,400 ocular patients have been treated with particle beams worldwide (1975–2020), mainly with proton beam with about 500 of these patients treated by helium and carbon-ion beams [1]. The physical characteristics of particle therapy allow for uniform dose distribution, minimal scatter, and sharp dose fall-off making it ideal for ocular tumors, which are in close proximity to critical structures. Dose optimization is designed to achieve local tumor control and minimize acute and late ocular morbidity for structures including the optic disc/nerve, macula, retina, lens, ciliary body, cornea, limbus/limbal stem cells, lacrimal gland, tear ducts, upper eyelid and eyelashes, lower eyelid, and bony orbit. Specialty centers and significant expertise have developed to provide a thoughtful and rigorous approach to advancing care for patients with rare ocular malignancies.

14.1 Uveal Melanoma

14.1.1 Anatomy and Epidemiology

UM is the most common adult primary intraocular malignancy and the most common indication for ocular proton beam radiation internationally. UMs arise in the choroid, ciliary body, and/or iris, which together constitute the uveal tract or vascular support layer of the eye (Figure 14.1a–d). Approximately 80% of UMs involve the choroid (the posterior uveal tract under the retina), 5–10% involve the iris, and 10–15% involve the ciliary body, which contains the muscle responsible for accommodation and lens movement. As choroidal lesions grow, Bruch's membrane (the membrane between choroid and retina) can stretch and rupture allowing tumor protrusion into the retina and creation of a characteristic "collar button" or mushroom-shaped tumor. Extraocular extension is significantly less common and may occur via aqueous channels, ciliary arteries, vortex veins, ciliary nerves, and the optic nerve [2].

The annual incidence of UM is estimated to be between 4 and 7 cases per million people in the United States, Canada, and Europe [3,4]. Approximately 1500–2000 new cases are diagnosed each year in the United States. Peak incidence is between 60 and 79 years of age, with <2% younger than 20 years old at diagnosis [5]. UM occurs more frequently in people with light-colored skin and eyes. Incidence rates are generally higher for males (RR = 1.3). Ocular melanomas (OM) represent ~3–5% of all melanomas, and OM includes 85% UMs, 5% conjunctival melanomas, and ~10% occur at other sites. This chapter is mainly focused on UMs as the most common primary eye tumor referred for definitive particle/proton beam therapy.

The etiology of UM is largely unknown and may include environmental, host, and genetic factors. It is extremely rare to have bilateral tumors, multiple UMs, or familial UM [6]. The lifetime risk of UM is estimated to be 1 in 400 in patients with oculodermal melanocytosis (also known as nevus of Ota, a condition of excessive melanocytes that cause hyperpigmentation of the eye and surrounding tissues). Other predisposing conditions are melanocytoma and the BAP1 tumor predisposition syndrome.

Risk factors, particularly for young patients, are challenging to delineate and may include factors such as skin/eye color, family history, sun/snow burn history, artificial UV light or other unusual solar event exposure, tanning bed use, hormonal exposure in pregnancy, and arc welding exposure [7–10]. A recent case series shows retinoid therapy use, which has been linked to various benign and reversible ocular effects, to be seen in a limited number of UM cases in young adults, though importantly no causal link is claimed [11–13]. Intermittent outdoor leisure, chronic occupational sunlight exposure, and birth latitude appear to be nonsignificant factors in meta-analyses. Further systematic study of UM patients for risk factors and genetics is required to provide relevant etiological data.

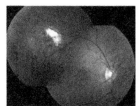 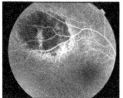 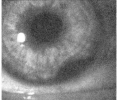 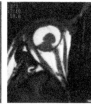

Figure 14.1 Uveal melanoma examples: (a) fundus photograph of right eye superotemporal choroidal melanoma, (b) fluoroscein angiogram, (c) iris melanoma, and (d) MRI of collar button choroidal melanoma.

14.1.2 Pathology and Genetics

In patients undergoing irradiation, enucleation, endoresection, or eye wall resection, several factors indicate increased risk of metastatic disease, which commonly involves the liver and portends poor life expectancy. These include (1) tumor clinical features, such as large tumor size (greater tumor diameter and height/thickness), ciliary body invasion, extraocular spread; (2) pathologic features, such as presence of epithelioid cells, high mitotic rate, large nucleolar size, tumor necrosis, lymphocytic infiltration, extravascular matrix patterns, such as closed loops; (3) genetic features, including chromosome 3 loss ("monosomy 3"), chromosome 8 gain, *BAP1* mutation, Class 2 gene expression profile (GEP), *PRAME* positivity; and (4) patient factors such as older age [6,14–19]. UM tumors are graded with pathologic patterns including spindle, mixed, and epithelioid types, with the presence of epithelioid cells being associated with a worse prognosis as noted.

Various molecular and genetic markers are under study with tools including gene expression profiling, multiplex ligation-dependent probe amplification (MLPA), and next-generation sequencing (NGS) [16,20]. Gene expression profiling via transcriptomic classification of UMs is based on RNA analysis of the primary tumor from a fine-needle biopsy or surgical sample [17]. The DecisionDx-UM Gene Expression Profile Test (Castle Biosciences, Friendswood, Texas, USA) provides a risk-stratification report by Class 1A, 1B, and 2 as well as *PRAME* status [18].

A "Class 1A" GEP signature is associated with an excellent prognosis, with 98% metastasis-free rate at 5 years. Patients with "Class 1B" tumors have a 79% metastasis-free rate at 5 years. Patients with "Class 2" tumors have a high risk of metastatic death, with a 28% metastasis-free rate at 5 years. The latter class is associated with other predictors of poor prognosis, including epithelioid cytology, looping extracellular matrix patterns, and chromosome 3 loss [17,18]. GEP class is not associated with differential local tumor response to proton RT. No difference has been noted in the mean change in tumor thickness 24 months after proton RT or in the overall rate of thickness change by GEP class [21].

PRAME (preferentially expressed antigen in melanoma) oncogene has been studied as an independent prognostic biomarker in UM that identifies increased metastatic risk in patients with GEP Class 1 or disomy 3 tumors [18]. Metastasis in Class 1 tumors is strongly associated with *PRAME* expression. Chromosome copy number changes associated with Class 1-*PRAME* + tumors include gain of 1q, 6p, 8q, and 9q, and loss of 6q and 11q. *PRAME* expression is also associated with larger tumor diameter and *SF3B1* mutations.

Tumor genetic information with chromosome 3 loss, *BAP1* mutation, and class 2 GEP correlate most strongly with metastatic death [19]. Chromosome 8 gain also confers increased mortality risk. Some studies show that both chromosome 3 loss and 8 gain must be present for metastasis to occur. Compared with monosomy 3 alone, survival is better when there is chromosome 6p gain. *GNAQ* or *GNA11* mutations are common (85% of UMs) and can be used in differentiating UM from other lesions, i.e., choroidal metastases [22,23]. *BAP1* tumor suppressor gene mutations on chromosome 3 are found in 49% of UM and are strongly correlated with metastasis. Mutations in *EIF1AX* and *SF3B1* are associated with low and intermediate risk, respectively. Other less common UM mutations include *SRSF2*, *U2AF1*, *PLCB4*, and *CYSLTR2* [19,22–25].

Currently, at the University of California, San Francisco, a next-generation genetic sequencing tool (the UCSF500 assay) is being used clinically to interrogate approximately 500 genes that are frequently mutated in cancers, including genes known to be altered in UM [19]. UCSF500 is used routinely on UM tumor samples and has detected chromosomal copy number changes and missense mutations that correlate strongly with metastasis predictors, including GEP. Continued development in genetic testing has provided clinically relevant data for prognostication and may potentially elucidate targets for personalized cancer therapy.

14.1.3 Staging

The current TNM (tumor, nodes, and metastases) staging system is based on the American Joint Committee on Cancer (AJCC) Staging Manual 8th edition [26]. The AJCC tumor (T) classification is defined according to a matrix of the tumor dimensions, including the largest basal diameter and the tumor thickness or height. The AJCC staging also subgroups tumors based on ciliary body involvement and extent of extrascleral extension. Of note, ciliary body and choroidal melanomas are staged differently from iris melanomas, which are often detected earlier and may be smaller in size as defined by clock hours and extension. T-stage for iris melanomas is based on size, presence of secondary glaucoma, extension into the ciliary body, and/or choroid, scleral, and extrascleral extension. Iris melanomas originate from the iris and are predominantly located in this region of the uvea. If less than half of the tumor volume is located within the iris, the tumor may have originated in the ciliary body, and classification may need to be adjusted accordingly [27].

Stage grouping is based on a matrix by T-classification for stages I–III. Any nodal or metastatic spread is considered stage IV disease. The staging system does not take tumor location within the various subsections of the uvea (i.e., peripapillary) or visual acuity (VA) into consideration, though this may certainly influence treatment modality choice and optimization.

14.2 Clinical Experience and Practical Considerations

14.2.1 Patient Presentation

Initial clinical presentation of UM can vary and approximately 33% of patients are asymptomatic at the time of diagnosis [6]. Usually these patients present to their local ophthalmologist or optometrist either for a routine examination or a refraction test. Symptomatic patients may present with visual symptoms, such as distortion, vision loss, floaters, scotomas, or flashing lights. Macular tumors can result in distorted central vision and larger tumors can produce an exudative retinal detachment and subretinal or vitreous hemorrhage also causing vision loss. Ciliary body or anterior choroidal melanomas can produce an overlying episcleral area of vascular engorgement, known as a "sentinel vessel." Iris melanomas may be noted by patients or providers visually. Less commonly, large intraocular melanomas can produce significant inflammation or necrosis to produce a unilateral cataract or severe intraocular pain.

Initial examination(s) may be performed by an optometrist, ophthalmologist, retinal specialist, emergency room physician, or other provider. Initial assessment may include clinical delineation of tumor size (diameter and thickness), location, geometry, coloration, and associated findings (i.e., subretinal fluid, orange pigment, exudative retinal detachment) as well as ocular imaging. UM pigmentation can be variable with as many as 25% of cases being amelanotic. Lesions that most commonly simulate UM include nevi, choroidal hemangiomas, rhegmatogenous retinal detachments, and choroidal metastases. Based on the initial clinical evaluation, patients may then be referred for further care to an ocular oncology center.

14.2.2 Ocular Oncology Work Up

Ocular oncology assessment includes establishing the diagnosis and determining the suitability of various treatment options. Slit-lamp examination, binocular indirect ophthalmoscopy, color fundus/iris photography, and ultrasonography (US) are performed. For posterior choroidal melanomas, fundus autofluorescence and optical coherence tomography (OCT) may be used. Ultrasound is used to measure tumor height and axial length. Ultrasonographer experience is important for accuracy and reproducibility, particularly for anterior tumors, or if there is extensive subretinal fluid. US and magnetic resonance imaging (MRI) may underestimate lesion diameters if there is a large area of relatively flat tumor extension. For pseudophakic patients, their pre-cataract surgery axial length can be retrieved and confirmed on MRI or CT as needed. Biopsy may be offered if there is diagnostic uncertainty or for survival prognostication.

MRI has been used in a limited fashion for UMs and may be of increasing utility for particle therapy centers in the future [28–30]. High-resolution MRI can be useful in the delineation of UM tumors, localized extraocular extension, and in the differentiation between UM and simulating lesions. MRI can also provide critical structure and postsurgical tantalum marker data which may improve tumor volume delineation for treatment planning purposes and is an area of active study.

Baseline metastatic screening is routinely performed as part of the initial cancer staging. The most common sites of metastatic spread are the liver, lung, and bone. Evaluation includes a thorough physical examination and imaging of the chest, abdomen, and pelvis with CT scan and/or MRI and PET scan.

Small pigmented uveal lesions (generally ≤3 mm in thickness and ≤10 mm in diameter) that appear inactive and have no clinical risk factors on examination may be considered for serial observation with close observation and imaging with serial photography and ultrasound [31,32]. Approximately two-thirds or more of these lesions may not grow and undergo "malignant transformation" and these patients hence may maintain good vision and no treatment effects in the affected eye. Treatment may be recommended; however, if there is documented growth, clinical, or visual changes, and/or associated risk factors, including tumors with larger bases, mushroom shape, thickness more than 2 mm, retinal detachment, subretinal fluid, orange pigment, diffuse (flat) configurations, ciliary body invasion, multifocal disease, potential concern for ring melanoma, and possible scleral or optic nerve penetration [31–33].

14.2.3 Therapeutic Decision-making

Overall, as UM is a rare tumor worldwide, there are various surgical and radiation-based therapeutic alternatives; however, no standardized care pathway has been defined. Prospective and retrospective studies demonstrate comparable survival rates between enucleation and irradiation [34,35]. Surgical options include local resection (with or without adjuvant radiation), enucleation or exenteration, and laser treatment, including transpupillary therapy, photodynamic therapy, and more recently, Aura AU-011 nanoparticle therapy [6,36,37]. Radiation modalities include charged particles (i.e., protons, helium, or carbon), plaque brachytherapy, and radiosurgery. Plaque brachytherapy and enucleation are the most commonly accessible UM treatment modalities worldwide.

Treatment outcomes and relative comparisons of particle/proton therapy with other treatment options are detailed later in this chapter. Tumor and patient parameters, provider and patient preference, and accessibility to specialized treatment facilities may be important to selecting the optimal radiation modality. Proton and particle beam radiation is considered the "gold standard" of care for UM given the high level of tumor control and overall eye preservation achieved [38–45]. The surgical and radiation techniques used in treatment of UMs with particle, most commonly proton therapy, are described in detail.

14.2.4 Marker Surgery and Biopsy

Standard clinical practice for UM patients who have decided to undergo proton beam therapy includes tantalum marker insertion. Tantalum markers (commonly referred to as "clips" or "rings") are radio-opaque, 2.5 mm diameter, 0.17 mm thickness, MRI-compatible, and an essential aspect of X-ray tumor localization for proton beam planning and daily image-guided treatment [29]. Most commonly, for choroidal and ciliary body tumors, these markers are surgically placed as close to the tumor edge as possible intraoperatively. Transillumination allows for tumor delineation and appropriate scleral marking of the tumor edge. Indirect ophthalmoscopy and scleral indentation may also be used to localize the markers as needed. Generally, four (range three to five) tantalum markers are sutured onto the sclera at the tumor margins. Marker-to-limbus, marker-to-marker, and marker-to-tumor measurements are taken.

For small, post-equatorial tumors, exposure may be enhanced by disinserting the overlying rectus muscles. To minimize risk of postoperative diplopia, the suture knot-to-limbus distance is measured and recorded before dividing the muscle. This allows precise muscle reinsertion to the original knot-to-limbus distance. For iris and small ciliary body melanomas with visible anterior chamber extension, proton beam radiotherapy may be administered without tantalum markers [46]. A final surgical assessment is reviewed with the radiation oncology team for use in proton planning and includes the following information (Figure 14.2a,b):

(a) posterior fundus or anterior iris drawing of the tumor and markers;

(b) intraoperative photograph for additional marker documentation;

(c) marker-to-limbus, marker-to-marker ("interclip"), marker-to-tumor measurements; markers given anatomic reference to delineate them on orthogonal X-ray imaging (i.e., superior or inferior, anterior or posterior, and temporal or nasal);

(d) tumor basal dimensions (circumferential and radial measurements), tumor height, distances of tumor margin to disc, tumor margin to fovea, anterior tumor margin to limbus if applicable, clock hours of tumor extension, and eye axial length;

(e) additional surgical notes for planning optimization, including potential areas of extension, extraocular spread, diffuse flat spread, pigmentation causing difficulty with transillumination (i.e., nevus of Ota, ocular melanocytosis), intraoperative procedures or complications (i.e., silicone oil tamponade [47], vitreous hemorrhage, exudative retinal detachment) which may affect treatment gaze angle options, etc.

At the time of marker insertion, tumor biopsy can be performed for diagnostic and/or prognostic purpose. Tumor sample can be evaluated for histopathology, gene expression profiling, MLPA, or next-generation genetic sequencing [19]. The tumor genetic data provide individual risk assessment for systemic disease, guidance for follow-up metastatic imaging, as well as potential molecular therapeutic targets for study.

There are a limited number of UM patients that may not undergo tantalum marker surgery due to comorbidities, visible iris/anterior tumor not requiring markers, extremely thin sclera, or rarely by preference. These patients may be aligned with clinical landmarks as well as visible tumor if present (i.e., iris) and confirmed by a "light field" replicating the radiation

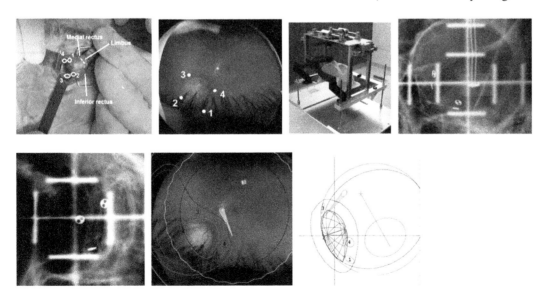

Figure 14.2 Patient pathway: (a) surgical tantalum clip placement, (b) fundus photograph clip assessment, (c) simulation head mask, (d) AP simulation film with clips, (e) lateral simulation film, (f) fundus view of treatment plan using EYEPLAN with disc and macular sparing techniques, and (g) beam's eye view of treatment plan.

beam entrance field. For posterior tumors not externally visible, this clinical "light-field" setup may require greater margin to account for lack of daily image guidance with markers [46].

The tantalum markers are inert and generally left in place even after RT is complete. In circumstances where patients experience discomfort due to markers, especially anterior ones, those may be removed after RT is completed. If a marker falls off on its own, the team must decide whether the marker must be replaced or if planning can continue with the available information.

Certain methods are being researched and thus far not in common practice worldwide. MRI-based planning is under study for clinical use with or without tantalum markers [28,30]. Feasibility studies have been done to test the placement of the tantalum markers away from the tumor edge due to the beam angle(s) used and/or angle of orthogonal X-ray imaging equipment in the treatment room [48]. In addition, initial testing of titanium markers, rather than tantalum, has shown benefit in minimizing distortion on CT scans for use in eye RT planning [49].

14.2.5 Radiation Consult and Simulation

Patients may be seen for consult in radiation oncology before or after tantalum marker surgery depending on clinic flow and decision-making needs. The most common international practices for proton ocular radiation care are detailed below.

Radiation oncology consult includes a thorough clinical history including symptoms, tumor details, risk factors, along with prior ocular history (i.e., cataract surgery, ocular trauma history, other eye disease or interventions), systemic disease with potential ocular risk (i.e., hypertension, diabetes, etc.), family history of cancer or ocular disease, prior history of radiation to the eye or surrounding tissues, medications and use of antioxidant/nutritional supplements, and other relevant history.

Comprehensive exam is performed, including as appropriate: (a) fundus exam; (b) external exam of any visible tumor (i.e., iris), conjunctival findings and sentinel vessels, postoperative changes; (c) supplementary pictures (i.e., additional views of iris/visible tumor for planning use or if change since last ophthalmologic picture); (d) extraocular movement/visual limitations and ability to gaze (i.e., for planning purpose/gaze angle); (e) interpupillary distance (in case healthy eye is needed for gaze fixation); and (f) any constitutional, nodal, pulmonary, or abdominal findings. Pregnancy status if applicable should be noted for appropriate precautions or therapy decisions.

During the simulation, a thermoplastic head mask and bite block or chin rest is made for head immobilization, most commonly in the seated position. During the COVID-19 pandemic, multiple safety precautions were implemented at certain institutions, including a chin rest alternative to the bite block (Figure 14.3a) [50]. The chin rest reduced salivary drip, increased patient comfort (reduced claustrophobia), and resulted in equivalent immobilization reproducibility.

The tantalum markers are imaged and serve as radiographic markers of the tumor for treatment planning and, ultimately, daily image-guided treatment delivery. Orthogonal images are taken at neutral gaze. If desired, two or more gaze angles can be imaged at simulation (Figure 14.2c–e), including potential treatment gaze angles. Data may be used for estimating torsion. Three-dimensional marker positioning is confirmed with operative notes/drawings. Specific CT/MRI imaging sequences can be utilized as noted in emerging literature [28–30].

14.3 Treatment Planning and Delivery

14.3.1 Eyeplan

Eyeplan treatment planning software (TPS) is the commonly used proton ocular RT planning system worldwide [51,52]. It includes eye and tumor modeling, gaze angle optimization, aperture design, beam parameter delineation, dose–volume histogram (DVH) analysis, marker alignment, and daily image-guided positioning assessment. The TPS uses a geometrical eye

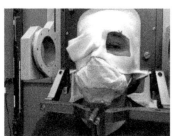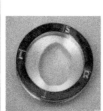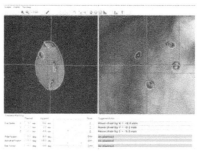

Figure 14.3 Treatment delivery (a) patient setup with chin rest in COVID-19 pandemic, (b) brass aperture, and (c) image guided daily treatment alignment with tantalum markers.

model scaled to the individual anatomy. Tumor measurements are based on clinical data from iris/fundus photography, ocular biometry, ultrasound images, CT/MRI, and intraoperative caliper measurements.

The following treatment planning inputs are used:

(a) tantalum marker spatial coordinates from orthogonal X-rays (simulation films);

(b) posterior fundus photograph (with disc and fovea for spatial calibration) for choroidal/ciliary body tumors, or anterior iris photograph for anterior iris tumors or ciliary body tumors with iris invasion;

(c) eye axial length;

(d) marker-to-limbus, marker-to-marker, marker-to-tumor distances;

(e) tumor dimensions, tumor-to-disc/fovea distances, anterior tumor margin-to-limbus if applicable, clock hours;

(f) specific tumor features, i.e., collar button, extraocular extension (drawn as a second tumor), location of tumor apex.

The fundus photograph image is oriented according to the macula-disc location. For anterior tumors, the image is oriented via the pupil center and iris edge. The tumor volume is drawn based on the clinical data, surgeon's intraoperative mapping/photograph, measurements, fundus photography, MRI images, and X-ray marker localization. The *Eyeplan* software schematically displays a three-dimensional model of the patient's eye and tumor (Figure 14.2f–g).

Of note, there is potential for geometric distortion of the fundus photograph for anterior tumors, since a 3D spherical surface is projected as a 2D image. Distortion is minimal near the posterior pole of the eye. The magnitude of this possible error at a distance of point 5 and 12 mm lateral to macula resulted in a distance error of ~0.2 and ~2.5 mm, respectively [53]. Such distortions are accounted for clinically in the fusion, tumor delineation, and modeling.

Once the tumor/eye model is confirmed, the optimal gaze fixation angle can be determined based on tumor coverage and critical structure dosing. Any limits due to patient vision loss or extraocular movement limits should be considered in gaze angle selection. Systematic rotation of the eye model around its central axis allows for visualization of target and critical structures and specific dose parameters are evaluated for normal tissue sparing. Gaze angle optimization is benefited by planner/physics team experience and automation of this process is being tested [54].

The tumor is centered on a single anterior entrance beam and an aperture is developed with a standard safety margin around the tumor profile. The aperture margin as drawn in *Eyeplan* represents the 50% circumferential isodose line. The aperture and distal margins are developed to encompass the following potential random or systematic uncertainties: (a)

geometrical eye model, i.e., eye length, tumor dimensions, marker positioning; (b) eye positioning and alignment throughout the treatment time; and (c) specific beam line parameters, i.e., range, penumbra, stopping power ratio [55].

The necessary beam range and modulation depth is calculated based on the appropriate depth of beam penetration and width of the spread-out-Bragg peak (SOBP) necessary to encompass the target volume and margin. The DVHs for each critical structure are calculated and the dose distribution is evaluated in the fundus view and multiple additional planes through the model. The relationship of the markers to the central beam axis and the collimator (aperture) are projected to ensure proper planned tumor coverage and daily treatment alignment. Figure 14.2g illustrates a beam's eye view with chosen gaze angle resulting in tumor coverage and normal tissue sparing of the lens, optic disc, and macula.

14.3.2 Planning Optimization and Dose–Volume Parameters

A rational tumor/critical structure dose evaluation is used to optimize treatment parameters, i.e., lateral margin, aperture shape, distal range, and gaze angle. Critical structures are systematically evaluated to minimize side effects, including to the (a) posterior structures, i.e., optic disc/nerve, macula, retina; (b) anterior structures, i.e., lens, ciliary body, cornea (particularly the limbus/limbal stem cells); and (c) other tissues, i.e., lacrimal gland, tear ducts, upper eyelid and eyelashes, lower eyelid, and bony orbit.

Apertures may vary between institutions and beamlines depending on lateral dose fall-off (Figure 14.3b) [56]. The aperture margin (50% isodose line) is commonly set at 2.5 mm around the tumor margin circumferentially and can be reduced focally to 2 mm near the macula, disc, or other critical structure as appropriate (Figure 14.4a). Some institutions increase the circumferential safety margin to 3 mm, particularly for ciliary body tumors.

The distal margin past the tumor posterior edge is commonly 2.5–3 mm The distal margin may be decreased to 2 mm in selected cases and depending on beam characteristics to minimize dose posteriorly to the disc/macula. Some centers increase distal margin to 4 mm particularly for ciliary body tumors (Table 14.1). Ciliary body tumors may be able to be treated without dose to the optic disc/macula, given sharp beam fall-off distally (Figure 14.4b).

Wedge filters may be used in a limited fashion to reduce the disc dose or treatment volume when appropriate (Figure 14.4c). For iris melanoma treatments, dilating drops may be used to reduce the target area.

Eyelid toxicity, particularly for the upper eyelid with potential keratinization of the palpebral conjunctiva, is reduced by gaze angle selection to minimize treating through the upper lid

(a)

(b)

(c)   (d)

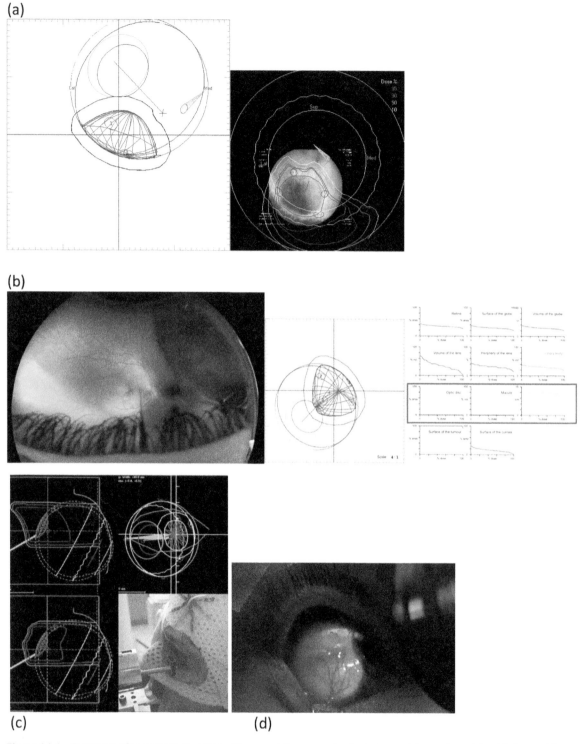

Figure 14.4 Examples of treatment planning with normal tissue sparing techniques: (a) macula notch with focused 2 mm aperture margin and fundus view showing macular sparing, (b) anterior ciliary body tumor with disc sparing using posterior beam fall-off, (c) wedge and compensator use for beam shaping, and (d) eyelid retraction and light field confirmation.

and retraction techniques (Figure 14.4d). Transpalpebral treatment may be used if the upper eyelid is in the field to minimize long-term complications by pulling the lash line out of the field and using the fellow eye for fixation [57]. Eyelid in the field can

be estimated within the planning model or at the time of set up, and range adjustments may be made accordingly.

DVH parameters can be utilized for data-informed ocular treatment planning optimization for normal tissue sparing

Table 14.1   Sample target volumes for primary proton RT for uveal melanoma.

Volume	Target
GTV	Gross tumor (by imaging, surgical markers, clinical data)
CTV-PTV	Aperture margin (defined as 50% isodose line) may vary across institutions, commonly 2.5 mm circumferential margin around "GTV" [56]. Consider focal reduction to 2 mm at critical structure (i.e., macula, disc) or increase to 3 mm particularly for ciliary body tumors, as appropriate and based on beam characteristics. Aperture margin <2 mm is not recommended [58]
	Accordingly, 90% isodose line may vary based on beamline and institutional preference, commonly ~1–2 mm margin on GTV [56,58]
	Distal margin beyond posterior tumor edge, commonly 2.5–3 mm. Consider 2–4 mm as appropriate per institutional preference

GTV = Gross tumor volume; CTV-PTV = clinical microscopic disease and planning margin.

(Table 14.2). Multiple reports identify volume of the macula and optic nerve length receiving 50% of total dose ("V50%" or ~28–30 GyE) as independent DVH predictors of post-PBRT vision loss [59–61].

For example, a relationship of V50% to the macula and optic nerve with time to first decrease in best corrected VA is shown in Figure 14.5a [59]. There is a dominant effect of the macular DVH parameter. Even when the most favorable patients with both low macular and nerve dose are excluded (i.e., V50% to 0% macula and ≤1 mm optic nerve), there is still a significant difference among remaining patients ($p = 0.001$) based on macular and nerve parameters. Hence, if the macula or disc/nerve can be relatively spared even despite the other receiving higher dose, there may be a visual advantage. Higher dose to both structures (i.e., V50% to >0% macula and >1 mm optic nerve) indicated highest probability of visual deterioration.

Another complication of PBRT is neovascular glaucoma (NVG). DVH analysis has shown that >30% of the lens or ciliary body receiving ≥50% dose (≥28 GyE) results in higher probability of NVG ($p < 0.0001$) [62]. In addition, V50–100% of the disc or macula also indicated higher NVG risk ($p < 0.0001$ and $p = 0.03$, respectively). If both anterior and posterior doses were above these specified thresholds, NVG risk was highest ($p < 0.0001$, Figure 14.5b). Multivariate analysis confirmed significant independent risk factors to include disc, lens, and optic nerve DVH parameters. Hence, DVH

parameters may be used to help optimize planning and better prognosticate risk of complications.

14.3.3   Dosing Regimens

UM proton radiation is delivered as a hypofractionated course over 4–5 days and the total dose across institutions worldwide is most commonly 60 GyE in four daily fractions [38]. Table 14.3 shows various dosing regimens for choroidal/ciliary body, iris, and conjunctival melanomas. At Massachusetts General Hospital (Boston, MA, USA), the standard dose is 70 GyE in five consecutive daily fractions and small posterior macular tumors may be given 50 GyE in five fractions [63]. Standard UM dose has been 56 GyE in four fractions at the University of California San Francisco (San Francisco, CA, USA) and 57.2 GyE in four fractions at the Clatterbridge Cancer Center (Clatterbridge, Wirral, UK) [38,64].

"Gray equivalent" is defined as Gray multiplied by the relative biological effectiveness, or RBE, for a type of radiation. The overall RBE for protons is commonly considered 1.1 times that of cobalt, so "GyE" = proton Gy × 1.1, across the SOBP.

However, RBE may be variable along the SOBP and higher with increasing depth [65–69]. Biological response may vary by tissue (eye as a CNS end-organ) as well as host, tumor, and treatment factors including dose fractionation [70–75]. For low-energy beams and small SOBP widths, dose-averaged

Table 14.2   Sample dose constraint guidelines for primary proton RT for uveal melanoma at UCSF.

OAR	For maximal sparing of certain ocular tissues	Partial sparing constraints*
Optic disc	$D_{max} = 0$ GyE	V50% to 0% (or ALARA**, <100%)
Optic nerve	$D_{max} = 0$ GyE	V50% to ≤1 mm (or ALARA)
Fovea/Macula	$D_{max} = 0$ GyE	V50% to 0% (or ALARA, <100%)
Ciliary body	V50% ≤ 30% (or ALARA)	V50% to ≤30% (or ALARA)
Lens	$D_{max} = 0$ GyE	V50% to ≤30% (or ALARA)

*V50% = Area/volume/length of structure receiving 50% of total dose (~28–30 GyE) [59-62].

**ALARA = As low as reasonably achievable.

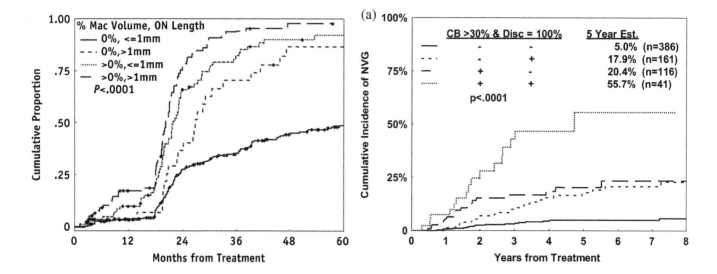

Figure 14.5 (a) Time to first best corrected visual acuity (BCVA) decline according to %macula volume or optic nerve length receiving 50% total dose (V50%) showing the dominant effect of the macular DVH parameter and that even when the most favorable subset is excluded (50% total dose to 0% macula and ≤1 mm ON), there remains a significant difference among the other three sets of patients (p = 0.001), indicating that relative sparing of either one of the nerve or macula results in VA benefit [59]. (b) Neovascular glaucoma (NVG) estimates after proton beam therapy as a function of anterior and posterior structure dose volume parameters with %volume of ciliary body (CB) and %disc receiving ≥50% dose (p < 0.0001). Anterior dose volume threshold "+" signifies >30% of the CB volume received ≥50% dose (28 GyE or higher). Posterior dose volume threshold "+" signifies that 100% of the optic disc received ≥50% dose. When both factors were at increased levels, NVG incidence was highest. When either anterior or posterior dose only was at or above the specified cut points, NVG occurrence was intermediate. When both structures were below threshold, then NVG incidence was lowest. The majority of patients had a 5% risk of developing NVG at 5 years [62].

Table 14.3 Type of eye melanoma treated with proton therapy and fractionation schemes worldwide. Adapted from international PTCOG-OPTIC survey of ocular proton therapy centers [38,48].

Type of eye tumor	Total dose (GyE)	Fractions	Number of institutions
Uveal melanoma (choroidal-ciliary body)	70	5	1
	60	4	7
	57.2–58.4	4	1
	56	4	1
	50	5	1
Iris melanoma	70	5	1
	60	4	4
	58.4	4	1
	56	4	1
	54–60	4	1
	50	4	1
Conjunctival melanoma*	70	5	1
	60	4	2
	60	8	1
	58.4	4	1
	56	4	1
	50	4 or 8	1
	45	8	1
	20.4–21.8	4	1

*Includes multimodality therapy with surgery, chemotherapy, and radiation.

linear energy transfer (LET$_d$) and thus RBE values may be higher. Some studies from low energy proton beamline (~65–68 MeV beam) have shown an RBE (cell line surviving fractions of 1–10%) of potentially of 1.19–1.27 at the distal part of the SOBP [69–72]. The LET$_d$ may also be slightly increased in the penumbra as compared to the center of the beam due to scattered and secondary protons [68,69]. Early biological data, at the time of initial charged particle therapy (CPT) at Lawrence-Berkeley Laboratory, was utilized to design beam-modulating propeller wheels to produce a negative slope for physical dose to account for the increased relative biological effect with depth for particles [76].

14.3.4 Imaging and Delivery

Most international proton ocular treatment centers use a dedicated passive scattering horizontal beamline. Low-energy eye beamlines in particular have unique beam characteristics critical for normal eye tissue sparing, based on sharp distal and lateral fall-off, high dose-homogeneity, excellent range precision, and short treatment time (~0.5–2 min) during which patients can hold gaze well [38,56].

Treatment is commonly delivered using a single anterior beam port. The patient is immobilized with a face mask and bite block or chin rest. Patient eye position is maintained with a visual target (small LED light) at the planned gaze direction. The treatment position is verified by daily digital radiography with orthogonal flat panel imaging and a clinical light field. The tantalum markers are imaged and verified against the plan and the patient position is adjusted accordingly (Figure 14.3c). Plan or aperture adjustments may be required depending on the patient setup, postoperative complications including eye torsion or swelling, gaze angle difficulty, visual loss requiring gaze fixation with the healthy eye, or other clinical situations.

Once the patient is in position, custom eyelid retractors are used to pull the eyelids outside of the beam path as much as possible. Local anesthetic eye drops and/or topical ophthalmic ointment is used for temporary numbing. The eyelids are carefully retracted to minimize patient discomfort and maximize potential preservation of the eyelid, tear duct, and eyelashes. The potential to retract is dependent on various factors, including postsurgical healing, natural skin stretch, eye socket anatomy, and choice of gaze angle. Different retractor sizes, multiple small retractors, and various techniques such as limited chin tilt and chair rotation can be utilized for effective retraction without affecting tumor and tantalum marker position. For small and medium tumors, the majority if not all of the eyelids can be retracted outside of the field. For larger tumors, the upper eyelid is preferentially removed to minimize complications where possible.

If it is not possible for the upper eyelid to be pulled out of the radiation path, then transpalpebral proton beam radiotherapy can be delivered. This technique avoids long-term upper eyelid margin and related ocular surface complications, without compromising local tumor control [57]. If a significant amount of eyelid remains in the field, then the distal range can be adjusted to compensate for the additional tissue.

The radiation delivery time is generally 30 s to about 1–2 min depending on institutional preference, beam characteristics, and dose rate. A magnified closed-circuit TV imaging during radiotherapy administration allows real-time gaze tracking. Treatment may be paused if there is gaze movement, though generally with appropriate coaching before and during treatment patients fare very well with gaze fixation particularly given the short treatment times. Following treatment, a temporary eye patch is placed until the effects of the anesthetic eye drop/ointment subside. An antibiotic/steroid ophthalmic ointment or drops may be used during the treatment week.

14.4 Treatment System Developments

14.4.1 Planning Systems

Additional software products are being used or tested worldwide, including commercial and in-house developed planning systems. These include *EOPP*-Eclipse Ocular Proton Planning® (Varian Medical Systems, Inc., Palo Alto, USA) [77]; *OCTOPUS*-Ocular Tumour Planning Utilities (German Cancer Research Centre DKFZ, Heidelberg, Germany in collaboration with Hahn-Meitner Institute, Berlin, Germany) [78]; *OPT'im-Eye-Tool/piDose* (HollandPTC, Delft, The Netherlands in collaboration with Leiden University Medical Center, Leiden, The Netherlands) [28]; and *RayOcular®* (RayStation®, RaySearch Laboratories, Stockholm, Sweden) [79]. While there remains significant overlap in various planning techniques across the systems, there are substantial differences as well. Further developments in CT/MRI imaging fusion, gaze angle optimization, critical structure and tumor modeling, radiograph handling, real-time eye tracking for gaze detection, MRI-based clipless planning, and pencil beam dose calculations, may influence relative future utility of these various planning system options in the proton ocular community [28,77–80].

14.4.2 Beamlines

Currently, most ocular proton treatment is delivered by dedicated passive scattering horizontal beam-lines with tight lateral and distal penumbra. The lateral fall-off (80–20%) is most commonly within a narrow range ~1.0–1.9 mm and distal fall-off (90–10%) ~0.7–2.3 mm [55,56]. New high-energy non-dedicated beam designs, which degrade energy to achieve the ranges required for superficial ocular treatment, may require significant adjustments to the beamline nozzles and treatment planning procedures to achieve adequate lateral and distal penumbra, dose rate, and other characteristics particularly for normal tissue sparing. Specifically, degraded beamlines have potential challenges, especially for critical structure dosing, such as greater dose inhomogeneity, range uncertainty, distal and lateral beam fall-off, treatment time for gaze fixation, dose rate variability, patient neutron dose, and displacement of a portable snout on nozzles.

The resultant impact on critical structure doses will require careful assessment along with applying the potential benefits of pencil beam technology, 3D imaging, and other developments under study. Further systematic study will be essential of critical structure doses, including but not limited to the optic disc/nerve, macula, retina, ciliary body, lens, cornea, limbus/limbal stem cells, lacrimal gland, eyelid, tear duct, and other critical structure doses.

14.4.3 MRI

Dedicated ocular particle centers have developed a comprehensive UM treatment approach over decades with clinical/surgical assessment, ocular photography, and ultrasound which can be incorporated into the widely utilized model-based eye TPS *Eyeplan*. Currently, this software does not allow MRI-based planning implementation. Imaging advances, novel TPS, and new proton centers will require surgical and planning expertise to develop. Increased MRI incorporation into the ocular planning systems may further improve the accuracy, reproducibility, and quality of care.

Specifically, 3- and 7-T high-resolution MRI may have increased utility for clip-based and/or clipless treatment [28–30]. MRI analysis could provide potential confirmation of surgical tantalum clip placement in relation to the tumor and eye and appear postoperatively as voids on MRI. This additional confirmation may be useful if tumors are more difficult to mark (i.e., far posterior) or for newer surgeons as a benchmark for surgical marker assessment. Some centers are exploring MRI-based planning without tantalum markers [28]. MRI has already served in conjunction with conventional techniques of fundus photography, ultrasound, and surgical assessment to delineate tumor and critical structure anatomy. MRI can also confirm vitreous hemorrhage, retinal detachment, and axial length in patients with cataract or if there is a discrepancy in axial measurements between eyes. MRI may not be well suited for large area, low height tumors with diffuse edges, and further study is required.

14.4.4 Other Delivery Developments

Most commonly a single anterior beam is used for ocular treatment given the conventional fixed beam setup for dedicated ocular beams and to minimize treatment angles through the brain or other surrounding orbital, lacrimal, or head and neck tissue. Gantry-based and incline beam setups have been reported [48]. If multiple beam angles are employed, then CT and MRI imaging may be utilized for planning to optimize geometry based on tumor location, size, and adjacent organs at risk. A smearing technique may need to be used to account for potential changes in anatomic position between supine and seated positions. At these centers, patients may undergo MRI and/or CT scans prior to tantalum marker surgery to determine potential treatment angles. In such cases, marker positioning may be based on expected beam angles, in-room imaging capacity, and surgical considerations. Markers sutured directly anterior to tumors may result in potential dose shadow effects for such set ups [81].

14.5 Clinical Outcomes

Particle therapy is well established as a "gold standard" treatment for UMs based on prospective [44], retrospective [58,82–96], and meta-analysis [39,40] data. The benefit of proton therapy includes improved tumor dose delivery and decreased collateral damage due to dose distribution, dose rate, linear energy transfer, and sharp dose fall-off outside the target region. Studies show the primary end point of tumor local control (LC) to be approximately 96% at 5 years and maintained at 10- and 15-year follow-up [39,58,82,83]. Eye preservation rates are approximately 90% at 5 years [82–85,97,98]. Short- and long-term LC rates are generally higher for charged particles compared with plaque brachytherapy [39,44,99]. Survival rates across studies are comparable between enucleation, plaque brachytherapy, and particle therapies [34,35,44]. Many patients are able to preserve their eye and maintain useful vision after proton therapy.

14.5.1 Local Control Outcomes

Multiple dedicated large volume ocular proton beam institutions report high LC for UM patients at 5 years of 96% (range 90.5–99%) [39,58,82–96]. For example, Massachusetts General Hospital described a LC of 97% at 5 years and 95% at 15 years [82,83]. The Paul Scherrer Institute (PSI, Villagen, Switzerland) reported a LC rate of 96% at 5 years and 95% at 10 years [58].

A meta-analysis comparing published studies of all radiation modalities used for choroidal melanomas showed that proton/particle beam resulted in the highest LC [39]. Of 6825 UM patients pooled worldwide, the average weighted local failure (LF) rate was 4.2% after proton beam RT. In comparison, plaque brachytherapy ($n = 3868$) resulted in a weighted mean LF of 9.5% in the meta-analysis. This is despite a somewhat smaller tumor diameter and height in the studies of plaques versus particles (11 vs. 14 mm and 4.5 vs. 5.5 mm, weighted mean tumor largest basal diameter and height, respectively) [39].

Another meta-analysis of 5040 patients (14 studies) comparing studies of CPT with iodine plaque therapy showed improved LC outcomes with CPT [40]. In this study, a significantly lower incidence of radiation retinopathy was noted with CPT and was hypothesized to be due to a more uniform dose distribution on average with a lower dose delivered to a smaller volume of retina. Furthermore, "late" radiation failures (beyond 5 years after treatment) have been noted more frequently after plaque brachytherapy than particle RT [99].

Of note, some early PSI patients (1984–1988) were treated with a reduced safety margin (less than 2 mm aperture margin, defining the 50% isodose line) due to proximity of the tumor to the fovea/disc. Those with a reduced aperture margin <2 mm had a much higher reported LF rate at 5 years of 28.7% (vs. only 3.7% LF for patients with standard safety margins) [58].

14.5.2 Trials

COMS: The early Collaborative Ocular Melanoma Study (COMS) reported on several long-term, multicenter clinical trials. The small tumors' cohort study of 204 patients (≤10 mm diameter, ≤3 mm height, no retinal detachment) with inactive appearing lesions was deemed suitable for close observation and had excellent 5-year cause-specific survival (CSS) of 99% and 5-year overall survival (OS) of 94%. The 2-year and 5-year tumor growth estimate were 21% and 31%, respectively [100,101]. Further studies of small lesions have shown that certain clinical features may be predictive of growth. Hence, select small lesions may be considered for early treatment, including those with documented growth, mushroom shape, presence of symptoms (i.e., photopsia, blurred vision), ciliary body involvement, >2 mm thickness, surface orange pigment, or subretinal fluid [102,103].

The early COMS medium tumor natural history arm (patients deferred or declined therapy) was noted to have a reduced 5-year OS of 70%, indicating that delayed care was detrimental for tumors of a certain size or characteristics [104]. The COMS medium tumor trial which enrolled 1317 patients and compared iodine-125 plaque brachytherapy versus enucleation showed a 5-year LC of 89.7% in the plaque arm; 5-year CSS of 91% (plaque arm) and 89% (enucleation arm); and 5-year OS was 82% and 81%, respectively (p = ns) [34,105]. The 12-year update similarly showed no difference in survival between the arms (12-year estimates OS 57–59% and CSS 79–83%) [35].

The COMS studies indicated comparable survival outcomes for radiation and surgery and suggested close follow-up such that any local recurrence would revert to re-treatment or enu-

cleation as needed. Of note, however, some have reasoned that the COMS data are inconclusive on the impact of failed local therapy on survival after iodine-125 plaque brachytherapy [106]. This is potentially due to the small subset of LFs, limited long-term follow-up, and possibility of micrometastic disease already present within the first five study years' post-eye treatment such that these early metastatic cases are not reflective of local therapy impact. Others have reported that LC is correlated with survival rates, i.e., with an overall 10-year CSS reported at 72.6% for patients with controlled tumors versus 47.5% for those with local recurrence [58].

UCSF-LBNL: A prospective randomized trial of helium ion versus iodine-125 plaque brachytherapy was conducted at UCSF and the Lawrence-Berkeley National Laboratory (LBNL) from 1985 to 1991 [44]. This trial included a total of 184 patients with tumors <15 mm diameter and <10 mm height, treated to 70 GyE. The particle arm dosing was over five fractions in 5–7 days delivered in <2 min fractions versus continuous low dose rate radiation in the I-125 arm (0.7–0.75 Gy/h at the tumor apex). Upon long-term follow-up, 12-year LC for particle versus plaque treatment was 98% versus 79%, respectively (p = 0.0006). Even if patients with tumors close to the disc (<2 mm) were excluded due to overall decreased control with plaques, 12-year LC remained better in the particle arm at 98% versus 86% in the plaque arm (p = 0.048). This is consistent with meta-analyses and other institutional data showing higher short and long-term LC post-particle therapy [44].

MGH-MEEI: In terms of dose comparison, a randomized dose trial evaluating doses of 50 GyE and 70 GyE in five fractions for proton beam therapy was conducted on 188 patients, with small/medium tumors <15 mm diameter and <5 mm height within four disc diameters of the disc or macula [63]. The study found no significant difference between dose regimens in terms of ocular toxicity or LC at 5 years. Follow-up for this study would allow long-term evaluation of LC outcomes at the 50-GyE dose regimen.

In a nonrandomized dose-searching study at Lawrence-Berkeley Laboratory of 347 patients receiving helium ion RT, dose was reduced from 80 GyE in five fractions to 48 GyE in four fractions (calculated with a helium RBE of 1.3, slightly greater than that of protons). LC in helium patients was 96% (at median follow-up 8.5 years), with no LC difference seen at 80, 70, 60, or 50 GyE in five fractions. At the lowest dose level of 48 GyE in four fractions, the LC rate fell to 87% [107].

14.5.3 Eye Preservation

Ocular proton beam RT allows for high rates of secondary clinical outcomes in terms of eye retention and functional vision preservation. Enucleation rate after proton therapy (secondary enucleation) at 5 years is approximately 10% (range 0–25%)

with small tumors ranging 2–3%, medium 7–8%, and large 22–25% [58,82–91,97,98]. Some large volume ocular proton centers have reported lower rates, with one study reporting enucleation rates of 0% for small, 0.3% for medium, and 10.5% for large tumors [97]. The overall rate at 15 years is approximately 15% [83,108]. Similarly, the COMS medium I-125 plaque study showed a 5-year enucleation of 12%; other series show a range of enucleation rates between 4% and 20% with plaques [6,109].

Approximately 60% of secondary enucleations following PBRT are performed for complications related to NVG. The remainder of secondary enucleations are done for local salvage after intraocular recurrence and as treatment of other complications, i.e., total exudative retinal detachment, severe intraocular inflammation, and a blind painful eye. Secondary enucleation rate varies based on risk factors including tumor height and diameter, tumor distance from optic disc/macula, retinal detachment, ciliary body involvement, baseline intraocular pressure, and VA. The majority of secondary enucleations occur between 0 and 3 years after proton therapy but can be required at longer follow-up as well [6,58,62,82–91].

Normal tissue toxicity should be carefully distinguished from "toxic tumor syndrome," in which the response of the irradiated tumor mass can lead to exudative retinal detachment, rubeosis and NVG after PBRT of a choroidal melanoma [110]. This can be treated with trans-scleral local resection of the irradiated tumor, with resultant preservation of the eye.

14.5.4 Visual Function

Useful vision preservation (>20/200 Snellen) with proton irradiation is reported at 3 years to be variable in the range of 40–65% [86,89,111]. Visual outcomes are directly related to patient, tumor, and treatment factors, including age, comorbidities such as diabetes, baseline VA, macular or peripapillary tumor location, tumor diameter and height, exudative retinal detachment, and radiation dose to the macula, nerve, and disc. The MGH-MEEI randomized dose study showed no difference in ocular toxicity and vision outcomes at 5 years despite somewhat lower normal tissue dose in the 50-GyE group. This was hypothesized to potentially be due potentially to a threshold for macular complications at ~40 GyE [63].

Large dataset visual analysis has shown that at 5-year follow-up, approximately half of PBRT-treated eyes with favorable pretreatment VA (20/40 or better) retained excellent VA (20/40 or better) post-treatment [59]. In those with initially unfavorable VA (20/50 or worse), 20% retained vision ≥20/100. DVH parameters at 50% total dose level to the macula and optic nerve can be used for treatment planning optimization and visual prognosis.

Comparing favorably with other radiation modalities, a nonrandomized study (*n* = 191) followed visual outcomes

after treatment with stereotactic radiosurgery (SRS) versus proton beam [112]. The report confirmed that more patients experienced significant visual loss (≥3 Snellen lines) at 65% with SRS versus 45% with protons at 3 years. The 5-year useful VA preservation (>20/200) was 37% on the I-125 arm of the COMS study; others report widely variable useful vision retention outcomes with brachytherapy, ranging between 23% and 73% [109].

14.5.5 Neovascular Glaucoma

NVG is a potential complication that can lead to enucleation in severe cases. A contemporary study using normal tissue dose optimization has shown a 5-year NVG rate of 13% post-PBRT compared with significantly higher historical rates [62]. The 5-year rate of enucleation due to NVG was 5%. Tumor height, diameter, and anterior as well as posterior critical structure dose–volume parameters may be used to predict NVG risk.

14.5.6 Carbon-ion Beam

A series of 116 patients were treated (2001–2012) with carbon-ion radiotherapy at the National Institute of Radiological Sciences in Chiba, Japan, for locally advanced or unfavorably located choroidal melanoma [113,114]. A total dose of 60–85 GyE in five fractions was used; RBE for carbon was estimated at 3.0 for the distal part of the SOBP. Initially NVG rate was elevated (40%) and so a two-port therapy was implemented in 2005 to reduce risk of NVG. Median follow-up was 4.6 years and LC, CSS, and OS were 93%, 82%, and 80%, respectively. The overall 5-year NVG incidence rate was 36%; the one-port group at 42% and the two-port group at 14% (*p* < 0.001). Similar to other studies noted, the DVH analysis showed that the average irradiated volume of the iris–ciliary body was significantly lower in the non-NVG group and in the two-port group.

14.5.7 Cost-effectiveness

A cost-analysis study showed that short course ocular proton therapy (4–5 fractions) may be more cost-effective than plaque brachytherapy based on current insurance schema [115]. Additional costs due to retinopathy, clinic visits, and lost vision are under study and may also impact cost-effectiveness evaluation favorably for proton beam compared with other radiation modalities [40,116]. Overall, optimal proton RT can potentially reduce complication risks and associated costs by delivering lower normal tissue dosing in the eye and peripheral head and neck compared with other techniques such as Gamma Knife, CyberKnife, and other stereotactic techniques [112,117].

14.5.8 Other RT Modalities

Briefly, alternative radiotherapeutic techniques using Gamma Knife, CyberKnife, and LINAC-based stereotactic photon therapy have been described [42,112,117–120]. These are often more readily available than other radiation techniques and hence may provide an opportunity for treatment of UM outside of specialized particle or brachytherapy centers. Overall, tumor dose inhomogeneity, extended treatment time, monitoring, and fixation of head position and gaze angle remain a challenge for SRS techniques. Invasive techniques including application of stereotactic frames and suturing of the extraocular muscles to achieve targeting generally limit the number of treatment fractions. Importantly, normal tissue doses tend to be higher with current sterotactic RT approaches compared with proton therapy [112,117].

Brachytherapy techniques are widely accessible worldwide. Issues of LC particularly for larger tumors or peripapillary tumors, the wider penumbra of certain isotopes such as iodine-125 and resultant increased normal ocular tissue dosing, radiation worker exposure, and risk for retinopathy and diplopia are considerations [39,40,109,115,116].

Meta-analyses and prospective randomized data comparing radiation modalities have consistently shown proton/particle beam to result in the highest LC overall [39,40,44]. Late radiation failures, beyond 5 years after treatment, have been noted less frequently after particle RT compared with other RT modalities [99]. Proton/Particle therapy has been shown to result in lower radiation retinopathy rates, potentially due to a more uniform dose distribution and lower doses to smaller retinal volumes overall [40,116]. Optic structure dosimetry, vision outcomes, and overall cost-effectiveness have been noted to be favorable after PBRT compared with other RT modalities [112,115,117]. Anterior eye complications are more common with CPT, however are significantly decreased with contemporary RT techniques in planning, dosing, and delivery, as well as advances in expert ophthalmologic care [62,97,110].

Contemporary prospective randomized trials and longer follow-up would allow further evaluation of different RT modalities regarding tumor control and, importantly, normal tissue complication rates.

14.6 Follow-Up and Toxicities

Patients' follow-up with ophthalmology at 3–6 month intervals initially for 2–3 years then may extend to 6–9-month intervals for 2–3 years and then at 9–12 month intervals. A thorough ocular examination with appropriate imaging is completed at each ophthalmology visit and patients will follow-up with a combination of the surgical, radiation, and medical oncologist, as appropriate. Frequency of metastatic surveillance may be further guided by clinical assessment and biopsy tumor genetics. Imaging may include liver MRI, CT, or ultrasound as well as chest CT at 3–12-month intervals depending on the oncology protocol, patient and tumor factors, and if a patient is on a clinical trial. Metastatic surveillance for intermediate or higher risk patients may follow every 3–6-month imaging for the first 2–5 years and then span to every 6–12 months. Patients with high-risk tumor genetics may also enroll in adjuvant clinical trials investigating novel therapeutics [121].

14.6.1 Local Recurrence

Local tumor recurrence may be treated with a second course of RT or enucleation. Proton re-irradiation for local relapse, particularly if there is a marginal failure, can be highly successful for salvage. A study reported on 48–70 CGE (for a total lifetime dose of 118–140 CGE) delivered to 31 patients with resultant 5-year rates for LC 69%, OS 64%, eye-retention 55%, and useful vision preservation in 27% [122]. Of note, the COMS study revealed that in 40% of eyes that underwent secondary enucleation for suspected LF after plaque brachytherapy, increased tumor size could not be histologically confirmed [123]. Ki-67 expression on immunohistochemistry and mitotic rate can be evaluated to determine viable tumor cells and true local recurrences in enucleated eyes.

Initially some tumors may continue to enlarge after proton beam RT due to an inflammatory response. Exudative retinal detachment or bleeding can cause the tumors to appear larger at follow-up examinations. Careful serial monitoring with examination, fundus photography, and ultrasound is required to distinguish tumor treatment response from potential local treatment failure or progression.

14.6.2 Metastatic Disease and Survival

A variety of current techniques can be utilized for metastatic risk assessment, including GEP, NGS (i.e., UCSF500), MLPA, and the Liverpool Uveal Melanoma Prognosticator Online tool, a multivariable analysis using anatomic, histologic, and genetic factors [16]. A Class 1A genetic profile on biopsy is associated with excellent survival prognosis at 5 years with a 98% metastasis-free rate [17]. Patients with Class 1B tumors have a 79% metastasis-free rate at 5 years, and Class 2 tumors have a low metastasis-free rate of 28% at 5 years. Before biopsy was standard practice, size criteria correlated to approximately 5-year OS of 80% across series (range 70–88%), with small tumors ranging 95–98%, medium 80–86%, and large 60% [58,83–89,97,98]. Additional factors adversely affecting survival prognosis include negative histopathologic and genetic markers, *PRAME* + status, older age, retinal detachment, large tumor diameter, increased tumor height, ciliary body involvement, and extrascleral extension.

Metastatic disease can develop most commonly in the liver, lung, and bone and can occur after a prolonged disease-free interval [124]. The COMS Group reported on 7541 patients screened for the COMS trials. While less than 1% had metastatic disease detected at the time of screening, the majority of eventual deaths on trial were associated with metastatic UM [125,126]. The mortality rate after diagnosis of metastatic disease at 1 year was 80% and at 2 years was 92%.

Of those diagnosed with metastatic disease, 91% had liver involvement, 28% lung, 18% bone, 12% skin and subcutaneous tissue, 11% lymph nodes, 5% brain, 1% spinal cord, and 1% fellow eye or orbit of either eye. A majority of patients had one site of metastatic involvement (52%), 25% two sites, and 24% had three or more sites [125,126].

Active therapeutic options are limited in the setting of metastatic disease treatment or prevention. Generally, UM metastases respond poorly to chemotherapy or targeted therapy and are usually fatal within 1 year of symptom onset. Long-term survival is rare except in patients with isolated liver metastases that are amenable to surgical resection. New combined systemic therapies and molecular targeted agents are currently being studied [16,121]. A randomized, phase III trial of Tebentafusp, a bispecific fusion protein (T cell receptor/anti-CD3), has shown potential OS benefit in patients with metastatic melanoma compared with investigator's choice of first-line therapy (1 year OS 73.2% vs. 57.5%, respectively) [127,128].

14.6.3 Toxicities

During the course of RT, patients may feel minor discomfort with eyelid retraction and may experience some anxiety or claustrophobia with the immobilization setup. This tends to be minimal and temporary.

Approximately 2–3 weeks post-RT patients may experience an eyelid epitheliitis reaction depending on extent of eyelid in the proton field. An antibiotic/steroid ophthalmic ointment is given for use twice daily while the reaction persists, usually 2–3 weeks. Most recover well and some may have persistent change in pigmentation or irritation of the skin. If the eyelid is in the field, there may be permanent madarosis (eyelash loss) in that region. If the upper eyelid is in the field, there can be resultant damage to the mucocutaneous junction and keratinization of the palpebral conjunctiva, which if not removed may abrade the cornea. Hence, upper eyelid retraction is purposefully carried out as much as possible in patient setup; alternatively, transpalpebral radiation delivery can curtail this effect [57].

Overall late toxicities may appear in approximately 5–30% of patients depending on risk factors and dosing. Common late toxicities after proton beam radiation include cataracts, NVG, and vision changes. All are highly correlated with dosing to certain normal tissues and tumor/DVH analysis can provide a rubric to evaluate risk of side effects for patients. Visually significant cataract may require surgery which may be recommended once tumor response is confirmed. Intra-ocular pressures may increase or patients may experience symptoms from NVG (vision loss, eye pain) which may require anti-VEGF injections or glaucoma surgery. In severe cases, enucleation may be required (overall low rate of secondary enucleation due to NVG post-PBRT, ~5% at 5 years, with contemporary normal tissue dosing techniques) [62].

Optic neuropathy, maculopathy, exudation, macular edema, retinal changes, or exudative detachment may be treated with laser, anti-VEGF, and steroid injections, as well as other treatments including surgery [129]. Toxic tumor syndrome (exudative retinal detachment, rubeosis, and NVG after UM PBRT) can be treated with trans-scleral local resection of the irradiated tumor [110].

Patients may experience dry eye and epiphora (abnormal overflow of tears due to excess secretion of tears or to obstruction of the lacrimal duct). Other changes due to surgical marker placement or radiation may include vitreous hemorrhage, eyelid edema, blood vessel changes (conjunctival telangectasias), acute or chronic pain or discomfort, iris rubeosis, scleral, corneal, conjunctival, or iris changes, light sensitivity, limbal stem cell deficiency, and rarely, diplopia. The patient is at risk of secondary enucleation due to complications that cannot be medically controlled or tumor progression, despite radiation.

14.7 Other Ocular Tumors

Along with treatment of UMs, secondary ocular malignancy (metastatic lesions to the uvea) and other diseases of the eye and orbit have also been successfully treated with proton ocular beamlines achieving high levels of LC. A similar setup as described above is used and dosing may be variable. For certain benign tumors or nonsurgical candidates, a clinical light field alignment may be required using anatomic landmarks (i.e., limbus) if no tantalum markers are placed. Dosing schemas for various malignant and benign eye conditions, as used by dedicated ocular centers worldwide, are listed in Tables 14.3 and 14.4 [38].

Conjunctival melanomas have been shown to respond well to multimodality treatment including excisional surgery, postsurgical topical chemotherapy eye drops (i.e., mitomycin C), and adjuvant radiation [130,131]. Conjunctival melanomas are generally treated to equivalent doses as UMs (Table 14.3). Additionally, conjunctival squamous cell carcinomas have been shown to have lower risk of local relapse with adjuvant proton irradiation. These can be treated with adjuvant proton dosing of 40–52 GyE post-excision [132].

Table 14.4 Type of other ocular cancers treated with proton therapy and fractionation schemes worldwide. Adapted from international PTCOG-OPTIC survey of large volume ocular proton therapy centers [38].

Type of eye tumor	Total dose (GyE)	Fractions	No. of institutions
Ocular hemangioma	20	8	4
	19.8	4	1
	16–22	4	1
	18	4	1
	15	4	1
Macular degeneration	24	2	2
	19.8	4	1
	18	2	1
Angioma	35	5	1
	20	4	1
	20	8	1
	19.8	4	1
	18	4	1
Choroidal metastasis	60	4	1
	45	4	1
	40	4	1
	20–40 (By histology)	4	1
	20–24	2	2
Retinoblastoma	45 (On gantry)	25	1
	31.6	6	1

Vascular tumors such as choroidal hemangiomas have been treated with dosing between 12and 20 GyE in four to eight fractions with either tantalum marker delineation or clinical light field setup [133,134]. At UCSF, hemangiomas are commonly treated with low dose ~16 GyE in four fractions. Macular degeneration has been treated to a total dose of 18–24 GyE in two to four fractions with clinical light field alignment [135]. Retinal angiomas have been given 18–35 GyE in four to eight fractions [38].

Choroidal metastases can be treated with proton beam therapy with dosing between 20 and 45 GyE in two to four fractions depending on histology, estimated radiosensitivity, and institutional protocols. Oligometastatic disease to the choroid can respond well to localized proton therapy, achieving high rates of LC while preserving function and avoiding contralateral eye dose [136,137].

Retinoblastoma has been treated with protons to 31.6 GyE in six fractions or on gantry-based systems with standard fractionation to 45 GyE [38]. Long-term follow-up of patients with retinoblastoma treated with PBRT demonstrated high LC rates, even in advanced cases, with retention of useful vision in the treated eye for many patients, and minimal other side effects. At a median follow-up of 8 years, no radiation-associated malignancies were observed in the children [138].

Lymphomas have been reported to be treated to very low dose, even as low as 4–8 GyE in two to four fractions, respectively, and can be retreated in the case of failure [139]. Commonly, lymphomas have been treated with 10–20 GyE total dose. A rare aggressive tumor, such as mucinous carcinoma of the periorbital tissue, has been treated with 56 GyE in the postoperative setting. Longer follow-up will allow for better outcomes characterization for these rare ocular tumors with proton beam therapy.

14.8 Conclusion

The treatment of ocular tumors with charged particle techniques has been extensively and rigorously evaluated over decades of scientific work. The approach requires specific clinical and physics expertise and great care in the application so that optimal LC and long-term eye preservation can be achieved. Acute and late ocular morbidity are dependent on patient, tumor, and treatment parameters, and further clinical exploration of techniques to maximize functional outcomes remain essential. Utilizing a thoughtful approach, proton and particle beam radiation can very successfully control tumor with the hope of preserving the eye and useful vision.

Acknowledgments

Thank you to Inder K. Daftari, PhD for his significant contributions to the science of proton ocular treatment and patient care. Thank you to our proton ocular and ocular oncology teams, UCSF/ UC Davis Crocker Laboratory team, Dr. Jeanne M. Quivey, and Dr. Theodore L. Phillips.

References

1 Jermann, M., PTCOG statistics, PTCOG Secretary & Treasurer c/o Paul Scherrer Institute (PSI). May 21, 2021 communication.

2 Coupland, S.E., Campbell, I., and Damato, B. (2008). Routes of extraocular extension of uveal melanoma: Risk factors and influence on survival probability. *Ophthalmology* Oct;115(10):1778–1785. doi: 10.1016/j.ophtha.2008.04.025. PMID: 18554722.

3 Singh, A.D. and Topham, A. (2003). Incidence of uveal melanoma in the United States: 1973-1997. *Ophthalmology* 110 (5): 956.

4 Virgili, G. et al. (2007). Incidence of uveal melanoma in Europe. *Ophthalmology* 114: 2309.

5 Barr, C.C., McLean, I.W., and Zimmerman, L.E. (1981). Uveal melanoma in children and adolescents. *Archives of Ophthalmology* 99: 2133.

6 Mishra, K.K., Quivey, J.M., Takamiya, R., Daftari, I., and Char, D.H. (2010). Uveal Melanoma. In: *Textbook of Radiation Oncology* (ed. S.A. Leibel and T.L. Phillips), 3rd ed, Philadelphia: Elsevier Inc.

7 Shah, C.P. et al. (2005). Intermittent and chronic ultraviolet light exposure and uveal melanoma: A meta-analysis. *Ophthalmology* 112 (9): 1599.

8 Weis, E., Shah, C.P., Lajous, M., Shields, J.A., and Shields, C.L. (2006). The association between host susceptibility factors and uveal melanoma: A meta-analysis. *Archives of Ophthalmology* 124 (1): 54–60.

9 Rodrigues, M., Koning, L., Coupland, S. et al. (2019). UM Cure 2020 Consortium. So close, yet so far: Discrepancies between uveal and other melanomas. A position paper from UM Cure 2020. *Cancers* 11 (7): E1032. https://doi.org/10.3390/cancers11071032.

10 Guenel, P., Laforest, L., Cyr, D. et al. (2001). Occupational risk factors, ultraviolet radiation, and ocular melanoma: A case-control study in France. *Cancer and Causes Control* 12: 451–459.

11 Fraunfelder, F.T., Fraunfelder, F.W., and Edwards, R. (2001). Ocular side effects possibly associated with isotretinoin usage. *American Journal of Ophthalmology* 132: 299–305.

12 Neudorfer, M., Goldshtein, I., Shamai-Lubovitz, O., Chodick, G., Dadon, Y., and Shalev, V. (2012). Ocular adverse effects of systemic treatment with isotretinoin. *Archives of Dermatology* 148 (7): 803–808.

13 Mishra, K.K., Scholey, J.E., Daftari, I.K., Afshar, A., Tsai, T., Park, S., Quivey, J.M., and Char, D.H. (2020). Oral isotretinoin and topical retinoid use in a series of young patients with ocular melanoma. *American Journal of Ophthalmology Case Reports* Sep; 19:100787.PMID: 32760850. PMCID: PMC7390773. 10.1016/j.ajoc.2020.100787.

14 Char, D.H., Kroll, S.M., Miller, T. et al. (1996). Irradiated uveal melanomas: Cytopathologic correlation with prognosis. *American Journal of Ophthalmology* 122: 509.

15 McLean, I.W., Saraiva, V.S., and Burnier, M.N. (2004). Pathological and prognostic features of uveal melanomas. *Canadian Journal of Ophthalmology. Journal Canadien D'ophthalmologie* 39: 343.

16 Jager, M.J., Shields, C.L., Cebulla, C.M., Abdel-Rahman, M.H., Grossniklaus, H.E., Stern, M.-H., Carvajal, R.D., Belfort, R.N., Jia, R., Shields, J.A., and Damato, B.E. (2020). Uveal melanoma. *Nature Reviews Disease Primers* Apr 9 6 (1): 24. 10.1038/s41572-020-0158-0.

17 Onken, M.D. et al. (2006). Prognostic testing in uveal melanoma by transcriptomic profiling of fine needle biopsy specimens. *The Journal of Molecular Diagnostics: JMD* 8 (5): 567.

18 Field, M.G., Decatur, C.L., Kurtenbach, S., Gezgin, G., Van Der Velden, P.A., Jager, M.J., Kozak, K.N., and Harbour, J.W. (2016). PRAME as an independent biomarker for metastasis in uveal melanoma. *Clinical Cancer Research: An Official Journal of the American Association for Cancer Research* March 1 22 (5): 1234–1242. 10.1158/1078-0432. CCR-15-2071.

19 Afshar, A.R., Damato, B.E., Stewart, J.M., Zablotska, L.B., Roy, R., Olshen, A.B., Joseph, N.M., and Bastian, B.C. (2019). Next-generation sequencing of uveal melanoma for detection of genetic alterations predicting metastasis. *Translational Vision and Science Technology* 8 (2): 18. https://doi.org/10.1167/tvst.8.2.18.

20 Schopper, V. and Correa, Z. (2016). Clinical application of genetic testing for posterior uveal melanoma. *International Journal of Retina and Vitreous* 2 (4): 10.1186/s40942-016-0030-2.

21 Chappell, M.C., Char, D.H., Cole, T.B., Harbour, J.W., Mishra, K.K., Weinberg, V.K., and Phillips, T.L. (2012). Uveal melanoma: Molecular pattern, clinical features, and radiation response. *American Journal of*

Ophthalmology Aug 154 (2): 227–232.e2. 10.1016/j.ajo.2012.02.022.

22 Van Raamsdonk, C.D., Bezrookove, V., Green, G. et al. (2009). Frequent somatic mutations of GNAQ in uveal melanoma and blue nevi. *Nature* 457: 599–602.

23 Van Raamsdonk, C.D., Griewank, K.G., Crosby, M.B. et al. (2010). Mutations in GNA11 in uveal melanoma. *The New England Journal of Medicine* 363: 2191–2199.

24 Harbour, J.W., Onken, M.D., Roberson, E.D. et al. (2010). Frequent mutation of BAP1 in metastasizing uveal melanomas. *Science* 330: 1410–1413.

25 Martin, M., Masshofer, L., Temming, P. et al. (2013). Exome sequencing identifies recurrent somatic mutations in EIF1AX and SF3B1 in uveal melanoma with disomy 3. *Nature Genetics* 45: 933–936.

26 Kivelä, T., Simpson, R.E., Grossniklaus, H.E. et al. (2016). Uveal melanoma. In: *AJCC Cancer Staging Manual*, 8th ed. New York, NY: Springer. 805–817.

27 Damato, B., Kacperek, A., Errington, D., and Heimann, H. (2013). Proton beam radiotherapy of uveal melanoma. *Saudi Journal of Ophthalmology* 27: 151–157.

28 Fleury, E., Trnkova, P., Erdal, E., Hassan, M., Stoel, B., Jaarma-Coes, M., Luyten, G., Herault, J., Webb, A., Beenakker, J.-W., and Pignol J-P, H.M. (2021). Three-dimensional MRI-based treatment planning approach for non-invasive ocular proton therapy. *Medical Physics* Mar 48 (3): 1315–1326. 10.1002/mp.14665. Epub 2021 Jan 17.

29 Oberacker, E., Paul, K., Huelnhagen, T., Oezerdem, C., Winter, L., Pohlmann, A., Boehmert, L., Stachs, O., Heufelder, J., Weber, A., Rehak, M., Seibel, I., and Niendorf, T. (2017). Magnetic Resonance Safety and Compatibility of Tantalum Markers Used in Proton Beam Therapy for Intraocular Tumors: A 7.0 Tesla Study. *Magnetic Resonance in Medicine* 78: 1533–1546.

30 Ferreira, T.A., Fonk, L.G., Jaarsma-Coes, M.G., Ggr, V.H., Marinkovic, M., and Beenakker, J.W.M. (2019). MRI of Uveal Melanoma. *Cancers (Basel)* Mar 17 11 (3): 377. 10.3390/cancers11030377.

31 Group COMS: Accuracy of diagnosis of choroidal melanomas in the Collaborative Ocular Melanoma Study. COMS Report No. 1. Arch Ophthalmol. 1990;108:1268.

32 Char, D.H. (1978). The management of small choroidal melanomas. *Survey of Ophthalmology* 22: 377.

33 Shields, C., Sioufi, K., Srinivasan, A., Di Nicola, M., Masoomian, B., Barna, L.E., Bekerman, V., Say, T., Mashayekhi, A., Emrich, J., Komarnicky, L., and Shields, J.A. (2018). Visual Outcome and Millimeter Incremental Risk of Metastasis in 1780 Patients with Small Choroidal Melanoma Managed by Plaque Radiotherapy. *JAMA Ophthalmology* 136 (12): 1325–1333. 10.1001/jamaophthalmol.2018.3881.

34 Diener-West, M. et al. (2001). The COMS randomized trial of iodine-125 brachytherapy for choroidal melanoma. III: Initial mortality findings. COMS Report No. 18. *Archives of Ophthalmology* 119: 969.

35 Collaborative Ocular Melanoma Study Group. (2006). Collaborative Ocular Melanoma Study Group: The COMS randomized trial of iodine 125 brachytherapy for choroidal melanoma: V. Twelve-year mortality rates and prognostic factors: COMS report no. 28. *Archives of Ophthalmology*. Dec; 124(12):1684–1693. doi: 10.1001/archopht.124.12.1684. PMID: 17159027

36 Shields, C.L., Lim, L.A.S., Dalvin, L.A., and Shields, J.A. (2019). Small choroidal melanoma: Detection with multimodal imaging and management with plaque radiotherapy or AU-011 nanoparticle therapy. *Current Opinion in Ophthalmology* May 30 (3): 206–214. 10.1097/ICU.0000000000000560.

37 National Cancer Institute. Phase 2 Trial to Evaluate Safety and Efficacy of AU-011 Via Suprachoroidal Administration in Subjects With Primary Indeterminate Lesions and Small Choroidal Melanoma. https://www.cancer.gov/about-cancer/treatment/clinical-trials/search/v?id=NCI-2020-04854&r=12021.

38 Hrbacek, J., Mishra, K.K., Kacperek, A. et al. (2016). Practice patterns analysis of ocular proton therapy centers: The international OPTIC survey. *International Journal of Radiation Oncology, Biology, Physics* 95: 336–343.

39 Chang, M.Y. and McCannel, T.A. (2013). Local treatment failure after globe-conserving therapy for choroidal melanoma. *Br J Ophthalmol* 97: 804–811.

40 Wang, Z., Nabhan, M., Schild, S.E. et al. (2013). Charged particle radiation therapy for uveal melanoma: A systematic review and meta-analysis. *International Journal of Radiation Oncology, Biology, Physics* 86: 18–26.

41 Mishra, K.K. (2016). Particle therapy is ideal for the treatment of ocular melanomas. *Medical Physics* Feb 43 (2): 631–634.

42 Weber, D.C. et al. (2005). Proton beam radiotherapy versus fractionated stereotactic radiotherapy for uveal melanomas: A comparative study. *International Journal of Radiation Oncology, Biology, Physics* 63 (2): 373.

43 Allen, A.M., Pawlicki, T., Dong, L. et al. (2012). An evidence based review of proton beam therapy: The report of ASTRO's emerging technology committee. *Radiotherapy and Oncology: Journal of the European Society for Therapeutic Radiology and Oncology* 103: 8–11.

44 Mishra, K.K., Quivey, J.M., Daftari, I.K., Weinberg, V., Cole, T.B., Patel, K., Castro, J.R., Phillips, T.L., and Char, D.H. (2015). Long-term Results of the UCSF-LBNL Randomized Trial: Charged Particle With Helium Ion Versus Iodine-125 Plaque Therapy for Choroidal and

Ciliary Body Melanoma. *International Journal of Radiation Oncology, Biology, Physics* Jun 1; 92(2):376–383. PMID: 25841624.

45 Toyama, S., Tsuji, H., Mizoguchi, N. et al. (2013). Long-term results of carbon ion radiation therapy for locally advanced or unfavorably located choroidal melanoma: Usefulness of CT-based 2-port orthogonal therapy for reducing the incidence of NVG. *International Journal of Radiation Oncology, Biology, Physics* 86: 270–276.

46 Oxenreiter, M.M., Lane, A.M., Aronow, M.B., Shih, H., Trofimov, A.V., Kim, I.K., and Gragoudas, E.S. (2020). Proton beam irradiation of uveal melanoma involving the iris, ciliary body and anterior choroid without surgical localisation (light field). *Br J Ophthalmol* Dec 21. 10.1136/bjophthalmol-2020-318063.

47 Daftari, I.K., Mishra, K.K., Seider, M., and Damato, B.E. (2018). Proton Beam Ocular Treatment in Eyes with Intraocular Silicone Oil: Effects on Physical Beam Parameters and Clinical Relevance of Silicone Oil in EYEPLAN Dose-Volume Histograms. *International Journal of Medical Physics, Clinical Engineering and Radiation Oncology* 7: 347–362. 10.4236/ijmpcero.2018.73029.

48 Hartsell, W.F., Kapur, R., Hartsell, S.O., Sweeney, P., Lopes, C., Duggal, A., Cohen, J., Chang, J., Polasani, R.S., Dunn, M., and Pankuch, M. (2016). Feasibility of Proton Beam Therapy for Ocular Melanoma Using a Novel 3D Treatment Planning Technique. *International Journal of Radiation Oncology • Biology • Physics* 95 (1): 353–359.

49 Daftari, I.K., Quivey, J.M., Chang, J.S., and Mishra, K.K. (2018). Feasibility study of titanium markers in choroidal melanoma localization for proton beam radiation therapy. *Medical Physics* 45 (3): March 1036–1039.

50 Mishra, K.K., Afshar, A., Thariat, J., Shih, H., Scholey, J., Daftari, I.K., Kacperek, A., Pica, A., Hrbacek, J., Dendale, R., Mazal, A., Heufelder, J., Char, D.H., Sauerwein, W., Weber, D.C., and Damato, B.E. (2020). Practice Considerations for Proton Beam Radiation Therapy of Uveal Melanoma During the Coronavirus Disease Pandemic: Particle Therapy Co-Operative Group Ocular Experience. *Advances in Radiation Oncology* Jul-Aug; 5(4):682–686. PMID: 32337386. PMCID: PMC7179507. https://doi.org/10.1016/j.adro.2020.04.010.

51 Goitein, M. and Miller, T. (1983). Planning proton therapy of the eye. *Medical Physics* 10: 275.

52 Sheen, M.A. Development of the eye proton therapy planning program. Proceedings of the 20th PTCOG Meeting, Vol. 10; Chester, England, 1994, pp. 16–18.

53 Daftari, I.K., Mishra, K.K., O'Brien, J.M., Tsai, T., Park, S.S., Sheen, M., and Phillips, T.L. (2010). Fundus image fusion in EYEPLAN software: An evaluation of a novel technique for ocular melanoma radiation treatment planning. *Medical Physics* Oct; 37(10):5199–5207. PMID: 21089753.

54 Hennings, F., Lomax, A., Pica, A., Weber, D.C., and Hrbacek, J. (2018). Automated treatment planning system for uveal melanomas treated with proton therapy: A proof-of-concept analysis. *International Journal of Radiation Oncology, Biology, Physics* 101: 724–731.

55 Slopsema, R.L., Mamalui, M., Zhao, T., Yeung, D., Malyapa, R., and Li, Z. (2013). Dosimetric properties of a proton beamline dedicated to the treatment of ocular disease. *Medical Physics* 41: 011707.

56 Kacperek, A. Ocular Proton Therapy Centers; 2012:149–177. https://doi.org/10.1007/978-3-642-21414-1_10

57 Konstantinidis, L., Roberts, D., Errington, R.D., Kacperek, A., Heimann, H., and Damato, B. (2015). Transpalpebral proton beam radiotherapy of choroidal melanoma. *Br J Ophthalmol* 99: 232–235. 10.1136/bjophthalmol-2014-305313.

58 Egger, E. et al. (2001). Maximizing local tumor control and survival after proton beam radiotherapy of uveal melanoma. *International Journal of Radiation Oncology, Biology, Physics* 51: 138–147.

59 Polishchuk, A.L., Mishra, K.K., Weinberg, V., Daftari, I.K., Nguyen, J.M., Cole, T.B., Quivey, J.M., Phillips, T.L., and Char, D.H. (2016). Temporal Evolution and Dose-Volume Histogram Predictors of Visual Acuity After Proton Beam Radiation Therapy of Uveal Melanoma. *International Journal of Radiation Oncology, Biology, Physics*. Jan 1; 97(1):91–97. doi: 10.1016/j.ijrobp.2016.09.019. Epub 2016 Sep 23. PMID: 27838186.

60 Caujolle, J.P., Mammar, H., Chamorey, E., Pinon, F., Herault, J., and Gastaud, P. (2010). Proton beam radiotherapy for uveal melanomas at nice teaching hospital: 16 years' experience. *International Journal of Radiation Oncology, Biology, Physics* 78: 98–103.

61 Thariat, J., Grange, J.D., Mosci, C. et al. (2016). Visual outcomes of parapapillary uveal melanoma following proton beam therapy. *International Journal of Radiation Oncology, Biology, Physics* 95: 328–335.

62 Mishra, K.K., Daftari, I.K., Weinberg, V., Cole, T., Quivey, J.M., Castro, J.R., Phillips, T.L., and Char, D.H. (2013). Risk factors for neovascular glaucoma after proton beam therapy of uveal melanoma: A detailed analysis of tumor and dose-volume parameters. *International Journal of Radiation Oncology, Biology, Physics* Oct 1; 87(2):330–336. PMID: 23886415.

63 Gragoudas, E.S. et al. (2000). A randomized controlled trial of varying radiation doses in the treatment of choroidal melanoma. *Archives of Ophthalmology* 118: 773.

64 Mishra, K.K., Kacperek, A., Daftari, I.K., Afshar, A., Scholey, J., Damato, B., Char, D., and Quivey, J. (2020). Proton Ocular Centers with Dedicated Fixed Low-Energy Beams: Key Concepts for New Centers. *IOVS* June 61 (7): page 3622.

65 Wouters, B., Skarsgard, L., Gerweck, L., Carabe-Fernandez, A., Wong, M., Durand, R.E., Nielson, D., Bussiere, M.R.,

Wagner, M., Biggs, P., Paganetti, H., and Suit, H.D. (2015). Radiobiological Intercomparison of the 160 MeV and 230 MeV Proton Therapy Beams at the Harvard Cyclotron Laboratory and at Massachusetts General Hospital. *Radiation Research* 183 (2): 174–187. http://dx.doi.org/10.1667/RR13795.1. https://bioone.org/journals/radiation-research/volume-183/issue-2/RR13795.1/Radiobiological-Intercomparison-of-the-160-MeV-and-230-MeV-Proton/10.1667/RR13795.1.short

66 Proton Relative, P.H. (2018). Biological Effectiveness – Uncertainties and Opportunities. *International Journal of Particle Theory* 5 (1): 2–14. 10.14338/IJPT-18-00011.1.

67 Haas-Kogan, D., Indelicato, D., Paganetti, H., Esiashvili, N., Mahajan, A., Yock, T., Flampouri, S., MacDonald, S., Fouladi, M., Stephen, K., Kalapurakal, J., Terezakis, S., Kooy, H., Grosshans, D., Makrigiorgos, M., Mishra, K.K., Young Poussaint, T., Cohen, K., Fitzgerald, T., Gondi, V., Liu, A., Michalski, J., Mirkovic, D., Mohan, R., Perkins, S., Wong, K., Vikram, B., Buchsbaum, J., and Kun, L. (2018). National Cancer Institute Workshop on Proton Therapy for Children: Considerations Regarding Brainstem Injury. *International Journal of Radiation Oncology • Biology • Physics* 101 (1): 152e168. https://doi.org/10.1016/j.ijrobp.2018.01.013.

68 Paganetti, H., Blakely, E., Carabe-Fernandez, A., Carlson, D.J., Das, I.J., Dong, L., et al. (2019). Report of the AAPM TG-256 on the relative biological effectiveness of proton beams in radiation therapy. *Medical Physics* 46: e53–78. https://doi.org/10.1002/mp.13390.

69 Blakely, E.A. (2020). The 20th Gray lecture 2019: Health and heavy ions. *The British Journal of Radiology* 93: 20200172. https://doi.org/10.1259/bjr.20200172.

70 Tang, J.T., Inoue, T., Inoue, T., Yamazaki, H., Fukushima, S., Fournier-Bidoz, N., et al. (1997). Comparison of radiobiological effective depths in 65-MeV modulated proton beams. *British Journal of Cancer* 76: 220–225. https://doi.org/10.1038/bjc.1997.365.

71 Courdi, A., Brassart, N., Hérault, J., and Chauvel, P. (1994). The depth-dependent radiation response of human melanoma cells exposed to 65 MeV protons. *The British Journal of Radiology* Aug 67 (800): 800–804. 10.1259/0007-1285-67-800-800.

72 Blakely, E.A., Bjornstad, K.A., Daftari, I.K., Renner, T.R., Nyman, M.A., Singh, R.P., Flocchini, R., Netherton, J., Verhey, L.J., Castro, J.R., and Char, D.H., 68 MeV proton radiobiology for treatment of uveal melanoma. (abstract) Radiation Research Society, 1996.

73 Tepper, J., Verhey, L., Goitein, M., and Suit, H.D. (1977). In vivo determinations of RBE in a high energy modulated proton beam using normal tissue reactions and fractionated dose schedules. *International Journal of Radiation Oncology, Biology, Physics* 2 (11-12): 1115–1122. https://doi.org/10.1016/0360-3016(77)90118-3.

74 Lühr, A., Von Neubeck, C., Pawelke, J., Seidlitz, A., Peitzsch, C., Bentzen, S.M., et al. (2018). "Radiobiology of Proton Therapy": Results of an international expert workshop. *Radiotherapy and Oncology: Journal of the European Society for Therapeutic Radiology and Oncology* 128: 56–67. https://doi.org/10.1016/j.radonc.2018.05.018.

75 Giovannini, G., Böhlen, T., Cabal, G., Bauer, J., Tessonnier, T., Frey, K., Debus, J., Mairani, A., and Parodi, K. (2016). Variable RBE in proton therapy: Comparison of different model predictions and their influence on clinical-like scenarios. *Radiation Oncology* May 17;11:68. doi: 10.1186/s13014-016-0642-6. PMID: 27185038; PMCID: PMC4869317: ...

76 Petti, P., Lyman, J.T., Renner, T.R., Castro, J.R., Collier, J.M., Daftari, I.K., and Ludewigt, B.A. (1991). Design of beam-modulating devices for charged-particle therapy. *Medical Physics* 18 (3): 513–518.

77 Varian Medical Systems. Planning Reference Guide for Eclipse Ocular Proton Planning Eclipse Ocular Proton Planning. 2007;(September):1–286.

78 Pfeiffer, K., Dobler, B., Rethfeldt, C., Schlegel, W., and Bendl, R. (2000). OCTOPUS, a planning tool for proton therapy of eye tumours. In: *The Use of Computers in Radiation Therapy*, Berlin, Heidelberg: Springer. 329–331. https://doi.org/10.1007/978-3-642-59758-9_124.

79 Raysearch Lab. https://www.raysearchlabs.com/media/press-releases/2020/new-release-of-groundbreaking-treatment-planning-system-raystation-provides-major-advances-for-proton-pbs-monte-carlo-with-gpu Accessed May 15, 2021.

80 Shin, D., Yoo, S.H., Moon, S.H., Yoon, M., Lee, S.B., and Park, S.Y. (2012). Eye tracking and gating system for proton therapy of orbital tumors. *Medical Physics* 39: 4265–4273.

81 Carnicer, A., Angellier, G., Thariat, J., Sauerwein, W., Caujolle, J.P., and Herault, J. (2013). Quantification of dose perturbations induced by external and internal accessories in ocular proton therapy and evaluation of their dosimetric impact. *Medical Physics* June 40 (6): https://aapm.onlinelibrary.wiley.com/doi/full/10.1118/1.4807090

82 Munzenrider, J.E. et al. (1989). Conservative treatment of uveal melanoma: Local recurrence after proton beam therapy. *International Journal of Radiation Oncology, Biology, Physics* 17: 493.

83 Gragoudas, E.S. (2006). Proton beam irradiation of uveal melanomas: The first 30 years. The Weisenfeld lecture. *Investigative Ophthalmology & Visual Science* 47 (11): 4666–4673.

84 Damato, B., Kacperek, A., Chopra, M. et al. (2005). Proton beam radiotherapy of choroidal melanoma: The Liverpool-

Clatterbridge experience. *International Journal of Radiation Oncology, Biology, Physics* 62: 1405–1411.

85 Char, D.H., Phillips, T., and Daftari, I. (2006). Proton teletherapy of uveal melanoma. *International Ophthalmology Clinics* 46: 41–49.

86 Dendale, R. et al. (2006). Proton beam radiotherapy for uveal melanoma: Results of Curie Institut-Orsay proton therapy center (ICPO). *International Journal of Radiation Oncology, Biology, Physics* 65 (3): 780–787.

87 Kodjikian, L. et al. (2004). Survival after proton-beam irradiation of uveal melanomas. *American Journal of Ophthalmology* 137: 1002.

88 Afshar, A.R., Stewart, J.M., Kao, A.A., Mishra, K.K., Daftari, I.K., and Damato, B.E. (2015). Proton beam radiotherapy for uveal melanoma. *Expert Review of Ophthalmology* 10: 577–585.

89 Fuss, M. et al. (2001). Proton radiation therapy for medium and large choroidal melanoma: Preservation of the eye and its functionality. *International Journal of Radiation Oncology, Biology, Physics* 49 (4): 1053–1059.

90 Courdi, A., Caujolle, J.P., Grange, J.D. et al. (1999). Results of proton therapy of uveal melanomas treated in Nice. *International Journal of Radiation Oncology, Biology, Physics* 45: 5–11.

91 Mosci, C., Mosci, S., Barla, A. et al. (2009). Proton beam radiotherapy of uveal melanoma: Italian patients treated in Nice, France. *European Journal of Ophthalmology* 19: 654–660.

92 Verma, V. and Mehta, M.P. (2016). Clinical outcomes of proton radiotherapy for uveal melanoma. *Clinical Oncology* 28: e17–e27.

93 Weber, B., Paton, K., Ma, R., and Pickles, T. (2016). Outcomes of proton beam radiotherapy for large non-peripapillary choroidal and ciliary body melanoma at TRIUMF and the BC cancer agency. *Ocular Oncology and Pathology* 2: 29–35.

94 Cirrone, G., Cuttone, G., Lojacono, P. et al. (2004). A 62-MeV proton beam for the treatment of ocular melanoma at Laboratori Nazionali del Sud-INFN. *IEEE Transactions on Nuclear Science* 51: 860–865.

95 Kacperek, A. (2009). Proton therapy of eye tumours in the UK: A review of treatment at Clatterbridge. *Applied Radiation and Isotopes: Including Data, Instrumentation and Methods for Use in Agriculture, Industry and Medicine* 67: 378–386.

96 Hocht, S., Bechrakis, N.E., Nausner, M. et al. (2004). Proton therapy of uveal melanomas in Berlin: 5 Years of experience at the Hahn-Meitner Institute. *Strahlentherapie Und Onkol* 180: 419–424.

97 Egger, E. et al. (2003). Eye retention after proton beam radiotherapy for uveal melanoma. *International Journal of Radiation Oncology, Biology, Physics* 55 (4): 867.

98 Egan, K.M. et al. (1989). The risk of enucleation after proton beam irradiation of uveal melanoma. *Ophthalmology* 96 (9): 1377.

99 Char, D.H. et al. (2002). Late radiation failures after iodine 125 brachytherapy for uveal melanoma compared with charged- particle (proton or helium ion) therapy. *Ophthalmology* 109: 1850.

100 The Collaborative Ocular Melanoma Study Group. (1997). Factors predictive of growth and treatment of small choroidal melanoma: COMS Report No. 5. *Archives of Ophthalmology* 115: 1537.

101 Mortality in patients with small choroidal melanoma. (1997). COMS report no. 4. The Collaborative Ocular Melanoma Study Group. *Archives of Ophthalmology* 115: 886.

102 Singh, A.D., Mokashi, A., Bena, J., Jacques, R., Rundle, P., and Rennie, I. (2006). Small Choroidal Melanocytic Lesions Features Predictive of Growth. *Ophthalmology* 113: 1032–1039.

103 Roelofs, K.A., O'Day, R.O., Al Harby, L., Arora, A.K., Cohen, V., Sagoo, M.S., and The, D.B. (2020). MOLES system for planning management of melanocytic choroidal tumors: Is it safe? *Cancers* 12: 1311. 10.3390/cancers12051311.

104 Straatsma, B.R. et al. (2003). Mortality after deferral of treatment or no treatment for choroidal melanoma. *American Journal of Ophthalmology* 136 (1): 47.

105 Jampol, L.M. et al. (2002). The COMS randomized trial of iodine 125 brachytherapy for choroidal melanoma: IV. Local treatment failure and enucleation in the first 5 years after brachytherapy. COMS report no. 19. *Ophthalmology* 109: 2197.

106 Damato, B. (2007). Legacy of the Collaborative Ocular Melanoma Study. *Arch Ophthalmol July* 125 (7): 966–968.

107 Castro, J.R., Char, D.H., Petti, P., Daftari, I.K., Quivey, J.M., Singh, R.P., Blakely, E., and Phillips, T.L. (1997). 15 years experience with helium ion radiotherapy for uveal melanoma. *IJROBP* 39 (5): 989–996.

108 Gragoudas, E. et al. (2002). Evidence-based estimates of outcome in patients irradiated for intraocular melanoma. *Archives of Ophthalmology* 120 (12): 1665.

109 Nag, S. et al. (2003). The American Brachytherapy Society recommendations for brachytherapy of uveal melanomas. *International Journal of Radiation Oncology, Biology, Physics* 56: 544.

110 Konstantinidis, L., Groenewald, C., Coupland, S., and Damato, B. (2014). Trans-scleral local resection of toxic choroidal melanoma after proton beam radiotherapy. *Br J Ophthalmol* 98 (6): 775–779.

111 Seddon, J.M. et al. (1986). Visual outcome after proton beam irradiation of uveal melanoma. *Ophthalmology* 93: 674.

112 Sikuade, M.J., Salvi, S., Rundle, P.A., Errington, D.G., Kacperek, A., and Rennie, I.G. (2015). Outcomes of treatment with stereotactic radiosurgery or proton beam therapy for choroidal melanoma. *Eye (Lond)* Sep;29(9):1194–1198. doi: 10.1038/eye.2015.109. Epub 2015 Jul 10. PMID: 26160531; PMCID: PMC4565940.

113 Tsuji, H. et al. (2007). Carbon-ion radiotherapy for locally advanced or unfavorably located choroidal melanoma: A phase I/II dose-escalation study. *International Journal of Radiation Oncology • Biology • Physics* 67: 857–862.

114 Toyama, S., Tsuji, H., Mizoguchi, N., Nomiya, T., Kamada, T., Tokumaru, S., Mizota, A., Ohnishi, Y., and Tsujii, H. (2013). and the Working Group for Ophthalmologic Tumors. Long-term Results of Carbon Ion Radiation Therapy for Locally Advanced or Unfavorably Located Choroidal Melanoma: Usefulness of CT-based 2-Port Orthogonal Therapy for Reducing the Incidence of Neovascular Glaucoma. *International Journal of Radiation Oncology • Biology • Physics* 86 (2): 270–276.

115 Moriarty, J.P., Borah, B.J., Foote, R.L., Pulido, J.S., and Shah, N.D. (2015). Cost-Effectiveness of Proton Beam Therapy for Intraocular Melanoma. *PLoS ONE* 10 (5): e0127814. https://doi.org/10.1371/journal.pone.0127814.

116 Mruthyunjaya, P. and Vail, D. (2019). Characterizing uveal melanoma treatment pathways in a large cohort of commercially insured patients. Abstract presentation, International Society of Ocular Oncology. March 23, 2019.

117 Zytkovicz, A. et al. (2007). Peripheral dose in ocular treatments with CyberKnife and Gamma Knife radiosurgery compared to proton radiotherapy. *Physics in Medicine and Biology* 52: 5957–5971.

118 Fakiris, A.J. et al. (2007). Gamma-knife-based stereotactic radiosurgery for uveal melanoma. *Stereotactic and Functional Neurosurgery* 85 (2-3): 106.

119 Liscak, R. and Vladyka, V. (2007). Radiosurgery in ocular disorders: Clinical applications. *Progress in Neurological Surgery* 20: 324.

120 Henderson, M.A. et al. (2006). Stereotactic radiosurgery and fractionated stereotactic radiotherapy in the treatment of uveal melanoma. *Technology in Cancer Research & Treatment* 5 (4): 411.

121 National Cancer Institute. Intraocular melanoma clinical trials. https://www.cancer.gov/about-cancer/treatment/clinical-trials/disease/intraocular-melanoma?pn=1. Accessed May 15, 2021.

122 Marucci, L. et al. (2006). Conservation treatment of the eye: Conformal proton reirradiation for recurrent uveal melanoma. *International Journal of Radiation Oncology, Biology, Physics* 64 (4): 1018.

123 Avery, R.B. et al. (2008). Histopathologic characteristics of choroidal melanoma in eyes enucleated after iodine-125 brachytherapy in the collaborative ocular melanoma study. *Archives of Ophthalmology* 126 (2): 207.

124 Kujala, E., Makitie, T., and Kivela, T. (2003). Very long-term prognosis of patients with malignant uveal melanoma. *Investigative Ophthalmology & Visual Science* 44 (11): 4651.

125 Diener-West, M. et al. (2004). Screening for metastasis from choroidal melanoma: The collaborative ocular melanoma study group report 23. *Journal of Clinical Oncology: Official Journal of the American Society of Clinical Oncology* 22: 2438.

126 Diener-West, M. et al. (2005). Development of metastatic disease after enrollment in the COMS trials for treatment of choroidal melanoma: COMS report no. 26. *Archives of Ophthalmology* 123 (12): 1639.

127 Middleton, M., McAlpine, C., Woodcock, V., Corrie, P., Infante, J., Steven, N., Evans, T., Anthoney, A., Shoushtari, A., Hamid, O., Gupta, A., Vardeu, A., Leach, E., Naidoo, R., Stanhope, S., Lewis, S., Hurst, J., O'Kelly, I., and Tebentafusp, S.M. (2020). A TCR/Anti-CD3 Bispecific Fusion Protein Targeting gp100, Potently Activated Antitumor Immune Responses in Patients with Metastatic Melanoma. *Clinical Cancer Research: An Official Journal of the American Association for Cancer Research* 26: 5869–5878.

128 Sophie Piperno-Neumann, J.C., Hassel, P.R., Jean-Francois Baurain, M.O., Butler, M.S., Sullivan, R.J., Ochsenreither, S., Reinhard Dummer, J.M., Kirkwood, A.M., Joshua, J.J., Sacco, A.N., Shoushtari, M.O., Carvajal, R.D., Omid Hamid, S.E., Abdullah, C.H., Goodall, H., and Nathan, P. (2021). Phase 3 randomized trial comparing tebentafusp with investigator's choice in first line metastatic uveal melanoma. April 10, abstract presentation. *American Association for Cancer Research* https://cancerres.aacrjournals.org/content/81/13_Supplement/CT002.abstract

129 Groenewald, C., Konstantinidis, L., and Damato, B. (2013). Effects of radiotherapy on uveal melanomas and adjacent tissues. *Eye* 27: 163–171.

130 Thariat, J., Salleron, J., Maschi, C., Fevrier, E., Lassalle, S., Gastaud, L., Baillif, S., Claren, A., Baumard, F., Herault, J., and Caujolle, J.P. (2019). Oncologic and visual outcomes after postoperative proton therapy of localized conjunctival melanomas. *Radiation Oncology* 14 (1): 239. 10.1186/s13014-019-1426-6.

131 Damato, B. and Coupland, S.E. (2009). Management of conjunctival melanoma. *Expert Review of Anticancer Therapy* 9 (9): 1227–1239. 10.1586/era.09.85.

132 Santoni, A., Thariat, J., Maschi, C., Herault, J., Baillif, S., Lassalle, S., Pevrichon, M.L., Salleron, J., and Caujolle, J.P. (2019). Management of invasive squamous cell carcinomas of the conjunctiva. *American Journal of Ophthalmology* April 200: 1–9. 10.1016/j.ajo.2018.11.024.

133 Chan, R.V., Yonekawa, Y., Lane, A.M. et al. (2010). Proton beam irradiation using a light-field technique for the treatment of choroidal hemangiomas. *Ophthalmologica* 224 (4): 209–216.

134 Levy-Gabriel, C., Rouic, L.L., Plancher, C. et al. (2009). Long-term results of low-dose proton beam therapy for circumscribed choroidal hemangiomas. *Retina* 29 (2): 170–175.

135 Mukkamala, L.K., Mishra, K.K., Daftari, I.K., Moshiri, A., and Park, S.S. (2020). Phase I/II randomized study of proton beam with anti-VEGF for exudative age-related macular degeneration: Long-term results. *Eye (Lond)* Dec 34 (12): 2271–2279.

136 Tsina, E.K., Lane, A., Zacks, D.N., Munzenrider, J.E., Collier, J.M., and Gragoudas, E.S. (2005). Treatment of metastatic tumors of the choroid with proton beam irradiation. *Ophthalmology* 112: 337–34.

137 Jardel, P., Sauerwein, W., Olivier, T., Bensoussan, E., Maschi, C., Lanza, F., Mosci, C., Gastaud, L., Angellier, G., Marcy, P.Y., Herault, J., Caujolle, J.P., Dendale, R., and Thariat, J. (2014). Management of choroidal metastases. *Cancer Treatment Reviews* 40: 1119–1128. http://dx.doi.org/10.1016/j.ctrv.2014.09.006.

138 Mouw, K.W., Sethi, R.V., Yeap, B.Y., MacDonald, S.M., Chen, Y.L., Tarbell, N.J., Yock, T.I., Munzenrider, J.E., Adams, J., Grabowski, E., Mukai, S., and Shih, H.A. (2014). Proton radiation therapy for the treatment of retinoblastoma. *International Journal of Radiation Oncology • Biology • Physics* 90 (4): 863–869.

139 Fasola, C.E., Jones, J.C., Huang, D.D., Le, Q.T., Hoppe, R., and Donaldson, S.S. (2013). Low-dose radiation therapy (2 Gy x 2) in the treatment of orbital lymphoma. *International Journal of Radiation Oncology • Biology • Physics* 86 (5): 930–935.

15

Brain, Skull Base, and Spinal Tumors

Dr. Kim Melanie Kraus & Univ. Prof. Dr. Stephanie E. Combs

Technical University of Munich (TUM), Department of Radiation Oncology, Ismaninger Straße 22, 81675 Munich, Germany

---

TABLE OF CONTENTS

15.1 Introduction

The physical and biological advantages of particle therapy, such as proton therapy or Carbon Ion Radiotherapy (CIRT), over conventional photon radiotherapy have already exploited for decades. In 1946 R. Wilson discovered the potential therapeutic effect of fast protons due to their favorable dose distribution in tissue [1]. This dose distribution is caused by the outstanding characteristic energy release of particles in matter. When charged particles such as protons or heavy ions travel through tissue they only release a small amount of energy after entering the tissue and deposit the largest amount of energy at the end of their path in tissue. This leads to a very steep dose fall off and a finite range of charged particles depending on their energy. This steep dose fall off is usually referred to as the Bragg-Peak. For protons, there is almost no dose deposition beyond the Bragg Peak; however, for heavy ions such as carbon ions, the nuclear fragmentation of the projectile can cause a small amount of unfavorable dose deposition beyond the Bragg Peak called fragmentation tail. However, at greater tissue depths heavy ions show a steeper lateral dose fall off compared to protons. Compared to photon beam dose distributions, these unique physical features of energy release of particles, however, allow for dose escalation within the tumor while sparing healthy surrounding tissue.

Additionally, besides the physical advantages, radiotherapy with heavy ions provides a superior relative biological effectiveness (RBE) compared to photon and proton beams [2]. The increased linear energy transfer (LET) of heavy ions in the tumor reveals in a more effective unrepairable deoxyribonucleic acid (DNA) damage and resulting cell death compared to low-LET radiation such as photons. Moreover, due to a reduced oxygen enhancement ration compared to photon beams, hypoxic tumors will be more sensitive to heavy particle treatment [3].

Besides the above mentioned advantages offered by heavy ion radiotherapy, for reaching therapeutic depths of tumors in human bodies, heavy charged particles have to be accelerated to energies of hundreds of MeV. For this, large and still expensive particle accelerators are required. Nowadays, only 12 centers in 5 countries (Japan, Germany, Italy, China, Austria) provide CIRT; worldwide only 2 centers are equipped with a gantry offering CIRT from all angles due to the size and expenses required.

Principles and Practice of Particle Therapy, First Edition. Edited by Timothy D. Malouff and Daniel M. Trifiletti.
© 2022 John Wiley & Sons Ltd. Published 2022 by John Wiley & Sons Ltd.

Since the first patient treatment in 1994 at The National Institute of Radiologic Sciences (NIRS) in Chiba, Japan, over 20,000 patients have been treated with carbon ions including a large variety of tumor sites.

Naturally, intracranial tumors are favorably suited for CIRT due to the necessity of sparing of vital surrounding tissue and thus maintaining neurological functions. Moreover, many primary brain tumors are characterized by radioresistance, and the biological properties of CIRT may overcome these properties and lead to increased local control and potentially overall survival. While most studies and clinical evaluations have been performed in gastrointestinal tumors, neurooncology focused groups have evaluated CIRT in different brain and skull base tumors.

15.2 Glioma

Gliomas are the most frequent primary brain malignancies graded by the World Health Organization (WHO) Grading system into low-grade (WHO I-II) and high-grade (WHO III-IV) tumors [4]. Prognostic relevant molecular markers such as mutations of the isocitrate dehydrogenase 1 and 2 genes (IDH1/IDH2) and loss of the chromosomal arms 1p and 19q further classify these tumors.

The rationale for CIRT of glioma might be diverse. Whereas low-grade glioma, such as pilocytic astrocytoma and oligodendroglioma, may preferably benefit in a decreased long-term morbidity from CIRT, high-grade gliomas could benefit from an improved tumor control and a resulting improved survival due to an increased biological effectiveness.

15.2.1 High-Grade Glioma

High-grade gliomas encompass anaplastic astrocytoma, anaplastic oligodendroglioma (WHO grade III), and glioblastoma multiforme (WHO grade IV). High-grade gliomas are the most frequent primary brain tumors with a poor prognosis and survival rates of less than one year and a strong dependence on grade and molecular signature [5-8]. Standard therapy comprises surgical resection followed by radio(chemo)therapy (RCT) [9-12]. Radiotherapy has shown to improve survival rates from a few months to approximately 14 months [13]. Despite these major improvements in outcomes, the majority of patients relapse early and median survival still ranged between 15 and 24 months, depending on molecular subtype. This forms the rationale of a more effective treatment. High-grade glioma are typically radio- and chemoresistant tumors requiring aggressive therapy and high radiation doses [12].

The combination of the conformal dose distribution and the increased RBE created the rationale to consider particle radiotherapy for administration of effective doses to high-grade gliomas.

To overcome the radioresistance and improve the unsatisfying outcome for treatment of high-grade glioma patients, high LET radiotherapy has been considered. In 1999, in a prospective phase II trial, Fitzek et al. [14] showed that a proton boost with doses up to 90 GyE was effective in preventing local tumor recurrences for patients suffering from glioblastoma multiforme. However, these high doses were associated with high rates of side effects, namely symptomatic necrosis. In 2001, Iwadate et al. [15] proved a superior effect on glioma cell death by high RBE CIRT compared to photon irradiation. In a small phase I/II trial with 48 patients, Mizoe et al. [16] investigated CIRT boost after RCT. Patients received RCT with nimustine hydrochloride (ACNU) given at a dose of 100 mg/m^2 during the first, fourth, and fifth weeks of irradiation. Patients received a radiation dose of 50 Gy in 25 fractions and a sequential carbon ion boost in 8 fractions with doses from 16.8 GyE to 24.8 GyE administered in 10% incremental steps. In the small patient cohort investigated, they found superior survival rates of 35 months for anaplastic astrocytoma patients and 17 months for patients suffering from glioblastoma multiforme.

Based on the patient cohort from the study above [16], Combs et al. investigated the cytotoxic effect of high LET CIRT on glioblastoma cell lines in combination with temozolomide chemotherapy in a preclinical retrospective in vitro analysis [17]. Combined RCT with temozolomide and CIRT showed to be more effective against glioblastoma cells compared to photon irradiation. Combination with temozolomide had an additive effect for both radiation types. After retrospective comparison of radiotherapy alone, RCT with temozolomide and CIRT for high-grade glioblastoma with a potential benefit for CIRT found [18]; this hypothesis is now being investigated in the CLEOPATRA trial investigating CIRT boost to the macroscopic tumor up to 18 GyE in 6 fractions after photon RCT with 48 Gy to 52 Gy in 24–26 fractions with temozolomide for primary glioblastoma compared to a proton boost with 10 GyE administered in 5 fractions. The study evaluated overall survival, and as secondary endpoints, progression-free survival, treatment toxicity, and safety. At the interim analysis after occurrence of 35 deaths (22 deaths in the intervention group and 13 in the control group) with a sample of 89 patients it was decided to stop the study since the hypothesis of superiority of carbon ion boost treatment over proton boots treatment could not be kept. Results are submitted for publication. Preliminary data from the investigators report a median overall survival of 18.1 vs. 16.23 months (p = 0.71) in the proton arm and carbon arm and a median progression-free survival of 6.2 and 6.6 (p = 0.69), respectively. Toxicity was acceptable; in particular, no grade ≥ 3 toxicity was detected.

Recently, data from Kong et al. [19] for 50 patients with anaplastic astrocytoma or glioblastoma was reported. Twenty-four patients received proton therapy with 60 GyE in 30 fractions and 26 patients received proton therapy plus a carbon ion boost with various dose escalation schemes with a total dose up to 12 GyE. Overall survival was 72.8% and local control rate was 59.8% at 18 months. No grade 3 or higher toxicities were observed.

The effect of an induction carbon ion boost followed by proton radiotherapy with concurrent temozolomide for high-grade glioma is investigated in a phase I/III study from the Shanghai Proton and Heavy Ion Center [20]. Patients with unifocal glioblastoma or anaplastic astrocytoma are enrolled. In phase I, the dose for the sequential carbon ion boost is determined by dose escalation from 3 to 18 GyE in 3 fractions. In phase III, patients are randomized to a carbon ion boost with the dose determined in phase I followed by 60 GyE proton therapy in 30 fractions with concurrent temozolomide at 75 mg/m^2, or to the control arm where proton therapy with temozolomide with the same doses will be applied without a carbon ion boost. The primary endpoints are overall survival and toxicity rates. The secondary endpoints that will be investigated are progression-free survival and tumor response.

In the recurrent or progressive state of high-grade glioma re-irradiation might often be required, either additional to surgery or definitive. However, due to suspected toxicities and limited effectiveness this can be challenging [21]. Nowadays, high-precision radiotherapy such as stereotactic radiotherapy and radiosurgery allow for dose escalation, thus treatment being more effective. However, particle therapy might offer additional benefits due to physical and biological properties.

In a recent analysis, retrospective analysis of 30 patients with recurrence of high-grade glioma safe reirradiation with carbon ions with 45 GyE in 15 fractions was reported. No grade 4 or higher toxicities were observed with a median overall survival of 13 months [22].

A randomized phase I/II study evaluating CIRT in case of recurrent glioma is the CINDERELLA trial [23]. The study compares CIRT with an escalating dose from 30 GyE in 10 fractions to 48 GyE in 16 fractions to fractionated photon radiotherapy with 36 Gy in 18 fractions. The primary endpoint of phase II of the study is the survival rate at 12 months after re-irradiation, and the secondary endpoint is progression-free survival. Preliminary results showed a median overall survival of 352 days with a beneficial impact of small target volumes (480 days [PTV < 75 ml] vs. 322 days [PTV > 75 ml], p = 0.06). No grade ≥ 3 toxicities were detected during follow up [24].

Treatment planning for low-grade gliomas should always include contrast-enhanced MRI, generally as T1-T2 and flair-weighted sequences (Table 15.1). If available, amino-acid PET imaging ishelpful.

15.2.2 Low-Grade Glioma

Low-grade gliomas, such differentiated astrocytoma andoligo-dendroglioma, are relatively rare brain tumors and mainly affect young adults [25]. Even though the prognosis of low-grade gliomas is satisfactory with a survival average of approximately 7 years for patients affected by astrocytomas and more than 15 years for those with oligodendrogliomas [26], low-grade gliomas are invasive and have the ability to progress to high-grade gliomas.

Clearly, intracranial radiotherapy can cause severe side effects. It has been proven that radiotherapy with particular sparing of the hippocampus can reduce therapy-associated neurocognitive impairment and improve the clinical outcome [27–29]. Moreover, intracranial radiotherapy for children and young adults has been shown to cause severe hormonal dysfunction depending on the administered dose [30]. Due to the increased radiosensitivity of normal tissue and expected patient life time, a challenge in radiotherapy of low-grade gliomas of children and young adults is the reduction of integral dose to prevent long-term side effects and secondary malignancies.

Thus, the rationale for the use of particle therapy for low-grade gliomas may be different compared to high-grade gliomas. An improved long-term morbidity due to more conformal dose delivery and successful sparing of intracranial structures could be the driving force to administer particle therapy.

The majority of clinical evidence is based on proton therapy [31–35]. Hug et al. [32] evaluated low-grade pediatric astrocytoma and found proton therapy to be a safe and highly conformal treatment modality with tolerable toxicity. In a dose escalation study by Fitzek et al. [34] for pediatric astrocytoma authors could not find superior local control or survival rates by dose escalation for combined proton and photon therapy for low- and high-grade tumors.

Several other studies from the Heidelberg Ion-Beam Therapy Center (HIT) and the Massachusetts General Hospital on proton therapy for low-grade gliomas confirmed the safety of proton therapy comparable to that of photon therapy [33,35–37].

Table 15.1 Recommended target volumes and radiation doses for treatment of high-grade gliomas.

Volume	Definitive	Postoperative	Dose
GTV	Visible tumor on T1-weighted MRI	Resection cavity and if available residual tumor	60 GyE with photons, potential for dose escalation with carbon or protons
CTV high risk	GTV + a few millimeters	GTV + 1–3 cm	60 GyE
PTV	CTV + 5 mm (institutional variability)	CTV + 3–5 mm (institutional variability)	60 GyE

Data for CIRT for low-grade glioma is rare compared to high-grade glioma.

CIRT for low-grade gliomas has been evaluated by Hasegawa et al. [38] in a phase I/II study at the National Institute of Radiological Sciences (NIRS) in Chiba, Japan. Fourteen patients with diffuse astrocytoma grade II were enrolled. The carbon ion dose was escalated from 50.4 GyE to 55.2 GyE in 24 fractions in phase I. Patients were divided into a low-dose and high-dose group. In the low-dose group a radiation dose of 46.2–50.4 GyE was applied and in the high-dose group a dose of 55.2 GyE was used. The median progression-free survival was significantly improved for the high dose group with 91 months compared to 18 months in the low dose group. The overall survival was 28 months in the low dose group and was not reached for the high dose group with a median follow up of 62 months. No grade 3 or higher toxicities were detected. The findings of this study demonstrate an association of a higher carbon ion dose with an improved outcome.

Limitations of particle therapy for brain tumors might be elevated rates of radiation-induced lesions within the white matter and radiation necrosis. For proton therapy of low-grade glioma, radiation-induced white matter lesions and necorsis were observed to appear at high LET regions with an increased RBE at the distal edge of the beam and also proximal to the ventricular system due to increased radiosensitivity [39,40]. However, in another study investigating intracranial proton therapy for children, no increased prevalence of symptomatic radiation necrosis were found [41].

Treatment planning for low-grade gliomas should always include contrast-enhanced MRI, generally as T1-T2 and flair-weighted sequences (Table 15.2). If available, amino-acid PET Imaging Is helpful.

15.3 Meningioma

Meningioma are primary central nervous system tumors, originating from the meningeal cells of the dura mater and commonly grow slowly. They can be located at the surface of the brain or spread along the cerebrospinal fluid. According to the WHO they are graded into: low-grade meningioma (grade I) that represent the majority of all meningiomas with a good prognosis, atypical meningiomas (grade II) which are associated with an increased recurrence rate, and anaplastic meningiomas (grade III) that are malignant and fast growing. Malignant meningiomas are associated with higher recurrence rates and worse survival compared to benign meningiomas [42]. Atypical and anaplastic meningiomas are associated with a five-year survival rate of 63.8% [4].

The primary treatment option for symptomatic grade I benign meningioma is surgery. However, in cases where complete resection might not be feasible due to an increased risk of impairment of critical neighboring structures, radiotherapy is an effective alternative for long-term tumor control [43]. Standard treatment for grade II and III meningiomas includes surgery followed by radiotherapy. High survival rates for meningiomas emphasize the need for maintaining neuronal functionality by sparing of organs at risk. However, high radiation doses are required for local tumor control and have been shown to improve patient survival despite of the radiation quality [44]. The rationale for particle radiation treatment is based on the opportunity to reduce these side effects due to a very conformal dose distribution, especially for meningioma in critical locations close to sensitive structures.

Several investigations have been performed to explore the application of proton therapy for meningioma at diverse locations with high local control rates and improved overall survival compared to photon therapy. Data from the Massachusetts General Hospital at Harvard University evaluating proton radiosurgery with a dose of 13 GyE for 50 patients with benign meningioma showed to be safe with a three-year local control rate of 94%. Tumor locations varied; 75% of the tumors were located at the cranial base [45].

In a study from Uppsala (Sweden), Gudjonsson reported clinical outcomes for 19 patients with skull base meningioma treated up to 24 GyE in 6 GyE single proton doses. The authors did not find any sign of tumor progression after 36 months and no severe toxicities were observed [46].

At the National Accelerator Center (NAC) (Republic of South Africa), fractionated or hypofractionated stereotactic proton therapy was investigated for 27 meningiomas, out of which 23 were located at the skull base. A total of 89% of the hypofractionated group were stable with tolerable toxicity in both groups [47].

Table 15.2 Recommended target volumes and radiation doses for treatment of low-grade gliomas.

Volume	Definitive	Postoperative	Dose
GTV	Visible tumor on T2-flair-weighted MRI	Resection cavity and if available residual tumor	54 GyE with photons, potential for dose escalation with carbon or protons
CTV high risk	GTV + a few millimeters	GTV + 5–10 mm	54 GyE
PTV	CTV + 5 mm (institutional variability)	CTV + 3–5 mm (institutional variability)	54 GyE

Data for 22 patients with atypical meningioma from the Indiana University Health Proton Therapy Center [48] between 2005 and 2013 showed that doses over 60 GyE were associated with a five-year local control rate of 88%. Doses lower than 60 GyE were shown to result in reduced local control rates of 50%. Patients in this study received fractionated proton therapy with prescription doses between 54 and 68.4 GyE and single fraction doses of 1.8–2GyE.

Safety and improved toxicity with promising clinical outcome for CIRT of meningiomas has been shown in multiple single institutional studies [36,49–52].

An early analysis for carbon ion boost for high-risk meningioma revealed a high local tumor control rate. In this study, 10 patients with anaplastic or atypical meningioma were enrolled. All received photon therapy with a median dose of 50.4 Gy followed by a carbon ion boost of 18 GyE to the macroscopic tumor residual. The results revealed a high local control rate of 86% at 5 years and 72% at 7 years without severe treatment-related side effects. Another prospective analysis of particle therapy for meningioma revealed a local control rate of 67% at 12 months after carbon ion boost for recurrent high-risk meningioma [53].

In the setting of reirradiation with either protons or carbon ions of recurrent meningiomas for 42 patients, particle therapy was shown to be safe [52]. No grade 4 or higher toxicity was observed. The progression-free survival was 71% after 1 year and 56.5% after 24 months with a significant impact of WHO grading.

At HIT, carbon ion boost therapy for subtotally resected high-risk meningiomas is evaluated in the MARCIE trial [54]. The MARCIE trial is an ongoing phase II study at HIT investigating a carbon ion boost with 16 GyE in 3 GyE fractions in combination with photon radiation therapy with a dose of 48 to 52 Gy after subtotal tumor resection (Simpson Grade 4–5). The primary endpoint is progression-free survival at 3 years.

Another trial also initiated at HIT is the PINOCHIO study that compares conventionally fractionated photon therapy, hypofractionated photon therapy, proton therapy, and CIRT for treatment of skull base meningioma (NCT01795300).

Obviously, the data on CIRT for meningioma is very limited. To date, there are very few data from prospective clinical trials. The majority of evidence is based on small retrospective studies with heterogeneous patient cohorts. However, the role of radiotherapy for meningioma is mostly limited to recurrent or residual tumors or those that are unresectable. Thus, patient characteristics might differ substantially. Long-term data of large prospective trials to answer questions on long-term morbidity and survival is mandatory.

15.3.1 Treatment Planning

Treatment planning for skull base meningioma is based on pre- and post-contrast T1-weighted and T2-weighted Magnetic Resonance Images (MRIs) to assure precise delineation of the target volume and organs at risk. Other MR sequences such as fluid attenuated inversion recovery (FLAIR) sequences can be helpful to distinguish the perilesional edema and the dural tail. In distinct cases also positron emission tomography (PET) with DOTATOC- and DOTANOC-tracers can supply additional information for large tumors infiltrating soft tissue or for those that cannot be distinguished on MRI and CT.

The gross tumor volume (GTV) for benign meningiomas is defined as the visible lesion on T1-contrast-enhanced MRIs with a slice thickness of 1–2 mm For clinical target volume definition (CTV) a few millimeters margin should be added to account for microscopic tumor infiltration.

For grade 2 and 3 meningioma postoperative the target volume includes the resection cavity and if available the residual tumor. The CTV is defined as the GTV plus 1–2 cm margin that can be smaller close to natural growth barriers such as the skull and the brain unless there is evidence of invasion.

The planning target volume (PTV) varies upon institutions but is typically defined as the CTV plus a 5 mm margin.

Typically, a dose of 54–60 GyE in 30–33 daily fractions of 1.8–2.0 GyE is prescribed to the target volume. For stereotactic radiosurgery typical doses used are 13–15 GyE given in a single fraction and 21–25 Gy given in 3–5 fractions (Table 15.3).

Table 15.3 Recommended target volumes and radiation doses for treatment of meningioma.

Volume	Definitive	Postoperative	Dose
GTV	Visible tumor on T1-weighted MRI	Resection cavity and if available residual tumor	54 GyE
CTV high risk	GTV + a few millimeters	GTV + 1–2 mm	54 GyE
CTV low risk			54 GyE
PTV	CTV + 5 mm (institutional variability)	CTV + 5 mm (institutional variability)	RT: 54–60 GyE at 1,8 GyE or fSRS: 21–25 GyE in 3–5 fractions or SRS: 13–15 GyE in a single fraction

15.4 Skull Base and Spinal Chordoma

15.4.1 Skull Base Chordoma

Chordoma are rare tumors that develop from remnants of the notochord of the skull base or the neural axis. Even though they typically grow slowly [55], they tend to be locally aggressive and show high rates of local recurrences. The primary treatment of chordomas is surgical resection. However, due to the very close proximity to sensitive structures, complete resection often cannot be achieved for chordomas of the clivus. Thus, adjuvant, or in case of unresectable tumors, definitive radiotherapy often is mandatory [56]. Due to their radioresistance, high radiation above 70 Gy is required to achieve high local tumor control rates [57]. The close proximity of nearby vital structures of the skull base necessitates highly conformal radiotherapy. Due to their preferable dose profiles, particle therapy with protons and carbon ions has been considered in a number of mostly retrospective studies with favorable results [58,59]. The majority of data accessible nowadays focuses on proton therapy.

In an early analysis with 169 patients receiving proton therapy with skull base chordomas at the Massachusetts General Hospital, Munzenrider et al. found local tumor control rates of 73% and 54% at 5 and 10 years, respectively [60]. Fung et al. investigated postoperative combined photon and proton therapy with doses between 68.4 GyE up to 73.8 GyE in fractions of 1,8 GyE at the Orsay Proton Therapy Center in France. Local control rates were even superior to the above mentioned American data. The found local control rates at 2, 4, and 5 years of 88.6%, 78.3%, and 75.1%, respectively.

Toxicity of CIRT for chordomas was found to be acceptable. Data on toxicity for CIRT was summarized in a recent metaanalysis [61]. The most common acute toxicities found were mucositits and local skin reactions [62,63] comparable with the results found for proton therapy [36]. Overall, grade 3 or higher toxicities were found in 0%–4%.

In a study with 96 patients treated with CIRT with a dose of 60–70 GyE in 20 fractions at the Gesellschaft für Schwerionenforschung (GSI) in Darmstadt (Germany) a local control rate of 70% at 5 years was found. About 4.1% developed optical neuropathy and 7.2% suffered from grade 1 and 2 temporal lobe injury [62]. In a small analysis of nine patients with skull base chordomas who underwent surgery and adjuvant CIRT the overall survival rate was 85.7%.

In a Japanese phase I/II study by Mizoe et al. from NIRS [64] CIRT with a dose up to 60.8 GyE in 16 fractions was investigated resulting in local control rates of 100% at 5 years. In an analysis of 155 patients with residual chordomas treated with CIRT at GSI with a dose of 60 GyE in 20 fractions, Uhl et al. reported local control rates of 82%, 72%, and 54% at 3, 5, and 10 years and overall survival rates of 95%, 85%, and 75% after 3, 5, and 10 years without the occurrence of higher grade toxicity [65].

Recently, long-term results of CIRT for skull base chordoma at NIRS in Japan were published by Koto et al. [66]. They analyzed 34 patients in a phase I/II trial. In the phase II study, patients were treated with 60.8 GyE in 16 fractions for inoperable skull base chordoma and found local control rates of 76.9% and 69.2% at 5 and 9 years. Overall survival was 93.5% and 77.4% at 5 and 9 years comparable to the data from a recent metaanalysis where overall survival rates were 100%, 94%, and 78% at 1, 5, and 10 years [61]. Interestingly, in the study from NIRS, authors reported in total 5 grade 3 or higher toxicities. One patient had grade 3 mucosal ulcer; two patients had grade 4 optical neuropathy and 1 grade 5 mucosal ulcer. Grade 2 brain injury was observed in three patients (9%). However, it has been shown before that doses over 50 GyE are associated with a higher risk of brain injury [67]. In this study, high fractional doses of 3.8 GyE were applied here compared to other studies [62]. Additionally, passive dose delivery was used, whereas more precise raster scanning approaches could improve the dose distribution.

An Italian study from CNAO in Pavia recently presented clinical outcome for 135 patients treated with protons or CIRT after surgical tumor resection [68]. They found local control rates at 5 years of 84% for proton therapy and 71% for CIRT with 12% grade 3 or higher toxicity irrespective of the particle used. The authors state that 87%–92% of local recurrences are located close at the interface of tumor and radiosensitive structures such as brain stem and optical structures. Thus, strict adherence to dose constraints most likely lead to underdosage of the tumor in these cases and might be reevaluated.

Due to the already promising results in clinical outcome for proton therapy of skull base chordomas, the potential benefit from CIRT is expected to be rather small. However, a few prospective trials try to elucidate the differences in clinical outcome between proton and carbon ion therapy. Proton therapy is currently being compared to CIRT in two studies from HIT. In the prospective randomized phase III HIT-1 study [69] (NCT01182779) proton therapy with a dose of 72 GyE is compared to CIRT with 63 GyE. The aim is to find out whether CIRT is superior to proton therapy with respect to local progression-free survival. Another trial initiated at HIT by Uhl et al. also evaluates hypofractionated CIRT versus proton therapy with a dose of 64 GyE in 16 fractions each in a randomized phase II trial [70]; however, this study focuses on chordoma of the sacrococcygeum.

Altogether, for chordoma and chondrosarcoma of the skull base, the clinical data for proton and photon therapy both show good results. However, for the challenging situations such as chordoma of the spine with post-operative metal implants, clinical results are worse [71,72]. The metal implants impact the application of particle therapy due to uncertainty in tumor delineation and range uncertainties [72]. Thus, other techniques such as image-guided and intensity-modulated radiotherapy (IGRT/IMRT) with photons [73] or stereotactic photon radiosurgery [74] with highly focused ablative radiation doses might be superior.

In summary, the treatment goal for chordoma focuses on high local control rates while sparing critical intracranial structures such as the brain stems or structures of the optic pathway. This can be optimally achieved by a multidisciplinary team offering a high grade of expertise in surgery and modern high-precision IGRT either with photons or particles [75].

15.4.2 Spinal Chordoma

The majority of spinal chordomas are located at the sacral spine. Due to their location they can also be associated with severe neurological morbidity such as bowel and urinary dysfunction. Thus, high-precision radiotherapy is mandatory for sacral chordomas.

Definitive proton therapy for unresectable spinal chordomas with the majority located at the sacral spine has been investigated by Chen et al. [76]. Median prescribed doses to the PTV was 77.4 GyE. Authors found a median overall survival of 91.7% and 78.1% at 3 and 5 years. A tumor volume of more than 500 cm^3 was associated with a worse overall survival.

Another study from Chiba (Japan) [77] evaluated CIRT for 188 patients with unresectable sacral chordomas with a maximum tumor volume of 345 cm^3. A total of 106 patients received a dose between 64.0 GyE and 73.6 GyE at 16 fractions. Authors found a five-year local control rate of 77.2% and a five-year overall survival of 81.1%. Six patients suffered from grade 3 peripheral nerve toxicity and two patients had grade 4 skin toxicity.

In a different study from HIT (Germany) [78] CIRT alone or in combination with photon IMRT for 56 patients with primary or recurrent sacral chordoma was investigated. Tumor volumes were between 5 and 1188 ml with a median of 244 ml. A dose between 60 and 74 GyE was prescribed to the tumor volume. The three-year local control probability was 53% and the overall survival rate after 25 months was 100% without higher grades of toxicities observed.

Differences in the outcome of proton and carbon ion therapy remain unclear. In an ongoing trial at HIT the difference between proton and carbon ion treatment for sacrococcygeal chordoma is explored [70].

15.5 Skull Base and Spinal Chondrosarcoma

Chondrosarcoma are rare malignant cartilaginous tumors with an estimated incidence of 1 in 200,000 per year [79] that account for less than 0.15% of all intracranial tumors. They develop from the skull bone and are locally destructive [80]. Due to their location close to sensitive vital structures, complete surgical resection is almost infeasible resulting in a high local recurrence rate. Thus, postoperative radiotherapy plays an important role in current treatment of chondrosarcoma [81]. The relative survival rate at 5 years based on a study of 9606 patient cases registered at the National Cancer Data Base of the American College of Surgeons was determined to be 75.2% [82].

Due to the similarity to chordomas chondrosarcomas face the same challenges with regard to treatment. Thus, the rationale for the application of particle therapy of chondrosarcoma of the skull base is similar to the one for chordomas. The majority of data available is based on studies on proton therapy. Survival rates of 75%–100% are reported.

In a study from the Paul Scherrer Institute (PSI) in Switzerland, proton therapy for skull base chondrosarcoma was investigated for 77 patients. Local control rates of 89.7% at 8 years and overall survival of 93.5% were found. Six out of 77 patients experienced higher grade toxicity [83] including hearing loss, brain and spinal cord necrosis, and optic neuropathy.

Simon et al. found an even higher local control rate of 100% at 5 years and 87.5% at 10 years after postoperative radiotherapy with protons with a clear benefit comparing to local control rates of 67.8% and 58.2% at 5 and 10 years after surgery alone [84].

In a dose escalation study, Palm et al. [85] showed that doses above 70 GyE improved the overall survival significantly up to 86.3% vs. 69.2% in favor of doses greater than 70 GyE. Definitive proton therapy was associated with improved overall survival at 5 years compared to conventional photon radiotherapy (75% vs. 19.1%). Perioperative proton therapy was also found to be associated with improved overall survival (97.1% vs. 69.4%).

These findings of high local control rates and overall survival rates for proton therapy almost hinder an escalation of these results for carbon ions.

A German study with 54 patients with low-grade and intermediate-grade chondrosarcomas of the skull base treated with carbon ions and a median dose of 60 GyE delivered in 3 GyE single fraction doses was conducted by Schulz-Ertner et al. They found local control rates of 96.2% at 3 years and 89.4% at 4 years with only one acute mucositis grade 3 and one late grade 3 toxicity in terms of worsening of a before known abducens nerve paresis. Overall survival was 98.2% at 5 years [63].

Uhl et al. [86] reported long-term results for 79 patients with skull base chondrosarcoma treated with a median total dose of 60 GyE at 3 GyE per fraction. Local control rates were 95.9%, 88%, and 88% and the corresponding overall survival rates were 96.1%, 96.1%, and 78.9% at 3, 5, and 10 years. They also found that age ≤ 45 years and a boost volume ≤ 55 ml was associated with a better local control rate. Moreover, they observed a reduction of cranial nerve deficits. As 73% of the patients suffered from cranial nerve deficits at baseline, the rate reduced to 45% to 53% at 7–10 years of follow up.

In the before-mentioned recent metaanalysis by Lu et al. [61], clinical outcome for 389 chordomas and 243 chondrosarcoma was assessed. Authors reported overall survival rates of 99%, 95%, and 79% and local control rates of 99%, 89%, and 88% at 1, 5, and 10 years.

A comparison of proton versus carbon ion therapy has been performed by Mattke et al. at HIT [87]. A total of 101 patients were included in the study. Authors compared proton therapy with a mean dose of 70 GyE at 2 GyE per fraction versus carbon ion therapy with 60GyE at 3 GyE per fraction for skull base chondrosarcoma. They showed local control rates of 100% vs. 90.5% and overall survival rates of 100% vs. 92.9% in favor of protons. However, these results were not statistically significant [87].

In order to evaluate the potential superiority of carbon ion irradiation to proton therapy a randomized phase III trial has been initiated at HIT [88] (NCT01182753). CIRT delivered with a dose of 60 GyE in 20 fractions is compared with 70 GyE in 35 fractions of proton therapy.

Limited data for spinal chondrosarcoma is available and mainly focuses on proton beam therapy. As chondrosarcoma are rather radioresistant high doses are required to achieve local control. Thus, a major challenge is reduction of dose to the spinal cord and critical surrounding structures to avoid toxicities.

Indelicato et al. [89] examined proton therapy for spinal chordoma and chondrosarcoma for 51 patients. A median dose of 70.2 GyE was prescribed and found a four-year overall survival rate of 72% and a local control rate of 58%. Patient age ≤ 58 years was associated with a higher rate of local recurrence.

The preliminary results for proton and carbon ion therapy for chordoma and chondrosarcoma of the skull base and cervi-cal spine from a study from China revealed that a lager tumor volume and reirradiation were associated with inferior survival [90]. Ninety-one patients were included in this study with a median tumor volume of 37.0 ml. Eight patients received proton therapy alone and 28 patients received combined proton and carbon ion therapy; 55 patients received CIRT alone. The two-year overall survival rate was 87.2%.

15.5.1 Treatment Planning

The GTV should be defined as the residual tumor on an CT fused with an MRI including T1-weighted, T2-weighted, and contrast-enhanced T1-weighted sequences with a slice thickness of 1–2 mm.

The CTV covers the GTV plus microscopic spread based on the preoperative tumor volume and residual postoperative tumor. For proton therapy, the CTV is often divided into the primary CTV and secondary CTV. The primary CTV is defined by the preoperative tumor volume including a margin of 10–20 mm plus residual tumor and resection margins excluding any normal tissue structures as well as edema. The posterior part of the sphenoidal sinus is included in the CTV in case patients receive a transsphenoidal resection. The secondary CTV includes the residual tumor and a margin of 5–10 mm plus the resection margins as locations with an increased risk for residual disease. For PTV delineation a margin of up to 5 mm is added to the CTV depending on the radiation technique and institutional positioning individuality.

Typically, a lower dose of 54 GyE is prescribed to the primary CTV and a higher dose of 74–76 GyE for the secondary CTV for chordoma and 70–72 GyE for chondrosarcoma (Table 15.4).

Table 15.4 Recommended target volumes and radiation doses for treatment of chordoma and chondrosarcoma.

Volume	Definitive	Postoperative	Dose
GTV	Visible tumor on T1-/T2-weighted and T1-weighted contrast enhanced MRI	Residual tumor on T1-/T2-weighted and T1-weighted contrast enhanced MRI	
CTV high risk		GTV + 5–10 mm + resection margins	74–76 GyE for chordoma 70–72 GyE for chondrosarcoma
CTV low risk		GTV + preoperative tumor volume + 10–20 mm + residual tumor + resection margins – any normal tissue structures/ edema	54 GyE
PTV	CTV + 5 mm (depending to radiation technique and institutional variability)	CTV + 5 mm (depending to radiation technique and institutional variability)	

References

1 Wilson, R.R. (1946). Radiological use of fast protons. *Radiology* 47: 487–491. https://doi.org/10.1148/47.5.487.

2 Krämer, M., Weyrather, W.K., and Scholz, M. (2003). The increased biological effectiveness of heavy charged particles: From radiobiology to treatment planning. *Technology in Cancer Research & Treatment* 2: 427–436. https://doi.org/10.1177/153303460300200507.

3 Tobias, C.A., Blakely, E.A., Alpen, E.L., Castro, J.R., Ainsworth, E.J., Curtis, S.B. et al. (1982). Molecular and cellular radiobiology of heavy ions. *International Journal of Radiation Oncology, Biology, Physics* 8: 2109–2120. https://doi.org/10.1016/0360-3016(82)90554-5.

4 Ostrom, Q.T., Gittleman, H., Liao, P., Vecchione-Koval, T., Wolinsky, Y., Kruchko, C. et al. (2017). CBTRUS statistical report: Primary brain and other central nervous system tumors diagnosed in the United States in 2010-2014. *Neuro-Oncology* 19: v1–88. https://doi.org/10.1093/neuonc/nox158.

5 Buckner, J.C. (2003). Factors influencing survival in high-grade gliomas. *Seminars in Oncology* 30: 10–14. https://doi.org/10.1053/j.seminoncol.2003.11.031.

6 Curran, W.J., Jr, Scott, C.B., Horton, J., Nelson, J.S., Weinstein, A.S., Fischbach, A.J. et al. (1993). Recursive partitioning analysis of prognostic factors in three radiation therapy oncology group malignant glioma trials. *Journal of the National Cancer Institute* 85: 704–710. https://doi.org/10.1093/jnci/85.9.704.

7 Adeberg, S., Harrabi, S.B., Verma, V., Bernhardt, D., Grau, N., Debus, J. et al. (2017). Treatment of meningioma and glioma with protons and carbon ions. *Radiation Oncology (London, England)* 12: 193. https://doi.org/10.1186/s13014-017-0924-7.

8 Wick, W., Weller, M., van Den Bent, M., Sanson, M., Weiler, M., Von Deimling, A. et al. (2014). MGMT testing–the challenges for biomarker-based glioma treatment. *Nature Reviews Neurology* 10: 372–385. https://doi.org/10.1038/nrneurol.2014.100.

9 Medical Research Council Brain Tumour Working Party (2001). Randomized trial of procarbazine, lomustine, and vincristine in the adjuvant treatment of high-grade astrocytoma: A medical research council trial. *Journal of Clinical Oncology* 19: 509–518. https://doi.org/10.1200/JCO.2001.19.2.509.

10 Shapiro, W.R., Green, S.B., Burger, P.C., Mahaley, M.S., Selker, R.G., VanGilder, J.C. et al. (1989). Randomized trial of three chemotherapy regimens and two radiotherapy regimens in postoperative treatment of malignant glioma: Brain tumor cooperative group trial 8001. *Journal of Neurosurgery* 71: 1–9. https://doi.org/10.3171/jns.1989.71.1.0001.

11 Chang, C.H., Horton, J., Schoenfeld, D., Salazer, O., Perez-Tamayo, R., Kramer, S. et al. (1983). Comparison of postoperative radiotherapy and combined postoperative radiotherapy and chemotherapy in the multidisciplinary management of malignant gliomas. A joint radiation therapy oncology group and eastern cooperative oncology group study. *Cancer* 52: 997–1007. https://doi.org/10.1002/1097-0142(19830915)52:6<997::AID-CNCR2820520612>3.0.CO;2-2.

12 Stupp, R., Mason, W.P., van Den Bent, M.J., Weller, M., Fisher, B., Taphoorn, M.J.B. et al. (2005). Radiotherapy plus concomitant and adjuvant temozolomide for glioblastoma. *The New England Journal of Medicine* 352: 987–996. https://doi.org/10.1056/NEJMoa043330.

13 Stupp, R., Hegi, M.E., Mason, W.P., van Den Bent, M.J., Taphoorn, M.J.B., Janzer, R.C. et al. (2009). Effects of radiotherapy with concomitant and adjuvant temozolomide versus radiotherapy alone on survival in glioblastoma in a randomised phase III study: 5-year analysis of the EORTC-NCIC trial. *The Lancet Oncology* 10: 459–466. https://doi.org/10.1016/S1470-2045(09)70025-7.

14 Fitzek, M.M., Thornton, A.F., Rabinov, J.D., Lev, M.H., Pardo, F.S., Munzenrider, J.E. et al. (1999). Accelerated fractionated proton/photon irradiation to 90 cobalt gray equivalent for glioblastoma multiforme: Results of a phase II prospective trial. *Journal of Neurosurgery* 91: 251–260. https://doi.org/10.3171/jns.1999.91.2.0251.

15 Iwadate, Y., Mizoe, J., Osaka, Y., Yamaura, A., and Tsujii, H. (2001). High linear energy transfer carbon radiation effectively kills cultured glioma cells with either mutant or wild-type p53. *International Journal of Radiation Oncology, Biology, Physics* 50: 803–808. https://doi.org/10.1016/s0360-3016(01)01514-0.

16 Mizoe, J.-E., Tsujii, H., Hasegawa, A., Yanagi, T., Takagi, R., Kamada, T. et al. (2007). Phase I/II clinical trial of carbon ion radiotherapy for malignant gliomas: Combined X-ray radiotherapy, chemotherapy, and carbon ion radiotherapy. *International Journal of Radiation Oncology, Biology, Physics* 69: 390–396. https://doi.org/10.1016/j.ijrobp.2007.03.003.

17 Combs, S.E., Bohl, J., Elsasser, T., Weber, K.-J., Schulz-Ertner, D., Debus, J. et al. (2009). Radiobiological evaluation and correlation with the local effect model (LEM) of carbon ion radiation therapy and temozolomide in glioblastoma cell lines. *International Journal of Radiation Biology* 85: 126–137. https://doi.org/10.1080/09553000802641151.

18 Combs, S.E., Bruckner, T., Mizoe, J.-E., Kamada, T., Tsujii, H., Kieser, M. et al. (2013). Comparison of carbon ion radiotherapy to photon radiation alone or in combination with temozolomide in patients with high-grade gliomas: Explorative hypothesis-generating retrospective analysis. *Radiotherapy and Oncology* 108: 132–135. https://doi.org/10.1016/j.radonc.2013.06.026.

19 Kong, L., Wu, J., Gao, J., Qiu, X., Yang, J., Hu, J. et al. (2020). Particle radiation therapy in the management of malignant glioma: Early experience at the Shanghai Proton and Heavy Ion Center. *Cancer* 126: 2802–2810. https://doi.org/10.1002/cncr.32828.

20 Kong, L., Gao, J., Hu, J., Lu, R., Yang, J., Qiu, X. et al. (2019). Carbon ion radiotherapy boost in the treatment of glioblastoma: A randomized phase I/III clinical trial. *Cancer communications (London, England)* 39: 5. https://doi.org/10.1186/s40880-019-0351-2.

21 Bauman, G.S., Sneed, P.K., Wara, W.M., Stalpers, L.J., Chang, S.M., McDermott, M.W. et al. (1996). Reirradiation of primary CNS tumors. *International Journal of Radiation Oncology, Biology, Physics* 36: 433–441. https://doi.org/10.1016/s0360-3016(96)00315-x.

22 Eberle, F., Lautenschläger, S., Engenhart-Cabillic, R., Jensen, A.D., Carl, B., Stein, M. et al. (2020). Carbon ion beam reirradiation in recurrent high-grade glioma. *Cancer Management and Research* 12: 633–639. https://doi.org/10.2147/CMAR.S217824.

23 Combs, S.E., Burkholder, I., Edler, L., Rieken, S., Habermehl, D., Jäkel, O. et al. (2010). Randomised phase I/II study to evaluate carbon ion radiotherapy versus fractionated stereotactic radiotherapy in patients with recurrent or progressive gliomas: The CINDERELLA trial. *BMC Cancer* 10: 533. https://doi.org/10.1186/1471-2407-10-533.

24 Combs, S.E., Bernhardt, D., Adeberg, S., Herfarth, K.K., Unterberg, A., Wick, W. et al. (2019). Carbon ion reirradiaton for patients with malignant gliomas: Toxicity and first results of the prospective dose-escalation phase I/II CINDERELLA trial. *Journal of Clinical Oncology* 37: 2059–2059. https://doi.org/10.1200/JCO.2019.37.15_suppl.2059.

25 Lin, Z., Yang, R., Li, K., Yi, G., Li, Z., Guo, J. et al. (2020). Establishment of age group classification for risk stratification in glioma patients. *BMC Neurology* 20: 310. https://doi.org/10.1186/s12883-020-01888-w.

26 Claus, E.B., Walsh, K.M., Wiencke, J.K., Molinaro, A.M., Wiemels, J.L., Schildkraut, J.M. et al. (2015). Survival and low-grade glioma: The emergence of genetic information. *Neurosurgical Focus* 38: E6. https://doi.org/10.3171/2014.10.FOCUS12367.

27 Gondi, V., Tomé, W.A., and Mehta, M.P. (2010). Why avoid the hippocampus? A comprehensive review. *Radiotherapy and Oncology* 97: 370–376. https://doi.org/10.1016/j.radonc.2010.09.013.

28 Gondi, V., Hermann, B.P., Mehta, M.P., and Tomé, W.A. (2012). Hippocampal dosimetry predicts neurocognitive function impairment after fractionated stereotactic radiotherapy for benign or low-grade adult brain tumors. *International Journal of Radiation Oncology, Biology, Physics* 83: e487–493. https://doi.org/10.1016/j.ijrobp.2011.10.021.

29 Marsh, J.C., Godbole, R.H., Herskovic, A.M., Gielda, B.T., and Turian, J.V. (2010). Sparing of the neural stem cell compartment during whole-brain radiation therapy: A dosimetric study using helical tomotherapy. *International Journal of Radiation Oncology, Biology, Physics* 78: 946–954. https://doi.org/10.1016/j.ijrobp.2009.12.012.

30 Merchant, T.E., Rose, S.R., Bosley, C., Wu, S., Xiong, X., and Lustig, R.H. (2011). Growth hormone secretion after conformal radiation therapy in pediatric patients with localized brain tumors. *Journal of Clinical Oncology* 29: 4776–4780. https://doi.org/10.1200/JCO.2011.37.9453.

31 McAllister, B., Archambeau, J.O., Nguyen, M.C., Slater, J.D., Loredo, L., Schulte, R. et al. (1997). Proton therapy for pediatric cranial tumors: Preliminary report on treatment and disease-related morbidities. *International Journal of Radiation Oncology, Biology, Physics* 39: 455–460. https://doi.org/10.1016/s0360-3016(97)00079-5.

32 Hug, E.B., Muenter, M.W., Archambeau, J.O., DeVries, A., Liwnicz, B., Loredo, L.N. et al. (2002). Conformal proton radiation therapy for pediatric low-grade astrocytomas. *Strahlentherapie und Onkologie* 178: 10–17. https://doi.org/10.1007/s00066-002-0874-2.

33 Combs, S.E., Ellerbrock, M., Haberer, T., Habermehl, D., Hoess, A., Jäkel, O. et al. (2010). Heidelberg Ion Therapy Center (HIT): Initial clinical experience in the first 80 patients. *Acta oncologica (Stockholm, Sweden)* 49: 1132–1140. https://doi.org/10.3109/0284186X.2010.498432.

34 Fitzek, M.M., Thornton, A.F., Harsh, G., Rabinov, J.D., Munzenrider, J.E., Lev, M. et al. (2001). Dose-escalation with proton/photon irradiation for Daumas-Duport lower-grade glioma: Results of an institutional phase I/II trial. *International Journal of Radiation Oncology, Biology, Physics* 51: 131–137. https://doi.org/10.1016/s0360-3016(01)01589-9.

35 Hauswald, H., Rieken, S., Ecker, S., Kessel, K.A., Herfarth, K., Debus, J. et al. (2012). First experiences in treatment of low-grade glioma grade I and II with proton therapy. *Radiation Oncology (London, England)* 7: 189. https://doi.org/10.1186/1748-717X-7-189.

36 Rieken, S., Habermehl, D., Haberer, T., Jaekel, O., Debus, J., and Combs, S.E. (2012). Proton and carbon ion radiotherapy for primary brain tumors delivered with active raster scanning at the Heidelberg Ion Therapy Center (HIT): Early treatment results and study concepts. *Radiation Oncology (London, England)* 7: 41. https://doi.org/10.1186/1748-717X-7-41.

37 Dennis, E.R., Bussiere, M.R., Niemierko, A., Lu, M.W., Fullerton, B.C., Loeffler, J.S. et al. (2013). A comparison of critical structure dose and toxicity risks in patients with low grade gliomas treated with IMRT versus proton radiation therapy. *Technology in Cancer Research & Treatment* 12: 1–9. https://doi.org/10.7785/tcrt.2012.500276.

38 Hasegawa, A., Mizoe, J.-E., Tsujii, H., Kamada, T., Jingu, K., Iwadate, Y. et al. (2012). Experience with carbon ion radiotherapy for WHO Grade 2 Diffuse astrocytomas. *International Journal of Radiation Oncology, Biology, Physics* 83: 100–106. https://doi.org/10.1016/j.ijrobp.2011.06.1952.

39 Bahn, E., Bauer, J., Harrabi, S., Herfarth, K., Debus, J., and Alber, M. (2020). Late contrast enhancing brain lesions in proton-treated patients with low-grade glioma: Clinical evidence for increased periventricular sensitivity and variable RBE. *International Journal of Radiation Oncology, Biology, Physics* 107: 571–578. https://doi.org/10.1016/j.ijrobp.2020.03.013.

40 Bauer, J., Bahn, E., Harrabi, S., Herfarth, K., Debus, J., and Alber, M. (2021). How can scanned proton beam treatment planning for low-grade glioma cope with increased distal RBE and locally increased radiosensitivity for late MR-detected brain lesions? *Medical Physics* n/a. https://doi.org/10.1002/mp.14739.

41 Bojaxhiu, B., Ahlhelm, F., Walser, M., Placidi, L., Kliebsch, U., Mikroutsikos, L. et al. (2018). Radiation necrosis and white matter lesions in pediatric patients with brain tumors treated with pencil beam scanning proton therapy. *International Journal of Radiation Oncology, Biology, Physics* 100: 987–996. https://doi.org/10.1016/j.ijrobp.2017.11.037.

42 Mahmood, A., Qureshi, N.H., and Malik, G.M. (1994). Intracranial meningiomas: Analysis of recurrence after surgical treatment. *Acta neurochirurgica (Wien)* 126: 53–58. https://doi.org/10.1007/BF01476410.

43 Debus, J., Wuendrich, M., Pirzkall, A., Hoess, A., Schlegel, W., Zuna, I. et al. (2001). High efficacy of fractionated stereotactic radiotherapy of large base-of-skull meningiomas: Long-term results. *Journal of Clinical Oncology* 19: 3547–3553. https://doi.org/10.1200/JCO.2001.19.15.3547.

44 Hug, E.B., Devries, A., Thornton, A.F., Munzenride, J.E., Pardo, F.S., Hedley-Whyte, E.T. et al. (2000). Management of atypical and malignant meningiomas: Role of high-dose, 3D-conformal radiation therapy. *Journal of Neuro-Oncology* 48: 151–160. https://doi.org/10.1023/a:1006434124794.

45 Halasz, L.M., Bussière, M.R., Dennis, E.R., Niemierko, A., Chapman, P.H., Loeffler, J.S. et al. (2011). Proton stereotactic radiosurgery for the treatment of benign meningiomas. *International Journal of Radiation Oncology, Biology, Physics* 81: 1428–1435. https://doi.org/10.1016/j.ijrobp.2010.07.1991.

46 Gudjonsson, O., Blomquist, E., Nyberg, G., Pellettieri, L., Montelius, A., Grusell, E. et al. (1999). Stereotactic irradiation of skull base meningiomas with high energy protons. *Acta Neurochirurgica (Wien)* 141: 933–940. https://doi.org/10.1007/s007010050399.

47 Vernimmen, F.J., Harris, J.K., Wilson, J.A., Melvill, R., Smit, B.J., and Slabbert, J.P. (2001). Stereotactic proton beam therapy of skull base meningiomas. *International Journal of Radiation Oncology, Biology, Physics* 49: 99–105. https://doi.org/10.1016/s0360-3016(00)01457-7.

48 McDonald, M.W., Plankenhorn, D.A., McMullen, K.P., Henderson, M.A., Dropcho, E.J., Shah, M.V. et al. (2015). Proton therapy for atypical meningiomas. *Journal of Neuro-Oncology* 123: 123–128. https://doi.org/10.1007/s11060-015-1770-9.

49 Combs, S.E., Hartmann, C., Nikoghosyan, A., Jäkel, O., Karger, C.P., Haberer, T. et al. (2010). Carbon ion radiation therapy for high-risk meningiomas. *Radiotherapy and Oncology* 95: 54–59. https://doi.org/10.1016/j.radonc.2009.12.029.

50 Combs, S.E., Kessel, K., Habermehl, D., Haberer, T., Jäkel, O., and Debus, J. (2013). Proton and carbon ion radiotherapy for primary brain tumors and tumors of the skull base. *Acta Oncologica (Stockholm, Sweden)* 52: 1504–1509. https://doi.org/10.3109/0284186X.2013.818255.

51 El Shafie, R.A., Czech, M., Kessel, K.A., Habermehl, D., Weber, D., Rieken, S. et al. (2018). Clinical outcome after particle therapy for meningiomas of the skull base: Toxicity and local control in patients treated with active rasterscanning. *Radiation Oncology (London, England)* 13: 54. https://doi.org/10.1186/s13014-018-1002-5.

52 El Shafie, R.A., Czech, M., Kessel, K.A., Habermehl, D., Weber, D., Rieken, S. et al. (2018). Evaluation of particle radiotherapy for the re-irradiation of recurrent intracranial meningioma. *Radiation oncology (London, England)* 13: 86. https://doi.org/10.1186/s13014-018-1026-x.

53 Combs, S.E., Welzel, T., Habermehl, D., Rieken, S., Dittmar, J.-O., Kessel, K. et al. (2013). Prospective evaluation of early treatment outcome in patients with meningiomas treated with particle therapy based on target volume definition with MRI and 68Ga-DOTATOC-PET. *Acta Oncologica (Stockholm, Sweden)* 52: 514–520. https://doi.org/10.3109/0284186X.2013.762996.

54 Combs, S.E., Edler, L., Burkholder, I., Rieken, S., Habermehl, D., Jäkel, O. et al. (2010). Treatment of patients with atypical meningiomas Simpson grade 4 and 5 with a carbon ion boost in combination with postoperative photon radiotherapy: The MARCIE Trial. *BMC Cancer* 10: 615. https://doi.org/10.1186/1471-2407-10-615.

55 Heffelfinger, M.J., Dahlin, D.C., MacCarty, C.S., and Beabout, J.W. (1973). Chordomas and cartilaginous tumors at the skull base. *Cancer* 32: 410–420. https://doi.org/10.1002/1097-0142(197308)32:2<410::aid-cncr2820320219>3.0.co;2-s.

56 Debus, J., Schulz-Ertner, D., Schad, L., Essig, M., Rhein, B., Thillmann, C.O. et al. (2000). Stereotactic fractionated radiotherapy for chordomas and chondrosarcomas of the skull base. *International Journal of Radiation Oncology, Biology, Physics* 47: 591–596. https://doi.org/10.1016/s0360-3016(00)00464-8.

57 Rackwitz, T. and Debus, J. (2019). Clinical applications of proton and carbon ion therapy. *Seminars in Oncology* 46: 226–232. https://doi.org/10.1053/j.seminoncol.2019.07.005.

58 Leeman, J.E., Romesser, P.B., Zhou, Y., McBride, S., Riaz, N., Sherman, E. et al. (2017). Proton therapy for head and neck cancer: Expanding the therapeutic window. *The Lancet Oncology* 18: e254–65. https://doi.org/10.1016/S1470-2045(17)30179-1.

59 Palm, A. and Johansson, K.-A. (2007). A review of the impact of *photon and proton external beam radiotherapy treatment mo*dalities on the dose distribution in field and out-of-field; implications for the long-term morbidity of cancer survivors. *Acta Oncologica (Stockholm, Sweden)* 46: 462–473. https://doi.org/10.1080/02841860701218626.

60 Munzenrider, J.E. and Liebsch, N.J. (1999). Proton therapy for tumors of the skull base. *Strahlentherapie und Onkologie* 175 (Suppl 2): 57–63. https://doi.org/10.1007/BF03038890.

61 Lu, V.M., O'Connor, K.P., Mahajan, A., Carlson, M.L., and Van Gompel, J.J. (2020). Carbon ion radiotherapy for skull base chordomas and chondrosarcomas: A systematic review and meta-analysis of local control, survival, and toxicity outcomes. *Journal of Neuro-Oncology* 147: 503–513. https://doi.org/10.1007/s11060-020-03464-1.

62 Schulz-Ertner, D., Karger, C.P., Feuerhake, A., Nikoghosyan, A., Combs, S.E., Jäkel, O. et al. (2007). Effectiveness of carbon ion radiotherapy in the treatment of skull-base chordomas. *International Journal of Radiation Oncology, Biology, Physics* 68: 449–457. https://doi.org/10.1016/j.ijrobp.2006.12.059.

63 Schulz-Ertner, D., Nikoghosyan, A., Hof, H., Didinger, B., Combs, S.E., Jäkel, O. et al. (2007). Carbon ion radiotherapy of skull base chondrosarcomas. *International Journal of Radiation Oncology, Biology, Physics* 67: 171–177. https://doi.org/10.1016/j.ijrobp.2006.08.027.

64 Mizoe, J., Hasegawa, A., Takagi, R., Bessho, H., Onda, T., and Tsujii, H. (2009). Carbon ion radiotherapy for skull base chordoma. *Skull Base* 19: 219–224. https://doi.org/10.1055/s-0028-1114295.

65 Uhl, M., Mattke, M., Welzel, T., Roeder, F., Oelmann, J., Habl, G. et al. (2014). Highly effective treatment of skull base chordoma with carbon ion irradiation using a raster scan technique in 155 patients: First long-term results. *Cancer* 120: 3410–3417. https://doi.org/10.1002/cncr.28877.

66 Koto, M., Ikawa, H., Kaneko, T., Hagiwara, Y., Hayashi, K., and Tsuji, H. (2020). Long-term outcomes of skull base chordoma treated with high-dose carbon-ion radiotherapy. *Head & Neck* 42: 2607–2613. https://doi.org/10.1002/hed.26307.

67 Koto, M., Hasegawa, A., Takagi, R., Fujikawa, A., Morikawa, T., Kishimoto, R. et al. (2014). Risk factors for brain injury after carbon ion radiotherapy for skull base tumors. *Radiotherapy and Oncology* 111: 25–29. https://doi.org/10.1016/j.radonc.2013.11.005.

68 Iannalfi, A., D'Ippolito, E., Riva, G., Molinelli, S., Gandini, S., Viselner, G. et al. (2020). Proton and carbon ion radiotherapy in skull base chordomas: A prospective study based on a dual particle and a patient-customized treatment strategy. *Neuro-Oncology* 22: 1348–1358. https://doi.org/10.1093/neuonc/noaa067.

69 Nikoghosyan, A.V., Karapanagiotou-Schenkel, I., Münter, M.W., Jensen, A.D., Combs, S.E., and Debus, J. (2010). Randomised trial of proton vs. carbon ion radiation therapy in patients with chordoma of the skull base, clinical phase III study HIT-1-Study. *BMC Cancer* 10: 607. https://doi.org/10.1186/1471-2407-10-607.

70 Uhl, M., Edler, L., Jensen, A.D., Habl, G., Oelmann, J., Röder, F. et al. (2014). Randomized phase II trial of hypofractionated proton versus carbon ion radiation therapy in patients with sacrococcygeal chordoma-the ISAC trial protocol. *Radiation Oncology* 9: 100. https://doi.org/10.1186/1748-717X-9-100.

71 DeLaney, T.F., Liebsch, N.J., Pedlow, F.X., Adams, J., Dean, S., Yeap, B.Y. et al. (2009). Phase II study of high dose photon/proton radiotherapy in the management of spine sarcomas. *International Journal of Radiation Oncology, Biology, Physics* 74: 732–739. https://doi.org/10.1016/j.ijrobp.2008.08.058.

72 Staab, A., Rutz, H.P., Ares, C., Timmermann, B., Schneider, R., Bolsi, A. et al. (2011). Spot-scanning-based proton therapy for extracranial chordoma. *International Journal of Radiation Oncology, Biology, Physics* 81: e489–496. https://doi.org/10.1016/j.ijrobp.2011.02.018.

73 Zabel-du Bois, A., Nikoghosyan, A., Schwahofer, A., Huber, P., Schlegel, W., Debus, J. et al. (2010). Intensity modulated radiotherapy in the management of sacral chordoma in primary versus recurrent disease. *Radiotherapy and Oncology* 97: 408–412. https://doi.org/10.1016/j.radonc.2010.10.008.

74 Yamada, Y., Laufer, I., Cox, B.W., Lovelock, D.M., Maki, R.G., Zatcky, J.M. et al. (2013). Preliminary results of high-dose single-fraction radiotherapy for the management of chordomas of the spine and sacrum. *Neurosurgery* 73: 673–680. discussion 680. https://doi.org/10.1227/NEU.0000000000000083.

75 Combs, S.E., Laperriere, N., and Brada, M. (2013). Clinical controversies: Proton radiation therapy for brain and skull base tumors. *Seminars in Radiation Oncology* 23: 120–126. https://doi.org/10.1016/j.semradonc.2012.11.011.

76 Chen, Y.-L., Liebsch, N., Kobayashi, W., Goldberg, S., Kirsch, D., Calkins, G. et al. (2013). Definitive high-dose photon/proton radiotherapy for unresected mobile spine and sacral chordomas. *Spine* 38: E930–936. https://doi.org/10.1097/BRS.0b013e318296e7d7.

77 Imai, R., Kamada, T., Araki, N., Abe, S., Iwamoto, Y., Ozaki, T. et al. (2016). Carbon ion radiation therapy for unresectable sacral chordoma: An analysis of 188 Cases. *International Journal of Radiation Oncology, Biology, Physics* 95: 322–327. https://doi.org/10.1016/j.ijrobp.2016.02.012.

78 Uhl, M., Welzel, T., Jensen, A., Ellerbrock, M., Haberer, T., Jäkel, O. et al. (2015). Carbon ion beam treatment in patients with primary and recurrent sacrococcygeal chordoma. *Strahlentherapie und Onkologie* 191: 597–603. https://doi.org/10.1007/s00066-015-0825-3.

79 Giuffrida, A.Y., Burgueno, J.E., Koniaris, L.G., Gutierrez, J.C., Duncan, R., and Scully, S.P. (2009). Chondrosarcoma in the United States (1973 to 2003): An analysis of 2890 cases from the SEER database. *The Journal of Bone and Joint Surgery (American)* 91: 1063–1072. https://doi.org/10.2106/JBJS.H.00416.

80 Kremenevski, N., Schlaffer, S.-M., Coras, R., Kinfe, T.M., Graillon, T., and Buchfelder, M. (2020). Skull Base Chordomas and Chondrosarcomas. *Neuroendocrinology* 110: 836–847. https://doi.org/10.1159/000509386.

81 Fernandez-Miranda, J.C., Gardner, P.A., Snyderman, C.H., Devaney, K.O., Mendenhall, W.M., Suárez, C. et al. (2014). Clival chordomas: A pathological, surgical, and radiotherapeutic review. *Head & Neck* 36: 892–906. https://doi.org/10.1002/hed.23415.

82 Damron, T.A., Ward, W.G., and Stewart, A. (2007). Osteosarcoma, chondrosarcoma, and Ewing's sarcoma: National Cancer Data Base Report. *Clinical Orthopaedics and Related Research®* 459: 40–47. https://doi.org/10.1097/BLO.0b013e318059b8c9.

83 Weber, D.C., Badiyan, S., Malyapa, R., Albertini, F., Bolsi, A., Lomax, A.J. et al. (2016). Long-term outcomes and prognostic factors of skull-base chondrosarcoma patients treated with pencil-beam scanning proton therapy at the Paul Scherrer Institute. *Neuro-Oncology* 18: 236–243. https://doi.org/10.1093/neuonc/nov154.

84 Simon, F., Feuvret, L., Bresson, D., Guichard, J.-P., El Zein, S., Bernat, A.-L. et al. (2018). Surgery and protontherapy in Grade I and II skull base chondrosarcoma: A comparative retrospective study. *PLoS ONE* 13. https://doi.org/10.1371/journal.pone.0208786.

85 Palm, R.F., Oliver, D.E., Yang, G.Q., Abuodeh, Y., Naghavi, A.O., and Johnstone, P.A.S. (2019). The role of dose escalation and proton therapy in perioperative or definitive treatment of chondrosarcoma and chordoma: An analysis of the National Cancer Data Base. *Cancer* 125: 642–651. https://doi.org/10.1002/cncr.31958.

86 Uhl, M., Mattke, M., Welzel, T., Oelmann, J., Habl, G., Jensen, A.D. et al. (2014). High control rate in patients with chondrosarcoma of the skull base after carbon ion therapy: First report of long-term results. *Cancer* 120: 1579–1585. https://doi.org/10.1002/cncr.28606.

87 Mattke, M., Vogt, K., Bougatf, N., Welzel, T., Oelmann-Avendano, J., Hauswald, H. et al. (2018). High control rates of proton- and carbon-ion-beam treatment with intensity-modulated active raster scanning in 101 patients with skull base chondrosarcoma at the Heidelberg Ion Beam Therapy Center. *Cancer* 124: 2036–2044. https://doi.org/10.1002/cncr.31298.

88 Nikoghosyan, A.V., Rauch, G., Münter, M.W., Jensen, A.D., Combs, S.E., Kieser, M. et al. (2010). Randomised trial of proton vs. carbon ion radiation therapy in patients with low and intermediate grade chondrosarcoma of the skull base, clinical phase III study. *BMC Cancer* 10: 606. https://doi.org/10.1186/1471-2407-10-606.

89 Indelicato, D.J., Rotondo, R.L., Begosh-Mayne, D., Scarborough, M.T., Gibbs, C.P., Morris, C.G. et al. (2016). A prospective outcomes study of proton therapy for chordomas and chondrosarcomas of the spine. *International Journal of Radiation Oncology, Biology, Physics* 95: 297–303. https://doi.org/10.1016/j.ijrobp.2016.01.057.

90 Guan, X., Gao, J., Hu, J., Hu, W., Yang, J., Qiu, X. et al. (2019). The preliminary results of proton and carbon ion therapy for chordoma and chondrosarcoma of the skull base and cervical spine. *Radiation oncology (London, England)* 14: 206. https://doi.org/10.1186/s13014-019-1407-9.

16

Head and Neck Cancers

Anna Lee, MD, MPH[1], Xingzhe Li, MD, MPH[2], and Nancy Lee, MD, FASTRO[2]

[1]*Department of Radiation Oncology, University of Texas MD Anderson Cancer Center, Houston, TX*
[2]*Department of Radiation Oncology, Memorial Sloan Kettering Cancer Center, New York, NY*
Corresponding author: *Nancy Y. Lee, MD, FASTRO Department of Radiation Oncology, Memorial Sloan Kettering Cancer Center, New York, NY1275 York Avenue New York, NY 10065*

16.1 Introduction

Radiation therapy has always been an integral part of multi-disciplinary management of head and neck cancer. Patients are either treated with definitive radiation in combination with chemotherapy or surgery followed by postoperative radiation with or without chemotherapy. Furthermore, focused radiation has been increasingly used in the settings of oligo-metastatic, oligoprogressive, or locoregional recurrent diseases to not only palliate symptoms and improve quality of life (QOL) but also to increase overall survival (OS). The improvement in OS despite metastatic disease is also likely attributed to improvements in systemic therapy.

Due to a combination of epidemiologic shifts toward more favorable or radiosensitive biology, such as Human Papilloma Virus (HPV)-related head and neck squamous cell carcinoma (SCC), as well as the improvement of radiation technology in many aspects, head and neck cancer patients are enjoying longer survival. Specifically, the adoption of intensity-modulated radiation therapy (IMRT) in the past two decades has been revolutionary in head and neck cancer treatment. IMRT has been shown to improve target coverage with better conformality and to spare critical normal tissues of high-dose radiation, causing less toxicities. However, due to the limitations in the physical properties of photon beam and the beam arrangement of IMRT, normal tissues are still exposed to low-to-moderate amount of radiation which could lead to toxicities. The chronic toxicities significantly affect QOL and may contribute to loss of productivity in these long-time survivors of head and neck cancer.

Particle therapy, and in particular, proton therapy, has been increasingly used in head and neck cancer treatment as the affordability and accessibility of this technology have improved steadily over the past decade. Other heavy particles in discussion primarily include neutrons, helium, carbon, and neon ions. Particle therapy offers potential advantages over photon-based radiation such as IMRT because of the unique physical characteristics of the particle beam. Most of the particle radiation dose is deposited across a very narrow range of depth, termed the "Bragg peak," reducing irradiation of normal tissues near the tumor. In head and neck cancer treatment, particle beam's advantage provides particular benefit in protecting major organs at risk (OARs) that are usually close to the tumor, including major salivary glands, oral cavity structures, pharyngeal mucosa, larynx, spinal cord, and brain tissue. The sparing of these OARs leads to significantly less toxicities, improving patients' QOL while potentially offering opportunities to dose-escalate for improved tumor control and longer survival. The prospect of expanding the therapeutic window of radiation treatment by particle therapy has led to exponentially increasing numbers of new particle centers opening or undergoing development across the United States and worldwide.

In this overview of particle therapy in head and neck cancer, we aim to provide a summary of recent development in treatment planning and delivery, the existing clinical evidence and ongoing prospective trials in major head and neck cancer subsites, and future directions that may further increase the therapeutic window of particle therapy in head and neck cancer.

16.2 Treatment Planning and Delivery

Particle therapy treatment planning is distinct from photon radiation planning due to differences in physical properties. Particles have a finite and defined depth of penetration with virtually no exit dose. Usually a spread-out Bragg peak (SOBP) is formed by using energy modulation technique to cover the range of the tumor target (Figure 16.1). Importantly, particle beam penetration is more affected by the type of tissue it traverses while the delivery affects dose distribution more than those with photons (Mohan and Grosshans, 2017).

Due to the sensitivity of particles to any materials in the beam's path as well as the use of tight margins, the process of CT simulation and immobilization requires close attention so that geometric uncertainties are accounted for. In most head and neck cases, patients are placed in the supine position with the neck in slight hyperextension. A five-point thermoplastic mask should be used for immobilization of the head, neck, and shoulders. If cervical nodes are not involved in treatment, a three-point mask can be considered. A bite block is used for oral cavity cancers, sinonasal cancers, and nasopharyngeal cancers. A custom bite block can be used to immobilize the oral tongue laterally to the contralateral side when unilateral treatment is planned. CT simulation with ≤3 mm slice thickness with and without IV contrast should be performed from the top of the head to the carina. Positron emission tomography (PET) is helpful for metabolically active gross disease and identification of involved or suspicious lymph nodes. Magnetic resonance imaging (MR) is recommended for accurate delineation of the extent of gross tumor in soft tissue as well as radiographic assessment of perineural spread. PET and MR images should be registered to the planning CT for accurate target delineation.

Our institution treats patients with proton therapy, so our main focus will be on protons; however, the same principles can be applied for other heavy particles. In general, fewer proton beams are needed in comparison to IMRT; thus, optimizing beam direction is important. The general goal is to minimize passage through complex tissue heterogeneities and have shorter paths to the distal tumor edge. The higher biological effectiveness at the end of the proton beam and the uncertainty in proton range mean critical structures (i.e., spinal cord) located just beyond the distal edge of the target should be avoided.

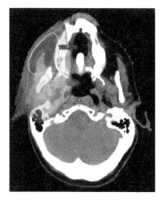 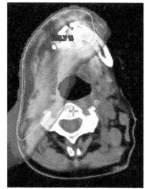 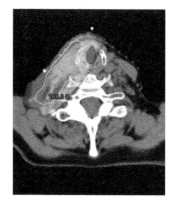

Figure 16.1 Example PBS plan (MFO-optimized) for patient with pT4aN0 squamous cell carcinoma of the right lower gingiva displaying the 50% isodose line. Green contour = CTV60.

During the planning process, heterogeneities along the beam path are taken into account to reflect the effects of varying tissue densities on the stopping power, while uncertainties of changes in the internal and external anatomy and setup errors are also considered. Artifacts such as dental hardware and surgical clips should be contoured and assigned the proper forced densities in order to ensure accurate beam calculation. All these effects are important as they can affect the potential shift of the Bragg peak location, whose terminal locations are the main loci of dose (Bortfeld, 1997) (Figure 16.1). These uncertainties are mitigated at the treatment planning stage utilizing robustness assessment.

The approach to dosing and fractionation can vary depending on the clinical scenario but in general, sequential cone downs are employed over dose painting as protons are more sensitive to changes in tumor response, thus allowing ease of adaptive planning. This method can also decrease hot spots in the plan. Furthermore, fraction sizes greater than 2 Gy are discouraged as the relative biological effectiveness (RBE) of protons is already higher, thus optimizing the toxicity profile. Details regarding dosing can be found under each subsection and sample constraints can be found in Table 16.1.

There are two main modes of proton delivery. In passive scatter, the lateral and longitudinal spread of the beam entering the nozzle can be shaped by customizing the field aperture, proton beamline and range compensator designs to ensure coverage of the tumor with appropriate three-dimensional margins. In pencil beam scanning, multiple beams from different directions are used to produce the desired pattern of dose. This latter mode enables the most advanced proton therapy used to date: intensity-modulated proton therapy (IMPT), which is especially useful in the head and neck where there is complex anatomic geometry and irregularity in target shapes (Ahn et al., 2014). IMPT coupled with multi-field optimization allows a high degree of conformality and intensity modulation to preferentially deposit proton dose with higher RBE in the target and away from normal tissues, improving the therapeutic window of proton therapy (Shen et al., 2015). Technical details of the planning process as well as special considerations for each subsite can be found in "Target Volume Delineation and Treatment Planning for Particle Therapy: A Practical Guide" (N. Y. Lee et al., 2018).

For daily treatment verification, daily orthogonal X-ray imaging is used in order to confirm setup accuracy. If available, in-room CT imaging (i.e., cone-beam CT) is ideally used for treatment verification on a weekly schedule. For sinonasal tumors, daily cone-beam CT is recommended as day-to-day variation in sinus mucous filling can impact the dose distribution. When in-room 3D imaging is not available, verification CT scans with the patient in the treatment position are recommended during the course of treatment to assess for changes in anatomy from weight loss or tumor shrinkage, which could lead to potential changes in the accuracy of the

Table 16.1 Sample dose constraint guidelines for primary radiation of the head and neck at MSK.

OAR	Constraint	Dose
Oral cavity	Mean dose	<10 Gy RBE
Oral cavity (for oropharyngeal cases)	Mean dose	35–40 Gy RBE
Spinal cord	Dose to 0.1 cm^3	<50 Gy RBE
	Surface max	64 Gy RBE[b]
Brainstem	Dose to 0.05 cm^3	<60 Gy RBE[a]
	Core max	53 Gy RBE
	Surface max	64 Gy RBE[b]
Cochlea[c]	Max dose	<50 Gy RBE
Optic nerves and chiasm	Dose to 0.05 cm^3	<60 Gy RBE
Ipsilateral parotid (for non-parotid cases)	Mean dose	25 Gy RBE
Ipsilateral parotid (for non-submandibular cases)	Mean dose	39 Gy RBE
Contralateral parotid and submandibular	Mean dose	0 Gy RBE
Larynx	Mean dose	<35 Gy RBE
Esophagus	Mean dose	<34 Gy RBE
Constrictors	Mean dose	<55 Gy RBE

[a]For plans with prescription dose ≤60 Gy RBE;
[b]Isodose line may touch structure surface;
[c]If ipsilateral hearing is absent, contralateral cochlea constraint is <35 Gy RBE.

dose distribution. At Memorial Sloan Kettering Cancer Center (MSK), verification scans are performed weekly for definitive cases and once halfway through treatment for postoperative cases, although the frequency can change depending on the clinical scenario.

16.3 Clinical Experiences and Practical Considerations

16.3.1 Oral Cavity Cancer

The most common subsites of oral cavity cancers are the oral tongue and floor of mouth. Known risk factors for the development of oral cavity cancer include tobacco, alcohol, and chewing of betel nut leaves. The typical management is surgical resection followed by risk-adapted therapy with radiation therapy and/or chemotherapy (Bernier et al., 2005).

Studies evaluating the use of proton therapy for oral cavity cancer alone are rare and the benefit of proton therapy for oral cavity cancer can be extrapolated from oropharyngeal cancer (see Section 16.3.2). For early stage, well-lateralized oral cavity cancers where the treatment target is unilateral, proton therapy can spare the contralateral side offering less side effects compared to IMRT (Kandula et al., 2013). As oral tongue cancers are difficult to control locally, the benefit of proton therapy is from potentially giving higher dose while minimizing toxicity. Furthermore, the higher RBE of protons may be beneficial when a tumor is unresectable or when a patient seeks a nonsurgical approach, especially in locally advanced cases where resection could be quite morbid and markedly reduce the QOL.

In Japan, a prospective trial of 33 patients with locally advanced oral tongue cancer was performed using a nonsurgical approach (Takayama et al., 2016). Treatment consisted of alternating chemoradiation, which included 5-fluorouracil (5-FU) and nedaplatin in week 1 followed by bilateral opposed photon fields to 36 Gy in 20 fractions to the bilateral neck and primary followed by another week of chemotherapy. Patients then received proton beam radiation to 28.6–39.6 Gy (RBE) in 13–18 fractions to the gross disease concurrently with intra-arterial cisplatin and sodium thiosulfate. At a median follow-up of 43 months, the 3-year local control (LC), regional control (RC) and OS were 86.6%, 83.9%, and 87%, respectively. Therapeutic end points were better than historical controls where surgery is typically employed. Furthermore, osteoradionecrosis (ORN) as a late effect was only seen in one patient as dose to the mandible was minimal. This is encouraging as the incidence of ORN after IMRT ranges from 2% to 16% (Gomez et al., 2011; Schuurhuis et al., 2011). Prospective studies evaluating a nonsurgical approach for oral cavity cancers may change the treatment paradigm by offering an organ-preserving approach without compromising cure.

While SCC of the oral cavity is already a challenging disease to control, non-squamous histologies are especially difficult in that they are relatively radioresistant. Ikawa and colleagues analyzed 76 patients with primarily T4 non-squamous oral cavity cancers treated at four different centers from 2004 to 2014 with carbon-ion therapy. With a median follow-up of 31.1 months, the 3-year LC was 86.6% and OS was 78.4%. Nine patients had grade 3 ORN and no grade 5 toxicities were observed (Ikawa et al., 2019). Interestingly, resectability did not affect LC perhaps highlighting the RBE potential of carbon ions.

Recommended target volumes and radiation doses for oral cavity cancer are in Table 16.2 and technical details regarding the planning process can be found in "Target Volume Delineation and Treatment Planning for Particle Therapy: A Practical Guide" (N. Y. Lee et al., 2018).

Table 16.2 Recommended target volumes and radiation doses for treatment of oral cavity cancer.

Volume	Definitive	Postoperative	Dose
GTV	Gross disease and involved regional lymph nodes	–	70 Gy (RBE)
High-risk CTV (CTV$_{70}$)	Include margin of 5 mm if there is uncertainty of gross disease extent	–	70 Gy (RBE)
High-risk CTV (CTV$_{66}$)	–	Include preoperative target volume and regions of extracapsular nodal extension, soft tissue invasion, bone invasion, and positive margins	66 Gy (RBE)
High-risk CTV (CTV$_{60}$)	Include up to a 10-mm margin for positive nodes, and high-risk ipsilateral or contralateral nodes	Include preoperative tumor volume and nodal disease, operative bed, and ipsilateral or contralateral nodes at high risk for subclinical disease	60 Gy (RBE)
Low-risk CTV (CTV$_{50}$)	Include ipsilateral and contralateral nodes at low risk for subclinical disease	Include uninvolved ipsilateral and contralateral lymph nodes at low risk for subclinical disease	50 Gy (RBE)

CTV = Clinical target volume; GTV = gross tumor volume; RBE = relative biological effectiveness.

16.3.2 Oropharyngeal Cancer

Radiation has been an integral part of the management of oropharyngeal cancer (OPC) in both definitive and adjuvant settings in addition to chemotherapy and surgery. IMRT has been employed to mitigate late toxicity such as xerostomia; however, adverse effects of treatments are still quite high especially in the setting of concurrent chemoradiation (Nguyen-Tan et al., 2014). With increasing numbers of younger and relatively healthy patients being diagnosed with HPV-positive OPC, further reduction of treatment related toxicities are necessary as these patients are expected to become long-term survivors after treatment (Nguyen-Tan et al., 2014). Multiple clinical trials are aimed at de-escalation of treatment intensity by reducing radiation dose or volume, using alternative radio-sensitizing agents, or integrating surgical resection of primary tumor in treatment of HPV-positive OPC with subsequent lower dose of RT. Proton therapy represents another promising measure for reducing treatment-related toxicities and improving long-term QOL.

Due to the anatomical complexity and large target volumes often seen in OPC, IMPT is generally recommended to enhance conformality and homogeneity of the radiation plan, while minimizing radiation to OARs. Early dosimetry studies have shown potential advantages of IMPT over IMRT in sparing of OARs (Blanchard et al., 2016; van de Water et al., 2012) and these dosimetry advantages could likely contribute to a favorable toxicity profile of proton therapy in OPC. Gunn et al. (2016) reported acute toxicities in 50 OPC patients (98% HPV+) treated with IMPT including grade 3 mucositis (58%), grade 3 dysphagia (24%), and grade 2 or worse xerostomia (25%), while no grade 4 or 5 toxicities were noted. In a separate report comparing the same 50 patients with 100 case matched OPC patients treated with IMRT, Blanchard et al. (2016) reported no statistical difference in OS or progression-free survival (PFS). Significant improvement in the preplanned composite end point of grade 3 weight loss or G-tube presence was noted at 3 months after treatment (odds ratio [OR] 0.44; 95% CI: 0.19–1; $p = 0.05$) and at 1 year after treatment (OR 0.23; 95% CI: 0.07–0.73; $p = 0.01$). Excellent disease control outcomes were reported with a 2-year OS of 94.5% and PFS of 88.6% for OPC patients treated with proton therapy.

Prospectively collected patient-reported outcomes (PROs) were reported by Sio et al. (2016) from 35 OPC patients treated by IMPT and 46 OPC patients treated by IMRT. Changes in taste and appetite in the subacute and chronic phases were significantly less with IMPT treatment. Collective symptom burden from the top 5 MDASI scores, generated from the MD Anderson Symptom Inventory for Head and Neck Cancer survey, was reportedly worse with IMRT only in the subacute phase. In another study investigating PROs of 64 patients after postoperative proton therapy (31 patients) versus IMRT (33 patients), Sharma et al. (2018) reported that patients receiving proton therapy had significantly less dose to many normal structures than those receiving IMRT, which was reflected by higher scores in both head and neck specific and general QOL measures, most notably less xerostomia at both 6 and 12 months after radiation.

OPC has recently become the most common HPV-related malignancy in the United States, stressing a compelling need to prospectively compare proton therapy to IMRT through multi-institutional randomized trial. An ongoing randomized phase III trial (NCT01893307) has been developed based on the above promising findings with IMPT with the schema of comparing IMPT versus IMRT for the treatment of OPC. The study aims to demonstrate at least non-inferiority of IMPT versus IMRT regarding oncologic outcomes, as well as to clarify the role of IMPT in mitigating treatment-related toxicities through secondary end points including PROs, physician-rated toxicity outcomes and cost–benefit analyses. Worldwide, two other prospective randomized trials have recently started recruiting, including the TORPEdO (TOxicity Reduction using Proton bEam therapy for Oropharyngeal cancer) trial by the UK National Health Service and the ARTSCAN V trial led by the Lund University Hospital in Sweden (Table 16.3). Recommended target volumes and radiation doses for oropharyngeal cancer are in Table 16.4 and technical details regarding the planning process can be found in "Target Volume Delineation and Treatment Planning for Particle Therapy: A Practical Guide" (N. Y. Lee et al., 2018) (Figure 16.2).

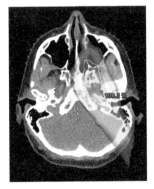 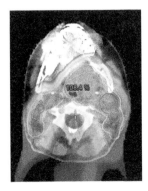 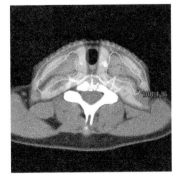

Figure 16.2 Example PBS plan (MFO-optimized) for patient with p16 + cT2N2 squamous cell carcinoma of the left tonsil displaying the 50% isodose line. Red contour = CTV70. Green contour = CTV30.

Table 16.3 Ongoing clinical trials investigating particle therapy in head and neck cancer.

	Institution	Trial name	Inclusion	Treatment	Primary end points	Study start
NCT04185974	University Hospital Heidelberg	Carbon Ion Re-Radiotherapy in Patients with Recurrent or Progressive Locally Advanced Head-and-Neck Cancer (CARE)	Locally recurrent HNC	Randomized to C12 vs. photon	Acute and subacute toxicity	August 2020
NCT03865277	Technische Universitat Dresden	Individualized Radiation Dose Prescription in HNSCC Based on F-MISO-PET Hypoxia-Imaging (INDIRA-MISO)	Locally advanced HNSCC	Randomized to standard CRT vs. dose-escalated CRT with carbon boost	Local control at 2 years	September 2019
NCT03829033	Lund University Hospital	Photon Therapy Versus Proton Therapy in Early Tonsil Cancer	Early stage SCC of the tonsil, unimodal and unilateral treatment	Randomized to PBT vs. conventional RT	Acute and late side effects	January, 2019
NCT03539198	Mayo Clinic	Study of Proton SBRT and Immunotherapy for Recurrent/Progressive Locoregional or Metastatic Head and Neck Cancer	Recurrent locoregional or recurrent metastatic HNC	Proton SBRT + nivolumab	Objective response rate	July 2018
NCT03274414	MSK	A Clinical Trial of Endoscopic Surgery Followed by Chemotherapy and Proton Radiation for the Treatment of Tumors in the Sinus and Nasal Passages	Cancer of the nasal cavity and/or paranasal sinuses	Endoscopic surgical resection and PBT	Local control at 1 year	September 2017
NCT03217188	MSK	A Phase II Study of Proton Re-irradiation for Recurrent Head and Neck Cancer	Recurrent or second primary HNC, previous head and neck radiation	PBT	Locoregional control at 1 year	July 2017
NCT03164460	MDA	Stereotactic Body Radiation Therapy or Intensity Modulated Radiation/ Proton Therapy in Treating Patients with Recurrent Head and Neck Cancer	Recurrent or second primary HNC, previous head and neck radiation (at least 30 Gy)	Randomized to SBRT vs. IMPT/ IMRT	Incidence of grade 3+ toxicity within 2 years post-RT	May 2017
NCT02923570	MSK, Mayo Clinic, Mount Sinai Hospital	A Phase II Randomized Study of Proton Beam Versus Photon Beam Radiotherapy in the Treatment of Unilateral Head and Neck Cancer	Unilateral head and neck targets (salivary, skin tumors)	Randomized to PBT vs. IMRT	Acute toxicity	October 2016
NCT02942693	Shanghai Proton and Heavy Ion Center	Trial Evaluating Particle Therapy with or without apatinib for H&N Adenoid Cystic Carcinoma	Inoperable or postop residual ACC of the head and neck	Randomized to apatinib followed by PBT + CIRT boost vs. particle therapy alone	Treatment response at 3 months	October 2016
NCT02795195	Shanghai Proton and Heavy Ion Center	Trial Evaluating Carbon Ion Radiotherapy (3 GyE Per Fraction) for Locally Recurrent NPC	Locally recurrent NPC	CIRT	Acute toxicity	June 2016
NCT02736786	Mayo Clinic	A Study of Mucosal Sparing Proton Beam Therapy (PBT) in Resected Oropharyngeal Tumors	Resected oropharyngeal tumors	Mucosal sparing PBT	Local control at 2 years	March 2016

Table 16.3 (Continued)

	Institution	Trial name	Inclusion	Treatment	Primary end points	Study start
NCT02663583	MDACC	Intensity-Modulated Proton Therapy (IMPT) or TransOral Robotic Surgery (TORS) for the Treatment of Low-Risk Oropharynx Squamous Cell	Stage I–III* previously untreated oropharyngeal squamous cell carcinoma	IMPT vs. transoral surgery	Functional outcome measured with patient-reported outcome and longitudinal digital wristband activity monitoring of study participants	January 2016
NCT01973179	Technische Universität Dresden	Re-irradiation of Recurrent Head and Neck Cancer	Previously irradiated head and neck cancer	PBT	Late toxicity within 24 months post-RT	July 2015
NCT01893307	MDACC, MGH, NCI, NIDCR	Phase II/III Randomized Trial of Intensity-Modulated Proton Beam Therapy (IMPT) Versus Intensity-Modulated Photon Therapy (IMRT) for the Treatment of Oropharyngeal Cancer of the Head and Neck	Stage III–IV* SCC of the oropharynx	Randomized to IMRT vs. IMPT	Rates of severe late toxicity 90 days to 2 years post-RT	August 2013
NCT01586767	MGH, NIH, NCI	A Phase II Study of Intensity-Modulated or Proton Radiation Therapy for Locally Advanced Sinonasal Malignancy	Locally advanced sinonasal tumors	PBT or IMRT	Local control at 2 years	July 2011
NCT01228448	MGH, NCI	In-Room PET in Proton Radiation Therapy	Brain, head and neck, and skull base tumors	PBT	Effectiveness of PBT quality assurance using in-room PET	October 2010
NCT03513042	Leiden University Medical Center	Early Response Evaluation of Proton Therapy by PET-imaging in Squamous Cell Carcinoma Located in the Head and Neck	Primary unresected HNSCC	IMPT	3-year local recurrence-free survival	Planned for June 2020
NCT03981068	Danish Head and Neck Cancer Group	A Phase II Study of Intensity Modulated Proton Therapy (IMPT) for Re-irradiation with Curative Intent for Recurrent or New Primary Head and Neck Cancer	Recurrent or second primary HNC, previous head and neck radiation	PBT	Any new grade ≥3 toxicity within 3 years post-RT	Planned for September 2019
NCT03450967	Samsung Medical Center	Durvalumab Plus Tremelimumab Combined with Proton Therapy for HNSCC	Recurrent or metastatic head and neck squamous cell carcinoma	PBT + durvalumab plus tremelimumab	Response rate	Planned for March 2018
	UK National Health Service Proton Service	A Phase III Trial of Intensity-modulated Proton Beam Therapy Versus Intensity-modulated Radiotherapy for Multi-toxicity Reduction in Oropharyngeal Cancer	Locally advanced OPSCC	Randomized to IMPT vs. IMRT	Patient-reported outcomes and feeding tube dependence or severe weight loss 12 months post-RT	Planned for January 2020

* AJCC 7th edition.
HNC = Head and neck cancer; HNSCC = head and neck squamous cell carcinoma; OPSCC = oropharyngeal squamous cell carcinoma; RT = radiation therapy; PBT = proton beam therapy; SBRT = stereotactic body radiation therapy; CIRT = carbon-ion radiation therapy; PET = positron emission tomography; MSK = Memorial Sloan Kettering Cancer Center; MDACC = MD Anderson Cancer Center; MGH = Massachusetts General Hospital; NCI = National Cancer Institute; NIDCR = National Institute of Dental and Craniofacial Research; NIH = National Institutes of Health.

Table 16.4   Recommended target volumes and radiation doses for treatment of oropharyngeal cancer.

Volume	Definitive	Postoperative	Dose
GTV	Gross disease and involved regional lymph nodes	–	70 Gy (RBE)
High-risk CTV (CTV$_{70}$)	Include margin of 5 mm if there is uncertainty of gross disease extent	–	70 Gy (RBE)
High-risk CTV (CTV$_{66}$)	–	Include preoperative target volume and regions of extracapsular nodal extension and/or positive margins	66 Gy (RBE)
High-risk CTV (CTV$_{60}$)	Include up to a 10-mm margin for positive nodes, and high-risk ipsilateral or contralateral nodes	Include preoperative tumor volume and nodal disease, operative bed, and ipsilateral or contralateral nodes at high risk for subclinical disease	60 Gy (RBE)
Low-risk CTV (CTV$_{50}$)	Include ipsilateral and contralateral nodes at low risk for subclinical disease	Include uninvolved ipsilateral and contralateral lymph nodes at low risk for subclinical disease	50 Gy (RBE)

For HPV positive disease, lower subclinical dosing may be considered

CTV = Clinical target volume; GTV = gross tumor volume; RBE = relative biological effectiveness.

16.3.3   Nasopharyngeal Cancer

Radiation with or without chemotherapy has been the standard of care for nasopharyngeal cancer (NPC) with IMRT often utilized to provide adequate tumor coverage given the complex anatomy of a tumor close to multiple OARs such as the pharyngeal constrictor muscles, major salivary glands, and skull base structures including cranial nerves, temporal lobes and the brain stem. IMRT has been shown to have excellent locoregional control (LRC) and minimal grade 3 or higher xerostomia (N. Lee et al., 2009). However, for more advanced disease such as T4 tumors, radioresistant diseases such as Epstein-Barr virus (EBV)-negative tumor, and locoregional recurrence after prior irradiation, IMRT results has been suboptimal (A. Chan et al., 2012; Huang et al., 2013; Stenmark et al., 2014). Proton therapy may provide better sparing of OARs and allow for potential dose-escalation to improve outcomes especially in such settings.

Chan et al. first reported the clinical outcomes from a phase II trial using combined proton/photon technique in 23 locally advanced NPC patients. At a median follow-up of 28 months, there was no local or regional relapse with two patients developing distant metastases. The disease-free survival (DFS) and OS at 2 years were 90% and 100%. No grade 4 or 5 toxicities were observed. The most common grade 3 or above toxicities included 29% hearing loss and 38% weight loss, while no grade 3 xerostomia was noted (A. Chan et al., 2012). In a matched case-control study of 10 NPC patients treated with IMPT and 20 matched patients treated with IMRT, Holliday et al. (2015) reported lower frequency of G-tube placement (20% vs. 65%, $p = 0.02$) in the IMPT cohort, likely attributed to lower mean dose to oral cavity. In another retrospective study of patients treated with proton therapy versus IMRT for NPC, nasal cavity or paranasal sinus cancers, McDonald et al. (2016) reported lower opioid require-

ment for pain and lower G-tube dependence rate likely related to lower mean dose to oral cavity and esophagus. We recently reviewed our institutional experience at MSK with one of the largest series of definitive NPC patients treated by IMPT ($n = 28$) in comparison with a matched IMRT ($n = 49$) cohort and found significantly better OAR sparing dosimetrically and fewer acute treatment related toxicities in the IMPT group such as fatigue, dysphagia, mucositis,, and weight loss.

Late toxicities from proton radiation in NPC have been reported in a study by Chan et al. (2004), in which 17 patients were treated with proton therapy for T4 NPC. Only one local failure was reported with median follow-up of 43 months. Late toxicities reported include five patients with radiographic temporal lobe changes, one with endocrine dysfunction, and one mandibular ORN. With longer follow-up of these single institution series and others that have recently been reported in abstract forms (Chou et al., 2018; X. Li, Lee, and Lee, 2020; Williams et al., 2019), more evidence will emerge in the near future to shed light on whether the dosimetry benefits and improvement in acute toxicities may translate into fewer late toxicities such as temporal lobe necrosis and ORN in NPC patients treated with proton therapy.

As the use of proton therapy is becoming more prevalent in NPC, carbon ion therapy has been employed as well, particularly in high-risk NPC where extent of disease encroaches upon critical structures. 26 patients with primarily stage III-IVB NPC were treated with IMRT followed by a carbon-ion boost in Heidelberg, Germany to median total dose of 74 Gy (RBE). At median follow-up of 40 months, complete response was seen in 60% and partial response in 20% per RECIST criteria. Only one patient showed a local in-field recurrence with estimated 5-year LC of 90% and OS of 86%. No toxicity greater than grade 3 was observed (Akbaba et al., 2019b). This approach allowed clinicians to offer dose-escalated treatment to optimize -control. The same group also reported outcomes of combined modality therapy with carbon boost for adenoid cystic carcinoma (ACC) of the nasopharynx ($n = 59$) and found similarly encouraging results as they were able to offer median total dose of 74 Gy (RBE) with 2-year LC of 83% and 2-year OS of 87% (Akbaba et al., 2019a). Cranial nerve palsy was observed in 14% of patients, which was less than reported series following photon RT although the authors note a likely increase with longer follow-up (Chew et al., 2001; Kong et al., 2011).

In summary, particle therapy for the treatment of NPC offers excellent locoregional control with less acute toxicities. Longer follow-up of existing series and updated prospective data are necessary to confirm the promising oncologic outcomes and the improvement in late toxicities such as neurological sequelae. The on-going NRG Oncology HN001, a phase II/III prospective randomized trial using plasma EBV DNA biomarker to direct therapy, allows proton therapy and collects QOL data. Recommended target volumes and radiation doses for nasopharyngeal cancer are in Table 16.5 and technical details regarding the planning process can be found in "Target Volume Delineation and Treatment Planning for Particle Therapy: A Practical Guide" (N. Y. Lee et al., 2018).

16.3.4 Sinonasal Cancer

Sinonasal cancer includes various histological subtypes such as SCC, ACC and olfactory neuroblastoma. Most sinonasal cancers are treated by surgical resection followed by radiation with or without chemotherapy. For very advanced disease, definitive chemoradiation is the treatment of choice. The complex anatomy involving multiple paranasal sinuses and the nasal cavity, and the proximity to skull base and other critical organs makes the treatment especially challenging with suboptimal outcomes (Waldron et al., 1998). Dosimetry comparison studies demonstrated that proton therapy, especially IMPT, may provide superior avoidance of critical structures compared to IMRT, which usually irradiate the ipsilateral optic structures beyond acceptable dose constraints (Lomax, Goitein, and Adams, 2003; Mock et al., 2004; Chera et al., 2009). Clinically, proton therapy has been utilized in the treatment of sinonasal cancer since early 2000s with encouraging oncologic outcomes (Fitzek et al., 2002; Pommier et al., 2006; Nishimura et al., 2007; Truong et al., 2009).

Zenda et al. (2015) reported late toxicities from proton radiation for sinonasal cancers in 90 patients, with a median follow-up 57.5 months, grade 3 late toxicities occurred in 17 patients (19%) and grade 4 toxicities in 6 patients (7%), including four events of optic nerve disorder. Russo et al. reported their institutional experience in treating locally advanced sinonasal SCC with proton therapy over two decades with a long median follow-up of living patients to 82 months. In 54 stage III or IV patients, LC rates at 2-year and 5-year were both 80% while 2-year OS and 5-year OS were 67% and 47%, respectively. Nine grade 3 and six grade 4 toxicities were reported with the majority being wound toxicities (Russo et al., 2016). Of note, both

Table 16.5 Recommended target volumes and radiation doses for definitive treatment of nasopharyngeal cancer.

Volume	Target	Dose
GTV	All gross disease identified on imaging and physical examination	70 Gy (RBE)
High-risk CTV (CTV$_{70}$)	GTV + 3 mm margin. At the interface with critical dose-limiting structures, a 1-mm margin is acceptable.	70 Gy (RBE)
High-risk CTV (CTV$_{59}$)	CTV$_{70}$ + 5 mm margin + regions at risk for microscopic disease:Entire nasopharynx Parapharyngeal space Anterior 1/3 of clivus (entire clivus if involved) Skull base (including coverage of foramen ovale and foramen rotundum) Posterior 1/4 of nasal cavity and maxillary sinuses (ensuring coverage of pterygopalatine fossa) Inferior sphenoid sinus (entire sphenoid sinus if involved) Pterygoid fossa Soft palate Retropharyngeal LN + retrostyloid space Bilateral nodal levels IB through V Cavernous sinus should be covered for advanced (T3–T4) lesions	59 Gy (RBE)
Low-risk CTV (CTV$_{56}$)	Level IV, VB, and supraclavicular nodes	56 Gy (RBE)

Notes:

1.All dosing is in 2 Gy/fraction and follow NRG-HN001 dosing and volume guidelines for IMPT treatment.

2.In select cases, level IB may be omitted in the node-negative neck and/or the lower risk node-positive neck (isolated retropharyngeal and/or isolated level IV adenopathy), at the discretion of the treating physician.

CTV = Clinical target volume; GTV = gross tumor volume; RBE = relative biological effectiveness.

studies showed toxicities developed more than 5 years after proton therapy, highlighting the need for long-term follow-up of these patients.

Yu et al. (2019) recently reported a multi-institutional experience from a registry study of the Proton Collaborative Group: 69 patients with sinonasal cancer were treated with curative intent proton radiation with IMPT including 27 treated for re-irradiation. In 42 patients who were treated with de novo proton radiation, 3-year freedom from locoregional recurrence rate and OS was 93% and 100%, widely exceeding any previously reported outcome in other series, likely because of the use of IMPT in all cases. Of note, no patients developed vision loss or symptomatic brain necrosis. Grade 3 or higher late toxicities occurred in 15% of patients, which is also quite favorable considering the inclusion of re-irradiation patients.

Most recently, we reported our experience treating 86 consecutive patients with sinonasal cancers with proton therapy. At a median follow-up of 23.4 months, the 2-year LC, DFS, and OS were 83%, 74%, and 81%, respectively, for radiation-native patients and 77%, 54%, and 66%, respectively, for reirradiated patients. IMPT significantly improved LC compared to 3D conformal proton techniques (91% vs. 72%, $p < 0.01$). Overall grade 3 toxicities were lower than historical controls (M. Fan et al., 2020b).

In one of the most compelling studies supporting the benefit of proton therapy in head and neck cancer patients, Patel and colleagues conducted a well-designed systematic review and meta-analysis of charged particle therapy (protons, carbon ions, helium ions, or other charged particles) versus photon therapy for paranasal sinus and nasal cavity malignant diseases. In this meta-analysis including 43 cohorts of patients (286 patients treated with charged particle therapy vs. 1186 treated with photon therapy), the authors reported significantly improved OS at 5 years with charged particle therapy. Specifically, in the subgroup analysis comparing patients treated with proton therapy vs. IMRT, the authors found improved LC and increased DFS at 5 years for proton therapy group. Such improvements in outcomes were likely due to better target coverage with charged particle therapy and potentially increased tumoricidal effect of charged particle therapy from higher RBEs, although the authors acknowledged potential biases from the heterogeneity of the cohorts and limited sample size in proton therapy versus IMRT comparison (Patel et al., 2014). Nevertheless, this meta-analysis provided high-level evidence that proton therapy may potentially improve the survival outcome in selected head and neck cancer patients.

Institutions that employ carbon-ion therapy have reported their outcomes in sinonasal cancers. Researchers from Heidelberg, Germany, retrospectively reviewed 16 patients with ACC of the head and neck who had skull base involvement and could not undergo complete resection. Primary

tumor sites included the maxillary sinus, nasopharynx, ethmoid sinus, upper jaw, parotid gland, and the orbit. Patients received photon fractionated stereotactic radiation followed by a carbon-ion boost to total median dose of 72 GyE. Actuarial LC at 3 years was 64.6% and OS was 83.3%. No patients developed grade 3 or higher late effects (Schulz-Ertner et al., 2003). Investigators from Japan also reported their outcomes using carbon ion in 22 patients with sinonasal adenocarcinoma using the same dosing regimen in their salivary gland patients (57.6 Gy/16 fractions and 64 Gy/16 fractions). Sixteen patients received definitive treatment. At a median follow-up of 43 months, the 3-year LC rate was 76.9% and OS was 59.1%. Grade 2 or higher toxicities including visual loss were observed in 31.8% of patients although this was considered acceptable given 63.6% of patients had T4b disease (Koto et al., 2014).

Other charged particles have been utilized, namely, from the University of California Lawrence Berkeley Laboratory. Castro et al. reported 10 patients treated with tumors of the paranasal sinus with doses ranging from 52 to 75 GyE with helium and neon ions. At mean follow-up of 29 months, LC was achieved in 6 out of 10 patients. Complications included brain injury, partial visual loss, and soft tissue and bone necrosis (Castro and Reimers, 1988). Given these patients were treated from 1975 to 1985, outcomes are as expected with the technological limitations for the time period.

Overall, it appears surgical resection remains the backbone of multidisciplinary management of sinonasal cancer with modern particle therapy, such as IMPT, offering excellent LC and OS with improved toxicity profile compared to traditional photon-based radiation. Recommended target volumes and radiation doses for sinonasal cancer are in Table 16.6 and technical details regarding the planning process can be found in "Target Volume Delineation and Treatment Planning for Particle Therapy: A Practical Guide" (N. Y. Lee et al., 2018).

16.3.5 Salivary Gland Cancer

In some cancers of the head and neck, such as salivary gland tumors if there is no involvement of midline structures, well-lateralized oral cavity, oropharynx, or skin cancers, the radiation treatment target could be limited to one side of the head and neck. Proton therapy offers excellent organ sparing with minimal exit dose in comparison to IMRT in treating unilateral head and neck targets (Kandula et al., 2013).

Dagan et al. prospectively evaluated the treatment related acute toxicities and nutritional status of a series of patients who received ipsilateral head and neck radiation for parotid tumors using proton therapy. They showed very low rates of mucosal toxicity and well-preserved weight and nutritional status throughout treatment (Dagan et al., 2016).

Table 16.6 Recommended target volumes and radiation doses for treatment of sinonasal cancer.

Volume	Definitive	Postoperative	Dose
GTV	Gross disease and involved regional lymph nodes	–	70 Gy (RBE)
High-risk CTV (CTV_{70})	Include margin of 5 mm if there is uncertainty of gross disease extent	–	70 Gy (RBE)
High-risk CTV (CTV_{66})	–	Include preoperative target volume and regions of extracapsular nodal extension, soft tissue invasion, bone invasion, and positive margins	66 Gy (RBE)
High-risk CTV (CTV_{60})	Include up to a 10-mm margin for positive nodes, and high-risk ipsilateral or contralateral nodes	Include preoperative tumor volume and nodal disease, operative bed, and ipsilateral or contralateral nodes at high risk for subclinical disease	60 Gy (RBE)
Low-risk CTV (CTV_{50})	Include ipsilateral and contralateral nodes at low risk for subclinical disease	Include uninvolved ipsilateral and contralateral lymph nodes at low risk for subclinical disease	50 Gy (RBE)

CTV = Clinical target volume; GTV = gross tumor volume; RBE = relative biological effectiveness.

Holliday and colleagues investigated ipsilateral head and neck radiation with IMPT in a relatively homogeneous population of patients with head and neck ACC in the postoperative setting. They reported a promising LC of 93.8% at a median follow-up of 2 years, with 25% acute and 6.3% chronic grade 3 or 4 toxicities (E. Holliday et al., 2016a).

Romesser and colleagues compared the toxic effects associated with unilateral proton therapy versus IMRT in 41 patients with major salivary gland tumors or cutaneous SCCs. Proton therapy provided similar tumor target coverage but with negligible radiation to the oral cavity, contralateral major salivary glands, and brainstem compared with IMRT. Reduced dose to these OARs resulted in decreased acute toxicities, including mucositis, dysgeusia, nausea or vomiting, and fatigue (Romesser et al., 2016a).

Chuong et al. (2019) from the Proton Collaborative Group reported acute toxicities from the largest series of patients with salivary gland tumors treated with unilateral proton beam radiation. One hundred and five patients (90 parotid, 15 submandibular) were included in the analysis. All except for one patient were treated to definitive dose either in the postoperative (70.5%) or definitive (29.5%) setting. Rates of acute side effects were considerably lower than historical IMRT outcomes: nausea (1.5%), dysgeusia (4.8%), xerostomia (7.6%), mucositis (10.5%), and dysphagia (10.5%).

The utilization of other heavy particles has been explored in salivary gland carcinomas. The University of Washington's experience of 545 patients treated for salivary gland malignancies with neutron therapy found 6- and 10-year LRC to be 84% and 79%, which was favorable compared to reported rates in photon radiation series. ORN developed in 3.4% of patients, which was comparable to rates in photon series (Timoshchuk et al., 2019). Another retrospective study by Huber et al. (2001) from Germany compared neutrons, photons and mixed beam

in 75 patients with advanced ACC and found 5-year locoregional control was 75% for neutron radiation and 32% for both photon and mixed beam; however, there was no difference in survival. One randomized study of 32 unresectable salivary gland carcinoma cases of photon versus neutron therapy found the neutron arm had 2-year locoregional control rate of 67% in comparison to 17% for photon-based RT leading to early closure due to the big differences (Griffin et al., 1988). A 10-year update of the trial showed 5-year LC was 56% for neutron therapy compared to 17% for photon RT despite no difference in OS. Neutron therapy did result in more severe toxicity such as pain and necrosis (Laramore et al., 1993). The authors do note that patients in this study were treated using low-energy neutron beams from relatively unsophisticated treatment facilities and since then high energy beams are employed, which are associated with less toxicity than older systems.

A prospective randomized trial (NCT02923570) is currently underway comparing proton therapy with IMRT for unilateral radiation in head and neck cancer, focusing on acute grade 2 or higher mucositis as the primary end point (Table 16.3). NRG Oncology/RTOG 1008, a phase II randomized trial of postoperative radiation with or without weekly cisplatin for salivary gland tumors has also allowed proton therapy.

Other particles such as carbon, neon, and helium have also been utilized in salivary gland carcinomas as they are relatively radioresistant and could benefit from the higher RBE of particle therapy. Clinicians from the Research Center for Charged Particle Therapy Hospital in Chiba, Japan treated 46 inoperable patients with locally advanced carcinomas of the parotid gland using carbon ion in the definitive setting. Histologies were varied with ACC (35%) being most common and 93% of the patients with T3+ disease. At a median follow-up of 62 months, 5-year LC and OS were 74.5% and 70.1%, respectively. Twenty-six patients were treated to 57.6 Gy and

20 patients received 64 Gy. Notable late effects include five patients with radiation-induced facial nerve palsy and five developed grade 2 brain injury (Koto et al., 2017). Another study from Japan conducted a multicenter analysis of 69 patients with major salivary gland carcinoma treated with carbon ion and found 3-year LC of 81% and OS of 94%, which was comparable to neutron series but improved compared to photon series. Ten percent of patients experienced grade 3 acute mucositis and acute dermatitis and late toxicities include 1% grade 3 dysphagia and 1% grade 3 brain abscess (K. Hayashi et al., 2018). These rates were improved over historical neutron series and comparable to photon series. Limited data regarding neon and helium ion have been reported. Investigators from the Lawrence Berkeley Laboratory reported nine patients with locally advanced salivary gland tumors treated with neon (eight) or helium (one) ions and found two local failures at a mean follow-up of 17 months (Castro and Reimers, 1988). One patient had moderately severe late skin changes 4 years post-

RT with neo ions, underscoring the high entrance dose seen with particle therapy.

Recommended target volumes and radiation doses for salivary gland cancer are in A and technical details regarding the planning process can be found in "Target Volume Delineation and Treatment Planning for Particle Therapy: A Practical Guide" (N. Y. Lee et al., 2018) (Figure 16.3).

16.3.6 Laryngeal and Hypopharyngeal Cancer

The utilization of particle therapy in laryngeal and hypopharyngeal cancer has been slow as early-stage laryngeal cancer is well controlled with 3D conformal radiation as well as IMRT. Furthermore, IMRT is able to spare critical structures reasonably well for more locally advanced disease. In the setting of T4 tumors, surgical resection is the standard of care; however, patients are increasingly seeking organ- and function-preserving treatments.

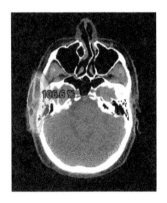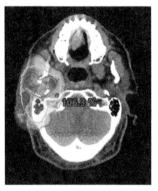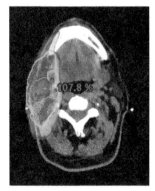

Figure 16.3 Example PBS plan (MFO-optimized) for patient with pT2N0 acinic cell carcinoma of the right parotid displaying the 50% isodose line. Red contour = CTV66. Green contour = CTV60.

Table 16.7 Recommended target volumes and radiation doses for treatment of salivary cancer.

Volume	Target	Dose
GTV	Gross unresected disease including primary tumor, involved nerves, and regional lymph nodes	70 Gy (RBE)
High-risk CTV (CTV$_{66}$)	Includes areas of extranodal extension or surgical margin positivity	66 Gy (RBE)
High-risk CTV (CTV$_{60}$)	Includes the postoperative bed, both at the primary tumor site and the ipsilateral neck (levels Ib–IV). Retropharyngeal and level V lymph nodes are typically not covered due to low risk of involvement and can be omitted at the physician's discretion	60 Gy (RBE)
Low-risk CTV (CTV$_{50}$)	Includes the undissected ipsilateral neck and should be treated based on estimated risk from risk factors	50 Gy (RBE)
Contralateral neck	Treatment of the contralateral neck should be considered in cases where tumor approaches midline (typically sublingual or minor salivary gland primaries) or when involved or suspicious lymph nodes are evident in the contralateral neck. In cases of large-volume ipsilateral nodal disease, where crossing lymphatic drainage to the opposite neck is possible, treatment of the contralateral neck can be considered as well. The decision to include the undissected node negative neck should be based on risk estimation for occult metastases	50 Gy (RBE)

CTV = Clinical target volume; GTV = gross tumor volume; RBE = relative biological effectiveness.

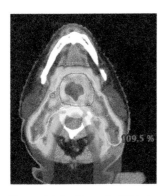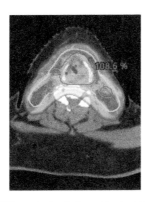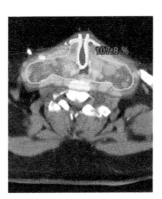

Figure 16.4 Example PBS plan (MFO-optimized) for patient with cT4N2c squamous cell carcinoma of the supraglottic larynx who refused total laryngectomy following induction chemotherapy displaying the 50% isodose line. Red contour = CTV70. Green contour = CTV50.

Table 16.8 Recommended target volumes and radiation doses for treatment of laryngeal and hypopharyngeal cancer.

Volume	Target	Dose
GTV	Gross primary tumor, involved surrounding structures, regional lymph nodes	70 Gy (RBE)
High-risk CTV (CTV$_{66}$)	Areas of positive surgical margin or shave excision or extranodal extension	66 Gy (RBE)
At-risk CTV (CTV$_{50-60}$)*	Areas at risk of microscopic disease Primary: include tracheoesophageal groove and >5 mm around GTV and CTV$_{66}$ In the postoperative setting include surgical bed. If tracheostomy performed include tracheostomy stoma	50–60 Gy (RBE)
	Neck: In node-positive disease include nodal levels II–VII and upper mediastinum to the level of the carina. Level V should be covered in the node-positive neck. Consider coverage of Level I and retropharyngeal nodes in setting of bulky neck disease	

*In select cases, the lateral necks can be omitted despite having pathologic lymph nodes. Please consult your surgeon.

CTV = Clinical target volume; GTV = gross tumor volume; RBE = relative biological effectiveness.

One retrospective study of 10 patients with cT1-2N0 SCC of the glottic larynx were planned with 3D conformal, IMRT, volumetric modulated arc therapy (VMAT), and proton therapy. Plans from the latter three modalities were superior to 3D conformal therapy with respect to superior planning target volume (PTV) coverage, degree of variation, and decreased mean dose to the thyroid and carotid arteries (Matthiesen et al., 2015). Another study from Sweden created three different plans with protons, IMRT, and 3D-CRT for five patients with T4N0M0 hyopharyngeal carcinoma. Protons and IMRT gave a significant tumor control probability increase compared to 3D-CRT; however, no difference between protons and IMRT was found. Proton therapy did provide lower nontarget doses than IMRT, which indicates a possibility for further dose escalation. In particular, there were large individual dose differences between protons and IMRT for the parotid glands (Johansson et al., 2004), indicating that with proper patient selection, the benefit of protons may be greater for certain cases. Our institution at MSK is offering patients with functional T4 laryngeal cancers an organ-preserving approach with proton therapy when available for patients who refuse total laryngectomy.

Recommended target volumes and radiation doses for laryngeal and hypopharyngeal cancer are in Table 16.8 and technical details regarding the planning process can be found in "Target Volume Delineation and Treatment Planning for Particle Therapy: A Practical Guide" (N. Y. Lee et al., 2018) (Figure 16.4).

16.3.7 Thyroid Cancer

Thyroid cancer is rare, representing only 1% of all diagnosed malignancies; however, the incidence is increasing due to the ability to detect early disease with advancements in diagnostic imaging studies (Davies and Welch, 2014). Thyroid cancer can be divided into four main subtypes including (1) well-differentiated malignancies (papillary, follicular, mixed, Hurthle cell), (2) medullary, (3) anaplastic, and (4) sarcomas and lymphomas. Papillary cancer is the most common histologic subtype comprising 80% of thyroid cancers followed by follicular cancer at 10% with the remainder being medullary, anaplastic, and others. The primary management is surgical resection followed by radioactive iodine (RAI); however, external beam radiation therapy (EBRT) is recommended for patients with differentiated thyroid cancer with gross residual or unresectable locoregional disease, except in those under 45 years of age with RAI avid disease (American Thyroid Association Guidelines Taskforce on Thyroid et al., 2009). The role for EBRT in more aggressive subtypes such as anaplastic is better established. Thus, thyroid cancer patients who require radiation therapy have more aggressive disease and as a result, local recurrence rates after radiation in these high-risk patients range from 15% to 25% in well-differentiated disease (Azrif et al., 2008; Brierley and Sherman, 2012) and 30% in medullary cancer (Nguyen et al., 1992).

In order to improve outcomes among patients requiring radiation therapy, high linear energy transfer radiation such as fast neutron have been explored as preclinical data showed improved cell killing for tumor cells in hypoxic or radioresistant phases (Britten, Peters, and Murray, 2001). The University of Washington reported 62 consecutive patients with advanced thyroid cancers of which 23 were treated with fast neutron (FNT) and 39 with photon RT. The majority (97%) had stage IV disease and 24 (39%) had anaplastic thyroid carcinoma. At a median follow-up of 14 months, there did not appear to be a survival benefit with FNT in patients with well-differentiated histologies compared to photon RT (median OS 17 vs. 69 months, $p = 0.04$) and there was a trend toward improved OS with medullary and anaplastic histologies. Locoregional control and toxicity were not assessed. The authors conclude that the use of fast neutrons in the more aggressive histologies warrants further investigation (Chapman et al., 2016). To date, there are no clinical reports on the use of proton therapy in the treatment of thyroid cancer; however, our center is using proton therapy to treat thyroid cancer patients with the goal of sparing midline structures posterior and superior to the target and will be reporting our experiences in the near future.

Recommended target volumes and radiation doses for thyroid cancer are in Table 16.9 and technical details regarding the planning process can be found in "Target Volume Delineation and Treatment Planning for Particle Therapy: A Practical Guide" (N. Y. Lee et al., 2018).

16.3.8 Non-melanomatous Skin Cancer

Non-melanomatous skin cancer (NMSC) is the most common cancer in the United States and includes basal cell and SCCs. Cutaneous SCCs that typically originate from the midface, scalp, or lateral surfaces of the face can present with clinical perineural invasion where the tumor involves nearby nerves and can spread proximally to the skull base (Feasel et al., 2001; Geist et al., 2008). Branches of cranial nerve V2 and VII are most commonly involved. Resection of the tumor in these situations can be difficult thus definitive radiation therapy is typically indicated.

In cases of NMSC with clinical perineural invasion, proton therapy can offer coverage to the target including the skull base while minimizing dose to critical structures nearby. Romesser et al. reported on the MSK experience of patients treated with proton therapy compared to IMRT for cases requiring ipsilateral radiation. This study included cutaneous SCC metastases to a major salivary gland. Those who received proton beam therapy (PBT) had significantly lower brainstem maximum (29.7 Gy vs. 0.62 Gy [RBE], $p < 0.001$), spinal cord maximum (36.3 Gy vs. 1.88 Gy [RBE], $p < 0.001$) and contralateral parotid gland mean doses (1.4 Gy vs. 0 Gy, $p < 0.001$), which translated into improved toxicity. Target coverage was not compromised with PBT (Romesser et al., 2016a).

Further benefit from proton therapy can be translated from studies where targets included the skull base region finding dosimetric benefits to normal OARs such as the temporal lobes (McDonald, Linton, and Calley, 2015), hippocampi, retina (Kennedy et al., 2015), and cornea (E. B. Holliday et al., 2016b). A review of proton therapy for clinical perineural invasion in cutaneous head and neck cancer suggest PBT as a means of dose intensification to improve the therapeutic ratio (Holtzman and Mendenhall, 2020).

Recommended target volumes and radiation doses for skin cancer are in Table 16.10 and technical details regarding the

---

Table 16.9 Recommended target volumes and radiation doses for treatment of thyroid cancer.

Volume	Target	Dose
GTV	Gross primary tumor, involved surrounding structures, regional lymph nodes	70 Gy (RBE)
High-risk CTV (CTV$_{66}$)	Areas of positive surgical margin or shave excision or extranodal extension	66 Gy (RBE)
At-risk CTV (CTV$_{50-60}$)*	Areas at risk of microscopic disease Primary: include tracheoesophageal groove and > 5 mm around GTV and CTV$_{66}$ In the postoperative setting include surgical bed. If tracheostomy performed include tracheostomy stoma Neck: In node positive disease include nodal levels II-VII and upper mediastinum to the level of the carina. Level V should be covered in the node-positive neck. Consider coverage of Level I and retropharyngeal nodes in setting of bulky neck disease	50–60 Gy (RBE)

*In select cases, the lateral necks can be omitted despite having pathologic lymph nodes. Please consult your surgeon.
CTV = Clinical target volume; GTV = gross tumor volume; RBE = relative biological effectiveness.

Table 16.10   Recommended target volumes and radiation doses for treatment of skin cancer.

Volume	Target	Dose
GTV	Gross disease seen on CT and/or MRI and on physical examination of a primary skin lesion	70 Gy (RBE)
High-risk CTV (CTV$_{66}$)	The gross disease with an isocentric 0.5-cm margin edited for anatomic boundaries to clinical spread. If a primary skin lesion is included in the target volume, a 1–2-cm margin on the skin surface should be provided	66–70 Gy (RBE) at 2 Gy (RBE) per fraction *or* 70.2 to 74.4 Gy (RBE) at 1.2 Gy (RBE) per fraction using twice-daily fractionation
At-risk CTV (CTV$_{54-60}$)*	The gross disease with an isocentric margin expansion of 0.5–1 cm edited for anatomic boundaries to clinical spread. If the nerve ganglion is involved, other proximal branches of the named nerve may be included. Also, the regional nodes at risk for spread should be included in this volume	50 Gy (RBE) at 2 Gy (RBE) per fraction *or* 50.4 Gy (RBE) at 1.2 Gy (RBE) per fraction using twice-daily fractionation

*In select cases, the lateral necks can be omitted despite having pathologic lymph nodes. Please consult your surgeon.
CTV = Clinical target volume; GTV = gross tumor volume; RBE = relative biological effectiveness.

planning process can be found in "Target Volume Delineation and Treatment Planning for Particle Therapy: A Practical Guide" (N. Y. Lee et al., 2018).

16.3.9   Re-irradiation for Recurrent Head and Neck Cancer

Local or regional recurrence of head and neck cancer after prior radiation treatment requires salvage therapy because uncontrolled local regional diseases can dramatically compromise patient's QOL and lead to inevitable mortality. Salvage therapy often includes surgery, followed by re-irradiation or in other cases, re-irradiation alone. These are highly challenging scenarios in which high doses of radiation are often necessary to achieve disease control for likely radioresistant tumors, yet the ability to deliver high doses of radiation is limited by nearby normal tissues which have already received significant amount of radiation from previous treatment. The most commonly utilized technique in re-irradiation for head and neck cancer has been IMRT. In the MSK experience reported by Riaz et al., 257 patients with recurrent head and neck cancer treated with IMRT re-irradiation showed a 2-year LRC of 47% and OS of 43%. Increased dose (>50 Gy) was independently associated with improved LRC (Riaz et al., 2014). Overall, the 1- to 2-year LRC rates in the available literature are approximately 50–60% with IMRT (Ho and Phan, 2018).

Proton therapy has been utilized in the re-irradiation settings with acceptable toxicity profile for recurrent or new primary head and neck cancer. Proton therapy can better avoid dose overlap with previously irradiated tissue, thereby reducing normal tissue toxicity as well as allowing dose escalation to achieve higher LRC. In a multi-institutional study on proton beam re-irradiation for recurrent head and neck cancer (*n* = 92), Romesser et al. reported a 1-year locoregional failure rate of 25.1% and OS of 65.2%, comparable to outcomes in

IMRT re-irradiation series, while risk of grade 3 or 4 toxicities was lower compared to IMRT re-irradiation. Specifically, there were relatively lower rates of late toxicity with only six cases of grade 3 or 4 skin complications (8.7%), four cases of grade 3 dysphagia (7.1%), and two cases of grade 5 bleeding (2.9%) (Romesser et al., 2016b). Phan et al. reported a retrospective analysis of 60 patients who received re-irradiation with proton therapy. In this study, LRC was 68% at 1 year with 30% of patients experienced acute grade 3 toxicities including 22% of patients requiring feeding tube at the end of proton radiation. However, the 1-year rate of late grade 3 toxicities decreased to 16.7% with only 2% of patients being feeding tube dependent. Three patients may have died of re-irradiation related toxicities (Phan et al., 2016). McDonald and colleagues reported a series of 61 patients receiving curative intent proton re-irradiation for primarily disease involving the skull base. The 2-year local failure rate was 19.7% with 14.7% acute and 24.6% late grade 3 or above toxicities reported including 3 treatment related deaths. In disease specific settings, a few smaller series of retrospective studies have demonstrated that proton re-irradiation can provide favorable LC and OS at the cost of acceptable rates of both acute and late toxicities in both nasopharyngeal cancer and oral cavity cancer (Dionisi et al., 2019; Y. Hayashi et al., 2017). These data supports the utilization of definitive proton re-irradiation for acceptable LC rate, although the 3–5% risk of treatment relate death also highlights the need for careful patient selection balancing the need for disease control and mitigating toxicity, especially in patients with larger retreatment volumes (J. Y. Lee et al., 2016).

For patients with locally recurrent head and neck cancer ineligible for definitive reirradiation as the local salvage therapy, the options are limited, and the prognosis is extremely guarded. Palliative Quad Shot (QS) reirradiation appears to be an effective last-line local therapy with minimal toxicity in patients with previously irradiated head and neck cancer. A recent study from MSK investigated last-line treatment with QS regimen (3.7 Gy twice daily over 2 consecutive days at 4-week intervals per cycle, up to 4 cycles) in such settings (D. Fan et al., 2020a). Among 166 patients, overall palliative response rate was 66% and symptoms improved in 60% of patients. On multivariate analysis, proton therapy, KPS > 70, presence of palliative response and 3–4 QS cycles were associated with improved local PFS and improved OS. The overall grade 3 toxicity rate was 10.8% and no grade 4–5 toxicities were reported. MSK has treated nearly 350 patients with proton reirradiation for head and neck malignancies, of which 300 had SCC histology. A review of these patients will be reported soon.

Carbon ion radiotherapy has also been used in the reirradiation setting. A review of 229 patients with recurrent disease in Germany treated with a median dose of 51 Gy in 3 Gy fractions showed at a median follow-up of 3.9 years, the median local PFS was 24.2 months with median OS of 26.1 months (Held et al., 2019). Serious acute toxicity included grade 4 laryngeal edema rate of 0.9%, grade 3 dysphagia of 1.3%, grade 3 fistula of 0.4%, and grade 3 impaired hearing of 0.4%. Late toxicities included grade 3 central nervous system (CNS) necrosis of 14.5%, grade 4 CNS necrosis of 0.8%, grade 3 ORN of 0.8%, and grade 4 carotid blowout of 0.8%. Their overall late severe toxicity rate of 14.5% was slightly higher than other reports from carbon-ion treatment in recurrent head and neck cancer which ranged from 10% to 12% (Jensen et al., 2015; Hu et al., 2018; Gao et al., 2019).

In summary, particle therapy demonstrated encouraging toxicity profiles and acceptable treatment outcomes in the re-irradiation setting. Ongoing prospective trials from Shanghai, Germany, MSK, Mayo Clinic, and MD Anderson will further assess for disease control, survival outcomes, long-term toxicity, and costs of particle therapy in locoregionally recurrent head and neck cancer (Table 16.3). Recommended target volumes and radiation doses for reirradiation are in Table 16.11 and technical details regarding the planning process can be found in "Target Volume Delineation and Treatment Planning for Particle Therapy: A Practical Guide" (N. Y. Lee et al., 2018).

16.4 Subacute and Late Toxicities

While particle therapy has a dosimetric advantage to photons by sparing of normal structures not in the treatment field, there is concern for toxicities related to tissues within or very close to the target, as multiple studies have demonstrated progressively higher RBE values at the distal edge of the Bragg peak (Britten et al., 2013; Cuaron et al., 2016), which may accidentally land in critical organs due to the combination of range uncertainly and suboptimal beam arrangement. Meanwhile, as particle therapy is often utilized in the re-irradiation setting for head and neck cancer patients, the intrinsic higher risks of normal tissue injury due to significant amount of radiation from previous treatment also contribute to potential subacute and late toxicities.

CNS toxicities after proton therapy could develop years later, be considerably symptomatic, and significantly affect the QOL in long-term survivors. Temporal lobe necrosis (TLN) is a form of CNS toxicity often observed after head and neck radiation to subsites such as skull base, nasopharynx and paranasal sinuses. In a series of 66 patients reported by McDonald and colleagues, any grade TLN approached 12.7% at 3 years with grade 2 or higher radiation necrosis happened in 5.7% of patients (McDonald, Linton, and Calley, 2015). A recent report from Kitpanit et al. (2020) found that among 234 patients treated with proton therapy to the skull base, the 2-year TLN rate was 4.6% with median time to TLN of 20.9 months. Another form of CNS toxicity is brainstem necrosis, especially in patients treated for skull base tumors. Substantial dosimetry data have been collected for brainstem injury after proton therapy in pediatric patients, contributing to guidelines defining parameters for safe delivery of proton radiation near the brainstem (Haas-Kogan et al., 2018). Japanese investigators have also studied radiation-induced brain changes (RIBC) on imaging as well as clinical symptoms such as vertigo, head and epilepsy in patients who were treated for skull base tumors and head and neck cancer (Miyawaki et al., 2009). They found that 17% of patients treated with proton therapy developed RIBC and 64% of patients treated with carbon-ion RT developed RIBC. The authors attribute some of the difference to higher

Table 16.11   Recommended target volumes and radiation doses for reirradiation.

Volume	Target	Dose
GTV	Gross tumor (by imaging or physical exam, including gross residual disease after resection)	66–72 Gy (RBE)
Microscopic residual disease	Positive margin or high-risk features present postresection, with no gross residual disease apparent by imaging or exam	60–70 Gy (RBE)

GTV = gross tumor volume; RBE = relative biological effectiveness.

dose per fraction (3.6 GyE vs. 2.5 GyE) of carbon ion compared to proton therapy; however, the physical properties of each particle may contribute to these differences as well.

Radiation-induced optic neuropathy (RION) may significantly affect patient's QOL. Kountouri et al. (2019) reported 6.5% risk of any grade of RION in 216 head and neck patients treated with pencil beam scanning proton therapy (Kountouri et al., 2019). In a large series of 514 patients treated over three decades at a single institution reported by P. C. Li et al. (2019), incidence of RION was 1% among patients who received less than 60 Gy (RBE), compared to 5.8% in patients receiving >60 Gy (RBE) to their optic pathways. Overall, it is reasonable to estimate about 5% risk of developing late CNS toxicities after proton radiation for head and neck cancer.

Non-CNS late toxicities after proton therapy have been reported. Owosho et al. (2016) reported favorable dosimetry parameters in contralateral tooth bearing mandible (at least 10-fold difference) using PBT in comparison with IMRT for patients receiving unilateral radiation treatment. Zhang et al. (2017) retrospectively reviewed over 500 OPC patient treated at MD Anderson (534 IMRT vs. 50 IMPT) and found lower mandibular doses for patient treated with IMPT (mean 25.6 vs. 41.2 Gy; $p < 0.001$) and lower rates of ORN in IMPT cases: 2% with IMPT versus 7.7% with IMRT. A potentially fatal toxicity of re-irradiation for head and neck cancer is carotid blowout (McDonald, Moore, and Johnstone, 2012). In a series of patients re-irradiated with particle therapy including proton therapy, the actuarial rate of carotid blowout was 2.7%, very similar to the rate reported in photon series (Dale et al., 2017). Improvement in other subacute or late toxicities after proton therapy versus IMRT such as xerostomia and dysphagia has

been discussed separately in previous sections regarding specific head and neck subsites.

Carbon-ion therapy, while particularly helpful for treating more radioresistant tumors such as ACC, adenocarcinoma, and mucosal malignant melanoma, presents with its own challenges with respect to toxicity given its relative higher RBE. Investigators from Japan reviewed 54 patients with head and neck cancer who were treated where the parotid gland received more than 5% of the prescribed dose. At a mean follow-up was 46.4 months, there was a dosimetric correlation with parotid gland atrophy with the volume receiving more than 5 Gy RBE (V5) as a significant risk factor (Morikawa et al., 2016).

Overall, particle therapy exhibited favorable subacute and late toxicity profile compared to photon-based radiotherapy in nonrandomized, retrospective studies. Ongoing prospective randomized trials will undoubtedly provide higher level evidence to support the observed benefit (Table 16.3).

16.5 Conclusion

Based on current evidence and promising trends, we have strong confidence that particle therapy and particularly proton therapy will become more accessible, more effective, and less toxic. The combination of improved patient selection, rapidly evolving technologies in proton radiation delivery, and deeper understanding of the biology should be able to further improve the therapeutic window of particle therapy, making it a cost-effective component of the contemporary management of head and neck cancer patients.

References

1 Ahn, P.H., Lukens, J.N., Teo, B.K., Kirk, M., and Lin, A. (2014). The use of proton therapy in the treatment of head and neck cancers. *Journal of Cancer* 20 (6): 421–426. 10.1097/PPO.0000000000000077.

2 Akbaba, S., Ahmed, D., Lang, K., Held, T., Mattke, M., Hoerner-Rieber, J., ... Adeberg, S. (2019a). Results of a combination treatment with intensity modulated radiotherapy and active raster-scanning carbon ion boost for adenoid cystic carcinoma of the minor salivary glands of the nasopharynx. *Oral Oncology* 91: 39–46. 10.1016/j.oraloncology.2019.02.019.

3 Akbaba, S., Held, T., Lang, K., Forster, T., Federspil, P., Herfarth, K., ... Adeberg, S. (2019b). Bimodal Radiotherapy with Active Raster-Scanning Carbon Ion Radiotherapy and Intensity-Modulated Radiotherapy in High-Risk Nasopharyngeal Carcinoma Results in Excellent Local Control. *Cancers (Basel)* 11 (3): 10.3390/cancers11030379.

4 American Thyroid Association Guidelines Taskforce on Thyroid, N., Differentiated Thyroid, C., Cooper, D.S., Doherty, G.M., Haugen, B.R., Kloos, R.T., ... Tuttle, R.M. (2009). Revised American Thyroid Association management guidelines for patients with thyroid nodules and differentiated thyroid cancer. *Thyroid* 19 (11): 1167–1214. 10.1089/thy.2009.0110.

5 Azrif, M., Slevin, N.J., Sykes, A.J., Swindell, R., and Yap, B.K. (2008). Patterns of relapse following radiotherapy for differentiated thyroid cancer: Implication for target volume delineation. *Radiotherapy and Oncology* 89 (1): 105–113. 10.1016/j.radonc.2008.05.023.

6 Bernier, J., Cooper, J.S., Pajak, T.F., Van Glabbeke, M., Bourhis, J., Forastiere, A., ... Lefebvre, J.L. (2005). Defining risk levels in locally advanced head and neck cancers: A comparative analysis of concurrent postoperative radiation plus chemotherapy trials of the EORTC (#22931) and RTOG (# 9501). *Head & Neck* 27 (10): 843–850. 10.1002/hed.20279.

7 Blanchard, P., Garden, A.S., Gunn, G.B., Rosenthal, D.I., Morrison, W.H., Hernandez, M., ... Frank, S.J. (2016). Intensity-modulated proton beam therapy (IMPT) versus intensity-modulated photon therapy (IMRT) for patients with oropharynx cancer - A case matched analysis. *Radiotherapy and Oncology: Journal of the European Society for Therapeutic Radiology and Oncology* 120 (1): 48–55. 10.1016/j.radonc.2016.05.022.

8 Bortfeld, T. (1997). An analytical approximation of the Bragg curve for therapeutic proton beams. *Medical Physics* 24 (12): 2024–2033. 10.1118/1.598116.

9 Brierley, J. and Sherman, E. (2012). The role of external beam radiation and targeted therapy in thyroid cancer. *Seminars in Radiation Oncology* 22 (3): 254–262. 10.1016/j.semradonc.2012.03.010.

10 Britten, R.A., Nazaryan, V., Davis, L.K., Klein, S.B., Nichiporov, D., Mendonca, M.S., ... Keppel, C. (2013). Variations in the RBE for cell killing along the depth-dose profile of a modulated proton therapy beam. *Radiation Research* 179 (1): 21–28. 10.1667/RR2737.1.

11 Britten, R.A., Peters, L.J., and Murray, D. (2001). Biological factors influencing the RBE of neutrons: Implications for their past, present and future use in radiotherapy. *Radiation Research* 156 (2): 125–135. 10.1667/0033-7587(2001)156[0125:bfitro]2.0.co;2.

12 Castro, J.R. and Reimers, M.M. (1988). Charged particle radiotherapy of selected tumors in the head and neck. *International Journal of Radiation Oncology, Biology, Physics* 14 (4): 711–720. 10.1016/0360-3016(88)90093-4.

13 Chan, A., Adams, J.A., Weyman, E., Parambi, R., Goldsmith, T., Holman, A., ... Delaney, T. (2012). A Phase II Trial of Proton Radiation Therapy With Chemotherapy for Nasopharyngeal Carcinoma. *International Journal of Radiation Oncology, Biology, Physics* 84 (3): S151–S152. 10.1016/j.ijrobp.2012.07.391.

14 Chan, A., Liebsch, L., Deschler, D., Adams, J., Vrishali, L., McIntyre, J., ... Busse, P. (2004). *Proton radiotherapy for T4 nasopharyngeal carcinoma.* Paper presented at the ASCO Annual Meeting Proceedings.

15 Chapman, T.R., Laramore, G.E., Bowen, S.R., and Orio, P.F., 3rd. (2016). *Neutron Radiation Therapy for Advanced Thyroid Cancers. Advanced Radiation Oncology* 1 (3): 148–156. 10.1016/j.adro.2016.05.001.

16 Chera, B.S., Malyapa, R., Louis, D., Mendenhall, W.M., Li, Z., Lanza, D.C., ... Mendenhall, N.P. (2009). Proton therapy for maxillary sinus carcinoma. *American Journal of Clinical Oncology* 32 (3): 296–303. 10.1097/COC.0b013e318187132a.

17 Chew, N.K., Sim, B.F., Tan, C.T., Goh, K.J., Ramli, N., and Umapathi, P. (2001). Delayed post-irradiation bulbar palsy in nasopharyngeal carcinoma. *Neurology* 57 (3): 529–531. 10.1212/wnl.57.3.529.

18 Chou, Y.C., Hung, S.P., Hsieh, C.E., Wu, Y.Y., and Chang, J.T.C. (2018). Intensity-Modulated Proton Therapy Reduces Acute Treatment-Related Toxicities for Patients with Nasopharyngeal Cancer: A Case-Control Propensity Score Match Study with Volumetric Modulated Arc Therapy. *International Journal of Radiation Oncology • Biology • Physics* 102 (3): e236–e237. 10.1016/j.ijrobp.2018.07.797.

19 Chuong, M., Bryant, J., Hartsell, W., Larson, G., Badiyan, S., Laramore, G.E., ... Vargas, C. (2019). Minimal acute toxicity from proton beam therapy for major salivary gland cancer. *Acta Oncology* 1–5. 10.1080/0284186x.2019.1698764.

20 Cuaron, J.J., Chang, C., Lovelock, M., Higginson, D.S., Mah, D., Cahlon, O., and Powell, S. (2016). Exponential Increase in Relative Biological Effectiveness Along Distal Edge of a Proton Bragg Peak as Measured by Deoxyribonucleic Acid Double-Strand Breaks. *International Journal of Radiation Oncology, Biology, Physics* 95 (1): 62–69. 10.1016/j.ijrobp.2016.02.018.

21 Dagan, R., Bryant, C.M., Bradley, J.A., Indelicato, D.J., Rutenberg, M., Rotondo, R., ... Mendenhall, W.M. (2016). A Prospective Evaluation of Acute Toxicity from Proton Therapy for Targets of the Parotid Region. *International Journal of Particle Theory* 3 (2): 285–290. 10.14338/ijpt-16-00010.2.

22 Dale, J.E., Molinelli, S., Ciurlia, E., Ciocca, M., Bonora, M., Vitolo, V., ... Fossati, P. (2017). Risk of carotid blowout after reirradiation with particle therapy. *Advances in Radiation Oncology* 2 (3): 465–474. 10.1016/j.adro.2017.05.007.

23 Davies, L. and Welch, H.G. (2014). Current thyroid cancer trends in the United States. *JAMA Otolaryngology-- Head & Neck Surgery* 140 (4): 317–322. 10.1001/jamaoto.2014.1.

24 Dionisi, F., Croci, S., Giacomelli, I., Cianchetti, M., Caldara, A., Bertolin, M., ... Amichetti, M. (2019). Clinical results of proton therapy reirradiation for recurrent nasopharyngeal carcinoma. *Acta Oncology* 58 (9): 1238–1245. 10.1080/0284186x.2019.1622772.

25 Fan, D., Kang, J.J., Fan, M., Wang, H., Lee, A., Yu, Y., ... Lee, N.Y. (2020a). Last-line local treatment with the Quad Shot regimen for previously irradiated head and neck cancers. *Oral Oncology* 104: 104641. 10.1016/j.oraloncology.2020.104641.

26 Fan, M., Kang, J.J., Lee, A., Fan, D., Wang, H., Kitpanit, S., ... Lee, N.Y. (2020b). Outcomes and toxicities of definitive radiotherapy and reirradiation using 3-dimensional conformal or intensity-modulated (pencil beam) proton therapy for patients with nasal cavity and paranasal sinus malignancies. *Cancer* 126 (9): 1905–1916. 10.1002/cncr.32776.

27 Feasel, A.M., Brown, T.J., Bogle, M.A., Tschen, J.A., and Nelson, B.R. (2001). Perineural invasion of cutaneous malignancies. *Dermatologic Surgery* 27 (6): 531–542. 10.1046/j.1524-4725.2001.00330.x.

28 Fitzek, M.M., Thornton, A.F., Varvares, M., Ancukiewicz, M., McIntyre, J., Adams, J., ... Amrein, P. (2002). Neuroendocrine tumors of the sinonasal tract. Results of a prospective study incorporating chemotherapy, surgery, and combined proton-photon radiotherapy. *Cancer* 94 (10): 2623–2634. 10.1002/cncr.10537.

29 Gao, J., Hu, J., Guan, X., Yang, J., Hu, W., Kong, L., and Lu, J.J. (2019). Salvage Carbon-Ion Radiation Therapy For Locoregionally Recurrent Head and Neck Malignancies. *Scientific Reports* 9 (1): 4259. 10.1038/s41598-019-39241-y.

30 Geist, D.E., Garcia-Moliner, M., Fitzek, M.M., Cho, H., and Rogers, G.S. (2008). Perineural invasion of cutaneous squamous cell carcinoma and basal cell carcinoma: Raising awareness and optimizing management. *Dermatologic Surgery* 34 (12): 1642–1651. 10.1111/j.1524-4725.2008.34341.x.

31 Gomez, D.R., Estilo, C.L., Wolden, S.L., Zelefsky, M.J., Kraus, D.H., Wong, R.J., ... Lee, N.Y. (2011). Correlation of osteoradionecrosis and dental events with dosimetric parameters in intensity-modulated radiation therapy for head-and-neck cancer. *International Journal of Radiation Oncology, Biology, Physics* 81 (4): e207–213. 10.1016/j.ijrobp.2011.02.003.

32 Griffin, T.W., Pajak, T.F., Laramore, G.E., Duncan, W., Richter, M.P., Hendrickson, F.R., and Maor, M.H. (1988). Neutron vs photon irradiation of inoperable salivary gland tumors: Results of an RTOG-MRC Cooperative Randomized Study. *International Journal of Radiation Oncology, Biology, Physics* 15 (5): 1085–1090. 10.1016/0360-3016(88)90188-5.

33 Gunn, G.B., Blanchard, P., Garden, A.S., Zhu, X.R., Fuller, C.D., Mohamed, A.S., ... Frank, S.J. (2016). Clinical Outcomes and Patterns of Disease Recurrence After Intensity Modulated Proton Therapy for Oropharyngeal Squamous Carcinoma. *International Journal of Radiation Oncology, Biology, Physics* 95 (1): 360–367. 10.1016/j.ijrobp.2016.02.021.

34 Haas-Kogan, D., Indelicato, D., Paganetti, H., Esiashvili, N., Mahajan, A., Yock, T., ... Kun, L. (2018). National Cancer Institute Workshop on Proton Therapy for Children: Considerations Regarding Brainstem Injury. *International Journal of Radiation Oncology*Biology*Physics* 101 (1): 152–168. https://doi.org/10.1016/j.ijrobp.2018.01.013.

35 Hayashi, K., Koto, M., Demizu, Y., Saitoh, J.I., Suefuji, H., and Okimoto, T. Japan Carbon-Ion Radiation Oncology Study, G. (2018). A retrospective multicenter study of carbon-ion radiotherapy for major salivary gland carcinomas: Subanalysis of J-CROS 1402 HN. *Cancer Science* 109 (5): 1576–1582. 10.1111/cas.13558.

36 Hayashi, Y., Nakamura, T., Mitsudo, K., Kimura, K., Yamaguchi, H., Ono, T., ... Tohnai, I. (2017). Re-irradiation using proton beam therapy combined with weekly intra-arterial chemotherapy for recurrent oral cancer. *Asia-Pacific Journal of Clinical Oncology* 13 (5): e394–e401. 10.1111/ajco.12502.

37 Held, T., Windisch, P., Akbaba, S., Lang, K., El Shafie, R., Bernhardt, D., ... Adeberg, S. (2019). Carbon Ion Reirradiation for Recurrent Head and Neck Cancer: A Single-Institutional Experience. *International Journal of Radiation Oncology, Biology, Physics* 105 (4): 803–811. 10.1016/j.ijrobp.2019.07.021.

38 Ho, J.C. and Phan, J. (2018). Reirradiation of head and neck cancer using modern highly conformal techniques. *40* 9: 2078–2093. 10.1002/hed.25180.

39 Holliday, E., Bhattasali, O., Kies, M.S., Hanna, E., Garden, A.S., Rosenthal, D.I., ... Frank, S.J. (2016a). Postoperative Intensity-Modulated Proton Therapy for Head and Neck Adenoid Cystic Carcinoma. *International Journal of Particle Theory* 2 (4): 533–543. 10.14338/ijpt-15-00032.1.

40 Holliday, E.B., Esmaeli, B., Pinckard, J., Garden, A.S., Rosenthal, D.I., Morrison, W.H., ... Frank, S.J. (2016b). A Multidisciplinary Orbit-Sparing Treatment Approach That Includes Proton Therapy for Epithelial Tumors of the Orbit and Ocular Adnexa. *International Journal of Radiation Oncology, Biology, Physics* 95 (1): 344–352. 10.1016/j.ijrobp.2015.08.008.

41 Holliday, E.B., Garden, A.S., Rosenthal, D.I., Fuller, C.D., Morrison, W.H., Gunn, G.B., ... Frank, S.J. (2015). Proton Therapy Reduces Treatment-Related Toxicities for Patients with Nasopharyngeal Cancer: A Case-Match Control Study of Intensity-Modulated Proton Therapy and Intensity-Modulated Photon Therapy. *International Journal of Particle Therapy* 2 (1): 19–28. 10.14338/ijpt-15-00011.1.

42 Holtzman, A.L. and Mendenhall, W.M. (2020). High-dose conformal proton therapy for clinical perineural invasion in cutaneous head and neck cancer. *Oral Oncology* 100: 104486. 10.1016/j.oraloncology.2019.104486.

43 Hu, J., Bao, C., Gao, J., Guan, X., Hu, W., Yang, J., ... Lu, J.J. (2018). Salvage treatment using carbon ion radiation in patients with locoregionally recurrent nasopharyngeal carcinoma: Initial results. *Cancer* 124 (11): 2427–2437. 10.1002/cncr.31318.

44 Huang, H.I., Chan, K.T., Shu, C.H., and Ho, C.Y. (2013). T4-locally advanced nasopharyngeal carcinoma: Prognostic influence of cranial nerve involvement in different radiotherapy techniques. *Scientific World Journal* 2013. 439073. 10.1155/2013/439073.

45 Huber, P.E., Debus, J., Latz, D., Zierhut, D., Bischof, M., Wannenmacher, M., and Engenhart-Cabillic, R. (2001). Radiotherapy for advanced adenoid cystic carcinoma: Neutrons, photons or mixed beam? *Radiotherapy and Oncology* 59 (2): 161–167. 10.1016/s0167-8140(00)00273-5.

46 Ikawa, H., Koto, M., Demizu, Y., Saitoh, J.I., Suefuji, H., Okimoto, T., ... Kamada, T. (2019). Multicenter study of carbon-ion radiation therapy for nonsquamous cell carcinomas of the oral cavity. *Cancer Medicine* 8 (12): 5482–5491. 10.1002/cam4.2408.

47 Jensen, A.D., Poulakis, M., Nikoghosyan, A.V., Chaudhri, N., Uhl, M., Munter, M.W., ... Debus, J. (2015). Re-irradiation of adenoid cystic carcinoma: Analysis and evaluation of outcome in 52 consecutive patients treated with raster-scanned carbon ion therapy. *Radiotherapy and Oncology* 114 (2): 182–188. 10.1016/j.radonc.2015.01.002.

48 Johansson, J., Blomquist, E., Montelius, A., Isacsson, U., and Glimelius, B. (2004). Potential outcomes of modalities and techniques in radiotherapy for patients with hypopharyngeal carcinoma. *Radiotherapy and Oncology* 72 (2): 129–138. 10.1016/j.radonc.2004.03.018.

49 Kandula, S., Zhu, X., Garden, A.S., Gillin, M., Rosenthal, D.I., Ang, K.K., ... Frank, S.J. (2013). Spot-scanning beam proton therapy vs intensity-modulated radiation therapy for ipsilateral head and neck malignancies: A treatment planning comparison. *Medical Dosimetry* 38 (4): 390–394. 10.1016/j.meddos.2013.05.001.

50 Kennedy, W.R., Dagan, R., Rotondo, R.L., Louis, D., Morris, C.G., and Indelicato, D.J. (2015). Proton therapy for pituitary adenoma. *Advances in Radiation Oncology* 15: 22–27.

51 Kitpanit, A., Lee, A., Pitter, K.L., Fan, D., Chow, J.C.H., Neal, B., ... Lee, N.Y. (2020 Spring). Temporal lobe necrosis in head and neck cancer patients after proton therapy to the skull base. *International Journal of Particle Theory*. 6(4):17–28. doi: 10.14338/IJPT-20-00014.1. Epub 2020 May 28. PMID: 32582816; PMCID: PMC7302730.

52 Kong, L., Lu, J.J., Liss, A.L., Hu, C., Guo, X., Wu, Y., and Zhang, Y. (2011). Radiation-induced cranial nerve palsy: A cross-sectional study of nasopharyngeal cancer patients after definitive radiotherapy. *International Journal of Radiation Oncology, Biology, Physics* 79 (5): 1421–1427. 10.1016/j.ijrobp.2010.01.002.

53 Koto, M., Hasegawa, A., Takagi, R., Ikawa, H., Naganawa, K., Mizoe, J.E., ... Neck, C. (2017). Definitive carbon-ion radiotherapy for locally advanced parotid gland carcinomas. *Head & Neck* 39 (4): 724–729. 10.1002/hed.24671.

54 Koto, M., Hasegawa, A., Takagi, R., Sasahara, G., Ikawa, H., and Mizoe, J.E. Organizing Committee for the Working Group for Head-and-Neck, C. (2014). Feasibility of carbon ion radiotherapy for locally advanced sinonasal adenocarcinoma. *Radiotherapy and Oncology* 113 (1): 60–65. 10.1016/j.radonc.2014.09.009.

55 Kountouri, M., Pica, A., Walser, M., Albertini, F., Bolsi, A., Kliebsch, U., ... Weber, D.C. (2019). Radiation-induced optic neuropathy after pencil beam scanning proton therapy for skull-base and head and neck tumours. *The British Journal of Radiology* 20190028. 10.1259/bjr.20190028.

56 Laramore, G.E., Krall, J.M., Griffin, T.W., Duncan, W., Richter, M.P., Saroja, K.R., ... Davis, L.W. (1993). Neutron versus photon irradiation for unresectable salivary gland tumors: Final report of an RTOG-MRC randomized clinical trial. Radiation Therapy Oncology Group. Medical Research Council. *International Journal of Radiation Oncology, Biology, Physics* 27 (2): 235–240. 10.1016/0360-3016(93)90233-l.

57 Lee, J.Y., Suresh, K., Nguyen, R., Sapir, E., Dow, J.S., Arnould, G.S., ... Eisbruch, A. (2016). Predictors of severe long-term toxicity after re-irradiation for head and neck cancer. *Oral Oncology* 60: 32–40. 10.1016/j.oraloncology.2016.06.017.

58 Lee, N., Harris, J., Garden, A.S., Straube, W., Glisson, B., Xia, P., ... Ang, K.K. (2009). Intensity-modulated radiation therapy with or without chemotherapy for nasopharyngeal carcinoma: Radiation therapy oncology group phase II trial 0225. *Journal of Clinical Oncology* 27 (22): 3684–3690. 10.1200/jco.2008.19.9109.

59 Lee, N.Y., Leeman, J.E., Cahlon, O., Sine, K., Jiang, G., Lu, J.J., and Both, S. (2018). *Target Volume Delineation and Treatment Planning for Particle Therapy.*

60 Li, P.C., Liebsch, N.J., Niemierko, A., Giantsoudi, D., Lessell, S., Fullerton, B.C., ... Shih, H.A. (2019). Radiation tolerance of the optic pathway in patients treated with proton and photon radiotherapy. *Radiotherapy and Oncology* 131: 112–119. https://doi.org/10.1016/j.radonc.2018.12.007.

61 Li, X., Lee, A., and Lee, N. (2020). Proton Therapy for Nasopharyngeal Cancer: A Matched Case-control Study of Intensity-Modulated Proton Therapy and Intensity-Modulated Photon Therapy. *International Journal of Radiation Oncology • Biology • Physics* 106 (5): 1138–1139. 10.1016/j.ijrobp.2019.11.198.

62 Lomax, A.J., Goitein, M., and Adams, J. (2003). Intensity modulation in radiotherapy: Photons versus protons in the paranasal sinus. *Radiotherapy and Oncology* 66 (1): 11–18. 10.1016/s0167-8140(02)00308-0.

63 Matthiesen, C., Herman Tde, L., Singh, H., Mascia, A., Confer, M., Simpson, H., ... Ahmad, S. (2015). Dosimetric and radiobiologic comparison of 3D conformal, IMRT, VMAT and proton therapy for the treatment of early-stage glottic cancer. *Journal of Medical Imaging and Radiation Oncology* 59 (2): 221–228. 10.1111/1754-9485.12227.

64 McDonald, M.W., Linton, O.R., and Calley, C.S. (2015). Dose-volume relationships associated with temporal lobe radiation necrosis after skull base proton beam therapy. *International Journal of Radiation Oncology, Biology, Physics* 91 (2): 261–267. 10.1016/j.ijrobp.2014.10.011.

65 McDonald, M.W., Liu, Y., Moore, M.G., and Johnstone, P.A. (2016). Acute toxicity in comprehensive head and neck radiation for nasopharynx and paranasal sinus cancers: Cohort comparison of 3D conformal proton therapy and intensity modulated radiation therapy. *Radiation Oncology* 11: 32. 10.1186/s13014-016-0600-3.

66 McDonald, M.W., Moore, M.G., and Johnstone, P.A. (2012). Risk of carotid blowout after reirradiation of the head and neck: A systematic review. *International Journal of Radiation Oncology, Biology, Physics* 82 (3): 1083–1089. 10.1016/j.ijrobp.2010.08.029.

67 Miyawaki, D., Murakami, M., Demizu, Y., Sasaki, R., Niwa, Y., Terashima, K., ... Sugimura, K. (2009). Brain injury after proton therapy or carbon ion therapy for head-and-neck cancer and skull base tumors. *International Journal of Radiation Oncology, Biology, Physics* 75 (2): 378–384. 10.1016/j.ijrobp.2008.12.092.

68 Mock, U., Georg, D., Bogner, J., Auberger, T., and Potter, R. (2004). Treatment planning comparison of conventional, 3D conformal, and intensity-modulated photon (IMRT) and proton therapy for paranasal sinus carcinoma. *International Journal of Radiation Oncology, Biology, Physics* 58 (1): 147–154. 10.1016/s0360-3016(03)01452-4.

69 Mohan, R. and Grosshans, D. (2017). Proton therapy - Present and future. *Advanced Drug Delivery Reviews* 109: 26–44. 10.1016/j.addr.2016.11.006.

70 Morikawa, T., Koto, M., Hasegawa, A., Takagi, R., Fujikawa, A., Tsuji, H., ... Kamada, T. (2016). Radiation-induced Parotid Gland Atrophy in Patients with Head and Neck Cancer After Carbon-ion Radiotherapy. *Anticancer Research* 36 (10): 5403–5407. 10.21873/anticanres.11116.

71 Nguyen, T.D., Chassard, J.L., Lagarde, P., Cutuli, B., Le Fur, R., Reme-Saumon, M., ... Chaplain, G. (1992). Results of postoperative radiation therapy in medullary carcinoma of the thyroid: A retrospective study by the French Federation of Cancer Institutes–the Radiotherapy Cooperative Group. *Radiotherapy and Oncology: Journal of the European Society for Therapeutic Radiology and Oncology* 23 (1): 1–5. 10.1016/0167-8140(92)90298-9.

72 Nguyen-Tan, P.F., Zhang, Q., Ang, K.K., Weber, R.S., Rosenthal, D.I., Soulieres, D., ... Le, Q.-T. (2014). Randomized phase iii trial to test accelerated versus standard fractionation in combination with concurrent cisplatin for head and neck carcinomas in the radiation therapy oncology group 0129 Trial: Long-term report of efficacy and toxicity. 32 (34): 3858–3867. 10.1200/jco.2014.55.3925

73 Nishimura, H., Ogino, T., Kawashima, M., Nihei, K., Arahira, S., Onozawa, M., ... Nishio, T. (2007). Proton-beam therapy for olfactory neuroblastoma. *International Journal of Radiation Oncology, Biology, Physics* 68 (3): 758–762. 10.1016/j.ijrobp.2006.12.071.

74 Owosho, A.A., Yom, S.K., Han, Z., Sine, K., Lee, N.Y., Huryn, J.M., and Estilo, C.L. (2016). Comparison of mean radiation dose and dosimetric distribution to tooth-bearing regions of the mandible associated with proton beam radiation therapy and intensity-modulated radiation therapy for ipsilateral head and neck tumor. *Oral Surgery, Oral Medicine, Oral Pathology and Oral Radiology* 122 (5): 566–571. 10.1016/j.oooo.2016.07.003.

75 Patel, S.H., Wang, Z., Wong, W.W., Murad, M.H., Buckey, C.R., Mohammed, K., ... Foote, R.L. (2014). Charged particle therapy versus photon therapy for paranasal sinus and nasal cavity malignant diseases: A systematic review and meta-analysis. *The Lancet Oncology* 15 (9): 1027–1038. 10.1016/S1470-2045(14)70268-2.

76 Phan, J., Sio, T.T., Nguyen, T.P., Takiar, V., Gunn, G.B., Garden, A.S., ... Frank, S.J. (2016). Reirradiation of Head and Neck Cancers With Proton Therapy: Outcomes and Analyses. *International Journal of Radiation Oncology, Biology, Physics* 96 (1): 30–41. 10.1016/j.ijrobp.2016.03.053.

77 Pommier, P., Liebsch, N.J., Deschler, D.G., Lin, D.T., McIntyre, J.F., Barker, F.G., 2nd, ... Chan, A.W. (2006). Proton beam radiation therapy for skull base adenoid cystic carcinoma. *Archives of Otolaryngology--head & Neck Surgery* 132 (11): 1242–1249. 10.1001/archotol.132.11.1242.

78 Riaz, N., Hong, J.C., Sherman, E.J., Morris, L., Fury, M., Ganly, I., ... Lee, N.Y. (2014). A nomogram to predict loco-regional control after re-irradiation for head and neck cancer. *Radiotherapy and Oncology: Journal of the European Society for Therapeutic Radiology and Oncology* 111 (3): 382–387. 10.1016/j.radonc.2014.06.003.

79 Romesser, P.B., Cahlon, O., Scher, E., Zhou, Y., Berry, S.L., Rybkin, A., ... Lee, N.Y. (2016a). Proton beam radiation therapy results in significantly reduced toxicity compared with intensity-modulated radiation therapy for head and neck tumors that require ipsilateral radiation. *Radiotherapy and Oncology: Journal of the European Society for Therapeutic Radiology and Oncology* 118 (2): 286–292. 10.1016/j.radonc.2015.12.008.

80 Romesser, P.B., Cahlon, O., Scher, E.D., Hug, E.B., Sine, K., DeSelm, C., ... Lee, N.Y. (2016b). Proton Beam Reirradiation for Recurrent Head and Neck Cancer: Multi-institutional Report on Feasibility and Early Outcomes. *International Journal of Radiation Oncology,*

Biology, Physics 95 (1): 386–395. 10.1016/j. ijrobp.2016.02.036.

81 Russo, A.L., Adams, J.A., Weyman, E.A., Busse, P.M., Goldberg, S.I., Varvares, M., ... Chan, A.W. (2016). Long-Term Outcomes After Proton Beam Therapy for Sinonasal Squamous Cell Carcinoma. *International Journal of Radiation Oncology, Biology, Physics* 95 (1): 368–376. 10.1016/j.ijrobp.2016.02.042.

82 Schulz-Ertner, D., Nikoghosyan, A., Jakel, O., Haberer, T., Kraft, G., Scholz, M., ... Debus, J. (2003). Feasibility and toxicity of combined photon and carbon ion radiotherapy for locally advanced adenoid cystic carcinomas. *International Journal of Radiation Oncology, Biology, Physics* 56 (2): 391–398. 10.1016/s0360-3016(02)04511-x.

83 Schuurhuis, J.M., Stokman, M.A., Roodenburg, J.L., Reintsema, H., Langendijk, J.A., Vissink, A., and Spijkervet, F.K. (2011). Efficacy of routine pre-radiation dental screening and dental follow-up in head and neck oncology patients on intermediate and late radiation effects. A retrospective evaluation. *Radiotherapy and Oncology: Journal of the European Society for Therapeutic Radiology and Oncology* 101 (3): 403–409. 10.1016/j. radonc.2011.09.018.

84 Sharma, S., Zhou, O., Thompson, R., Gabriel, P., Chalian, A., Rassekh, C., ... Lin, A. (2018). Quality of Life of Postoperative Photon versus Proton Radiation Therapy for Oropharynx Cancer. *International Journal of Particle Theory* 5 (2): 11–17. 10.14338/ijpt-18-00032.1.

85 Shen, J., Liu, W., Anand, A., Stoker, J.B., Ding, X., Fatyga, M., ... Bues, M. (2015). Impact of range shifter material on proton pencil beam spot characteristics. *Medical Physics* 42 (3): 1335–1340. 10.1118/1.4908208.

86 Sio, T.T., Lin, H.K., Shi, Q., Gunn, G.B., Cleeland, C.S., Lee, J.J., ... Frank, S.J. (2016). Intensity Modulated Proton Therapy Versus Intensity Modulated Photon Radiation Therapy for Oropharyngeal Cancer: First Comparative Results of Patient-Reported Outcomes. *International Journal of Radiation Oncology, Biology, Physics* 95 (4): 1107–1114. 10.1016/j.ijrobp.2016.02.044.

87 Stenmark, M.H., McHugh, J.B., Schipper, M., Walline, H.M., Komarck, C., Feng, F.Y., ... Carey, T.E. (2014). Nonendemic HPV-positive nasopharyngeal carcinoma: Association with poor prognosis. *International Journal of Radiation Oncology, Biology, Physics* 88 (3): 580–588. 10.1016/j.ijrobp.2013.11.246.

88 Takayama, K., Nakamura, T., Takada, A., Makita, C., Suzuki, M., Azami, Y., ... Fuwa, N. (2016). Treatment results of alternating chemoradiotherapy followed by proton beam therapy boost combined with intra-arterial infusion chemotherapy for stage III-IVB tongue cancer.

Journal of Cancer Research and Clinical Oncology 142 (3): 659–667. 10.1007/s00432-015-2069-0.

89 Timoshchuk, M.A., Dekker, P., Hippe, D.S., Parvathaneni, U., Liao, J.J., Laramore, G.E., and Dillon, J.K. (2019). The efficacy of neutron radiation therapy in treating salivary gland malignancies. *Oral Oncology* 88: 51–57. 10.1016/j. oraloncology.2018.11.006.

90 Truong, M.T., Kamat, U.R., Liebsch, N.J., Curry, W.T., Lin, D.T., Barker, F.G., 2nd, ... Chan, A.W. (2009). Proton radiation therapy for primary sphenoid sinus malignancies: Treatment outcome and prognostic factors. *Head & Neck* 31 (10): 1297–1308. 10.1002/hed.21092.

91 van de Water, T.A., Lomax, A.J., Bijl, H.P., Schilstra, C., Hug, E.B., and Langendijk, J.A. (2012). Using a reduced spot size for intensity-modulated proton therapy potentially improves salivary gland-sparing in oropharyngeal cancer. *International Journal of Radiation Oncology, Biology, Physics* 82 (2): e313–319. 10.1016/j. ijrobp.2011.05.005.

92 Waldron, J.N., O'Sullivan, B., Warde, P., Gullane, P., Lui, F.F., Payne, D., and Cummings, B. (1998). Ethmoid sinus cancer: Twenty-nine cases managed with primary radiation therapy. *International Journal of Radiation Oncology, Biology, Physics* 41 (2): 361–369. 10.1016/ s0360-3016(98)00018-2.

93 Williams, V.M., Sasidharan, B., Aljabab, S., Parvathaneni, U., Laramore, G.E., Wong, T.P., and Liao, J.J. (2019). Proton Radiotherapy for Locally Advanced Nasopharyngeal Carcinoma: Early Clinical Outcomes From a Single Institution. *International Journal of Radiation Oncology • Biology • Physics* 105 (1): E397. 10.1016/j.ijrobp.2019.06.1576.

94 Yu, N.Y., Gamez, M.E., Hartsell, W.F., Tsai, H.K., Laramore, G.E., Larson, G.L., ... Patel, S.H. (2019). A Multi-Institutional Experience of Proton Beam Therapy for Sinonasal Tumors. *Advances in Radiation Oncology* 4 (4): 689–698. 10.1016/j.adro.2019.07.008.

95 Zenda, S., Kawashima, M., Arahira, S., Kohno, R., Nishio, T., Tahara, M., ... Akimoto, T. (2015). Late toxicity of proton beam therapy for patients with the nasal cavity, para-nasal sinuses, or involving the skull base malignancy: Importance of long-term follow-up. *International Journal of Clinical Oncology* 20 (3): 447–454. 10.1007/s10147-014-0737-8.

96 Zhang, W., Zhang, X., Yang, P., Blanchard, P., Garden, A.S., Gunn, B., ... Frank, S.J. (2017). Intensity-modulated proton therapy and osteoradionecrosis in oropharyngeal cancer. *Radiotherapy and Oncology: Journal of the European Society for Therapeutic Radiology and Oncology* 123 (3): 401–405. 10.1016/j.radonc.2017.05.006.

17

Thoracic Malignancies

Proton Beam and Carbon-ion Therapy for Thoracic Cancers and Recurrent Disease

Matthew S. Ning, MD MPH*, Vivek Verma, MD, and Steven H. Lin, MD PhD

Department of Radiation Oncology, The University of Texas MD Anderson Cancer Center, Houston, TX, USA
*Corresponding Author: Matthew S. Ning, MD, MPH, Department of Radiation Oncology, The University of Texas MD Anderson Cancer Center, 1515 Holcombe Blvd., Houston, TX 77030

Conflicts of Interest: Support was provided in part by NCI/NIH Cancer Center Support Grant (CA16672). Otherwise, the authors have no relevant disclosures to declare with respect to this work.

17.1   Introduction

Thoracic malignancies represent a heterogeneous spectrum of primary cancers and metastatic disease. Radiation plays an essential role in management, as local ablation and cytoreduction of disease are directly associated with improved outcomes. Over the past decade, therapeutic advancements have led to a growing population of long-term survivors as well as an increasing number of patients susceptible to treatment-related toxicities. As such, novel strategies to further optimize the therapeutic ratio remain an active area of research. Particle therapy has correspondingly emerged as an exciting treatment strategy for many thoracic cancers, exemplified by dosimetric and clinical advantages over photon radiotherapy. This chapter discusses the evolving indications and rationale for utilizing particle therapy among this unique patient population. Following a comprehensive review of the clinical data, we discuss

patient selection and safety considerations, technical challenges, and economic and operational factors as a practical guide for clinicians. We then close by exploring future directions currently under investigation. Taken together, this focused examination highlights the promise of particle therapy for improving thoracic patient outcomes and further expanding the field.

17.2   Clinical Applications: Review of the Retrospective and Prospective Data to Date

17.2.1   Non-small Cell Lung Cancer: Definitive Treatment

Lung cancer kills more people each year than colon, breast, and prostate cancer combined, with non-small cell lung cancer

Principles and Practice of Particle Therapy, First Edition. Edited by Timothy D. Malouff and Daniel M. Trifiletti.
© 2022 John Wiley & Sons Ltd. Published 2022 by John Wiley & Sons Ltd.

(NSCLC) accounting for 85% of new cases annually. The 5-year survival rates range from 92% in early-stage disease to 13% for locally advanced cases. However, systemic therapy has dramatically improved over the last decade, delaying distant progression among these patients and thus placing greater emphasis on the role of local therapy. The standard of care for unresected NSCLC involves radiotherapy: alone for early-stage tumors or concurrent with chemotherapy for locally advanced disease.

Due to their location, these neoplasms naturally originate and invade in proximity to critical structures such as the heart, cord, esophagus, and uninvolved lung. Thus, chemoradiation may be accompanied by significant toxicities; however, particle therapy has emerged as a new modality to further optimize the management of these patients. Numerous dosimetric comparative studies have demonstrated theoretical advantages of particle therapy for NSCLC [1], notably with respect to lung parameters, esophageal, heart, and spinal cord doses [2]

(Figure 17.1). The reduction in low-dose bath [3] from highly conformal particle therapy techniques has potential clinical relevance particularly in the setting of concurrent chemotherapy [4]. Furthermore, the relative differences in biologic effectiveness noted with particle therapies have the potential for differential tumoricidal effects.

The reduced dose exposure to various organs-at-risk (OARs) has since been supported by favorable clinical and safety outcomes (Table 17.1), even in the setting of greater target doses [5]. One of the earliest studies from Loma Linda reported outcomes of high-dose hypofractionated proton beam therapy (PBT) for early-stage tumors [6]. Over their 12-year experience, 111 patients (median tumor size 3.6 cm) were treated with doses ranging from 51 to 70 Gy in 10 daily fractions over 2 weeks. Patients with peripheral T1 tumors exhibited 4-year local control (LC), disease-specific survival, and overall survival (OS) rates of 96%, 88%, and 60%, respectively, at 4 years. The incidence of radiation pneumonitis was found to be

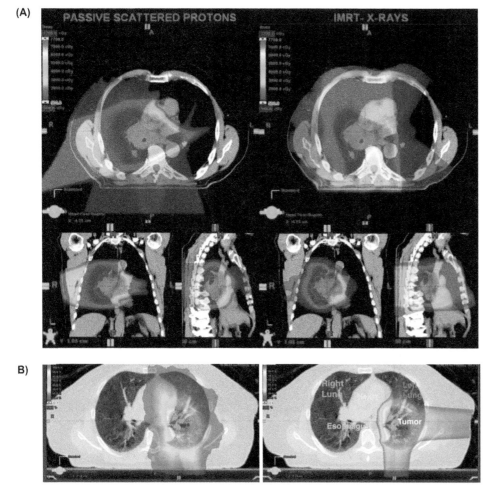

Figure 17.1 Example comparisons between proton beam radiotherapy versus photon IMRT for the definitive treatment of lung cancer. (A) Note that the contralateral lung is almost completely spared with protons *(reproduced from open access source)* [127]. (B) At the high dose region near the tumor, the photon IMRT plan *(left panel)* is more conformal than the proton plan *(right panel)* due to extra margin accounting for range uncertainty; however, there is superior sparing of organs well outside the field *(reproduced from open access source)* [128].

Table 17.1 Selected published and anticipated studies of particle beam therapy in the definitive treatment of non-small cell lung cancer [7–11,18–20,123,124].

Reference	Type	Indication	Modality	Chemo	Prescription (median)	Follow-up(months)	Outcomes	Toxicity (nonheme)
Ohnishi et al. [7]	Retrospective	Stage I (T1–2a) T2a 29% Central 13%	PSPT	None	BED_{10} 110 GyE	38	3-year OS 80% 3-year PFS 64% 3-year LC 90%	Grade 2 ≥ 10% Grade 3 ≥ 1% Grade 5 1%
Chang et al. [8]	Phase I/II	IA–IIB (T1–T3) T2/3 57%/9% IIA/B 11%/9%	PSPT	None	87.5 GyE in 35 fxs	83	5-year OS 28% 5-year LC 85%	Grade 2 ≥ 51% Grade 3 ≥ 3%
Chang et al. [9]	Phase II	Stage IIIA 47% Stage IIIB 53%	PSPT	Concurrent ± induction (31%) Adjuvant (28%)	74 GyE	27	5-year OS 29% 5-year PFS 22% 5-year LRF 28%	Grade 2 ≥ 34% (acute) ≥16% (late) Grade 3 ≥ 9% (acute) ≥12% (late) Grade 4 ≥ 2% (late)
Remick et al. [10]	Retrospective	Adjuvant PORT N2 (67%) R1–2 (48%)	PSPT (81%) IMPT (19%)	Neoadjuvant (7%) Sequential (70%) Concurrent (22%)	50.4 GyE in 28 fxs	23	2-year OS 78% 2-year LC 93%	Grade 2 ≥ 37% (acute) Grade 3 7% (acute)
Liao et al. [11]	Phase II RCT	IIA–IV (M1b) and recurrent	PSPT	Concurrent ± induction (74%)	66 or 74 GyE	26	1-year LF 11% OS 26 months	Grade 3 ≥ 11%
Saitoh et al. [18]	Phase II	Stage I (T1–2a) peripheral	CIRT	None	53–60 GyE in 4 fxs	56	5-year PFS 51% 5-year OS 75% 5-year LC 88%	Grade 2 5% Grade 3 3%
Karube et al. [19]	Phase I/II	Stage I (T1–2) peripheral Age ≥ 80 years	CIRT	None	28–50 GyE in single fx	43	5-year OS 40% 5-year LC 86%	Grade 2 ≥ 4% (acute) ≥7% (late)
Takahashi et al. [20]	Phase I/II	Stage IIA–IIIA N0–N1 79% Single-N2 21%	CIRT	Induction (8%)	68–72 GyE in 16 fxs	25	2-year OS 52% 2-year LC 93%	Grade 2 ≥ 16% (acute) ≥10% (late) Grade 3 3–5% (acute) 3–5% (late)
RTOG 1308 [123]	Phase III RCT	Stages II–IIIB	PBT	Concurrent	70 GyE in 35 fxs	Enrolling	OS (primary)	Cardiopulmonary and hematologic AEs
NCT01629498 [124]	Phase I/II RCT	Recurrent and stages II–IIIB	IMPT	Concurrent	Up to 78 GyE in 30 fxs	Enrolling	LPFS (primary)	Grade 3+ AEs (coprimary)

N (#): Ohnishi 669; Chang [8] 35; Chang [9] 64; Remick 27; Liao 57; Saitoh 37; Karube 70; Takahashi 62; RTOG 1308 330 (estimate); NCT01629498 100 (estimate) minimal, with no patients requiring steroid therapy, even with total doses of 70 Gy.

A much larger retrospective series from Japan evaluated the efficacy and safety of protons among 682 patients with stage I (clinical T1a–T2a) NSCLC treated to a median biological effective dose of 110 GyE [7]. At a median follow-up of 38 months, the 3-year OS, progression-free survival (PFS), and LC rates were 79.5%, 64%, and 90%, respectively. The incidence of grade ≥3 pneumonitis and dermatitis were 1.7% and 0.4%, respectively, indicating acceptable outcomes and low toxicity among these patients. Further supporting these findings, MD Anderson subsequently published long-term follow-up of a phase I/II study of dose-escalated PBT for early-stage NSCLC [8]. A total of 35 patients with T1–3 node-negative disease were treated to 87.5 Gy in 35 daily fractions. At a noteworthy median follow-up of 83 months, the 5-year local recurrence-free, regional recurrence-free, and distant metastasis-free survival rates were 85%, 89%, and 54%, respectively, with the incidence of Grade 3+ toxicities <5%. Taken together, these series indicate that PBT to ablative doses is well tolerated and effective for early-stage NSCLC.

With respect to locally advanced disease, a single-arm phase II study also by MD Anderson evaluated PBT with concurrent chemotherapy for unresected stage IIIA/B disease. The 5-year report described 64 patients treated to 74 GyE with passively scattered technique and concurrent carboplatin/paclitaxel. At a median follow-up of 27 months, the 5-year OS, PFS, actuarial distant metastasis, and locoregional recurrence (LRR) rates were 29%, 22%, 54%, and 28%, respectively [9]. Local and regional treatment failures were noted among 16% and 14% of patients, with nearly half failing distantly. Rates of grade 3 acute esophagitis and late pneumonitis were 8% and 12%, respectively. Late toxicity was uncommon; although rates of grade 4 esophagitis and bronchial fistula were both 2%, with no grade 4 pneumonitis noted. Additionally, in the postoperative setting, a retrospective study reported outcomes among 61 patients treated for positive microscopic margins and/or positive N2 disease to a median dose of 50.4 Gy (of whom 27 received PBT) [10], also reporting favorable short-term outcomes and high tolerance at a median follow-up of 23 months for the proton cohort.

Yet, despite the promising clinical and toxicity outcomes observed in these single-arm prospective and retrospective reports, the only randomized (phase II) trial to date was negative with respect to a benefit with PBT over photon therapy for advanced NSCLC [11]. In this trial, conducted by MD Anderson and Massachusetts General Hospital, unresected patients (including stage IIB through oligometastatic disease) were adaptively randomized to definitive treatment with either PBT ($n = 57$) or intensity-modulated photon radiotherapy (IMRT) ($n = 92$) to 60–74 GyE with concurrent chemotherapy. Both primary co-end points, locoregional control

(LRC) and grade 3+ radiation pneumonitis, were similar between arms. While protons reduced the lung V5, lung V10, and heart dose, there was no significant difference in outcomes: local failure (~11% in both arms) and grade 3+ pneumonitis (10.5% PBT vs. 6.5% IMRT).

However, these negative outcomes were likely attributable to several criticisms with respect to trial design. The largest criticism is with respect to the dosimetric screening inclusion criterion. Patients were only deemed eligible for randomization after generation and review of comparison IMRT and PBT plans, and only patients with acceptable plans for either modality were included. This stringency likely mitigated any signal of benefit that would have been observed with protons, as patients who may have benefited from its utilization (as opposed to photon therapy) were excluded prior to randomization. The second major caveat was the treatment era for particle therapy during which this trial was conducted. During this early phase of protons, the modern advances in planning, delivery, and technology were underdeveloped. Consistent with most existing data on protons, this randomized trial also utilized passive scatter technique (due to the low widespread availability of pencil beam technology at the time). However, the latter is ideal for anatomically complex disease, including central tumors and cases with involvement of the contralateral lung, hilum, and/or extensive mediastinal adenopathy [12]. Pencil beam scanning technique, permitting intensity-modulated PBT (IMPT), has been demonstrated to yield statistically significant reductions in maximum spinal cord, mean heart, and numerous lung dose parameters when compared with IMRT or even passive scatter PBT (PSPT) [2]; and the greater target conformality and dose painting ability versus passive scatter techniques [13] makes IMPT a more analogous comparison to IMRT (Figure 17.2).

Furthermore, the general quality of PBT (even PSPT) has continued to improve with greater planning and delivery experience over time, as demonstrated by the learning curve noted over the course of the study: pneumonitis rates for trial patients decreased by half (31–13%) over the enrollment timeframe. Thus, this greater collective experience and the widespread adoption of IMPT are expected to correlate with reductions in treatment-related toxicities and improved therapeutic ratio among patients with NSCLC [2]. PBT in general has continued to improve at a rapid pace, now with the widespread adoption of robust planning techniques and 4D-image guided motion management strategies, and dramatic improvements in outcomes and toxicity are expected as newer techniques are increasingly employed.

In addition to PBT, carbon-ion radiotherapy (CIRT) has gained increased interest as a definitive modality for NSCLC over recent years. High linear energy transfer (LET) radiation theoretically offers advantages with respect to biological effectiveness: as compared to photon and PBT, CIRT may yield

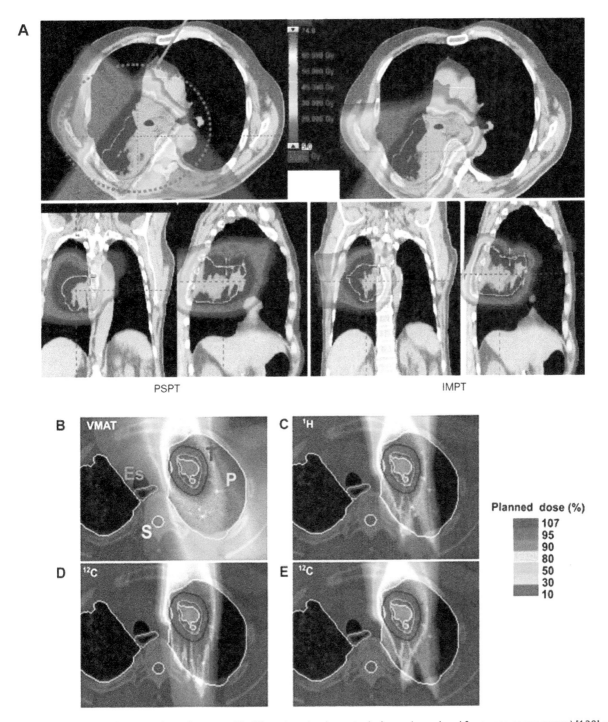

Figure 17.2 Example comparisons between (A) different proton beam techniques *(reproduced from open access source)* [128] and among (B–E) different charged particles *(reproduced from open access source)* [129]. (A) As compared to passive scatter technique *(left panel)*, pencil beam scanning permits intensity-modulated proton therapy *(right panel)*, with greater target conformality and sparing of normal structures as well as simultaneous integrated boost. (B) Photon IMRT imparts greater non-prescription radiation dose to adjacent structures such as esophagus and cord than particle therapy counterparts: (C) proton beam, (D) single-field carbon ion, and (E) dual-field carbon ion.

stronger sterilization effects on intrinsically radioresistant tumors, with greater killing of hypoxic, G0, and S-phase cells. By efficiently eradicating hypoxic tumor cells [14], carbon ions may offer a solution to hypoxia-induced radioresistance, which constitutes a major obstacle in curative cancer treatment for many sites.

Initial dosimetric comparisons of CIRT with photon therapy indicated more homogeneous target dose and lower OAR doses with CIRT plans for both stage I [15] and stage III [16] NSCLC (Figure 17.2). Due to these DVH benefits, CIRT has been demonstrated to be a feasible alternative for NSCLC patients with interstitial lung disease (ILD), a frequent complication which may limit patient eligibility for definitive radiotherapy [17].

Clinically, prospective single-arm trials of CIRT have already been conducted among both the early-stage and locally advanced settings, with outcomes at least comparable to those of PBT (Table 17.1). A phase II study of hypofractionated CIRT for stage I (cT1–T2a) NSCLC encompassed 37 patients with peripheral tumors treated to 52.8–60 Gy in four fractions within a single week. With a median follow-up of 56 months, the 5-year actuarial LC and OS rates were 88% and 75%, respectively; and the incidence of grade 2+ was roughly 5% [18]. Another phase I/II trial confirmed the efficacy and safety of single-fraction dose-escalation among 70 octogenarians [19], with 5-year LC, cause-specific survival, and OS rates of 86%, 65%, and 40% at a median follow-up of 43 months, and no grade 3+ toxicities observed.

In the locally advanced setting (stage III), a phase I/II study treated 62 patients (most of whom had N0–1 disease) to prescription doses of 68–76 GyE in 16 fractions over 4 weeks. At a median follow-up of 25 months, the 2-year LC and OS for the entire cohort were 93% and 52%, and these excellent outcomes were maintained even among the cT3-4N0 subset [20]. Grade 3 adverse events (AEs) (radiation pneumonitis and tracheoesophageal fistula) occurred among ≤5%, and only among patients receiving 76 GyE (with no grade 3+ toxicities noted with 72 GyE).

For definitive CIRT alone (without chemotherapy), 72 GyE in 16 fractions has been reinforced as a standard option by multiple retrospective series from Japan ($n = 64$–141), with median follow-up times ranging between 18.5 and 29 months [21–23]. Altogether, these have reported 2-year OS, PFS, and LC rates of 55–62%, 39–42%, and 74–82%, respectively [21–23], with grade 3+ toxicity rates of roughly 5% (including mediastinal hemorrhage, radiation pneumonitis, and bronchial fistula events) [21–23] along with the incidence of grade 2 radiation pneumonitis closer to 10% [24].

Collectively, these data support the feasibility of definitive CIRT alone for inoperable stages II–III NSCLC with acceptable toxicity rates, recognizing that these study populations mainly comprised a relatively lower burden of nodal disease (mostly N0-1, with single-station N2 also noted) and were treated in the absence of concurrent chemotherapy. Therefore, additional studies are warranted to further define the utility of CIRT in a more "clinically routine" setting.

As a final important point, irradiation of a moving organ with particle beam therapy (either PBT or CIRT) can easily result in over- and underdosages of the target volume [25]. As such, the planning and delivery of particle therapy requires comprehensive physics expertise and dosimetric experience with 4D-robustness optimization techniques [26], as well as vigilant quality assurance measures to mitigate errors and ensure conformality of actual dose, even under interfractional variations [27]. Although IMPT is ideal for anatomically complex disease, such as very central tumors or those with involvement of the contralateral lung, hilum, and/or extensive mediastinal adenopathy [12], the associated higher target conformality comes at the expense of the baseline plan robustness appreciated by simpler passive scatter techniques [13]. Notable anatomical changes and target motion in this setting can lead to marginal misses if unaccounted for, and there is concern for interplay effects, referring to degradation in dose distribution based on simultaneous relative motion between the target and the beam.

However, such limitations may be avoided by employing technical planning and treatment delivery techniques. Regarding planning, 4D (versus 3D) robust optimization produces significantly more interplay-effect-resistant plans for target coverage, while maintaining comparable dose to normal tissues [28]. Additionally, analytic pencil beam algorithms are poorly suited for particle dose calculations in the lung and can overpredict target dose by nearly 50% [29], while underestimating the dose to normal lung tissue [30]. Instead, Monte Carlo algorithms can significantly improve treatment quality by better reflecting delivered dose distributions [29]. These advancements have been made possible over the last several years due to technological improvements in computational power, which permit once time-intensive complex dose calculations and inverse planning algorithms to be completed within a standard clinical workflow. Additionally, novel methods to more accurately reduce range margins can improve confidence in the plan and further decrease treatment-related toxicity [30]. As an example, implementation of dual-energy CT has been found to improve estimates by up to 50% with respect to range uncertainty.

With respect to treatment delivery, patient setup to tumor (in lieu of bone) unsurprisingly ensures optimal dose distribution, further supporting the significance of volumetric imaging (versus 2D radiographs) for particle therapy in lung cancer [31,32]. Adaptive planning can reduce normal tissue doses and prevent target misses, particularly in the setting of large tumors that decrease markedly in size during therapy [33]. Other strategies to potentially enhance CTV dose homogeneity for moving targets include extending fractionation and/or the number of treatment fields [34]. These are just a few examples of the continuous improvements in particle therapy since inception that will continue to improve radiotherapy planning, treatment delivery, and patient outcomes.

17.2.2 Locoregionally Recurrent and Oligometastatic Disease: Thoracic Re-Irradiation

LRRs are common following the initial treatment of lung cancer, occurring in more than 25% of patients upon follow-up (and not uncommonly in-field), yet management of these thoracic recurrences remains a challenge. Re-irradiation may be a treatment option for some patients in efforts to achieve durable tumor control but can be associated with considerable risk of high-grade toxicities. The fear of excessive and potentially life-threatening toxicities to previously irradiated organs often limits the inability to safely deliver definitive (≥60 Gy) doses in the recurrent setting. However, particle therapy can help shift the balance toward efficacy and acceptable toxicities due to physical advantages such as the limited exit dose. If utilized correctly, particle therapy can help achieve favorable outcomes for recurrent lung cancer [35] (Figure 17.3).

MD Anderson published one of the first series demonstrating the feasibility of PBT for re-irradiation of LRR NSCLC [36] (Table 17.2). In this early report, 33 patients underwent retreatment to a median dose of 66 GyE in 32 fractions (following initial treatment to 63 Gy in 33 fractions roughly 3 years prior), 8 of whom also received concurrent chemotherapy for recurrence. At a median follow-up of 11 months, the 1-year rates of OS, PFS, LRC,

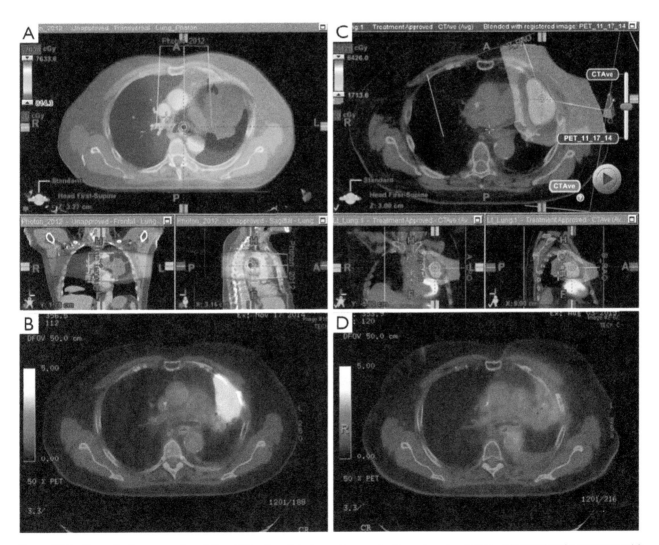

Figure 17.3 Example demonstration of the utility of particle beam therapy for thoracic re-irradiation of locoregional recurrence with definitive intent. This patient was initially treated with (A) concurrent chemoradiotherapy to 70 Gy with photon therapy, then developed (B) local recurrence at 2-year follow-up, for which he underwent (C) salvage intensity-modulated proton beam therapy to 66 Gy with concurrent chemotherapy. He tolerated treatment well, with (D) no evidence of disease or significant toxicity as of last follow-up *(reproduced from open access source)* [128].

Table 17.2 Overview of studies on particle beam therapy for salvage re-irradiation of locoregionally recurrent lung cancer [21,36–41]

Reference	Type	Re-radiotherapy interval	Histology	Location	Modality	Concurrent Chemo	N (#)	Prescription (median)	Follow-up (months)	Outcomes	Toxicity (non-heme)
McAvoy et al. [36]	Retrospective	36 months	NSCLC	Central 85% In-field 58% Marginal 6%	PSPT	24%	33	66 GyE in 32 fxs (prior EQD2 62 Gy)	11	2-year OS 33% / 2-year PFS 14% / 2-year LRC 24% / Drop-out 6%	Grade 2–4 ≤55% (acute) ≤21% (late) / Grade 2 ≥27% (any) / Grade 3 ≥15% (any) / Grade 4 9% (any)
Chao et al. [37]	Prospective multicenter	19 months	NSCLC	Varies	PBT	68%	57	66.6 GyE	8	2-year OS 43% / 2-year PFS 38% / LRC 75% / Drop-out 9%	Grade 3–4 33% (acute) 7% (late) / Grade 3 25% (any) / Grade 4 7% (any) / Grade 5 5% (acute) 5% (late)
Badiyan et al. [38]	Prospective multicenter	20 months	NSCLC 91% SCLC 9%	Varies	PBT (5% IMPT)	30%	79	60 GyE (prior EQD2 60–83 Gy)	11	1-year OS 60% (median 15 months) / 1-year PFS 43% (median 11 months) / 1-year LRFS 56% (median 13 months)	Grade 2 ≥11% (acute) ≥5% (late) / Grade 3 6% (acute) 1% (late) / Grade 5 1–3% (acute) 1% (late)
Ho et al. [39]	Retrospective	30 months	NSCLC 81%	Central 81% In-field 85% Marginal 11%	IMPT	48%	27	66 GyE in 30 fxs (prior EQD2 60 Gy)	11	1-year OS 54% (median 18 mos) / 1-year LC 78% / 1-year LRC 61% / 1-year PFS 51%	Grade 2 ≥26% / Grade 3 7% (late)
Shirai et al. [40]	Retrospective	16 months	NSCLC	Regional recurrences	CIRT	None	8	53 GyE in 12 fxs (hypo-frac)	28	2-year LC 86% / 2-year PFS 50% / 2-year OS 71%	Grade 2 13% (acute) 13% (late)
Karube et al. [21]	Retrospective	20 months	NSCLC	In-field	CIRT	None	29	66 GyE in 12 fxs (prior 46 GyE in single fx)	29	2-year LC 67% / 2-year PFS 52% / 2-year OS 69%	Grade 2 24% (any) / 7% (acute) / 21% (late) / Grade 3 3% (any)
Hayashi et al. [41]	Prospective	17 months	77% Primaries 23% Mets	Central 18% In-field 75% Marginal 25%	CIRT	None	95	66 GyE in 12 fxs (prior 53 GyE in 4 fxs)	18	2-year LC 54% / 2-year OS 62%	Grade 2 ≥5% (acute) ≥5% (late) / Grade 3 2% (late) / Grade 4 1% (acute) / Grade 5 1% (late)

and distant metastasis-free survival were 47%, 28%, 54%, and 39%, respectively. Rates of grade ≥3 toxicity included 9% esophageal (with one grade 4 cases) and 21% pulmonary (with two grade 4 cases), and two patients (6%) failed to complete re-treatment.

Shortly thereafter, a multi-institutional prospective study evaluated PBT for the same population, reporting outcomes among 57 patients treated at three different proton therapy centers (68% of whom received concurrent systemic therapy) [37]. The median time between the initial and re-irradiation course was 19 months, and the median prescription dose in the re-irradiation setting was 66.6 Gy, with 68% of patients receiving concurrent chemotherapy. LRC was 75%, and the 1-year rates of OS and PFS were 59% and 58%, respectively. Grade 3+ toxicity developed in 42% of patients (39% acute; 12% late), with grade 5 toxicities observed among 10.5%, and again 5 patients (7%) failed to complete re-irradiation. These severe toxicities were associated with increased composite dose overlap of the central airway region, mean esophagus and heart doses, and receipt of concurrent chemotherapy, with decreased survival corresponding to increased mean esophagus dose.

Another multi-institutional prospective collaboration reported their registry outcomes of 79 recurrent lung cancer patients re-irradiated with PBT at 8 separate institutions. The median time from prior treatment was 19.9 months, and 30% received concurrent chemotherapy. At a follow-up of 10.7 months, median OS and PFS were 15.2 and 10.5 months, respectively. Acute and late grade 3 toxicities occurred in 6% and 1%, with all patients completing treatment but three succumbing to possible radiation toxicity during follow-up [38].

These initial studies conveyed the utility of PBT as a definitive salvage modality with promising efficacy for the LRR setting, while emphasizing the importance of appropriate patient selection and continued vigilance for toxicity. Taking these educational points into account, MD Anderson published an updated retrospective series of 27 patients who specifically received IMPT for re-irradiation, to a median dose of 66 GyE at a median of 29.5 months following the initial course. At a follow-up of 11.2 months, the median survival was 18 months, with a 1-year OS of 54%. In-field LC was 85%, with 1-year freedom from locoregional failure (LRF) and 1-year PFS rates of 61% and 51%, respectively. However, re-irradiation was relatively well tolerated, with only 7% experiencing late grade 3 pulmonary toxicity, and no grade 4–5 toxicities, suggesting that IMPT may further improve outcomes with minimizing potential toxicities in this setting [39].

In addition to PBT, several studies from Japan have also evaluated the efficacy and safety of re-irradiation with CIRT, demonstrating favorable disease outcomes without producing severe toxicities in well-selected patients (Table 17.2). One retrospective study evaluated the utility of hypofraction-

ated CIRT among 15 patients with isolated regional metastases after initial definitive therapy. Most patients received 52.8 GyE in 12 fractions over 3 weeks in the absence of systemic therapy, demonstrating 2-year LC, PFS, and OS rates of 92%, 47%, and 75%, respectively, at a median follow-up of 28 months. No grade 3+ AEs were noted [40]. Another study investigated its utility among 29 patients with in-field recurrences of stage I NSCLC (which were initially treated with CIRT). The median prescribed dose in this setting was 66 GyE in 12 fractions (following initial treatment doses of 46 GyE). At a median follow-up of 29 months, 2-year OS, LC, and PFS rates after re-irradiation were 69.0%, 67%, and 52%, respectively, again with no grade 3+ radiotherapy-induced adverse effects noted [21].

Expanding upon these smaller works, a prospective study evaluated carbon-ion re-irradiation among 95 patients with LRR, metastatic, or secondary lung tumors. The median dose in this setting was 66 Gy (following an initial dose of 52.8 Gy), in the absence of concurrent chemotherapy. Outcomes were less impressive than the prior series but demonstrated moderate efficacy at a follow-up of 18 months, with 2-year LC and OS rates of 54% and 62%, respectively, which remained noteworthy given the heterogeneous population (e.g., 23% with metastatic lung tumors of nonpulmonary origin). The rate of grade ≥3 toxicity was less than 5%, although isolated cases of grade 4 pneumonitis and grade 5 bronchopleural fistula were observed [41]. Nevertheless, these studies have collectively laid the foundation for CIRT as a feasible and safe modality for definitive salvage treatment of recurrent disease.

As suggested by the broad inclusion criteria of the prior prospective study, the rationale of definitive salvage therapy is similar in some ways to that of local consolidative therapy for oligometastatic disease (or stage IV disease involving only a limited number of distant sites) [42]. In either scenario, the goal of treatment is to improve outcomes through ablation or cytoreduction of gross disease. While stereotactic ablative techniques have emerged as a standard modality to address oligometastatic sites, SABR with photons may not always be a feasible option. For some cases, particularly in the setting of thoracic re-irradiation, hypofractionated particle therapy could afford more favorable dose profiles to previously irradiated OARs adjacent to the target field, with potential utility in the setting of photon radioresistance.

To this end, another study from Japan analyzed the efficacy and feasibility of CIRT and PBT for the treatment of oligometastatic lung tumors, reporting outcomes on a total of 47 patients who received particle therapy for 59 pulmonary lesions to a median dose of 60 GyE in 8 fractions. At a median follow-up time of 17 months, the 2-year LC, OS, and PFS rates were 79%, 54%, and 27%, respectively. Observed toxicities were mild: 13% grade 2 and 13% grade 3 toxicity. Additionally, an older study evaluated efficacy specifically among 34 patients with oligo-recurrent colorectal cancer metastatic to lung (total 44 pulmonary lesions) treated with CIRT to a higher BED of 60 GyE (but in median daily doses of 15 GyE) [43]. At a median follow-up of 23.7 months, the LC rates remained at 85% at 2 and 3 years, while the OS was 65% and 50%, respectively. There were no grade 3+ toxicities. Taken together, these studies demonstrate that particle therapy is well tolerated and effective in the treatment of oligometastatic lung tumors, as well as safely delivered via high-dose prescriptions (BED10 ≥ 110 GyE10) to optimize LC in this setting [44].

17.2.3 Limited-Stage Small Cell Lung Cancer (LS-SCLC)

As the prognosis of limited-stage small cell lung cancer (LS-SCLC) continues to improve—particularly with the promise of immunotherapeutic innovations—treatment-related toxicities merit reconsideration for this patient population [45,46]. Traditional chemoradiotherapy (with concurrent platinum agent and etoposide) is the standard of care for LS-SCLC, but accompanied by high toxicity rates, particularly acute grade 3+ esophagitis and pneumonitis. Particle therapy, however, could potentially reduce the incidence of AEs with treatment.

Yet, the data on particle therapy for this population are extremely limited, with just two series evaluating the utility of PBT in their management. The University of Florida published the earliest case series of six patients with LS-SCLC treated via passively scattered PBT, most commonly to 60–66 GyE in 30–34 daily fractions with concurrent chemotherapy [47]. At a median follow-up of 12 months, the 1-year OS and PFS were 83% and 66%, respectively. Treatment was well tolerated with no acute grade 3+ esophagitis or acute grade 2+ pneumonitis, corresponding to the superior lung and esophageal sparing noted dosimetrically on IMRT plan comparisons).

More recently, a prospective registry was published of 30 patients with LS-SCLC treated concurrently with PBT to a median of 63.9 GyE (45–66.6) in 33–37 fractions (daily or twice-daily) [48]. At median follow-up of 14 months, the 1- and 2-year LC, recurrence-free survival, and OS were 85% and 69%, 63% and 42%, and 72% and 58%, respectively. High-grade toxicities were also limited, but not as low as observed with the University of Florida series, with grade 2 pneumonitis and esophagitis reported among 10% and 43% of patients, respectively, and grade 3+ toxicity rates less than 5%. Notably, one case of grade 4 esophagitis occurred in a patient receiving twice-daily PBT.

These clinical findings were consistent with IMRT plan comparisons, which demonstrated significant reductions in the cord, heart (V30, V45, and mean), and lung (V5 and mean) with PBT, but not with respect to esophagus mean or lung V20 [48]. Only a minority of treatments in this study

(13%) were delivered via IMPT, which would have yielded higher conformality over traditional passive scatter methods for bulky mediastinal disease near OARs (such as the esophagus). IMPT would have likely resulted in better toxicity outcomes than those observed in this historical series and should be included for legitimate and modern comparisons with IMRT, given the ubiquitous adoption of IMPT now across treatment centers [45].

17.2.4 Esophageal Cancer

The standard of care for locally advanced esophageal cancer is radiotherapy with concurrent chemotherapy (e.g., cisplatin/5-fluorouracil, carboplatin/paclitaxel, etc.) in either the definitive or pre-esophagectomy setting, with 3-year OS rates ranging from 30% to 60%. Given the central location of the esophagus proximal to critical thoracic structures, such as the heart and lungs, radiotherapy can result in clinically significant toxicities such as pneumonitis, pericarditis, and coronary artery disease. However, particle therapy could help minimize the collateral dose to these OARs and thus decrease the incidence of cardiopulmonary and other AEs (including surgical complications for trimodality patients), with initial dosimetric comparison studies demonstrating considerable reductions in dose to the lung [49] (mean reduced by 51% [50]), heart [49,51] (mean reduced by 41% [50]), and liver (Figure 17.4) [49].

As with many other indications and sites, treatment of esophageal cancer with PBT seems to have continuously improved with time and experience (Table 17.3). The first published clinical report with concurrent chemotherapy was an analysis of 62 patients treated to a median dose of 50.4 GyE on a MD Anderson prospective trial. Initial disease outcomes were quite encouraging with a median follow-up of 20.1 months, but the authors observed two grade 5 toxicities, conveying the potential for severe toxicities with this relatively novel radiotherapy modality [52]. Several years thereafter, a subsequent retrospective analysis by the same institution compared outcomes among 132 PBT patients versus 211 IMRT patients, with much more encouraging results. PBT was associated with significantly better OS and PFS, and no differences were observed in treatment-related toxicity [53]. PBT has since been reported as a safe treatment for elderly patients with esophageal cancer [54], and prospective registry studies have noted superiority in patient-reported health-related quality-of-life measures as compared to photon radiotherapy [55].

Most recently, these positive results were again supported by a randomized phase IIB trial comparing PBT to IMRT for treatment of locally advanced esophageal cancer to 50.4 Gy. A total of 145 patients were randomized, with 107 (61 IMRT vs. 46 PBT) available for analysis with a median follow-up of 44.1 months. The 3-year PFS and OS rates were similar

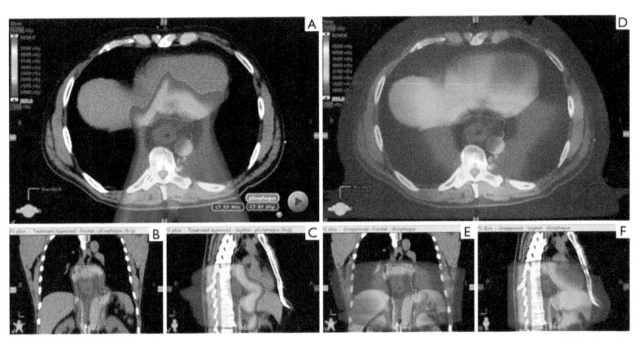

Figure 17.4 Comparison of intensity-modulated proton therapy versus photon radiotherapy for definitive treatment of distal esophageal adenocarcinoma. Note that target coverage is well preserved, but the proton beam plan benefits from relatively lower dose to the heart and lungs as compared to the photon plan *(reproduced from open access source)* [130].

among groups, at roughly 51% and 44.5%, respectively. However, PBT (80% of which was delivered via PSPT) significantly reduced the risk and severity of AEs as compared to IMRT [56]. This study underwent early closure upon activation of the ongoing NRG-GI006 randomized controlled trial, but the positive signal suggests that PBT is an effective treatment for esophageal cancer, with less toxicity as compared to photon radiotherapy.

Interestingly, PBT for combined chemoradiation has also been found to minimize the risk of severe lymphopenia, which is associated with immune suppression and poor prognosis in the setting of locally advanced thoracic malignancies. Since circulating lymphocytes are exquisitely sensitive to radiation exposure, even the low scattered doses from photon chemoradiation may result in lymphopenia. A propensity matched analysis of 480 PBT versus 136 photon patients treated with neoadjuvant chemoradiotherapy found a greater proportion of grade 4 lymphopenia among IMRT patients (40.4% vs. 17.6%), and PBT was associated with a significant risk reduction in grade 4 lymphopenia on multivariable analysis (OR 0.29) [57]. Another propensity matched retrospective analysis of 220 bimodality patients treated at MD Anderson also found treatment with IMRT to be associated with increased risk of grade 4 lymphopenia as compared to PBT (OR 2.13) [58].

Corroborating these findings, a separate report of patients treated with concurrent carboplatin/paclitaxel at the Mayo Clinic yielded similar results, with higher risk of grade 4 lymphopenia (56% vs. 22%) among 79 photon patients versus 65

PBT patients (all of whom were treated with pencil-beam scanning technique). The potential for PBT to minimize hematologic toxicities is further supported by dosimetric comparison studies, which demonstrate the high potential for bone marrow sparing [59]. Moreover, densely ionizing radiation is proposed to have additional immunobiological advantages secondary to distinct cell death pathways [60,61], with preliminary *in-vitro* studies indicating increased release of immune-stimulating inflammatory cytokines following heavy-ion exposure [62] and perhaps different timing of their release clinically [63].

CIRT is notably still under development for the management of esophageal cancer (Table 17.3). However, its utility was exemplified by an early phase I/II clinical trial of preoperative short-course treatment, enrolling 31 patients treated to doses escalating from 28.8 GyE up to 36.8 GyE, followed by surgery 4–8 weeks thereafter. Disease outcomes were encouraging with excellent LC, and the incidence of acute and/or late toxicity was <5%, suggesting that CIRT is also an effective neoadjuvant modality with the potential avoidance of severe events when utilized judiciously [64].

While prior studies have failed to demonstrate a benefit in LC or survival with dose-escalation, up to 75% of treatment failures following definitive chemoradiotherapy can occur within the intact target volume; therefore, questions remain regarding the potential utility of dose escalation in further enhancing disease control in the modern era. IMRT, for example, can facilitate dose escalation to the gross tumor without

Table 17.3 Selected published and anticipated studies of charged particle beam therapy in the definitive treatment of esophageal cancer [52,53,56,64,66–68,125]

Reference	Type	Indication	Modality	Chemo	N (#)	Prescription (median)	Follow-up (months)	Outcomes	Toxicity (non-heme)
Lin et al. [52]	Prospective	Definitive (53%) Pre-op (47%)	PSPT	Concurrent ± induction (42%)	62	50.4 GyE in 28 fxs	20	pCR 28% / 3-year OS 52% / 3-year LRC 57%	Grade 2 ≥ 37% / Grade 3 ≥ 10% / Grade 5 3% / *Drop-out 3%*
Xi et al. [53]	Retrospective	Definitive	PSPT (95%) IMPT (5%)	Concurrent ± induction (29%)	132	50.4 GyE in 28 fxs	45	5-year OS 42% / 5-year PFS 35% / 5-year LRC 60%	Grade 3 38% / Grade 5 1%
Lin et al. [56]	Phase IIB RCT	Definitive (54%) Pre-op (46%)	PSPT (80%) IMPT (20%)	Concurrent ± induction (7%)	46	50.4 GyE in 28 fxs	44	pCR 30% / 3-year PFS 45% / 3-year OS 51%	Grade 2–4 ≥ 11% / *Drop-out 4%*
Akutsu et al. [64]	Phase I/II	Neoadjuvant	CIRT	None	31	28.8–36.8 GyE in 8 fxs (hypo)	>36	*Drop-out 5%* / pCR 39% / 5-year PFS 62%	Grade 2 ≥ 39% *(acute)* / Grade 3 3% *(acute)*
Mizumoto et al. [66]	Retrospective	Definitive	Photon + PBT boost	None	19	78 GyE in 48 days	111	5-year OS 43% / 5-year LC 84%	Grade 2 ≥ 26% *(acute)* / Grade 3 ≥ 5% *(acute)* / ≥5% *(late)*
Fernandes et al. [67]	Prospective	Salvage re-radiotherapy (interval 32 months)	PSPT (93%) IMPT (7%)	Concurrent (79%)	14	54 GyE in 30 fxs (prior 54 Gy)	10	1-year OS 71% (median 13 mos) / *Drop-out 7%*	Grade 2 64% *(acute)* / ≥14% *(late)* / Grade 3 29% *(acute)* / ≥7% *(late)* / Grade 5 7% *(acute)* / 7% *(late)*
DeCesaris et al. [68]	Retrospective	Salvage re-radiotherapy (interval 38 months)	IMPT	Concurrent (89%) Induction (6%)	17	53.4 GyE in 29–30 fxs (prior 50 Gy)	12	1-year OS 69% (median 20 months) / 1-year LC 75% (median 22 months)	Grade 3 12% *(acute)* / 11% *(late)* / Grade 4 12% *(late)* / Grade 5 7% *(late)*
NRG GI006 [125]	Phase III RCT	Definitive and neoadjuvant	PBT	Concurrent	300 *(estimate)*	50.4 GyE in 28 fxs	Enrolling	OS *(coprimary)*	Grade 3+ cardiopulm AEs *(coprimary)*

necessitating an increase in normal tissue dose via simultaneous integrated boost (SIB) technique [65]. Moreover, due to its physical properties, particle therapy may permit even further dose escalation safely without significantly increasing toxicity. A recent Japanese study evaluated the safety of hyperfractionated concomitant boost via PBT among 19 esophageal cancer patients treated to a median dose of 78 GyE (ranging up to 83 GyE) in less than 7 weeks. The response rate was an impressive 100% (89% complete), with 5-year LC and OS rates of 84% and 43%, respectively. Only two grade 3 esophageal toxicities were noted (one acute and one late), with otherwise no hematologic, pulmonary, or cardiac events noted; and there were no treatment interruptions [66].

Extrapolating from this concept, particle therapy may improve the feasibility of re-irradiation for LRR esophageal cancers, even potentially for those in-field, albeit with inherent risks (Table 17.3). University of Pennsylvania investigators conducted a prospective clinical trial of PBT re-irradiation for esophageal cancers, treating 14 patients to a median dose of 54 GyE (cumulative 110 GyE), frequently with concurrent chemotherapy, at a median interval of 32 months from the initial radiotherapy course. At 10 months of follow-up, two grade 5 toxicities were observed (one acute esophagopleural fistula and one late esophageal ulcer), along with several grade 3 toxicities. The median OS and time to local failure were 13 months and 10 months, respectively [67]. More recently, University of Maryland researchers published a series of 17 patients with esophageal and gastroesophageal junction cancers re-irradiated with IMPT technique. At a median follow-up of 11.6 months, 1-year LC and OS were 75% and 69%, respectively; the incidence of grade 3+ late toxicities was 28% [68]. Taken together, these studies indicate that esophageal re-irradiation is feasible with PBT, although the risk of severe toxicity is non-negligible, and patients should be counseled accordingly. At the same time, particle therapy offers a potential modality for this high-risk population with limited management options, many of whom would not have been treatable with conventional IMRT plans [68].

As a final note, it should be mentioned that organ and target motion pose a major challenge in particle treatment planning, with range deviations reported to reduce target coverage [50] considerably on 4D-CT plans (V95 range 50–95%) [69] and even magnify dose to critical structures during the breathing cycle (e.g., up to 3.5× higher maximum spinal cord dose) [69]. Thus, as with lung cancer, individual 4D-robustness optimization is recommended to ensure adequate target coverage by accounting for the potential impact of intrafractional dose deviations, particularly from respiratory and diaphragmatic motion during free breathing [70].

17.2.5 Thymic Cancers

Despite the relatively limited indications for radiotherapy in thymic malignancies, they represent the most common primary tumors of the anterior mediastinum. Patients can also present at young ages and experience long-term survivorship following treatment (and thus longer intervals to encounter late effects). Therefore, if radiotherapy is indicated, particle therapy may offer benefit with respect to late complications of the heart, lungs, esophagus, and breast (particularly with respect to secondary malignancies).

Most studies have again involved planning comparisons of PBT versus IMRT, demonstrating significant dose reductions to critical structures (with consistent reductions in irradiated volumes and/or mean doses to the lung, esophagus, and heart) without compromising target volume coverage [71–73]. One analysis noted average reductions of 36.5%, 33.5%, and 60% in mean dose to the heart, lungs, and esophagus, respectively [74]. In particular, a substantial reduction of the risk of cardiac failure and secondary cancer development has been hypothesized with robust PBT planning techniques [75], hypothetically translating to an estimated 5 excess secondary malignancies avoided per 100 patients treated with PBT (for patients diagnosed at the median age) [72]. Similar benefits with respect to OAR sparing have also been simulated for carbon-ion therapy [73].

These dosimetric advantages are expected to reduce toxicity; however, their actual clinical significance warrants further investigation. To this end, there have been a handful of clinical series on thymic patients treated with adjuvant and/or definitive PBT, though limited with respect to patient numbers and follow-up periods (ranging from 5.5 months [71] to 2.6 years [74]). Nevertheless, these studies have collectively reported outcomes comparable to historical data and very few radiation-induced acute toxicities following median doses of 54–61.2 GyE, with no mention of grade ≥3 toxicities for *de-novo* disease [71,74,76,77]. The most relevant acute grade 2 toxicity appeared to be dermatitis, reported as high as 37% among one of the larger cohorts treated at the University of Pennsylvania [76,77]. Longer follow-up with larger study populations will help confirm these findings and further elucidate the role particle therapy for thymic cancers.

17.2.6 Mesothelioma

Malignant pleural mesothelioma (MPM) is a cancer of the pleural cavity that typically presents at an advanced stage. Multidisciplinary management of these cases remains a challenge but select cases may benefit from hemithoracic irradiation of the entire affected pleura for potential enhancement of locoregional control, most commonly following macroscopic resection (either extrapleural pneumonectomy or pleurectomy/decortication). As such, the circumferential target volumes are large and complex, abutting several critical organs which limit the ability to safely deliver definitive doses. However, particle therapy has the potential to overcome these geometric challenges and minimize the collateral dose to proximal organs (and hence influence the treatment-related morbidity) during hemithoracic irradiation.

Indeed, dosimetric comparison studies of adjuvant PBT versus IMRT plans indicate superior OAR sparing with PBT [78,79], mainly for the liver (with mean dose reductions of 9.5 Gy [78] or by more than 50%), ipsilateral kidney (with V20 Gy reductions of 50–60% [78]), and contralateral lung (limiting mean dose to <1.5 Gy and V5 Gy to <10%) [80], along with benefits noted for the contralateral kidney [78,79], spinal cord [79], esophagus [78], and heart (with mean doses decreased by ≥50%) [80], as compared with standard IMRT. These studies also indicate improvements in target coverage, dose conformity, and dose homogeneity with PBT [78,79]; and the application of normal tissue complication probability (NTCP) models in one analysis translated to hypothetical reductions in radiation-induced liver disease, kidney injury, and acute esophagitis [78].

Admittedly, clinical experiences have been limited to small single institution series but have thus far corroborated these dosimetric predictions with respect to feasibility and safety. One of the earliest series by MD Anderson compared their experience of 4 IMPT patients with 3 IMRT patients treated for lung-intact MPM [81], demonstrating lower mean doses to the contralateral lung, heart, esophagus, liver, and ipsilateral kidney, with superior contralateral lung sparing in the setting of mediastinal nodal boost. Clinically, all patients receiving IMPT fared well without treatment breaks, and daily treatment time was under an hour (half setup; half delivery) for patients [81]. Supporting these findings, the University of Maryland reported a larger series of 10 patients treated via PBT to a median total dose of 55 GyE following extended pleurectomy/decortication. All patients received chemotherapy, and treatment was again well tolerated, with no patient experiencing grade ≥2 toxicity. Two-year LC was 90%, with distant and regional failure rates of 50% and 30%, respectively. Median survival was 19.5 months, and 1- and 2-year OS rates were 58% and 29% [82].

When prescribing PBT for MPM, close attention must be paid to range uncertainty, organ motion, anatomical changes, beam path tissue heterogeneity, and limitations in image guidance, all of which pose challenges to optimal irradiation with PBT. At least two separate treatment fields should be utilized; and given the complex and irregular hemithoracic target, IMPT may be the optimal technique, delivered via opposed (AP/PA) or slightly oblique beam arrangement. Multi-field optimization should be exercised to maximally spare normal tissues, and plan robustness (for dose perturbances from isocenter offsets, range variations, etc.) should be evaluated for all plans.

While there have not been any clinical studies of carbon-ion therapy conducted in MPM, emerging *in-vitro* data suggest that these particle beams are effective against mesothelioma cells and serve as a potential solution to further optimize LRC [83,84]. With respect to charged particle therapy in general, further outcome data are necessary before routine adoption in patient care.

17.3 Practical Considerations

17.3.1 Patient Selection: Clinical Characteristics, Safety, and Toxicity

The inherent heterogeneity within each specific type of thoracic neoplasm discussed above necessitates questions regarding whether all such patients would benefit to the same degree from particle therapy. Numerous variables contributing to this heterogeneity will be further explored, recognizing that carefully and judiciously selecting patients for particle therapy can better address the fine line between dosimetric advantages and economic burden. Because particle therapy has been touted to benefit patients largely by means of toxicity reduction (rather than LC- and/or survival-related end points), a logical starting point to optimizing patient selection begins with an evaluation of which patients are most likely to experience treatment-related toxicities.

The most notable variables associated with the likelihood of developing severe AEs are dosimetric factors, which in turn often depend on the location and/or extent of disease with respect to OARs. Owing to the unique physical properties of particle therapy modalities (e.g., rapid dose falloff), particle therapy may provide the greatest proportional benefit when compared to IMRT in "dosimetrically high-risk" patients. Although this term does not have an objective definition, it often refers to disease closely abutting any number of OARs—especially the esophagus, lung, and heart, which are the three main OARs contributing to the vast majority of intrathoracic AEs.

The risk for severe esophageal AEs correlates with dosimetric factors (e.g., mean dose or maximum point dose), which in turn relates to the volume of disease in closer proximity to the esophagus [85]. Hence, lung cancer cases with increasing levels of esophageal-abutting primary and/or nodal disease (or both) may benefit to a greater degree from particle therapy. Similarly, pulmonary toxicity is exquisitely sensitive to the overall volume of disease [86,87]; this can be mathematically explained (assuming that the volume of a thoracic neoplasm is spheroid or ovoid) by the volume of irradiated lung being very sensitive to small incremental increases in tumor diameter. Thus, larger tumors (resulting in greater irradiated volumes of normal lung) are also expected to proportionally benefit to a greater degree from particle therapy.

Lastly, cardiac toxicity is just beginning to be explored as a means of both radiation-induced AEs as well as potentially impacting survival [88]. Given that thoracic tumors are associated with higher cardiac dose than other anatomical sites (with associated risk of severe cardiac events, especially among patients with preexisting cardiac disease) [89], it is reasonable to surmise that these cases may benefit from particle therapy-mediated cardiac dose reduction. Additionally, the emerging notion of lymphopenia caused by low-dose radiation may also impact outcomes, since lymphocytes are needed to mount an antitumoral immune response [90]. Although particle therapy reduces the volumes of heart or lung receiving low-dose radiation, it is currently unknown which patients benefit most from a reduction in low-dose radiation (e.g., those with higher baseline lymphocyte counts, or irrespective of baseline lymphocyte counts).

There are several other factors associated with the propensity to develop any of the aforementioned AEs. For instance, studies have correlated smoking status with the risk of radiation pneumonitis [91], pretherapy dysphagia to radiation esophagitis [85], and preexisting cardiac disease with radiation-induced cardiotoxicity [92]. These factors should be taken into account independently of dosimetric factors when evaluating a patient's proportional benefit from particle therapy. Modeling studies encompassing these, as well as volumetric anatomical factors, have been proposed as a means to better perform patient selection for particle therapy in lung cancers [92,93] but require further validation.

In addition to these variables, age and/or performance status have been associated with the risk of developing many types of radiation-induced AEs [94,95]. It has been a relatively longstanding belief that younger patients may benefit to a greater degree from particle therapy (given that age is a powerful risk factor for survival) because the putative toxicity-reducing effects of particle therapy may not be actualized in older patients owing to the lack of longer term survival. However, the first completed randomized trial showing a benefit to PBT over IMRT, performed in esophageal cancer patients, has taken a major step toward challenging this notion [56]. This trial comprised a relatively older population (median age 69), and the PBT arm had a statistically greater proportion of patients with poorer performance status. Yet, patients who received PBT experienced fewer and less severe AEs, which were largely driven by a reduction in postoperative complications in the trimodality patients. This implies that, despite the aforementioned dogma, older patients have a substantial proclivity to develop treatment-related AEs, which can be effectively addressed by particle therapy. Hence, this finding underscores that patient selection for particle therapy should ideally be measured based on the baseline risk of developing AEs (both acute and late), which should supersede singular factors such as age and performance status.

Taken together, it is acknowledged that—similar to any oncologic intervention—there are patients who will benefit from particle therapy to a greater extent than others. These notions regarding optimizing patient selection for particle therapy are essential in order to ensure adequate reduction in treatment-related AEs yet maintain cost-effective care.

17.3.2 Technical Aspects: Planning and Delivery

Although the unique physical properties of heavy particles lead to high target conformity and very low (or no) exit dose, these factors also give rise to unique technical challenges regarding the fidelity and accuracy of adequate dose delivery. Although a complete discussion of these issues is beyond the scope of this chapter, a few challenges in the context of thoracic cancers will be discussed herein. These will be subdivided into factors specific to the treatment planning process, along with patient-specific (including anatomic) factors. Guidelines for the delineation of target volumes are described in Table 17.4.

There are numerous inaccuracies associated with the treatment planning process for particle therapy, which result in range uncertainties. Dose calculations for treatment planning rely on the imperfect process of converting Hounsfield units on the planning CT scan into stopping power values. Inaccuracies in this conversion can be caused by a variety of sources including the presence of CT artifacts, uncertainties in beam profiles (including beam hardening), estimation of the radiologic thickness of compensator/bolus material, and background CT "noise." Additionally, dose calculation algorithms can independently cause range uncertainties; for instance, some dose calculation platforms such as the pencil-beam algorithm can be less accurate for certain beam angles (e.g., those oblique to the patient surface), a fact that is the most pronounced in the thorax as opposed to other anatomic areas [96,97]. Because few areas of the body are associated with as marked differences in tissue densities as the thorax, range uncertainties can directly result in spatially inaccurate dose information, tumor misdosing, and/or OAR overdosing (especially with IMPT plans) [98]. These limitations are often remedied by utilizing high-quality onboard imaging (discussed subsequently), Monte Carlo algorithms for dose calculation, the use of additional target margins to account for uncertainties, and/or prudent selection of beam angles (such as selecting a greater number of adequately robust beam angles).

Anatomic factors associated with the thorax can result in unique sources of technical errors. For instance, respiratory motion can result in spatial inaccuracies. This is especially true if scanning beams are used, which do not uniformly treat the target, but rather in a piecemeal fashion (e.g., voxel by voxel with IMPT). The presence of an additional variable, respiration-associated target motion, can cause a portion of the target to be over- or underdosed. This stems from an interaction between two "moving parts": respiration-associated tumor movement and the dynamic movement of a beam over the target volume, a phenomenon is known as the interplay effect. Although a potentially serious issue, there are several proposed methods with which to mitigate its occurrence. These include patient selection strategies—as larger tumors, relatively small respiratory amplitudes, and/or more regular breathing patterns are associated with attenuation of the interplay effect, preferential delivery of scanning beams for these cases may be relatively more advantageous [99]. Technical strategies include increasing the spot size of an IMPT beam [100] and spreading out the delivered dose by means of multiple rounds of scanning (termed re-scanning) [101]. Respiratory motion management strategies such as breathhold [102] or gated [103] beam delivery are also essential, along with the use of four-dimensional imaging-based robust optimization, which incorporates the motion, shape, and position of both the target and pertinent OARs into the beam-specific optimization algorithm [104–106].

Lastly, interfractional anatomic changes in the thorax have the potential to cause large dose differences given the large tissue density differences within the thorax. Interfractional anatomic changes can occur from a variety of sources, such as patient-related (e.g., organ filling, fluid/air build-up) and disease-related (e.g., tumor shrinkage) factors. In order to address these challenges, volumetric onboard imaging to guide the delivery of particle therapy is becoming increasingly mandatory. Whereas the initial generation of particle therapy facilities utilized two-dimensional image guidance (e.g., orthogonal X-rays), the most modern centers most often utilize three-dimensional imaging (e.g., cone-beam computed tomography). It may be argued that the lack of contemporary high-quality image guidance can in itself be a deterrent to receiving particle therapy [107]. The presence of contemporary volumetric image-guided approaches can best allow for adaptive planning, a method which involves constructing an "updated" treatment plan based on anatomical changes, in efforts to improve OAR doses and/or target coverage [108]. The frequency of required adaptive planning depends on the particular type of thoracic neoplasm, along with a clinician-defined (subjective) willingness to do so. Some publications have reported relatively lower instances of requiring adaptive planning [48], whereas others have implemented it in the majority of patients [109]. Nevertheless, this method remains an important tool to address the unique challenges of interfractional changes, not limited to thoracic cancers or even particle therapy.

In summary, several factors—related to both the treatment planning process as well as anatomic issues specific to the thorax—present unique challenges for the delivery of particle therapy. In practice, strong coordination between clinicians, physicists, and dosimetrists are required to thoroughly address these limitations while being cognizant of the additional time and resources required to execute these processes. In the modern era of particle therapy, the increasing availability of technology to address these limitations has allowed for an expansion in the use of particle therapy.

17.3.3 Economic Factors and Operational Sustainability

Despite the potential benefits associated with particle therapy, a large gap remains between the number of patients who receive PBT versus the number who could potentially benefit or enroll in research trials. Insurance authorization, while a critical component of the United States health-care system, persists as a resource-intensive barrier to patient access. Shedding light on this issue, an investigation of 903 patients (553 with thoracic cancers) who entered the prior authorization process for PBT revealed denial rates as high as 70% with managed care (private) payors [110]. Most of these patients were subsequently overturned, but the appeal process was associated with significant time delays of 3 weeks to final decision. Such delays are particularly relevant to cancer patients, for whom interrupted treatments can result in poor outcomes. And while third-party payors deny coverage due to lack of level 1 evidence, the very trials necessary to generate data cannot accrue due to coverage denials [107,111].

To better address such obstacles for patients, treatment centers can integrate business solutions to help streamline navigation through the multilayered authorization steps [112]. These payor-focused operational strategies can improve patient access while decreasing time and administrative burden, at least in the short term. However, United States health care is a complex adaptive system with multiple stakeholders dynamically evolving in response to another's actions. Thus, the key for sustainability is increased transparency and collaboration among stakeholders to promote timely patient care and research. In the context of particle therapy, the justification for restrictive coverage policies is rooted in payor concerns regarding cost and utilization. Particle therapy is admittedly more expensive up-front, due to higher unit-related technological expenses as compared to photon radiotherapy.

However, objective evidence-based coverage policies can help ensure appropriate patient selection, and the actual impact of particle therapy on payor reimbursement can dramatically differ from model cost estimates. For example, our proton therapy center collaborated directly with stakeholders on an insurance coverage pilot, ensuring pre-authorized coverage of PBT in prospective trials and evidence-supported anatomical sites for nearly 200,000 plan enrollees. This entailed a comprehensive cost-of-care analysis evaluating total medical charges among case-matched PBT versus IMRT patients, demonstrating no significant differences with respect to average medical costs [113]—a surprising result (among a prospective clinical cohort) which diverged significantly from anticipated cost estimates. At three years of follow-up, this coverage pilot demonstrated that appropriate access to particle therapy does not necessitate overutilization or significantly increased comprehensive medical costs. Stakeholder collaboration to develop objective, transparent medical policies up-front (with clinician input) can streamline patient access to care while reducing administrative burden for all parties.

With respect to upfront investment and operational expenses, technological advancements have actually resulted in dramatic cost reductions associated with PBT equipment over time [114,115]. The industrial-sized centers of the prior era have slowly transitioned toward smaller compact units that are readily incorporable within existing real estate and associated with significantly less capital investment cost: from $100–250 million down to $25–30 million per new treatment facility [114,116,117]. These same innovations have also been accompanied by improvements in plan robustness [118] and delivery efficiency [119], which further decrease the threshold for operational sustainability [114,116,117], leading to greater provider adoption and patient access.

On a final note, current costing methodologies have overlooked the full benefits associated with particle therapy utilization. While associated with higher upfront costs, particle therapy has the potential of superior long-term value over time, due to fewer toxicities and decreased costs over a full cycle of care (including posttreatment follow-up) [120]. In addition to the direct costs of care (e.g., medical and pharmaceutical expenses), there are indirect costs with respect to patient disability and productivity [121], for which particle therapy also offers benefit. Only longer follow-up can define the full extent of these direct and indirect cost advantages associated with particle therapy utilization. Furthermore, most cost analyses fail to take quality-of-life data into account, which often favors particle therapy [122]. Taking all these factors into consideration, along with the positive changes in contemporary cost figures, will certainly enhance the value of particle therapy relative to historical cost-effectiveness models and support its sustainability as a treatment modality moving forward.

17.4 Future Directions: Research Areas under Active Investigation

Similar to the case for many other disease sites, particle therapy for thoracic malignancies remains in its infancy. Although to date there are no randomized trials of particle therapy versus photon radiotherapy for oligometastatic disease, SCLC, re-

irradiation, and thymoma, this section will discuss the immediate forefront of future discovery: the currently accruing phase III trials for locally advanced NSCLC, esophageal cancer, and mesothelioma.

The RTOG 1308 trial (NCT01993810) [123] is randomizing patients with unresected stage II-IIIB NSCLC to IMRT versus PBT. Both arms utilize a prescription dose up to 70 Gy and are delivered with concurrent chemotherapy (along with adjuvant durvalumab following a protocol amendment). This trial is nearing accrual and has primary end points of OS as well as cardiotoxicity/lymphopenia.

An analogous partially randomized phase I/II trial is also ongoing at MD Anderson but specifies IMPT utilization along with a SIB component (NCT01629498) [124]. Prescription doses are as high as 78 Gy to the GTV (maintaining 60 Gy to the surrounding CTV), conventionally delivered in 30 daily fractions over 6 weeks with concurrent weekly chemotherapy. Primary end points also differ from RTOG 1308, instead focusing on CTCAE-defined grade 3+ toxicity and local PFS (to evaluate the effect of SIB on tumor control). Both trials are important steps necessary to understand the role of PBT in a general (unselected) locally advanced NSCLC population.

The recently launched NRG GI006 trial (NCT03801876) [125] is evaluating the PBT versus IMRT question in esophageal cancer (comprising both the definitive and trimodality populations). This trial is built on the aforementioned promising phase IIB randomized data for esophageal cancer showing a reduction in total toxicity burden (a quantitative amalgamation of 11 AEs) but no preliminary differences in OS. The primary end points are OS and CTCAE-defined grade 3+ cardiopulmonary AEs.

The NRG LU006 trial (NCT04158141) [126], also recently activated, is addressing a broader question in mesothelioma regarding the controversial utility of postoperative radiotherapy. Both IMRT and PBT are allowed for this study; although the trial is not powered for a separate comparison of either modality, analyzing outcomes and toxicities by modality will provide much-needed prospective data on the safety and efficacy of PBT for mesothelioma.

There are several noteworthy aspects regarding each of the aforementioned randomized trials. First, only one trial has made a prespecified stratification for IMPT, and given its dosimetric superiority compared to PSPT, the utility of IMPT for these neoplasms will remain unaddressed even following publications of these trials. The vast majority of patients on RTOG 1308 [123] received PSPT, whereas the other contemporary trials are expected to enroll a higher proportion of IMPT cases. Second, subgroup analyses (planned or unplanned) from these trials will be critical to optimize patient selection for PBT, and for this purpose, these trials should ideally collect an array of anatomic and/

Table 17.4 Example target volumes and prescription doses for treatment of thoracic malignancies with proton beam radiotherapy. Note that all contours (iGTV, iCTV) should account for full respiratory cycle motion via 4D-CT Simulation, utilizing either the maximal intensity projection (MIP) image set for free-breathing treatments or encompassing motion among several (≥3) breath-hold image sets for respiratory gating

Indication	Target volumes	Prescription (RBE)
Locally advanced NSCLC [9,11]	iGTV: primary tumor and involved regional lymphatics (via CT, PET/CT, and EBUS) iCTV: above plus 6–10 mm anatomically-tailored margin for microscopic extension	60–74 GyE in 30–37 fxs
Postoperative NSCLC[10]	iGTV: gross residual disease on post-operative restaging imaging (if indicated) iCTV: initial sites of disease, including bronchial stump, ipsilateral hilum, involved nodal stations (per path report), and mediastinal pleura adjacent to surgical bed	R0: 50–54 GyE in 25–30 fxs R1: 54–60 GyE in 27–30 fxs R2: 60–70 GyE in 30–35 fxs
Limited stage SCLC [47,48]	iGTV: primary tumor and involved regional nodal disease (no elective coverage) iCTV: above plus 6–10 mm anatomically tailored margin for microscopic extension	45 GyE in 30 fxs (BID) or 66–70 GyE in 30–35 fxs (QD)
Thymic malignancies [71,73–77]	iGTV: gross disease (on postoperative or post-induction imaging as appropriate) iCTV: surgical bed/clips (encompassing entire preoperative tumor extent) and/or iGTV plus 6–20 mm anatomically tailored margin (e.g., for definitive cases) + entire thymus if not already incorporated (e.g., definitive case or partial resection)	R0: 45–50.4 GyE in 25–28 fxs R1: 54–60 GyE in 27–30 fxs R2/Definitive:60–70 GyE in 30–35 fxs
Locoregionally recurrent lung cancer [36,39]	iGTV: active gross disease (aided by FDG-avidity on fused restaging PET/CT) iCTV: above plus 5–8 mm anatomically tailored margin for microscopic extension	60–66 GyE in 30–33 fxs (with concurrent chemo) or hypo-frac 45–52.5 GyE in 15 fxs (for radiotherapy alone)
Esophageal cancer [56,125]	iGTV: primary tumor and involved regional lymphatics (via PET/CT and EGD/EUS) iCTV: primary tumor with 10–15 mm radial and 3–4 cm craniocaudal expansion along length of esophagus and cardia + involved lymph nodes with 5–15 mm radial margin + elective nodal coverage depending on primary location, if node-positive status (e.g., celiac for distal and GEJ tumors, or supraclavicular for upper thoracic tumors)	50–50.4 GyE in 25–28 fxs
Malignant pleural mesothelioma [80,81]	iGTV: gross residual disease on post-operative restaging imaging iCTV: entire hemithoracic external pleural surface, encompassing 5-mm rind from lung apex/thoracic inlet down through diaphragm insertion posteriorly (T1 to T12-L2) + involved nodal stations (no elective regional coverage recommended) + surgical clips/incisions and procedural tracks as appropriate	iGTV: 60–66 GyE (boost) iCTV: 45–54 GyE in 25–30 fxs

or dosimetric information (e.g., the size of tumor volumes). Third, evaluation of non-OS end points from these trials will also be essential given that the rate of treatment-related deaths is generally quite low for each neoplasm, which affords PBT little room for OS improvement. As such, AE reduction parameters and quality-of-life metrics should be considered considerably more important when evaluating the utility PBT for these neoplasms. Fourth, as none of these trials encompass other heavy particles such as carbon ions,

their evidence-based utility for these malignancies remains relatively scant.

The expansion of particle therapy for thoracic cancers is expected to substantially continue over the coming years. The eventual publication of randomized data, as well as the launch of additional trial concepts, will undoubtedly influence the rate of this expansion, as well as better address the unique advantages and pitfalls of particle therapy for a heterogeneous variety of thoracic malignancies.

References

1 Anderle, K., Stroom, J., Pimentel, N., Greco, C., Durante, M., and Graeff, C. (2016). In silico comparison of photons versus carbon ions in single fraction therapy of lung cancer. *Medical Physics* 32 (9): 1118–1123. doi:10.1016/j.ejmp.2016.08.014.

2 Berman, A.T., Teo, B.-K.-K., Dolney, D., et al. (2013). An in-silico comparison of proton beam and IMRT for postoperative radiotherapy in completely resected stage IIIA non-small cell lung cancer. *Radiation Oncology* 8: 144. doi:10.1186/1748-717X-8-144.

3 Hoppe, B.S., Huh, S., Flampouri, S., et al. (2010). Double-scattered proton-based stereotactic body radiotherapy for

stage I lung cancer: A dosimetric comparison with photon-based stereotactic body radiotherapy. *Radiotherapy and Oncology : Journal of the European Society for Therapeutic Radiology and Oncology* 97 (3): 425–430. doi:10.1016/j.radonc.2010.09.006.

4 Vogelius, I.R., Westerly, D.C., Aznar, M.C., et al. (2011). Estimated radiation pneumonitis risk after photon versus proton therapy alone or combined with chemotherapy for lung cancer. *Acta Oncologica* 50 (6): 772–776. doi:10.3109/0284186X.2011.582519.

5 Wang, X.S., Shi, Q., Williams, L.A., et al. (2016). Prospective study of patient-reported symptom burden in patients with non-small-cell lung cancer undergoing proton or photon chemoradiation therapy. *Journal of Pain and Symptom Management* 51 (5): 832–838. doi:10.1016/j.jpainsymman.2015.12.316.

6 Bush, D.A., Cheek, G., Zaheer, S., et al. (2013). High-dose hypofractionated proton beam radiation therapy is safe and effective for central and peripheral early-stage non-small cell lung cancer: Results of a 12-year experience at Loma Linda University Medical Center. *International Journal of Radiation Oncology, Biology, Physics* 86 (5): 964–968. doi:10.1016/j.ijrobp.2013.05.002.

7 Ohnishi, K., Nakamura, N., Harada, H., et al. (2020). Proton beam therapy for histologically or clinically diagnosed stage I non-small cell lung cancer (NSCLC): The first nationwide retrospective study in Japan. *International Journal of Radiation Oncology, Biology, Physics* 106 (1): 82–89. doi:10.1016/j.ijrobp.2019.09.013.

8 Chang, J.Y., Zhang, W., Komaki, R., et al. (2017). Long-term outcome of phase I/II prospective study of dose-escalated proton therapy for early-stage non-small cell lung cancer. *Radiotherapy and Oncology : Journal of the European Society for Therapeutic Radiology and Oncology* 122 (2): 274–280. doi:10.1016/j.radonc.2016.10.022.

9 Chang, J.Y., Verma, V., Li, M., et al. (2017). Proton beam radiotherapy and concurrent chemotherapy for unresectable stage III non-small cell lung cancer: Final results of a phase 2 study. *JAMA Oncology* 3 (8): e172032. doi:10.1001/jamaoncol.2017.2032.

10 Remick, J.S., Schonewolf, C., Gabriel, P., et al. (2017). First clinical report of proton beam therapy for postoperative radiotherapy for non-small-cell lung cancer. *Clinical Lung Cancer* 18 (4): 364–371. doi:10.1016/j.cllc.2016.12.009.

11 Liao, Z., Lee, J.J., Komaki, R., et al. (2018). Bayesian adaptive randomization trial of passive scattering proton therapy and intensity-modulated photon radiotherapy for locally advanced non-small-cell lung cancer. *Journal of Clinical Oncology : Official Journal of the American Society of Clinical Oncology* 36 (18): 1813–1822. doi:10.1200/JCO.2017.74.0720.

12 Register, S.P., Zhang, X., Mohan, R., and Chang, J.Y. (2011). Proton stereotactic body radiation therapy for clinically challenging cases of centrally and superiorly located stage I non-small-cell lung cancer. *International Journal of Radiation Oncology, Biology, Physics* 80 (4): 1015–1022. doi:10.1016/j.ijrobp.2010.03.012.

13 Zhu, Z., Liu, W., Gillin, M., et al. (2014). Assessing the robustness of passive scattering proton therapy with regard to local recurrence in stage III non-small cell lung cancer: A secondary analysis of a phase II trial. *Radiation Oncology* 9: 108. doi:10.1186/1748-717X-9-108.

14 Klein, C., Dokic, I., Mairani, A., et al. (2017). Overcoming hypoxia-induced tumor radioresistance in non-small cell lung cancer by targeting DNA-dependent protein kinase in combination with carbon ion irradiation. *Radiation Oncology* 12 (1): 208. doi:10.1186/s13014-017-0939-0.

15 Wink, K.C.J., Roelofs, E., Simone, C.B., et al. (2018). Photons, protons or carbon ions for stage I non-small cell lung cancer—Results of the multicentric ROCOCO in silico study. *Radiotherapy and Oncology : Journal of the European Society for Therapeutic Radiology and Oncology* 128 (1): 139–146. doi:10.1016/j.radonc.2018.02.024.

16 Kubo, N., Saitoh, J.-I., Shimada, H., et al. (2016). Dosimetric comparison of carbon ion and X-ray radiotherapy for Stage IIIA non-small cell lung cancer. *Journal of Radiation Research* 57 (5): 548–554. doi:10.1093/jrr/rrw041.

17 Nakajima, M., Yamamoto, N., Hayashi, K., et al. (2017). Carbon-ion radiotherapy for non-small cell lung cancer with interstitial lung disease: A retrospective analysis. *Radiation Oncology* 12 (1): 144. doi:10.1186/s13014-017-0881-1.

18 Saitoh, J.-I., Shirai, K., Mizukami, T., et al. (2019). Hypofractionated carbon-ion radiotherapy for stage I peripheral nonsmall cell lung cancer (GUNMA0701): Prospective phase II study. *Cancer Medicine* 8 (15): 6644–6650. doi:10.1002/cam4.2561.

19 Karube, M., Yamamoto, N., Nakajima, M., et al. (2016). Single-fraction carbon-ion radiation therapy for patients 80 years of age and older with stage I non-small cell lung cancer. *International Journal of Radiation Oncology, Biology, Physics* 95 (1): 542–548. doi:10.1016/j.ijrobp.2015.11.034.

20 Takahashi, W., Nakajima, M., Yamamoto, N., et al. (2015). A prospective nonrandomized phase I/II study of carbon ion radiotherapy in a favorable subset of locally advanced non-small cell lung cancer (NSCLC). *Cancer* 121 (8): 1321–1327. doi:10.1002/cncr.29195.

21 Karube, M., Yamamoto, N., Shioyama, Y., et al. (2017). Carbon-ion radiotherapy for patients with advanced stage non-small-cell lung cancer at multicenters. *Journal of Radiation Research* 58 (5): 761–764. doi:10.1093/jrr/rrx037.

22 Hayashi, K., Yamamoto, N., Nakajima, M., et al. (2019). Clinical outcomes of carbon-ion radiotherapy for locally advanced non-small-cell lung cancer. *Cancer Science* 110 (2): 734–741. doi:10.1111/cas.13890.

23 Anzai, M., Yamamoto, N., Hayashi, K., et al. (2020). Safety and efficacy of carbon-ion radiotherapy alone for stage III

non-small cell lung cancer. *Anticancer Research* 40 (1): 379–386. doi:10.21873/anticanres.13963.

24 Hayashi, K., Yamamoto, N., Karube, M., et al. (2017). Prognostic analysis of radiation pneumonitis: Carbon-ion radiotherapy in patients with locally advanced lung cancer. *Radiation Oncology* 12 (1): 91. doi:10.1186/s13014-017-0830-z.

25 Mori, S., Furukawa, T., Inaniwa, T., et al. (2013). Systematic evaluation of four-dimensional hybrid depth scanning for carbon-ion lung therapy. *Medical Physics* 40 (3): 031720. doi:10.1118/1.4792295.

26 Stuschke, M., Kaiser, A., Pöttgen, C., Lübcke, W., and Farr, J. (2012). Potentials of robust intensity modulated scanning proton plans for locally advanced lung cancer in comparison to intensity modulated photon plans. *Radiotherapy and Oncology : Journal of the European Society for Therapeutic Radiology and Oncology* 104 (1): 45–51. doi:10.1016/j.radonc.2012.03.017.

27 Graeff, C. (2017). Robustness of 4D-optimized scanned carbon ion beam therapy against interfractional changes in lung cancer. *Radiotherapy and Oncology : Journal of the European Society for Therapeutic Radiology and Oncology* 122 (3): 387–392. doi:10.1016/j.radonc.2016.12.017.

28 Liu, W., Schild, S.E., Chang, J.Y., et al. (2016). Exploratory study of 4D versus 3D robust optimization in intensity modulated proton therapy for lung cancer. *International Journal of Radiation Oncology, Biology, Physics* 95 (1): 523–533. doi:10.1016/j.ijrobp.2015.11.002.

29 Taylor, P.A., Kry, S.F., and Followill, D.S. (2017). Pencil beam algorithms are unsuitable for proton dose calculations in lung. *International Journal of Radiation Oncology, Biology, Physics* 99 (3): 750–756. doi:10.1016/j.ijrobp.2017.06.003.

30 Grassberger, C., Daartz, J., Dowdell, S., Ruggieri, T., Sharp, G., and Paganetti, H. (2014). Quantification of proton dose calculation accuracy in the lung. *International Journal of Radiation Oncology, Biology, Physics* 89 (2): 424–430. doi:10.1016/j.ijrobp.2014.02.023.

31 Sakai, M., Kubota, Y., Saitoh, J.-I., et al. (2018). Robustness of patient positioning for interfractional error in carbon ion radiotherapy for stage I lung cancer: Bone matching versus tumor matching. *Radiotherapy and Oncology : Journal of the European Society for Therapeutic Radiology and Oncology* 129 (1): 95–100. doi:10.1016/j.radonc.2017.10.003.

32 Li, Y., Kubota, Y., Kubo, N., et al. (2020). Dose assessment for patients with stage I non-small cell lung cancer receiving passive scattering carbon-ion radiotherapy using daily computed tomographic images: A prospective study. *Radiotherapy and Oncology : Journal of the European Society for Therapeutic Radiology and Oncology* 144: 224–230. doi:10.1016/j.radonc.2020.01.003.

33 Koay, E.J., Lege, D., Mohan, R., Komaki, R., Cox, J.D., and Chang, J.Y. (2012). Adaptive/nonadaptive proton radiation planning and outcomes in a phase II trial for locally advanced non-small cell lung cancer. *International Journal of Radiation Oncology, Biology, Physics* 84 (5): 1093–1100. doi:10.1016/j.ijrobp.2012.02.041.

34 Wölfelschneider, J., Friedrich, T., Lüchtenborg, R., et al. (2016). Impact of fractionation and number of fields on dose homogeneity for intra-fractionally moving lung tumors using scanned carbon ion treatment. *Radiotherapy and Oncology : Journal of the European Society for Therapeutic Radiology and Oncology* 118 (3): 498–503. doi:10.1016/j.radonc.2015.12.011.

35 Verma, V., Rwigema, J.-C.M., Malyapa, R.S., Regine, W.F., and Simone, C.B. (2017). Systematic assessment of clinical outcomes and toxicities of proton radiotherapy for reirradiation. *Radiotherapy and Oncology : Journal of the European Society for Therapeutic Radiology and Oncology* 125 (1): 21–30. doi:10.1016/j.radonc.2017.08.005.

36 McAvoy, S.A., Ciura, K.T., Rineer, J.M., et al. (2013). Feasibility of proton beam therapy for reirradiation of locoregionally recurrent non-small cell lung cancer. *Radiotherapy and Oncology : Journal of the European Society for Therapeutic Radiology and Oncology* 109 (1): 38–44. doi:10.1016/j.radonc.2013.08.014.

37 Chao, -H.-H., Berman, A.T., Simone, C.B., et al. (2017). Multi-institutional prospective study of reirradiation with proton beam radiotherapy for locoregionally recurrent non-small cell lung cancer. *Journal of Thoracic Oncology : Official Publication of the International Association for the Study of Lung Cancer* 12 (2): 281–292. doi:10.1016/j.jtho.2016.10.018.

38 Badiyan, S.N., Rutenberg, M.S., Hoppe, B.S., et al. (2019). Clinical outcomes of patients with recurrent lung cancer reirradiated with proton therapy on the Proton Collaborative Group and University of Florida Proton Therapy Institute Prospective Registry Studies. *Practical Radiation Oncology* 9 (4): 280–288. doi:10.1016/j.prro.2019.02.008.

39 Ho, J.C., Nguyen, Q.-N., Li, H., et al. (2018). Reirradiation of thoracic cancers with intensity modulated proton therapy. *Practical Radiation Oncology* 8 (1): 58–65. doi:10.1016/j.prro.2017.07.002.

40 Shirai, K., Kubota, Y., Ohno, T., et al. (2019). Carbon-ion radiotherapy for isolated lymph node metastasis after surgery or radiotherapy for lung cancer. *Frontiers in Oncology* 9: 731. doi:10.3389/fonc.2019.00731.

41 Hayashi, K., Yamamoto, N., Karube, M., et al. (2018). Feasibility of carbon-ion radiotherapy for re-irradiation of locoregionally recurrent, metastatic, or secondary lung tumors. *Cancer Science* 109 (5): 1562–1569. doi:10.1111/cas.13555.

42 Ning, M.S., Gomez, D.R., Heymach, J.V., and Swisher, S.G. (2019). Stereotactic ablative body radiation for oligometastatic and oligoprogressive disease. *Translational Lung Cancer Research* 8 (1): 97–106. doi:10.21037/tlcr.2018.09.21.

43 Takahashi, W., Nakajima, M., Yamamoto, N., et al. (2014). Carbon ion radiotherapy for oligo-recurrent lung metastases from colorectal cancer: A feasibility study. *Radiation Oncology* 9: 68. doi:10.1186/1748-717X-9-68.

44 Sulaiman, N.S., Fujii, O., Demizu, Y., et al. (2014). Particle beam radiation therapy using carbon ions and protons for oligometastatic lung tumors. *Radiation Oncology* 9: 183. doi:10.1186/1748-717X-9-183.

45 Verma, V., Choi, J.I., and Simone, C.B. (2018). Proton therapy for small cell lung cancer. *Translational Lung Cancer Research* 7 (2): 134–140. doi:10.21037/tlcr.2018.04.02.

46 Verma, V., Fakhreddine, M.H., Haque, W., Butler, E.B., Teh, B.S., and Simone, C.B. (2018). Cardiac mortality in limited-stage small cell lung cancer. *Radiotherapy and Oncology : Journal of the European Society for Therapeutic Radiology and Oncology* 128 (3): 492–497. doi:10.1016/j.radonc.2018.06.011.

47 Colaco, R.J., Huh, S., Nichols, R.C., et al. (2013). Dosimetric rationale and early experience at UFPTI of thoracic proton therapy and chemotherapy in limited-stage small cell lung cancer. *Acta Oncologica* 52 (3): 506–513. doi:10.3109/0284186X.2013.769063.

48 Rwigema, J.-C.M., Verma, V., Lin, L., et al. (2017). Prospective study of proton-beam radiation therapy for limited-stage small cell lung cancer. *Cancer* 123 (21): 4244–4251. doi:10.1002/cncr.30870.

49 Welsh, J., Gomez, D., Palmer, M.B., et al. (2011 Dec 1). Intensity-modulated proton therapy further reduces normal tissue exposure during definitive therapy for locally advanced distal esophageal tumors: A dosimetric study. *International Journal of Radiation Oncology, Biology, Physics* 81 (5): 1336–1342. doi:10.1016/j.ijrobp.2010.07.2001. Epub 2011 Apr 4. PMID: 21470796; PMCID: PMC4086056.

50 Warren, S., Partridge, M., Bolsi, A., et al. (2016 May 1). An analysis of plan robustness for esophageal tumors: Comparing volumetric modulated arc therapy plans and spot scanning proton planning. *International Journal of Radiation Oncology, Biology, Physics* 95 (1): 199–207. doi:10.1016/j.ijrobp.2016.01.044. Epub 2016 Jan 30. PMID: 27084641; PMCID: PMC4838670.

51 Shiraishi, Y., Xu, C., Yang, J., Komaki, R., and Lin, S.H. (2017 Oct). Dosimetric comparison to the heart and cardiac substructure in a large cohort of esophageal cancer patients treated with proton beam therapy or Intensity-modulated radiation therapy. *Radiotherapy and Oncology: Journal of the European Society for Therapeutic Radiology and Oncology* 125 (1): 48–54. doi:10.1016/j.radonc.2017.07.034. Epub 2017 Sep 13. PMID: 28917586.

52 Lin, S.H., Komaki, R., Liao, Z., et al. (2012). Proton beam therapy and concurrent chemotherapy for esophageal cancer. *International Journal of Radiation Oncology, Biology, Physics* 83 (3): e345–351. doi:10.1016/j.ijrobp.2012.01.003.

53 Xi, M., Xu, C., Liao, Z., et al. (2017). Comparative outcomes after definitive chemoradiotherapy using proton beam therapy versus intensity modulated radiation therapy for esophageal cancer: A retrospective, single-institutional analysis. *International Journal of Radiation Oncology, Biology, Physics* 99 (3): 667–676. doi:10.1016/j.ijrobp.2017.06.2450.

54 Ono, T., Nakamura, T., Azami, Y., et al. (2015 Nov 27). Clinical results of proton beam therapy for twenty older patients with esophageal cancer. *Radiology and Oncology* 49 (4): 371–8. doi:10.1515/raon-2015-0034. PMID: 26834524; PMCID: PMC4722928.

55 Garant, A., Whitaker, T.J., Spears, G.M., et al. (2019 Nov). A comparison of patient-reported health-related quality of life during proton versus photon chemoradiation therapy for esophageal cancer. *Practical Radiation Oncology* 9 (6): 410–417. doi: 10.1016/j.prro.2019.07.003. Epub 2019 Jul 13. PMID: 31310815.

56 Lin, S.H., Hobbs, B.P., Verma, V., et al. (2020). Randomized phase IIB trial of proton beam therapy versus intensity-modulated radiation therapy for locally advanced esophageal cancer. *Journal of Clinical Oncology : Official Journal of the American Society of Clinical Oncology* 38 (14): 1569–1579. doi:10.1200/JCO.19.02503.

57 Shiraishi, Y., Fang, P., Xu, C., et al. (2018). Severe lymphopenia during neoadjuvant chemoradiation for esophageal cancer: A propensity matched analysis of the relative risk of proton versus photon-based radiation therapy. *Radiotherapy and Oncology : Journal of the European Society for Therapeutic Radiology and Oncology* 128 (1): 154–160. doi:10.1016/j.radonc.2017.11.028.

58 Fang, P., Shiraishi, Y., Verma, V., et al. (2018). Lymphocyte-sparing effect of proton therapy in patients with esophageal cancer treated with definitive chemoradiation. *International Journal of Peptide Research and Therapeutics* 4 (3): 23–32. doi:10.14338/IJPT-17-00033.1.

59 Warren, S., Hurt, C.N., Crosby, T., Partridge, M., and Hawkins, M.A. (2017 Nov 1). Potential of proton therapy to reduce acute hematologic toxicity in concurrent chemoradiation therapy for esophageal cancer. *International Journal of Radiation Oncology, Biology, Physics* 99 (3): 729–737. doi:10.1016/j.ijrobp.2017.07.025. Epub 2017 Jul 29. PMID: 29280467; PMCID: PMC5612280.

60 Dong, C., He, M., Tu, W., et al. (2015). The differential role of human macrophage in triggering secondary bystander effects after either gamma-ray or carbon beam irradiation. *Cancer Letters* 363 (1): 92–100. doi:10.1016/j.canlet.2015.04.013.

61 Keta, O.D., Todorović, D.V., Bulat, T.M., et al. (2017). Comparison of human lung cancer cell radiosensitivity after irradiations with therapeutic protons and carbon ions. *Experimental Biology and Medicine (Maywood, N.J.)* 242 (10): 1015–1024. doi:10.1177/1535370216669611.

62 Durante, M. and Formenti, S. (2020 Mar). Harnessing radiation to improve immunotherapy: Better with particles?*The British Journal of Radiology*93 (1107): 20190224. doi:10.1259/bjr.20190224. Epub 2019 Jul 22. PMID: 31317768; PMCID: PMC7066943.

63 Li, Y., Dykstra, M., Best, T.D., et al. (2019). Differential inflammatory response dynamics in normal lung following stereotactic body radiation therapy with protons versus photons. *Radiotherapy and Oncology : Journal of the European Society for Therapeutic Radiology and Oncology* 136: 169–175. doi:10.1016/j.radonc.2019.04.004.

64 Akutsu, Y., Yasuda, S., Nagata, M., et al. (2012). A phase I/II clinical trial of preoperative short-course carbon-ion radiotherapy for patients with squamous cell carcinoma of the esophagus. *Journal of Surgical Oncology* 105 (8): 750–755. doi:10.1002/jso.22127.

65 Chen, D., Menon, H., Verma, V., et al. (2019). Results of a phase 1/2 trial of chemoradiotherapy with simultaneous integrated boost of radiotherapy dose in unresectable locally advanced esophageal cancer. *JAMA Oncology*. Published online September 17. doi:10.1001/jamaoncol.2019.2809.

66 Mizumoto, M., Sugahara, S., Okumura, T., et al. (2011). Hyperfractionated concomitant boost proton beam therapy for esophageal carcinoma. *International Journal of Radiation Oncology, Biology, Physics* 81 (4): e601–606. doi:10.1016/j.ijrobp.2011.02.041.

67 Fernandes, A., Berman, A.T., Mick, R., et al. (2016). A prospective study of proton beam reirradiation for esophageal cancer. *International Journal of Radiation Oncology, Biology, Physics* 95 (1): 483–487. doi:10.1016/j.ijrobp.2015.12.005.

68 DeCesaris, C.M., McCarroll, R., Mishra, M.V., et al. (2020). Assessing outcomes of patients treated with re-irradiation utilizing proton pencil-beam scanning for primary or recurrent malignancies of the esophagus and gastroesophageal junction. *Journal of Thoracic Oncology : Official Publication of the International Association for the Study of Lung Cancer* 15 (6): 1054–1064. doi:10.1016/j.jtho.2020.01.024.

69 Haefner, M.F., Sterzing, F., Krug, D., et al. (2016). Intrafractional dose variation and beam configuration in carbon ion radiotherapy for esophageal cancer. *Radiation Oncology (London, England)*11, 150. https://doi.org/10.1186/s13014-016-0727-2.

70 Yu, J., Zhang, X., Liao, L., et al. (2016 Mar). Motion-robust intensity-modulated proton therapy for distal esophageal cancer. *Medical Physics.* 43 (3): 1111–1118. doi:10.1118/1.4940789. PMID: 26936698.

71 Parikh, R.R., Rhome, R., Hug, E., et al. (2016). Adjuvant proton beam therapy in the management of thymoma: A dosimetric comparison and acute toxicities. *Clinical Lung Cancer* 17 (5): 362–366. doi:10.1016/j.cllc.2016.05.019.

72 Vogel, J., Lin, L., Litzky, L.A., Berman, A.T., and Simone, C.B. (2017). Predicted rate of secondary malignancies following adjuvant proton versus photon radiation therapy for thymoma. *International Journal of Radiation Oncology, Biology, Physics* 99 (2): 427–433. doi:10.1016/j.ijrobp.2017.04.022.

73 Haefner, M.F., Verma, V., Bougatf, N., et al. (2018). Dosimetric comparison of advanced radiotherapy approaches using photon techniques and particle therapy in the postoperative management of thymoma. *Acta Oncologica* 57 (12): 1713–1720. doi:10.1080/0284186X.2018.1502467.

74 Zhu, H.J., Hoppe, B.S., Flampouri, S., et al. (2018). Rationale and early outcomes for the management of thymoma with proton therapy. *Translational Lung Cancer Research* 7 (2): 106–113. doi:10.21037/tlcr.2018.04.06.

75 Franceschini, D., Cozzi, L., Loi, M., et al. (2020). Volumetric modulated arc therapy versus intensity-modulated proton therapy in the postoperative irradiation of thymoma. *Journal of Cancer Research and Clinical Oncology* 146 (9): 2267–2276. doi:10.1007/s00432-020-03281-z.

76 Mercado, C.E., Hartsell, W.F., Simone, C.B., et al. (2019). Proton therapy for thymic malignancies: Multi-institutional patterns-of-care and early clinical outcomes from the proton collaborative group and the university of Florida prospective registries. *Acta Oncologica* 58 (7): 1036–1040. doi:10.1080/0284186X.2019.1575981.

77 Vogel, J., Berman, A.T., Lin, L., et al. (2016). Prospective study of proton beam radiation therapy for adjuvant and definitive treatment of thymoma and thymic carcinoma: Early response and toxicity assessment. *Radiotherapy and Oncology : Journal of the European Society for Therapeutic Radiology and Oncology* 118 (3): 504–509. doi:10.1016/j.radonc.2016.02.003.

78 Lorentini, S., Amichetti, M., Spiazzi, L., et al. (2012). Adjuvant intensity-modulated proton therapy in malignant pleural mesothelioma. A comparison with intensity-modulated radiotherapy and a spot size variation assessment. *Strahlentherapie Und Onkologie : Organ Der Deutschen Rontgengesellschaft [Et Al]* 188 (3): 216–225. doi:10.1007/s00066-011-0038-3.

79 Krayenbuehl, J., Hartmann, M., Lomax, A.J., Kloeck, S., Hug, E.B., and Ciernik, I.F. (2010). Proton therapy for malignant pleural mesothelioma after extrapleural pleuropneumonectomy. *International Journal of Radiation Oncology, Biology, Physics* 78 (2): 628–634. doi:10.1016/j.ijrobp.2009.11.006.

80 Zeng, J., Badiyan, S.N., Garces, Y.I., et al. (2020). Consensus statement on proton therapy in mesothelioma. *Practical*

Radiation Oncology. Published online May 24. doi:10.1016/j. prro.2020.05.004.

81 Pan, H.Y., Jiang, S., Sutton, J., et al. (2015). Early experience with intensity modulated proton therapy for lung-intact mesothelioma: A case series. *Practical Radiation Oncology* 5 (4): e345–353. doi:10.1016/j.prro.2014.11.005.

82 Rice, S.R., Li, Y.R., Busch, T.M., et al. (2019). A novel prospective study assessing the combination of photodynamic therapy and proton radiation therapy: Safety and outcomes when treating malignant pleural mesothelioma. *Photochemistry and Photobiology* 95 (1): 411–418. doi:10.1111/php.13065.

83 Sai, S., Suzuki, M., Kim, E.H., et al. (2018). Effects of carbon ion beam alone or in combination with cisplatin on malignant mesothelioma cells in vitro. *Oncotarget* 9 (19): 14849–14861. doi:10.18632/oncotarget.23756.

84 Yamauchi, Y., Safi, S., Orschiedt, L., et al. (2017). Low-dose photon irradiation induces invasiveness through the SDF-1α/CXCR4 pathway in malignant mesothelioma cells. *Oncotarget* 8 (40): 68001–68011. doi:10.18632/ oncotarget.19134.

85 Werner-Wasik, M., Yorke, E., Deasy, J., Nam, J., and Marks, L.B. (2010). Radiation dose-volume effects in the esophagus. *International Journal of Radiation Oncology, Biology, Physics* 76 (3 Suppl): S86–93. doi:10.1016/j.ijrobp.2009.05.070.

86 Graham, M.V., Purdy, J.A., Emami, B., et al. (1999). Clinical dose-volume histogram analysis for pneumonitis after 3D treatment for non-small cell lung cancer (NSCLC). *International Journal of Radiation Oncology, Biology, Physics* 45 (2): 323–329. doi:10.1016/s0360-3016(99)00183-2.

87 Hernando, M.L., Marks, L.B., Bentel, G.C., et al. (2001). Radiation-induced pulmonary toxicity: A dose-volume histogram analysis in 201 patients with lung cancer. *International Journal of Radiation Oncology, Biology, Physics* 51 (3): 650–659. doi:10.1016/s0360-3016(01)01685-6.

88 Bradley, J.D., Hu, C., Komaki, R.R., et al. (2020). Long-term results of NRG oncology RTOG 0617: Standard- versus high-dose chemoradiotherapy with or without cetuximab for unresectable stage III non-small-cell lung cancer. *Journal of Clinical Oncology : Official Journal of the American Society of Clinical Oncology* 38 (7): 706–714. doi:10.1200/JCO.19.01162.

89 Wang, X., Palaskas, N.L., Yusuf, S.W., et al. (2020). Incidence and onset of severe cardiac events after radiotherapy for esophageal cancer. *Journal of Thoracic Oncology : Official Publication of the International Association for the Study of Lung Cancer* 15 (10): 1682–1690. doi:10.1016/j. jtho.2020.06.014.

90 Tucker, S.L., Liu, A., Gomez, D., et al. (2016). Impact of heart and lung dose on early survival in patients with non-small cell lung cancer treated with chemoradiation. *Radiotherapy and Oncology : Journal of the European Society for Therapeutic Radiology and Oncology* 119 (3): 495–500. doi:10.1016/j.radonc.2016.04.025.

91 Tucker, S.L., Xu, T., Paganetti, H., et al. (2019). Validation of effective dose as a better predictor of radiation pneumonitis risk than mean lung dose: Secondary analysis of a randomized trial. *International Journal of Radiation Oncology, Biology, Physics* 103 (2): 403–410. doi:10.1016/j. ijrobp.2018.09.029.

92 Teoh, S., Fiorini, F., George, B., Vallis, K.A., and Van Den Heuvel, F. (2019). Proton vs photon: A model-based approach to patient selection for reduction of cardiac toxicity in locally advanced lung cancer. *Radiotherapy and Oncology : Journal of the European Society for Therapeutic Radiology and Oncology*. Published online August 17. doi:10.1016/j.radonc.2019.06.032.

93 McNamara, A.L., Hall, D.C., Shusharina, N., et al. (2020). Perspectives on the model-based approach to proton therapy trials: A retrospective study of a lung cancer randomized trial. *Radiotherapy and Oncology : Journal of the European Society for Therapeutic Radiology and Oncology* 147: 8–14. doi:10.1016/j.radonc.2020.02.022.

94 Koga, K., Kusumoto, S., Watanabe, K., Nishikawa, K., Harada, K., and Ebihara, H. (1988). Age factor relevant to the development of radiation pneumonitis in radiotherapy of lung cancer. *International Journal of Radiation Oncology, Biology, Physics* 14 (2): 367–371. doi:10.1016/0360-3016(88)90445-2.

95 Ahn, S.-J., Kahn, D., Zhou, S., et al. (2005). Dosimetric and clinical predictors for radiation-induced esophageal injury. *International Journal of Radiation Oncology, Biology, Physics* 61 (2): 335–347. doi:10.1016/j.ijrobp.2004.06.014.

96 Saini, J., Maes, D., Egan, A., et al. (2017). Dosimetric evaluation of a commercial proton spot scanning Monte-Carlo dose algorithm: Comparisons against measurements and simulations. *Physics in Medicine and Biology* 62 (19): 7659–7681. doi:10.1088/1361-6560/aa82a5.

97 Huang, S., Souris, K., Li, S., et al. (2018). Validation and application of a fast Monte Carlo algorithm for assessing the clinical impact of approximations in analytical dose calculations for pencil beam scanning proton therapy. *Medical Physics* 45 (12): 5631–5642. doi:10.1002/ mp.13231.

98 Seco, J., Panahandeh, H.R., Westover, K., Adams, J., and Willers, H. (2012). Treatment of non-small cell lung cancer patients with proton beam-based stereotactic body radiotherapy: Dosimetric comparison with photon plans highlights importance of range uncertainty. *International Journal of Radiation Oncology, Biology, Physics* 83 (1): 354–361. doi:10.1016/j.ijrobp.2011.05.062.

99 Li, Y., Kardar, L., Li, X., et al. (2014). On the interplay effects with proton scanning beams in stage III lung cancer. *Medical Physics* 41 (2): 021721. doi:10.1118/1.4862076.

100 Dowdell, S., Grassberger, C., Sharp, G.C., and Paganetti, H. (2013). Interplay effects in proton scanning for lung: A 4D Monte Carlo study assessing the impact of tumor and beam delivery parameters. *Physics in Medicine and Biology* 58 (12): 4137–4156. doi:10.1088/0031-9155/58/12/4137.

101 Schätti, A., Zakova, M., Meer, D., and Lomax, A.J. (2013). Experimental verification of motion mitigation of discrete proton spot scanning by re-scanning. *Physics in Medicine and Biology* 58 (23): 8555–8572. doi:10.1088/0031-9155/58/23/8555.

102 Dueck, J., Knopf, A.-C., Lomax, A., et al. (2016). Robustness of the voluntary breath-hold approach for the treatment of peripheral lung tumors using hypofractionated pencil beam scanning proton therapy. *International Journal of Radiation Oncology, Biology, Physics* 95 (1): 534–541. doi:10.1016/j.ijrobp.2015.11.015.

103 Matsuura, T., Miyamoto, N., Shimizu, S., et al. (2013). Integration of a real-time tumor monitoring system into gated proton spot-scanning beam therapy: An initial phantom study using patient tumor trajectory data. *Medical Physics* 40 (7): 071729. doi:10.1118/1.4810966.

104 Casares-Magaz, O., Toftegaard, J., Muren, L.P., et al. (2014). A method for selection of beam angles robust to intra-fractional motion in proton therapy of lung cancer. *Acta Oncologica* 53 (8): 1058–1063. doi:10.3109/02841 86X.2014.927586.

105 Engwall, E., Fredriksson, A., and Glimelius, L. (2018). 4D robust optimization including uncertainties in time structures can reduce the interplay effect in proton pencil beam scanning radiation therapy. *Medical Physics*. Published online July 16. doi:10.1002/mp.13094.

106 Meijers, A., Knopf, A.-C., Crijns, A.P.G., et al. (2020). Evaluation of interplay and organ motion effects by means of 4D dose reconstruction and accumulation. *Radiotherapy and Oncology : Journal of the European Society for Therapeutic Radiology and Oncology* 150: 268–274. doi:10.1016/j.radonc.2020.07.055.

107 Nantavithya, C., Gomez, D.R., Wei, X., et al. (2018). Phase 2 study of stereotactic body radiation therapy and stereotactic body proton therapy for high-risk, medically inoperable, early-stage non-small cell lung cancer. *International Journal of Radiation Oncology, Biology, Physics* 101 (3): 558–563. doi:10.1016/j.ijrobp.2018.02.022.

108 Van Der Laan, H.P., Anakotta, R.M., Korevaar, E.W., et al. (2019). Organ sparing potential and inter-fraction robustness of adaptive intensity modulated proton therapy for lung cancer. *Acta Oncologica* 58 (12): 1775–1782. doi:10. 1080/0284186X.2019.1669818.

109 Hoffmann, L., Alber, M., Jensen, M.F., Holt, M.I., and Møller, D.S. (2017). Adaptation is mandatory for intensity modulated proton therapy of advanced lung cancer to ensure target coverage. *Radiotherapy and Oncology : Journal of the European Society for Therapeutic Radiology and Oncology* 122 (3): 400–405. doi:10.1016/j. radonc.2016.12.018.

110 Ning, M.S., Gomez, D.R., Shah, A.K., et al. (2019). The insurance approval process for proton radiation therapy: A significant barrier to patient care. *International Journal of Radiation Oncology, Biology, Physics* 104 (4): 724–733. doi:10.1016/j.ijrobp.2018.12.019.

111 Hoppe, B.S., Henderson, R., Pham, D., et al. (2016). A phase 2 trial of concurrent chemotherapy and proton therapy for stage III non-small cell lung cancer: Results and reflections following early closure of a single-institution study. *International Journal of Radiation Oncology, Biology, Physics* 95 (1): 517–522. doi:10.1016/j.ijrobp.2015.11.004.

112 Brooks, E.D., Ning, M.S., Palmer, M.B., Gunn, G.B., Frank, S.J., and Shah, A.K. (2020). Strategic operational redesign for successfully navigating prior authorization barriers at a large-volume proton therapy center. *JCO Oncology Practice*. Published online July 8:JOP1900533. doi:10.1200/ JOP.19.00533.

113 Ning, M.S., Palmer, M.B., Shah, A.K., et al. (2020). Three-year results of a prospective statewide insurance coverage pilot for proton therapy: Stakeholder collaboration improves patient access to care. *JCO Oncology Practice*. Published online April 17:JOP1900437. doi:10.1200/JOP.19.00437.

114 Schippers, J.M., Lomax, A., Garonna, A., and Parodi, K. (2018). Can technological improvements reduce the cost of proton radiation therapy? *Seminars in Radiation Oncology* 28 (2): 150–159. doi:10.1016/j.semradonc.2017.11.007.

115 Goitein, M. and Jermann, M. (2003). The relative costs of proton and X-ray radiation therapy. *Clinical Oncology (The Royal College of Radiologists)* 15 (1): S37–50. doi:10.1053/ clon.2002.0174.

116 Loeffler, J.S. and Durante, M. (2013). Charged particle therapy–optimization, challenges and future directions. *Nature Reviews. Clinical Oncology* 10 (7): 411–424. doi:10.1038/nrclinonc.2013.79.

117 Mansur, D.B. (2014). Incorporating a compact proton therapy unit into an existing National Cancer Institute-designated comprehensive cancer center. *Expert Review of Anticancer Therapy* 14 (9): 1001–1005. doi:10.1586/1473714 0.2014.948857.

118 Mohan, R. and Bortfeld, T. (2011). Proton therapy: Clinical gains through current and future treatment programs. *Frontiers of Radiation Therapy and Oncology* 43: 440–464. doi:10.1159/000322509.

119 Van De Water, S., Kooy, H.M., Heijmen, B.J.M., and Hoogeman, M.S. (2015). Shortening delivery times of intensity modulated proton therapy by reducing proton energy layers during treatment plan optimization. *International Journal of Radiation Oncology, Biology, Physics* 92 (2): 460–468. doi:10.1016/j.ijrobp.2015.01.031.

120 Verma, V., Mishra, M.V., and Mehta, M.P. (2016). A systematic review of the cost and cost-effectiveness studies of proton radiotherapy. *Cancer* 122 (10): 1483–1501. doi:10.1002/cncr.29882.

121 Smith, G.L., Lopez-Olivo, M.A., Advani, P.G., et al. (2019). Financial burdens of cancer treatment: A systematic review of risk factors and outcomes. *Journal of the National Comprehensive Cancer Network : JNCCN* 17 (10): 1184–1192. doi:10.6004/jnccn.2019.7305.

122 Verma, V., Simone, C.B., and Mishra, M.V. (2018). Quality of life and patient-reported outcomes following proton radiation therapy: A systematic review. *Journal of the National Cancer Institute* 110: 4. doi:10.1093/jnci/djx208.

123 Comparing photon therapy to proton therapy to treat patients with lung cancer - Full text view - ClinicalTrials.gov. Accessed September 11, 2020. https://clinicaltrials.gov/ct2/show/NCT01993810

124 Image-guided, intensity-modulated photon or proton beam radiation therapy in treating patients with stage II-IIIB non-small cell lung cancer - Full text view - ClinicalTrials.gov. Accessed September 11, 2020. https://clinicaltrials.gov/ct2/show/NCT01629498

125 Comparing proton therapy to photon radiation therapy for esophageal cancer - Full text view - ClinicalTrials.gov. Accessed September 11, 2020. https://clinicaltrials.gov/ct2/show/NCT03801876

126 Testing the addition of targeted radiation therapy to surgery and the usual chemotherapy treatment (Pemetrexed and Cisplatin [or Carboplatin]) for stage I-IIIA malignant pleural mesothelioma - Full text view - ClinicalTrials.gov. Accessed September 11, 2020. https://clinicaltrials.gov/ct2/show/NCT04158141

127 Skinner, H.D. and Komaki, R. (2012). Proton radiotherapy in the treatment of lung cancer. *Translational Cancer Research* 1 (4): 264–270. doi:10.21037/787. with permission of AME Publishing Company.

128 Giap, H., Roda, D., and Giap, F. (2015). Can proton beam therapy be clinically relevant for the management of lung cancer? *Translational Cancer Research* 4 (4): E3–E15. doi:10.21037/5403. with permission of AME Publishing Company.

129 Dokic, I., Mairani, A., Niklas, M., et al. (2016). Next generation multi-scale biophysical characterization of high precision cancer particle radiotherapy using clinical proton, helium-, carbon- and oxygen ion beams. *Oncotarget* 7 (35): 56676–56689. doi:10.18632/oncotarget.10996.

130 Jethwa, K.R., Haddock, M.G., Tryggestad, E.J., and Hallemeier, C.L. (2020). The emerging role of proton therapy for esophagus cancer. *Journal of Gastrointestinal Oncology* 11 (1): 144–156. doi:10.21037/jgo.2019.11.04. with permission of AME Publishing Company.

18

Gastrointestinal Tumors

Daniel K Ebner MD MPH, Makoto Shinoto MD PhD, Shigeru Yamada MD PhD

Hospital of the National Institutes of Quantum and Radiological Science and Technology (QST Hospital), Chiba, Japan 4-9-1 Anagawa, Inage-kuChiba-shi Chiba 263-8555 Japan

---

TABLE OF CONTENTS

18.1   Introduction

Particle radiotherapy offers distinctive advantages over conventional radiotherapy, notably regarding enhanced tumor dose delivery with concurrent reduction in normal tissue dose. With heavy-ion radiotherapy, this enhanced dose delivery is coupled with increased biological effect within the target tumor, owing to a larger amount of energy being delivered to tissue per unit length, or so-called high linear energy transfer (LET). Initial forays into the usage of particles began with neutron radiotherapy in 1936 [1,2], which demonstrates high-LET but conventional dose distribution. Proton beam radiotherapy (PBT) exhibits the Bragg peak, discussed elsewhere in this book, and its first clinical use occurred at the Lawrence Berkeley National Laboratory in 1954. Heavy-ion irradiation, combining both the enhanced dose distribution of PBT with the high-LET exhibited by neutron therapy, followed in 1957 [3]. The first center for dedicated heavy-ion radiotherapy was constructed at the National Institute of Radiological Sciences (NIRS) in Japan, now the National Institutes of Quantum and Radiological Science and Technology (QST). NIRS began dedicated clinical application of carbon-ion radiotherapy (CIRT) at the Heavy Ion Medical Accelerator in Chiba (HIMAC) in 1994 [4].

Principles and Practice of Particle Therapy, First Edition. Edited by Timothy D. Malouff and Daniel M. Trifiletti.
© 2022 John Wiley & Sons Ltd. Published 2022 by John Wiley & Sons Ltd.

The unique properties of particle therapy and particularly heavy-ion radiotherapy have been demonstrated at length over the intervening decades, with major research and development occurring in Japan, Germany, Italy, Austria, and others, concurrent with efforts by the United States principally in advancing proton radiotherapy [5,6]. Gastrointestinal malignancies offer unique challenges related to radioresistant diseases surrounded by radiosensitive structures, combined with the risk of severe reduction in quality of life with treatment toxicity. The enhanced distribution of particle therapy enables better sparing of surrounding structures, while enhanced relative biological effect (RBE) offers potential for increased control of tumor. CIRT, for instance, demonstrates a RBE at the distal portion of its Bragg peak of ~3 in comparison with ~1.1 for proton, versus photon irradiation [4]. CIRT and heavy-ion radiotherapy more generally have demonstrated other radiobiological advantages, including diminishment of oxygen effect, enhanced ratio of double-stranded DNA breaks with subsequent tumor destruction, lack of (sublethal damage) SLD repair, and reduction in sensitivity to cell-cycle chronicity [7].

Here, a review of modern particle therapy for gastrointestinal disease is conducted, with focus on esophageal, pancreatic, (recurrent) rectal, anal, and colon cancers, though the latter two have a paucity of data in particle therapy. Modern data in all sites almost exclusively employ proton or carbon-ion irradiation, informed by preliminary data generated using neutron, helium, neon, pion, and other beams in the 1970–1990s [8]. More exotic forms of particulate irradiation, such as antiproton radiotherapy, have been theorized and demonstrated unique promise *in vitro*, owing to proton–antiproton annihilation within the Bragg peak amplifying biological effect [9,10], but with complications in their physical dose distribution [11]; they have not been clinically deployed to date. Multi-ion radiotherapy remains experimental [12].

Of note, modern dose convention for particle therapy uses Gray standardized by RBE, abbreviated Gy. Conventions across previous papers vary considerably, with numerous proton papers reporting dose simply using Gy, and others Gray Equivalent (GyE). In most papers using Gy alone, it is difficult to ascertain as to whether the reported value is standardized by the expected RBE of proton in target tissue, an assumed RBE value of 1.1, or a reporting of physical dose delivered. Except where noted, the abbreviations within each paper were maintained, though the underlying comparability of these dose models may require careful examination. Additionally, dose values listed between centers incorporating differing dose models (heavy-ion radiotherapy centers in Europe or Japan, for instance) cannot be directly compared; efforts to reconcile these differences are underway [13].

18.2 Esophageal Cancer

Esophageal cancer is the seventh most common cancer, with notably high prevalence in East Asia. Ninety-five percent of cases consist of squamous cell carcinoma or adenocarcinoma. It is the sixth most common cause of cancer death in the world [14]. Survival ranges from 15% to 25% worldwide, with endoscopic resection or surgery performed with curative intent. Neoadjuvant chemotherapy and chemoradiotherapy (CRT) following surgery, particularly in more advanced stages of disease, are standard.

Cancer of the esophagus offers significant challenges with regard to impact on patient quality of life, impacting the ability to eat and drink and thereby exacerbating treatment toxicity concerns. The esophagus lies in close proximity to radiosensitive organs; significant late cardiopulmonary toxicity has historically limited achievement of significant control, though improvements in chemotherapeutic treatment and the advent of intensity modulated radiotherapy (IMRT) have contributed to improved outcomes [15,16]. RTOG 85-01 first established that CRT yielded better overall survival (OS) than radiotherapy alone, and this has become standard treatment.

Notably, bulky, unresectable disease can be difficult to treat with conventional radiotherapy due to proximity of the tumor to both the spinal cord as well as the heart and lungs. Owing to these toxicity limitations, particle therapy was considered for its potential to reduce toxicity, with further opportunity for dose escalation and theoretical improvements in treatment outcome. Dose–volume histogram (DVH) comparisons demonstrated initial promise, with the physical dose distribution offered by PBT enabling reduction in organs at risk (OAR) doses without affecting planning treatment volume (PTV) prescription coverage [17]. Employment of a left lateral plus posterior-anterior (PA) beam approach with 1:2 weighting has been demonstrated superior to IMRT in lowering mean heart and lung doses and informs current approaches for treatment planning (Table 18.1) [18,19].

18.2.1 Treatment Planning

For proton irradiation of esophageal cancer as part of a trimodal approach, one common method involves delineation of the GTV as all diseases seen on PET and on esophagogastroduodenoscopy. CTV involves irradiation of all areas of potential spread, with PTV constituting a 1–1.5-cm margin around the CTV. Dose delivered was 50.4 Gy (RBE) in 28 fractions [20].

For definitive proton irradiation of locally advanced esophageal cancer, a common treatment regimen involves delineation of the primary tumor and clinically positive lymph nodes

Table 18.1 Recommended target volumes and radiation doses for treatment of esophageal cancer.

Volume	Proton – trimodality	Proton – locally advanced/ nonsurgical	Carbon – presurgical	Carbon – definitive (T1BN0)
Gross tumor volume	All diseases seen on positron emission tomography (PET) and esopha gogastroduo denoscopy (EGD)	Primary tumor and clinically positive lymph nodes	Gross disease	All gross disease seen on endoscopy
Clinical target volume	All areas of potential disease spread	Subclinical tumor expansion, with 2 cm craniocaudal and 3 mm radial expansion of the primary lesion		GTV and prophylactic regional lymph nodes. Boost CTV 3 cm above and below the tumor, with lateral, anterior, and posterior borders >1 cm from the primary
Planning target volume	1–1.5 cm margin around CTV	5 mm margin	GTV plus 3 cm craniocaudal margin, plus metastatic lymph nodes(LNs) with 1 cm margin	CTV plus 1 cm margin, dose delivered with respiratory gating
Dose	50.4 Gy (RBE) in 28 fractions	60 GyE in 30 fractions	36.8 GyE in 8 fractions	50.4 Gy (RBE) in 12 fractions
Reference	Lin et al. [20]	Hirano et al. [18]	Akutsu et al. [21]	

CTV: Clinical target volume; EGD: esophagogastroduodenoscopy; LN: lymph nodes; PET: positron emission tomography; RBE: relative biological effect.

as the gross tumor volume (GTV), with subclinical tumor expansion additionally included as to the clinical target volume (CTV). The primary lesion is thereby expanded by 2 cm craniocaudally and 3 mm radially. An additional 5-mm expansion is placed on the entire CTV, constituting the PTV for treatment. Normal tissue constraints include V20 GyE < 20%, heart V30 GyE <46% and mean dose <26 GyE, and spinal cord D_{max} of 48 GyE, using a proton RBE of 1.1 [18].

For preoperative short-course carbon irradiation at the NIRS, trials involved the use of passive-scattering irradiation. Iridium seeds were implanted endoscopically to the esophageal wall at the proximal and when possible distal edges of the primary tumor. Five-millimeter thick CT images were used for treatment planning on the HIPLAN treatment software. The PTV included the entire primary tumor (GTV) plus a 3-cm craniocaudal margin, as well as metastatic LNs with a 1-cm margin. Respiratory gating was used during CT image acquisition as well as during treatment [21].

Definitive carbon-ion irradiation is currently under investigation via clinical trial, treating to 50.4 Gy (RBE) in 12 fractions. GTV constitutes all gross disease seen on endoscopy, with CTV encompassing both primary lesion as well as prophylactic regional lymph node areas: for the upper thoracic esophagus, the supraclavicular fossae and superior mediastinum; for the middle thoracic esophagus, the supraclavicular fossae, mediastinum, and perigastric region; for the lower thoracic esophagus, the mediastinum and perigastric region. Boost CTV is defined as 3 cm craniocaudal to the tumor. Lateral, anterior, and posterior margins were extended to 1+ cm beyond the primary tumor. The PTV is defined as the CTV plus a 1-cm margin for inter- and intrafractional motion, and treatment is delivered using respiratory gating (Table 18.2) [22].

18.2.2 Proton

Proton beam therapy (PBT) has been employed as a boost therapy, amplifying a base photon dose. Sugahara et al. at the University of Tsukuba in 2005 reported results from 40 patients receiving a combined photon/proton treatment regimen employing 48 Gy of photon amplified by 31.7 GyE proton boost, delivering a total median of 76 Gy. Six patients received protons only to a median dose of 82 Gy. Five patients experienced grade 3 esophagitis, with 15% developing post-RT ulceration. Three patients experienced late grade 3 esophagus morbidity, with two patients experiencing grade 5 toxicity. Globally, survival and local control (LC) were superior to conventional radiotherapy at that time [23].

Mizumoto et al. reported in 2011 a retrospective evaluation of hyperfractionated boost PBT for patients treated between 1990 and 2007, with focus on late toxicity. Median dose was 78 GyE (70–83 GyE) delivered over a median 48 days (38–53 days), with 10 patients having T3–4 disease. One- and 5-year actuarial survival was 79% and 42.8%, respectively, with 1- and 5-year LC of 93.8% and 84.4%. One grade 3 late esophageal toxicity was noted [19].

Takeda and colleagues conducted a similar evaluation of PBT with CRT for stage I–III esophageal cancer, reporting on 47 patients enrolled between 2009 and 2012. Patients received two cycles of systemic 5-fluorouracil (5-FU) with nedaplatin. Photon irradiation for the first half of treatment was followed by PBT. With a median follow-up of 29 months for all patients and 40 months for survivors, the 3-year OS, progression-free survival (PFS), and LC were 59.2%, 56.3%, and 69.8%, respectively. Two patients experienced esophageal stenosis, one a fistula, and two radiation pneumonitis, for five grade 3–4 late toxicities [24].

Table 18.2 Particle therapy for esophageal cancer.

Study	Modality	Patient number	Stage	Median dose (fx)	Local control			Overall survival		
					1 year	3 years	5 years	1 year	3 years	5 years
Combination										
Sugahara 2005	Photon + proton	40	cT1–4N0–1M0	48 Gy + 31.7 GyE			T1 83%, T2–4 29%	(2 years) 81.8%	T1 55%, T2–4 13%	
	Proton	6	cT1–4N0–1M0	82 GyE						
Mizumoto 2011	Photon + proton	19	cT1–4N0–1M0, 10 with T3–4 disease	78 GyE over 48 days	93.80%		84.40%	79%		42.80%
Takeda 2016	Photon, proton, chemotherapy	47	Stages I–III	36 Gy photon + 33–39.6 GyE proton, 5-fluorouracil + nedaplatin		67.70%			59.20%	
Proton										
Wang 2013	Proton, chemotherapy, surgery	72	Stages I–IVa (no metastases)	50.4 Gy, 28 fx						
Ishikawa 2015	Proton, chemotherapy	40	Stages I–III	60 GyE, 30 fx + 4–10 GyE if residual suspected; cisplatin and 5-fluorouracil	66% (2 years)			77% (2 years, disease-specific)		
Xi 2017	Proton (scattering and IMPT)	132	Stages I–III	45.0–63.0 Gy			59.90%			41.60%
Hirano 2018	Proton, chemotherapy	27	Stage III	60 GyE, 30 fx + cisplatin + FU	PFS: 40.6%			90.80%		
Ono 2020	Proton, chemotherapy	54 seniors	Stages I–IV (70% inoperable, 40% III/IV)	72–90.8 Gy (RBE), variable including: cisplatin, 5-FU, nedaplatin, tegafur, gimeracil, oteracil-potassium		71.50%	61.80%	74.9% (2 years)	66%	56%
Lin 2020: Phase IIB	Proton, chemotherapy	46	Stages II–III	50.4 Gy					44.50%	

Carbon						
Akutsu 2011	Carbon + surgery	31	Stages I–IVa	28.8–36.8 GyE, 8 fx		St1 61%, St2 77%, St3 29%
Ongoing trials						
Mayo Clinic NCT02452021	Proton trimodality	30				
Loma Linda NCT01684904	Proton plus paclitaxel/ cisplatin	38				
NRG Phase III NCT03801876	Proton vs. IMRT	300				
WashU Phase II NCT03482791	Proton boost					
MGH Phase II NCT04656041	Proton with liposomal irinotecan	40				
Isozaki 2020	Carbon ion	38	T1bN0	43.2–50.4 Gy (RBE)	Cause specific	97%
Isozaki 2020	Carbon ion		Stage II–III	33.6–36.8 Gy (RBE)	50+% noting pathologic complete response to date	91%

Wang and colleagues evaluated trimodal therapy for esophageal cancer in 2013, evaluating 444 patients treated between 1998 and 2011 who received chemoradiation and surgical resection; 72 of these patients received PBT, with the rest receiving either 3DCRT or IMRT [25]. Pulmonary and GI complications were reduced in the IMRT and PBT cohorts in comparison with 3DCRT, with PBT demonstrating the lowest rates of complication. PBT was noted on analysis to have the lowest average total lung DVH curve.

Ishikawa and colleagues at the University of Tsukuba presented an initial retrospective evaluation of combination PBT with cisplatin and 5-FU in 2015 [26]. Forty patients with stage I–III disease were treated between 2008 and 2012, receiving a total of 60 GyE in 30 fractions. An additional 4–10 GyE was delivered if residual disease was suspected. With a median 24-month follow-up, no grade 3+ cardiopulmonary toxicity was observed. Two-year disease-specific survival and locoregional control were 77% and 66%, respectively. No patient with stage I–II disease had disease-specific death at time of last follow-up.

Xi and colleagues retrospectively evaluated patients who received definitive CRT with either PBT ($n = 132$) or IMRT ($n = 211$), building off initial work by Lin et al. [20,27] PBT demonstrated significantly better OS, PFS, distant metastasis-free survival, and marginally better locoregional failure-free survival (LRFFS), without differences in toxicity between groups. On multivariate analysis, PBT had improved OS and LRFFS, with clinical stage subgroup analysis revealing considerably higher 5-year OS and PFS rates in the PBT group for stage III disease, though not for stage I/II patients. The authors concluded that prospective evaluation was warranted, with observed differences in age, race, and insurance coverage between cohorts.

In 2018, Hirano and colleagues dosimetrically evaluated PBT versus 3D conformal RT (3DCRT) and IMRT for locally advanced esophageal squamous cell carcinoma (ESCC) in 27 patients with stage III disease between October 2012 and December 2015 [18]. In comparison with 3DCRT, PBT demonstrated significantly lower dose excepting lung V10 GyE and V15 GyE and significantly lower heart dose; dose to healthy tissue was significantly lower in all variables versus IMRT.

Ono and colleagues in 2020 reported on PBT in the setting of senior patients with ESCC, retrospectively reviewing 54 patients aged 75 and older treated with PBT from January 2009 to December 2013. Thirty eight (70.4%) were inoperable and over 40% had stage III/IV ESCC. The 5-year OS and cancer-specific survival rates were 56.2% and 71.7%, respectively. Five-year LC was 61.8%, with three cases of grade 3 esophageal ulceration [28].

Lin and colleagues reported in 2020 a randomized phase IIB trial of PBT versus IMRT for locally advanced esophageal cancer [29]. Patients were randomly assigned to either PBT or IMRT for 50.4 Gy, with stratification for histology, resectability, induction chemotherapy, and stage. The trial was notable for incorporating a Bayesian group sequential design, closing prior to the planned 67% interim analysis. One-hundred and forty-five patients were randomly assigned, with 107 evaluable and a median follow-up of 44.1 months. Of note, 80% of PBT was conducted using the passive scattering method. The posterior mean total toxicity burden was 2.3 times higher for IMRT than PBT, with a postoperative complication score 7.6 times higher for IMRT. The 3-year PFS rate and 3-year OS rates were not significantly different.

Multiple clinical trials incorporating PBT in esophageal cancer are currently in progress. The Mayo Clinic is conducting an observational study of pencil-beam scanning PBT as a component of trimodality therapy for esophageal cancer in 30 patients, evaluating for grade 3+ adverse events (NCT02452021). Loma Linda University is accruing a phase II trial of PBT plus chemotherapy incorporating paclitaxel with cisplatin for resectable esophageal or esophagogastric junction cancer, with an expected recruitment of 38 patients (NCT01684904). NRG Oncology with the National Cancer Institute is conducting a phase III randomized trial of 300 participants, evaluating PBT versus IMRT in esophageal cancer (NCT03801876). Washington University School of Medicine is conducting a phase II trial of PBT for both resectable (to 50 or 50.4 Gy) and unresectable (to 59.4 or 60 Gy) disease, with standard chemotherapy, evaluating predominantly toxicity and patient-reported outcomes (NCT03482791). MD Anderson is conducting a phase I/II trial evaluating simultaneous integrated proton boost in esophageal cancer in combination with chemotherapy, evaluating first for maximum tolerated dose and then to evaluate control and pathological response (NCT01102088). Massachusetts General Hospital (MGH) is including proton irradiation in a phase II trial evaluating in 40 patients with liposomal irinotecan in combination with standard chemotherapeutic regimens for gastroesophageal junction or esophagogastric cancer (NCT04656041).

18.2.3 Carbon

The combination of dose distribution and radiobiologic advantages inherent to CIRT allows for hypofractionated regimens for treatment of esophageal cancer. A representative treatment distribution is shown in Figure 18.1.

Akutsu and colleagues published in 2011 the first phase I/II dose-escalation clinical trial for preoperative short-course CIRT in resectable esophageal carcinoma, conducted between 2004 and 2008 at NIRS. Thirty-one patients of stage I–IVa were treated with a total dose of 28.8–36.8 GyE in eight fractions over 2 weeks, with esophagectomy and LN dissection performed 1–2 months following irradiation. Pathologic response was 100% in T1 cases, 87.5% in T2 cases, and 45.5% in T3 cases, with 5-year OS for stages I, II, and III of 61%, 77%, and 29%, respectively. CIRT alone achieved a complete response in 39% of patients with noted improved survival, and 60% of T1 and T2 cases achieved pathologic complete responses (pCR). One case exhibited grade 3 postoperative acute respiratory distress syndrome which was considered unrelated to CIRT [21]. This trial was continued

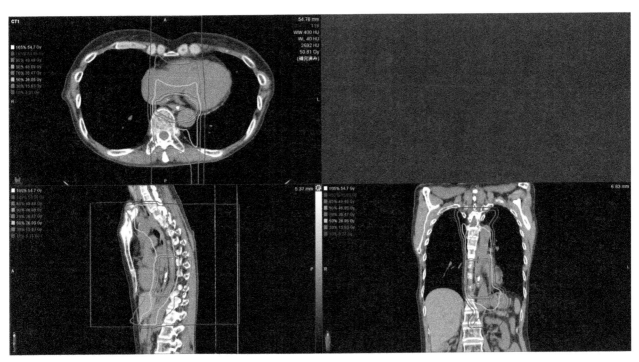

Figure 18.1   Representative esophagus treatment plan with CIRT.

in two separate trials, one a phase I/II CIRT monotherapy course for T1bN0 esophageal cancer from 2007 and another a phase I/II preoperative short-course combination CIRT and chemotherapy trial for stage II/III resectable esophageal cancer from 2012.

The former trial for T1bN0 esophageal cancer employed 12 fractions in 3-week course targeting a 43.2–50.4-Gy (RBE) dose regimen, with 38 patients treated to date; the trial is ongoing. Thirteen patients were deemed at high risk for surgery or CRT due to age or comorbidity. Grade 3 acute esophagitis and grade 3 acute hematotoxicity were observed in four and three cases, respectively, with one late grade 3+ case reported secondary to aspiration pneumonitis, felt to be not directly related to CIRT. Thirty-two cases (84.2%) demonstrated a complete response, with local recurrence in 11 patients successfully salvaged with surgical or endoscopic resection. At a median 43-month follow-up, 3- and 5-year OS were 86% and 81%, respectively; cause-specific survivals were 97% and 91%, respectively. This was favorably compared with surgical results from Japan, which yielded 3- and 5-year survival of T1bN0 esophageal cancer of 85% and 76.8% [22].

The latter trial for stage II/III resectable esophageal carcinoma excluded those with T4 disease and is ongoing. Dose escalation has been performed from 33.6 Gy (RBE) in 5% increments, with escalation occurring when no severe adverse events are noted; 19 cases have been treated to date, with dose now 36.8 Gy (RBE). Thirteen cases involved stage III disease, and eight cases T3 disease, with over half achieving pCR. An update is anticipated as the trial accrues [22].

Isolated lymph node recurrences have similarly been treated with CIRT. Isozaki and colleagues retrospectively evaluated 48 Gy (RBE) in 12 fraction regimen achieving 2-, 3-, and 5-year LC of 92.4%, with 2-, 3-, and 5-year OS of 70%, 58.3%, and 21.9%, respectively. No grade 3+ toxicities were reported [30].

18.2.4   Neutron and Other Particles

Given the proximity of the esophagus to sensitive tissues, neutron therapy, combining high-LET irradiation with a conventional dose distribution, has not proven promising in the treatment of esophageal cancer. A 1983 phase I RTOG trial for neutron therapy with and without photon treatment for inoperable esophageal cancer demonstrated poor response and median survival of less than 10 months, with complication rates exceeding 50% "severe" late side effects [31]. Modern trials incorporating neutron or other ion therapy do not appear to exist at time of writing.

Collectively, particle irradiation for esophageal cancer appears notably promising, enabling higher dose delivery with improved sparing of normal tissue and toxicity in comparison with conventional irradiation.

18.3   Pancreatic Cancer

Pancreatic ductal adenocarcinoma remains one of the most lethal cancers known, with OS at 5 years only 5–10%. It represents the fourth most common cause of cancer death [32]. As early disease is generally asymptomatic, the majority of patients are ineligible for curative surgical resection at time of presentation; even with resection, 5-year survival remains low owing to common metachronous metastasis and disease recurrence [33,34]. Advancements in adjuvant and neoadjuvant treatment notably via FOLFIRINOX [35] have improved outcomes somewhat, but the role of radiotherapy for pancreatic cancer has to date been limited, following numerous negative trials [36] in the setting of the disease inherently being radioresistant, likely due to hypoxia. Other than surgery, radiotherapy is the only technique that has demonstrated improved LC [37], and dose-escalation strategies have proven promising [36].

The optimal management of borderline and unresectable, locally advanced pancreatic cancer (LAPC) is poorly defined, with sequential and concurrent conventional CRT failing to improve survival outcomes. Given a high rate of local recurrence with chemoradiation, improved LC has been suggested as one method by which survival benefit may be achieved, leading to testing of IMRT and stereotactic body radiotherapy to deliver escalated doses to the tumor bed. To date, however, meaningful survival improvement has not been seen. Conventional radiotherapeutic regimens are limited by the proximity of the pancreas to surrounding radiosensitive gastrointestinal tissue. The ability for particle radiotherapy to offer dose escalation in target tissue through the enhanced dose distribution of the particle beam, added with the enhanced RBE of the carbon-ion beam

(suggested as high as 4.5 in pancreatic cells [38], with notable increase in cancer stem cells), informed initial trials of particle therapy for pancreatic cancer (Table 18.3).

18.3.1 Treatment Planning

In locally advanced and borderline resectable disease, proton therapy has been employed as part of a combined neoadjuvant regimen with FOLFIRINOX. GTV is delineated on post-chemotherapy CT imaging, including all visible disease. CTV adds a 1-cm margin with elective nodal coverage of celiac, porta hepatis, superior mesenteric artery and vein, and para-aortic groups. The PTV is expanded as necessary for setup variability and internal motion, with 25 GyE in five fractions delivered [39,40].

For definitive proton irradiation of LAPC, all gross disease is delineated as the GTV. CTV constitutes the GTV plus 0.5–1.5-cm margins, with exclusions provided for OAR. If needed, the PTV is extended for expected setup variability but was noted used in a recent definitive study. Treatment involves 60 GyE in 20 fractions to the GTV, and 40 GyE in 20 fractions to the CTV, in one notable trial [41].

For neoadjuvant CIRT, CTV was defined as the GTV plus a 5-mm margin, with the locoregional elective lymph nodes and neuroplexus regions included, comprising the celiac, superior mesenteric, peripancreatic, portal, and para-aortic

Table 18.3 Recommended target volumes and radiation doses for treatment of pancreatic cancer.

Volume	Neoadjuvant proton	Definitive proton (LAPC)	Neoadjuvant carbon	Definitive carbon (LAPC)
Gross tumor volume	Post-chemotherapy CT scan, including all tumor visible on imaging	All gross disease	All gross disease	Primary tumor and metastatic lymph nodes as diagnosed by CT, MRI, ^{18}F-FDG-PET) imaging
Clinical target volume	Added 1-cm margin with elective nodal coverage of celiac, porta hepatis, superior mesenteric artery and vein, and para-aortic groups	GTV + 0.5–1.5-cm margins, excluding OAR	GTV + 5-mm margins, excluding OARs. For pancreatic head disease, includes the elective lymph nodes (celiac, superior mesenteric, peripancreatic, portal, and para-aortic regions; for body or tail disease, includes the splenic region) and neuroplexus	GTV + 5-mm margin, neuroplexus, and prophylactic nodal areas around pancreas (celiac, superior mesenteric, peri-pancreatic, portal, para-aortic for pancreatic head cancer and splenic region for pancreatic body and tail cancer)
Planning target volume	As necessary for setup variability and internal motion		CTV + 5-mm margins, excluding OARs	CTV with 5-mm margin to compensate for setup errors
Dose	25 GyE in 5 fractions	60 GyE in 20 fractions to GTV, 40 GyE in 20 fractions to CTV		52.8 Gy (RBE) or 55.2 Gy (RBE) in 12 fractions
Reference	Murphy et al. [39]	Kawashiro et al. [44]		Hattori et al. [41]

regions for pancreatic head, and the splenic region for body and tail cancers. The PTV included the CTV plus a 5-mm margin for positioning error. Margins were reduced for those patients with disease too close to critical organs, and GTV was delineated using a combination of CT, MRI, and PET imaging. Treatment involves delivery of 36.8 Gy (RBE) CIRT [42,43].

For definitive CIRT treatment of unresectable LAPC, GTV was defined as the primary tumor and metastatic lymph nodes as diagnosed by CT, MRI, and ^{18}F-FDG-PET imaging. The CTV encompassed the GTV with a 5-mm margin, as well as the neuroplexus and prophylactic nodal areas around pancreas (celiac, superior mesenteric, peri-pancreatic, portal, para-aortic for pancreatic head cancer, and splenic region for pancreatic body and tail cancer). PTV encompassed the CTV with 5-mm margin to compensate for setup errors. Dose delivered was 52.8 Gy (RBE) or 55.2 Gy (RBE) in 12 fractions (Table 18.4) [44].

18.3.2 Proton

Hong and colleagues at the MGH published a phase I/II trial in 2014 on preoperative short-course PBT and capecitabine for resectable pancreatic cancer. Forty-eight patients were enrolled in total. Thirty-five patients treated in the phase II portion of the trial received 25 GyE in five fractions, with two experiencing a grade 3+ toxicity. Eleven of the 48 patients did not ultimately undergo resection, with two due to metastatic progression and eight deemed unresectable upon surgical exploration. Locoregional failure occurred in 16% of resected patients, with 73% developing distant metastasis; median survival was 17.3 months, with 42% alive at 2 years. For the 37 patients able to undergo resection, median survival time was 27 months [45].

For LAPC, in 2012, Terashima and colleagues at the Hyogo Ion Beam Medical Center presented a prospective phase I/II study of gemcitabine-concurrent PBT treatment of T3–T4 disease, enrolling 50 patients [46]. PBT dose was increased from 50 to 70.2 GyE in 25–26 fractions. At a median follow-up of 12.5 months, 1-year OS was 76.8%, with grade 3+ gastric ulcer and hemorrhage seen in five patients, including grade 5 toxicity. Takitori et al. conducted a separate evaluation of 91 patients treated at Hyogo, with endoscopic examination before and after gemcitabine-concurrent proton irradiation. A percentage of 49.4 of patients were observed to have radiation-induced ulceration of the stomach and duodenum [47].

Sachsman and colleagues at the Florida Proton Therapy Institute in 2014 reported preliminary results for 11 patients with unresectable pancreatic cancer treated with 59.4 Gy (RBE) in 33 fractions and concomitant oral capecitabine. Only gross disease was targeted. At a median follow-up of 14 months (23 months for survivors), 1- and 2-year OS were 61% and 31%, with freedom from local progression of 86% and 69%, respectively. No grade 2+ toxicity was noted [48].

Notably promising results were published in 2017. Hattori and colleagues at the Nagoya Proton Therapy Center presented 18 patients with inoperable LAPC (cStage III per UICC 7th classification) receiving concurrent chemotherapy and proton irradiation; here, S-1 chemotherapy was used [41]. PBT was delivered at 60 GyE in 20 fractions to the GTV, with 40 GyE to the CTV, employing a field-in-field technique. With a median follow-up of 12 months, LC and OS at 1 year were 100% and 80%, respectively. One grade 4 depression, one grade 3 thrombocytopenia, and one grade 3 liver abscess and cholangitis were noted.

In 2018 and 2019, Murphy and colleagues at MGH evaluated total neoadjuvant therapy with FOLFIRINOX followed by CRT, including proton irradiation, for both locally advanced and borderline resectable pancreatic adenocarcinoma in two single-arm phase II trials [39,40]. The primary end point in both trials was R0 resection. Short and long-course proton and photon irradiation was employed depending on tumor restaging following 8 cycles of preoperative FOLFIRINOX, with 27 receiving short-course proton irradiation. In borderline disease, 31 of 48 eligible patients achieved R0 resection, with median PFS of 14.7 months, and 2-year PFS of 43%. Median OS was 37.7 months, with a 2-year OS of 56%. Resected patients achieved a median PFS of 48.6 months, with 2-year PFS and OS of 55% and 72%, respectively. In LAPC and with a similar protocol, 7 patients of 49 were eligible to receive short-course proton irradiation, while the rest received long-course photon irradiation. R0 resection was achieved in 34 of 49 patients, with median PFS of 17.5 months and median OS of 31.4 months; among those patients who achieved resection, median PFS was 21.3 months with median OS 33.0 months.

A number of clinical trials are in progress for proton radiotherapy at time of writing. A phase II trial of high-dose PBT with elective nodal irradiation and concomitant chemotherapy was initiated at the University of Florida, targeting an accrual of 60 patients with unresectable, borderline, or medically inoperable pancreatic adenocarcinoma. About 40.5 Gy (RBE) in 18 fractions will be delivered to gross disease and elective nodal volume, followed by 22.5 Gy (RBE) in a 10 fraction boost, targeting a total dose of 63 Gy (RBE) in 28 fractions, with concomitant capecitabine (NCT02598349). MGH in collaboration with the NCI have an active trial evaluating proton irradiation combined with FOLFIRINOX-losartan, evaluating the number of patients able to achieve R0 resection (NCT01821729). Georgetown University has a phase I trial in active recruitment, evaluating proton therapy with mFOLFIRINOX, with a planned irradiation dosage of 5 GyE in five doses (NCT03885284). The University of Maryland Baltimore is recruiting a phase I study of concurrent Nab-Paclitaxel and gemcitabine with hypofractionated ablative proton therapy for LAPC, maximum tolerated dosage. Patients will receive 67.5 Gy in 15 fractions (NCT03652428). The Mayo Clinic is evaluating moderately hypofractionated photon and proton CRT as definitive versus neoadjuvant therapy in pancreatic cancer, assessing treatment response utilizing molecular biomarkers. Primary outcome is grade 3+ GI acute events (NCT03902600).

18.3.3 Carbon Ion

Carbon ion was first utilized at the NIRS, Japan, from 2000 to 2003, with 22 patients with localized, resectable pancreatic cancer treated. Doses between 44.8 and 48 Gy (RBE) were delivered at 2.8–3.0 Gy (RBE) per fraction, achieving LC of 100% at 1 year and 87% at 2 years, with OS of 59% at 1 year. This led to development of initial clinical trials. A representative treatment distribution dose distribution is shown in Figure 18.2.

For preoperative short-course CIRT, a phase I trial was reported by Shinoto and colleagues in 2013 [42], after which the trial was extended to phase II; the phase I/II results were updated by Ebner et al. in 2017 [43]. The phase I trial consisted of a dose-escalation study from 30 Gy (RBE), with 36.8 Gy (RBE) ultimately established for phase II, both delivered in eight fractions over 2 weeks. Thirty-eight patients were available for analysis at time of publication: dose included 30 Gy (RBE) in 6, 31.6 Gy (RBE) in 5, 33.6 Gy (RBE) in 4, 35.2 Gy (RBE) in 7, and 36.8 Gy (RBE) in 24 patients, with surgery following 4–6 weeks after chemoradiation. Six cases were found at the time of surgery to be unresectable. At a median follow-up of 30.9 months, LC for resectable patients at

1, 3, and 5 years was estimated at 100%, 92.3%, and 92.3%, with OS of 78%, 54%, and 40%, respectively. Sixty-five percent of patients developed distant metastasis. In resectable cases, OS extended to 87%, 65%, and 49%, respectively, while the unresectable cases had a median survival of 11.7 months. One patient had an acute grade 3 liver reaction, and one a late grade 4 portal vein stenosis. One noted advantage by the authors was the 2-week course of CIRT, with hypofractionation viewed as favorable for minimizing risk of disease progression prior to surgery.

A phase II trial was initiated in 2012 at NIRS (UMIN000010120), delivering a total dose of 36.8 Gy (RBE) in eight fractions with concurrent gemcitabine. This is recruiting at current [49]. The PIOPPO trial in Italy was initiated in 2018 (NCT03822936) as a multicenter phase II trial in which patients with resectable or borderline pancreatic cancer will undergo three cycles FOLFIRINOX following by 38.4 Gy (RBE) CIRT over 2 weeks. Final results are expected in 2023 [50].

For LAPC, Shinoto et al. at NIRS in 2016 reported a phase I/II clinical trial using combination gemcitabine and CIRT from 2007 to 2012 [51]. Dose escalation was performed in two steps, with CIRT fixed at 43.2 GyE and gemcitabine increased stepwise from 400 mg/m^2 to 1000 mg/m^2. Thereafter, CIRT was increased by 5% increments to 55.2 GyE. Seventy-two patients were enrolled. Locoregional elective nodal regions were included in the CTV, and follow-up incorporated both CT scans as well as FDG-PET-CT scans. Grade 3–4 hematologic toxicity was seen in 53% of patients, with dose-limiting toxicity seen only in three patients;

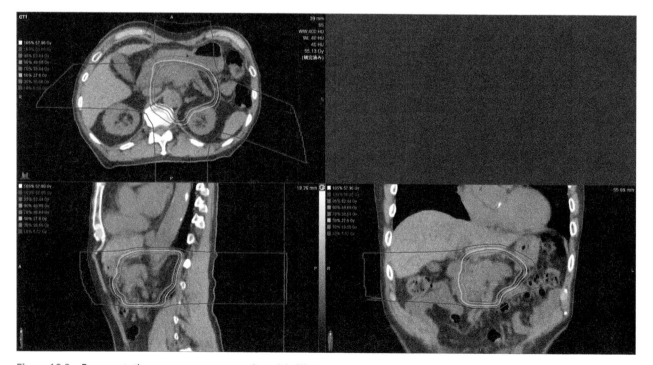

Figure 18.2 Representative pancreas treatment plan with CIRT.

two patients suffered from grade 4 neutropenia at 43.2 Gy (RBE), and grade 3 intratumoral infection was seen in one patient treated with 50.4 Gy (RBE). With regard specifically to radiotherapy, one grade 3 gastric ulcer with hemorrhage was noted at 50.4 Gy (RBE). Median OS was 19.6 months. OS for the entire cohort at 1 and 2 years were 73% and 35%, respectively; for the high-dose group with stage III disease, the 2-year FFLP and OS were 40% and 48%, compared with 9% and 23% in the low dose cohort. LC at 2 years was 83% based on CT imaging; incorporating FDG-PET criteria, however, LC was 30%. Dose was capped at 55.2 Gy (RBE) due to perceived risk of severe late toxicity.

Kawashiro et al. retrospectively pooled and analyzed the use of CIRT for LAPC across the Japan Carbon-Ion Radiation Oncology Study Group (J-CROS), comprising three institutions and 72 patients treated from 2012 to 2014 [52]. Either 52.8 Gy (RBE) or 55.2 Gy (RBE) were delivered in 12 fractions, with 78% of patients receiving concurrent gemcitabine at 1,000 mg/m^2. Median survival was 21.5 months, with 1- and 2-year OS of 73% and 46%, respectively. The authors described that while no difference in LC was detected between low- and high-dose cohorts, distant metastasis-free survival appeared improved in patients receiving high-dose CIRT; of note, the high-dose cohort also was more likely to receive concurrent chemotherapy. Twenty-six percent of patients experienced grade 3–4 hematologic toxicity secondary to gemcitabine, with one patient developing a grade 3 duodenal ulcer.

Kawashiro et al. further conducted a retrospective evaluation of CIRT for locoregionally recurrent pancreatic cancer, encompassing 30 patients [53]. Thirty percent received 52.8 Gy (RBE) and 70% received 55.2 Gy (RBE) in 12 fractions, with 57% receiving either S-1 or gemcitabine. Median OS was 25.9 months, with 1- and 2-year OS of 79% and 51%, respectively. No grade 3 toxicity was noted.

Incorporation of respiratory gating with scanning-beam irradiation has shown promise for delivering a simultaneous, integrated boost [54], and it is important to note that technological development of the CIRT apparatus is ongoing. Theoretical advantages have been suggested with LET painting of the target tumor or incorporation of multi-ionic treatment [12,55–58]. Modern analysis of LAPC patients receiving CIRT and concurrent chemotherapy have continued to see improvements in survival with advancement of treatment technique, with a reported 2-year OS of 60% [22]; full exploration of this data is forthcoming.

A number of trials are ongoing at time of publication with regard to evaluation of heavy-ion radiotherapy in LAPC, including two international collaborations (Table 18.4). Albert Einstein College of Medicine and the Shanghai Proton and Heavy Ion Center (SPHIC) have collaborated to form a phase I dose-escalation trial for CIRT in LAPC, beginning in 2016 (Trial NCT03403049), incorporating combination photon and CIRT irradiation. Dose escalation involves de-escalation of

photon irradiation and escalation of CIRT, respectively. Maximum dosage was 56 Gy (RBE) carbon-ion monotherapy in 14 fractions. Recruitment was reported as finished as of January 2018, though results have not yet reached publication. The University of Texas Southwestern initiated a phase III trial for CIRT in LAPC with the NIRS in Japan in May 2019 (Trial NCT03536182), planning for 110 patients to be randomly assigned chemoradiation incorporating either photon or CIRT. CIRT is to be delivered with 55.2 Gy (RBE) in 12 fractions, while photon will consist of IMRT of 50.4–56.0 Gy in 28 fractions. Chemotherapy will include gemcitabine with CIRT, and gemcitabine or capecitabine for photons, with sequential chemotherapy incorporating gemcitabine + nab-paclitaxel or FOLFIRINOX. Recent reports are that this trial is to be discontinued without patient accrual [49]. Within Japan, a multi-institutional prospective phase II trial was initiated by J-CROS (Trial J-CROS 1502 Pancreas), to a target of 55.2 Gy (RBE) in 12 fractions with concurrent gemcitabine.

SPHIC had additionally developed a trial combining PBT and CIRT in LAPC, enrolling 10 patients between 2015 and 2019 (Trial NCT03949933). Patients were to be treated with a dose of 50.4 GyE in 28 fractions to the CTV, with CIRT boost of 12–18 GyE delivered to the GTV. Recruitment status was listed as completed in March 2020; results are forthcoming.

The Heidelberg Ion Beam Therapy Center (HIT) in 2013 initiated a phase I trial of raster scanning CIRT with weekly gemcitabine and adjuvant gemcitabine for LAPC, termed the PHOENIX-1 trial [59]. This trial aimed to evaluate treatment safety from 42 GyE/14 fractions to 54 GyE in 18 fractions but is currently on hold. A separate trial was initiated at HIT evaluating CIRT for LAPC or locally recurrent pancreatic cancer (Trial NCT04194268), termed the PACK-trial. This is a prospective single-center phase I/II trial utilizing fixed 48 Gy (RBE) in 12 fractions; locoregional lymph node regions are not included in the CTV if deemed unaffected, with concurrent gemcitabine. Target accrual is 25 patients, with anticipated publication around 2023. The trial protocol is forthcoming [49].

18.3.4 Neutron and Other Particles

Limited modern data exist for other particle irradiation for the treatment of pancreatic cancer; a brief review of older literature is presented here. Similar to esophageal cancer, the proximity of the pancreas to OARs has limited the utility of neutron therapy in treatment. A 1989 RTOG trial evaluated 49 inoperable patients treated with neutrons ± photons, with median survival reduced from 8.3 months in the photon arm to 5.6 months in the neutron arm [60]. The largest trial reported was conducted at Fermilab between 1977 and 1994, enrolling 173 patients with unresectable exocrine pancreatic adenocarcinoma. They treated 106 with neutron monotherapy and 67 with concomitant fluorouracil (5-FU), with median survival of 6 months for

Table 18.4 Particle therapy for pancreatic cancer.

Study	Modality	Patient number	Stage	Median dose (fx)	Local control 1 year	Local control 2 years	Local control 5 years	Overall survival 1 year	Overall survival 2 years	Overall survival 5 years
Preoperative										
Hong 2014	Proton + capecitabine	48	Resectable	25 GyE, 5 fx		84% (resected patients)			42%	
Ebner 2015 + Shinoto 2013	Carbon	38		30.0–36.8 Gy (RBE) in 8 fx	100%	3 years; 92.3%	92.30%	78% (resectable: 87%)	3 years; 54% (resectable: 65%)	40% (resectable: 49%)
Locally advanced										
Terashima 2012	PBT + gemcitabine	50	T3–T4	50–70.2 GyE, 25–26 fx				76.80%		
Sachsman 2014	Proton + capecitabine	11	T3–T4	59.4 Gy (RBE), 33 fx, only gross disease	FFLP: 86%	FFLP: 69%		61%	31%	
Hattori 2017	Proton + S-1	18	cStage III	GTV: 60 GyE, CTV: 40 GyE, 20 fx	100%			80%		
Murphy 2018	Proton + FOLFIRINOX	27	Borderline	25 Gy/5 fx or 30 Gy/10 fx		PFS: 43% (resected: 55%)			56% (resected: 72%)	
			LAPC	25 Gy/5 fx or 30 Gy/10 fx		Median PFS 17.5 months (resected: 21.3)			Median OS 31.4 month (resected 33.0)	
Shinoto 2016	Carbon + gemcitabine	72	LAPC	43.2 GyE–55.2 GyE/12 fx		30% (using PET)		73%	35% (48% high dose)	
Kawashiro 2018	Carbon + gemcitabine	72	LAPC	52.8 or 55.2 Gy (RBE)/12 fx	84%	76%		73%	46%	
Isozaki 2020	Carbon + concurrent chemotherapy	Ongoing trial	LAPC					DMFS: 41%	60%	FMFS: 28%
Recurrent										
Kawashiro 2018	Carbon + gemcitabine or S-1	30	Recurrent	52.8 or 55.2 Gy (RBE)/12 fx				79%	51%	
Other										
Los Alamos 1987	Pion	33		21–41 Gy	0%					
Lawrence Berkeley 1988	Helium			60–70 GyE					Median OS: 7.8 month	
Fermilab 1996	Neutron	106	Unresectable						(3-year) 0%	
	Neutron + 5-FU	67	Unresectable						(3-year) 7%	

Clinical trials

Proton

Phase II high-dose PBT with nodal irradiation	NCT02598349	University of Florida	Unresectable, borderline, inoperable	40.5 Gy (RBE)/18 fx to GTV+ and elective nodes + 22.5 Gy (RBE)/10 fx boost, with capecitabine
Proton and FOLFIRINOX-Losartan	NCT01821729	MGH and NCI	LAPC	Combination proton and FOLFIRINOX-Losartan
Phase I of Proton and mFOLFIRINOX	NCT03885284	Georgetown University	Adjuvant	25 GyE in 5 fx + mFOLFIRINOX for 12 cycles
Phase 1 of proton and concurrent nab-paclitaxel + gemcitabine	NCT03652428	University of Maryland—Baltimore	LAPC	67.5 Gy in 15 fx to max tolerated dosage
Definitive vs. Neoadjuvant hypofractionation photon/proton CRT	NCT03902600	Mayo Clinic	T1-4 N0-2 M0	45 Gy/15 fx with 5-FU or capecitabine

Carbon

CIRT for LAPC	UMIN000010120	NIRS/QST	Neoadjuvant	36.8 Gy (RBE) in 8 fractions with gemcitabine
CIPHER	NCT03536182	UT Southwestern with QST Hospital	Unresectable Pancreatic Cancer	A: CIRT in 12 fractions with concurrent gemcitabine, adjuvant gemcitabine and nab-paclitaxel B: IMRT in 28 fractions with concurrent gemcitabine, adjuvant gemcitabine and nab-paclitaxel
PIOPPO	NCT03822936	CNAO	Resectable or borderline resectable pancreatic adenocarcinoma	Neoadjuvant FOLFIRONX followed by 38.4 GyE/8 fractions CIRT. Resection and adjuvant gemcitabine
Proton and carbon ion radiotherapy for locally advanced pancreatic cancer	NCT03949933	SPHIC	LAPC	Proton therapy to 50.4 GyE/28 fractions with a carbon boost (12–18 GyE in 3 GyE per fraction)
Shanghai and Albert Einstein Trial	NCT03403049	Albert Einstein College of Medicine and the Shanghai Proton and Heavy Ion Center	LAPC	Phase I dose escalation involving photon de-escalation and carbon dose escalation. Results forthcoming
PACK-trial	NCT04194268	Heidelberg	LAPC/Recurrent	Phase I/II for 48 Gy (RBE) in 12 fractions with gemcitabine

DMFS = Distant metastasis-free survival; FFLP = freedom from local progression; PFS = progression-free survival.

monotherapy and 9 months for the combination arm, respectively; 3-year survival was 0% and 7% for each arm. Grade 3 toxicities of 18% and 25% were reported in each arm, as well as grade 4 toxicity of 5% and 6% [61].

Pion radiotherapy has been attempted in varying cancers; for pancreatic cancer, one 33-patient cohort was reported in 1987 by the Los Alamos Meson Physics Facility. Patients treated with pions alone received 21–41 Gy, with a subset receiving combination photon/pion irradiation. LC was 0% in all patients [62].

The Lawrence Berkeley Laboratory conducted one randomized trial of helium-ion radiotherapy in LAPC in 1988, comparing 60 Gy photon therapy versus 60–70 GyE of helium. Both groups survival was 6.5 months in the photon arm, and 7.8 months in the helium-ion arm, with 21% and 27% of patients experiencing moderate-to-severe GI toxicity [63].

Collectively, particle irradiation for pancreatic cancer has demonstrated unique promise, with significant achievements in LC noted using the heavy-ion beam. Randomized trials are forthcoming.

18.4 Colorectal and Recurrent Rectal Cancer

Colorectal cancer encompasses two distinct clinical entities with different standard treatment regimens, and the use of particle therapy in both is uncommon relative to other GI cancers. Conventional colon cancer treatment includes surgical resection with adjuvant chemotherapy without radiotherapy, while rectal cancer includes chemoradiation followed by total mesenteric resection, with ongoing evaluation of promising "watch and wait" results in organ preservation [64,65]. To our knowledge, particle therapy has not been used in colon cancer.

Interest has focused on the utilization of particulate irradiation to reduce toxicity in treating rectal cancers, particularly with bulky disease. RT and chemotherapy improve sphincter preservation, LC, and survival, and standard of care for stage II or III rectal adenocarcinoma includes neoadjuvant chemoradiation with 50.4 Gy in 28 fractions with 5-FU or capecitabine, total mesorectal excision, then adjuvant FOLFOX for 4-6 months. LC and survival remain poor for unresectable T4 or cT3 tumors with lateral extension or involvement of the mesorectal fascia. Postoperative recurrence rates are still 5–15%, with 5-year survival of locally recurrent rectal cancer (LRRC) treated with conventional chemoradiation ranging from 20% to 25%; surgical re-resection, if possible, may improve rates to 30–45% [22].

Conventional radiotherapy results in 25+% of patients developing grade 3+ acute toxicity during neoadjuvant treatment [66]. PBT has demonstrated dosimetric advantages over photon irradiation, reducing dosage to bone marrow, small bowel, and bladder, and potentially offering dose escalation

so as to increase possibility of achieving clinical complete response given modern "wait and see" nonsurgical approaches to disease management. Informed by preclinical data demonstrating severe hypoxia in locally recurrent disease, CIRT has been employed with the aim of achieving improved LC in recurrent disease, as well as improving long-term survival, leveraging its high LET and lower OER (Table 18.5) [4]. Recommended target volumes are discussed in Table 18.6.

18.4.1 Treatment Planning

There are no current standardized methodologies for treatment of colorectal disease using proton or carbon-ion irradiation; predominantly, recurrent (colo)rectal cancer has been treated, and a majority of this has been limited to case series. The largest proton cohort, reported by Ogi and colleagues, delivered 70 Gy RBE in 25 fractions to 23 patients with LRRC. This was an abstract update to an original publication by Hamauchi and colleagues [67], itself appearing to be an abstract without details of planning. From Berman et al.'s seven-patient case series, the method involved a double-scattering proton beam, and adjustments to the beam-design algorithm for range uncertainties. They used the water equivalent path length (WEPL) to the CTV distal margin plus 3.5% of the WEPL to account for CT uncertainty, with an additional 3 mm to account for uncertainty in the beam energy, beamline component thickness, and range compensator design, with additional changes made to the compensator to ensure proper coverage [68]. CTV included the recurrent tumor or tumor bed with a margin left to the judgement of the treating physician, and including all diseases noted on PET/CT at time of simulation. A PTV accounting for lateral uncertainties of 0.5–1 cm was employed.

For carbon-ion irradiation of recurrent rectal cancer, the GTV incorporates all diseases seen on CT, MRI, and PET images. The CTV incorporates a 5-mm margin, with internal margin referencing 4D CT imaging for evaluation of tumor movement. The PTV summates the CTV plus internal margin, plus additional setup margin as needed. A dose of 73.6 Gy (RBE) is thereby administered in 16 fractions over 4 weeks (Table 18.7).

18.4.2 Proton

Dosimetric studies have demonstrated significant theoretical reduction in toxicity with PBT in comparison to conventional irradiation modalities [69]. However, clinical outcomes for the use of PBT in colorectal disease remain limited.

Preliminary evidence has been published, predominantly from Japan. In 2015 Mokutani and colleagues at Osaka University retrospectively evaluated two LRRC patients treated with proton irradiation and one with CIRT at Hyogo Ion Beam Medical Center. One patient underwent abdomin-

Table 18.5 Particle therapy for colorectal cancer.

Study	Modality	Patient number	Stage	Median dose (fx)	Local control			Overall survival		
					1 year	3 years	5 years	1 year	3 years	5 years
Mokutani 2015	Proton	2	LRRC	74 GyE/37 fx	100%	50%		100%	100%	50%
	Carbon	1	LRRC	70.4 GyE/16 fx	100%	100%				
Berman 2014	Combination photon/proton	7	LRRC	Photon 50.4 Gy, proton 45–64.8 Gy (RBE)	6 complete response, 2 local recurrence@14 mo			~57%		
Murata 2016	Proton	1	LRRC	67.5 GyE/25 fx	Partial response for 25 months achieved					
Ogi 2018	Proton	23	LRRC	70 Gy RBE/25 fx			39.00%			47.60%
Kawamura 2019	Proton	4	Adjuvant					75%	25%	
Yamada 2016	Carbon	180	LRRC	67.2–73.6 Gy (RBE)			88% (high dose)			59% (high dose)
Shiba 2019 (GUNMA 0801)	Carbon	28	LRRC	73.6 Gy (RBE)/16 fx		86%			92%	
Shinoto 2019	Carbon	224	LRRC	70.4–73.6 Gy (RBE)/16 fx		93%	88%		73%	51%
Shinoto 2016	Carbon	23	LRRC Post-RT Salvage	70.4 GyE/16 fx				83%	65%	
Cai 2020	Carbon	25	LRRC	48–72 Gy (RBE)	High dose: 100%	High dose: 100%		82.90%	65.10%	
Clinical trials										
Proton										
PBT Reirradiation of LRRC	NCT03098108	Samsung Medical Center	LRRC	70.4 Gy (RBE) in 16 fx to GTV, 44.8 to CTV, with capecitabine ± resection or spacer insertion						
Phase II Dose-escalated PBT for pelvic recurrence from rectal cancer	NCT04695782	University of Aarhus		Neoadjuvant PBT 55 Gy (RBE)/44 fx, twice daily, vs. definitive PBT 57.5–65 Gy (RBE) in 46–52 fx, twice daily						
PRORECT: Preoperative Short-Course Radiation Therapy with PROtons Compared to Photons in High-Risk RECTal Cancer	NCT04525989	Karolinska		5 Gy/5 fx PBT vs. 5 Gy/5 fx photon, with CAPOX and surgery						
Carbon										
PANDORA-01: Recurrent and inoperable rectal cancer	NCT02672449	Heidelberg	Recurrent and inoperable rectal cancer	Dose Escalation (36–54 GyE in 3 GyE fractions)						

LRRC = Locally recurrent rectal cancer, either unresectable or patients refused surgery.

Table 18.6 Recommended target volumes and radiation doses for treatment of recurrent rectal cancer

Volume	Proton	Carbon
Gross tumor volume	All gross disease	All gross disease
Clinical target volume	To determination of treating physician, with 3.5% of WEPL to distal edge of CTV plus 3-mm included	5-mm margin
Planning target volume	Additional 0.5–1 cm for lateral uncertainties	CTV + internal margin for movement + any additional setup margin felt needed
Dose	61.2 Gy (RBE)	73.6 Gy (RBE)
Reference	Berman et al. [68]	Shiba et al. [78]

WEPL = Water equivalent path length.

operineal excision in 2002, recurring in 2004 with tegafur-uracil administered for 2 years before receiving PBT with acute grade 1 dermatitis, receiving 74 GyE in 37 fractions in 2006. Distant metastasis was noted in 2008 with local recurrence, ultimately succumbing to disease in 2012. A second patient underwent low anterior resection in 2005, with local recurrence 6 years later. He received 74 GyE in 37 fractions in 2012 and had remained tumor free at time of publication in 2015. A third case underwent endoscopic mucosal resection, requiring additional surgical treatment which was refused. He received

CIRT (70.4 GyE in 16 fractions), with distant but no local recurrence. Murata and colleagues at Suita Municipal Hospital similarly reported a single case in which rectal cancer recurred 8.5 years after primary resection, with interval distant metastasis [70]. About 67.5 GyE in 25 fractions were delivered, with partial response achieved for 2 years and 1 month.

Berman and colleagues at the University of Pennsylvania reported in 2014 a preliminary cohort of seven patients with LRRC who received PBT to 6,120 cGy (RBE) (range 4,500–6,480 cGy), following a median prior photon dose of 5,040 cGy

Table 18.7 Particle therapy for anal cancer

Study	Modality	Patient number	Stage	Median dose (fx)	Local control			Overall survival		
					1 year	3 years	5 years	1 year	3 years	5 years
Ie 2014	Proton	1	Recurrent	70 Gy (RBE)/25 fx			100%			100%
Wo 2019	Proton + chemotherapy	25	T1-4 N0-3	T1-2N0: 50.4 Gy CTV, 42 Gy elective LNs	100%			87%		
				T3 + N +: 54 Gy CTV, 50.4–54 Gy involved LN, 45 Gy elective LNs						
Clinical trials										
LET-optimized IMPT with 5-FU and cisplatin for stage I–III anal cancer	NCT03690921		MD Anderson							
SWANCA: Swedish Anal Carcinoma Study	NCT04462042		Umeå University	Randomized photon vs. proton irradiation						
IMPT for anal cancer	NCT03018418		University of Cincinnati	50.4–54 CGE in 28–30 fx, nodal volumes 42–54 CGE, with 5-FU and mitomycin						

[68]. With a median follow-up of 14 months, there were three acute grade 3 and three late grade 4 toxicities; four patients were alive at time of follow-up. Six had a metabolic complete response, with two subsequently experiencing local recurrence. Three patients had complete pain resolution, and three partial.

Ogi and colleagues at the Shizuoka General Hospital Cancer Center updated Hamauchi and colleagues in 2018 [67] with an abstracted retrospective evaluation of 23 patients with LRRC who received PBT, involving patients with a single lesion who refused radical surgical therapy or were otherwise unable to undergo surgery [71]. About 70 Gy (RBE) was delivered in 25 fractions. At a median of 28.9 months, 5-year OS and LC were 47.6% and 39.0%, respectively, with 15 patients experiencing recurrence or progression. Ten patients (43.4%) demonstrated regrowth at the proton beam irradiation site. Three patients experienced late grade 3 adverse events (2× ileum fistula, 1× urinary tract obstruction).

Kawamura and colleagues reported on four patients undergoing PBT following surgical debulking [72]. During the debulking procedure, the tumor was wrapped in omentum, serving as a makeshift spacer to enable irradiation. Three of the four died following distant metastasis to lungs or lymph nodes at 11, 24, and 31 months, respectively, with one remaining alive without recurrence at 43 months.

Numerous trials have evaluated proton irradiation for oligometastatic liver disease involving CRC. Colbert and colleagues in 2017 retrospectively evaluated five patients with bilateral metastases treated with entire right hemiliver ablative irradiation, with four patients receiving a biologic equivalent dose greater than 89.6 Gy with either partial or complete radiographic response. Of these, two patients died of distant progression, and two were alive at time of review [73]. Hong and colleagues published a single-arm phase II study (Trial NCT01239381) giving 89 patients with limited extrahepatic disease, 800 mL or greater of uninvolved liver, and without cirrhosis (or were Child–Pugh *A*) PBT to one to four liver metastases of 30–50 GyE in five fractions, dependent on effective volume to be irradiated. Thirty four of these metastases constituted colorectal cancer. One- and 3-year LC were 71.9% and 61.2%, respectively, with no grade 3+ toxicity noted [74]. Kang and colleagues at the Loma Linda University Medical Center in 2018 published a phase I study on maximum tolerated hypofractionated proton dose for liver metastasis, treating nine patients up to a dose of 60 Gy. No dose-limiting toxicity was noted, with no grade 3 or higher adverse events [75]. Notably, two patients experienced local recurrence and were re-irradiated without escalated toxicity noted.

Three trials are ongoing in South Korea evaluating PBT with concurrent chemotherapy for previously irradiated LRRC. One, a single-arm prospective study at Samsung Medical Center (Trial NCT03098108) plans a dose of 70.4 Gy (RBE) in 16 fractions to the GTV with 44.8 Gy (RBE) to the CTV along with concurrent capecitabine and provisions for resection and

spacer insertion. Two studies based at the National Cancer Center in Korea are prospective single-organ phase II clinical trials evaluating 7,200 cGy in 15 fractions of proton irradiation for pulmonary (Trial NCT03566355) or liver (Trial NCT03577665) metastases from colorectal cancer. A prospective phase II nonrandomized observational study of dose-escalated PBT for pelvic recurrences from rectal cancer at the University of Aarhus (Trial NCT04695782) was posted in 2021, planning an enrollment of 65 patients to one of two arms: (1) neoadjuvant PBT with 55 Gy (RBE) in 44 fractions, delivered twice daily, or (2) definitive PBT of 57.5–65 Gy (RBE) in 46–52 fractions, include R0-resection and 1-year LC, with an estimated 7.5 years until study completion. The Preoperative Short-Course Radiation Therapy with PROtons Compared to Photons in High-Risk RECTal Cancer (PRORECT) trial at Karolinska (Trial NCT04525989) proposes an enrollment of 254 participants randomized to either 5 Gy in 5 fractions PBT or 5 Gy in 5 fractions photon irradiation. Patients will receive at least four courses of CAPOX, with plan for surgery between weeks 17 and 20.

There do not appear to be any current trials evaluating PBT in colon cancer at time of writing.

18.4.3 Carbon Ion

Heavy-ion irradiation of rectal cancer occurs predominantly in the recurrent or inoperative setting, with the majority of disease surgically resected. A representative treatment dose distribution is shown in Figure 18.3.

Initial therapy for LRRC began at NIRS in 2001. Yamada and colleagues demonstrated the potential for CIRT for pelvic recurrence of rectal cancer, conducting a phase I/II dose-escalation study on 180 patients with 186 lesions accrued between April 2001 and August 2012 [76]. Seventy-one relapses occurred in the presacral region, with 82 in the pelvic sidewalls, 28 in the perineum, and 5 near the colorectal anastomosis. Treatment consisted of 16 fractions in 4 weeks with a total dose between 67.2 and 73.6 Gy (RBE) administered. About 73.6 Gy (RBE) resulted in no grade 3+ acute reactions, with 5-year LC and OS at this dose level of 88% and 59%, respectively. These compared favorably with contemporary 5-year survival rates with conventional RT and re-resection of 0–40%. Notably, no difference in survival was observed between those patients who did and did not receive chemotherapy.

Shinoto and colleagues, as well as Isozaki and colleagues, have noted that during initial trialing for CIRT in LRRC many were excluded due to presence of GI tract in the irradiation field. As such, at NIRS, a surgical spacer is implanted so as to separate the GI tract from target tumor, with equivalent results noted with and without spacer [4,77]. Modern data suggest a slight increased risk of pelvic infection in treatment paradigms incorporating the spacer. A new trial has been initiated at NIRS/QST to remove irradiated large

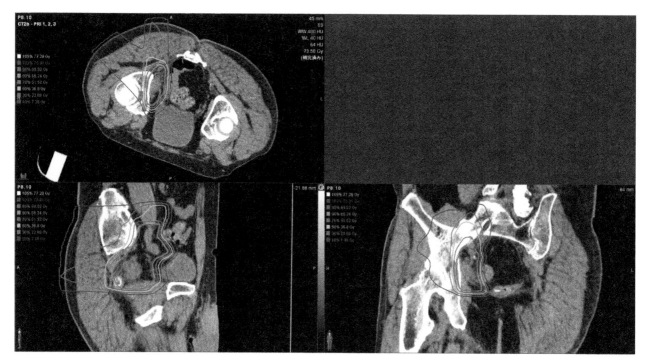

Figure 18.3 Representative recurrent rectal treatment plan with CIRT.

and small bowel shortly after CIRT, instead of doing the spacer procedure [22].

The GUNMA 0801 prospective study at the University of Gunma evaluated rectal cancer patients treated with primary curative intent therapy to a dose of 73.6 Gy (RBE) in 16 fractions, encompassing 28 patients. At a median follow-up of 38.9 months, 3-year OS and LC were 92% and 86%, respectively. No patients developed grade 3+ acute toxicities, while two patients developed late grade 3 pelvic infections [78].

J-CROS conducted a pooled retrospective evaluation of patients treated with 70.4 Gy (RBE) or 73.6 Gy (RBE) in 16 fractions, evaluating 224 patients treated across 3 institutions in Japan. At a median follow-up of 62 months, 3- and 5-year OS were 73% and 51%, respectively, with LC of 93% and 88%. Three patients experienced grade 3 acute toxicity and 12 patients late toxicity, predominantly pelvic infection.

CIRT has demonstrated unique promise in pelvic re-irradiation, offering palliation of symptoms with improved LC. Standard treatment generally involves preoperative chemoradiation to 50+ Gy followed by total mesorectal excision, limiting the potential for further conventional irradiation. Shinoto and colleagues reported on 23 patients treated with 70.4 GyE in 16 fractions who had received prior pelvic irradiation. Grade 3 toxicities occurred in six patients, with major late toxicities predominantly involving peripheral neuropathy and infection. One- and 3-year OS were 83% and 65%, respectively [77].

Cai and colleagues at the SPHIC published their institutional experience in mid-2020, evaluating 25 patients with unresectable LRRC. At a median follow-up of 19.6 months and median dose of 72 Gy (RBE) (range 48–75.6 Gy [RBE]), LC at 1 and 2 years were 90.4% and 71.8%; notably, for nine patients receiving less than 66 Gy (RBE), LC was 76.2% and 30.5%, respectively. In the high-dose cohort, LC was 100% at 2 years. OS at 1 and 2 years were 82.9% and 65.1%, respectively, with no grade 3+ acute toxicity. Three grade 3 late toxicities were reported: one each for gastrointestinal toxicity, neuropathy, and pelvic infection [79].

At HIT, Combs and colleagues initiated the PANDORA-01 trial (Trial NCT01528683) in 2012, a phase I/II dose-escalation CIRT trial for recurrent and inoperable rectal cancer. The protocol has been published, involving increasing doses from 36 to 54 GyE given in 3 GyE fractions, in the setting of patients having received 20–60 Gy of photon irradiation during their primary treatment course. Results are still forthcoming [80].

Though substantial clinical evidence demonstrates the tumoricidal capacity of CIRT in recurrent rectal cancer, additional laboratory evidence has demonstrated the *in-vitro* and *in-vivo* capacity of combination chemo(carbon)radiotherapy on destroying colorectal cancer stem cells. Koom and colleagues evaluated human colorectal cancer cell lines HCT116 and HT29, demonstrating a synergistic, dose-dependent response to CIRT cell killing effect when combined with 5-FU. Though CIRT monotherapy-induced expression of apoptotic and autophagy-related genes (*Bax*, *Bcl2*, *Beclin1*, *ATG7*), combination therapy further enhanced this response, while CIRT served to disrupt the spheroid-forming capacity of CD133+ cell subpopulations [81].

With regard to colon cancer, to our knowledge no trials incorporating heavy-ion radiotherapy have been performed to date. Makishima and colleagues conducted a retrospective trial evaluating single-fraction CIRT for colorectal metastasis to the liver, performed as a dose-escalation study. Thirty-one patients were enrolled in the study, with 29 receiving single-fraction CIRT, with dose escalated from 36 Gy (RBE) to 58 Gy (RBE). Dose-limiting toxicity was not observed, but at 53 Gy (RBE) two patients with disease lying close to the hepatic portal region experienced late grade 3 liver toxicity due to biliary obstruction. Escalation to 58 Gy (RBE) was limited to those patients with peripheral disease. Three-year OS was 78%, with LC of 82% in doses of 53 Gy (RBE) or greater; lower doses had LC of 28% [82]. Isozaki and colleagues further evaluated CIRT for treatment of isolated para-aortic lymph node recurrence from colorectal cancer [83], with 52.8 Gy (RBE) in 12 fractions achieving a LC rate at 2- and 3 years of 70.1%, and 2- and 3-year OS of 83.3% and 63%, respectively. No grade 3+ adverse events occurred. Ebner and colleagues noted an abscopal-like event amongst these cases, likely the first reported in the literature for colorectal cancer [84].

18.4.4 Neutron and Other Particles

Neutron irradiation has been explored in rectal cancer, though results have been limited. Batterman in 1982 reported a pilot study employing a six-field neutron treatment plan for inoperable or recurrent rectal cancer. Twenty-five patients were enrolled, receiving 17 or 19 Gy in 20 fractions with neutrons. Though toxicity was superior to two-field irradiation, OS was at best comparable to 50 Gy photon irradiation [85,86]. Duncan and colleagues followed in 1987 with two randomized trials on inoperable and recurrent rectal tumors in Edinburgh, with a statistically insignificant increase in LC. OS did not differ between populations, though neutron therapy yielded increased skin toxicity [87].

Combination therapy achieved some measure of improvement: Eising et al. published an interim analysis of combination photon/fast neutron therapy for rectal cancer recurrence in 1989, evaluating 20 patients with either residual disease following surgery (2) or with recurrence (18) [88]. Thirty to 40 Gy of photons in 2 Gy fractions were combined with 5–10 Gy of neutrons at 0.7–1.6 Gy, across three to five treatment fields. At 9 months, pain relief was achieved in 73% of patients, and 56% OS noted in the setting of six patients presenting with distant metastasis at the time of treatment. Side effects were limited.

The conformal nature of particle irradiation offers unique advantage when treating locoregional recurrent disease within the gastrointestinal tract, including enabling repeated reirradiation of recurrent disease without intolerable toxicity. Further evaluation of reirradiation is needed, though CIRT appears to show unique promise.

18.5 Anal Cancer

Distinct from colorectal cancer, squamous cell carcinoma of the anal canal is definitively treated with 5-FU and mitomycin-C in combination with radiotherapy, while residual and recurrent disease is managed with surgery [89]. Early stage disease generally offers good locoregional control with relapse-free survival and colostomy-free survival notably lower in advanced, T3–4 disease [90]. With conventional radiotherapy, generally 60 Gy or higher, toxicity is a significant barrier to treatment with hematologic toxicity amplified by conventional irradiation of the pelvic bone marrow in the setting of chemotherapy; in the Intergroup trial, for instance, 18% of patients developed grade 4+ hematologic toxicity along with dermatitis secondary to perianal irradiation [91].

In conventional radiotherapy, RTOG 0529 [92] demonstrated promise for dose-painted IMRT in reducing treatment toxicity, generating significant sparing of acute grade 2+ hematologic and grade 3+ dermatologic and gastrointestinal toxicity. This informs forays into the usage of PBT, with the principal goal of reducing toxicity and potential dose escalation.

18.5.1 Treatment Planning

Multiple proton irradiation methodologies are under evaluation at this time. In the published literature, one methodology by Wo and colleagues incorporates the guidelines of RTOG 0529 and with specific dose–volume targets for small bowel, large bowel, femoral heads, iliac crests, external genitalia, and bladder, available at https://doi.org/10.1016/j.ijrobp.2019.04.040. Per RTOG 0529, oral and IV contrast were used to better allow visualization of bowel, iliac, and inguinal vessels, with a radio-opaque marker placed at the anal verge with wire to outline the caudad extent of the anal tumor. All tissues were contoured on CT slices, with GTV contoured using a combination of examination, imaging, and endoscopic findings. GTV_A encompassed the primary anal tumor, $GTVN_{50}$ the metastatic nodal regions ≤3 cm, and $GTVN_{54}$ the metastatic nodal regions >3 cm. The CTV encompassed the GTV plus areas of potential disease, with a 2.5-cm and 1-cm expansion applied to the primary and nodal GTVs, subject to manual editing and review. Elective nodal CTVs including mesorectum, presacrum, bilateral internal and external iliac, and bilateral inguinal nodal areas were additionally included. PTVs constituted a 1-cm expansion around all CTVs and were edited solely to avoid overlap with the skin. T1-2N0 disease received 50.4 Gy to primary CTV, 42 Gy to elective LNs; T3 + or N + disease received 54 Gy to primary CTV, 50.4–54 Gy to involved LN, and 45 Gy to elective LNs.

No definitive treatment methodology exists for CIRT in anal cancer.

18.5.2 Proton

Dosimetric studies for scanning PBT have demonstrated reduced mean doses to key organs of interest within the pelvis beyond matched plans with IMRT and VMAT [93,94]. Pencil-beam scanning PBT via oblique posterior fields favorably compared with 7-field IMRT plans, reducing V15 for small bowel from 151 to 81 cm^3 with IMRT and PBT, respectively. This has been verified in additional studies, with PBT showing reduced dose across numerous OARs [69,95]. However, owing to the geometry employed with PBT, lumbosacral bone marrow dose was notably higher.

Clinical translation of these dosimetry studies is limited to date, with initial studies focusing principally on recurrent disease. Initial data includes a 2014 case report on locally recurrent anorectal cancer by Ie and colleagues at Shizuoka Cancer Center Hospital [96]. One patient treated with 70 Gy (RBE) in 25 fractions over 5 weeks experienced a clinically complete, durable response lasting 7 years.

Wo and colleagues conducted a multi-institutional pilot feasibility study on definitive concurrent chemoradiation, combining PBT with 5-FU and mitomycin-c for T1-4N03 squamous cell carcinoma of the anal canal (Trial NCT01858025). RTOG 0529 RT schema were used: T1-2N0 disease received 50.4 Gy to primary CTV, 42 Gy to elective LNs; T3+ or N+ disease received 54 Gy to primary CTV, 50.4–54 Gy to involved LN, and 45 Gy to elective LNs. Twenty-five patients were enrolled between 2014 and 2017, with 23 patients completing the protocol. Grade 3+ radiation dermatitis was 24% at median follow-up of 17.6 months, with 1-year LC and OS of 100% and 87%, respectively. Compared to DP-IMRT, grade 3+ hematologic toxicity decreased 24% while grade 3+ dermatologic toxicity increased 4%, while GI toxicity increased 71%. The authors advocated for study in a larger population [97].

Three trials are under development on clinicaltrials.gov incorporating proton irradiation. One trial based at MD Anderson Cancer Center in collaboration with the National Cancer Institute incorporates LET-optimized IMPT with standard chemotherapy (fluorouracil, cisplatin) for the treatment of newly diagnosed stage I–III anal cancer (Trial NCT03690921). The primary outcome is acute grade 3+ GI, GU, or hematologic toxicity. Recruitment began in 2018. The Swedish Anal Carcinoma Study, termed SWANCA, is a comparative study under development at Umeå University (NCT04462042) which will be a randomized phase II study of 100 patients randomized to either photon or proton irradiation. Recruitment has yet to begin. A pilot study of IMPT with goal of reducing toxicity in anal cancer is in recruitment at the University of Cincinnati (Trial NCT03018418) and aims to identify the rates of grade 3+ hematologic, GI, GU, or dermatological acute toxicity. About 50.4–54 CGE will be delivered in 28–30 fractions, with nodal volumes 42–54 CGE, in addition to concurrent 5-FU and mitomycin.

18.5.3 Carbon and Other Particle Radiotherapy

There is limited preclinical or clinical evidence in other forms of particulate radiotherapy. Franklin reported in 1980 on Hammersmith Hospital's experience treating ten anal cancer patients with fast neutron irradiation [98]. All patients received a temporary colostomy prior to treatment. Three patients had extension of the disease into their pelvis at time of irradiation and were treated palliatively; all died within 1 year of treatment. For the remaining seven, four were reported as having normal function without evidence of recurrence, while two developed radionecrosis and one local recurrence. A colostomy was required in one patient, and two others required abdominoperineal resection, but it was noted that the majority were able to avoid permanent colostomy.

With regard to CIRT, anal cancer is not treated at NIRS/QST; one case of metastatic anal cancer to the lung has been described, experiencing local failure at 10.7 months [99]. A dosimetric evaluation of CIRT boost for anal carcinoma was performed by Kraus and colleagues in 2017 [100], comparing recalculated CIRT boost plans with photon-boosted IMRT through 54 treatment fractions in 3 different patients. Similar dosimetric results were generated, and the authors encouraged potential clinical exploration of carbon ion in anal cancer.

Current experience with particle irradiation in anal cancer is limited, and more evidence will be needed before a recommendation can be clearly made. The results of the ongoing trials are anticipated.

18.6 Conclusion

Particle therapy has demonstrated unique promise in the treatment of gastrointestinal disease, offering improved dose distribution and consequent reductions in toxicity versus conventional radiotherapy, while also affording potential dose escalation in difficult to treat disease. Though historical trials with neutron and helium were limited, modern CIRT has appeared promising, offering the dose distribution benefits of PBT combined with the enhanced RBE of high LET irradiation. Numerous trials in gastrointestinal disease are ongoing. Notably, development of heavy-ion irradiation remains under development, particularly with regard to incorporation of LET optimization in target tumor tissue. Consequently, significant development that remains before a mature literature with robust prospective trials can be developed, or modalities with equivalent levels of development compared with one another. Based on these findings thus far, however, current results are promising for the future of particle therapy.

Bibliography

1 Curtis, S.B. (1980). The new particles and their application in medicine. In: *Advances in Radiation Protection and Dosimetry in Medicine*5–25. Lawrence Berkeley National Laboratory, Springer.

2 Halperin, E.C. (2006). Particle therapy and treatment of cancer. *Lancet Oncology* 7: 676–685.

3 Castro, J.R. and Quivey, J.M. (1977). Clinical experience and expectations with helium and heavy ion irradiation. *International Journal of Radiation Oncology, Biology, Physics* 3: 127–131.

4 Tsujii, H. , Kamada, T., Shirai, T., Noda, K., Tsuji, H., and Karasawa. (2014). Carbon-ion radiotherapy. In: *Carbon-Ion Radiother*. Springer, Japan.

5 Kamada, T. et al. (2015). Carbon ion radiotherapy in Japan: An assessment of 20 years of clinical experience. *Lancet Oncology* 16: e93–e100.

6 Loeffler, J.S. and Durante, M. (2013). Charged particle therapy – Optimization, challenges and future directions. *Nature Reviews Clinical Oncology* 10: 411–424.

7 Ohno, T. (2013). Particle radiotherapy with carbon ion beams. *EPMA Journal* 4: 9.

8 Meyer, J.J., Czito, B.G., and Willett, C.G. (2007). Particle radiation therapy for gastrointestinal malignancies. *Gastrointest. Cancer Research GCR* 1: S50–59.

9 Kovacevic, S. et al. (2009). V-79 Chinese hamster cells irradiated with antiprotons, a study of peripheral damage due to medium and long range components of the annihilation radiation. *International Journal of Radiation Oncology, Biology, Physics* 85: 1148–1156.

10 Bassler, N. et al. (2008). Antiproton radiotherapy. *Radiotherapy and Oncology. European Journal of Social Theory Radiology and Oncology* 86: 14–19.

11 Paganetti, H., Goitein, M., and Parodi, K. (2010). Spread-out antiproton beams deliver poor physical dose distributions for radiation therapy. *Radiotherapy and Oncology. European Journal of Social Theory. Radiology and Oncology* 95: 79–86.

12 Ebner, D.K., Frank, S.J., Inaniwa, T., Yamada, S., and Shirai, T. (2021). The emerging potential of multi-ion radiotherapy. *Frontier in. Oncology* 11: 624786.

13 Fossati, P., Matsufuji, N., Kamada, T., and Karger, C.P. (2018). Radiobiological issues in prospective carbon ion therapy trials. *Medical Physics* 45: e1096–e1110.

14 Ono, T. (2021). Review of clinical results of charged-particle therapy for esophageal cancer. *Esophagus, The Official journal of The Japan Esophageal Society* 18: 33–40.

15 Kole, T.P., Aghayere, O., Kwah, J., Yorke, E.D., and Goodman, K.A. (2012). Comparison of heart and coronary artery doses associated with intensity-modulated radiotherapy versus three-dimensional conformal radiotherapy for distal esophageal cancer. *International Journal of Radiation Oncology*. 83: 1580–1586.

16 Lin, S.H. et al. (2012). Propensity score-based comparison of long-term outcomes with 3-dimensional conformal radiotherapy vs intensity-modulated radiotherapy for esophageal cancer. *International Journal of Radiation Oncology* 84: 1078–1085.

17 Zhang, X. et al. (2008). Four-dimensional computed tomography-based treatment planning for intensity-modulated radiation therapy and proton therapy for distal esophageal cancer. *International Journal of Radiation Oncology-Biology-Physics* 72: 278–287.

18 Hirano, Y. et al. (2018). Dosimetric comparison between proton beam therapy and photon radiation therapy for locally advanced esophageal squamous cell carcinoma. *Radiation Oncology London England*13: 23.

19 Makishima, H. et al. (2015). Comparison of adverse effects of proton and X-ray chemoradiotherapy for esophageal cancer using an adaptive dose-volume histogram analysis. *The Journal of Radiation Research(Tokyo)* 56: 568–576.

20 Lin, S.H. et al. (2012). Proton beam therapy and concurrent chemotherapy for esophageal cancer. *International Journal of Radiation Oncology-Biology-Physics* 83: e345–351.

21 Akutsu, Y. et al. (2012). A phase I/II clinical trial of preoperative short-course carbon-ion radiotherapy for patients with squamous cell carcinoma of the esophagus: Carbon-ion therapy for esophageal cancer. *Journal of Surgical Oncology* 105: 750–755.

22 Isozaki, Y. et al. (2020). Heavy charged particles for gastrointestinal cancers. *The Journal of Gastroenterology* 11: 203–211.

23 Sugahara, S. et al. (2005). Clinical results of proton beam therapy for cancer of the esophagus. *International Journal of Radiation Oncology* 61: 76–84.

24 Takada, A. et al. (2016). Preliminary treatment results of proton beam therapy with chemoradiotherapy for stage I–III esophageal cancer. *Cancer Medicine* 5: 506–515.

25 Wang, J. et al. (2013). Predictors of postoperative complications after trimodality therapy for esophageal cancer. *International Journal of Radiation Oncology* 86: 885–891.

26 Ishikawa, H. et al. (2015). Proton beam therapy combined with concurrent chemotherapy for esophageal cancer. *Anticancer Research* 35: 1757–1762.

27 Xi, M. et al. (2017). Comparative outcomes after definitive chemoradiotherapy using proton beam therapy versus intensity modulated radiation therapy for esophageal cancer: A retrospective, single-institutional analysis. *International Journal of Radiation Oncology-Biology-Physics* 99: 667–676.

28 Ono, T., Wada, H., Ishikawa, H., Tamamura, H., and Tokumaru, S. (2020 Aug). Proton beam therapy is a safe and

effective treatment in elderly patients with esophageal squamous cell carcinoma. *Thoracic Cancer* , 11(8):2170–2177. doi: 10.1111/1759-7714.13524. Epub 2020 Jun 8. PMID: 32510875; PMCID: PMC7396394.

29 Lin, S.H. et al. (2020). Randomized Phase IIB trial of proton beam therapy versus intensity-modulated radiation therapy for locally advanced esophageal cancer. *Journal of Clinical Oncology Off. Journal American Society of Clinical Oncology* 38: 1569–1579.

30 Isozaki, Y. et al. (2018). Salvage carbon-ion radiotherapy for isolated lymph node recurrence following curative resection of esophageal cancer. *Anticancer Research* 38: 6453–6458.

31 Laramore, G.E. et al. (1983). RTOG Phase I study on fast neutron teletherapy for squamous cell carcinoma of the esophagus. *International Journal of Radiation Oncology-Biology-Physics* 9: 465–473.

32 Rawla, P., Sunkara, T., and Gaduputi, V. (2019). Epidemiology of pancreatic cancer: Global trends, etiology and risk factors. *World Journal of Oncology* 10: 10–27.

33 Ryan, D.P., Hong, T.S., and Bardeesy, N. (2014). Pancreatic adenocarcinoma. *The New England Journal of Medicine* 371: 1039–1049.

34 Oettle, H. et al. (2007). Adjuvant chemotherapy with gemcitabine vs observation in patients undergoing curative-intent resection of pancreatic cancer: A randomized controlled trial. *JAMA* 297: 267.

35 Conroy, T. *et al.* (2018). FOLFIRINOX or gemcitabine as adjuvant therapy for pancreatic cancer. *The New England Journal of Medicine* 379: 2395–2406.

36 Bouchart, C. et al. (2020). Novel strategies using modern radiotherapy to improve pancreatic cancer outcomes: Toward a new standard? *Therapeutic Advances in Medical Oncology* 12: 175883592093609.

37 Loehrer, P.J. et al. (2011). Gemcitabine alone versus gemcitabine plus radiotherapy in patients with locally advanced pancreatic cancer: An Eastern Cooperative Oncology Group trial. *Journal of Clinical Oncology Off Journal American Society of Clinical Oncology* 29: 4105–4112.

38 Sai, S. et al. (2015). Combination of carbon ion beam and gemcitabine causes irreparable DNA damage and death of radioresistant pancreatic cancer stem-like cells *in vitro* and *in vivo*. *Oncotarget* 6: 5517–5535.

39 Murphy, J.E. et al. (2019). Total neoadjuvant therapy with FOLFIRINOX in combination with losartan followed by chemoradiotherapy for locally advanced pancreatic cancer: A phase 2 clinical trial. *JAMA Oncology* 5: 1020.

40 Murphy, J.E. et al. (2018). Total neoadjuvant therapy with FOLFIRINOX followed by individualized chemoradiotherapy for borderline resectable pancreatic adenocarcinoma: A phase 2 clinical trial. *JAMA Oncology* 4: 963.

41 Hattori, Y. et al. (2017). Image-guided hypofractionated proton therapy and concurrent chemotherapy for inoperable locally advanced pancreatic cancer: Toxicities and preliminary outcomes. *International Journal of Radiation Oncology* 99: E153.

42 Shinoto, M. et al. (2013). Phase 1 trial of preoperative, short-course carbon-ion radiotherapy for patients with resectable pancreatic cancer. *Cancer* 119: 45–51.

43 Ebner, D.K. et al. (2017). Phase 1/2 trial of preoperative short-course carbon-ion radiation therapy for patients with resectable pancreatic cancer. *International Journal of Radiation Oncology-Biology-Physics* 99: S144.

44 Kawashiro, S. et al. (2018). Multi-institutional study of carbon-ion radiotherapy for locally advanced pancreatic cancer: Japan carbon-ion radiation oncology study group (J-CROS) study 1403 pancreas. *International Journal of Radiation Oncology* 101: 1212–1221.

45 Hong, T.S. et al. (2014). A phase 1/2 and biomarker study of preoperative short course chemoradiation with proton beam therapy and capecitabine followed by early surgery for resectable pancreatic ductal adenocarcinoma. *International Journal of Radiation Oncology-Biology-Physics* 89: 830–838.

46 Terashima, K. et al. (2012). A phase I/II study of gemcitabine-concurrent proton radiotherapy for locally advanced pancreatic cancer without distant metastasis. *Radiotherapy Oncology Journal of European Society of Therapy. Radiology and Oncology* 103: 25–31.

47 Takatori, K. et al. (2014). Upper gastrointestinal complications associated with gemcitabine-concurrent proton radiotherapy for inoperable pancreatic cancer. *The Journal of Gastroenterology* 49: 1074–1080.

48 Sachsman, S. *et al.* (2014). Proton therapy and concomitant capecitabine for non-metastatic unresectable pancreatic adenocarcinoma. *International Theory of Praticle Theory* 1: 692–701.

49 Liermann, J. et al. (2020). Carbon ion radiotherapy in pancreatic cancer: A review of clinical data. *Radiotherapy and Oncology* 147: 145–150.

50 Vitolo, V. et al. (2019). Preoperative chemotherapy and carbon ions therapy for treatment of resectable and borderline resectable pancreatic adenocarcinoma: A prospective, phase II, multicentre, single-arm study. *BMC Cancer* 19: 922.

51 Shinoto, M. et al. (2016). Carbon ion radiation therapy with concurrent gemcitabine for patients with locally advanced pancreatic cancer. *International Journal of Radiation Oncology-Biology-Physics* 95: 498–504.

52 Kawashiro, S. et al. (2018). Multi-institutional study of carbon-ion radiotherapy for locally advanced pancreatic cancer: Japan carbon-ion radiation oncology study group

(J-CROS) study 1403 pancreas. *International Journal of Radiation Oncology-Biology-Physics* 101: 1212–1221.

53 Kawashiro, S. et al. (2018). Carbon-ion radiotherapy for locoregional recurrence after primary surgery for pancreatic cancer. *Radiother. Oncol* 129: 101–104.

54 Kawashiro, S. et al. (2017). Dose-escalation study with respiratory-gated carbon-ion scanning radiotherapy using a simultaneous integrated boost for pancreatic cancer: Simulation with four-dimensional computed tomography. *The British Journal of Radiology* 90: 20160790.

55 Bassler, N., Jäkel, O., Søndergaard, C.S., and Petersen, J.B. (2010). Dose- and LET-painting with particle therapy. *Acta Oncol* 49: 1170–1176.

56 Inaniwa, T. et al. (2020). Experimental validation of stochastic microdosimetric kinetic model for multi-ion therapy treatment planning with helium-, carbon-, oxygen-, and neon-ion beams. *Physics in Medicine and Biology* 65: 045005.

57 Okonogi, N. (2020). et al. Dose-averaged linear energy transfer per se does not correlate with late rectal complications in carbon-ion radiotherapy. *Radiotherapy and Oncology*153, december 2020, 272–278.

58 Hagiwara, Y. et al. (2019). Influence of dose-averaged linear energy transfer on tumour control after carbon-ion radiation therapy for pancreatic cancer. *Clinical and Translational Radiation Oncology* 21: 19–24.

59 Combs, S.E. et al. (2013). Phase I study evaluating the treatment of patients with locally advanced pancreatic cancer with carbon ion radiotherapy: The PHOENIX-01 trial. *BMC Cancer* 13: 419.

60 Thomas, F.J. et al. (1989). Evaluation of neutron irradiation of pancreatic cancer. Results of a randomized radiation therapy oncology group clinical trial. *American Journal of Clinical Oncology* 12: 283–289.

61 Cohen, L. et al. (1996). Pancreatic cancer: Treatment with neutron irradiation alone and with chemotherapy. *Radiology* 200: 627–630.

62 Von Essen, C.F., Bagshaw, M.A., Bush, S.E., Smith, A.R., and Kligerman, M.M. (1987). Long-term results of pion therapy at Los Alamos. *International Journal of Radiation Oncology-Biology-Physics* 13: 1389–1398.

63 Linstadt, D. et al. (1988). Comparison of helium-ion radiation therapy and split-course megavoltage irradiation for unresectable adenocarcinoma of the pancreas. Final report of a Northern California Oncology Group randomized prospective clinical trial. *Radiology* 168: 261–264.

64 Habr-Gama, A. et al. (2004). Operative versus nonoperative treatment for stage 0 distal rectal cancer following chemoradiation therapy: Long-term results. *Transactions of the Meeting of the American Surgical Association* CXXII: 309–316.

65 Habr-Gama, A. et al. (2014). Local recurrence after complete clinical response and watch and wait in rectal cancer after neoadjuvant chemoradiation: Impact of salvage therapy on local disease control. *International Journal of Radiation Oncology* 88: 822–828.

66 Sauer, R. *et al.* (2004). Preoperative versus postoperative chemoradiotherapy for rectal cancer. *The New England Journal of Medicine* 351: 1731–1740.

67 Hamauchi, S. *et al. (2012). Safety and efficacy of proton-beam radiation therapy for patients with locally recurrent rectal cancer. Annals of Oncology* 23: xi160.

68 Berman, A.T. et al. (2014). Proton reirradiation of recurrent rectal cancer: dosimetric comparison, toxicities, and preliminary outcomes. *International Journal of Praticle Theory* 1: 2–13.

69 Vaios, E.J. and Wo, J.Y. (2020). Proton beam radiotherapy for anal and rectal cancers. *Journal of Gastrointestinal Oncology* 11: 176–186.

70 Murata, K. et al. (2016). [An 85-year-old man with lymph node metastasis of recurrent rectal cancer treated usingproton beam therapy]. *Gan To Kagaku Ryoho* 43: 1473–1475.

71 Ogi, Y. et al. (2018). Effect and safety of proton beam therapy for locally recurrent rectal cancer. *Journal of Clinical Oncology* 36: 743–743.

72 Kawamura, H. et al. (2019). [Four patients who underwent proton beam therapy after debulking surgery and omental wrapping of the residual tumor as a spacer for unresectable local recurrence of rectal cancer]. *Gan To Kagaku Ryoho* 46: 79–82.

73 Colbert, L.E., Cloyd, J.M., Koay, E.J., Crane, C.H., and Vauthey, J.-N. (2017). Proton beam radiation as salvage therapy for bilateral colorectal liver metastases not amenable to second-stage hepatectomy. *Surgery* 161: 1543–1548.

74 Hong, T.S. et al. (2017). Phase II study of proton-based stereotactic body radiation therapy for liver metastases: Importance of tumor genotype. *The Journal of the National Cancer Institute* 109.

75 Kang, J.I. et al. (2018). A phase I trial of Proton stereotactic body radiation therapy for liver metastases. *Journal of Gastrointestinal Oncology* 10: 112–117.

76 Yamada, S. et al. (2016). Carbon-ion radiation therapy for pelvic recurrence of rectal cancer. *International Journal of Radiation Oncology – Biology - Physics* 96: 93–101.

77 Shinoto, M., Ebner, D.K., and Yamada, S. (2016). Particle radiation therapy for gastrointestinal cancers. *Current Oncology Reports* 18: 17.

78 Shiba, S. et al. (2019). Prospective Observational Study of High-Dose Carbon-Ion Radiotherapy for Pelvic Recurrence of Rectal Cancer (GUNMA 0801. *Frontier in Oncology* 9: 702.

79 Cai, X. et al. (2020). The role of carbon ion radiotherapy for unresectable locally recurrent rectal cancer: A single institutional experience. *Radiation Oncology (London, England)* 15: 209.

80 Combs, S.E. et al. (2012). Phase I/II trial evaluating carbon ion radiotherapy for the treatment of recurrent rectal cancer: The PANDORA-01 trial. *BMC Cancer* 12: 137.

81 Koom, W.S. et al. (2020). Superior effect of the combination of carbon-ion beam irradiation and 5-fluorouracil on colorectal cancer stem cells in vitro and in vivo. *Oncology Targets Therapy* 13: 12625–12635.

82 Makishima, H. et al. (2019). Single fraction carbon ion radiotherapy for colorectal cancer liver metastasis: A dose escalation study. *Cancer Science* 110: 303–309.

83 Isozaki, Y. et al. (2017). Carbon-ion radiotherapy for isolated para-aortic lymph node recurrence from colorectal cancer. *Journal of Surgical Oncology* 116: 932–938.

84 Ebner, D.K., Kamada, T., and Yamada, S. (2017). Abscopal effect in recurrent colorectal cancer treated with carbon-ion radiation therapy: 2 case reports. *Advanced Radiational Oncology* 2: 333–338.

85 Battermann, J.J. (1982). Results of d + T fast neutron irradiation on advanced tumors of bladder and rectum. *International Journal of Radiation Oncology – Biology - Physics* 8: 2159–2164.

86 Battermann, J.J., Hart, G.A., and Breur, K. (1981). Dose-effect relations for tumour control and complication rate after fast neutron therapy for pelvic-tumours. *British Journal of Surgery* 54: 899–904.

87 Duncan, W. et al. (1987). Results of two randomised clinical trials of neutron therapy in rectal adenocarcinoma. *Radiotherapy Oncology Journal of European Society of Therapy. Radiology and Oncology* 8: 191–198.

88 E, E., R, P., U, H. & E, S (1990). Neutron therapy (dT, 14 MeV) for recurrence of rectal cancer: Interim analysis from Münster. *Strahlenther. Onkol. Organ Dtsch. Rontgengesellschaft Al* 166: 90–94.

89 Northover, J. et al. (2010). Chemoradiation for the treatment of epidermoid anal cancer: 13-year follow-up of the first randomised UKCCCR Anal Cancer Trial (ACT I. *British Journal of Surgery* 102: 1123–1128.

90 Gunderson, L.L. et al. (2012). Long-term update of US GI intergroup RTOG 98-11 phase III trial for anal carcinoma: Survival, relapse, and colostomy failure with concurrent chemoradiation involving fluorouracil/mitomycin versus fluorouracil/cisplatin. *Journal of Clinical Oncology Off. Journal of American Society of Clinicaal Oncology* 30: 4344–4351.

91 Flam, M. et al. (1996). Role of mitomycin in combination with fluorouracil and radiotherapy, and of salvage chemoradiation in the definitive nonsurgical treatment of epidermoid carcinoma of the anal canal: Results of a phase III randomized intergroup study. *Journal of Clinical Oncology* 14: 2527–2539.

92 Kachnic, L.A. et al. (2013). RTOG 0529: A Phase 2 evaluation of dose-painted intensity modulated radiation therapy in combination with 5-fluorouracil and mitomycin-C for the reduction of acute morbidity in carcinoma of the anal canal. *International Journal of Radiation Oncology* 86: 27–33.

93 Anand, A. et al. (2015). Scanning proton beam therapy reduces normal tissue exposure in pelvic radiotherapy for anal cancer. *Radiotherapy and Oncology Journal of the European Society for Radiotherapy and Oncology* 117: 505–508.

94 Kronborg, C. et al. (2018). Prospective evaluation of acute toxicity and patient reported outcomes in anal cancer and plan optimization. *Radiotherapy and Oncology* 128: 375–379.

95 Ojerholm, E. et al. (2015). Pencil-beam scanning proton therapy for anal cancer: A dosimetric comparison with intensity-modulated radiotherapy. *Acta Oncologica* 54: 1209–1217.

96 Ie, M. et al. (2014). [Complete response of locally recurrent anorectal cancer to proton beam therapy alone–a case report]. *Gan To Kagaku Ryoho* 41: 2623–2625.

97 Wo, J.Y. et al. (2019). Pencil beam scanning proton beam chemoradiation therapy with 5-fluorouracil and mitomycin-C for definitive treatment of carcinoma of the anal canal: A multi-institutional pilot feasibility study. *International Journal of Radiation Oncology* 105: 90–95.

98 Franklin, A. (1980). Anal cancer treated by fast neutron radiation. *British Journal of Surgery* 67: 469–472.

99 Ebner, D.K. et al. (2017). Respiration-gated fast-rescanning carbon-ion radiotherapy. *Japanese Journal of Clinical Oncology* 47: 80–83.

100 Kraus, K.M., Pfaffenberger, A., Jäkel, O., Debus, J., and Sterzing, F. (2016). Evaluation of dosimetric robustness of carbon ion boost therapy for anal carcinoma. *International Theory of Praticle Theory* 3: 382–391.

19

Hepatobiliary Cancers

Krishan R. Jethwa[1], Christopher L. Hallemeier[2]

[1] Department of Therapeutic Radiology, Yale University School of Medicine, New Haven, CT
[2] Department of Radiation Oncology, Mayo Clinic, Rochester, MN

Corresponding authors: Krishan R. Jethwa, MD, Department of Therapeutic Radiology, Yale University School of Medicine, New Haven, CT. 15 York Street, PO Box 208040, New Haven, CT, 0652-0. Christopher L. Hallemeier, MD, Department of Radiation Oncology, Mayo Clinic, 200 First St. SW, Rochester, MN 55905.

TABLE OF CONTENTS

Principles and Practice of Particle Therapy, First Edition. Edited by Timothy D. Malouff and Daniel M. Trifiletti.
© 2022 John Wiley & Sons Ltd. Published 2022 by John Wiley & Sons Ltd.

19.1 Introduction

Hepatobiliary cancers include hepatocellular carcinoma (HCC), gallbladder cancer (GBCA), extrahepatic cholangiocarcinoma (EHCC), and intrahepatic cholangiocarcinoma (IHCC). Hepatobiliary cancers are the fifth most common cancer and second leading cause of cancer-related death worldwide with an estimated 1,060,500 cases and 946,718 deaths in 2018 [1]. Within the United States alone, there will be an estimated 54,790 cases and 34,250 deaths during 2020 [2]. The preferred treatment for patients with localized hepatobiliary cancers is surgical resection; however, the minority of patients are suitable for surgery due to the extent of disease at diagnosis or underlying comorbidities, including baseline liver dysfunction. Radiotherapy is emerging as a treatment option for patients, largely driven by the development of more conformal radiotherapy technologies which facilitate the delivery of tumoricidal radiotherapy doses while sparing adjacent normal tissues.

Charged particle therapy, namely proton therapy or carbon-ion radiotherapy, is one such technology that has a distinct physical advantage over photon-based techniques as it is capable of delivering the same radiotherapy dose to the target volume but with significantly lower entrance and exit doses of radiation passing through surrounding normal organs. A charged particle, such as a proton or carbon ion, deposits small amounts of energy along its entrance path; however, as the particle slows down, the energy deposition rises rapidly and results in most of the energy being deposited at the end of the ionization track. This peak of the deposition of energy at a specified depth is known as the Bragg peak. These physical characteristics and dosimetric phenomena are particularly pertinent for patients with liver tumors, as the most critical normal tissue is the uninvolved liver which is highly sensitive to even low-intermediate radiation doses [3–6]. Therefore, particle therapy has the potential to reduce the risk of radiation-induced liver disease (RILD) without compromising the ability to deliver tumoricidal radiation doses.

While multiple charged particle techniques have been investigated, proton therapy and carbon-ion radiotherapy (CIRT) form the vast majority of data for patients with liver tumors and will be specifically discussed. In terms of physical dose distribution, these modalities are highly similar but with slightly lower entrance doses for CIRT. Biologically, there are considerable differences. The relative biological effectiveness (RBE) is thought to be dependent on multiple factors including radiation dose per fraction, oxygen concentration, tissue radiosensitivity, and the specific clinical or biological end point [7–10]. The current clinical convention for proton therapy is to use a fixed RBE value of 1.1 in order to correct the physical dose relative to photon therapy, although it is hypothesized to be higher near the Bragg peak. Considering the mod-estly increased RBE of 1.1 for proton therapy, the potential benefits when compared with photon techniques are predominately due to the physical dosimetric advantages rather than biologic differences.

The RBE of carbon ions is estimated to be between 2 and 5. It is relatively higher than proton therapy due to the higher linear energy transfer, and comparatively more DNA double-strand breaks which are difficult to repair and often "lethal" events, produced by heavier ions [11–13]. While these radiobiological characteristics of carbon ions may be most beneficial for radioresistant tumor histologies, the slightly more favorable dose distribution of CIRT compared with proton therapy combined with these biological aspects could theoretically further improve the therapeutic ratio.

Herein, we discuss the evaluation, management, role of radiotherapy, and the evolving role of particle therapy for patients with hepatobiliary cancers.

19.2 Hepatocellular Carcinoma

19.2.1 Epidemiology and Etiology

The most common primary liver cancers are HCC, which comprises 7–5% of cases, and IHCC, which comprises 1–5% of cases [1,2,14,15]. Liver cancer is predicted to be the sixth most common and fourth leading cause of cancer-related death worldwide in 2018 with an estimated 841,000 new cases and 782,000 deaths. The incidence of liver cancer is increasing rapidly, and is predicted to be the sixth most common and fourth leading cause of cancer-related death worldwide in 2018 with an estimated 841,000 new cases ad 782,000 deaths. The 5-year survival for patients with liver cancer is estimated at 18%, thus making it the second most lethal cancer after pancreatic cancer. There is substantial geographical heterogeneity with high-risk areas in Northern and Western Africa and Eastern and South-Eastern Asia, likely reflective of differences in environmental exposures rather than genetic predisposition [14].

The majority occur in patients with underlying cirrhosis, most commonly related to chronic infection with hepatitis B virus (HBV) or hepatitis C virus (HCV). Chronic HBV infection is the most common etiology in most developing countries. Within developed countries, cirrhosis secondary to chronic HCV infection remains the predominant risk factor, with low rates of chronic HBV infection due to primary prevention with HBV vaccination.

Other risk factors include aflatoxin exposure, alcohol use, hemochromatosis, primary biliary cirrhosis, autoimmune hepatitis, Wilson's disease, and alpha-1 antitrypsin deficiency.

The rising incidences of obesity, type 2 diabetes mellitus, and metabolic syndrome are associated with a rising incidence of nonalcoholic fatty liver disease (NAFLD) and nonalcoholic steatohepatitis (NASH), which can cause cirrhosis. Within the United States, the incidence of NAFLD-associated HCC is expected to increase by 122% between 2016 and 2030 [16]. Up to 30% of HCCs in patients with a non-cirrhotic liver appear to arise from hepatic adenomas [17].

19.2.2 Pathology

Primary liver tumors often resemble and arise from the major cells of origin which compose the liver, including hepatocytes (HCC), biliary epithelial cells (IHCC), endothelial cells (angiosarcoma, epithelioid hemangioendothelioma), or combinations of each (hepatoblastoma) [18]. Benign tumors comprise approximately 12% of all primary liver tumors, including dysplastic nodules, hepatic adenomas, focal nodule hyperplasia, liver cysts, hamartomas, hemangiomas, lipomas, and fibromas. HCC and IHCC comprise approximately 85% of primary liver tumors.

The 2019 World Health Organization (WHO) classification categorizes HCC into several subtypes: fibrolamellar, scirrhous, clear cell, steatohepatitic, macrotrabecular, chromophobe, neutrophil rich, and lymphocyte rich [18]. Fibrolamellar HCC is a distinct histopathologic subtype of HCC, which tends to present in young patients (mean age in their 20s) with no history of chronic liver disease. Fibrolamellar HCC is associated with a more indolent natural history and better prognosis. It is recognized that primary liver tumors may represent a continuum, with HCC and IHCC at the two ends of the spectrum and a range of tumors in between with variable differentiation along the two different cell lineages (e.g., combined hepatocellular-cholangiocarcinoma).

On gross pathology, HCC may form solitary, well-circumscribed nodules, or in the presence of cirrhosis, may be multinodular within the liver, or may diffusely infiltrate throughout the liver without forming circumscribed nodules [19]. Portal vein, hepatic vein, inferior vena cava, or hepatic arterial invasion may occur and is increasingly common with larger tumors. Invasion of major biliary ducts is less common. Lymph node metastasis occurs in 25.5% of patients, most commonly to the periportal or hepatic artery lymph nodes and less commonly to hilar, hepatoduodenal, inferior phrenic, and paracaval lymph nodes [20,21]. At diagnosis, approximately 1–5% of patients will have distant metastasis, most commonly to the lung, nonregional lymph nodes, bone, or adrenal gland [22,23].

19.2.3 Clinical Presentation

In patients with known cirrhosis, HCC is often diagnosed through routine screening ultrasound (US) imaging and blood alpha-fetoprotein (AFP) measurement. In early stages, HCC may be asymptomatic except for symptoms and signs related to a patient's underlying liver disease. Patients may have symptoms of abdominal pain, weight loss, malaise, fatigue, fever, early satiety, or diarrhea. In some instances, HCC may manifest as an acute decompensation of liver cirrhosis with worsening ascites, encephalopathy, jaundice, or variceal bleeding. Occasionally, patients with HCC may develop paraneoplastic syndromes, such as hypoglycemia, erythrocytosis, hypercalcemia, or diarrhea. Cutaneous manifestations may include dermatomyositis, pemphigus foliaceus, pityriasis rotunda, or the sign of Leser-Trélat.

19.2.4 Diagnostic Evaluation

Diagnostic evaluation should include comprehensive history, physical examination, laboratory evaluation including complete blood count, metabolic panel, liver function, viral hepatitis panel, coagulation studies, AFP, and serum CA 19-9. In conjunction with clinical factors, these laboratory studies may help characterize the severity of liver dysfunction and assist in patient prognostication through the use of the Child–Turcotte–Pugh (CP) Classification (most commonly used in this context) or Albumin–Bilirubin (ALBI) grade for HCC (Table 19.1). The Model for End-Stage Liver Disease (MELD) may also be utilized as a prognostic tool for patients with cirrhosis.

Diagnostic imaging may include multiphasic dynamic contrast-enhanced computed tomography (CT), magnetic resonance imaging (MRI), or abdominal US. CT of the chest, abdomen, and pelvis is recommended to evaluate for extrahepatic spread or distant metastasis, and a bone scan may be considered.

The diagnosis of HCC can often be made based upon underlying clinical suspicion and per CT or MRI imaging findings without the need for a biopsy. Imaging features used to diagnose HCC include tumor size, pattern of contrast enhancement, and growth on serial imaging and may be classified as per the American College of Radiology (ACR) Liver Imaging Reporting and Data System (LI-RADS) which ranges from LIRADS-1 (definitely benign—HCC likelihood 0%), LIRADS-2 (probably benign—HCC likelihood 13%), LIRADS-3 (intermediate risk—HCC likelihood 38%), LIRADS-4 (probably HCC—HCC likelihood 74%), or LIRADS-5 (definitely HCC—HCC likelihood 94%) [24,25]. Characteristic features of HCC include tumor size ≥ 1 cm, non-rim hepatic arterial phase hyperenhancement relative to liver parenchyma, non-peripheral hypoenhancement (i.e., wash out) relative to liver parenchyma in the portal venous phase, smooth peripheral enhancement ("capsular enhancing appearance") in the portal venous or delayed arterial phase, and $\geq 50\%$ increase in size within 6 months (demonstrated in Figure 19.1).

Patient subgroups at high risk for developing HCC include those with cirrhosis or those without cirrhosis who have HBV infection with either active hepatitis, family history of HCC, or

Table 19.1 Prognostic scores for hepatobiliary tumors.

Child–Pugh score (CP)

Bilirubin (mg/dL)	<2	2–3	>3
Albumin (g/dL)	>3.5	2.8–3.5	<2.8
Prothrombin time (s)	<4	4–6	>6
Encephalopathy	None	1–2	3–4
Ascites	None	Mild	Severe
Sum score	CP-A	CP-B	CP-C
	5–6	7–9	>9

Albumin–Bilirubin Grade (ALBI)

Log 10 Bilirubin (μmol/L) × 0.66 + Albumin (g/dL) × –0.085

ALBI grade	Grade 1	Grade 2	Grade 3
	≤–2.60	>–2.60 to ≤–1.39	>–1.39

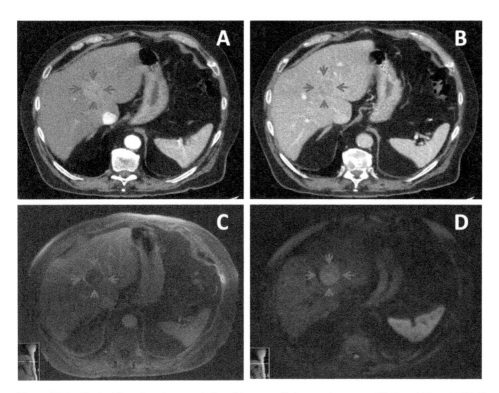

Figure 19.1 Typical imaging characteristics of hepatocellular carcinoma on CT (A and B) and MRI (C and D), including enhancement on early (arterial) phase (A), contrast washout and pseudocapsule on delayed (portal) phase (B and C), and restricted diffusion on diffusion weighted imaging (D).

high-risk demographics such as Africans, African-Americans, Asian males over age 40, or Asian females over age 50. Imaging surveillance at 3–6-month intervals is recommended for high-risk patients or patients with chronic, nonviral liver disease without cirrhosis and an AFP >400 ng/mL who have liver lesions measuring <1 cm on screening US [26]. For lesions measuring ≥1 cm on US, a CT or MRI is indicated. A biopsy may

not be required for diagnosis for high-risk patient subgroups or patients with chronic, nonviral liver disease without cirrhosis and an AFP >400 ng/mL if LIRADS-5 imaging criteria are identified. However, if the imaging criteria are suspicious but uncertain (e.g., LIRADS-4), and the result would affect patient management, a biopsy may be indicated. In patients without underlying liver disease, liver malignancies are more commonly related to metastatic disease and diagnostic evaluation should proceed to identify occult, undiagnosed liver disease or to assess for the possibility of extrahepatic malignancy. Liver biopsy may then be considered based upon subsequent findings.

19.2.5 Staging

HCC staging is based upon the eighth edition of the American Joint Commission on Cancer (AJCC) staging manual (Table 19.2) [27]. The Barcelona Clinic Liver Cancer (BCLC) staging system (Figure 19.2) is a widely utilized staging and prognostication system which assists in patient management decisions [28].

19.2.6 General Management

The majority of patients with HCC will have comorbid liver disease, and thus the benefits of treating the liver cancer must be balanced with the potential morbidities of treatment and the competing risks of morbidity or death from the underlying liver disease. The

BCLC staging system is the most widely utilized staging system which incorporates extent of tumor burden, baseline liver function, and performance status in order to differentiate patients amongst 1 of 5 stages and subsequently provide treatment recommendations. Multidisciplinary management, including hepatology, hepatobiliary surgery, transplant surgery, pathology, radiology (diagnostic and interventional), medical oncology, and radiation oncology, is essential in these often-complex clinical scenarios.

19.2.6.1 BCLC Stage 0-A
Patients with BCLC stage 0-A tumors may be amenable to curative-intent local therapy in the form of resection, liver transplantation, ablation, and in some select circumstances, radiotherapy.

Most studies have defined patients with resectable HCC as those with one to three unilobar lesions (most ideal candidate having a solitary lesion), no evidence of extrahepatic disease or macrovascular invasion, good performance status, preserved liver synthetic function (CP-A, highly select CP-B), and no clinically significant evidence of portal hypertension [26,29]. Clinically significant portal hypertension has been associated

Table 19.2 American Joint Committee on Cancer Staging eighth edition for hepatobiliary cancers [28].

Primary tumor: liver	
T0	No evidence of primary tumor
T1a	Solitary tumor ≤2 cm
T1b	Solitary tumor >2 cm without vascular invasion
T2	Solitary tumor >2 cm with vascular invasion or multiple tumors, none >5 cm
T3	Multiple tumors, at least one of which is >5 cm
T4	Single tumor or multiple tumors of any size involving a major branch of the portal vein or hepatic vein, or tumor(s) with direct invasion of adjacent organs other than the gallbladder or with perforation of visceral peritoneum
N0	No regional lymph node metastasis
N1	Regional lymph node metastasis
Primary tumor: intrahepatic bile duct	
T0	No evidence of primary tumor
Tis	Carcinoma *in situ* (intraductal tumor)
T1a	Solitary tumor ≤5 cm without vascular invasion
T1b	Solitary tumor >5 cm without vascular invasion
T2	Solitary tumor with intrahepatic vascular invasion or multiple tumors, with or without vascular invasion
T3	Tumor perforating the visceral peritoneum
T4	Tumor involving local extrahepatic structures by direct invasion
N0	No regional lymph node metastasis
N1	Regional lymph node metastasis present

(Continued)

Table 19.2 (Continued)

Primary tumor: proximal or perihilar cholangiocarcinoma	
T0	No evidence of primary tumor
Tis	Carcinoma *in situ* or high-grade dysplasia
T1	Tumor confined to the bile duct, with extension up to the muscle layer or fibrous tissue
T2a	Tumor invades beyond the wall of the bile duct to surrounding adipose tissue
T2b	Tumor invades adjacent hepatic parenchyma
T3	Tumor invades unilateral branches of the portal vein or hepatic artery
T4	Tumor invades the main portal vein or its branches bilaterally, or the common hepatic artery; or unilateral second-order biliary radicals with contralateral portal vein or hepatic artery involvement
N0	No regional lymph node metastasis
N1	One to three positive lymph nodes typically involving the hilar, cystic duct, common bile duct, hepatic artery, pancreatoduodenal, and portal vein lymph nodes
N2	Four or more positive lymph nodes from the sites described for N1

Primary tumor: distal cholangiocarcinoma	
Tis	Carcinoma *in-situ* or high-grade dysplasia
T1	Tumor invades the bile duct wall with a depth less than 5 mm
T2	Tumor invades the bile duct wall with a depth of 5–12 mm
T3	Tumor invades the bile duct wall with a depth greater than 12 mm
T4	Tumor involves the celiac axis, superior mesenteric artery, and/or common hepatic artery
N0	No regional lymph node metastasis
N1	Metastasis in one to three regional lymph nodes
N2	Metastasis in four or more regional lymph nodes

Primary tumor: gallbladder	
T0	No evidence of primary tumor
Tis	Carcinoma *in situ*
T1a	Tumor invades the lamina propria
T1b	Tumor invades the muscular layer
T2a	Tumor invades the perimuscular connective tissue on the peritoneal side, without involvement of the serosa (visceral peritoneum)
T2b	Tumor invades the perimuscular connective tissue on the hepatic side, with no extension into the liver
T3	Tumor perforates the serosa (visceral peritoneum) and/or directly invades the liver and/or one other adjacent organ or structure, such as the stomach, duodenum, colon, pancreas, omentum, or extrahepatic bile ducts
T4	Tumor invades the main portal vein or hepatic artery or invades two or more extrahepatic organs or structures
N0	No regional lymph node metastasis
N1	Metastases to one to three regional lymph nodes
N2	Metastases to four or more regional lymph nodes
Distant metastasis	
M0	No distant metastasis
M1	Distant metastasis

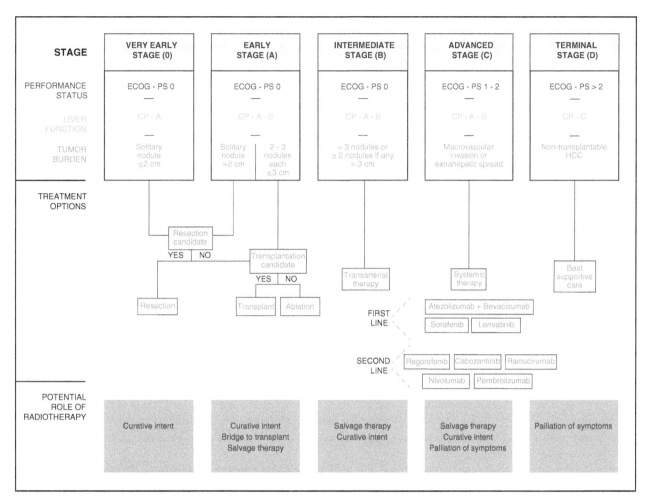

Figure 19.2   Adapted Barcelona Clinic Liver Cancer Staging System. Based on [28].

with poorer 3- and 5-year overall survival (OS) and increased rates of postoperative clinical decompensation [30]. Preoperative imaging may also be utilized to estimate the future liver remnant (FLR) volume in relation to the total liver volume. In patients without cirrhosis, the ratio of FLR to total liver volume is preferred to be ≥25% [31,32]. For patients who do not meet this criteria, preoperative portal vein embolization of the involved liver segment may be considered to induce hypertrophy of the portion of liver that will remain after surgery [33]. In patients deemed suitable for an operation, resection is associated with a 5-year OS of approximately 60% and low postoperative mortality (<3%). However, approximately 70% will experience tumor recurrence by 5 years—a rate which unfortunately has not been reduced with cancer-directed adjuvant therapy [34–36]. Data do suggest that antiviral therapy for HBV or HCV after curative-intent therapy for HBV- or HCV-associated HCC may improve OS [37–40].

Liver transplantation can be performed in patients with a limited tumor burden who are not candidates for resection due to poor baseline liver function or anatomic tumor location. The added advantage of this approach is that the underlying liver disease may be cured. The Milan Criteria for liver

transplantation has been adopted by the United Network for Organ Sharing (UNOS) and defined appropriate candidates as those with a single tumor nodule measuring ≤5 cm, or 2–3 nodules each ≤3 cm, and no evidence of macrovascular tumor invasion or extrahepatic spread [41]. Amongst this select cohort, transplantation is associated with 5-year OS of 60–80%, 10-year OS of 50%, and tumor recurrence rates less than 15% [42,43]. Liver transplantation in patients who do not meet Milan criteria is generally associated with poorer outcomes [44]. However, the use of neoadjuvant therapy in an effort to down-stage tumors which do not meet the Milan criteria is accepted by UNOS as a way of converting patients to being potential transplant candidates [45–47]. Additionally, neoadjuvant local therapy may be considered for patients who are on the transplant waiting list to decrease the risk of tumor progression and dropout. This practice may be most beneficial for patients with solitary tumors measuring 2–5 cm or those with two to three tumors with an anticipated wait time of over 6 months because the historical rates of dropout have been as high as 25% and 58% at 6 and 12 months [26,45,48,49].

Ablative therapies can induce local tumor necrosis through chemical ablation (percutaneous ethanol ablation [PEI] or acetic acid) or thermal ablation (radiofrequency ablation [RFA], microwave ablation [MWA], or cryoablation) and may be utilized in patients who are not candidates for surgery or as a bridging therapy prior to resection or transplantation [50]. RFA has demonstrated improved response rates and local control when compared to PEI [51,52]. MWA is a more recently developed ablative technique which has demonstrated comparable efficacy to RFA but potentially improved local tumor control when treating larger tumors [53]. Poorer candidates for ablative therapies include patients with tumors measuring >3 cm, tumors adjacent to major bile ducts, intraabdominal organs, or the diaphragm, or patients with tumors adjacent to vasculature which may serve as a "heat sink" and result in poorer efficacy [54]. In select circumstances, patients with a solitary HCC measuring 3–5 cm may be considered for combination transarterial therapy (discussed below) plus ablation [55]. There have been at least four prospective randomized studies in addition to meta-analyses comparing surgical resection versus RFA for HCC which suggest improved OS with surgical resection, although there is a lower incidence of complications after RFA [50,56–63]. Liu et al. compared surgical resection versus RFA plus TACE and similarly demonstrated improved outcomes with surgical resection [64].

Prior data have suggested that tumor size is strongly associated with outcomes after either surgery or ablation, with a suggestion that tumor control and survival may be more comparable after either intervention in patients with solitary, small tumors (≤3 cm, with best outcomes <2 cm) [65–68]. There has been no randomized study to date comparing surgery versus ablation for patients with solitary tumors measuring ≤3 cm, although Pompili et al. performed a multi-institutional retrospective comparison of 544 patients and identified comparable 4-year OS (74% vs. 66%, $p = 0.353$), HCC recurrence (56% vs. 57%, $p = 0.765$), and rates of major complication (4.5% vs. 2.0%, $p = 0.101$) [67]. These data support the use of ablative therapies as a potential alternative to resection in well-selected patients with small tumors in locations anatomically amenable to ablation.

19.2.6.2 BCLC Stage B

Patients with BCLC stage B, and in some instances stage C, disease may be amenable to transarterial therapies, and in select cases, ablative therapy or radiotherapy. Transarterial therapies take advantage of the vascular supply of HCC, which typically derives 80% of blood supply from the hepatic artery in comparison to normal liver parenchyma which derives the majority of its blood supply from the portal venous system. Transarterial therapies include transarterial "bland" embolization (TAE), transarterial chemoembolization (TACE), and transarterial radioembolization (TARE)/selective internal radiotherapy (SIRT). Transarterial therapies may increase the risk of liver failure, hepatic necrosis, and liver abscess so they

are contraindicated in patients with CP-C cirrhosis and relatively contraindicated in patients with biliary obstruction with a bilirubin >3 mg/mL or with portal vein thrombosis.

TACE involves the hepatic arterial infusion of the chemotherapeutic agent followed by bland embolization of the feeding vessels and has demonstrated an improvement in OS when compared to supportive care alone. Lo et al. randomized patients predominately with HBV-related HCC to TACE versus supportive care and identified 2-year OS of 31% versus 11% ($p = 0.002$), while Llovet et al. performed a similar randomization amongst patients predominately with HCV-related HCC and identified 2-year OS of 63% versus 27% ($p = 0.009$) [69,70]. Subsequent meta-analysis and systematic review have similarly identified improved OS with TACE, objective response rates of approximately 50%, and <1% risk of TACE-related mortality [71,72]. TACE delivery with the use of drug-eluting beads (DEB-TACE) has demonstrated comparable efficacy with potentially less toxicity when compared with conventional TACE [73,74]. There is some debate regarding the added benefit of TACE when compared with TAE. Brown et al. randomized 101 patients with BCLC stage A-C HCC to doxorubicin-eluting microsphere TACE versus microsphere-alone TAE and did not find any differences in PFS or OS [75]. Similarly, a meta-analysis including 676 patients amongst 6 clinical trials demonstrated increased toxicity with TACE compared with TAE, and no improvements in OS, PFS, or objective response rates [76]. There has also been exploration of combination therapies, such as TACE + RFA [55,77,78] or TACE + radiotherapy [79,80], with data suggesting potential benefits of combination therapy in select patients.

SIRT involves the hepatic arterial infusion of microspheres embedded with radioactive isotopes—most commonly with the beta-emitter, yttrium-90 (^{90}Y). There are no published randomized phase III trials to date comparing TACE versus SIRT for patients with BCLC stage B disease, although there are data suggesting its safety with response rates and survival comparable to or better than TACE [81–84]. The SARAH phase III trial randomized patients to either SIRT or sorafenib and identified comparable OS but more favorable quality of life and treatment tolerance in the cohort receiving SIRT [85]. Similarly, the SIRveNIB trial randomized patients with locally advanced HCC to SIRT versus sorafenib and identified comparable OS with significantly less toxicity in the SIRT cohort [86].

While there is still controversy regarding the optimal management of patients with BCLC stage B disease, the generally preferred approach remains transarterial therapy.

19.2.6.3 BCLC Stage C

Patients with BCLC stage C disease or those with earlier stage disease who have progressed after prior therapy are typically managed with systemic therapy. For select patients with favorable baseline liver function (preferably CP-A or ≤CP-B7), there may be a role for local therapy such as TACE, TACE + radiotherapy [87], or radiotherapy alone [88,89].

Sorafenib, an oral multi-kinase inhibitor that suppresses tumor cell proliferation and angiogenesis, has demonstrated an improvement in OS when compared with observation for patients with advanced or metastatic HCC [90,91]. The Sorafenib Hepatocellular Carcinoma Assessment Randomized Protocol (SHARP) trial included 602 patients with advanced HCC and randomized them to sorafenib versus best supportive care [91]. Approximately 70% had macroscopic vascular invasion, extrahepatic spread, or both, and 97% had CP-A cirrhosis. The sorafenib cohort had improved median OS compared with those receiving best supportive care (10.7 versus 7.9 months, $p < 0.001$). Similarly, Cheng et al. reported on 271 patients from the Asia-Pacific region with advanced, predominately HBV-related, HCC (97% CP-A) who were randomized to sorafenib versus best supportive care [90]. The median OS was 6.5 versus 4.2 months ($p = 0.014$) in favor of sorafenib. These data established sorafenib as the standard-of-care systemic therapy and it remained the sole proven systemic option for almost a decade. Lenvatinib, another multi-kinase inhibitor, was subsequently compared with sorafenib as first-line therapy within the phase III randomized REFLECT trial and demonstrated non-inferior OS (13.6 vs. 12.3 months, HR: 0.92, 95% CI: 0.79–1.06) [92]. More recently, a combined regimen of atezolizumab, a PDL-1 inhibitor, plus bevacizumab, a VEGF inhibitor, has demonstrated an improvement in OS, PFS, and quality of life when compared to sorafenib, thereby supporting its use as a standard first-line treatment option for patients with advanced HCC [93]. After disease progression, multiple agents, including regorafenib (multi-kinase inhibitor) [94], cabozantinib (tyrosine kinase inhibitor) [95], ramucirumab (VEGF inhibitor) [96,97], and PD-1 inhibitors, nivolumab [98] and pembrolizumab [99], have each demonstrated favorable responses predominately in patients with CP-A cirrhosis. Other agents, including FOLFOX cytotoxic chemotherapy [100], VEGF and PDGF inhibitors (e.g., linifanib, axitinib) [101,102], and MET inhibitors (i.e., tivantinib) [103] are also being explored.

19.2.6.4 BCLC D

Patients with BCLC stage D disease have a poor prognosis with a median survival of 3–6 months due to the underlying comorbid liver disease. Generally, best supportive care is recommended, although if performance status or liver function improve, local or systemic treatment options may be considered. In select instances, radiotherapy may be utilized to palliate symptoms such as abdominal pain, discomfort, nausea, or fatigue [104].

19.2.7 Definitive Radiotherapy for Hepatocellular Carcinoma

Historically, radiotherapy has not been considered a standard therapy for early stage or locally advanced HCC. Despite data suggesting HCC is a radiosensitive tumor, it is located in a highly radiosensitive organ, and thus technical limitations of radiotherapy initially precluded safe tumoricidal radiotherapy delivery. Investigators from the University of Michigan were amongst the first to demonstrate that durable local control could be safely achieved with 3D conformal radiotherapy with dosing based upon volume of spared liver [105–108]. In a cohort of 35 patients with unresectable HCC without portal vein invasion, they demonstrated that a regimen of 40–90 Gy (median, 60.75 Gy) in 1.5 Gy fractions twice daily with hepatic arterial floxuridine was associated with a 1-year local control (LC) and OS of 81% and 57%, respectively, and a 4% risk of RILD.

Improvements in simulation, motion management, treatment planning, image-guidance, and the advent of particle therapy and stereotactic body radiotherapy (SBRT) have allowed further improvement in the therapeutic ratio of liver irradiation. Multiple prospective phase I and II trials have demonstrated that photon SBRT is associated with excellent local control and acceptable rates of liver toxicity for well-selected patients predominately with CP-A or CP-B cirrhosis [88,109–111]. Bujold et al. reported a sequential phase I/II trial of 102 patients with HCC and CP-A cirrhosis treated with photon SBRT to a dose of 24–54 Gy in 6 fractions (median 36 Gy) [88]. The median tumor size was 7.2 cm and 55% had vascular involvement. The 1-year LC and OS were 87% and 55%, respectively. Seven patients had grade 5 toxicity, including liver failure in five patients. Takeda et al. reported a phase II trial of 90 patients with early-stage HCC, CP-A (91%) or CP-B (9%) cirrhosis, and solitary tumors measuring ≤4 cm in size [111]. The median dose was 40 Gy in 5 fractions. Three-year LC was 96% and 3-year OS was 67%. Eight (9%) patients had CP scores that worsened by two points. To date, there are no reported randomized phase III trials comparing photon SBRT to other forms of local therapy, although multiple are ongoing [112–116].

For patients with large tumors or for patients with tumors closely approximating GI luminal organs or the porta hepatis, hypofractionated radiotherapy incorporating similar motion management strategies and treatment planning techniques as SBRT may be effectively utilized. Hong et al. reported a prospective phase II trial including 44 patients with HCC and CP-A or CP-B liver function who received up to 67.5 GyE in 15 fractions (median 58.05 GyE) while limiting the mean liver dose (MLD) to ≤24 GyE [117]. The 2-year LC and OS were 95% and 63%, respectively, and 5% of patients experienced a grade 3+ toxicity.

Radiotherapy has also been combined with other forms of local therapy, such as TACE, to further improve local tumor control. Huo et al. reported a meta-analysis including 25 trials and 2,577 patients comparing TACE alone versus TACE plus radiotherapy [80]. They reported that TACE plus radiotherapy had significantly improved 1-year (OR: 1.36; 95% CI: 1.19–1.54), 3-year (OR: 1.91; 95% CI: 1.55–2.35), and 5-year (OR: 3.98; 95% CI: 1.86–8.51) OS and improved complete response rates (OR: 2.73; 95% CI: 1.95–3.81) when compared to TACE alone. Yoon et al. reported a randomized phase III trial of 90 patients with CP-A cirrhosis and liver-confined HCC with macroscopic vascular invasion who were randomized to either sorafenib or TACE plus radiotherapy to a dose of 45 Gy in 2.5–3.0 Gy fractions [87]. The TACE plus radiotherapy cohort had significantly improved radiologic response (33.3% vs. 2.2%, $p < 0.001$), median time to progression (31.0 vs. 11.7 weeks, $p < 0.001$), and OS (55.0 vs. 43.0 weeks, $p = 0.04$), when compared to the sorafenib cohort despite 91% of patients receiving sorafenib crossing over to receive TACE and RT by 24 weeks. While these data are promising, further confirmatory results in the context of large randomized phase III trials are warranted. The RTOG 1112 trial is comparing sorafenib alone versus sequential SBRT followed by sorafenib for patients with HCC [118].

19.2.8 Clinical Outcomes of Particle Therapy for Hepatocellular Carcinoma

19.2.8.1 Proton Therapy

Early dosimetric comparisons suggest that particle therapy may offer significantly lower mean, low-, and intermediate-radiation doses to the normal liver when compared with photon techniques [3–6]. Table 19.3 summarizes the current clinical data evaluating the use of proton therapy for patients with HCC.

In 1992, Tanaka et al. from the University of Tsukuba reported one of the earliest prospective experiences of proton therapy for a cohort of 11 patients with inoperable HCC [119]. No patients experienced severe adverse effects and 1-year LC was achieved in 80–86% of patients. Since then, many series, predominately from Asia, have demonstrated the feasibility, safety, and efficacy of proton therapy for HCC.

Mizumoto et al. from the University of Tsukuba reported a prospective series consisting of 266 patients with predominately CP-A (76%) or CP-B (23%) cirrhosis and HCC with a median tumor size of 3.4 cm (range 0.6–13.0) [120]. Patients received radiotherapy doses adapted based upon tumor location with peripheral tumors receiving a dose of 66 GyE in 10 fractions, tumors located within 2 cm of the porta hepatis receiving a dose of 72.6 GyE in 22 fractions, and tumors within 2 cm of GI luminal organs receiving a dose of 77 GyE in 35 fractions. The 3-year OS and LC were 61% and 87%. Grade 3 or higher acute or late GI toxicity occurred in 5% and 1% of patients, respectively. A recent update from the University of Tsukuba further stratified outcomes by BCLC stage for 129 patients treated per this proton therapy regimen [121]. The 5-year OS was 69%, 66%, and 25% and 5-year LC was 94%, 87%, and 75% for patients with BCLC 0-A, BCLC B, and BCLC C disease, respectively. Interestingly, these outcomes for patients with BCLC 0-A disease are comparable to that of hepatectomy series, thus suggesting a potential surgical alternative for select patients.

Comparable results have also been reported amongst other Asian institutions. Komatsu et al. from Kobe University reported on 242 patients with predominately CP-A (76%) or CP-B (23%) cirrhosis [122]. The majority (71%) of patients had tumors measuring less than 5 cm in size and 26% had evidence of vascular invasion. Patients received proton therapy with a dose of 52.8–84.0 GyE in 4–38 fractions, depending on proximity to critical normal tissues. The 5-year OS and LC were 38% and 90%, respectively. Kawashima et al. from the National Cancer Center Hospital East in Chiba prospectively assessed 30 patients with HCC and CP-A (67%) or CP-B (33%) cirrhosis treated with proton therapy [123]. The median tumor size was 4.5 cm (range 2.5–8.2 cm) and 40% of patients had vascular invasion. Patients were treated to a dose of 76 GyE in 20 fractions. The 2-year LC was 96% and 2- and 3-year OSs were 66% and 62%, respectively. Kim et al. from the Center for Liver Cancer in Korea reported on 41 patients with HCC and vascular involvement, predominately CP-A (93%) cirrhosis, and a median tumor size of 5.8 cm (range 2.0–16.0 cm) treated to a dose of 50–66 GyE in 10 fractions adapted per the proximity to GI luminal organs [124]. The 2-year OS was 51% and 2-year LC was 81%. Amongst these series, acute grade 3 or higher adverse events ranged from 0% to 5%, 0% to 1% experienced classic RILD, and 0% to 25% experienced CP-class progression or an increased in CP score by at least 2 points within 3–6 months.

There are also data supporting the role of proton therapy from Western countries. Bush et al. from Loma Linda reported the first experience in 2004 with a subsequent update in 2011 of a prospective phase II trial including 76 patients with HCC, a mean tumor size of 5.5 cm, and CP-A (29%), CP-B (47%), or CP-C (24%) cirrhosis [125,126]. Patients were treated to a dose of 63 GyE in 15 fractions. The crude rate of LC was 80%. The median OS was 34, 13, and 12 months for patients with CP-A, CP-B, and CP-C cirrhosis, respectively. No patient experienced a grade 3 or higher acute toxicity or RILD. Hong et al. reported a multi-institutional prospective trial from Massachusetts General Hospital, MD Anderson Cancer Center, and the University of Pennsylvania which included 44 patients with HCC, a median tumor size of 5.0 cm (1.9–18.0 cm), 30% had vascular involvement, and CP-A (73%) or CP-B (21%) cirrhosis [117]. Patients were treated to a maximum dose of 67.5 GyE

Table 19.3 Select series of proton therapy for hepatocellular carcinoma.

References	Study design	Patients (n)	CP status A/B/C (%)	Median tumor size (cm) (range)	TVT/ PVTT (%)	Dose (GyE)	Fractions	OS	LC	Liver toxicity	Toxicity
[125]	Prospective phase 2	34	CP-5–6: 41% CP-7–8: 21% CP-9–10: 21%	5.6 (1.0–10.0)	–	63	15	OS2: 55%	LC2: 75%	0% RILD by 6 months	3% G2 + late toxicity
[298]	Retrospective	162	51/36/6	3.8 (1.5–14.5)	6	72 (50–88) EQD2: 63–95	Oct 24	OS5: 24%	LC5: 87%	10% had transient 3× ULN AST/ALT elevation	
[123]	Prospective phase 2	30 ≤10 cm	67/33/0	4.5 (2.5–8.2)	4	76	20	OS1: 77% OS2: 66% OS3: 62%	LC2: 96%	27% treatment-related hepatic insufficiency by 6 months	
[299]	Retrospective	19	0/0/100	4.0 (2.5–8.0)	–	72 (50–84)	16 (10–24)	OS1: 53% OS2: 42%	Crude 95%	0% RILD 0% CP progression (14, 74%, had CP improvement)	0% G3 + acute toxicity
[300]	Retrospective	21 Age ≥80 years	71/24/5	4.0 (1.0–13.5)	–	Peripheral: 60 Central: 66 Adjacent to GI luminal organ: 70	Peripheral: 10 Central: 22 Adjacent to GI luminal organ: 35	OS1: 84% OS3: 62%	Crude: 100%	0% RILD 0% CP progression by 6 months	0% G3 + acute non-hematologic toxicity 0% G3 + late toxicity
[301]	Retrospective	53 ≤2 cm from porta hepatis	87/11/2	4.3 (1.0–13.0)	28	72.6	22	OS2: 57% OS3: 45%	LC2: 94% LC3: 86%	8% CP progression by 2 points	0% G3 acute toxicity
[302]	Retrospective	35	80/20/0	6.0 (2.5–13.0)	100	72.6 (55–77)	Oct 35	OS2: 48% OS5: 21%	LC2: 91% LC5: 91%	11% CP class progression (A–B) by 3 months 0% treatment related late liver failure	–

(Continued)

Table 19.3 (Continued)

References	Study design	Patients (n)	CP status A/B/C (%)	Median tumor size (cm) (range)	TVT/PVTT (%)	Dose (GyE)	Fractions	OS	LC	Liver toxicity	Toxicity
[303]	Prospective	51 ≥2 cm from porta hepatis of GI organs	80/20/0	2.8 (0.8–9.3)	–	66	10	OS3: 49% OS5: 39%	LC3: 95% LC5: 88%	16% CP class progression (A–B)	6% rib fracture
[304]	Retrospective	318	74/24/2	–	14	Peripheral: 66 ≤2 cm from porta hepatis: 72.6 ≤2 cm from GI luminal organ: 77	Peripheral: 10 ≤2 cm from porta hepatis: 22 ≤2 cm from GI luminal organ: 35	OS1: 90% OS3: 65% OS5: 45%	–	–	2% G3 acute toxicity (n = 4 dermatologic, n = 1 GI)
[305]	Retrospective	22 >10 cm tumors	50/50/0	CP-A: 11 CP-B: 10–14	50	CP-A: 72.6 CP-B: 47.3–89.1	CP-A: 22 CP-B: 10–35	OS1: 64% OS2: 36%	LC2: 87%	23% died of liver failure, 14% with no viable HCC	0% G3 acute toxicity
[306]	Retrospective	150 Single lesion < 5 cm 105 PBT 45 CIRT	83/17/0	–	–	PBT: 52.8–76 CIRT: 52.8	PBT: 4–20 CIRT: 4–8	OS5: PBT: 49% CIRT: 68%	LC5: PBT: 93% CIRT: 92%	–	5% G3 + acute toxicity
[122]	Retrospective	242	76/23/1	<5 (71%) 5–10 (23%) >10 (6%)	26	52.8–84.0	Apr 38	OS5: 38%	LC5: 90%	0.4% G3 + transaminase elevation	3% G3 + late toxicity
[120]	Prospective	266	76/23/1	3.4 (0.6–13.0)	–	Peripheral: 66 ≤2 cm from porta hepatis: 72.6 ≤2 cm from GI luminal organ: 77	Peripheral: 10 ≤2 cm from porta hepatis: 22 ≤2 cm from GI luminal organ: 35	OS1: 87% OS3: 61% OS5: 48%	LC1: 98% LC3: 87% LC5: 81%	–	5% G3 acute skin toxicity 1% G3 late GI toxicity

Ref	Study type	N	Ratio	Tumor size	%	Dose	Fractions	mOS/OS	LC/Crude	RILD/CP progression	Toxicity
[126]	Prospective phase 2	76	29/47/24	5.5 (Mean)	5	63	15	mOS CPA: 34 m CPB: 13 m CPC: 12 m	Crude: 80%	0% RILD	0% G3 acute toxicity
[307]	Retrospective	27	67/33/0	7.0 (3.0–16.0)	100	50–66	20–22	OS2: 33%	Crude: 67%	15% CP progression by 1 point at 3 months	0% G3 + late toxicity
[308]	Prospective pilot	15 11 HCC 3 IHCC 1 Metastasis	60/40/0	–	–	60 (45–75)	15	OS1: 53% OS2: 40% OS3: 33%	Crude: 93%	0% RILD	–
[4]	Phase 1 prospective trial	27	89/11	≤5 (81%)	–	60–72	20–24	OS3: 56% OS5: 42%	LC3: 80% LC5: 64%	4% CP progression of 1 point by 3 months; 15% CP improvement of 1 point by 3 months, remainder stable	0% G3 + acute toxicity
[117]	Prospective phase 2	44	73/21/0	5.0 (1.9–12.0)	30	Peripheral: 67.5 ≤2 cm from porta hepatis: 58.05	15	OS2: 63%	LC2: 95%	4% CP class progression (A–B) by 6 months	6% G3 + acute toxicity
[309]	Retrospective	24	100/0/0	9.0 (5.0–18.0)	83	72.6 (60.8–85.8)	22	OS2: 52%	LC2: 87%	25% CP class progression (A–B), half of which attributed to out of field tumor progression	

(Continued)

Table 19.3 (Continued)

References	Study design	Patients (n)	CP status A/B/C (%)	Median tumor size (cm) (range)	TVT/ PVTT (%)	Dose (GyE)	Fractions	OS	LC	Liver toxicity	Toxicity
[124]	Retrospective	41	93/7/0	5.8 (2.0–16.0)	100	≤1 cm from GI luminal organs: 50; 1–1.9 cm from GI luminal organs: 60; ≥2 cm from GI luminal organs: 66	10	OS2: 51%	LC2: 88%	2% CP progression by 1 point at 3 months	0% G3 + acute non-hematologic toxicity
[121]	Retrospective	129	78/22	3.9 (1.0–13.5)	13	Peripheral: 66; ≤2 cm from porta hepatis: 72.5; ≤2 cm from GI luminal organ: 77	Peripheral: 10; ≤2 cm from porta hepatis: 22; ≤2 cm from GI luminal organ: 35	OS5: ; BCLC 0-A: 69%; BCLC B: 66%; BCLC C: 25%	LC5: ; BCLC 0-A: 94%; BCLC B: 87%; BCLC C: 75%		
[310]	Retrospective	83; 58 PBT; 25 CIRT	75/25/0; BCLC 0/A/B/C 10/46/16/30	3.0 (1.0–14.1)	–	PBT: 72.6 (50–74); CIRT: 45.0 (45–52.8)	PBT: 10–37; CIRT: 2–4	Overall cohort: OS1: 83%; OS3: 55%; OS5: 39%	LC1: 86%; LC2: 85%; LC3: 85%; No difference between PBT or CIRT cohorts	Overall cohort 36% CP progression at 6 months; 19% 1 point increase; 17% 2 point increase; 0% ≥ 3 point increase	–
[311]	Retrospective	101	89/10/1	2.5 (1.0–16.0)	29	48; 50–66	6; 10	–	–	4% CP progression ≥ 2 points at 3 months	–

Ref	Study type	N	Ratio	Follow-up		Dose	Fractions	OS	LC	CP progression	Toxicity
[127]	Retrospective	46	83/17/0	6.0 (1.5–21.0)	28	67.5 (24–91) Most common Peripheral: 67.5 Central: 58–60	6–25 Most common Peripheral: 15 Central: 15–20	OS1: 73% OS2: 62%	LC1: 95% LC2: 81%	CP progression at 4 months: 13%, ≥2 points 9%	13% G3 acute toxicity
[312]	Systematic review	~900	–	–	–	–	–	OS5: 32%	LC3–5: ~80%	–	–
[128]	Systematic review	5,204 1,627 particle therapy 1,473 SBRT 2,104 conventional photons	73/–/–	4.5	19						
[313]	Meta-analysis	16 studies, 1516 1,135 PBT 99 PBT or CIRT 282 CIRT	72/26/3	4.75 (2.5–9.0)	–	BED10: 96.4 (68.75–122.5)	–	OS1: 86% OS2: 62% OS5: 35%	LC1: 86% LC2: 89% LC5: 89%	0.7% Acute G3 + liver toxicity 0.7% late G3 + liver toxicity	7% G3 + acute toxicity

(median dose 58.05 GyE) in 15 fractions depending upon proximity to the porta hepatis. The 2-year OS and LC were 63% and 95%, respectively, and 4% experienced CP-class progression (A–B) by 6 months. Chadha et al. later reported a retrospective series from MD Anderson Cancer Center including 46 patients treated with a similar dosing scheme [127]. The 2-year OS and LC were 62% and 81%, respectively, and 9% of patients experienced CP progression by ≥2 points by 4 months after radiotherapy.

Qi et al. reported a systematic review comparing particle therapy, conventional photon radiotherapy, or photon SBRT for HCC [128]. They identified improved 1-, 3-, and 5-year OS, locoregional control, acute toxicity, and late toxicity with the use of particle therapy versus conventional photons, in addition to less late toxicity for the particle therapy cohort when compared with the photon SBRT cohort.

19.2.8.2 Carbon-ion Radiotherapy

CIRT has also demonstrated safety and efficacy in the treatment of patients with HCC, with the majority of data coming from institutions in Japan and Germany (demonstrated in Table 19.4). Kato et al. from the National Institute of Radiologic Sciences (NIRS) reported an early prospective phase I/II trial including 24 patients treated with stepwise escalating doses of 49.5–79.5 GyE in 15 fractions [129]. Patients had either CP-A (67%) or CP-B (33%) cirrhosis and had HCC with a median tumor size of 5.0 cm (range 2.1–8.5 cm). The 1-, 3-, and 5-year LC were 92%, 81%, and 81%, and 1-, 3-, and 5-year OS were 92%, 50%, and 25%, respectively. LC was 100% in the subgroup of patients treated to a dose of 72.0 GyE or higher. No patient experienced CP progression ≥2 points.

Imada et al. reported a subsequent experience from NIRS including 64 patients treated with a dose of 52.8 GyE in 4 fractions [130]. For patients with peripheral tumors, LC was 96% at both 3 and 5 years, and the 3- and 5-year OS were 61% and 35%, respectively. For patients with tumors within 2 cm of the porta hepatis, LC was 88% at both 3 and 5 years, and the 3- and 5-year OS were 44% and 22%, respectively. Kasuya et al. reported a combined analysis of prospective trials from NIRS evaluating CIRT regimens ranging from 48 to 52.8 GyE in 4 fractions, 48 to 58 GyE in 8 fractions, and 54 to 69.6 GyE in 12 fractions [131]. The LC at 1, 3, and 5 years were 95%, 91%, and 90%, and the 1-, 3-, and 5-year OS rates were 90%, 50%, and 25%, respectively. The safety and efficacy of CIRT in 12, 8, and 4 fractions were confirmed, and from these data, 52.8 GyE in 4 fractions was established as the NIRS institutional recommended regimen. Shibuya et al. reported a relatively large multi-institutional retrospective series including 174 patients treated with doses of 48 GyE in 2 fractions or 52.8–60 GyE in 4 fractions [132]. The 2-year LC and OS were 92% and 80% with no patients experiencing an acute grade 3 or higher toxicity. Yasuda et al. reported on 57 patients with a longer-term

median follow-up of 54 months treated with CIRT to a dose of 45 GyE in 2 fractions. The 5-year LC and OS were 91% and 45%, respectively, and no patient experienced CP progression ≥2 points [133].

Habermehl et al. reported an initial experience of six patients treated with CIRT at the Heidelberg Ion-Beam Therapy Center in Germany [11]. Patients were treated to a dose of 40 GyE in four fractions and the median OS was 11 months with a crude LC rate of 100% and 0% grade 3 toxicity. These data provided the background for the prospective phase I PROMETHEUS-01 trial which will be investigating CIRT delivered with intensity-modulated raster-scanning for the treatment of HCC with a primary end point of toxicity and secondary end points of progression-free survival and response [134]. A prospective comparison of CIRT versus proton therapy for patients with HCC is currently underway, although an interim analysis with a median follow-up of 12.5 months has been presented in abstract form [135]. The 1- and 2-year LC, OS, and treatment-related toxicities have thus far been comparable between both treatment cohorts. More mature results published in manuscript form are eagerly anticipated.

19.3 Intrahepatic Cholangiocarcinoma

19.3.1 Epidemiology and Etiology

Cholangiocarcinomas arise from the bile duct epithelium and can be differentiated based upon location as GBCA, EHCC, and IHCC, in order of decreasing frequency. IHCCs are primary liver tumors arising from the bile duct epithelium within the liver proximal to the secondary biliary branches and can be divided into small duct type (peripheral cholangiocarcinomas) or large duct type proximal to the bifurcation of the right and left hepatic ducts [27]. IHCC make up approximately 10–15% of primary liver tumors, although they represent only 5–10% of cholangiocarcinomas.

The incidence of IHCC has been rising by approximately 2.3% per year between 1973 and 2012, potentially related to a misclassification of perihilar tumors as IHCC rather than EHCC. The incidence of IHCC has increased even more rapidly at a rate of 4.36% per year between 2003 and 2012, potentially related to improved evaluation of carcinoma of unknown primary and the increasing recognition of occult IHCC [136].

Within Western countries, the main risk factors for cholangiocarcinoma are primary sclerosing cholangitis (PSC), ulcerative colitis even in the absence of identifiable PSC, and chronic hepatolithiasis. PSC is the single most common risk factor in Western countries and is associated with approximately a 10% lifetime risk and as high as 30% in autopsy series, with a third of cases diagnosed within 2 years after initial PSC diagnosis [137]. Other less common risk factors include fibropolycystic

Table 19.4 Select series of carbon-ion radiotherapy for hepatocellular carcinoma.

Author (year)	Study design	Patients (n)	CP status A/B/C (%)	Median tumor size (cm) (range)	TVT/ PVTT (%)	Dose (GyE)	Fractions	OS	LC	Liver toxicity	Toxicity
[129]	Prospective phase 1/2	24	67/33/0	5.0 (2.1–8.5)	13	49.5–79.5	15	OS1: 92%	LC1: 92%	78% CP progression of 1 point ≤3 months after CIRT	–
								OS3: 50%	LC3: 81%	75% CP progression of 1 point >3 months after CIRT	
								OS5: 25%	LC5: 81%	0% CP progression of 2 points	
[130]	Prospective phase 1/2	64	77/23/0	4.0 (1.2–12.0)	70	52.8	4	Peripheral	Peripheral	84% CP progression of 1 point >3 months after CIRT	
		Peripheral: 46						OS3: 61%	LC3: 96%	16% CP progression of 2 points >3 months after CIRT	
		≤2 cm from porta hepatis: 18						OS5:35%	LC5: 96%		
								≤2 cm from porta hepatis:	≤2 cm from porta hepatis:		
								OS3: 44%	LC3: 88%		
								OS5: 22%	LC5: 88%		
[122]	Retrospective	101	77/20/3	<5 (75%)	18	52.8–76.0	Apr 20	OS5: 36%	LC5: 93%	3% G3 + transaminase elevation	
				5–10 (20%)						16% CP progression of 2 points >3 months after CIRT	
				>10 (5%)							
[11]	Retrospective	6	80/20	3.5 (0.9–4.5)	–	40	4	mOS: 11 m	Crude 100%	–	0% G3 acute toxicity
[131]	Prospective phase 1/2	126	77/23/0	4.0 (1.0–12.0)	17	48–52.8	4	OS1: 90%	LC1: 95%	33% CP progression ≥1 point at 3 months	20% G3 + acute toxicity
						48–58	8	OS3: 50%	LC3: 91%	4% CP progression ≥2 points at 3 months	
						54–69.6	12	OS5: 25%	LC5: 90%	27% CP progression ≥1 point at 6 months	
										5% CP progression ≥2 points at 6 months	

(Continued)

Table 19.4 (Continued)

Author (year)	Study design	Patients (n)	CP status A/B/C (%)	Median tumor size (cm) (range)	TVT/PVTT (%)	Dose (GyE)	Fractions	OS	LC	Liver toxicity	Toxicity
[314]	Retrospective	31 Age ≥ 80 years	87/13/0	4.5 (1.5–9.3)	20	Peripheral: 52.8–60 Adjacent to GI organs: 60	Peripheral: 4 Adjacent to GI organs: 12	OS2: 82%	LC2: 89%	3% CP progression (A to B) by 3 months 13% CP progression of 1 point by 3 months 3% CP progression of 2 points by 3 months 16% CP progression of 1 point by >3 months 3% CP progression of 2 points by > 3 months	0% G2 + acute toxicity 10% G3 late encephalopathy
[310]	Retrospective	83 58 PBT 25 CIRT	75/25/0 BCLC 0/A/B/C 10/46/16/30	3.0 (1.0–14.1)	–	PBT: 72.6 (50–74) CIRT: 45.0 (45–52.8)	PBT: 10–37 CIRT: 2–4	Overall cohort OS1: 83% OS3: 55% OS5: 39%	LC1: 86% LC2: 85% LC3: 85% No difference between PBT or CIRT cohorts	Overall cohort 36% CP progression at 6 months 19% 1 point increase 17% 2 point increase 0% ≥3 point increase	
[132]	Multi-institutional retrospective	174	88/12/0	3.0 (0.8–10.3)	–	48 52.8–60	2 4	OS1: 95% OS2: 83% OS3: 73%	LC1: 95% LC2: 88% LC3: 81%	2% RILD	6% (5.2% skin or chest wall) G3 + acute toxicity

Ref	Study type	N	Location	CP/fraction	Median size		Dose (Gy)	Fractions	OS	LC	CP progression	Toxicity
[315]	Retrospective PSM	31		93/7/0	3.4 (1.1–7.8)	–	52.8–60	04 Dec	OS3: 88%	LC3: 80%	7% progression of CP score (A–B) at 3 months	
[316]	Phase 1 prospective trial	21		100/0/0 CPA5: 62% CPA6: 38%	4.8 (3.0–7.8)	0	60	4	OS1: 91% OS2: 80%	LC1: 100% LC2: 92%	10% CP progression at 3 months 16% CP progression at 6 months	0% G3 + acute toxicity 19% G2 + acute toxicity
[133]	Retrospective	57 >1 cm from GI organs		89/11/0	3.3 (1.3–9.5)	0	45	2	OS1: 97% OS3: 67% OS5: 45%	LC1: 98% LC3: 91% LC5: 91%	0% progression of CP by ≥2 points	4% G3 acute skin toxicity

liver disease (e.g., choledochal cysts), bile duct adenomas, multiple biliary papillomatosis, Caroli's disease, cystic fibrosis, exposure to the radiopaque medium thorium dioxide, and tobacco smoking. In some parts of Asia, parasitic infestation with *Clonorchis sinensus* (liver fluke) or *Opisthorchis viverrini* is associated with a 25–50 times increased risk of cholangiocarcinoma. IHCC is also associated with cirrhosis, and HBV or HCV infection. However, despite these known risk factors, many cases of cholangiocarcinoma occur without an obvious cause.

19.3.2 Pathology—Intrahepatic and Extrahepatic Cholangiocarcinoma

Over 90% of cholangiocarcinomas are adenocarcinoma, with squamous cell carcinoma or adenosquamous carcinoma compromising most of the remainder. Morphologically, both IHCC and EHCC can be sclerosing, nodular, or papillary subtypes. Sclerosing tumors are most common and are characterized by an intense desmoplastic reaction, early bile-duct wall invasion, and hence, poorer resectability and cure rates [138]. Nodular tumors develop as constricting annular lesions, are highly invasive, and similarly are associated with poor outcomes. Papillary tumors are least common, but due to their presentation as bulky masses within the common bile duct with early biliary obstruction, they are often diagnosed earlier and associated with a more favorable prognosis [139]. Cholangiocarcinomas may be further classified according to macroscopic growth pattern, such as mass-forming type (approximately 60%) which develop as a distinct mass within the liver parenchyma, periductal-infiltrating type with longitudinal extension along the bile duct, or intraductal growth type with a papillary or tumor-thrombus type growth-pattern [140]. Up to 7% of patients will have multi-centric tumors at diagnosis [138]. Lymph node involvement is identified in 30–50% of patients, most commonly within hilar, cystic, choledochal, periportal, hepatic arterial, posterior pancreaticoduodenal, hepatoduodenal, or celiac lymph nodes, and is more frequent in patients with EHCC when compared to patients with IHCC [27,141]. At diagnosis, approximately 30% of patients will have distant metastasis, most commonly to the liver, peritoneum, non-regional lymph nodes, or lung.

19.3.3 Clinical Presentation

IHCC most commonly occurs in patients aged 50–70 years. Disease may be identified in asymptomatic patients incidentally on imaging or during screening for HCC in high-risk patients with liver cirrhosis. The most common symptoms include dull right upper quadrant abdominal pain, weight loss, or fatigue. It is relatively less common to manifest as obstructive jaundice when compared with patient with EHCC.

19.3.4 Diagnostic Evaluation

Diagnostic evaluation should include comprehensive history, physical examination, and laboratory evaluation including complete blood count, metabolic panel, liver function, viral hepatitis panel, and coagulation studies. CA 19-9 may serve as a useful tumor marker for patients with IHCC, although AFP may assist in differentiating IHCC from HCC, and CEA or CA 125 is occasionally elevated and can be used in patient monitoring [142]. Similarly to patients with HCC, the CP, MELD, or ALBI classifications may assist with management decisions.

Diagnostic imaging may include multiphasic dynamic contrast-enhanced CT, MRI, or US. Classically, IHCC may be differentiated from HCC by identifying characteristics of a hypodense hepatic lesion during the portal venous phase, peripheral enhancement throughout both arterial and venous phases, delayed arterial phase enhancement, biliary dilatation, and in some cases, capsular retraction due to the dense fibrotic nature of the tumor [143]. On gadoxetate-enhanced MRI, IHCC appear as hypointense lesions on T1-weighted images and are heterogeneously hyperintense on T2-weighted images [144]. On dynamic MR images, IHCC shows moderate peripheral enhancement followed by progressive and concentric filling in the tumor. Identification of this "target appearance" on dynamic imaging or diffusion-weighted imaging may help differentiate a peripheral mass-forming IHCC from HCC [145].

Some intrahepatic tumors may contain both elements of HCC and cholangiocarcinoma (i.e., mixed hepatocellular-cholangiocellular carcinoma) and exhibit a distinct appearance on cross-sectional imaging with a strong enhancing rim and an irregular shape on gadoxetate-enhanced MRI [146]. In the absence of classic imaging features and supportive information for HCC or cholangiocarcinoma, biopsy may be needed for confirmation of the diagnosis.

Magnetic resonance cholangiopancreatography (MRCP) is a noninvasive technique for evaluating the intrahepatic and extrahepatic bile ducts and the pancreatic duct which may provide information about disease extent and potential resectability comparable to that obtained using CT and invasive techniques like angiography or endoscopic retrograde cholangiopancreatography (ERCP) [147,148].

Invasive imaging techniques, such as endoscopic ultrasound (EUS), may offer local tumor assessment and assessment of regional lymphadenopathy while also allowing fine-needle aspiration of suspicious lymph nodes [149]. ERCP may also be performed for local tumor or stricture assessment and permit brush cytology, biopsy, or interventions to alleviate biliary obstruction.

CT of the chest, abdomen, and pelvis is recommended to evaluate for extrahepatic spread or distant metastasis. Positron emission tomography-computed tomography (PET-CT) is not routinely performed.

Histologic diagnosis of cholangiocarcinoma prior to surgical resection can be challenging. A suspicious mass with typical imaging characteristics in the appropriate clinical context should be considered malignant. IHCC may be amenable to percutaneous US or CT-guided biopsy. In some instances, histologic or cytologic confirmation may be obtained through EUS-guided biopsy of regional lymph nodes, or through ERCP with biopsy or brushing demonstrating malignant cells or abnormal cytogenetics [150]. Transperitoneal fine-needle aspiration or EUS-guided biopsy of the primary tumor is not recommended because of the potential for tumor seeding and may preclude the possibility of subsequent liver transplant [151].

19.3.5 Staging

IHCC staging is based upon the eighth edition of the AJCC staging manual (Table 19.2) [27].

19.3.6 General Management

19.3.6.1 Localized Disease

The only proven potentially curative therapy for patients with IHCC is surgical resection, although only about 20% of patients are candidates for resection at the time of diagnosis [152]. Margin-negative (R0) surgical resection is associated with improved survival and lower rates of recurrence [153–160]. Rates of recurrence after surgery are approximately 50–70% and 5-year OS is approximately 40% (~40–60% after R0 resection) [141,159]. Apart from surgical margin status, other variables associated with recurrence and poorer survival after surgery include poorly differentiated tumor grade, larger tumor size, multifocal disease, vascular invasion, perineural invasion, lymphovascular space invasion, and regional lymph node metastasis [141,161–164]. Radical resection with liver transplantation is generally not recommended for patients with IHCC because of the high rates of relapse and 5-year OS of only 20–30% [165].

Data guiding adjuvant therapy for patients with resected biliary tract cancers have some limitations with the bulk of data coming from retrospective series, and even amongst the phase III randomized trials, there is considerable patient heterogeneity with inclusion of patients with IHCC, EHCC, and GBCA—all known to have different biology and disease natural histories. In the BILCAP trial, 447 patients with resected biliary tract or GBCA were randomized to receive either adjuvant capecitabine or observation [166]. In the per-protocol analysis, median OS was found to be improved with adjuvant capecitabine (median OS 51.1 vs. 36.4 months; HR: 0.75, 95% CI: 0.58–0.97, $p = 0.028$). Contrary to these findings, the PRODIGE 12-ACCORD 18 Trial included 196 patients with resected biliary tract cancer and randomized them to adjuvant gemcitabine plus oxaliplatin versus observation and did not demonstrate any improvements in relapse-free survival or OS [167]. The phase II SWOG S0809 trial, which included 79 patients with resected EHCC or GBCA, evaluated an adjuvant regimen of sequential capecitabine plus gemcitabine chemotherapy followed by capecitabine-based chemoradiotherapy to a dose of 52.5–54 Gy for patients after an R0 resection or 55–59.4 Gy for patients who underwent an R1 resection [168]. The results were promising with 2-year OS of 65% and no differences in OS for those who underwent an R0 versus R1 resection, potentially indicating that postoperative chemoradiotherapy may mitigate the adverse impact of a positive margin. Furthermore, Horgan et al. reported a meta-analysis of 6,712 patients assessing the role of postoperative therapy for patients with resected biliary tract or GBCA [169]. Chemotherapy or chemoradiotherapy was associated with a significantly greater benefit than radiotherapy alone, with the greatest benefit of adjuvant therapy seen in those with lymph-node involvement or positive surgical margins. Based upon these data, consensus guidelines suggest offering 6 months of adjuvant capecitabine for patients with resected biliary tract or GBCA, with consideration for postoperative chemoradiotherapy for patients with IHCC, EHCC, or GBCA who have undergone an R1 resection [170].

19.3.6.2 Locally Advanced, Unresectable, or Metastatic Disease

The ABC-02 trial included 410 patients with unresectable or metastatic biliary tract cancer and randomized them to gemcitabine plus cisplatin versus gemcitabine alone and demonstrated an improvement in median OS (12 vs. 8 months) with combination chemotherapy, thus establishing the standard-of-care treatment [171]. However, despite the improvement in median OS, only five (1%) of patients were alive and disease free at 2 years. Multiple locoregional surgical alternatives have been evaluated including radiotherapy (discussed separately), RFA, TACE, or SIRT with the goal of extending survival for patients with unresectable, locoregionally confined disease. RFA has demonstrated a median OS of 38.5 months and 5-year OS of 15% for a well-selected cohort of 13 patients with IHCC measuring less than 5 cm [172]. TACE has demonstrated median OS of 11–15 months and 2- and 3-year OS of 27% and 8%, respectively [173,174]. In a systematic review including 298 patients amongst 12 studies, SIRT was associated with median OS of 15.5 months [175].

19.3.7 Definitive Radiotherapy for Intrahepatic Cholangiocarcinoma

A number of prospective and retrospective reports have indicated favorable LC rates and OS after radiotherapy for patients with IHCC who were deemed unsuitable for surgical resection. Tse et al. reported a phase I trial including 10 patients with IHCC treated with SBRT to a dose of 24–60 Gy (median dose 36 Gy) in 6 fractions [176]. The median OS was 15.0 months and 1-year LC was 65%. Tao et al. reported on a cohort of 79 patients with inoperable IHCC treated with definitive radiotherapy to doses of 35–100 Gy (median 58.05 Gy) in 3–30 fractions [177]. The median OS was 30 months and 3-year OS was 44%. Treatment with a BED >80.5 Gy_{10} was associated with significantly improved 3-year OS (73% vs. 38%, $p = 0.017$) and 3-year LC (78% vs. 45%, $p = 0.04$). Hong et al. reported a prospective phase II trial including 37 patients with inoperable IHCC who were treated with definitive proton therapy to a median dose of 58.05 GyE (range 58.05–67.5 GyE) in 15 fractions [117]. The 2-year LC and OS were 94% and 47%, respectively, and 8% of patients experienced grade 3 toxicity.

The recently closed NRG GI-001 phase III trial randomized patients with inoperable IHCC to gemcitabine plus cisplatin versus sequential gemcitabine plus cisplatin followed by radiotherapy to a dose of 37.5–67.5 Gy in 15 fractions [178]. The primary end point is OS. Unfortunately, the trial closed due to poor accrual. The UK ABC-07 trial is a phase II trial randomizing patients who do not demonstrate disease progression after an initial six cycles of gemcitabine plus cisplatin to either two additional cycles of chemotherapy or focal ablative radiotherapy in 5–15 fractions [179].

19.3.8 Clinical Outcomes of Particle Therapy for Cholangiocarcinoma and Gallbladder Cancer

19.3.8.1 Proton Therapy
Similarly to experiences with HCC, there are a few series evaluating the role of proton therapy for patients with either IHCC or EHCC with the similar goal of reducing acute and late toxicities without compromising tumor control (demonstrated in Table 19.5).

Hong et al. reported a multi-institutional prospective phase II trial of hypofractionated proton therapy for patients with HCC or IHCC [117]. A total of 37 patients had IHCC and were treated to a dose of 67.5 GyE in 15 fractions if peripherally located or a dose of 58.05 GyE in 15 fractions if located within 2 cm of the porta hepatis. The 2-year OS was 47% and the 2-year LC was 94%. Each of the six patients who experienced local progression were treated to doses less than 60 GyE. Grade 3 or higher treatment-related toxicity occurred in 6% of the overall cohort and 4% experienced CP-class progression from CP-A to CP-B within 6 months.

Ohkawa et al. reported a retrospective experience of 20 patients with IHCC treated with proton therapy to a median dose of 72.6 GyE (range 55–79.2) in 10–22 fractions [180]. Local control at 1, 2, and 3 years was 88%, 60%, and 60%, and

the 1-, 2-, and 3-year OS were 82%, 61%, and 38%, respectively. No patient experienced a grade 3 or higher non-hematologic acute toxicity. Similarly, Makita et al. reported a retrospective series of 28 patients with either IHCC, EHCC, or GBCA treated with curative intent proton therapy to a dose of 50.6–80.0 GyE in 2.0–3.2 GyE fractions [181]. The 1-year LC and OS were 68% and 49%, respectively. Grade 3 or higher acute toxicities occurred in 4% of patients and no patient experienced a grade 3 or higher late toxicity.

19.3.8.2 Carbon-ion Radiotherapy
There is a relatively limited experience with use of CIRT or other heavy particles in the treatment of patients with cholangiocarcinoma (demonstrated in Table 19.5). Abe et al. from Gunma University in Japan reported on seven patients with either IHCC ($n = 7$) or perihilar EHCC ($n = 1$) [182]. Patients received a dose of 52.8–60 GyE delivered in 4 fractions for peripherally located tumors or 12 fractions for more centrally located IHCC or perihilar EHCC. The median OS was 16 months, and at a median follow-up of 16 months (range 7–29 months), the crude rate of LC was 71%. No patients experienced an acute grade 3 or higher toxicity. Kasuya et al. reported one of the largest multi-institutional retrospective series from the Japan Carbon-Ion Radiation Oncology Study Group including 56 patients with either IHCC ($n = 29$) or perihilar EHCC ($n = 27$) [183]. Patients received CIRT to a dose of 52.8–76 GyE in 4–26 fractions. For patients with IHCC, the 1- and 2-year OS were 78% and 53%, while for patients with perihilar EHCC, the rates were 61% and 26%, respectively. One patient experienced a grade 5 liver toxicity and one patient experienced late grade 3 bile duct stenosis.

19.4 Extrahepatic Cholangiocarcinoma and Gallbladder Cancer

19.4.1 Epidemiology and Etiology

Extrahepatic biliary tract cancers comprised GBCA and EHCC which arise within the extrahepatic biliary tree distal to the secondary biliary branches. EHCC may be further differentiated as perihilar which represent 50–70% of EHCC and can be classified anatomically per the Bismuth-Corlette classification, or as distal EHCC with the anatomical transition occurring just proximal to the insertion of the cystic duct to form the common bile duct. Worldwide, there were an estimated 219,420 cases of GBCA during 2018 [1]. Within the United States, there will be an estimated 8,000 cases of GBCA and approximately 3,000–4,000 cases of EHCC diagnosed during 2020 predominately occurring in patients older than 60 years [2]. There is considerable geographic variability in GBCA incidence which correlates with the prevalence of cholelithiasis and/or *Salmonella typhi* prevalence with particularly high

Table 19.5 Select series of particle therapy for cholangiocarcinoma or gallbladder cancer.

References	Study design	Patients (n)	CP status A/B/C (%)	Median tumor size (cm) (range)	TVT/ PVTT (%)	Dose (GyE)	Fractions	OS	LC	Liver toxicity	Toxicity
Proton therapy											
[181]	Retrospective	28	–	2.0–17.5	–	50.6–80.0	2.0–3.2 GyE fractions	OS1: 49%	LC1: 68%	–	4% G3 + acute toxicity
		6 IHCC									0% G3 + late toxicity
		6 PHCC									14% G2 + late duodenal toxicity
		3 Distal EHCC									
		3 gall bladder									
[180]	Retrospective	20	70/30/0	5.0 (1.5–14.0)	–	72.6 (55–79.2)	Oct 22	OS1: 82%	LC1: 88%	–	0% G3 + acute non-hematologic toxicity
		12 curative intent						OS2: 61%	LC2: 60%		
								OS3: 38%	LC3: 60%		
[117]	Prospective phase 2	37 IHCC	87/10/10	6.0 (2.2–10.9)	28%	Peripheral: 67.5	15	OS2: 47%	LC2: 94%	4% CP class progression (A–B) by 6 months	Overall cohort 6% G3 + acute toxicity
						≤2 cm from porta hepatis: 58.05					
Carbon-ion therapy											
[182]	Retrospective	7	–	3.3–7.6	–	52.8–60	Peripheral: 4	mOS: 16 m		–	
		6 IHCC					Central/ PHCC: 12				
		1 PHCC									
[183]	Retrospective	56	93/7/0	3.7 (1.5–11.0)	–	52.8–76	Apr 26	OS1: 70%	Crude: 71%	1 G5 liver toxicity	0% G3 + acute toxicity
		29 IHCC						OS2: 41%		1 G3 bile duct stenosis	
		27 PHCC						IHCC OS1: 78%			
								OS2: 53%			
								PHCC OS1: 61%			
								OS2: 26%			

rates in South America and Northern India [184]. While North America is considered a low-incidence area, there may be an increasing incidence in younger individuals [185].

Risk factors for GBCA include chronic cholelithiasis (especially if symptomatic), female gender (2–6 times more frequent in women than men), obesity, diabetes mellitus, high carbohydrate intake, chronic biliary infection or inflammation, gallbladder polyps, calcification of the gallbladder wall (porcelain gallbladder), or an anomalous pancreaticobiliary ductal junction [186–189]. The combination of chronic infection with *S. typhi* and cholelithiasis is strongly associated with GBCA [190]. However, the increased risk of GBCA in patients with asymptomatic cholelithiasis is so low that prophylactic resection of the gallbladder is not recommended.

Risk factors for EHCC are as mentioned for IHCC, although there is a lesser association with cirrhosis, HBV infection, or HCV infection.

19.4.2 Pathology—Gallbladder Cancer

Over 90% of GBCA are adenocarcinomas. Other less common histologies may include adenosquamous carcinoma, squamous cell carcinoma, small cell neuroendocrine tumors, lymphomas, or sarcomas [189,191]. Carcinogenesis of GBCA is thought to follow a progressive sequence over approximately 20 years of chronic inflammation leading to gastric-type or intestinal-type metaplasia, low-grade dysplasia, dysplastic progression, high grade carcinoma *in-situ*, and ultimately, invasive GBCA. These step-wise changes can be found in the mucosa-adjacent GBCA in 90% of cases [189].

Grossly, GBCA can be infiltrative, nodular, papillary, mucinous, or a combination. Histology, grade, stage of disease, vascular invasion, and location (hepatic surface vs. peritoneal surface) are strongly associated with survival [192,193]. Papillary carcinomas, which comprise approximately 5% of GBCA, have the most favorable prognosis. The thin-walled gallbladder and lack of a well-defined muscular layer allow early invasion and extension outside of the gallbladder to involve neighboring organs, such as the liver, and early vascular and lymphatic dissemination. Approximately 50% of patients with GBCA will have lymph node involvement at the time of surgical resection, although this rate is strongly associated with T-stage with reported rates of 17–40% for T2 tumors and as high as 80% for T4 tumors. Lymph node dissemination is most frequently within cystic, hilar, choledochal, periportal, hepatic arterial, hepatoduodenal, pancreaticoduodenal, celiac, or superior mesenteric regions, although lymph node regions beyond the hepatoduodenal ligament (e.g., celiac or superior mesenteric) are considered non-regional [193,194]. At diagnosis, approximately 40% of patients will have distant metastasis, most commonly to the liver or peritoneum and with lesser frequency to the lungs [185].

19.4.3 Clinical Presentation

Patients with early GBCA are most commonly asymptomatic or have symptoms which mimic cholelithiasis or cholecystitis. Despite improved recognition and imaging techniques, only 50% of GBCAs are identified prior to surgery [191]. Amongst symptomatic patients, the most common symptoms include abdominal pain, anorexia, nausea, vomiting, and when advanced, may present with malaise, weight loss, or biliary obstruction.

In contrast to IHCC, patients with EHCC usually become symptomatic when the tumor obstructs the biliary system. Symptoms may include obstructive jaundice, pruritus, clay-colored stools, dark urine, dull right upper quadrant abdominal pain, weight loss, or fever [149].

19.4.4 Diagnostic Evaluation

Diagnostic evaluation including physical examination, laboratory evaluation, and diagnostic imaging for both GBCA and EHCC is similar to that for HCC and IHCC. CA 19-9 has generally been less specific for EHCC and GBCA as it may be elevated due to biliary stasis or biliary infection, although it remains helpful in the evaluation of indeterminate biliary strictures [149].

US is usually the initial diagnostic study to evaluate for presumed gallstone-related disease and can identify biliary stricture with associated proximal biliary ductal dilatation in patients with EHCC, although it has limited sensitivity for the detection of GBCA [195]. If suspicious US features are identified or a patient has incidentally diagnosed GBCA at the time of cholecystectomy, cross-sectional imaging with either CT, MRI, or MRCP is indicated to assess for the location, extent, regional spread, and feasibility of oncologic surgical resection. ERCP may also be indicated for biliary decompression/stenting, biopsy, or brushing cytologic confirmation.

EHCC may not be clearly visible on cross-sectional imaging, especially for small non-mass forming tumors, although ductal dilatation (>6 mm) with or without hepatic atrophy may be suggestive of the diagnosis. Proximal EHCC may cause dilation of the intrahepatic ducts alone, while both intrahepatic and extrahepatic ducts are dilated with more distal lesions [196]. In the context of unilobar biliary obstruction, contralateral hepatic lobe hypertrophy and ipsilateral hepatic lobe atrophy (hypertrophy–atrophy complex) may be identified [149]. MRCP may be used to assess local tumor extent and resectability and in some series has been reported to have comparable accuracy to ERCP [197]. Considering most patients present with biliary obstruction, therapeutic ERCP is commonly utilized to alleviate biliary obstruction and can also be used to characterize the location of the stricture(s), help distinguish the cause of the obstruction (e.g., focal pattern for EHCC vs.

diffuse-patchy "beads on a string" pattern for PSC), and can be used for biopsy or brushings with cytology and cytogenetics.

CT of the chest, abdomen, and pelvis is recommended to evaluate for regional spread or distant metastasis. PET-CT is not routinely performed, although it may complement conventional imaging in identifying regional or distant metastatic disease, and if a diagnosis remains uncertain after standard evaluation, it may assist in clinical diagnosis and subsequent decision making [149].

GBCA is often histologically confirmed incidentally after simple cholecystectomy for presumed symptomatic cholelithiasis or cholecystitis. Establishing a tissue diagnosis of EHCC can be much more challenging, particularly for perihilar tumors. Due to the limited number of cells collected during ERCP with brushing, the sensitivity of conventional cytology is approximately 20% [198]. Chromosomal analysis with fluorescent *in-situ* hybridization (FISH) is associated with improved sensitivity of 47% and specificity of 97% [199]. In FISH analysis, three subsets of chromosomal amplification can occur: trisomy 7, tetrasomy or duplication of all chromosomes labeled, and polysomy or amplification of at least two chromosomes beyond tetrasomy. Polysomy is observed in up to 77% of patients with cholangiocarcinoma and when identified in combination with a dominant stricture can satisfy the diagnostic criteria for this disease [149,200]. As mentioned previously, transperitoneal fine-needle aspiration or EUS-guided biopsy of the primary tumor is not recommended [151].

19.4.5 Staging

GBCA and EHCC are staged per the AJCC eighth edition staging manual, with unique staging systems for GBCA, perihilar (proximal) EHCC, and distal EHCC (Table 19.2) [27].

19.4.6 General Management — Gallbladder Cancer

19.4.6.1 Localized Disease

Complete resection with negative margins is the only proven potentially curative treatment for patients with GBCA [201]. Considering most patients are incidentally diagnosed after simple cholecystectomy, referral to a surgical oncologist for consideration of re-resection is indicated in most cases. Patients with T1a disease may be adequately managed with simple cholecystectomy with long-term survival approaching 100% [202]. For patients with T2 or higher disease, the optimal surgery is cholecystectomy with limited resection of hepatic segments IVB and V in addition to a porta hepatis, gastrohepatic, and retroduodenal lymphadenectomy, although more extended hepatic resections may be required to achieve negative margins in some patients [201,203]. Surgical management

of patients with T1b disease is controversial, although extended resection is generally recommended because some series demonstrate that a significant proportion of patients will have residual disease in the liver, common bile duct, or regional lymph nodes at the time of re-resection after prior simple cholecystectomy [191,202,204–208]. Common bile-duct resection is associated with increased perioperative morbidity and, therefore, is typically only recommended for those with adherent porta hepatic lymph node disease or for those with locally invasive disease in order to obtain negative margins [209]. Lymph node involvement, which is present in approximately 50% of patients at surgical resection, is the most important prognostic factor. Five-year OS is approximately 60% for patients with T1bN0 disease, 50% for T2N0 disease, but only 20% for patients with lymph node involvement [210].

19.4.6.2 Locally Advanced, Unresectable, or Metastatic Disease

For patients with unresectable GBCA, management may include systemic therapy alone, radiotherapy with palliative or curative intent (if locoregionally confined), or best supportive care with palliation of biliary obstruction.

19.4.7 General Management — Extrahepatic Cholangiocarcinoma

19.4.7.1 Localized Disease

Potentially curative options for patients with perihilar EHCC include surgical resection or neoadjuvant chemoradiotherapy followed by radical resection with liver transplantation, although less than 50% of patients are amenable to curative intent therapy at diagnosis [211–213]. Surgical resection involving bile-duct resection combined with a modified hepatic resection has demonstrated improved R0 resection rates, OS, and hepatic recurrence when compared to bile-duct resection alone [141,214–219]. R0 resection is possible in approximately 20–40% of patients explored with curative intent but may be as high as 75% when combined with hepatic resection. Major prognostic factors are margin status, vascular invasion, tumor grade, and lymph node metastasis [220]. The 5-year OS is approximately 30–50% after R0 resection and approximately 10–25% after R1 resection.

Neoadjuvant chemoradiotherapy followed by liver transplantation has demonstrated promising outcomes for select patients with perihilar EHCC who are not suitable for conventional surgical resection [221,222]. Initial series evaluated liver transplantation alone and identified relapse rates of approximately 80%, with approximately half occurring in the liver allograft, and 5-year OS of 25–30%. Neoadjuvant chemoradiotherapy with a regimen of 45 Gy in 1.5 Gy, twice daily, fractions with concurrent 5-FU or capecitabine followed by biliary brachytherapy prior to transplantation was subsequently explored to improve upon these outcomes. A multi-center report from 12 transplantation centers including 287 patients reported that neoadjuvant chemoradiotherapy followed by transplantation was associated with a 5-year OS of 53% (intent to treat) and a 5-year recurrence-free survival of 65% amongst those who underwent transplantation [221]. Tumor size greater than 3 cm and prior transperitoneal biopsy were identified as adverse prognostic factors. These data have established this regimen as a potentially curative option with promising outcomes amongst a patient cohort typically considered incurable by conventional surgical techniques.

Surgery, typically with a pancreaticoduodenectomy, is the only proven potentially curative treatment option for patients with a distal EHCC. Isolated bile-duct excision with frozen section analysis may be attempted in patients with mid bile-duct tumors without involvement of the liver or pancreas; however, this situation is uncommon. R0 resection may be achievable in approximately 80% of patients with localized disease [141]. The 5-year OS is approximately 20–50% but may be as high as 50–60% for patients who undergo R0 resection and does not have lymph node involvement [141,223–227]. Lymph node involvement is identified in approximately 60% of patients and is associated with a 5-year OS of approximately 20% [225–227].

Adjuvant therapy with chemotherapy or chemoradiotherapy is often considered in patients with EHCC or GBCA due to the high rates of compromised surgical margins, risk of locoregional recurrence, and its impact on OS [138,166,168]. As described previously, the BILCAP trial demonstrated an improvement in OS with the delivery of capecitabine compared with observation for patients with resected biliary tract or GBCA. However, there is considerable heterogeneity in disease biology and patterns of failure amongst these disease entities, with locoregional recurrence being the predominant pattern of relapse for patients with EHCC. While there are no prospective randomized trials evaluating postoperative radiotherapy for patients with resected EHCC, multiple retrospective studies support its use [228–230]. Kim et al. reported on 168 patients with resected EHCC, of which 115 received postoperative chemoradiotherapy to a median dose of 45 Gy in 25 fractions. The 5-year OS was significantly improved (37% vs. 28%) with the addition of chemoradiotherapy [229]. Similarly, Im et al. reported on 336 patients, 168 of which received adjuvant therapy, and demonstrated that both adjuvant chemotherapy (HR: 0.62, 95% CI: 0.44–0.89) and chemoradiotherapy (HR: 0.46, 95% CI: 0.28–0.77) were associated with improved OS [228]. As previously mentioned, the SWOG S0809 trial prospectively evaluated postoperative chemotherapy followed by chemoradiotherapy for patients with resected EHCC or GBCA and demonstrated favorable 2-year OS of 65% [168].

19.4.7.2 Locally Advanced, Unresectable, or Metastatic Disease

For patients with unresectable EHCC, management may include systemic therapy alone, radiotherapy with palliative or curative intent (if locoregionally confined), or best supportive care. Patients will often have significant biliary obstruction, and therefore all should be evaluated for the need for biliary decompression.

19.4.8 Definitive Radiotherapy for Extrahepatic Cholangiocarcinoma or Gallbladder Cancer

The majority of data describing curative-intent radiotherapy for patients with EHCC or GBCA are limited to relatively small, single institution series. Crane et al. reported on 52 patients treated with radiotherapy doses of 30–85 Gy with concurrent 5-FU chemotherapy in 73% of patients [231]. They demonstrated a median OS of 10 months and 2-year OS of 13%. Bisello et al. reported on 76 patients treated with a median radiotherapy dose of 50 Gy, biliary brachytherapy in 51%, and concurrent 5-FU or gemcitabine-based chemotherapy in 78% of patients [232]. They demonstrated a median OS of 13.5 months, 2-year OS of 26%, and 3-year OS of 11%. Yoshioka reported on 209 patients treated between 2000 and 2011 with radiotherapy to a dose of 50 Gy with concurrent chemotherapy in 78% of patients plus biliary brachytherapy in 27% [233]. Two-year OS was approximately 30%. LC in these series was approximately 60%.

To assess the potential benefit of the addition of radiotherapy to chemotherapy for this cohort of patients, Torgeson et al. performed a propensity score-matched National Cancer Database analysis of 2,996 patients with unresectable EHCC or GBCA treated with chemotherapy alone versus chemoradiotherapy [234]. Chemoradiotherapy was associated with better median OS (14.5 vs. 12.6 months, HR: 0.84, $p < 0.001$). Similarly, Shinohara et al. performed a propensity-score matched analysis using the Surveillance, Epidemiology, and End Results database and demonstrated a median OS of 9 versus 4 months (HR: 0.61; 95% CI: 0.54–0.70, $p < 0.0001$) in favor of radiotherapy versus no radiotherapy or surgery [235].

The Fédération Francophone de Cancérologie Digestive 9902 phase II randomized trial compared treatment with 6 months of gemcitabine plus oxaliplatin versus 5-FU and cisplatin-based chemoradiotherapy to a dose of 50 Gy [236]. The study closed early due to slow accrual, but amongst the 36 accrued patients (anticipated accrual of 72 patients), there was no difference in median PFS (5.8 vs. 11.0 months, HR: 0.65, 95% CI: 0.32–1.33) or median OS (13.5 vs. 19.9 months, HR: 0.69, 95% CI: 0.31–1.55) and acute grade 3–4 toxicity (47% vs. 75%) for the chemoradiotherapy versus chemotherapy alone cohorts, respectively. Therefore, the role of radiotherapy for patients with unresectable EHCC or GBCA remains controversial.

19.5 Liver Metastasis

19.5.1 Clinical Outcomes of Particle Therapy for Liver Metastasis

There are a few series reporting results of proton therapy for patients with liver metastasis which demonstrate the early feasibility, safety, and efficacy of this strategy (demonstrated in Table 19.6). Hong et al. reported a prospective phase II trial of 89 patients with liver metastasis most commonly from colorectal (38%), pancreas (15%), or gastroesophageal (13%) primary tumors [237]. The median tumor size was 2.5 cm (range 0.5–11.9 cm). Patients were treated to a median dose of 40 GyE (range 30–50 GyE) in five fractions. The 1- and 3-year LC were 72% and 61%, and 1- and 3-year OS were 66% and 21%. No patient experienced grade 3 or higher acute toxicity. The largest experience of proton therapy for patients with liver metastasis was reported by Fukumitsu et al. and included 140 patients with predominately colorectal (43%), pancreas (14%), gastric (9%), or breast cancer (9%) [238]. Patients were treated to a dose of 72.6 GyE in 10–35 fractions. The 5-year LC and OS were 53% and 25%, respectively.

Colbert et al. reported an experience of right hemi-liver ablative radiotherapy in five patients who had bilobar colorectal liver metastasis but were not candidates for second stage right hepatectomy [239]. Treatment was delivered to the entire right lobe of the liver to a median dose of 100 GyE in 25 fractions. Follow-up ranged from 8 to 24 months for the treated patients, and the crude rates of LC and OS were 80% and 60%, respectively. All four patients treated with a BED greater than 89.6 Gy_{10} achieved partial or complete radiographic response and in-field LC at last follow-up.

Makishima et al. conducted a phase I dose-escalation study of single fraction CIRT for patients with colorectal liver metastases unsuitable for resection [240]. Twenty-nine patients were treated with 36–58 GyE in one fraction. No acute grade 3 or higher dose limiting toxicities were observed; however, two patients (of 11) developed late grade 3 biliary obstruction at a dose of 53–58 Gy/L fraction. The 3-year OS was 78% for all patients. The 3-year actuarial local control was 82% in patients receiving 53–58 Gy/L fraction.

19.6 Particle Therapy Planning

19.6.1 Simulation

Prior to simulation, most patients with intrahepatic tumors will have placement of MRI compatible peritumoral fiducial markers to assist with daily image guidance. High-Z fiducials provide excellent radiographic contrast for imaging; as such, gold fiducials have been used most commonly. One potential downside to high-Z fiducials is that they may cause dose perturbations for particle therapy. Fiducials made from lower Z materials such as titanium, or composite materials such as carbon-coated zirconium dioxide, may provide more acceptable particle therapy dosimetry [241].

Patients are most commonly simulated supine, arms above their head, in a custom immobilization device. Ideally, multiphasic CT and/or MRI should be obtained to assist with target delineation. Respiratory motion should be assessed at the time of simulation, typically with a 4D CT. Tumors with movement greater than 1 cm in any direction may be considered for respiratory motion management strategies to allow improved sparing of non-tumor liver from the target volume. Techniques may include abdominal compression or beam gating strategies such as voluntary breath-hold (BH), respiratory-phase, or amplitude-based gating. However, this must be balanced with the potential for introduction of additional uncertainties, increased technical and process complexity, and overall practice efficiency decreases associated with extending the treatment delivery time.

19.6.2 Target Volumes

Suggestions for radiotherapy target volumes and dose are demonstrated in Table 19.7. The internal gross target volume (iGTV) should be delineated based upon the planning CT, accounting for potential tumor motion throughout the respiratory cycle, and all registered diagnostic studies including multiphasic CT and/or MRI. The clinical target volume (CTV) should include the iGTV plus adjacent regions considered at risk for harboring microscopic disease. For patients with HCC, IHCC, or liver metastasis typically being considered for ablative radiotherapy techniques, the CTV can often include the iGTV with no additional margin [242]. However, consideration of a marginal expansion of approximately 0.5 cm may be considered for patients with tumors >5 cm, portal vein vascular thrombus, or those with ambiguous tumor borders.

The CTV for patients with EHCC or GBCA may require considerably larger expansions due to the risk of microscopic disease extension locally and within regional lymph nodes. The proximity to organs such as the liver, duodenum, and stomach and the recommended target volumes often precludes ablative radiotherapy strategies due to risk of toxicity to closely adjacent organs at risk. An expansion of 0.5–2.0 cm upon the iGTV may be considered to account for subclinical spread along the biliary tree. Highest risk regional lymph node regions include the hepatoduodenal ligament, celiac artery, superior mesenteric artery, or retroperitoneal/para-aortic lymph nodes [243–246].

Typical planning target volume (PTV) expansions are 4–10 mm but depend upon patient, setup, immobilization, respiratory motion management, and daily image guidance factors. Daily image guidance may be a particular concern with

Table 19.6 Select series of particle therapy for liver metastasis.

References	Study design	Patients (n)	CP status A/B/C (%)	Tumor histology	Median tumor size (cm) (range)	Dose (GyE)	Fractions	OS	LC	Liver toxicity	Toxicity
Proton therapy											
[238]	Retrospective	140	86/6/1	Colorectal: 43% Pancreas: 14% Stomach: 9% Breast: 9%	4.0 (1.0–18.0)	72.6 (9–77)	Oct 35	OS5: 24%	LC5: 53%	–	–
[237]	Prospective phase 2	89	No cirrhosis or CPA	Colorectal: 38% Pancreas: 15% Esophagogastric: 13% Other: 34%	2.5 (0.5–11.9)	40 (30–50)	5	mOS: 18 m OS1: 66% OS3: 21%	LC1: 72% LC3: 61%		0% G3 acute toxicity
[239]	Retrospective	5	–	Colorectal: 100%	Right hemiliver	100	25	Crude: 60%	Crude: 80%	–	–
[317]	Retrospective	8	–	Breast: 100%	4.0 (1.2–7.0)	66 / 72.6	10 / 22	OS1: 88% OS3: 73% OS5: 58%	LC1: 86% LC3: 86% LC5: 86%	0% RILD	0% G3 acute toxicity 0% G3 late toxicity
[318]	Retrospective	9	–	Gastric: 100%	3.0 (2.0–6.0)	64–77	Oct 35	OS1: 100% OS3: 78% OS5: 56%	LC1: 89% LC3: 71% LC5: 71%	0% RILD 0% CP progression of >2 points	0% G4 + acute toxicity 0% G3 late toxicity
[319]	Prospective phase 1	9	–	Colorectal: 56%	3	36–60	3	Crude: 33%	Crude: 86%	0% RILD	0% G3 acute toxicity 0% G3 late toxicity
[240]	Prospective phase 1	29 / 14 lesions	–	Colorectal: 100%	2.5 (1.2–10.2)	36–58	1	OS3: 78%	≥53 GyE LC3: 82% ≤48 GyE LC3: 28%	7% Late G3 biliary obstruction	0% Dose-limiting toxicity

Table 19.7   Recommended target volumes and radiotherapy dose for hepatobiliary cancers.

Disease(s)	Target volume	Definitive	Postoperative	Dose (GyE)
Hepatocellular carcinoma Intrahepatic cholangiocarcinoma Liver metastasis	GTV	Gross liver tumor	–	Peripheral tumors: 30–60 GyE in 5–6 fractions. Goal liver mean dose ≤13 GyE Central tumors: 58.05–67.5 Gy in 15 fractions Goal liver mean dose <24 Gy
	CTV	Gross liver tumor. May consider 0–0.5 cm margin to encompass potential microscopic disease	–	Peripheral tumors: 30–60 GyE in 5–6 fractions. Goal liver mean dose ≤13 GyE Central tumors: 58.05–67.5 Gy in 15 fractions Goal liver mean dose <24 Gy
Extrahepatic cholangiocarcinoma Gallbladder cancer	GTV	Gross primary tumor and involved regional lymph nodes	Gross residual disease	50–60 GyE in 25–33 fractions Goal liver mean dose <30 Gy
	CTV high	Gross primary tumor plus 0.5–2.0 cm along biliary tree or within hepatic parenchyma to encompass potential microscopic disease Grossly involved lymph nodes plus 0.5–1.0 cm	Pre-operative tumor volume and operative bed plus 0.5–2.0 cm margin to encompass potential microscopic disease	50–60 GyE in 25–33 fractions Goal liver mean dose <30 Gy
	CTV low	Lymph node regions at risk for microscopic disease, potentially including hepatoduodenal ligament, celiac artery, superior mesenteric artery, or retroperitoneal/para-aortic lymph nodes	Lymph node regions at risk for microscopic disease, potentially including hepatoduodenal ligament, celiac artery, superior mesenteric artery, or retroperitoneal/para-aortic lymph nodes	45 GyE in 25 fractions Goal liver mean dose <30 Gy

particle therapy as onboard image guidance technology is not as mature when compared with modern photon radiotherapy platforms [247].

19.6.3   Radiotherapy Dose

For patients with HCC, IHCC, or liver metastasis, the radiotherapy dose is often a balance between achieving tumoricidal dose while maintaining acceptable liver dosimetric constraints; however, further consideration should also be given for tumors closely approximating the porta hepatis, central biliary tree, or GI luminal organs. For patients suitable for SBRT, RTOG 1112 provides dosing recommendations for 5–6 fraction regimens: ideally MLD (excluding the GTV) ≤13 Gy should be a goal. If this cannot be achieved, then the prescription dose should be decreased, with a maximum allowed MLD of up to 17 Gy [118]. Patients with tumors measuring >5–10 cm, centrally located, or within 2 cm of GI luminal organs may be more suitable for moderately hypofractionated regimens. An acceptable dosing regimen may include 67.5 Gy in 15 fractions, with consideration of reducing the dose to 58.05 Gy or offering non-homogeneous tumor coverage adjacent to the porta hepatis or GI luminal organs in order to meet acceptable dosimetric constraints to critical organs at risk [117]. The radiotherapy dose and coverage may be adjusted to achieve an MLD of ≤24–27 Gy. Figure 19.3 demonstrates representative photon volumetrically modulated arc therapy and pencil beam scanning proton therapy plans for a patient with a large HCC involving the right lobe of the liver treated to a dose of 58.05 GyE in 15 fractions. Figure 19.4 demonstrates a representative pencil beam scanning proton therapy plan for a patient with a large, unresectable, IHCC treated to a dose of 58.05 GyE along with a 9-month post-treatment CT of the abdomen showing a significant reduction in tumor size and enhancement.

Patients with EHCC or GBCA are more routinely treated with conventionally fractionated radiotherapy regimens due to the close proximity to liver, stomach, and duodenum and hence the concern for potentially life-threatening toxicity if treating with ablative regimens. For EHCC or GBCA in the adjuvant setting, most studies have reported doses ranging from 45 to 54 Gy at 1.8 to 2.0 Gy per fraction. In the unresectable or definitive setting, most studies have reported doses of 45–60 Gy at 1.8–2.0 Gy per fraction. At risk elective lymph node regions may be treated to a dose of approximately 45 Gy in 1.8 Gy fractions. Moderately hypofractionated 15-fraction regimens may be considered with an effort to safely deliver modest tumor dose escalation while placing greatest priority on meeting acceptable dosimetric constraints for critical organs at risk.

19.6.4 Planning Techniques and Considerations

Particle therapy treatment planning adds considerable complexity when compared to photon therapy treatment planning. Herein we discuss a number of the uncertainties of particle therapy treatment planning for hepatobiliary tumors and existing techniques to help mitigate these uncertainties.

Uncertainty in particle range, or the depth in tissue or material where the particle will stop, remains a significant concern. During the planning process, particle relative stopping power is determined using the stoichiometric method, which is the adopted standard in CT image Hounsfield unit (HU) to relative stopping power calibration [248]. However, HU has a nonlinear and potentially degenerate relationship with relative stopping power, particularly in the context of various tissues or material types

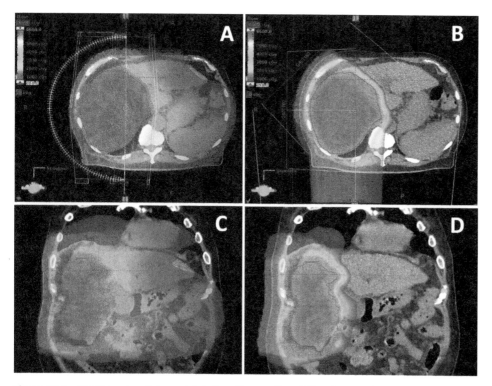

Figure 19.3 Photon volumetric modulated arc therapy (A and C) and proton beam radiotherapy (B and D) plans for a patient with a large hepatocellular carcinoma involving most of the right lobe of the liver. The prescription dose is 58.05 GyE in 15 fractions. Note significantly improved sparing of the left lobe of the liver with proton beam radiotherapy.

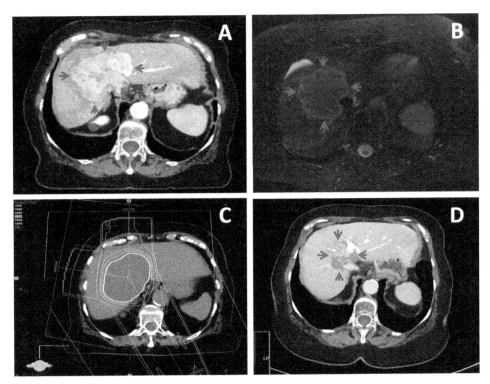

Figure 19.4 Eighty-year-old female with biopsy proven intrahepatic cholangiocarcinoma, unresectable due to vascular involvement, shown on CT (A) and MRI (B). She received proton beam radiotherapy, 58.05 GyE in 15 fractions over 3 weeks (C). The isodose lines are 5,805 cGy (white), 5,000 (cyan), 4,000 cGy (green), 3,000 cGy (blue), 2,000 cGy (yellow), 1,000 cGy (cyan), and 500 cGy (magenta). CT at 9 months after treatment shows significant reduction in size and enhancement of the mass.

which are relevant to particle therapy. The use of dual energy CT as part of the HU-relative stopping power calibration process may reduce this uncertainty [249,250]. In the context of proton therapy, a range uncertainty planning margin of approximately 3.5% + 1 mm expansion along the beam direction has been suggested [251]. The use of Monte-Carlo dose calculation may improve this uncertainty margin. In the context of liver radiotherapy, this margin may be excessive as there is less tissue heterogeneity compared with other sites involving more bone–tissue, bone–air, or tissue–lung interfaces [252].

The accuracy of particle therapy range predictions is directly related to the water-equivalent thickness (WET) along the beam path. Inter-fractional variation in patient anatomy which can occur in the context of set-up variability, weight loss, pleural effusions, ascites, stomach or bowel variable filling, medical devices, or tumor changes may have a dramatic impact upon the particle therapy dose distribution.

Structures which are subject to variable filling with different density materials such as food, water, stool, gas, or medical devices may generate additional uncertainty in dose distribution. If these are nontarget tissues, the simplest solutions would be to avoid beam entrance through this region of uncer-

tainty, and in the instance of stomach or bowel filling, to have more restrictive patient dietary or meal timing instructions. If this is not feasible or is deemed undesirable, these structures may be contoured and a HU override derived from sampling of neighboring HU within the organ and outside of the region of uncertainty (e.g., gas) may be applied.

Plastic stents, particularly biliary, are often constructed with a radiopaque material to assist with imaging identification and thereby provide relatively high HU. Because these stent walls are thin, a common practice is to override the HU to water-equivalent. Metallic objects, like fiducials or metallic stents, generate additional uncertainty because the integrity of the CT scan is affected by reconstruction artifact with higher HU streaking and lower HU shadowing around the object and the object often appearing larger than true size. The use of extended HU reconstruction scales and iterative reconstruction techniques may allow for improved metal object identification and contouring and improve CT image quality [253–255]. These techniques may mitigate the need to address streaking artifact with manual contouring and HU overrides, but this decision would need to be made for the individual patient. Metallic object dose perturbations and their impact on plan quality are an additional concern [256]. These perturbations may prove negligible with realistic "spread out Bragg peak" beams. The use of multiple beams from various angles would further mitigate this issue by better dispersing the potential hot or cold spots [257].

Intra-fraction anatomical changes which occur due to periodic tumor motion with respiration and the associated "interplay effect" may cause considerable plan degradation if not accounted for. Typical tumor motion in the liver can range from 1 to 19 mm, most significantly along the superior–inferior direction [258–260]. To account for this, patients should undergo 4D CT simulation to characterize respiratory motion of the target and adjacent normal structures [261,262]. Choosing beam angles which minimize the change in WET throughout the respiratory cycle, for instance limiting beam entrance through the lung, diaphragm, or pleural effusions, will offer maximum robustness [263–265]. Active motion management strategies such as abdominal compression to reduce diaphragmatic excursion have been successfully employed [266]. For pencil beam scanning proton therapy specifically, several techniques have been utilized to minimize dosimetric plan degradation due to motion interplay. Repainting strategies have commonly been used to better disperse delivered proton spots across the breathing cycle and thereby dampen dosimetric heterogeneity [265,267–272]. Beam-gating strategies have also been used, which can include free-breathing treatment with respiratory phase- or amplitude-based gating or treatment with image-guided BH techniques [43]. In some circumstances, beam-gating may be combined with repainting strategies, although this may pose additional treatment efficiency concerns [268,273,274].

Because of the added sensitivity of particle therapy plans to degradation due to range uncertainties and anatomical variability, robust plan evaluation has been adopted as the standard of practice. Robust evaluation of positional or set-up uncertainties is achieved by moving the plan isocenter or beam location along the three Cartesian axes (x, y, z) by a positional offset (e.g., 5 mm) appropriate for the clinical context and image guidance strategy and recalculating the dose on the planning CT. Robust evaluation of range uncertainty involves systematic scaling of the CT-HU inferred relative stopping power by percentages deemed consistent with the anticipated range fluctuation, for example, ±3%. For patients in which HU overrides were utilized to account for potential variable bowel gas filling or medical devices, dose recalculation assuming CT-HU relative stopping power extremes may improve plan robustness. Furthermore, to account for variability during the respiratory cycle, recalculation of the plan on the extreme motion phases (e.g., phase 0 and phase 50) may be performed. In some circumstances, calculation of the 4D dynamic dose may be done to better estimate the magnitude of interplay effects [275–281].

Plan robustness may also be monitored throughout the course of treatment. This can be accomplished by obtaining repetitive CT scans in the radiotherapy treatment position and assessing the dose distribution on the new image data set. Based upon dosimetric criteria, the treatment plans can be "adapted" to accommodate observed imaging changes.

As discussed previously, the current clinical convention is to use a fixed relative RBE value to correct the physical dose relative to photon therapy. However, in regions surrounding the Bragg peak, the RBE is hypothesized to be significantly higher and could theoretically lead to substantially increased dose to normal tissues. In the context of hepatobiliary radiotherapy, treatment fields should be designed not only to minimize exposure to organs at risk, mitigate the uncertainties described above, but also to limit multiple beams from having overlapping end of range segments (i.e., overlapping Bragg peaks) adjacent to critical structures like bowel, thereby dispersing potentially biologically "hot" segments of the plan.

19.7 Acute and Late Complications

Classic RILD was historically the dose-limiting toxicity of liver radiotherapy, typically occurring approximately 2 weeks to 4 months after radiotherapy and being pathologically characterized as a veno-occlusive phenomenon secondary to fibrosis [282,283]. Classic RILD is characterized by anicteric hepatomegaly, ascites, and elevated liver enzymes, particularly alkaline phosphatase. The estimated rate of classic RILD is approximately 5% or less after conventionally fractionated whole liver radiation to a dose of 28–30 Gy but rises sharply to approximately 50% at MLDs of 36–42 Gy. Apart from radiation dose, other risk factors include severity of underlying liver cirrhosis, primary liver cancer (vs. metastasis), male gender, and hepatic intra-arterial chemotherapy.

In the contemporary era of more conformal radiotherapy techniques, classic RILD is relatively infrequent. Non-classic RILD is more common, particularly in patients with comorbid underlying liver disease, typically manifesting as acute or subacute liver decompensation. In patients with underlying cirrhosis, RILD is most commonly characterized by an increase in CP score by 2 or more points within 3–6 months of completion of radiotherapy, while in non-cirrhotic patients, RILD is more commonly characterized by an increase in serum transaminases by 5 times the upper limit of normal. The predominant risk factors for non-classic RILD include the severity of underlying liver disease and liver radiation exposure, including MLD and the ability to spare a critical volume of normal liver (e.g., 700 cm^3 or 800 cm^3) from doses above a threshold dose [283–285]. Recent data do suggest that the volume of liver receiving low-intermediate radiation doses (2.5–

10 Gy) may also be associated with non-classic RILD [110,282,286,287].

For patients with CP-A cirrhosis, it is recommended to limit the mean normal liver dose to less than 28 Gy for conventionally fractionated radiotherapy. For SBRT, it is recommended to limit the mean normal liver dose to less than 13–18 Gy in 3–6 fractions. Additionally, the dose delivered to a threshold volume of liver should be minimized, for example, >800 cm^3 to receive <18 Gy in 3–6 fractions [288] or ≥700 cm^3 to receive less than 15 Gy in 3–5 fractions [283]. Patients with CP-B or CP-C cirrhosis are at higher risk of liver toxicity after radiotherapy. Therefore, more conservative recommendations for this cohort would include a mean normal liver dose of less than 6 Gy with an absolute constraint of less than 16 Gy [283,285].

GI luminal organs are highly sensitive to radiotherapy and may limit safe delivery of tumoricidal radiotherapy doses in some patients. When delivering conventionally fractionated radiotherapy over 25–30 fractions, a dose of approximately 55 Gy is associated with a risk of severe duodenal or stomach complications (e.g., ulceration, bleeding, or fistula) of approximately 5–10% [289–293]. This risk may rise to approximately 30% with doses above 55 Gy [289].

Patients receiving radiotherapy for cholangiocarcinoma are at considerable risk of cholangitis predominately due to tumor related obstruction, with rates of severe infection reported as high as 60% after radiotherapy [294]. Late complications of biliary stricture may occur in patients receiving SBRT adjacent to the central biliary tract. Toesca et al. reported that when contouring the central biliary tract as the portal vein plus a 1.5-cm isotropic expansion, the strongest dosimetric associates with grade 3 or higher hepatobiliary toxicity were the volumes receiving a BED of 40 Gy$_{10}$ ≥ 37 cm^3 and 30 Gy$_{10}$ ≥ 45 cm^3 [295].

Mild-to-moderate skin and chest-wall toxicity may be more common in patients receiving particle therapy when compared to patients receiving photon-based radiotherapy techniques, particularly for thinner patients with peripherally located tumors. However, it is relatively uncommon to have severe grade 3 or higher skin toxicity. This risk may be reduced by using multiple treatment fields to disperse entrance dose, the use of pencil beam scanning proton therapy relatively to passively scattered techniques, and with the use of CIRT when compared with proton therapy. To minimize the risk of severe chest wall pain or rib fracture, the chest wall volume receiving a dose of 30 Gy or higher in 3–5 fractions should be limited to less than 30 cm^3 [296].

Severe kidney injury is uncommon after radiotherapy for hepatobiliary cancers. It is recommended to maintain a mean dose to both kidneys of less than 18 Gy and to limit a dose of 18–20 Gy to less than 32% to achieve a risk of kidney injury of 5% or less [297].

References

1 Bray, F., et al. (2018). Global cancer statistics 2018: GLOBOCAN estimates of incidence and mortality worldwide for 36 cancers in 185 countries. *CA: A Cancer Journal for Clinicians* 68 (6): 394–424.

2 Siegel, R.L., Miller, K.D., and Jemal, A. (2020). Cancer statistics, 2020. *CA: A Cancer Journal for Clinicians* 70 (1): 7–30.

3 Gandhi, S.J., et al. (2015). Clinical decision tool for optimal delivery of liver stereotactic body radiation therapy: Photons versus protons. *Practical Radiation Oncology* 5 (4): 209–218.

4 Kim, J.Y., et al. (2015). Normal liver sparing by proton beam therapy for hepatocellular carcinoma: Comparison with helical intensity modulated radiotherapy and volumetric modulated arc therapy. *Acta Oncologica* 54 (10): 1827–1832.

5 Toramatsu, C., et al. (2013). What is the appropriate size criterion for proton radiotherapy for hepatocellular carcinoma? A dosimetric comparison of spot-scanning proton therapy versus intensity-modulated radiation therapy. *Radiation Oncology* 8: 48.

6 Wang, X., et al. (2008). Proton radiotherapy for liver tumors: Dosimetric advantages over photon plans. *Medical Dosimetry : Official Journal of the American Association of Medical Dosimetrists* 33 (4): 259–267.

7 Beltran, C., et al. (2020). Radiation biology considerations of proton therapy for gastrointestinal cancers. *Journal of Gastrointestinal Oncology* 11 (1): 225–230.

8 Giovannini, G., et al. (2016). Variable RBE in proton therapy: Comparison of different model predictions and their influence on clinical-like scenarios. *Radiation Oncology* 11: 68.

9 Paganetti, H. (2014). Relative biological effectiveness (RBE) values for proton beam therapy. Variations as a function of biological endpoint, dose, and linear energy transfer. *Physics in Medicine and Biology* 59 (22): R419–72.

10 Paganetti, H., et al. (2002). Relative biological effectiveness (RBE) values for proton beam therapy. *International Journal of Radiation Oncology, Biology, Physics* 53 (2): 407–421.

11 Habermehl, D., et al. (2013). Hypofractionated carbon ion therapy delivered with scanned ion beams for patients with hepatocellular carcinoma - feasibility and clinical response. *Radiation Oncology* 8: 59.

12 Habermehl, D., et al. (2014). The relative biological effectiveness for carbon and oxygen ion beams using the raster-scanning technique in hepatocellular carcinoma cell lines. *PLoS One* 9 (12): e113591.

13 Shinoto, M., Ebner, D.K., and Yamada, S. (2016). Particle Radiation Therapy for Gastrointestinal Cancers. *Current Oncology Reports* 18 (3): 17.

14 Marrero, J.A., et al. (2018). Diagnosis, Staging, and Management of Hepatocellular Carcinoma: 2018 Practice Guidance by the American Association for the Study of Liver Diseases. *Hepatology* 68 (2): 723–750.

15 Villanueva, A. (2019). Hepatocellular Carcinoma. *The New England Journal of Medicine* 380 (15): 1450–1462.

16 Estes, C., et al. (2018). Modeling NAFLD disease burden in China, France, Germany, Italy, Japan, Spain, United Kingdom, and United States for the period 2016-2030. *Journal of Hepatology* 69 (4): 896–904.

17 Liu, T.C., et al. (2014). Noncirrhotic hepatocellular carcinoma: Derivation from hepatocellular adenoma? Clinicopathologic analysis. *Modern Pathology : An Official Journal of the United States and Canadian Academy of Pathology, Inc* 27 (3): 420–432.

18 Board, W.C.T.E. (2019). *Digestive System Tumours*. International Agency for Research on Cancer.

19 Okuda, K., Peters, R.L., and Simson, I.W. (1984). Gross anatomic features of hepatocellular carcinoma from three disparate geographic areas. Proposal of new classification. *Cancer* 54 (10): 2165–2173.

20 Primary Liver Cancer in Japan. (1990). Clinicopathologic features and results of surgical treatment. *Annals of Surgery* 211 (3): 277–287.

21 Watanabe, J., Nakashima, O., and Kojiro, M. (1994). Clinicopathologic study on lymph node metastasis of hepatocellular carcinoma: A retrospective study of 660 consecutive autopsy cases. *Japanese Journal of Clinical Oncology* 24 (1): 37–41.

22 Uka, K., et al. (2007). Clinical features and prognosis of patients with extrahepatic metastases from hepatocellular carcinoma. *World Journal of Gastroenterology : WJG* 13 (3): 414–420.

23 Yi, J., et al. (2013). Screening for extrahepatic metastases by additional staging modalities is required for hepatocellular carcinoma patients beyond modified UICC stage T1. *Hepatogastroenterology* 60 (122): 328–332.

24 Claudon, M., et al. (2013). *Guidelines and good clinical practice recommendations for Contrast Enhanced Ultrasound (CEUS) in the liver - update 2012: A WFUMB-EFSUMB initiative in cooperation with representatives of AFSUMB, AIUM, ASUM, FLAUS and ICUS. Ultrasound in Medicine & Biology* 39 (2): 187–210.

25 Van Der Pol, C.B., et al. (2019). Accuracy of the Liver Imaging Reporting and Data System in Computed Tomography and Magnetic Resonance Image Analysis of Hepatocellular Carcinoma or Overall Malignancy-A Systematic Review. *Gastroenterology* 156 (4): 976–986.

26 Heimbach, J.K., et al. (2018). AASLD guidelines for the treatment of hepatocellular carcinoma. *Hepatology* 67 (1): 358–380.

27 Amin, M.B., Edge, S., Greene, F., Byrd, D.R., Brookland, R.K., Washington, M.K., Gershenwald, J.E., Compton, C.C.,

Hess, K.R., Sullivan, D.C., Jessup, J.M., Brierley, J.D., Gaspar, L.E., Schilsky, R.L., and Balch, C.M. (2017). *AJCC Cancer Staging Manual*, 8th. Springer International Publishing: American Joint Commission on Cancer.

28 Llovet, J.M., Brú, C., and Bruix, J. (1999). Prognosis of hepatocellular carcinoma: The BCLC staging classification. *Seminars in Liver Disease* 19 (3): 329–338.

29 Roayaie, S., et al. (2015). The role of hepatic resection in the treatment of hepatocellular cancer. *Hepatology* 62 (2): 440–451.

30 Berzigotti, A., et al. (2015). Portal hypertension and the outcome of surgery for hepatocellular carcinoma in compensated cirrhosis: A systematic review and meta-analysis. *Hepatology* 61 (2): 526–536.

31 Kubota, K., et al. (1997). Measurement of liver volume and hepatic functional reserve as a guide to decision-making in resectional surgery for hepatic tumors. *Hepatology* 26 (5): 1176–1181.

32 Shoup, M., et al. (2003). Volumetric analysis predicts hepatic dysfunction in patients undergoing major liver resection. *Journal of Gastrointestinal Surgery : Official Journal of the Society for Surgery of the Alimentary Tract* 7 (3): 325–330.

33 Glantzounis, G.K., et al. (2017). The role of portal vein embolization in the surgical management of primary hepatobiliary cancers. A systematic review. *European Journal of Surgical Oncology : The Journal of the European Society of Surgical Oncology and the British Association of Surgical Oncology* 43 (1): 32–41.

34 Bruix, J., et al. (2015). *Adjuvant sorafenib for hepatocellular carcinoma after resection or ablation (STORM): A phase 3, randomised, double-blind, placebo-controlled trial. The Lancet Oncology* 16 (13): 1344–1354.

35 Ishizawa, T., et al. (2008). Neither multiple tumors nor portal hypertension are surgical contraindications for hepatocellular carcinoma. *Gastroenterology* 134 (7): 1908–1916.

36 Wang, J., et al. (2013). A meta-analysis of adjuvant therapy after potentially curative treatment for hepatocellular carcinoma. *Canadian Journal of Gastroenterology* 27 (6): 351–363.

37 Huang, G., et al. (2015). Antiviral therapy improves postoperative survival in patients with hepatocellular carcinoma: A randomized controlled trial. *Annals of Surgery* 261 (1): 56–66.

38 Xia, B.W., et al. (2015). Efficacy of antiviral therapy with nucleotide/nucleoside analogs after curative treatment for patients with hepatitis B virus-related hepatocellular carcinoma: A systematic review and meta-analysis. *Clinics and Research in Hepatology and Gastroenterology* 39 (4): 458–468.

39 Xu, J., et al. (2015). Effect of adjuvant interferon therapy on hepatitis b/c virus-related hepatocellular carcinoma after curative therapy - meta-analysis. *Advances in Clinical and Experimental Medicine : Official Organ Wroclaw Medical University* 24 (2): 331–340.

40 Yin, J., et al. (2013). Effect of antiviral treatment with nucleotide/nucleoside analogs on postoperative prognosis of hepatitis B virus-related hepatocellular carcinoma: A two-stage longitudinal clinical study. *Journal of Clinical Oncology : Official Journal of the American Society of Clinical Oncology* 31 (29): 3647–3655.

41 Martin, A.P., et al. (2007). Overview of the MELD score and the UNOS adult liver allocation system. *Transplantation Proceedings* 39 (10): 3169–3174.

42 Mazzaferro, V., et al. (2011). Milan criteria in liver transplantation for hepatocellular carcinoma: An evidence-based analysis of 15 years of experience. *Liver Transplantation : Official Publication of the American Association for the Study of Liver Diseases and the International Liver Transplantation Society* 17 (Suppl 2): S44–57.

43 Mazzaferro, V., et al. (1996). Liver transplantation for the treatment of small hepatocellular carcinomas in patients with cirrhosis. *The New England Journal of Medicine* 334 (11): 693–699.

44 Mazzaferro, V., et al. (2018). Metroticket 2.0 Model for Analysis of Competing Risks of Death After Liver Transplantation for Hepatocellular Carcinoma. *Gastroenterology* 154 (1): 128–139.

45 Kulik, L., et al. (2018). Therapies for patients with hepatocellular carcinoma awaiting liver transplantation: A systematic review and meta-analysis. *Hepatology* 67 (1): 381–400.

46 Parikh, N.D., Waljee, A.K., and Singal, A.G. (2015). Downstaging hepatocellular carcinoma: A systematic review and pooled analysis. *Liver Transplantation : Official Publication of the American Association for the Study of Liver Diseases and the International Liver Transplantation Society* 21 (9): 1142–1152.

47 Mazzaferro, V., et al. (2020). Liver transplantation in hepatocellular carcinoma after tumour downstaging (XXL): A randomised, controlled, phase 2b/3 trial. *The Lancet Oncology* 21 (7): 947–956.

48 Park, S.J., et al. (2012). Risk factors for liver transplant waitlist dropout in patients with hepatocellular carcinoma. *Clinical Transplantation* 26 (4): E359–64.

49 Yao, F.Y., et al. (2003). A follow-up analysis of the pattern and predictors of dropout from the waiting list for liver transplantation in patients with hepatocellular carcinoma: Implications for the current organ allocation policy. *Liver Transplantation : Official Publication of the American Association for the Study of Liver Diseases and the International Liver Transplantation Society* 9 (7): 684–692.

50 Weis, S., et al. (2013 Dec 19). Radiofrequency (thermal) ablation versus no intervention or other interventions for hepatocellular carcinoma. *Cochrane Library: Cochrane Reviews* (12): Cd003046 doi: 10.1002/14651858.CD003046.pub3. PMID: 24357457.

51 Lin, S.M., et al. (2005). Randomised controlled trial comparing percutaneous radiofrequency thermal ablation, percutaneous ethanol injection, and percutaneous acetic acid injection to treat hepatocellular carcinoma of 3 cm or less. *Gut* 54 (8): 1151–1156.

52 Shiina, S., et al. (2005). A randomized controlled trial of radiofrequency ablation with ethanol injection for small hepatocellular carcinoma. *Gastroenterology* 129 (1): 122–130.

53 Chinnaratha, M.A., et al. (2016). Percutaneous thermal ablation for primary hepatocellular carcinoma: A systematic review and meta-analysis. *Journal of Gastroenterology and Hepatology* 31 (2): 294–301.

54 Kim, N., et al. (2020). Stereotactic body radiation therapy vs. radiofrequency ablation in Asian patients with hepatocellular carcinoma. *Journal of Hepatology* 73 (1): 121–129.

55 Peng, Z.W., et al. (2013). Radiofrequency ablation with or without transcatheter arterial chemoembolization in the treatment of hepatocellular carcinoma: A prospective randomized trial. *Journal of Clinical Oncology : Official Journal of the American Society of Clinical Oncology* 31 (4): 426–432.

56 Cai, H., et al. (2014). Radiofrequency ablation versus reresection in treating recurrent hepatocellular carcinoma: A meta-analysis. *Medicine (Baltimore)* 93 (22): e122.

57 Chen, M.S., et al. (2006). A prospective randomized trial comparing percutaneous local ablative therapy and partial hepatectomy for small hepatocellular carcinoma. *Annals of Surgery* 243 (3): 321–328.

58 Feng, K., et al. (2012). A randomized controlled trial of radiofrequency ablation and surgical resection in the treatment of small hepatocellular carcinoma. *Journal of Hepatology* 57 (4): 794–802.

59 Feng, Q., et al. (2015). Efficacy and safety of percutaneous radiofrequency ablation versus surgical resection for small hepatocellular carcinoma: A meta-analysis of 23 studies. *Journal of Cancer Research and Clinical Oncology* 141 (1): 1–9.

60 Huang, J., et al. (2010). A randomized trial comparing radiofrequency ablation and surgical resection for HCC conforming to the Milan criteria. *Annals of Surgery* 252 (6): 903–912.

61 Jia, J.B., et al. (2017). Radiofrequency ablation versus resection for hepatocellular carcinoma in patients with Child-Pugh A liver cirrhosis: A meta-analysis. *Clinical Radiology* 72 (12): 1066–1075.

62 Ng, K.K.C., et al. (2017). Randomized clinical trial of hepatic resection versus radiofrequency ablation for early-stage hepatocellular carcinoma. *The British Journal of Surgery* 104 (13): 1775–1784.

63 Xu, G., et al. (2012). Meta-analysis of surgical resection and radiofrequency ablation for early hepatocellular carcinoma. *World Journal of Surgical Oncology* 10: 163.

64 Liu, H., et al. (2016). Randomized clinical trial of chemoembolization plus radiofrequency ablation versus

partial hepatectomy for hepatocellular carcinoma within the Milan criteria. *The British Journal of Surgery* 103 (4): 348–356.

65 Livraghi, T., et al. (2008). Sustained complete response and complications rates after radiofrequency ablation of very early hepatocellular carcinoma in cirrhosis: Is resection still the treatment of choice? *Hepatology* 47 (1): 82–89.

66 Peng, Z.W., et al. (2012). Radiofrequency ablation versus hepatic resection for the treatment of hepatocellular carcinomas 2 cm or smaller: A retrospective comparative study. *Radiology* 262 (3): 1022–1033.

67 Pompili, M., et al. (2013). Long-term effectiveness of resection and radiofrequency ablation for single hepatocellular carcinoma ≤3 cm. Results of a multicenter Italian survey. *Journal of Hepatology* 59 (1): 89–97.

68 Ruzzenente, A., et al. (2012). Surgical resection versus local ablation for HCC on cirrhosis: Results from a propensity case-matched study. *Journal of Gastrointestinal Surgery : Official Journal of the Society for Surgery of the Alimentary Tract* 16 (2): 301–311. discussion 311.

69 Llovet, J.M., et al. (2002). Arterial embolisation or chemoembolisation versus symptomatic treatment in patients with unresectable hepatocellular carcinoma: A randomised controlled trial. *Lancet* 359 (9319): 1734–1739.

70 Lo, C.M., et al. (2002). Randomized controlled trial of transarterial lipiodol chemoembolization for unresectable hepatocellular carcinoma. *Hepatology* 35 (5): 1164–1171.

71 Lencioni, R., et al. (2016). Lipiodol transarterial chemoembolization for hepatocellular carcinoma: A systematic review of efficacy and safety data. *Hepatology* 64 (1): 106–116.

72 Llovet, J.M. and Bruix, J. (2003). Systematic review of randomized trials for unresectable hepatocellular carcinoma: Chemoembolization improves survival. *Hepatology* 37 (2): 429–442.

73 Golfieri, R., et al. (2014). Randomised controlled trial of doxorubicin-eluting beads vs conventional chemoembolisation for hepatocellular carcinoma. *British Journal of Cancer* 111 (2): 255–264.

74 Lammer, J., et al. (2010). Prospective randomized study of doxorubicin-eluting-bead embolization in the treatment of hepatocellular carcinoma: Results of the PRECISION V study. *Cardiovascular and Interventional Radiology* 33 (1): 41–52.

75 Brown, K.T., et al. (2016). Randomized trial of hepatic artery embolization for hepatocellular carcinoma using doxorubicin-eluting microspheres compared with embolization with microspheres alone. *Journal of Clinical Oncology : Official Journal of the American Society of Clinical Oncology* 34 (17): 2046–2053.

76 Facciorusso, A., et al. (2017). Transarterial chemoembolization vs bland embolization in hepatocellular carcinoma: A meta-analysis of randomized trials. *United European Gastroenterology Journal* 5 (4): 511–518.

77 Kim, J.H., et al. (2011). Medium-sized (3.1-5.0 cm) hepatocellular carcinoma: Transarterial chemoembolization plus radiofrequency ablation versus radiofrequency ablation alone. *Annals of Surgical Oncology* 18 (6): 1624–1629.

78 Wang, W., Shi, J., and Xie, W.F. (2010). Transarterial chemoembolization in combination with percutaneous ablation therapy in unresectable hepatocellular carcinoma: A meta-analysis. *Liver International : Official Journal of the International Association for the Study of the Liver* 30 (5): 741–749.

79 Abdel-Rahman, O. and Elsayed, Z. (2017). External beam radiotherapy for unresectable hepatocellular carcinoma. *Cochrane Library: Cochrane Reviews* 3 (3): Cd011314.

80 Huo, Y.R. and Eslick, G.D. (2015). Transcatheter arterial chemoembolization plus radiotherapy compared with chemoembolization alone for hepatocellular carcinoma: A systematic review and meta-analysis. *JAMA Oncology* 1 (6): 756–765.

81 Lobo, L., et al. (2016). Unresectable hepatocellular carcinoma: Radioembolization versus chemoembolization: A systematic review and meta-analysis. *Cardiovascular and Interventional Radiology* 39 (11): 1580–1588.

82 Salem, R., et al. (2016). Y90 radioembolization significantly prolongs time to progression compared with chemoembolization in patients with hepatocellular carcinoma. *Gastroenterology* 151 (6): 1155–1163.e2.

83 Soydal, C., et al. (2016). Comparison of survival, safety, and efficacy after transarterial chemoembolization and radioembolization of Barcelona Clinic Liver Cancer stage B-C hepatocellular cancer patients. *Nuclear Medicine Communications* 37 (6): 646–649.

84 Zhang, Y., et al. (2015). Transarterial Y90 radioembolization versus chemoembolization for patients with hepatocellular carcinoma: A meta-analysis. *Bioscience Trends* 9 (5): 289–298.

85 Vilgrain, V., et al. (2017). Efficacy and safety of selective internal radiotherapy with yttrium-90 resin microspheres compared with sorafenib in locally advanced and inoperable hepatocellular carcinoma (SARAH): An open-label randomised controlled phase 3 trial. *The Lancet Oncology* 18 (12): 1624–1636.

86 Chow, P.K.H., et al. (2018). SIRveNIB: Selective internal radiation therapy versus sorafenib in Asia-Pacific patients with hepatocellular carcinoma. *Journal of Clinical Oncology : Official Journal of the American Society of Clinical Oncology* 36 (19): 1913–1921.

87 Yoon, S.M., et al. (2018). Efficacy and safety of transarterial chemoembolization plus external beam radiotherapy vs sorafenib in hepatocellular carcinoma with macroscopic vascular invasion: A randomized clinical trial. *JAMA Oncology* 4 (5): 661–669.

88 Bujold, A., et al. (2013). Sequential phase I and II trials of stereotactic body radiotherapy for locally advanced hepatocellular carcinoma. *Journal of Clinical Oncology : Official Journal of the American Society of Clinical Oncology* 31 (13): 1631–1639.

89 Culleton, S., et al. (2014). Outcomes following definitive stereotactic body radiotherapy for patients with Child-Pugh B or C hepatocellular carcinoma. *Radiotherapy and Oncology : Journal of the European Society for Therapeutic Radiology and Oncology* 111 (3): 412–417.

90 Cheng, A.L., et al. (2009). Efficacy and safety of sorafenib in patients in the Asia-Pacific region with advanced hepatocellular carcinoma: A phase III randomised, double-blind, placebo-controlled trial. *The Lancet Oncology* 10 (1): 25–34.

91 Llovet, J.M., et al. (2008). Sorafenib in advanced hepatocellular carcinoma. *The New England Journal of Medicine* 359 (4): 378–390.

92 Kudo, M., et al. (2018). Lenvatinib versus sorafenib in first-line treatment of patients with unresectable hepatocellular carcinoma: A randomised phase 3 non-inferiority trial. *Lancet* 391 (10126): 1163–1173.

93 Finn, R.S., et al. (2020). Atezolizumab plus Bevacizumab in unresectable hepatocellular carcinoma. *The New England Journal of Medicine* 382 (20): 1894–1905.

94 Bruix, J., et al. (2017). Regorafenib for patients with hepatocellular carcinoma who progressed on sorafenib treatment (RESORCE): A randomised, double-blind, placebo-controlled, phase 3 trial. *Lancet* 389 (10064): 56–66.

95 Abou-Alfa, G.K., et al. (2018). Cabozantinib in patients with advanced and progressing hepatocellular carcinoma. *The New England Journal of Medicine* 379 (1): 54–63.

96 Zhu, A.X., et al. (2019). Ramucirumab after sorafenib in patients with advanced hepatocellular carcinoma and increased α-fetoprotein concentrations (REACH-2): A randomised, double-blind, placebo-controlled, phase 3 trial. *The Lancet Oncology* 20 (2): 282–296.

97 Zhu, A.X., et al. (2015). Ramucirumab versus placebo as second-line treatment in patients with advanced hepatocellular carcinoma following first-line therapy with sorafenib (REACH): A randomised, double-blind, multicentre, phase 3 trial. *The Lancet Oncology* 16 (7): 859–870.

98 El-Khoueiry, A.B., et al. (2017). Nivolumab in patients with advanced hepatocellular carcinoma (CheckMate 040): An open-label, non-comparative, phase 1/2 dose escalation and expansion trial. *Lancet* 389 (10088): 2492–2502.

99 Zhu, A.X., et al. (2018). Pembrolizumab in patients with advanced hepatocellular carcinoma previously treated with sorafenib (KEYNOTE-224): A non-randomised, open-label phase 2 trial. *The Lancet Oncology* 19 (7): 940–952.

100 Qin, S., et al. (2013). Randomized, multicenter, open-label study of oxaliplatin plus fluorouracil/leucovorin versus doxorubicin as palliative chemotherapy in patients with advanced hepatocellular carcinoma from Asia. *Journal of Clinical Oncology : Official Journal of the American Society of Clinical Oncology* 31 (28): 3501–3508.

101 Cainap, C., et al. (2015). Linifanib versus Sorafenib in patients with advanced hepatocellular carcinoma: Results of a randomized phase III trial. *Journal of Clinical Oncology : Official Journal of the American Society of Clinical Oncology* 33 (2): 172–179.

102 Kang, Y.K., et al. (2015). Randomized phase II study of axitinib versus placebo plus best supportive care in second-line treatment of advanced hepatocellular carcinoma. *Annals Of Oncology : Official Journal Of The European Society For Medical Oncology / ESMO* 26 (12): 2457–2463.

103 Rimassa, L., et al. (2018). *Tivantinib for second-line treatment of MET-high, advanced hepatocellular carcinoma (METIV-HCC): A final analysis of a phase 3, randomised, placebo-controlled study*. *The Lancet Oncology* 19 (5): 682–693.

104 Soliman, H., et al. (2013). Phase II trial of palliative radiotherapy for hepatocellular carcinoma and liver metastases. *Journal of Clinical Oncology : Official Journal of the American Society of Clinical Oncology* 31 (31): 3980–3986.

105 Ben-Josef, E., et al. (2005). Phase II trial of high-dose conformal radiation therapy with concurrent hepatic artery floxuridine for unresectable intrahepatic malignancies. *Journal of Clinical Oncology : Official Journal of the American Society of Clinical Oncology* 23 (34): 8739–8747.

106 Dawson, L.A., et al. (2000). Escalated focal liver radiation and concurrent hepatic artery fluorodeoxyuridine for unresectable intrahepatic malignancies. *Journal of Clinical Oncology : Official Journal of the American Society of Clinical Oncology* 18 (11): 2210–2218.

107 McGinn, C.J., et al. (1998). Treatment of intrahepatic cancers with radiation doses based on a normal tissue complication probability model. *Journal of Clinical Oncology : Official Journal of the American Society of Clinical Oncology* 16 (6): 2246–2252.

108 Robertson, J.M., et al. (1997). A phase I trial of hepatic arterial bromodeoxyuridine and conformal radiation therapy for patients with primary hepatobiliary cancers or colorectal liver metastases. *International Journal of Radiation Oncology, Biology, Physics* 39 (5): 1087–1092.

109 Kang, J.K., et al. (2012). Stereotactic body radiation therapy for inoperable hepatocellular carcinoma as a local salvage treatment after incomplete transarterial chemoembolization. *Cancer* 118 (21): 5424–5431.

110 Lasley, F.D., et al. (2015). Treatment variables related to liver toxicity in patients with hepatocellular carcinoma, Child-Pugh class A and B enrolled in a phase 1-2 trial of stereotactic body radiation therapy. *Practical Radiation Oncology* 5 (5): e443-e449.

111 Takeda, A., et al. (2016). Phase 2 study of stereotactic body radiotherapy and optional transarterial chemoembolization

for solitary hepatocellular carcinoma not amenable to resection and radiofrequency ablation. *Cancer* 122 (13): 2041–2049.

112 Randomized trial comparing stereotactic body radiation therapy to microwave ablation for the treatment of localized hepatocellular carcinoma.

113 Duke Cancer Institute. Trial comparing PLA to HIGRT therapy (PROVE-HCC).

114 Transarterial chemoembolization versus stereotactic body radiation therapy for hepatocellular carcinoma (TRENDY).

115 A trial on SBRT after incomplete TAE or TACE versus exclusive TAE or TACE for treatment of inoperable HCC.

116 Transarterial Chemoembolization Compared with Stereotactic Body Radiation Therapy or Stereotactic Ablative Radiation Therapy in Treating Patients with Residual or Recurrent Liver Cancer Undergone Initial Transarterial Chemoembolization.

117 Hong, T.S., et al. (2016). Multi-institutional phase II study of high-dose hypofractionated proton beam therapy in patients with localized, unresectable hepatocellular carcinoma and intrahepatic cholangiocarcinoma. *Journal of Clinical Oncology : Official Journal of the American Society of Clinical Oncology* 34 (5): 460–468.

118 RTOG 1112: Sorafenib tosylate with or without stereotactic body radiation therapy in treating patients with liver cancer.

119 Tanaka, N., et al. (1992). Proton irradiation for hepatocellular carcinoma. *Lancet* 340 (8831): 1358.

120 Mizumoto, M., et al. (2011). Proton beam therapy for hepatocellular carcinoma: A comparison of three treatment protocols. *International Journal of Radiation Oncology, Biology, Physics* 81 (4): 1039–1045.

121 Fukuda, K., et al. (2017). Long-term outcomes of proton beam therapy in patients with previously untreated hepatocellular carcinoma. *Cancer Science* 108 (3): 497–503.

122 Komatsu, S., et al. (2011). Clinical results and risk factors of proton and carbon ion therapy for hepatocellular carcinoma. *Cancer* 117 (21): 4890–4904.

123 Kawashima, M., et al. (2005). Phase II study of radiotherapy employing proton beam for hepatocellular carcinoma. *Journal of Clinical Oncology : Official Journal of the American Society of Clinical Oncology* 23 (9): 1839–1846.

124 Kim, D.Y., et al. (2017). Risk-adapted simultaneous integrated boost-proton beam therapy (SIB-PBT) for advanced hepatocellular carcinoma with tumour vascular thrombosis. *Radiotherapy and Oncology : Journal of the European Society for Therapeutic Radiology and Oncology* 122 (1): 122–129.

125 Bush, D.A., et al. (2004). High-dose proton beam radiotherapy of hepatocellular carcinoma: Preliminary results of a phase II trial. *Gastroenterology* 127 (5 Suppl 1): S189–93.

126 Bush, D.A., et al. (2011). The safety and efficacy of high-dose proton beam radiotherapy for hepatocellular carcinoma: A phase 2 prospective trial. *Cancer* 117 (13): 3053–3059.

127 Chadha, A.S., et al. (2019). Proton beam therapy outcomes for localized unresectable hepatocellular carcinoma. *Radiotherapy and Oncology : Journal of the European Society for Therapeutic Radiology and Oncology* 133: 54–61.

128 Qi, W.X., et al. (2015). Charged particle therapy versus photon therapy for patients with hepatocellular carcinoma: A systematic review and meta-analysis. *Radiotherapy and Oncology : Journal of the European Society for Therapeutic Radiology and Oncology* 114 (3): 289–295.

129 Kato, H., et al. (2004). Results of the first prospective study of carbon ion radiotherapy for hepatocellular carcinoma with liver cirrhosis. *International Journal of Radiation Oncology, Biology, Physics* 59 (5): 1468–1476.

130 Imada, H., et al. (2010). Comparison of efficacy and toxicity of short-course carbon ion radiotherapy for hepatocellular carcinoma depending on their proximity to the porta hepatis. *Radiotherapy and Oncology : Journal of the European Society for Therapeutic Radiology and Oncology* 96 (2): 231–235.

131 Kasuya, G., et al. (2017). Progressive hypofractionated carbon-ion radiotherapy for hepatocellular carcinoma: Combined analyses of 2 prospective trials. *Cancer* 123 (20): 3955–3965.

132 Shibuya, K., et al. (2018). Short-course carbon-ion radiotherapy for hepatocellular carcinoma: A multi-institutional retrospective study. *Liver International : Official Journal of the International Association for the Study of the Liver* 38 (12): 2239–2247.

133 Yasuda, S., et al. (2020). Long-term results of high-dose 2-fraction carbon ion radiation therapy for hepatocellular carcinoma. *Advances in Radiation Oncology* 5 (2): 196–203.

134 Combs, S.E., et al. (2011). Phase I study evaluating the treatment of patients with hepatocellular carcinoma (HCC) with carbon ion radiotherapy: The PROMETHEUS-01 trial. *BMC Cancer* 11: 67.

135 Demizu, Y., et al. (2015). A prospective comparison between proton and carbon ion therapy for hepatocellular carcinoma: An interim analysis. Proceedings to the 54th annual meeting for the particle therapy cooperative group (PTCOG) and the 2nd annual meeting of PTCOG – North America. *International Journal of Particle Therapy* 2 (1): 55–365.

136 Saha, S.K., et al. (2016). Forty-year trends in cholangiocarcinoma incidence in the U.S.: Intrahepatic disease on the rise. *Oncologist* 21 (5): 594–599.

137 Rosen, C.B., et al. (1991). Cholangiocarcinoma complicating primary sclerosing cholangitis. *Annals of Surgery* 213 (1): 21–25.

138 Nakeeb, A., et al. (1996). Cholangiocarcinoma. A spectrum of intrahepatic, perihilar, and distal tumors. *Annals of Surgery* 224 (4): 463–473. discussion 473-5.

139 Jarnagin, W.R., et al. (2005). Papillary phenotype confers improved survival after resection of hilar cholangiocarcinoma. *Annals of Surgery* 241 (5): 703–712. discussion 712-4.

140 Yamasaki, S. (2003). Intrahepatic cholangiocarcinoma: Macroscopic type and stage classification. *Journal of Hepato-biliary-pancreatic Surgery* 10 (4): 288–291.

141 DeOliveira, M.L., et al. (2007). Cholangiocarcinoma: Thirty-one-year experience with 564 patients at a single institution. *Annals of Surgery* 245 (5): 755–762.

142 Malaguarnera, G., et al. (2011). Markers of bile duct tumors. *World Journal of Gastrointestinal Oncology* 3 (4): 49–59.

143 Valls, C., et al. (2000). Intrahepatic peripheral cholangiocarcinoma: CT evaluation. *Abdominal Imaging* 25 (5): 490–496.

144 Manfredi, R., et al. (2004). Magnetic resonance imaging of cholangiocarcinoma. *Seminars in Liver Disease* 24 (2): 155–164.

145 Chong, Y.S., et al. (2012). Differentiating mass-forming intrahepatic cholangiocarcinoma from atypical hepatocellular carcinoma using gadoxetic acid-enhanced MRI. *Clinical Radiology* 67 (8): 766–773.

146 Potretzke, T.A., et al. (2016). Imaging features of biphenotypic primary liver carcinoma (Hepatocholangiocarcinoma) and the potential to mimic hepatocellular carcinoma: LI-RADS analysis of CT and MRI features in 61 Cases. *AJR. American Journal of Roentgenology* 207 (1): 25–31.

147 Park, H.S., et al. (2008). Preoperative evaluation of bile duct cancer: MRI combined with MR cholangiopancreatography versus MDCT with direct cholangiography. *AJR. American Journal of Roentgenology* 190 (2): 396–405.

148 Rösch, T., et al. (2002). A prospective comparison of the diagnostic accuracy of ERCP, MRCP, CT, and EUS in biliary strictures. *Gastrointestinal Endoscopy* 55 (7): 870–876.

149 Blechacz, B., et al. (2011). Clinical diagnosis and staging of cholangiocarcinoma. *Nature Reviews. Gastroenterology & Hepatology* 8 (9): 512–522.

150 Van Beers, B.E. (2008). Diagnosis of cholangiocarcinoma. *HPB : The Official Journal of the International Hepato Pancreato Biliary Association* 10 (2): 87–93.

151 Levy, M.J., Heimbach, J.K., and Gores, G.J. (2012). Endoscopic ultrasound staging of cholangiocarcinoma. *Current Opinion in Gastroenterology* 28 (3): 244–252.

152 Endo, I., et al. (2008). Intrahepatic cholangiocarcinoma: Rising frequency, improved survival, and determinants of outcome after resection. *Annals of Surgery* 248 (1): 84–96.

153 Farges, O., et al. (2011). Influence of surgical margins on outcome in patients with intrahepatic cholangiocarcinoma: A multicenter study by the AFC-IHCC-2009 study group. *Annals of Surgery* 254 (5): 824–829. discussion 830.

154 Konstadoulakis, M.M., et al. (2008). Fifteen-year, single-center experience with the surgical management of intrahepatic cholangiocarcinoma: Operative results and long-term outcome. *Surgery* 143 (3): 366–374.

155 Lang, H., et al. (2009). Operations for intrahepatic cholangiocarcinoma: Single-institution experience of 158 patients. *Journal of the American College of Surgeons* 208 (2): 218–228.

156 Murakami, Y., et al. (2011). Prognostic factors after surgical resection for intrahepatic, hilar, and distal cholangiocarcinoma. *Annals of Surgical Oncology* 18 (3): 651–658.

157 Nakagohri, T., et al. (2003). Aggressive surgical resection for hilar-invasive and peripheral intrahepatic cholangiocarcinoma. *World Journal of Surgery* 27 (3): 289–293.

158 Paik, K.Y., et al. (2008). What prognostic factors are important for resected intrahepatic cholangiocarcinoma? *Journal of Gastroenterology and Hepatology* 23 (5): 766–770.

159 Ribero, D., et al. (2012). Surgical approach for long-term survival of patients with intrahepatic cholangiocarcinoma: A multi-institutional analysis of 434 patients. *Archives of Surgery* 147 (12): 1107–1113.

160 Tamandl, D., et al. (2008). Influence of hepatic resection margin on recurrence and survival in intrahepatic cholangiocarcinoma. *Annals of Surgical Oncology* 15 (10): 2787–2794.

161 Fisher, S.B., et al. (2012). Lymphovascular and perineural invasion as selection criteria for adjuvant therapy in intrahepatic cholangiocarcinoma: A multi-institution analysis. *HPB : The Official Journal of the International Hepato Pancreato Biliary Association* 14 (8): 514–522.

162 Hyder, O., et al. (2013). Recurrence after operative management of intrahepatic cholangiocarcinoma. *Surgery* 153 (6): 811–818.

163 Hyder, O., et al. (2014). A nomogram to predict long-term survival after resection for intrahepatic cholangiocarcinoma: An Eastern and Western experience. *JAMA Surgery* 149 (5): 432–438.

164 Spolverato, G., et al. (2015). Conditional probability of long-term survival after liver resection for intrahepatic cholangiocarcinoma: A multi-institutional analysis of 535 patients. *JAMA Surgery* 150 (6): 538–545.

165 Rana, A. and Hong, J.C. (2012). Orthotopic liver transplantation in combination with neoadjuvant therapy: A new paradigm in the treatment of unresectable intrahepatic cholangiocarcinoma. *Current Opinion in Gastroenterology* 28 (3): 258–265.

166 Primrose, J.N., et al. (2019). Capecitabine compared with observation in resected biliary tract cancer (BILCAP): A randomised, controlled, multicentre, phase 3 study. *The Lancet Oncology* 20 (5): 663–673.

167 Edeline, J., et al. (2019). Gemcitabine and oxaliplatin chemotherapy or surveillance in resected biliary tract cancer (PRODIGE 12-ACCORD 18-UNICANCER GI): A randomized phase III study. *Journal of Clinical Oncology : Official Journal of the American Society of Clinical Oncology* 37 (8): 658–667.

168 Ben-Josef, E., et al. (2015). SWOG S0809: A phase II intergroup trial of adjuvant capecitabine and gemcitabine followed by radiotherapy and concurrent capecitabine in extrahepatic cholangiocarcinoma and gallbladder carcinoma. *Journal of Clinical Oncology : Official Journal of the American Society of Clinical Oncology* 33 (24): 2617–2622.

169 Horgan, A.M., et al. (2012). Adjuvant therapy in the treatment of biliary tract cancer: A systematic review and meta-analysis. *Journal of Clinical Oncology : Official Journal of the American Society of Clinical Oncology* 30 (16): 1934–1940.

170 Shroff, R.T., et al. (2019). Adjuvant therapy for resected biliary tract cancer: ASCO clinical practice guideline. *Journal of Clinical Oncology : Official Journal of the American Society of Clinical Oncology* 37 (12): 1015–1027.

171 Valle, J., et al. (2010). Cisplatin plus gemcitabine versus gemcitabine for biliary tract cancer. *The New England Journal of Medicine* 362 (14): 1273–1281.

172 Kim, J.H., et al. (2011). Radiofrequency ablation for the treatment of primary intrahepatic cholangiocarcinoma. *AJR. American Journal of Roentgenology* 196 (2): W205–9.

173 Kiefer, M.V., et al. (2011). Chemoembolization of intrahepatic cholangiocarcinoma with cisplatinum, doxorubicin, mitomycin C, ethiodol, and polyvinyl alcohol: A 2-center study. *Cancer* 117 (7): 1498–1505.

174 Kuhlmann, J.B., et al. (2012). Treatment of unresectable cholangiocarcinoma: Conventional transarterial chemoembolization compared with drug eluting bead-transarterial chemoembolization and systemic chemotherapy. *European Journal of Gastroenterology & Hepatology* 24 (4): 437–443.

175 Al-Adra, D.P., et al. (2015). Treatment of unresectable intrahepatic cholangiocarcinoma with yttrium-90 radioembolization: A systematic review and pooled analysis. *European Journal of Surgical Oncology : The Journal of the European Society of Surgical Oncology and the British Association of Surgical Oncology* 41 (1): 120–127.

176 Tse, R.V., et al. (2008). Phase I study of individualized stereotactic body radiotherapy for hepatocellular carcinoma and intrahepatic cholangiocarcinoma. *Journal of Clinical Oncology : Official Journal of the American Society of Clinical Oncology* 26 (4): 657–664.

177 Tao, R., et al. (2016). Ablative radiotherapy doses lead to a substantial prolongation of survival in patients with inoperable intrahepatic cholangiocarcinoma: A retrospective dose response analysis. *Journal of Clinical Oncology : Official Journal of the American Society of Clinical Oncology* 34 (3): 219–226.

178 NRG GI001: Radiation therapy vs. observation following gemcitabine and cisplatin for inoperable localized liver cancer.

179 A trial looking at stereotactic body radiotherapy and chemotherapy for people with locally advanced bile duct cancer (ABC-07).

180 Ohkawa, A., et al. (2015). Proton beam therapy for unresectable intrahepatic cholangiocarcinoma. *Journal of Gastroenterology and Hepatology* 30 (5): 957–963.

181 Makita, C., et al. (2014). Clinical outcomes and toxicity of proton beam therapy for advanced cholangiocarcinoma. *Radiation Oncology* 9: 26.

182 Abe, T., et al. (2016). Initial Results of Hypofractionated Carbon Ion Radiotherapy for Cholangiocarcinoma. *Anticancer Research* 36 (6): 2955–2960.

183 Kasuya, G., et al. (2019). Carbon-ion radiotherapy for cholangiocarcinoma: A multi-institutional study by and the Japan carbon-ion radiation oncology study group (J-CROS). *Oncotarget* 10 (43): 4369–4379.

184 Randi, G., Franceschi, S., and La Vecchia, C. (2006). Gallbladder cancer worldwide: Geographical distribution and risk factors. *International Journal of Cancer. Journal International Du Cancer* 118 (7): 1591–1602.

185 Kiran, R.P., Pokala, N., and Dudrick, S.J. (2007). Incidence pattern and survival for gallbladder cancer over three decades–an analysis of 10301 patients. *Annals of Surgical Oncology* 14 (2): 827–832.

186 De Groen, P.C., et al. (1999). Biliary tract cancers. *The New England Journal of Medicine* 341 (18): 1368–1378.

187 Lazcano-Ponce, E.C., et al. (2001). Epidemiology and molecular pathology of gallbladder cancer. *CA: A Cancer Journal for Clinicians* 51 (6): 349–364.

188 Strom, B.L., et al. (1995). Risk factors for gallbladder cancer. An international collaborative case-control study. *Cancer* 76 (10): 1747–1756.

189 Wistuba, I.I. and Gazdar, A.F. (2004). Gallbladder cancer: Lessons from a rare tumour. *Nature Reviews. Cancer* 4 (9): 695–706.

190 Nagaraja, V. and Eslick, G.D. (2014). Systematic review with meta-analysis: The relationship between chronic Salmonella typhi carrier status and gall-bladder cancer. *Alimentary Pharmacology & Therapeutics* 39 (8): 745–750.

191 Duffy, A., et al. (2008). Gallbladder cancer (GBC): 10-year experience at Memorial Sloan-Kettering Cancer Centre (MSKCC). *Journal of Surgical Oncology* 98 (7): 485–489.

192 Henson, D.E., Albores-Saavedra, J., and Corle, D. (1992). Carcinoma of the gallbladder. Histologic types, stage of disease, grade, and survival rates. *Cancer* 70 (6): 1493–1497.

193 Shindoh, J., et al. (2015). Tumor location is a strong predictor of tumor progression and survival in T2 gallbladder cancer: An international multicenter study. *Annals of Surgery* 261 (4): 733–739.

194 Tsukada, K., et al. (1997). Lymph node spread from carcinoma of the gallbladder. *Cancer* 80 (4): 661–667.

195 Pandey, M., et al. (2000). Carcinoma of the gallbladder: Role of sonography in diagnosis and staging. *Journal of Clinical Ultrasound : JCU* 28 (5): 227–232.

196 Saini, S. (1997). Imaging of the hepatobiliary tract. *The New England Journal of Medicine* 336 (26): 1889–1894.

197 Vogl, T.J., et al. (2006). Staging of Klatskin tumours (hilar cholangiocarcinomas): Comparison of MR cholangiography, MR imaging, and endoscopic retrograde cholangiography. *European Radiology* 16 (10): 2317–2325.

198 Hattori, M., et al. (2011). Prospective study of biliary cytology in suspected perihilar cholangiocarcinoma. *The British Journal of Surgery* 98 (5): 704–709.

199 Halling, K.C. and Kipp, B.R. (2007). Fluorescence in situ hybridization in diagnostic cytology. *Human Pathology* 38 (8): 1137–1144.

200 DeHaan, R.D., et al. (2007). An assessment of chromosomal alterations detected by fluorescence in situ hybridization and p16 expression in sporadic and primary sclerosing cholangitis-associated cholangiocarcinomas. *Human Pathology* 38 (3): 491–499.

201 Dixon, E., et al. (2005). An aggressive surgical approach leads to improved survival in patients with gallbladder cancer: A 12-year study at a North American Center. *Annals of Surgery* 241 (3): 385–394.

202 Lee, S.E., et al. (2011). Systematic review on the surgical treatment for T1 gallbladder cancer. *World Journal of Gastroenterology : WJG* 17 (2): 174–180.

203 Foster, J.M., et al. (2007). Gallbladder cancer: Defining the indications for primary radical resection and radical re-resection. *Annals of Surgical Oncology* 14 (2): 833–840.

204 Downing, S.R., et al. (2011). Early-stage gallbladder cancer in the Surveillance, Epidemiology, and End Results database: Effect of extended surgical resection. *Archives of Surgery* 146 (6): 734–738.

205 Jensen, E.H., et al. (2009). A critical analysis of the surgical management of early-stage gallbladder cancer in the United States. *Journal of Gastrointestinal Surgery : Official Journal of the Society for Surgery of the Alimentary Tract* 13 (4): 722–727.

206 Pawlik, T.M., et al. (2007). Incidence of finding residual disease for incidental gallbladder carcinoma: Implications for re-resection. *Journal of Gastrointestinal Surgery : Official Journal of the Society for Surgery of the Alimentary Tract* 11 (11): 1478–1486. discussion 1486-7.

207 Shirai, Y., et al. (2012). "Extended" radical cholecystectomy for gallbladder cancer: Long-term outcomes, indications and limitations. *World Journal of Gastroenterology : WJG* 18 (34): 4736–4743.

208 You, D.D., et al. (2008). What is an adequate extent of resection for T1 gallbladder cancers? *Annals of Surgery* 247 (5): 835–838.

209 D'Angelica, M., et al. (2009). Analysis of the extent of resection for adenocarcinoma of the gallbladder. *Annals of Surgical Oncology* 16 (4): 806–816.

210 Zaydfudim, V., et al. (2008). The impact of tumor extent (T stage) and lymph node involvement (N stage) on survival after surgical resection for gallbladder adenocarcinoma. *HPB : The Official Journal of the International Hepato Pancreato Biliary Association* 10 (6): 420–427.

211 Cameron, J.L., et al. (1990). Management of proximal cholangiocarcinomas by surgical resection and radiotherapy. *American Journal of Surgery* 159 (1): 91–97. discussion 97-8.

212 Fortner, J.G., Vitelli, C.E., and Maclean, B.J. (1989). Proximal extrahepatic bile duct tumors. Analysis of a series of 52 consecutive patients treated over a period of 13 years. *Archives of Surgery* 124 (11): 1275–1279.

213 Langer, J.C., et al. (1985). Carcinoma of the extrahepatic bile ducts: Results of an aggressive surgical approach. *Surgery* 98 (4): 752–759.

214 Burke, E.C., et al. (1998). Hilar Cholangiocarcinoma: Patterns of spread, the importance of hepatic resection for curative operation, and a presurgical clinical staging system. *Annals of Surgery* 228 (3): 385–394.

215 Cheng, Q.B., et al. (2012). Resection with total caudate lobectomy confers survival benefit in hilar cholangiocarcinoma of Bismuth type III and IV. *European Journal of Surgical Oncology : The Journal of the European Society of Surgical Oncology and the British Association of Surgical Oncology* 38 (12): 1197–1203.

216 Ito, F., et al. (2008). Resection of hilar cholangiocarcinoma: Concomitant liver resection decreases hepatic recurrence. *Annals of Surgery* 248 (2): 273–279.

217 Matsuo, K., et al. (2012). The Blumgart preoperative staging system for hilar cholangiocarcinoma: Analysis of resectability and outcomes in 380 patients. *Journal of the American College of Surgeons* 215 (3): 343–355.

218 Nishio, H., Nagino, M., and Nimura, Y. (2005). Surgical management of hilar cholangiocarcinoma: The Nagoya experience. *HPB : The Official Journal of the International Hepato Pancreato Biliary Association* 7 (4): 259–262.

219 Van Gulik, T.M., et al. (2011). Multidisciplinary management of hilar cholangiocarcinoma (Klatskin tumor): Extended resection is associated with improved survival. *European Journal of Surgical Oncology : The Journal of the European Society of Surgical Oncology and the British Association of Surgical Oncology* 37 (1): 65–71.

220 Groot Koerkamp, B., et al. (2015). Survival after resection of perihilar cholangiocarcinoma-development and external validation of a prognostic nomogram. *Annals Of Oncology : Official Journal Of The European Society For Medical Oncology / ESMO* 26 (9): 1930–1935.

221 Darwish Murad, S., et al. (2012). Efficacy of neoadjuvant chemoradiation, followed by liver transplantation, for perihilar cholangiocarcinoma at 12 US centers. *Gastroenterology* 143 (1): 88–98.e3. quiz e14.

222 Rosen, C.B., Heimbach, J.K., and Gores, G.J. (2010). Liver transplantation for cholangiocarcinoma. *Transplant International : Official Journal of the European Society for Organ Transplantation* 23 (7): 692–697.

223 Bortolasi, L., et al. (2000). Adenocarcinoma of the distal bile duct. A clinicopathologic outcome analysis after curative resection. *Digestive Surgery* 17 (1): 36–41.

224 Cheng, Q., et al. (2007). Distal bile duct carcinoma: Prognostic factors after curative surgery. A series of 112 cases. *Annals of Surgical Oncology* 14 (3): 1212–1219.

225 Fong, Y., et al. (1996). Outcome of treatment for distal bile duct cancer. *The British Journal of Surgery* 83 (12): 1712–1715.

226 Murakami, Y., et al. (2007). Pancreatoduodenectomy for distal cholangiocarcinoma: Prognostic impact of lymph node metastasis. *World Journal of Surgery* 31 (2): 337–342. discussion 343-4.

227 Yoshida, T., et al. (2002). Prognostic factors after pancreatoduodenectomy with extended lymphadenectomy for distal bile duct cancer. *Archives of Surgery* 137 (1): 69–73.

228 Im, J.H., et al. (2016). Surgery alone versus surgery followed by chemotherapy and radiotherapy in resected extrahepatic bile duct cancer: Treatment outcome analysis of 336 patients. *Cancer Research and Treatment : Official Journal of Korean Cancer Association* 48 (2): 583–595.

229 Kim, T.H., et al. (2011). Role of adjuvant chemoradiotherapy for resected extrahepatic biliary tract cancer. *International Journal of Radiation Oncology, Biology, Physics* 81 (5): e853–9.

230 Nakeeb, A., et al. (2002). Improved survival in resected biliary malignancies. *Surgery* 132 (4): 555–563. discussion 563-4.

231 Crane, C.H., et al. (2002). Limitations of conventional doses of chemoradiation for unresectable biliary cancer. *International Journal of Radiation Oncology, Biology, Physics* 53 (4): 969–974.

232 Bisello, S., et al. (2019). Radiotherapy or chemoradiation in unresectable biliary cancer: A retrospective study. *Anticancer Research* 39 (6): 3095–3100.

233 Yoshioka, Y., et al. (2014). Impact of intraluminal brachytherapy on survival outcome for radiation therapy for unresectable biliary tract cancer: A propensity-score matched-pair analysis. *International Journal of Radiation Oncology, Biology, Physics* 89 (4): 822–829.

234 Torgeson, A., et al. (2017). Chemoradiation therapy for unresected extrahepatic cholangiocarcinoma: A propensity score-matched analysis. *Annals of Surgical Oncology* 24 (13): 4001–4008.

235 Shinohara, E.T., et al. (2009). Radiotherapy is associated with improved survival in adjuvant and palliative treatment of extrahepatic cholangiocarcinomas. *International Journal of Radiation Oncology, Biology, Physics* 74 (4): 1191–1198.

236 Phelip, J.M., et al. (2014). Gemcitabine plus cisplatin versus chemoradiotherapy in locally advanced biliary tract cancer: Fédération Francophone de Cancérologie Digestive 9902 phase II randomised study. *European Journal of Cancer (Oxford, England : 1990)* 50 (17): 2975–2982.

237 Hong, T.S., et al. (2017). Phase II study of proton-based stereotactic body radiation therapy for liver metastases: Importance of tumor genotype. *Journal of the National Cancer Institute* 109 (9).

238 Fukumitsu, N., et al. (2015). Proton beam therapy for metastatic liver tumors. *Radiotherapy and Oncology : Journal of the European Society for Therapeutic Radiology and Oncology* 117 (2): 322–327.

239 Colbert, L.E., et al. (2017). Proton beam radiation as salvage therapy for bilateral colorectal liver metastases not amenable to second-stage hepatectomy. *Surgery* 161 (6): 1543–1548.

240 Makishima, H., et al. (2019). Single fraction carbon ion radiotherapy for colorectal cancer liver metastasis: A dose escalation study. *Cancer Science* 110 (1): 303–309.

241 Gleeson, F.C., et al. (2018). Knowledge of endoscopic ultrasound-delivered fiducial composition and dimension necessary when planning proton beam radiotherapy. *Endoscopy International Open* 6 (6): E766-e768.

242 Hong, T.S., et al. (2014). Interobserver variability in target definition for hepatocellular carcinoma with and without portal vein thrombus: Radiation therapy oncology group consensus guidelines. *International Journal of Radiation Oncology, Biology, Physics* 89 (4): 804–813.

243 Choi, H.S., et al. (2018). Patterns of failure after resection of extrahepatic bile duct cancer: Implications for adjuvant radiotherapy indication and treatment volumes. *Radiation Oncology* 13 (1): 85.

244 Jarnagin, W.R., et al. (2003). Patterns of initial disease recurrence after resection of gallbladder carcinoma and hilar cholangiocarcinoma: Implications for adjuvant therapeutic strategies. *Cancer* 98 (8): 1689–1700.

245 Koo, T.R., et al. (2014). Patterns of failure and prognostic factors in resected extrahepatic bile duct cancer: Implication for adjuvant radiotherapy. *Radiation Oncology Journal* 32 (2): 63–69.

246 Zhou, W., et al. (2020). Prognostic factors and patterns of recurrence after curative resection for patients with distal cholangiocarcinoma. *Radiotherapy and Oncology : Journal* of the European Society for Therapeutic Radiology and Oncology 147: 111–117.

247 Tryggestad, E.J., et al. (2020). Managing treatment-related uncertainties in proton beam radiotherapy for gastrointestinal cancers. *Journal of Gastrointestinal Oncology* 11 (1): 212–224.

248 Schneider, U., Pedroni, E., and Lomax, A. (1996). The calibration of CT Hounsfield units for radiotherapy treatment planning. *Physics in Medicine and Biology* 41 (1): 111–124.

249 Michalak, G., et al. (2017). A comparison of relative proton stopping power measurements across patient size using dual- and single-energy CT. *Acta Oncologica* 56 (11): 1465–1471.

250 Taasti, V.T., et al. (2017). Validation of proton stopping power ratio estimation based on dual energy CT using fresh tissue samples. *Physics in Medicine and Biology* 63 (1): 015012.

251 Goitein, M. (1985). Calculation of the uncertainty in the dose delivered during radiation therapy. *Medical Physics* 12 (5): 608–612.

252 Schuemann, J., et al. (2014). Site-specific range uncertainties caused by dose calculation algorithms for proton therapy. *Physics in Medicine and Biology* 59 (15): 4007–4031.

253 Andersson, K.M., et al. (2018). Evaluation of two commercial CT metal artifact reduction algorithms for use in proton radiotherapy treatment planning in the head and neck area. *Medical Physics* 45 (10): 4329–4344.

254 Axente, M., et al. (2015). Clinical evaluation of the iterative metal artifact reduction algorithm for CT simulation in radiotherapy. *Medical Physics* 42 (3): 1170–1183.

255 Kim, Y.J., et al. (2019). Dual-energy and iterative metal artifact reduction for reducing artifacts due to metallic hardware: A loosening hip phantom study. *AJR. American Journal of Roentgenology* 212:5, 1106–1111.

256 Tryggestad, E., Storm, A., Remmes, N., Beltran, C., Haddock, M.G., Kruse, J., Topazian, M., and Hallemeier, C.L. (2018). Experimental study of proton dose perturbations due to self-expanding metallic stents-Proceedings of the 57(th) annual meeting of the particle therapy cooperative group (PTCOG). *International Journal of Particle Therapy* 5 (2): 58–229.

257 Jalaj, S., et al. (2015). Proton radiotherapy dose perturbations caused by esophageal stents of varying material composition are negligible in an experimental model. *Endoscopy International Open* 3 (1): E46–50.

258 Kitamura, K., et al. (2003). Tumor location, cirrhosis, and surgical history contribute to tumor movement in the liver, as measured during stereotactic irradiation using a real-time tumor-tracking radiotherapy system. *International Journal of Radiation Oncology, Biology, Physics* 56 (1): 221–228.

259 Shirato, H., et al. (2004). Intrafractional tumor motion: Lung and liver. *Seminars in Radiation Oncology* 14 (1): 10–18.

260 Von Siebenthal, M., et al. (2007). Systematic errors in respiratory gating due to intrafraction deformations of the liver. *Medical Physics* 34 (9): 3620–3629.

261 Yaremko, B.P., et al. (2008). Determination of respiratory motion for distal esophagus cancer using four-dimensional computed tomography. *International Journal of Radiation Oncology, Biology, Physics* 70 (1): 145–153.

262 Zhang, X., et al. (2008). Four-dimensional computed tomography-based treatment planning for intensity-modulated radiation therapy and proton therapy for distal esophageal cancer. *International Journal of Radiation Oncology, Biology, Physics* 72 (1): 278–287.

263 Mori, S. and Chen, G.T. (2008). Quantification and visualization of charged particle range variations. *International Journal of Radiation Oncology, Biology, Physics* 72 (1): 268–277.

264 Mori, S., et al. (2008). Quantitative assessment of range fluctuations in charged particle lung irradiation. *International Journal of Radiation Oncology, Biology, Physics* 70 (1): 253–261.

265 Yu, J., et al. (2016). Motion-robust intensity-modulated proton therapy for distal esophageal cancer. *Medical Physics* 43 (3): 1111–1118.

266 Lin, L., et al. (2017). Evaluation of motion mitigation using abdominal compression in the clinical implementation of pencil beam scanning proton therapy of liver tumors. *Medical Physics* 44 (2): 703–712.

267 Furukawa, T., et al. (2010). Moving target irradiation with fast rescanning and gating in particle therapy. *Medical Physics* 37 (9): 4874–4879.

268 Gelover, E., et al. (2019). Clinical implementation of respiratory-gated spot-scanning proton therapy: An efficiency analysis of active motion management. *Journal Of Applied Clinical Medical Physics / American College of Medical Physics* 20 (5): 99–108.

269 Knopf, A.C., Hong, T.S., and Lomax, A. (2011). Scanned proton radiotherapy for mobile targets-the effectiveness of re-scanning in the context of different treatment planning approaches and for different motion characteristics. *Physics in Medicine and Biology* 56 (22): 7257–7271.

270 Mori, S., et al. (2014). Amplitude-based gated phase-controlled rescanning in carbon-ion scanning beam treatment planning under irregular breathing conditions using lung and liver 4DCTs. *Journal of Radiation Research* 55 (5): 948–958.

271 Schatti, A., et al. (2013). Experimental verification of motion mitigation of discrete proton spot scanning by re-scanning. *Physics in Medicine and Biology* 58 (23): 8555–8572.

272 Seco, J., et al. (2009). Breathing interplay effects during proton beam scanning: Simulation and statistical analysis. *Physics in Medicine and Biology* 54 (14): N283–94.

273 Johnson, J.E., Herman, M.G., and Kruse, J.J. (2019). Optimization of motion management parameters in a synchrotron-based spot scanning system. *Journal Of Applied Clinical Medical Physics / American College of Medical Physics* 20 (9): 69–77.

274 Schätti, A., et al. (2014). The effectiveness of combined gating and re-scanning for treating mobile targets with proton spot scanning. An experimental and simulation-based investigation. *Physics in Medicine and Biology* 59 (14): 3813–3828.

275 Botas, P., et al. (2018). Density overwrites of internal tumor volumes in intensity modulated proton therapy plans for mobile lung tumors. *Physics in Medicine and Biology* 63 (3): 035023.

276 Boye, D., Lomax, T., and Knopf, A. (2013). Mapping motion from 4D-MRI to 3D-CT for use in 4D dose calculations: A technical feasibility study. *Medical Physics* 40 (6): 061702.

277 Li, H., et al. (2012). Dynamically accumulated dose and 4D accumulated dose for moving tumors. *Medical Physics* 39 (12): 7359–7367.

278 Liu, C., et al. (2019). Dosimetric comparison of distal esophageal carcinoma plans for patients treated with small-spot intensity-modulated proton versus volumetric-modulated arc therapies. *Journal Of Applied Clinical Medical Physics / American College of Medical Physics* 20 (7): 15–27.

279 Liu, W., et al. (2016). Exploratory study of 4D versus 3D robust optimization in intensity modulated proton therapy for lung cancer. *International Journal of Radiation Oncology, Biology, Physics* 95 (1): 523–533.

280 Pepin, M.D., et al. (2018). A Monte-Carlo-based and GPU-accelerated 4D-dose calculator for a pencil beam scanning proton therapy system. *Medical Physics* 45 (11): 5293–5304.

281 Pfeiler, T., et al. (2018). Experimental validation of a 4D dose calculation routine for pencil beam scanning proton therapy. *Zeitschrift Fur Medizinische Physik* 28 (2): 121–133.

282 Dawson, L.A., et al. (2002). Analysis of radiation-induced liver disease using the Lyman NTCP model. *International Journal of Radiation Oncology, Biology, Physics* 53 (4): 810–821.

283 Pan, C.C., et al. (2010). Radiation-associated liver injury. *International Journal of Radiation Oncology, Biology, Physics* 76 (3 Suppl): S94–100.

284 Rusthoven, K.E., et al. (2009). Multi-institutional phase I/II trial of stereotactic body radiation therapy for liver metastases. *Journal of Clinical Oncology : Official Journal of the American Society of Clinical Oncology* 27 (10): 1572–1578.

285 Velec, M., et al. (2017). Predictors of liver toxicity following stereotactic body radiation therapy for hepatocellular carcinoma. *International Journal of Radiation Oncology, Biology, Physics* 97 (5): 939–946.

286 Mizumoto, M., et al. (2012). Evaluation of liver function after proton beam therapy for hepatocellular carcinoma. *International Journal of Radiation Oncology, Biology, Physics* 82 (3): e529–35.

287 Pursley, J., et al. (2020 Aug 1). Dosimetric analysis and normal-tissue complication probability modeling of Child-Pugh score and albumin-bilirubin grade increase after hepatic irradiation. *International Journal of Radiation Oncology, Biology, Physics*107(5):986–995. doi: 10.1016/j.ijrobp.2020.04.027. Epub 2020 Apr 27. PMID: 32353390; PMCID: PMC7381375.

288 Son, S.H., et al. (2010). Stereotactic body radiotherapy for patients with unresectable primary hepatocellular carcinoma: Dose-volumetric parameters predicting the hepatic complication. *International Journal of Radiation Oncology, Biology, Physics* 78 (4): 1073–1080.

289 Buskirk, S.J., et al. (1992). Analysis of failure after curative irradiation of extrahepatic bile duct carcinoma. *Annals of Surgery* 215 (2): 125–131.

290 Kelly, P., et al. (2013). Duodenal toxicity after fractionated chemoradiation for unresectable pancreatic cancer. *International Journal of Radiation Oncology, Biology, Physics* 85 (3): e143–9.

291 Sachsman, S., Nichols, C., Jr, Morris, C.G., et al. (2014). Proton therapy and concomitant capecitabine for non-metastatic unresectable pancreatic adenocarcinoma. *International Journal of Particle Therapy* 1 (3): 692–701.

292 Stanic, S. and Mayadev, J.S. (2013). Tolerance of the small bowel to therapeutic irradiation: A focus on late toxicity in patients receiving para-aortic nodal irradiation for gynecologic malignancies. *International Journal of Gynecological Cancer : Official Journal of the International Gynecological Cancer Society* 23 (4): 592–597.

293 Verma, J., et al. (2014). Dosimetric predictors of duodenal toxicity after intensity modulated radiation therapy for treatment of the para-aortic nodes in gynecologic cancer. *International Journal of Radiation Oncology, Biology, Physics* 88 (2): 357–362.

294 Tsujino, K., et al. (1995). Definitive radiation therapy for extrahepatic bile duct carcinoma. *Radiology* 196 (1): 275–280.

295 Toesca, D.A., et al. (2017). Central liver toxicity after SBRT: An expanded analysis and predictive nomogram. *Radiotherapy and Oncology : Journal of the European Society for Therapeutic Radiology and Oncology* 122 (1): 130–136.

296 Dunlap, N.E., et al. (2010). Chest wall volume receiving >30 Gy predicts risk of severe pain and/or rib fracture after lung stereotactic body radiotherapy. *International Journal of Radiation Oncology, Biology, Physics* 76 (3): 796–801.

297 Dawson, L.A., et al. (2010). Radiation-associated kidney injury. *International Journal of Radiation Oncology, Biology, Physics* 76 (3 Suppl): S108–15.

298 Chiba, T., et al. (2005). Proton beam therapy for hepatocellular carcinoma: A retrospective review of 162 patients. *Clinical Cancer Research : An Official Journal of the American Association for Cancer Research* 11 (10): 3799–3805.

299 Hata, M., et al. (2006). Proton beam therapy for hepatocellular carcinoma patients with severe cirrhosis. *Strahlentherapie Und Onkologie : Organ Der Deutschen Rontgengesellschaft. [Et Al]* 182 (12): 713–720.

300 Hata, M., et al. (2007). Proton beam therapy for aged patients with hepatocellular carcinoma. *International Journal of Radiation Oncology, Biology, Physics* 69 (3): 805–812.

301 Mizumoto, M., et al. (2008). Proton beam therapy for hepatocellular carcinoma adjacent to the porta hepatis. *International Journal of Radiation Oncology, Biology, Physics* 71 (2): 462–467.

302 Sugahara, S., et al. (2009). Proton-beam therapy for hepatocellular carcinoma associated with portal vein tumor thrombosis. *Strahlentherapie Und Onkologie : Organ Der Deutschen Rontgengesellschaft. [Et Al]* 185 (12): 782–788.

303 Fukumitsu, N., et al. (2009). A prospective study of hypofractionated proton beam therapy for patients with hepatocellular carcinoma. *International Journal of Radiation Oncology, Biology, Physics* 74 (3): 831–836.

304 Nakayama, H., et al. (2009). Proton beam therapy for hepatocellular carcinoma: The University of Tsukuba experience. *Cancer* 115 (23): 5499–5506.

305 Sugahara, S., et al. (2010). Proton beam therapy for large hepatocellular carcinoma. *International Journal of Radiation Oncology, Biology, Physics* 76 (2): 460–466.

306 Komatsu, S., et al. (2011). Risk factors for survival and local recurrence after particle radiotherapy for single small hepatocellular carcinoma. *The British Journal of Surgery* 98 (4): 558–564.

307 Lee, S.U., et al. (2014). Effectiveness and safety of proton beam therapy for advanced hepatocellular carcinoma with portal vein tumor thrombosis. *Strahlentherapie Und Onkologie : Organ Der Deutschen Rontgengesellschaft. [Et Al]* 190 (9): 806–814.

308 Hong, T.S., et al. (2014). A prospective feasibility study of respiratory-gated proton beam therapy for liver tumors. *Practical Radiation Oncology* 4 (5): 316–322.

309 Kimura, K., et al. (2017). Clinical results of proton beam therapy for hepatocellular carcinoma over 5 cm. *Hepatology Research : The Official Journal of the Japan Society of Hepatology* 47 (13): 1368–1374.

310 Sorin, Y., et al. (2018). Effectiveness of particle radiotherapy in various stages of hepatocellular carcinoma: A pilot study. *Liver Cancer* 7 (4): 323–334.

311 Yu, J.I., et al. (2018). Initial clinical outcomes of proton beam radiotherapy for hepatocellular carcinoma. *Radiation Oncology Journal* 36 (1): 25–34.

312 Dionisi, F., et al. (2014). Is there a role for proton therapy in the treatment of hepatocellular carcinoma? A systematic review. *Radiotherapy and Oncology : Journal of the European Society for Therapeutic Radiology and Oncology* 111 (1): 1–10.

313 Spychalski, P., et al. (2019). Patient specific outcomes of charged particle therapy for hepatocellular carcinoma - A systematic review and quantitative analysis. *Radiotherapy and Oncology : Journal of the European Society for Therapeutic Radiology and Oncology* 132: 127–134.

314 Shiba, S., et al. (2017). Carbon ion radiotherapy for 80 years or older patients with hepatocellular carcinoma. *BMC Cancer* 17 (1): 721.

315 Shiba, S., et al. (2019). A comparison of carbon ion radiotherapy and transarterial chemoembolization treatment outcomes for single hepatocellular carcinoma: A propensity score matching study. *Radiation Oncology* 14 (1): 137.

316 Shibuya, K., et al. (2019). A feasibility study of high-dose hypofractionated carbon ion radiation therapy using four fractions for localized hepatocellular carcinoma measuring 3 cm or larger. *Radiotherapy and Oncology : Journal of the European Society for Therapeutic Radiology and Oncology* 132: 230–235.

317 Fukumitsu, N., et al. (2017). Follow-up study of liver metastasis from breast cancer treated by proton beam therapy. *Molecular and Clinical Oncology* 7 (1): 56–60.

318 Fukumitsu, N., et al. (2017). Proton beam therapy for liver metastases from gastric cancer. *Journal of Radiation Research* 58 (3): 357–362.

319 Kang, J.I., et al. (2019). A phase I trial of Proton stereotactic body radiation therapy for liver metastases. *Journal of Gastrointestinal Oncology* 10 (1): 112–117.

20

Breast Cancer

Julie A. Bradley, MD and Xiaoying Liang, PhD

From the Department of Radiation Oncology, University of Florida College of Medicine, Jacksonville, FL
Corresponding Author: Julie A. Bradley, MD Department of Radiation Oncology, University of Florida, 2015 North Jefferson St., Jacksonville, FL 32206

TABLE OF CONTENTS

20.1 Introduction

The simultaneous goals of breast cancer therapy consist of maximizing disease control and minimizing toxicity, while preserving quality of life. Achieving these goals requires (1) covering the at-risk regions with the appropriate radiation dose, (2) protecting the normal healthy tissue adjacent to the target volume from incidental radiation exposure, and (3) maintaining cosmesis of the breast or reconstructed breast and functional capacity, including arm mobility and the ability to exercise, while reducing the likelihood of arm edema. These goals are realized by personalizing the treatment to the individual. In radiotherapy, factors to consider include use of radiotherapy, treatment volume, dose, fractionation, patient positioning, type of beam, and delivery method.

Dosimetric analysis guides the radiotherapy treatment planning process. Dosimetric criteria can determine patient positioning as well as beam choices such as electrons, photons, protons, or a combination of these. In daily practice, patient- and disease-specific decisions are made to prioritize target coverage or organ-at-risk (OAR) sparing. The dose–volume metrics and isodose line distributions are key determinants in plan selection.

Principles and Practice of Particle Therapy, First Edition. Edited by Timothy D. Malouff and Daniel M. Trifiletti.
© 2022 John Wiley & Sons Ltd. Published 2022 by John Wiley & Sons Ltd.

The treatment planning process is an essential part of radiotherapy. While radiotherapy yields significant improvements in disease control and survival, it also has been associated with cardiopulmonary morbidity and mortality [1]. Mean heart dose (MHD) has been the primary planning parameter used in breast cancer radiotherapy. Darby et al. reported on a linear relationship between MHD and major coronary events and were unable to identify any threshold without an increased risk [2]. Similarly, evaluating individual patient datasets, van den Bogaard et al. found a linear relationship between MHD and acute coronary events [3]. These investigators also reported that the volume of the left ventricle exposed to 5 Gy correlated with acute coronary events. In a study by Taylor et al., dose to all of the left ventricle subsegments correlated with cardiac injury [4]. Other cardiac subsegments have been analyzed for contributory effects to radiation-induced cardiac disease, including exposure of the coronary arteries [4]. However, a direct dose–volume relationship has yet to be defined. Complementing the series on cardiac structures, investigators found that right ventricle exposure to radiation reduces right ventricular systolic function, expanding the view that MHD alone is likely insufficient to understanding cardiac injury after radiotherapy [5]. In regards to the lungs, Gokula et al. reported higher rates of radiation pneumonitis when the ipsilateral lung V20 exceeded 30% or the mean lung dose exceeded 15 Gy, and on the effects of age and smoking status on the rate of radiation pneumonitis [6]. Radiotherapy lung doses and the effect of a low dose to a large area versus a high dose to a small area, which varies by technique—3D conformal photons versus photon-based intensity-modulated radiation therapy (IMRT)—also remain an area of research.

Over the last decade, dosimetric comparisons between protons and photons have increased interest in the use of protons in breast cancer radiotherapy as radiation oncologists search for avenues to improving the therapeutic ratio while achieving optimal target coverage and OAR sparing. Data quantifying the theoretical improvement in the therapeutic ratio with proton therapy continue to emerge, including through a Patient-Centered Outcomes Research Institute-sponsored randomized trial comparing protons and photons [7]. The potential and value of proton therapy in breast cancer radiotherapy continue to be defined and optimized. This chapter focuses primarily on proton therapy, which is the particle therapy with the most investigation to date.

20.2 Dosimetric Analyses

The earliest reports on proton therapy for breast cancer emerged at the turn of the century. In 2002, Johansson et al. published a dosimetric study of women with node-positive left-sided breast cancer [8]. Treatment plans were designed for 11 patients using 4 techniques each: passive-scatter proton therapy, IMRT, 3D conformal tangential radiotherapy, and 3D conformal mixed electron-photon radiotherapy. Normal-tissue complication probability (NTCP) models were evaluated based on the dosimetric parameters and demonstrated a decrease in mean cardiac mortality from 2.1% with the best photon plans (mixed electron–photon) to 0.5% with the proton plans. Another dosimetric study with multiple plans designed on a single computed tomography (CT) dataset from an anonymized patient found that, while IMRT could decrease the dose to adjacent organs, there was a limit beyond which further decrease in OAR dose compromised target coverage [9]. In contrast, the pencil-beam scanning (PBS) proton therapy plan achieved a greater reduction in OAR doses without a deterioration in target coverage. The study was updated in 2010 to include 20 patients with left-sided breast cancer, with a 3D photon, IMRT, and PBS proton plan designed for each patient, and their results corroborated their earlier findings [10]. A dosimetric comparison of free-breathing scanning proton therapy plans to enhanced-inspiration gating photon plans showed a decrease in heart, lung, and integral dose with the proton plans, with the greatest absolute difference in the cases requiring regional nodal irradiation (RNI) [11]. Additional dosimetric reports have compared proton therapy to IMRT and 3D conformal photons in the setting of bilateral implant reconstruction after mastectomies [12], unfavorable chest-wall anatomy without reconstruction [12], combination proton–photon planning [13], and proton therapy to tomotherapy and volumetric modulated arc therapy (VMAT) [14].

Mast et al. conducted a comparative dosimetric analysis for treatment of the whole breast alone (no nodal irradiation) in 20 women with left-sided breast cancer. Free-breathing and deep-inspiration breath-hold (DIBH) IMRT and intensity-modulated proton therapy (IMPT) plans were designed for each patient. DIBH IMRT decreased OAR doses compared to free-breathing IMRT, but the heart, left-anterior descending artery (LAD), and lung doses neared zero with IMPT (free breathing and DIBH). Lin et al. reported similar findings, with proton radiation achieving the lowest dose to the LAD compared to IMRT with DIBH [15]. In these studies and others, the ability with proton therapy to contain the radiation exposure within the target organ has been remarkable.

Comparative proton–photon dosimetric analyses were also performed for partial-breast volumes. In a dosimetric study comparing techniques for partial-breast irradiation (PBI), Wang et al. found that both passive scattering and IMPT improved the dosimetry compared to 3D conformal photon therapy [15]. Between the two proton techniques, IMPT afforded a lower skin dose and higher conformality, while passive scattering achieved minimal low-dose exposure and less uncertainty. They also compared en face to tangential beams for IMPT. A single tangential field demonstrated significant loss of clinical target volume (CTV) coverage with respiratory motion, and they concluded that the use of en face and multiple beams reduces range uncertainty as well as rib dose. Moon et al. analyzed dosimetry for 30 patients undergoing PBI [16]. Four plans were designed for each patient: 3D conformal photons, IMRT, tomotherapy, and proton therapy. The heart and lung doses were lowest with the proton plans (cardiac V10 = 0%; average ipsilateral lung V20 = 0.4%), as was the nontarget breast volume. Bush et al. compared dosimetry for 10 women treated in the prone position with passive-scatter proton therapy [17]. Compared to the proton plan, both photon plans (multifield and reduced tangents) resulted in more exposure of the skin and the nontarget breast to both low and high doses.

Evaluating PBI in a definitive rather than adjuvant setting, Lischalk et al. reported on comparative dosimetry for 15 women with early-stage breast cancer [18]. With a prescription dose of 50 Gy over five fractions, the plans for each patient were designed using stereotactic ablative radiotherapy (SABR), PBS proton therapy, and 3D conformal photon therapy. While all three modalities achieved target coverage, the SABR and proton plans better spared the adjacent OARs compared to the photon plans. Of note, the planning target volume (PTV) margin differed with each treatment technique, measuring 2, 5, and 10 mm for SABR, proton therapy, and 3D photon therapy, respectively.

20.3 Clinical Analyses

20.3.1 Partial-breast Irradiation

PBI with proton therapy was investigated as a means to minimize the ipsilateral breast dose as well as heart, lung, and contralateral breast exposure compared to external-beam photon therapy, with the benefit of being a noninvasive modality compared to brachytherapy options. In 2006, Kozak et al. reported on the early outcomes of 20 women with stage I breast cancer who underwent adjuvant accelerated PBI with passive-scatter proton therapy to a total dose of 32 Gy at 4 Gy per fraction twice daily (BID) [19]. One to three fields were used, but only one field per fraction. In this phase I/II trial with a median 12-month follow-up, no patients experienced recurrent disease. Acute dermatitis was common, with most patients experiencing moderate-to-severe erythema and/or hyperpigmentation. Despite this acute toxicity, the cosmetic ratings were good or excellent by 85% of physicians and 100% of patients at last follow-up, although changes in pigmentation remained present in approximately 50%. One patient developed moderate-to-severe fibrosis and one developed clinical fat necrosis. Three patients developed rib pain, one of whom had a documented rib fracture. Overall patient satisfaction

was 95%. Using the same dose-fractionation schedule, Galland-Girodet et al. analyzed 98 patients treated with accelerated PBI (19 with passively scattered protons and 79 with photons or photons/electrons) with a median follow-up of 82.5 months [20]. The 7-year local recurrence rate was 11% in the proton cohort compared to 4% in the photon cohort, but this difference did not reach statistical significance ($p = 0.22$). Physician-rated good/excellent cosmesis was higher for patients treated with photons (94% vs. 62% with protons), and similarly high for patient-reported good/excellent cosmesis (96% photons vs. 92% protons; $p = 0.95$). While a difference in late cutaneous toxicity was seen between the photon and proton cohorts, there were no differences in noncutaneous toxicity including rib fracture, fat necrosis, and breast pain.

Using daily fractionation (40 Gy in 10 fractions) and a minimum of two fields per fraction, Bush et al. conducted a phase II trial of passive-scatter prone PBI [21]. For the 50 women enrolled in this study, planning goals included minimizing the skin volume (3-mm subtraction from the body surface) receiving 90% of the prescription dose, which was achieved by using primarily lateral and anterior beams and modifying apertures to decrease the dose to the skin. With a median follow-up of 48 months, the 5-year overall survival rate was 96% and the disease-free survival rate was 92%. In total, four patients developed recurrent disease: one with ipsilateral axillary recurrence 12 months after radiation that was successfully salvaged with mastectomy and chemotherapy and three with distant recurrences (brain, bone, chest wall, and mediastinum). One patient developed an in-breast out-of-field tumor 66 months after proton PBI, which was considered a new primary. Dermatitis comprised the only acute toxicity, and no patients developed fat necrosis, pneumonitis, cardiac events, or rib fracture during the follow-up period. Overall, 90% of patients rated cosmesis as good or excellent. In an update published in 2014 on 100 patients with a median follow-up of 60 months, the 5-year ipsilateral breast tumor recurrence-free, disease-free, and overall survival rates were 97%, 94%, and 95%, respectively [22]. No patients developed an in-field recurrence. In another phase II study, Chang et al. also used once-daily fractionation but with a prescription of 30 Gy over five consecutive fractions, with the patient in a supine position [23]. With a slightly longer follow-up (median, 59 months), no local, regional, or distant recurrences developed in the 30 patients enrolled in the study. The initial 15 patients were treated with a single field, but planning was then transitioned to 2 fields for the subsequent 15 patients in an effort to decrease skin doses. One patient developed moist desquamation. Two patients developed rib fractures (7%) at 6 months and 2 years after radiation. Both received treatment with a single field.

Ovalle et al. applied the RTOG external-beam fractionation regimen used for photon therapy and delivered 34 Gy at 3.4 Gy per fraction BID using passive-scatter proton therapy with two

Table 20.1 Clinical studies for partial-breast irradiation with proton therapy.

Study	No. of pts.	Prescription dose	Modality	Median follow-up, months	Disease outcomes	Toxicity (no. of pts.)	Physician- and patient-reported good/excellent cosmesis rates
Kozak et al. [19]	20	32 Gy in 8 fx BID	PS PT	12	No LR	Severe fibrosis (1); fat necrosis (1); rib fracture (1)	85% and 100%
Chang et al. [23]	30	30 Gy in 5 fx QD	PS PT	59	No LR, regional or distant recurrence	Rib fracture (2)	Not reported
Galland-Girodet et al. [20]	98	32 Gy in 8 fx BID	PS PT, n = 19; photons or electrons, n = 79	82.5	7-year LR 6%	Rib fracture (4); fat necrosis (12)	62% and 92% for PT; 94% and 96% for photon/ electron therapy
Bush et al. [22]	100	40 Gy in 10 fx QD	PS PT (prone)	60	5-year breast tumor recurrence-free survival 97%; DFS 94%; OS 95%	Fat necrosis (1); rib fracture, pneumonitis, cardiac events (0)	90%
Ovalle et al. [24]	43	34 Gy in 10 fx BID	PS PT	≥6	Not reported	Fat necrosis (1); mild (1), moderate (2), and severe (3) retraction/ asymmetry	Not reported
Mutter et al. [25]	76	21.9 Gy in 3 fx QD	PBS PT	12	Not reported	No grade ≥2 toxicity	98% (patient-reported)

BID: Twice daily; fx: fractions; no.: number; PBS: pencil-beam scanning; PS: passive-scattering; PT: proton therapy; pts: patients; QD: once daily.

or three fields per fraction [24]. In an assessment of 43 women with a minimum of 6 months of follow-up, >90% of patients developed acute dermatitis, which improved with time, and moderate hyperpigmentation was present in only 5% of patients at 6 months. Given the limitations of the Common Terminology Criteria of Adverse Events (CTCAE) scale in assessing skin toxicity, the investigators developed a modified scale by subcategorizing the observed skin changes.

A unique hypofractionated approach was recently reported by Mutter et al. [25]. Using PBS, they delivered a prescription dose of 21.9 Gy over 3 fractions to 76 women. The study's primary end point was cosmesis, specifically the difference in fair/poor cosmesis at 3 years compared to baseline. With a median follow-up of 12 months, the highest toxicity observed was grade 1 and good/excellent cosmesis was reported by 98% of patients.

For proton PBI, dose fractionation, number of fields per fraction, and skin-sparing planning techniques are important variables to consider in order to maximize favorable cosmetic outcomes. In Table 20.1, the clinical studies for PBI with proton therapy are summarized [19,22,23,24,25].

20.3.2 Whole-Breast or Chest-Wall ± Regional Nodal Irradiation

Most of the clinical studies to date have focused on RNI. While no studies have yet evaluated whole-breast irradiation alone as a primary focus of investigation, some have included a small subset of women with treatment directed to only the whole breast. As discussed in Section 20.2, the dosimetry of treating the whole breast with proton therapy is outstanding. However, in many cases, the dosimetry is also very good with photon therapy. Cardiac-sparing techniques, such as prone positioning, DIBH, gating, and in some cases VMAT or IMRT, can achieve low heart and lung doses in many patients [26,27,28–33]. Because the absolute dosimetric differences between protons and photons are greatest when the regional lymphatics are targeted, most studies have explored the application of proton therapy in this setting.

In a prospective phase I/II feasibility trial, MacDonald et al. evaluated 12 women with breast cancer treated with mastectomy and undergoing chest wall and RNI (laterality: n = 1 right, n = 11 left) using passive-scatter proton therapy to a dose of 45–50.4 Gy [28]. Primary objectives included evaluation of grade ≥3 pneumonitis or any toxicity grade ≥4 within 3 months of completing radiotherapy. Doses to the adjacent OARs were low, with an average MHD of 0.44 Gy (range, 0.1–1.2 Gy), mean heart V20 of 0.01% (range, 0–2.4%), and mean ipsilateral lung V20 of 12.7% (range, 4.4–22.1%). The study successfully met its end points, and, with a median follow-up of 6 months (range, 3.5–11.2 months), no patients developed radiation pneumonitis or grade 4 or 5 toxicity. Another prospective feasibility study by Bradley et al. included 18 women with stage IIA-IIIB breast cancer (9 left-sided and 9 right-sided) [29]. All patients received breast or chest wall and RNI to 50.4 Gy RBE in 28 fractions, including the internal mammary nodes. Treatments were delivered with passive-scatter proton therapy, and 50% of patients had mixed proton–photon plans. The median follow-up was 20 months. All patients had comparison photon-only plans, which resulted in inferior dosimetry for all patients compared to the proton or proton–photon plans. With the proton plans, the median MHD was 0.6 Gy for patients with left-sided and 0.5 Gy for those with right-sided disease.

In 2015, Cuaron et al. reported on 30 prospectively followed women who were treated with uniform-scanning proton therapy to 50.4 Gy RBE (45 Gy RBE to the chest wall and lymph nodes with a 5.4-Gy chest wall boost), with similar dosimetric parameters achieved as in the MacDonald trial (average MHD, 1 Gy; mean heart V20, 1.16%; mean ipsilateral lung V20, 16.5%) [30]. In 90% of women, the cancer was in the left breast, 87% underwent mastectomy, and 93% received breast/chest wall and RNI that included the internal mammary nodes. With a median follow-up of 9.3 months, one patient developed liver metastasis and no patients developed a local–regional recurrence. While no grade 4–5 toxicities developed, 28.6% of patients developed acute moist desquamation, considered grade 2. In 2019, this series was updated to include 42 women who had undergone mastectomy [31]. The median MHD for the cohort was 0.7 Gy. One patient developed an in-field chest-wall recurrence 2.5 years after completing radiation. With a median follow-up of 35 months, no other patients developed a local recurrence. The 3-year local–regional disease-free survival was 84.1% and the overall survival was 97.2%. A larger series of 91 patients treated with uniform scanning (77%) or PBS (23%) demonstrated a primary pattern of failure of distant metastases ($n = 10$), including 2 with simultaneous local–regional recurrence [32]. The vast majority of patients (90%) had node-positive disease. With a median follow-up of 15.5 months, two patients experienced an isolated local–regional recurrence.

With a focus on acute toxicities, Thorpe et al. reported on 82 women in a multi-institutional prospective registry treated with breast conservation and proton therapy (PBS and uniform scanning) [33]. The median dose delivered was 50.4 Gy over 28 fractions, and most patients had left-sided breast cancer (74%) and received RNI (83%, including 66% with internal mammary node irradiation) and a lumpectomy bed boost (90%). With a median follow-up of 8.1 months, <10% experienced a grade 3 toxicity and none had grade 4–5 toxicity. Local recurrence in the tumor bed occurred in two patients at 4.2 and 14.1 months after radiotherapy.

Another series focused on women in a prospective registry who had undergone mastectomy with immediate reconstruction with tissue expanders. The investigators found that 51 women received PBS proton therapy to the chest wall and regional lymphatics with either standard fractionation (73%; 50 Gy in 25 fractions) or hypofractionation (27%; 40.5 Gy in 15 fractions) [34]. This is the first study to report the use of hypofractionation with RNI using proton therapy. Some patients received a simultaneous integrated boost to undissected lymph nodes. No patients received a boost to the chest wall. The breast cancer was left-sided in 69% of women. The median MHD was 0.7 Gy for left-sided and 0.4 Gy for right-sided tumors and median ipsilateral lung V20 was 14%. The median follow-up was 19 months. Rates of infection, unplanned reoperations, and reconstruction failures were all higher in the patients who received hypofractionation ($p \leq 0.03$).

Jimenez et al. conducted a phase II study with the primary end points of (1) incidence of ≥grade 3 radiation pneumonitis or (2) any grade 4 toxicity within 3 months of RT [35]. Eligibility criteria included treatment of the regional lymphatics, including the internal mammary nodes, and dosimetric measure of inadequate target coverage, or V20 ≥ 5% or LAD ≥ 20 Gy, with conventional radiation. The study enrolled 70 women: 91% with a left-sided primary and 94% with stage II or III disease. The prescribed dose was 50.4 Gy in 28 fractions to the chest wall, 45 Gy in 25 fractions to the breast with a 14.4-Gy boost to the lumpectomy bed over 8 fractions and 45–50.4 Gy in 25–28 fractions to the regional nodes using PBS (67%) or passive scattering (33%). With a median follow-up of 55 months, the 5-year local–regional recurrence and overall survival were 1.5% and 91%, respectively. Of the patients who underwent mastectomy with immediate reconstruction, 32% experienced post-radiation complications; the 5-year unplanned reoperation actuarial rate was 33%. No grade 4–5 toxicity developed, and grade 3 toxicity was rare. Cardiac strain echocardiogram, amino-terminal pro-B-type natriuretic peptide, and ultrasensitive troponin I were obtained prior to radiation and at 4 and 8 weeks after radiation, with no significant changes at the selected time points.

The early results of these clinical studies consistently demonstrate full target coverage with low OAR doses. The median or average MHD was <1 Gy in these series, including in women with left-sided breast cancers with internal mammary node irradiation. While results on disease control are still limited, the 5-year data from Jimenez et al. demonstrate a high rate of local–regional control and overall survival. No studies reported grade 4 or 5 toxicity. Grade 3 toxicity was limited overall and usually acute dermatitis. Table 20.2 summarizes the clinical studies on proton therapy for breast cancer [28,36–41,35]. A randomized study comparing protons and photons is underway, with a primary end point of major cardiovascular events [7].

20.3.3 Carbon-ion Therapy

The use of carbon-ion therapy for breast cancer is in its early stages of development. Compared to proton therapy, the sharper penumbra of carbon-ion therapy [36] may improve sparing of

Table 20.2 Clinical studies for breast/chest wall ± regional nodal irradiation with proton therapy.

Study	No. of patients (laterality)	Mastectomy/ BCS	Regional nodal irradiation	Prescription dose, initial phase	Modality	Dosimetry	Median follow-up, mos.	Disease outcomes (no. of pts.)	Toxicity (no. of pts.)
MacDonald et al. [28]	12 (92% left)	100%/0%	100%	45–50.4 Gy at 1.8 Gy/fx	PS PT	Median MHD, 0.44 Gy; ipsilateral mean V20, 12.7%	6	Not reported	Grade 3 fatigue (1)
Bradley et al. [29]	18 (50% left)	61%/39%	100%	50.4 Gy at 1.8 Gy/fx	PS PT (matched photon fields, 9 pts.)	Median MHD, 0.6 Gy left and 0.5 Gy right; median IL V20, 22%	20	Not reported	Grade 2 pneumonitis (1); grade 3 acute dermatitis (4); grade 3 cellulitis (1)
Cuaron et al. [30]	30 (90% left)	87%/13%	100%	45–50.4 Gy at 1.8 Gy/fx	US PT	Median MHD, 1 Gy; median IL V20, 16.5%	9.3	No LRR; DM (4)	No acute grade 3; grade 3 reconstruction complication (1); No rib fracture
Verma et al. [32]	91 (62% left, 2% bilateral)	71%/29%	100%	44.8–50.4 Gy at 1.8 Gy/fx	US (77%) and PBS (23%) PT	Not reported	15.5	Isolated LRR (2) with DM (1) and with simultaneous LRR (2)	Grade 3 dermatitis (5); grade 3 chest wall pain (1); cellulitis (7); rib fracture (2)
Luo et al. [31]	42 (86% left)	100%/0%	100%	45–50.4 Gy at 1.8 Gy/fx	US PT	Median MHD, 0.8 Gy left and 0.1 Gy right; median IL V20, 16%	35	3-year LR-DFS 96%; DM-free survival, 84%; OS, 97%; CW in-field failure,	No acute grade 3; grade 3 pneumonitis (1) 27% reconstruction complications; No rib fracture
Smith et al. [34]	51 (69% left, 4% bilateral)	100%/0%	100%	50 Gy at 2 Gy/fx (73%) or 40.5 at 2.7 Gy/fx (27%)	PBS PT	Median MHD, 0.6 Gy; median IL V20, 13.9%	19	Not reported	Grade 3 dermatitis (2); reconstruction failure (8)
Jimenez et al. [35]	70 (91% left)	93%/7%	100%	45–50.4 Gy at 1.8 Gy/fx	PS (33%) and PBS (67%) PT	Median MHD, 0.5 Gy; median IL V20, 15%	55	5-year LRR, 1.5%; OS, 91%	Grade 3 dermatitis (2); grade 3 seroma (1); grade 3 infection (1); grade 1 and 2 pneumonitis (4 and 1); rib fracture (5)
Thorpe et al. [33]	82 (74% left)	0%/100%	83%	42.5–54 Gy in 16–30 fx	US (67%) and PBS (22%) PT	Not reported	8.1	LR in tumor bed (2)	Grade 3 dermatitis (5); grade 3 breast pain (5)

BCS: Breast-conserving surgery; CW: chest wall; DFS: disease-free survival; DM: distant metastasis; fx: fraction; IL: ipsilateral lung; LR: local recurrence; LRR: local–regional recurrence; MHD: mean heart dose; OS: overall survival; PBS: pencil-beam scanning; PS: passive-scattering; PT: proton therapy; US: uniform scanning.

the esophagus and thyroid, if carbon ion is used for RNI in breast cancer. It is hypothesized that carbon-ion therapy may prove advantageous in locally advanced, chemotherapy-resistant breast cancer and unresected gross nodal disease, such as disease in the internal mammary and supraclavicular locations [36,37].

Several *in-vitro* studies have demonstrated a significant reduction in the surviving fraction of breast cancer cell lines using carbon ions compared to photons. One *in-vitro* study using human triple-negative breast cancer cell lines irradiated with photons versus carbon ions, with and without cisplatin, demonstrated increased cell kill with carbon ions [38]. Similarly, an *in-vitro* study evaluating Her2-positive breast cancer cell lines found the highest efficacy for carbon-ion therapy with concurrent lapatinib compared to photons [39]. Zhang et al. measured increased G2/M phase arrest, DNA lesions, and apoptosis/necrosis with carbon ions compared to photons for the same prescription dose [40].

Clinically, carbon-ion therapy has been explored in the preoperative setting for breast cancer. The treatment of gross tumor maximizes the radiobiological and physical advantages of carbon ions compared to the treatment of microscopic disease in the postoperative setting [36]. A phase I study in seven patients aged ≥60 years with stage I hormone receptor-positive breast cancer to evaluate safety and efficacy of three dose levels (48, 52.8, and 60 Gy) given in 4 fractions over 4 days to the tumor bed using robust immobilization, fiducial markers, and 3,290-MeV carbon-ion fields [41]. The only acute side effect reported was grade 1 dermatitis, which occurred in four patients. After 3 months, patients underwent lumpectomy and sentinel lymph node biopsy. Pathologic assessment found a treatment response in six of seven patients, including two patients with a complete response (defined as nonviable cells). With follow-up ranging from 37 to 48 months, all patients experienced disease control, excellent cosmesis, and no late effects. The investigators have since commenced with a phase II study using 60 Gy. The time period to achieve pathologic response requires further investigation. While in this phase I trial few patients had a pCR at 3 months after radiation, in an earlier case report of a patient who declined surgery, definitive carbon-ion irradiation to 52.8 Gy in four fractions using respiratory gating was delivered, with tumor response at 3 months but complete radiographic response occurring after 12 months [41,42]. Another case report describes the use of carbon-ion therapy for oligometastatic breast cancer, treating a patient with a 6-cm liver metastasis to 36 Gy in one fraction, with sustained local control over 8 years [43]. Passive-scatter carbon-ion therapy was used in these clinical studies. In a dosimetric comparison between passive scattering and active scanning for PBI with carbon ions, with the tumor intact, target coverage and skin sparing were similar between the two modalities [44].

Preoperative radiotherapy is undergoing increasing investigation as a treatment approach with photon therapy [45]. If the treatment paradigm shifts from adjuvant radiotherapy to preoperative or definitive radiotherapy paradigms, carbon-ion therapy may enhance efficacy given its high linear energy transfer (LET). The initial clinical experiences highlight the importance of rigorous patient immobilization and daily tumor localization. Clinical trials are necessary to evaluate the indications, techniques, and treatment safety and efficacy of this promising radiotherapy modality.

20.3.4 Male Breast Cancer

Male breast cancer is uncommon, comprising 1% of breast cancers, with an increasing incidence and decreasing mortality in the United States [46,47]. Although clinical studies have predominately included women with breast cancer, that does not mean that men do not receive the same benefits from particle therapy. The thoracic anatomy of males and females is similar, and the challenges of optimal target coverage while minimizing heart and lung dose exist for both sexes. Giap et al. published a case report of a man who received radiation to 50 Gy for a thymic carcinoma and subsequently developed a medial breast cancer 20 years later [48]. His comorbidities included coronary artery disease, cardiomyopathy, and congestive heart failure. He underwent lumpectomy followed by adjuvant PBS proton therapy to 50.4 Gy to the whole breast with a simultaneous integrated boost to the lumpectomy cavity of 58 Gy, all in 28 fractions. Compared to photon planning, the proton plan decreased the dose to the heart (mean, 3.1 vs. 0.02 Gy), the left lung (mean, 7.9 vs. 0.04 Gy), and the esophagus (maximum, 6.8 vs. 0.01 Gy).

20.3.5 Re-irradiation

Thorpe et al. reported the results of a prospective multi-institutional registry study using proton therapy for re-irradiation in the treatment of women with recurrent breast cancer [49]. The median follow-up time from re-irradiation was 12.7 months (range, 0–41.8 months) for the 50 women who were treated to a median dose of 55.1 Gy (range, 45.1–76.3 Gy); the median cumulative dose was 110.6 Gy (range, 70.6–156.8 Gy). Uniform scanning was the most common technique used (in 52%) followed by PBS (24%), with 24% not reported. For most patients, several years had elapsed from their prior course of radiation (median, 103.8 months; range, 5.5–430.8 months). The 1-year local recurrence-free survival was 93%, with variation seen for those who had gross disease at the time of RT (84%) and those with only microscopic disease (100%; $p = 0.06$). Grade 3 acute toxicities included pain in 4%, dermatitis in 2%, lymphedema in 2%, and anorexia in 2%. Late grade 3 toxicities were also infrequent (8%) with no grade 4 or 5 toxicities, although the short follow-up limits full evaluation of late effects. In a small retrospective review, Gabani et al. reported on 16 women with breast cancer who underwent re-irradiation with passive-scatter proton therapy [50]. While the median follow-up was slightly longer than that of Thorpe et al., at 18.7 months it was still insufficient to fully characterize late toxicities. With a median re-irradiation dose of 50.4 Gy in 28 fractions (plus 10–16-Gy boost in 81%) and a median of 10.2 years (range, 0.7–20.2 years) from the prior course of radiation, 31% experienced acute grade 3–4 dermatitis and 25% developed a chest wall infection. Pneumonitis developed in two patients, rib fracture in one (asymptomatic, found incidentally), brachial plexopathy in one, and late grade 3–4 fibrosis in three patients. One patient developed metastatic disease, and no patients experienced a local or regional recurrence. Ten patients (62.5%) received concurrent hyperthermia, a notable difference from the study by Thorpe et al., and a possible contributory factor to the higher rates of acute toxicity due to the radiosensitizing effect of hyperthermia.

These initial reports of re-irradiation were published in 2019 and it is anticipated that additional reports will follow over the next several years. Moreover, maturation of these data for further evaluation of late toxicities and disease control will be important in evaluating proton therapy for salvage treatment and in counseling patients. It is hypothesized that carbon-ion therapy may provide benefit for re-irradiation of breast cancer, but clinical data have not yet been published [36].

20.4 Overview of Treatment Planning

20.4.1 CT Simulation

While one institution has reported on prone positioning for PBI [17], proton therapy is most commonly developed in the supine position with arms overhead. Care with positioning to minimize skin folds in the low neck, axilla, and inframammary region is necessary, as it is with photon planning, to minimize increased dermatitis in areas that are self-bolused. If the breast is large and displays more than minimal overlap onto the upper abdomen, 3D conformal photons may provide a better option over proton therapy, due to the challenges of establishing a reproducible setup daily for a large, ptotic, mobile breast [48].

When planning for proton therapy, there is an option to treat with the arms down and akimbo (Figure 20.1A), which is preferred by many patients, particularly those with arthritis or prior shoulder injury. With the current technology, the arms-

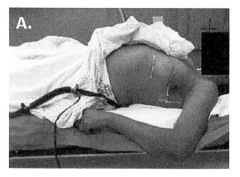
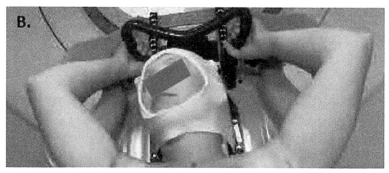
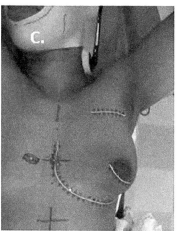
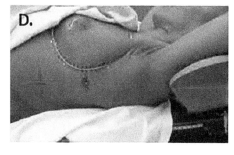
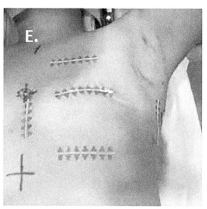

Figure 20.1 Images from computed tomography (CT) simulation illustrating (A) positioning with arms down and akimbo to maximally open the axilla; (B) open-face mask to immobilize the chin and head position in the setting of supraclavicular nodal irradiation; (C and D) wire placement extending from the 3:00 to the 9:00 positions of the breast, superior extent of the breast, and lumpectomy incision to assist in clinical target volume (CTV) delineation; and (E) wire placement on the mastectomy incision and lateral, superior, medial, and inferior borders of the chest wall to assist in CTV delineation.

down position can interfere with the use of cone-beam computed tomography (CBCT) due to collision factors, and particular attention to reproducibility of the arm position is necessary. A face mask or chin strap can assist in immobilization of the supraclavicular lymph nodes (Figure 20.1B) with the head turned toward the contralateral side. For bilateral breast or chest-wall irradiation, particularly with nodal irradiation, the head is best positioned in the midline with neck extension.

DIBH is typically not indicated with proton therapy, even with left-sided tumors, as the heart exposure is low with free-breathing and not measurably improved with DIBH [51,52] or with cardiac gating [11,53].

Metallic wires are used to delineate the breast or chest wall, to provide a reference between visual clinical evaluation of the anatomy in relation to the anatomy on the chest CT images. For an intact breast, a wire is placed extending from the 3:00 to the 9:00 positions of the breast, with an additional piece of wire placed at the superior aspect of the breast tissue (Figure 20.1C,D). A wire is placed on the lumpectomy incision, which can be helpful in contouring the lumpectomy cavity, particularly if the surgeon omitted placement of clips in the surgical bed. After the mastectomy (with or without reconstruction), a wire is placed on the mastectomy incision, and separate pieces of wire are placed to mark each of the lateral, superior, medial, and inferior borders (Figure 20.1E). These metallic wires must have an override during the proton planning, as they distort the beam and will not be present at the time of treatment.

Axial CT images are obtained at 1–2-mm increments. If contrast is used to assist in delineation of the nodal regions and cardiac substructures, a second noncontrast CT should also be obtained and used for planning. At our institution, 4D CT is acquired, from which the average intensity projection CT is reconstructed and used for planning and generating a digitally reconstructed radiograph. The average CT is considered a more realistic reference for daily setup given the respiratory motion.

20.4.2 Contouring

Most of the contours for proton planning share the same definition of those used with photon planning, as the target regions are the same.

Although radiation is typically delivered after the gross disease has been surgically excised, the nomenclature for the tumor bed still includes a gross tumor volume (GTV). The GTV TumorBed is defined as the surgical clips placed by the surgeon to denote the edges of the surgical cavity and seroma, if present. A 1–1.5-cm expansion on GTV TumorBed is performed to create the CTV TumorBed, which is edited to within the confines of the CTV breast. CTV TumorBed is then expanded by 0.5–1 cm to yield the PTV TumorBed, also edited to stay within the CTV Breast.

PBI: In the prone phase II trial, the expansions for CTV and PTV were 1 and 0.2 cm, respectively, and daily kV orthogonal image guidance was used, with the surgical clips in the lumpectomy bed serving as fiducial markers [22]. The CTV was edited to exclude the skin and chest wall. Using a similar image guidance approach but supine position, Kozak et al. defined the lumpectomy bed as the CTV and expanded this by 1.5–2 cm to create a PTV, which was edited to exclude the chest wall and 5-mm from the skin [19]. A nonuniform PTV margin was used by Chang et al., with the PTV margin determined by the width of the negative surgical resection margin (e.g., "2, 1.5, and 1 cm [PTV margin] for resection margins <1, 1–2 , and >2 cm, respectively"), with the PTV edited from the pectoralis muscle and 3 mm from the skin [23].In contrast,Ovalle et al. defined the tumor bed (including surgical clips and seroma) and then expanded this volume by 1.5 cm, excluding the chest wall and 5 mm from the skin; PTV use was not specified [24].

Whole-breast irradiation: The contours for whole-breast irradiation with protons mirror that with photons [54]. The contour is subtracted 5 mm from the body surface anteriorly and reaches the anterior edge of the pectoralis major posteriorly. The superior and inferior aspects of the breast may be easily visible or can be determined based on the wires placed at CT simulation and by comparison to the contralateral breast when present.

With 3D conformal photon therapy, the low axilla receives dose even when it is not defined as a target due to the typical tangent beam arrangement in which radiation passes through the low axilla to reach the breast (Figure 20.2A). In contrast, with proton therapy, the low axilla will only receive radiation if a target is contoured in that region. Owing to the en face beam arrangement and the sharp dose fall off attributable to the Bragg peak, the incidental dose to the low axilla is minimal with protons, even when the adjacent breast tissue is fully covered (Figure 20.2B). Therefore, if the photon treatment includes high tangents to cover the low axilla, then that portion of the axilla should be contoured and intentionally targeted with proton therapy.

RNI: Contouring atlases, of which there are many, provide useful guidance for both proton and photon planning. The original Radiation Therapy Oncology Group (RTOG) contouring atlas, developed after a study demonstrating variance among experts, relies primarily on muscle and bony anatomy definitions [54,55]. Other atlases expanded these guidelines, employing the location of vasculature to assist in contour definition [56,57,64]. Investigators have evaluated recurrence patterns in relation to these contouring guidelines, with some reporting that a proportion of local–regional recurrences develop outside of the guideline regions [58,59,67]. Kowalski et al. delineated multiple sets of contours on a single CT dataset, then planned with several radiation techniques including

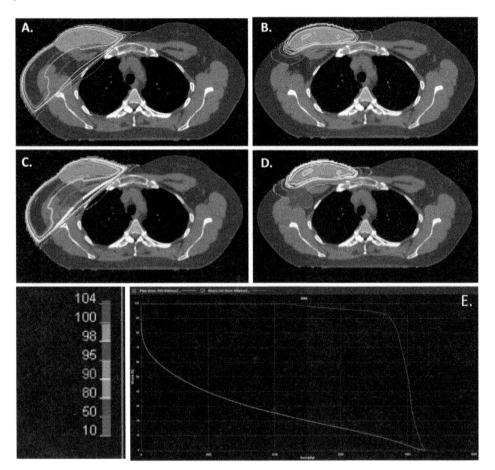

Figure 20.2   In treatment of the whole breast only, the low axilla receives (A) measurable dose with 3D conformal photon tangent fields by nature of the beam arrangement and (B) minimal dose with pencil-beam scanning (PBS) if the low axilla is not contoured for intentional targeting. (C and D) A volume for the low axilla is drawn in pink, highlighting the difference in incidental dose to this area. (E) The dose–volume histogram for the low axilla with 3D photons (dashed line) and PBS (solid line), when the low axilla is not contoured and included as a target.

3D conformal photons, VMAT, and proton therapy [60]. In overlaying PET scans from patients with gross nodal disease, they found that nodal coverage fell below 95% using the European Society for Radiotherapy and Oncology (ESTRO) and RTOG contouring guidelines when planning with VMAT or proton therapy. This study highlights the importance of target delineation when using highly conformal radiotherapy. The RadComp atlas was designed specifically with proton therapy in mind. This atlas includes an optional volume to consider when treatment is delivered with protons, which is located posterior to the traditional supraclavicular region [54]. With photons, this region receives exit dose and sometimes entrance dose from a posterior axillary field; yet, with protons, the dose to this region is negligible unless the contour is intentionally extended to include this region. Regardless of the contouring guidelines utilized, in patients with gross nodal disease at diagnosis, fusion of the diagnostic imaging with the CT simulation imaging is recommended to accurately identify and tailor the at-risk region for an individual patient (Figure 20.3).

In the setting of a retropectoral implant, the ESTRO Advisory Committee on Radiation Oncology Practice (ACROP) contouring guideline recommends the posterior aspect of the chest wall CTV extend to the pectoralis major, except in cases of T3 or T4 disease, locally advanced breast cancer with an incomplete response to chemotherapy, or pectoralis muscle or chest wall invasion [61]. Otherwise, the contour excludes the expander/implant. With photon techniques, the tissue posterior to the expander/implant will receive some radiation, although perhaps not a full dose, while in proton therapy the dose to this region is close to zero. The optimal target in this setting, particularly when proton therapy is used, remains an area of controversy.

Targeting of the dissected axilla is another controversial topic in proton radiotherapy treatment planning. As discussed in regards to the whole breast and the low axilla, the undissected axilla will receive minimal to no dose with proton therapy if it is not contoured for intentional targeting. In photon-based planning, the dissected axilla still receives some

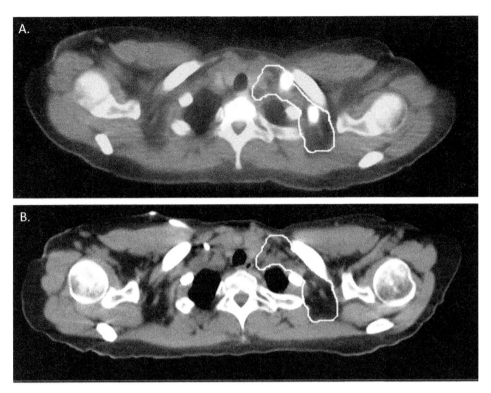

Figure 20.3 The (A) positron emission tomography imaging taken at diagnosis, demonstrating extensive supraclavicular disease, was fused with the (B) computed tomography simulation images with the clinical target volume (in yellow) extended posteriorly to cover the area at risk for residual microscopic disease.

dose, even if it is not the full prescription dose [62]. The question remains: is no dose to the dissected axilla acceptable? Some physicians will include the dissected axilla as a target in proton planning given the concern for complete absence of dose to this region.

The PTV provides the classic solution in photon therapy to address setup uncertainty by geometric expansion from the CTV. However, the PTV cannot do the same in proton therapy. The static dose approximation is invalid for proton therapy since the dose distribution can be significantly perturbed when the water equivalent thickness (WET) changes along the beam path due to setup errors [63,64]. To account for organ motion, setup uncertainties, and range uncertainty, the beam-specific PTV (BsPTV) structure may be created. The BsPTV [65] involves three parts: (1) expanding CTV laterally relative to the beam direction to mitigate a geometric miss due to setup error and organ motion, (2) adding distal and proximal margins to account for range uncertainty, and (3) adding extra margins to account for the WET variation along the beam path introduced by misalignment of heterogeneous tissues due to setup errors. Thus, for breast cancer treatment, a conventional uniform PTV expansion along the beam axis is not routinely performed. Rather, a 0.5-cm lateral expansion of the CTV is performed, edited to exclude the esophagus and thyroid. The range uncertainty and potential variations in radiological path

length are accounted for by either robust optimization for PBS or a smearing margin for passive scattering.

OARs: The heart and each lung should be contoured in all cases. Substructure delineation of the heart is especially useful in proton therapy, where contouring of the ventricles and the coronary arteries (primarily the LAD for left-sided and the right coronary artery for right-sided) allows those regions to be selectively avoided. While intravenous contrast on the simulation scan helps with these delineations, these substructures can be identified on noncontrast-enhanced CT scans.

For PBI, the ipsilateral breast should be contoured for all cases. The target is the lumpectomy bed, and the remainder of the breast becomes a relative avoidance structure to maximize cosmesis. For RNI, the esophagus, thyroid, ipsilateral brachial plexus, and ipsilateral humeral head should be delineated. While contouring of the contralateral breast is important in photon cases to ensure avoidance, particularly with IMRT and VMAT plans, proton plans rarely create exposure of the contralateral breast.

For patients with an expander with a metal port, if the proton beam travels through the high-density magnet, the magnet must be contoured and assigned the appropriate density value and relative stopping power (RSP) based on its physical properties. There are several techniques for contouring and accounting for this magnet [66,67,76].

20.4.3 Prescription Dose

The prescription dose for PBI with protons varies from 3 to 10 fractions and daily and BID regimens. The studies discussed previously provide additional detail on the recommended prescription doses. For whole-breast irradiation, the hypofractionated regimens that have been widely adopted for photon therapy are also employed with proton therapy (40.05 Gy in 15 fractions or 42.4 Gy in 16 fractions [68,69], with a 3–5-fraction boost ranging from 2 to 2.65 Gy per fraction).

At present, for both proton and photon radiotherapy, 1.8–2 Gy per fraction to total doses of 45–50.4 Gy to the breast or chest wall and regional lymphatics remains the standard regimen in the United States. While hypofractionation studies in the United States are being conducted on this topic, level I evidence is currently lacking. In the setting of radiation for postmastectomy expander reconstruction, Smith et al. demonstrated higher rates of infection and reconstruction toxicity with hypofractionation compared to standard fractionation [69]. Thus, hypofractionation for RNI should be used cautiously until further evidence supporting this approach is available.

20.4.4 Target Coverage

Historically with 2D and 3D photon radiotherapy for breast cancer, a prescription of 50 Gy to a point resulted in 40–45 Gy coverage of ≥95% of the target region. Thus, with proton planning, to achieve similar target coverage to traditional photon plans, investigators at some centers prescribe 50 Gy and accept 95% coverage to 95% of the target volume. This approach creates plans with lower hot spots. Alternatively, some investigators prescribe a lower dose of 45 Gy, with the intention of 100% of the dose covering ≥95% of the target region. As the internal mammary nodes are readily covered with proton therapy, the goal target coverage need not be reduced to 90% of the dose to 90% of the volume, as it often is in photon planning [70].

20.4.5 OAR Constraints

PBI: In a multi-institutional prospective phase I/II trial, Galland-Girodet et al. used treatment planning guidelines consisting of ≤50% of the prescription dose to the nontarget breast tissue (defined as the ipsilateral breast minus the PTV TumorBed) and dose inhomogeneity <15% [20]. While some proton PBI studies did not report the use of heart or lung constraints in their methods, the heart and lung doses achieved neared zero [20,22]. Ovalle et al. adhered to the National Surgical Adjuvant Breast and Bowel Project (NSABP) B-39/RTOG 0413 guidelines, asserting that all cases met these constraints [24], which include (1) <60% and <35% of the ipsilateral breast (PTV TumorBed not excluded) receiving ≥50% of the prescribed dose and 100% of the prescription dose, respectively; (2) maximum 3% of the prescription dose to the contralateral breast; (3) ipsilateral lung volume receiving 30% of the prescription dose <15%; (4) contralateral lung volume receiving 5% of the prescription dose <15%; (5) heart V5 (Rx) <5% for right-sided and <40% for left sided disease; and (6) maximum 3% of the prescription dose to the thyroid [71].

Whole-breast irradiation: The normal tissue constraints used in RTOG 1005 provide a standard reference for dose constraints in the setting of hypofractionation for breast-only radiation with photons. The goal and acceptable criteria were as follows, respectively: MHD, ≤3.2 Gy and ≤4 Gy, heart D5%, ≤16 Gy and ≤20 Gy; and heart V8, ≤30% and ≤35% (with lower parameters for right-sided breast cancer) [72]. For the ipsilateral lung, the goal and acceptable criteria were, respectively, V16, ≤15% and ≤20%; V8, ≤35% and ≤40%; V4, ≤50% and ≤55%.

For standard fractionation (2 Gy) treatment of the whole breast with photons, arm 1 of RTOG1304/NSABPB51 provides guidelines on OAR constraints labeled as "per protocol" and "variation acceptable," with a dose exceeding "variation acceptable" considered a deviation [70]. For the ipsilateral lung, these were, respectively, V5, ≤50% and 55%; V10, ≤35% and 40%; and V20, ≤15% and 20%. V5 ≤10% is the per protocol constraint for the contralateral lung, with up to 15% an acceptable variation. Regarding plan maximum dose, ≤115% is per protocol, with acceptable variation up to 120% and a conformity index (95% prescription dose to the breast PTV) per protocol of 0.95 ≤ CI ≤ 2.0, with 0.85 ≤ CI ≤ 2.5 an acceptable variation. Dose constraints for the contralateral breast include a maximum dose of 3.1 Gy (per protocol; 4.96-Gy variation acceptable) and less than 5% receiving 1.86 Gy (per protocol; 3.1-Gy variation acceptable). The per protocol MHD is ≤4 Gy, with up to 5 Gy an acceptable variation. The per protocol and variation acceptable D5% are 20 Gy and 25 Gy for patients with left-sided breast cancer, while per protocol and acceptable variation maximum doses are 20 Gy and 25 Gy for patients with right-sided breast cancer. The per protocol cardiac V10 Gy is 30% for patients with left-sided breast cancer and 10% for right-sided, while variation acceptable criteria are 35% and 15% for left- and right-sided, respectively.

RNI: Similarly, for breast or chest wall and RNI, the RTOG1304/NSABPB51 protocol provides guidance on normal tissue constraints [70]. For arm 2, which includes RNI, the MHD per protocol constraint is ≤4 Gy and variation acceptable criterion is ≤5 Gy. The other cardiac parameters for D5% and V15 differ based on laterality of the breast cancer; the per protocol constraint and variation acceptable criterion are as follows, respectively: left-sided D5%, ≤25 Gy and ≤30 Gy; right-sided D0%, ≤25 Gy and 30 Gy; left-sided V15, ≤30% and ≤35%; and right-sided V15, ≤10% and ≤15%. With proton therapy, these cardiac constraints are often easily met. Many support an additional constraint on the LAD with proton therapy (varying from <3 to <10 Gy to 0.1 cm^3 of the coronary artery) to maximize cardiac-sparing, although the selection of this constraint is not based on empirical dose–volume data. The lung constraints from this cooperative group protocol are applicable to proton therapy planning: ipsilateral lung V20, ≤30% and ≤35%; V10, ≤35% and ≤40%; and V5, ≤50% and 55%; contralateral lung V5, ≤10% and ≤15%, per protocol and variation acceptable, respectively. The protocol does not provide constraints on esophagus, thyroid, or brachial plexus.

It is important to constrain the dose to the esophagus, as there is no crisp block edge at the border of the esophagus with proton therapy (or photon IMRT) as there is with 3D conformal photons. Therefore, the esophagus is at risk of increased dose exposure with proton therapy. While no consensus exists to define the esophagus constraint with proton therapy, our institutional constraint is 0.1 cm^3 ≤95% of the prescription dose. Others use esophagus D0.01 cm^3 ≤ 36 Gy [66], and 70% prescription dose to ≤1 cm^3 [73], or D_{max} ≤40 Gy (R Jimenez, MD, email communication, September 2020).

Similarly, a standard constraint has not been employed for the thyroid or the brachial plexus. In other disease sites, maximum dose to the brachial plexus of 60–66 Gy is a common constraint [74]. In breast cancer, these doses near the brachial plexus are not reached unless a nodal boost in the high axilla or supraclavicular region is indicated. In analyzing the effect of RBE heterogeneity on the brachial plexus during proton planning, Mutter et al. recommend a physical constraint of 0.01 cm^3 brachial plexus ≤102% based on relative biological effectiveness (RBE) biologic planning [75]. At our institution, we limit 0.1 cm^3 of the brachial plexus to ≤95% of the prescription dose in low-risk cases and ≤100% in high-risk cases such as N3 disease for PBS plans.

While the humeral head typically does not have a set constraint, it is considered a structure to avoid in PBS planning and blocked using the aperture shape in passive scattering. Regarding dose heterogeneity, it is recommended that the hot spot remain <107% for the ideal, with up to 110% considered acceptable.

With PBS, the dose to the skin rind can be adjusted to reduce radiation dermatitis. While current practice patterns vary, at our institution, we limit the 5-mm skin rind to 45 Gy for intact breast and 47.5 Gy for the chest wall. For inflammatory disease, no limit is set on the skin rind. When using passive scattering, Liang et al. found that V52.5CGE and D10 cm^3 for the skin rind (body minus 5 mm) and smoking were associated with acute grade 3 dermatitis [76].

Lower OAR doses can typically be achieved with proton therapy compared to photon techniques. Thus, while one should be familiar with the constraints used in photon planning, proton plans should be designed to minimize normal tissue doses in order to obtain the maximum benefit from this modality, rather than accepting a plan that meets photon constraints but does not fully yield the maximal OAR sparing afforded by protons [48]. Figures 20.4–20.6 demonstrate target contours and dose distributions for representative cases for partial-breast and ipsilateral breast and RNI, and bilateral chest wall and RNI, respectively.

20.4.6 Image Guidance

Daily image guidance is a standard of care in proton therapy delivery, with alignment goals of ≤2 mm. Several options exist to achieve this low tolerance on daily setup errors. kV orthogonal imaging is a common approach, with alignment focused on bony anatomy. Contours of bony landmarks are used for daily alignment, including the humeral head, clavicle, sternum, and vertebral column. While bony anatomy is useful, the breast or chest wall is composed of soft tissue and therefore not well visualized on kV imaging. CBCT is a tool that has been used with photons for >15 years but has only recently become more available in proton gantries. Challenges with field of view and collision still limit its functionality as the primary method of daily imaging for breast cancer. To avoid collision with the gantry and or imaging panel, the couch is required to offset laterally from the target isocenter to reach a more central position. The typical field of view may prohibit imaging of the entire breast, so alignment still occurs based

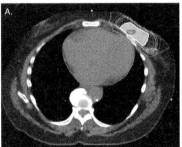
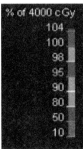
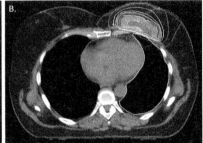

Figure 20.4 Target contours in colorwash (GTV in red and CTV in yellow) with isodose distribution shown for partial breast irradiation to 40 Gy RBE in 10 daily fractions using (A) three-field passive-scatter and (B) two-field PBS techniques.

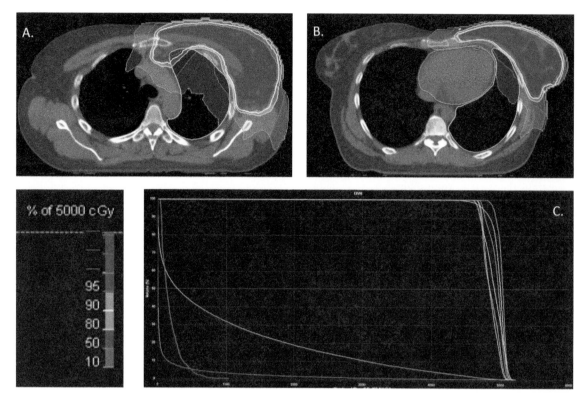

Figure 20.5 (A, B) Isodose distribution for a pencil-beam scanning plan for treatment of the breast and comprehensive regional lymphatics. (C) The dose–volume histogram for the clinical target volume targets (all > 95%/95%) and heart (orange; mean dose, 1.1 Gy; V5, 5.2%; V25, 1%), left anterior descending artery (dark purple, 0.1 cm³, 5.1 Gy), and left lung (light purple, V5 42.7%, V20 18.9%).

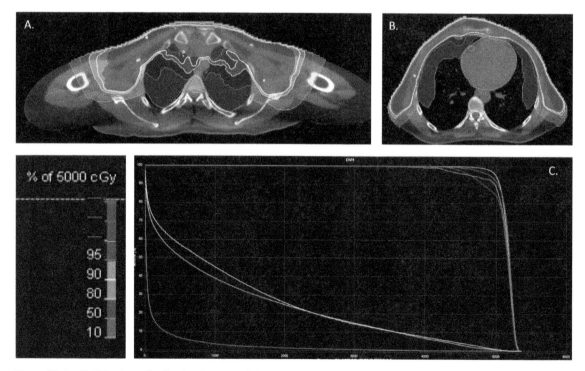

Figure 20.6 (A,B) Isodose distribution for a pencil-beam scanning plan for treatment of the bilateral chest wall and bilateral comprehensive regional lymphatics including bilateral internal mammary chains for five intercostal spaces due to gross internal mammary lymph node involvement at diagnosis. (C) The dose–volume histogram for the clinical target volume targets (yellow, orange, and red) and heart (orange; mean dose, 1.4 Gy; V5, 10.5%; V25, 0.9%), left lung (purple; V5, 50.6%; V20, 24.8%), and right lung (light blue; V5, 57.4%; V20, 25.9%).

primarily on bony anatomy. This problem is solved with the latest compact IBA ProteusOne CBCT system (Ion Beam Applications, Belgium), which allows acquisition of CBCT images using a large field of view. However, this large field of view CBCT doubles the time of acquisition as it requires an additional set of data with the imaging panel offset and with no imaging panel offset.

In recent years, surface-guided radiation therapy (SGRT) has been applied to many treatment sites, including the breast, in photon therapy. SGRT provides the potential advantage of directly evaluating the surface of the soft tissue location and reproducibility. Studies on the use for SGRT in photon therapy for breast cancer treatment have demonstrated that SGRT enables a reduction of the initial setup variability and effectively reduces the setup error on skin [77,78,88,89]. However, others have shown that while SGRT showed marked improvements over laser and tattoo setup, the system did not prove accurate enough to replace the daily orthogonal kV images aligned to bony anatomy [79]. In addition, the setup accuracy for surface imaging is sensitive to the region of interest selection [80]. Therefore, extra caution must be exercised when using SRGT to setup a patient, especially for proton therapy, as the dose distribution of proton therapy is very sensitive to WET changes along the beam path. Batin et al. reported on a small series of women undergoing postmastectomy proton therapy [81]. In a comparison of kV orthogonal X-rays with surface imaging (AlignRT by VisionRT, London, UK), the vertical, longitudinal, and lateral translations were smaller with surface imaging, ranging from 2.6 to 3.2 mm with orthogonal X-rays compared to 0.8–1.5 mm with surface imaging. The setup time also decreased by nearly 50%, from an average of 11 min with orthogonal X-rays to 6 min with surface imaging. After further evaluation of the surface imaging setup technique, the

investigators reported on a cohort of 28 women who had undergone mastectomy, including those with and without immediate reconstruction [82]. As noted in this study evaluating image guidance methods, the expander and/or implant can potentially shift between CT simulation and the start of radiotherapy, or during the course of radiotherapy (Figure 20.7), and this shift cannot be readily identified by surface imaging.

20.4.7 Beam Angle Selection

For both the passive-scattering and PBS techniques, en face fields angled between 0° and 60° align with the axis of respiratory motion (Figure 20.8). Thus, the effect of respiration is minimized as the direction of motion is along the radiologic path length throughout the respiratory cycles. Beam angles >5° apart are recommended to improve dose homogeneity and robustness. Non-overlapping beams are recommended for PBI and tumor bed or nodal boosts. With en face to slightly oblique beams, respiratory motion has a negligible effect on dose distribution [83].

20.4.8 Passive Scattering

With this 3D proton technique, brass apertures and range compensators are used to establish the field size and achieve the appropriate depth of the proton beam as it changes throughout the treatment volume. The aperture margin is 10 mm from the CTV to account for the penumbra and setup uncertainties lateral to the beam direction. A smearing margin of 6–8 mm is applied to the range compensator to account for potential variations in radiologic path length. Two beam

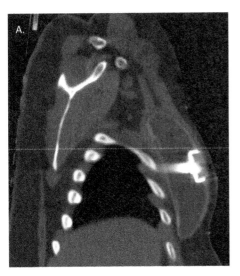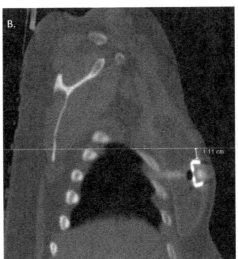

Figure 20.7 Sagittal computed tomography simulation image for a patient at (A) initial planning and (B) verification computed tomography imaging on treatment day 3 showing a 1-cm shift in the port position, requiring replanning.

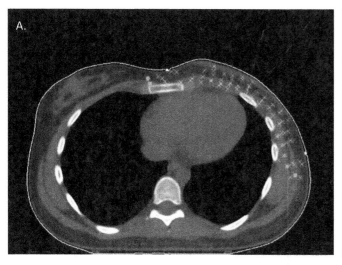 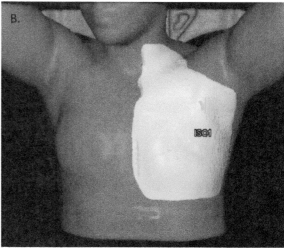

Figure 20.8 For treatment of the chest wall and comprehensive regional lymphatics with pencil-beam scanning, (A) two en face beams were used, shown in blue and orange (gantry 40° and couch 15°; gantry 15° and couch 0°) with spots displayed on an axial slice of the planning computed tomography imaging and (B) 45 Gy RBE dose cloud shown on skin rendering with the isocenter marked.

angles are recommended to decrease the skin dose and the hot spot and increase the robustness of the plan. For partial-breast or whole-breast irradiation, the target volume typically fits into a single 25-cm snout. For RNI, often matched fields are needed due to the larger target size. As the depth of the supraclavicular region typically differs from the depth of the chest wall/breast, a separate supraclavicular field is recommended to allow optimization of this field separately, which helps decrease the skin dose in this region [48]. The shape of this supraclavicular field resembles the standard field shape used when treating with 3D conformal photons. Matchlines should be shifted throughout the course of radiotherapy to minimize hot and cold spots at the field junctions. The fields for each set of matchlines should be adjusted by >5°, and each with its own aperture and compensator. A minimum of two matchlines is recommended, separated by ≥1 cm. Fields are matched on skin, with the light fields confirmed daily to verify alignment.

20.4.9 Pencil-beam Scanning

Pencil-beam scanning (PBS) uses magnets to scan the proton pencil beam across the target volume, allowing continuous variation in the fluence applied at each Bragg position, thereby enabling the delivery of IMPT. The conformal dose achieved at both the distal and the proximal ends results in better skin sparing compared with the passive-scattering technique. In IMPT planning, the beam selection follows the same principles as the passive-scattering plans. A range shifter is required to reduce the beam energy to deliver dose to a shallow depth target. In addition, a relatively large air gap exists between the range shifter and the patient surface to avoid collision. With the combined use of a range shifter and a relatively large air gap, a dose calculation algorithm capable of accurately modeling the large-angle scattered particles is essential [84]. Studies have shown that pencil-beam algorithms may lead to clinically meaningful dose-distribution calculation errors for IMPT breast plans [85,86,98,99]. Therefore, use of Monte Carlo algorithms is recommended. To account for the setup and range uncertainties, robust optimization with 5-mm setup uncertainties and 3.5% range uncertainties are typically used. Robustness evaluation is recommended to ensure the desired dose distribution can be achieved despite perturbation. Liang et al. demonstrated that plans using these planning parameters are able to maintain adequate target coverage despite the inter-fractionation motion and setup errors [87].

20.4.10 Technique for Implants and Expanders

For breast or chest wall implants, the density of the implant material (most commonly saline or silicone) requires consideration in the treatment planning process. The implant made from silicone should be contoured and overridden with proper density and RSP [67]. Failure to do this could result in excess dose to the underlying OAR.

In the treatment of patients with tissue expanders, the filling of the expander should remain the same from the time of CT simulation until the completion of radiation treatment. The expander shall be full or near full to optimize reproducibility and dose distribution. Breast tissue expanders typically consist of a silicon rubber wall with a metallic injection port. The metallic injection port includes a thin metal shell and a magnetic core. The metal shell of the port is usually a submillimeter in thickness and, therefore, causes negligible dose perturbation. The magnet inside the port has a high RSP (>5) and creates substantial artifacts on the CT images. Therefore, particular attention is needed for the high-density magnet. The artifacts produced by the high-density magnet must be overridden by the corresponding saline (inside the saline solution). If the proton beams pass through the magnet, the magnet must be contoured using the proper window level to match the dimensions to the vendor's specifications and, thereafter,

assign it with the corresponding RSP (Figure 20.9A). For passive-scatter plans, proton beams must treat through the magnet. To decrease and smear the range uncertainties, ≥3 en face beams are used. The beam angles are chosen to maximize the angular distance between the beams and, therefore, maximize the distance between the magnet shadow to the chest wall. If matched fields are used, the match line should be ≥2 cm from the expander port. Figure 20.9B shows an example of a DS

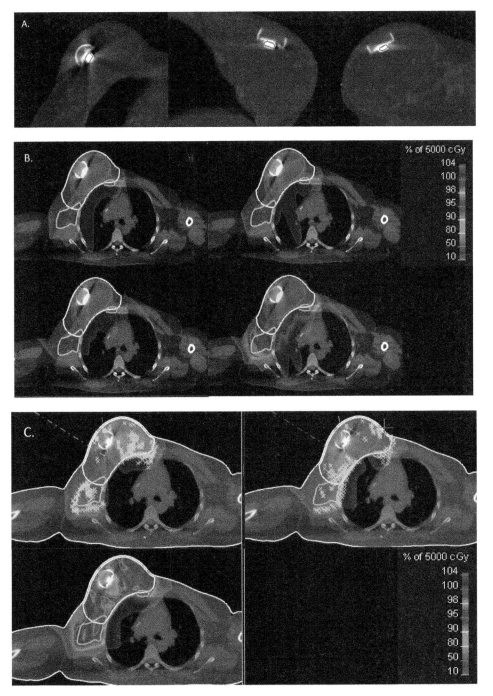

Figure 20.9   (A) Contour of the magnet that resides in the port of the expander in axial, sagittal, and coronal views, respectively.

plan using three beams with gantry angles of 355°, 340°, and 315° treating through the magnet. Each beam delivering one-third of the dose achieved a composite dose of 50 Gy. With PBS, one can choose to either treat through or treat around the port [66]. Our institution uses the latter technique (Figure 20.9C), which utilizes multifield optimization to eliminate proton spots that potentially pass through the port. Two beam angles with a hinge angle of 60°–70° are chosen to complement each other so that the target shadowed by one field can be supplemented by doses delivered by the other field. A cumulative uniform dose to the target around the port is achieved. With this technique that treats around the magnet, no spots pass through the magnet, thereby obviating the need to contour and override the magnet. The cold area in the vicinity of the metal within the saline solution of the expander is not a concern, as the expander itself is not considered a target at risk of harboring microscopic disease.

20.4.11 Adaptive Planning

Given the sensitivity of the proton beam to changes in anatomy, verification CTs are commonly used during the course of proton radiotherapy to ensure stability of the dose distribution [34,66]. Variables such as change in patient weight, breast edema from the radiotherapy, change in seroma, and movement of the metal port of the expander can influence the dose distribution. At our institution, for a 5–6-week course of proton radiotherapy, verification CTs are performed during weeks 2 and 4, while for a 3–4-week course, a verification CT is completed during week 2. Verification CTs are not utilized in PBI, unless >2 weeks elapse between CT simulation and radiation start.

When replanning is indicated, deformable registration is used to transfer the contours to the verification CT, and the contours are reviewed by the physician. The dosimetrist embarks on replanning, using the same techniques, target coverage, and OAR constraints used for the original plan. Smith et al. reported that 5 of 51 patients required replanning based on surveillance verification CTs, "most commonly to reduce inhomogeneity and improve target coverage within the CTV" [34].

20.5 Toxicity

20.5.1 Acute Toxicity

During PBI, symptoms during the 1–2-week course are typically minimal, with focal breast erythema, possible desquamation, and fatigue developing within 6 weeks after completing radiation. Kozak et al. reported moderate-to-severe erythema/hyperpigmentation in 79% at 4 weeks and moist desquamation in 22% of patients 6–8 weeks after radiation using passive-scatter proton therapy to 32 Gy in 8 fractions given BID [19]. In the series by Bush et al., the only acute toxicity was dermatitis [21]. Chang et al. reported 1 patient out of 30 (regimen 30 Gy in 5 daily fractions) and Ovalle et al. reported 1 out of 43 (regimen 34 Gy in 10 BID fractions) with moist desquamation, although 93% had skin changes including 16% with dry desquamation in the latter study [23,24]. The peak skin reaction occurred 6 weeks after radiation.

Grade ≥3 acute toxicity was uncommon in the clinical studies assessing breast or chest wall irradiation with or without RNI. MacDonald et al. reported a single-grade 3 toxicity in a patient experiencing severe fatigue during radiotherapy. In the passive-scatter series by Bradley et al., 22% experienced acute grade 3 dermatitis and no other ≥grade 3 toxicity developed [29]. In Cuaron et al., the single-grade 3 toxicity was a case of post-mastectomy reconstruction failure associated with cellulitis [30]. Grade 3 toxicity occurred in 7.3% of women in the study by Thorpe et al. and in 6% of women in the study by Verma et al., consisting of dermatitis and breast pain [32,33]. In the prospective phase II study by Jimenez et al., grade 3 toxicity included 3% with acute dermatitis and 1% each for seroma and infection [35]. No series reported grade 4 or 5 toxicity.

DeCesaris et al. compared acute skin toxicity per CTCAE, version 4.0, among patients who had received standard fractionation radiotherapy for locoregional control between 2015 and 2017 [88]. In this single-institution retrospective analysis, 45% of women received treatment with PBS proton therapy and 55% photon therapy. There was a statistically significant difference in both race and smoking, with more black patients (64%) and people who previously smoked (51%) in the photon cohort compared to the proton cohort (28% black and 28% former smoking use; $p = 0.004$ and $p = 0.032$, respectively). While grade 3 radiation dermatitis was the similar between the two groups (4.3% with photons vs. 5.1% with protons), patients treated with protons experienced more grade 2 dermatitis (25.5% with photons vs. 64.1% with protons). The planning process for skin dose with PBS was not outlined in the methods.

Grade 2 esophagitis has been reported across several series in which patients received RNI. Cuaron et al. noted that in some of their cases there was overlap between the PTV of the medial supraclavicular nodes and the esophagus [30]. They adjusted their practice to exclude the medial supraclavicular nodes from the field except in high-risk cases. Smith et al. describe their approach of "limiting the medial extent of the supraclavicular CTV to the lateral border of the internal carotid artery," resulting in only 2% of patients experiencing grade 2 esophagitis [34]. Overall, the rates of grade 2 esophagitis ranged from 2% to 33% [29,32,34,37,38]. With increased attention to the esophagus in treatment planning, the rates of esophagitis are expected to decrease.

Radiation pneumonitis was uncommon. In the series by Luo et al., one patient experienced grade 3 pneumonitis, which developed 1 year after radiation [31]. She had a history of contralateral chest wall and nodal radiation as well as stem cell transplant. She was treated with steroids and supplemental oxygen for the dyspnea, and she was then diagnosed with early pulmonary fibrosis. One patient in the cohort of 18 reported by Bradley et al. developed grade 2 pneumonitis, and this patient had received concurrent chemotherapy with the proton radiation [29]. In the series by Jimenez et al., three patients (4%) developed grade 1 and one patient (1%) developed grade 2 pneumonitis [35]. Other studies reported no diagnoses of radiation pneumonitis [28,30,32,33].

20.5.2 Late Toxicity

Cosmesis was the primary long-term outcome evaluated in the PBI studies. In a report on 5-year outcomes among 109 women treated with proton PBI, Bush et al. report >90% patient and physician-reported good or excellent cosmesis, with grade 1 telangiectasias in 7% of patients [22]. Teichman et al. performed a survey of women who had undergone proton PBI and photon whole-breast irradiation [89]. With a median follow-up of 6.5 years, the proton PBI cohort reported less difference in breast size, texture, pain, shape, and swelling.

When the treatment field is expanded to include the whole breast or chest wall and regional lymphatics, additional adjacent organs receive radiation dose compared to treatment of just a portion of the breast. No studies have reported late toxicity related to the esophagus, thyroid, or brachial plexus [31,34]. While, theoretically, proton therapy may reduce the risk of second malignancies [90], follow-up is currently too short to assess this end point. The contributory effect of radiation on lymphedema in the setting of axillary nodal surgery is difficult to determine. Only a few series using proton therapy for RNI have reported rates of lymphedema, primarily grade 1, ranging from 3% to 29% and commonly presenting postoperatively before radiation [31,32,35]. In the series by Verma et al., 8% of patients developed a post-radiation skin infection requiring antibiotics, including 1 with sepsis, and one patient required a latissimus flap closure for a non-healing wound [32].

Based on the significant dosimetric improvement in cardiac exposure, proton therapy is expected to reduce the rate of post-radiation cardiac disease and mortality. However, long-term follow-up is necessary to evaluate this late toxicity. With short median follow-up, cardiac disease is rare, as expected in these clinical studies with median follow-ups <5 years. One patient experienced an acute grade 2 pericardial effusion, which was attributed to trastuzumab [33], and a patient with right-sided breast cancer with an MHD of 0 Gy developed congestive heart failure during radiation, which was attributed to doxorubicin

[29]. To date, no unexpected cardiac toxicity has occurred in these clinical studies, all of which used en face beam arrangements, with the end of range in or near cardiac tissue. Stick et al. applied the Darby model to a cohort of 41 patients with left-sided breast cancer requiring internal mammary radiation treated with photons, followed by a PBS proton plan analysis [91]. The median MHD for the photon plans was 1.9 Gy (range, 0.5–7.6 Gy) compared to 0.3 Gy (range, 0.04–0.9 Gy) for the proton plans. The median excess absolute risk at age 80 years, without and with cardiac risk factors, respectively, was 0.5% (range, 0.03–1.0%) and 1.0% (range, 0.2–2.9%) for the photons plans compared to 0.06% (range, 0.004–0.3%) and 0.13% (range, 0.02–0.5%) for the proton plans. The excess cardiac risk is known to be affected by treatment and patient variables, including MHD, left ventricle exposure age, smoking, and other comorbidities [2,3].

Reconstruction complications are known to occur with postoperative radiotherapy, including capsular contracture and loss of the expander or implant. In a photon series of 1,415 patients with immediate reconstruction and expander-implant exchange prior to photon radiation, 6.9% of patients developed grade IV capsular contracture and 9.1% required removal of the expander or implant [92]. In the Luo et al. proton series, an overall rate of 27% (7/26) of patients reported reconstruction complications: six with capsular contracture and one with an infection of the implant [31]. The implant was removed in five of these patients. One of 15 patients experienced a grade 3 reconstructive complication requiring removal of implant and bilateral reconstruction in the setting of recurrent cellulitis and implant asymmetry; and another patient developed a grade 1 toxicity without further specification in the series by Cuaron et al. [30]. In a postmastectomy proton cohort in which most patients had bilateral mastectomies with reconstruction, the rate of reconstruction complications was compared between the irradiated and unirradiated sides [34]. Reconstruction failure developed in 16% (8/51 patients) and 5% (2/42 patients) of the irradiated and unirradiated sides, respectively, with hypofractionation and older age associated with significantly higher risks of reconstruction failure. The rate of ≥1 complication was threefold higher in the irradiated sides (39% [20/51] vs. 12% [5/42]). These complications included infection, seroma, contracture, hematoma, and flap necrosis. Jimenez et al. reported outcomes for three subgroups [35]. First, in those with a single-stage implant, 12 of 39 patients developed post-radiation complications including three with loss of the implant (of whom two had subsequent successful autologous reconstruction) and nine with revisions for loss of symmetry or contracture. In 11 patients who underwent expander to implant reconstruction, 3 required additional surgery for cosmetic revision due to contracture. Among 14 patients who did not undergo immediate reconstruction, 1 underwent delayed expander to implant and 2 underwent autologous reconstruction. In the latter group, 1 experienced failure of the flap requiring additional surgical intervention for implant placement. Based on these results, the risk of complications in the setting of breast reconstruction resembles photon series, with particular caution needed in the setting of hypofractionation.

Overall, the incidence of rib fractures following proton therapy for breast cancer has been low, ranging from 0% to 7%. As with the other late toxicities, continued follow-up is necessary to assess for additional post-radiation events over time. Several series, with follow-up ranging from 9 to 35 months, have reported no development of rib fractures [30,31] while another series with 15.5-month median follow-up had 2% of patients experience rib fractures at 13 and 39 months after radiation [32]. Jimenez et al. reported a rib fracture rate of 7%, all grade 1, with a median time to rib fracture of 15.9 months, and concern for an end-of-range effect [35,93]. This rate of rib fracture has yet to be demonstrated in other series to date, and it may be a function of treatment planning approach, patient population, and/or length of follow-up. However, patients should be counseled about the risk and monitored for this late toxicity, and >1 beam should be considered to minimize the end-of-range effect.

20.6 Future Directions

Radiation dose to OARs correlates with toxicity, but the interplay of cardiotoxic systemic therapy and host factors, such as age and comorbidities, on these relationships remains an area of active investigation. For example, Taylor et al. reported higher rates of cardiac mortality and lung cancer after radiotherapy for breast cancer in long-term active smokers compared to nonsmokers [94]. Another report highlights concern for higher rates of cardiac injury from systemic therapy in those with a BRCA mutation [95]. In both the studies by Darby et al. and van den Bogaard et al., age and cardiac risk factors were associated with higher rates of cardiac toxicity for the same given dose to the heart [2,3]. OAR constraints are not routinely objectively altered for such risk factors, although the treating radiation oncologist may subjectively select to achieve a lower OAR dose in such situations. Advancements are also underway in genomic analysis for radiosensitivity of both tumor and healthy tissue [96,97, 108–111]. Through identification of radiosensitive versus radioresistant tumors and patient susceptibility to radiation injury of healthy tissue, personalized radiotherapy

can be delivered, including selection of radiation dose, modality, and technique, based on the genomic findings [98].

In proton therapy, a constant RBE of 1.1 is used as a standard practice; however, increasing LET with increasing depth in a pristine Bragg curve, with the RBE exceeding 1.1 at the Bragg peak and distal falloff have been reported. As a result, the dose estimated with a constant RBE of 1.1 is likely an underestimation of the biological dose to the critical structures immediately beyond the target area [99]. The variable RBE is increasingly recognized in proton therapy as an important factor that might affect clinical outcomes [100,101,112]. A recently published American Association of Physicists in Medicine Task Group Report-256 [102] reviewed the RBE variations and discussed the current clinical use of RBE and the clinical relevance of RBE variations. In regard to proton treatment for breast cancer, studies have shown a biological dose increase in the brachial plexus [75] and ribs [93]. A recently published dose-averaged LET-weighted biological dose study on 20 breast patients (10 post-mastectomy and 10 post-lumpectomy) [103] demonstrated enhanced biological dose compared to standard dose with an assumed RBE of 1.1 for the heart, ribs, esophagus, and brachial plexus. The study by Underwood et al. investigated follow-up CT scans for 10 proton and 10 photon patients and discovered a significant difference between the proton and photon cohorts in qualitative radiologic scoring of changes in the pulmonary tissue [104]. This finding supports the hypothesis that the proton RBE for lung-density changes exceeds 1.1. Wang et al. published the first paper on clinical evidence of rib fractures after proton treatment for breast cancer, indicating the increased dose-averaged LET and RBE at the distal edge of proton beams [93].

RBE varies with LET, dose, the biological end point, and the intrinsic radiosensitivity of the tissue [105]. Significant variations exist on the estimated RBE among different models [106,107]. Therefore, caution is needed when applying RBE models for plan optimization and/or evaluation. It is important to conduct clinical outcome studies to correlate the clinical toxicities with the reconstructed RBE doses.

Investigation into these matters is ongoing, with the goals of optimizing outcomes through minimization of exposure to adjacent healthy tissue, reduction in clinical toxicity, maintenance of high levels of tumor control, and personalization of radiotherapy using biology and genomics.

References

1 Clarke, M., Collins, R., Darby, S. et al. (2005). Effects of radiotherapy and of differences in the extent of surgery for early breast cancer on local recurrence and 15-year survival: An overview of the randomised trials. *Lancet (London, England)* Dec 17 366 (9503): 2087–2106.

2 Darby, S.C., Ewertz, M., McGale, P. et al. (2013). Risk of ischemic heart disease in women after radiotherapy for breast cancer. *The New England Journal of Medicine* Mar 14 368 (11): 987–998.

3 van den Bogaard, V.A., Ta, B.D., van der Schaaf, A. et al. (2017). Validation and modification of a prediction model for acute cardiac events in patients with breast cancer treated with radiotherapy based on three-dimensional dose distributions to cardiac substructures. *Journal of Clinical Oncology: Official Journal of the American Society of Clinical Oncology* Apr 10 35 (11): 1171–1178.

4 Taylor, C., McGale, P., Brønnum, D. et al. (2018). Cardiac structure injury after radiotherapy for breast cancer: Cross-sectional study with individual patient data. *Journal of Clinical Oncology: Official Journal of the American Society of Clinical Oncology* Aug 1 36 (22): 2288–2296.

5 Tuohinen, S.S., Skyttä, T., Virtanen, V., Luukkaala, T., Kellokumpu-Lehtinen, P.L., and Raatikainen, P. (2015). Early effects of adjuvant breast cancer radiotherapy on right ventricular systolic and diastolic function. *Anticancer Research* Apr 35 (4): 2141–2147.

6 Gokula, K., Earnest, A., and Wong, L.C. (2013). Meta-analysis of incidence of early lung toxicity in 3-dimensional conformal irradiation of breast carcinomas. *Radiation Oncology (London, England)* Nov 14 8: 268.

7 Bekelman, J.E., Lu, H., Pugh, S. et al. (2019). Pragmatic randomised clinical trial of proton versus photon therapy for patients with non-metastatic breast cancer: The radiotherapy comparative effectiveness (RadComp) consortium trial protocol. *BMJ Open* Oct 15 9 (10): e025556.

8 Johansson, J., Isacsson, U., Lindman, H., Montelius, A., and Glimelius, B. (2002). Node-positive left-sided breast cancer patients after breast-conserving surgery: Potential outcomes of radiotherapy modalities and techniques. *Radiotherapy and Oncology: Journal of the European Society for Therapeutic Radiology and Oncology* Nov 65 (2): 89–98.

9 Lomax, A.J., Cella, L., Weber, D., Kurtz, J.M., and Miralbell, R. (2003). Potential role of intensity-modulated photons and protons in the treatment of the breast and regional nodes. *International Journal of Radiation Oncology, Biology, Physics* Mar 1 55 (3): 785–792.

10 Ares, C., Khan, S., Macartain, A.M. et al. (2010). Postoperative proton radiotherapy for localized and locoregional breast cancer: Potential for clinically relevant improvements? *International Journal of Radiation Oncology, Biology, Physics* Mar 1 76 (3): 685–697.

11 Flejmer, A.M., Edvardsson, A., Dohlmar, F. et al. (2016). Respiratory gating for proton beam scanning versus photon 3D-CRT for breast cancer radiotherapy. *Acta Oncologica (Stockholm, Sweden)* May 55 (5): 577–583.

12 MacDonald, S.M., Jimenez, R., Paetzold, P. et al. (2013). Proton radiotherapy for chest wall and regional lymphatic radiation; dose comparisons and treatment delivery. *Radiation Oncology (London, England)* Mar 24 8: 71.

13 Xu, N., Ho, M.W., Li, Z., Morris, C.G., and Mendenhall, N.P. (2014). Can proton therapy improve the therapeutic ratio in breast cancer patients at risk for nodal disease? *American Journal of Clinical Oncology* Dec 37 (6): 568–574.

14 Fagundes, M., Hug, E.B., Pankuch, M. et al. (2015). Proton Therapy for Local-regionally Advanced Breast Cancer Maximizes Cardiac Sparing. *International Journal of Particle Therapy* 1 (4): 827–844.

15 Lin, L.L., Vennarini, S., Dimofte, A. et al. (2015). Proton beam versus photon beam dose to the heart and left anterior descending artery for left-sided breast cancer. *Acta Oncologica (Stockholm, Sweden)* Jul 54 (7): 1032–1039.

16 Moon, S.H., Shin, K.H., Kim, T.H. et al. (2009). Dosimetric comparison of four different external beam partial breast irradiation techniques: Three-dimensional conformal radiotherapy, intensity-modulated radiotherapy, helical tomotherapy, and proton beam therapy. *Radiotherapy and Oncology: Journal of the European Society for Therapeutic Radiology and Oncology* Jan 90 (1): 66–73.

17 Bush, D.A., Slater, J.D., Garberoglio, C., Yuh, G., Hocko, J.M., and Slater, J.M. (2007). A technique of partial breast irradiation utilizing proton beam radiotherapy: Comparison with conformal x-ray therapy. *Cancer Journal* Mar-Apr 13 (2): 114–118.

18 Lischalk, J.W., Chen, H., Repka, M.C. et al. (2018). Definitive hypofractionated radiation therapy for early stage breast cancer: Dosimetric feasibility of stereotactic ablative radiotherapy and proton beam therapy for intact breast tumors. *Advances in Radiation Oncology* Jul-Sep 3 (3): 447–457.

19 Kozak, K.R., Smith, B.L., Adams, J. et al. (2006). Accelerated partial-breast irradiation using proton beams: Initial clinical experience. *International Journal of Radiation Oncology, Biology, Physics* Nov 1 66 (3): 691–698.

20 Galland-Girodet, S., Pashtan, I., MacDonald, S.M. et al. (2014). Long-term cosmetic outcomes and toxicities of proton beam therapy compared with photon-based 3-dimensional conformal accelerated partial-breast irradiation: A phase 1 trial. *International Journal of Radiation Oncology, Biology, Physics* Nov 1 90 (3): 493–500.

21 Bush, D.A., Slater, J.D., Garberoglio, C., Do, S., Lum, S., and Slater, J.M. (2011). Partial breast irradiation delivered with proton beam: Results of a phase II trial. *Clinical Breast Cancer* Aug 11 (4): 241–245.

22 Bush, D.A., Do, S., Lum, S. et al. (2014). Partial breast radiation therapy with proton beam: 5-year results with cosmetic outcomes. *International Journal of Radiation Oncology, Biology, Physics* Nov 1 90 (3): 501–505.

23 Chang, J.H., Lee, N.K., Kim, J.Y. et al. (2013). Phase II trial of proton beam accelerated partial breast irradiation in breast cancer. *Radiotherapy and Oncology: Journal of the European Society for Therapeutic Radiology and Oncology* Aug 108 (2): 209–214.

24 Ovalle, V., Strom, E.A., Shaitelman, S. et al. (2018). Proton partial breast irradiation: Detailed description of acute clinico-radiologic effects. *Cancers* Apr 7 10 (4).

25 Mutter, R.W., Jethwa, K.R., Gonuguntla, K. et al. (2019). 3 fraction pencil-beam scanning proton accelerated partial breast irradiation: Early provider and patient reported

outcomes of a novel regimen. *Radiation Oncology (London, England)* Nov 21 14 (1): 211.

26 Hjelstuen, M.H., Mjaaland, I., Vikström, J., and Dybvik, K.I. (2012). Radiation during deep inspiration allows loco-regional treatment of left breast and axillary-, supraclavicular- and internal mammary lymph nodes without compromising target coverage or dose restrictions to organs at risk. *Acta Oncologica (Stockholm, Sweden)* Mar 51 (3): 333–344.

27 Ranger, A., Dunlop, A., Hutchinson, K. et al. (2018). A Dosimetric Comparison of Breast Radiotherapy Techniques to Treat Locoregional Lymph Nodes Including the Internal Mammary Chain. *Clinical Oncology (Royal College of Radiologists (Great Britain))* Jun 30 (6): 346–353.

28 MacDonald, S.M., Patel, S.A., Hickey, S. et al. (2013). Proton therapy for breast cancer after mastectomy: Early outcomes of a prospective clinical trial. *International Journal of Radiation Oncology, Biology, Physics* Jul 1 86 (3): 484–490.

29 Bradley, J.A., Dagan, R., Ho, M.W. et al. (2016). Initial report of a prospective dosimetric and clinical feasibility trial demonstrates the potential of protons to increase the therapeutic ratio in breast cancer compared with photons. *International Journal of Radiation Oncology, Biology, Physics* May 1 95 (1): 411–421.

30 Cuaron, J.J., Chon, B., Tsai, H. et al. (2015). Early toxicity in patients treated with postoperative proton therapy for locally advanced breast cancer. *International Journal of Radiation Oncology, Biology, Physics* Jun 1 92 (2): 284–291.

31 Luo, L., Cuaron, J., Braunstein, L. et al. (2019). Early outcomes of breast cancer patients treated with post-mastectomy uniform scanning proton therapy. *Radiotherapy and Oncology: Journal of the European Society for Therapeutic Radiology and Oncology* Mar 132: 250–256.

32 Verma, V., Iftekaruddin, Z., Badar, N. et al. (2017). Proton beam radiotherapy as part of comprehensive regional nodal irradiation for locally advanced breast cancer. *Radiotherapy and Oncology: Journal of the European Society for Therapeutic Radiology and Oncology* May 123 (2): 294–298.

33 Thorpe, C.S., Niska, J.R., Anderson, J.D. et al. (2020).Acute toxicities after proton beam therapy following breast-conserving surgery for breast cancer: Multi-institutional prospective PCG registry analysis. *The Breast Journal* Apr 15.

34 Smith, N.L., Jethwa, K.R., Viehman, J.K. et al. (2019). Post-mastectomy intensity modulated proton therapy after immediate breast reconstruction: Initial report of reconstruction outcomes and predictors of complications. *Radiotherapy and Oncology: Journal of the European Society for Therapeutic Radiology and Oncology* Nov 140: 76–83.

35 Jimenez, R.B., Hickey, S., DePauw, N. et al. (2011). Phase II study of proton beam radiation therapy for patients with breast cancer requiring regional nodal irradiation. *Journal of Clinical Oncology: Official Journal of the American Society of Clinical Oncology* Oct 20 37 (30): 2778–2785.

36 Malouff, T.D., Mahajan, A., Mutter, R.W. et al. (2020). Carbon ion radiation therapy in breast cancer: A new frontier. *Breast Cancer Research and Treatment* Jun 181 (2): 291–296.

37 Schlaff, C.D., Krauze, A., Belard, A., O'Connell, J.J., and Camphausen, K.A. (2014). Bringing the heavy: Carbon ion therapy in the radiobiological and clinical context. *Radiation Oncology (London, England)* Mar 28 9 (1): 88.

38 Sai, S., Vares, G., Kim, E.H. et al. (2015). Carbon ion beam combined with cisplatin effectively disrupts triple negative breast cancer stem-like cells in vitro. *Molecular Cancer* Sep 4 14: 166.

39 Sai, S., Kim, E.H., Vares, G. et al. (2020). Combination of carbon-ion beam and dual tyrosine kinase inhibitor, lapatinib, effectively destroys HER2 positive breast cancer stem-like cells. *American Journal of Cancer Research* 10 (8): 2371–2386.

40 Zhang, Q., Kong, Y., Yang, Z. et al. (). Preliminary study on radiosensitivity to carbon ions in human breast cancer. *Journal of Radiation Research* May 22 61 (3): 399–409.

41 Karasawa, K., Omatsu, T., Arakawa, A. et al. (2019). A Phase I clinical trial of carbon ion radiotherapy for Stage I breast cancer: Clinical and pathological evaluation. *Journal of Radiation Research* May 1 60 (3): 342–347.

42 Akamatsu, H., Karasawa, K., Omatsu, T., Isobe, Y., Ogata, R., and Koba, Y. (2014). First experience of carbon-ion radiotherapy for early breast cancer. *Japanese Journal of Radiology* May 32 (5): 288–295.

43 Harada, M., Karasawa, K., Yasuda, S., Kamada, T., and Nemoto, K. (2015). One shot of carbon-ion radiotherapy cured a 6-cm chemo-resistant metastatic liver tumor: A case of breast cancer. *Japanese Journal of Radiology* Sep 33 (9): 598–602.

44 Matsubara, H., Karasawa, K., Furuichi, W. et al. (2018). Comparison of passive and scanning irradiation methods for carbon-ion radiotherapy for breast cancer. *Journal of Radiation Research* Sep 1 59 (5): 625–631.

45 Lightowlers, S.V., Boersma, L.J., Fourquet, A. et al. (2017). Preoperative breast radiation therapy: Indications and perspectives. *European Journal of Cancer (Oxford, England: 1990)* Sep 82: 184–192.

46 Miao, H., Verkooijen, H.M., Chia, K.S. et al. (2011). Incidence and outcome of male breast cancer: An international population-based study. *Journal of Clinical Oncology: Official Journal of the American Society of Clinical Oncology* Nov 20 29 (33): 4381–4386.

47 Konduri, S., Singh, M., Bobustuc, G., Rovin, R., and Kassam, A. (2020). Epidemiology of male breast cancer. *Breast (Edinburgh, Scotland)* Aug 22 54: 8–14.

48 Bradley, J.A., Ho, M.W., Li, Z. et al. (2017). A technical guide for passive scattering proton radiation therapy for breast cancer. *International Journal of Particle Therapy. Spring* 3 (4): 473–484.

49 Thorpe, C.S., Niska, J.R., Girardo, M.E. et al. (2020). Proton beam therapy reirradiation for breast cancer: Multi-institutional prospective PCG registry analysis. *The Breast Journal* Nov 25 (6): 1160–1170.

50 Gabani, P., Patel, H., Thomas, M.A. et al. (2019). Clinical outcomes and toxicity of proton beam radiation therapy for re-irradiation of locally recurrent breast cancer. *Clinical and Translational Radiation Oncology* Nov 19: 116–122.

51 Patel, S.A., Lu, H.M., Nyamwanda, J.A. et al. (2017). Postmastectomy radiation therapy technique and cardiopulmonary sparing: A dosimetric comparative analysis between photons and protons with free breathing versus deep inspiration breath hold. *Practical Radiation Oncology. Nov - Dec* 7 (6): e377–e384.

52 Yu, J., Park, S.S., Herman, M.G., Langen, K., Mehta, M., and Feigenberg, S.J. (2017). Free breathing versus breath-hold scanning beam proton therapy and cardiac sparing in breast cancer. *International Journal of Particle Therapy. Winter* 3 (3): 407–413.

53 Dasu, A., Flejmer, A.M., Edvardsson, A., and Witt Nystrom, P. (2018). Normal tissue sparing potential of scanned proton beams with and without respiratory gating for the treatment of internal mammary nodes in breast cancer radiotherapy. *Physica Medica: PM: An International Journal Devoted to the Applications of Physics to Medicine and Biology: Official Journal of the Italian Association of Biomedical Physics (AIFB)* Aug 52: 81–85.

54 RTOG. (2020). Breast Cancer Atlas. *Countouring Atleses.* http://www.rtog.org/corelab/contouringatlases/breastcanceratlas.aspx. November 12, 2020.

55 Li, X.A., Tai, A., Arthur, D.W. et al. (2009). Variability of target and normal structure delineation for breast cancer radiotherapy: An RTOG Multi-Institutional and Multiobserver Study. *International Journal of Radiation Oncology, Biology, Physics* Mar 1 73 (3): 944–951.

56 Nielsen, M.H., Berg, M., Pedersen, A.N. et al. (2013). Delineation of target volumes and organs at risk in adjuvant radiotherapy of early breast cancer: National guidelines and contouring atlas by the Danish Breast Cancer Cooperative Group. *Acta Oncologica (Stockholm, Sweden)* May 52 (4): 703–710.

57 Offersen, B.V., Boersma, L.J., Kirkove, C. et al. (2015). ESTRO consensus guideline on target volume delineation for elective radiation therapy of early stage breast cancer. *Radiotherapy and Oncology: Journal of the European Society for Therapeutic Radiology and Oncology* Jan 114 (1): 3–10.

58 Brown, L.C., Diehn, F.E., Boughey, J.C. et al. (2015). Delineation of Supraclavicular Target Volumes in Breast Cancer Radiation Therapy. *International Journal of Radiation Oncology, Biology, Physics* Jul 1 92 (3): 642–649.

59 Chang, J.S., Lee, J., Chun, M. et al. (2018). Mapping patterns of locoregional recurrence following contemporary treatment with radiation therapy for breast cancer: A multi-institutional validation study of the ESTRO consensus guideline on clinical target volume. *Radiotherapy and Oncology: Journal of the European Society for Therapeutic Radiology and Oncology* Jan 126 (1): 139–147.

60 Kowalski, E.S., Feigenberg, S.J., Cohen, J. et al. (2020). Optimal target delineation and treatment techniques in the era of conformal photon and proton breast and regional nodal irradiation. *Practical Radiation Oncology* May-Jun 10 (3): 174–182.

61 Kaidar-Person, O., Vrou Offersen, B., Hol, S. et al. (2019). ESTRO ACROP consensus guideline for target volume delineation in the setting of postmastectomy radiation therapy after implant-based immediate reconstruction for early stage breast cancer. *Radiotherapy and Oncology: Journal of the European Society for Therapeutic Radiology and Oncology* Aug 137: 159–166.

62 Mayinger, M., Borm, K.J., Dreher, C. et al. (2019). Incidental dose distribution to locoregional lymph nodes of breast cancer patients undergoing adjuvant radiotherapy with tomotherapy - is it time to adjust current contouring guidelines to the radiation technique? *Radiation Oncology (London, England)* Aug 1 14 (1): 135.

63 Lomax, A.J. (2008). Intensity modulated proton therapy and its sensitivity to treatment uncertainties 2: The potential effects of inter-fraction and inter-field motions. *Physics in Medicine and Biology* Feb 21 53 (4): 1043–1056.

64 Engelsman, M. and Kooy, H.M. (2005). Target volume dose considerations in proton beam treatment planning for lung tumors. *Medical Physics* Dec 32 (12): 3549–3557.

65 Park, P.C., Zhu, X.R., Lee, A.K. et al. (2012). A beam-specific planning target volume (PTV) design for proton therapy to account for setup and range uncertainties. *International Journal of Radiation Oncology, Biology, Physics* Feb 1 82 (2): e329–336.

66 Mutter, R.W., Remmes, N.B., Kahila, M.M. et al. (2017). Initial clinical experience of postmastectomy intensity modulated proton therapy in patients with breast expanders with metallic ports. *Practical Radiation Oncology* Jul-Aug; 7 (4): e243–e252.

67 Moyers, M.F., Mah, D., Boyer, S.P., Chang, C., and Pankuch, M. (2014). Use of proton beams with breast prostheses and tissue expanders. *Medical Dosimetry: Official Journal of the American Association of Medical Dosimetrists. Spring* 39 (1): 98–101.

68 Haviland, J.S., Owen, J.R., Dewar, J.A. et al. (2013). The UK Standardisation of Breast Radiotherapy (START) trials of radiotherapy hypofractionation for treatment of early breast cancer: 10-year follow-up results of two randomised controlled trials. *The Lancet Oncology* Oct 14 (11): 1086–1094.

69 Whelan, T.J., Pignol, J.P., Levine, M.N. et al. (2010). Long-term results of hypofractionated radiation therapy for breast cancer. *The New England Journal of Medicine* Feb 11 362 (6): 513–520.

70 NRG Oncology. (2016). NSABP B-51 RTOG 1304: A Randomized Phase III Clinical Trial Evaluating Post-mastectomy Chestwall and Regional Nodal XRT and Post-lumpectomy Regional Nodal XRT in Patients with Positive Axillary Nodes Before Neoadjuvant Chemotherapy Who Convert to Pathologically Negative Axillary Nodes after Neoadjuvant Chemotherapy. https://www.nrgoncology.org/Clinical-Trials/Protocol/nsabp-b-51-rtog-1304?filter=nsabp-b-51-rtog-1304. November 12, 2020.

71 NRG Oncology. (2019) NSABP B-39 RTOG 0413: A randomized phase III study of conventional whole breast irradiation (WBI) versus partial breast irradiation (PBI) for women with stage 0, I, or II breast cancer.

72 NRG Oncology. (2014). RTOG-1005: A phase III trial of accelerated whole breast irradiation with hypofractionation plus concurrent boost versus standard whole breast irradiation plus sequential boost for early-stage breast cancer. https://www.nrgoncology.org/Clinical-Trials/Protocol/rtog-1005?filter=rtog-1005. November 12, 2020.

73 DeCesaris, C.M., Pollock, A., Zhang, B., et al. (2020). Assessing the need for adjusted organ-at-risk planning goals for patients undergoing adjuvant radiation therapy for locally advanced breast cancer with proton radiation. Practical Radiation Oncology. Oct 15.

74 Yan, M., Kong, W., Kerr, A., and Brundage, M. (2019). The radiation dose tolerance of the brachial plexus: A systematic review and meta-analysis. *Clinical and Translational Radiation Oncology* Sep 18: 23–31.

75 Mutter, R.W., Jethwa, K.R., Wan Chan Tseung, H.S. et al. (2020). Incorporation of biologic response variance modeling into the clinic: Limiting risk of brachial plexopathy and other late effects of breast cancer proton beam therapy. *Practical Radiation Oncology* Mar-Apr 10 (2): e71–e81.

76 Liang, X., Bradley, J.A., Zheng, D. et al. (2018). Prognostic factors of radiation dermatitis following passive-scattering proton therapy for breast cancer. *Radiation Oncology (London, England)* Apr 19 13 (1): 72.

77 Cravo, S.A., Fermento, A., Neves, D. et al. (2018). Radiotherapy setup displacements in breast cancer patients: 3D surface imaging experience. *Reports of Practical Oncology and Radiotherapy: Journal of Greatpoland Cancer Center in Poznan and Polish Society of Radiation Oncology* Jan-Feb 23 (1): 61–67.

78 Laaksomaa, M., Sarudis, S., Rossi, M. et al. (2019). AlignRT(®) and Catalyst™ in whole-breast radiotherapy with DIBH: Is IGRT still needed? *Journal of Applied Clinical Medical Physics* Mar 20 (3): 97–104.

79 Hattel, S.H., Andersen, P.A., Wahlstedt, I.H., Damkjaer, S., Saini, A., and Thomsen, J.B. (2019). Evaluation of setup and intrafraction motion for surface guided whole-breast cancer radiotherapy. *Journal of Applied Clinical Medical Physics* Jun 20 (6): 39–44.

80 Guo, B., Shah, C.S., Magnelli, A. et al. (2017).Surface Guided Radiation Therapy (SGRT): The Sensitivity of the Region of Interest (ROI) Selection on the Translational and Rotational Accuracy for Whole Breast Irradiation. *International Journal of Radiation Oncology*Biology*Physics* 2017/10/01 99 (2,Supplement): E666–E667.

81 Batin, E., Depauw, N., MacDonald, S., and Lu, H.M. (2016). Can surface imaging improve the patient setup for proton postmastectomy chest wall irradiation? *Practical Radiation Oncology* Nov - Dec 6 (6): e235–e241.

82 Batin E, Depauw N, Jimenez RB, MacDonald S, Lu HM. Reducing. (2018). X-ray imaging for proton postmastectomy chest wall patients. *Practical Radiation Oncology* Sep-Oct; 8 (5): e266–e274

83 Ödén, J., Toma-Dasu, I., Eriksson, K., Flejmer, A.M., and Dasu, A. (2017). The influence of breathing motion and a variable relative biological effectiveness in proton therapy of left-sided breast cancer. *Acta Oncologica (Stockholm, Sweden)* Nov 56 (11): 1428–1436.

84 Saini, J., Maes, D., Egan, A. et al. (2017). Dosimetric evaluation of a commercial proton spot scanning Monte-Carlo dose algorithm: Comparisons against measurements and simulations. *Physics in Medicine and Biology* Sep 12 62 (19): 7659–7681.

85 Liang, X., Li, Z., Zheng, D., Bradley, J.A., Rutenberg, M., and Mendenhall, N. (2019). A comprehensive dosimetric study of Monte Carlo and pencil-beam algorithms on intensity-modulated proton therapy for breast cancer. *Journal of Applied Clinical Medical Physics* Jan 20 (1): 128–136.

86 Liang, X., Bradley, J.A., Zheng, D. et al. (2019). The impact of dose algorithms on tumor control probability in intensity-modulated proton therapy for breast cancer. *Physica Medica: PM: An International Journal Devoted to the Applications of Physics to Medicine and Biology: Official Journal of the Italian Association of Biomedical Physics (AIFB)* May 61: 52–57.

87 Liang, X., Mailhot Vega, R.B., Li, Z., Zheng, D., Mendenhall, N., and Bradley, J.A. (2020). Dosimetric consequences of image guidance techniques on robust optimized intensity-modulated proton therapy for treatment of breast Cancer. *Radiation Oncology (London, England)* Feb 27 15 (1): 47.

88 DeCesaris, C.M., Rice, S.R., Bentzen, S.M., Jatczak, J., Mishra, M.V., and Nichols, E.M. (2019). Quantification of acute skin toxicities in patients with breast cancer undergoing adjuvant proton versus photon radiation therapy: a single institutional experience. *International Journal of Radiation Oncology, Biology, Physics* Aug 1 104 (5): 1084–1090.

89 Teichman, S.L., Do, S., Lum, S. et al. (2018). Improved long-term patient-reported health and well-being outcomes of early-stage breast cancer treated with partial breast proton therapy. *Cancer Medicine* Dec 7 (12): 6064–6076.

90 Raptis, A., Ödén, J., Ardenfors, O., Flejmer, A.M., Toma-Dasu, I., and Dasu, A. (2017). Cancer risk after breast proton therapy considering physiological and radiobiological uncertainties. *Physica Medica: PM: An International Journal Devoted to the Applications of Physics to Medicine and Biology: Official Journal of the Italian Association of Biomedical Physics (AIFB)* Aug 76: 1–6.

91 Stick, L.B., Yu, J., Maraldo, M.V. et al. (2017). Joint Estimation of Cardiac Toxicity and Recurrence Risks After Comprehensive Nodal Photon Versus Proton Therapy for Breast Cancer. *International Journal of Radiation Oncology, Biology, Physics* Mar 15 97 (4): 754–761.

92 Cordeiro, P.G., Albornoz, C.R., McCormick, B., Hu, Q., and Van Zee, K. (2014). The impact of postmastectomy radiotherapy on two-stage implant breast reconstruction: An analysis of long-term surgical outcomes, aesthetic results, and satisfaction over 13 years. *Plastic and Reconstructive Surgery* Oct 134 (4): 588–595.

93 Wang, C.C., McNamara, A.L., Shin, J. et al. (2020). End-of-range radiobiological effect on rib fractures in patients receiving proton therapy for breast cancer. *International Journal of Radiation Oncology, Biology, Physics* Jul 1 107 (3): 449–454.

94 Taylor, C., Correa, C., Duane, F.K. et al. (2017). Estimating the Risks of Breast Cancer Radiotherapy: Evidence From Modern Radiation Doses to the Lungs and Heart and From Previous Randomized Trials. *Journal of Clinical Oncology: Official Journal of the American Society of Clinical Oncology* May 20 35 (15): 1641–1649.

95 Sajjad, M., Fradley, M., Sun, W. et al. (2017). An Exploratory Study to Determine Whether BRCA1 and BRCA2 Mutation Carriers Have Higher Risk of Cardiac Toxicity. *Genes* Feb 2 8 (2).

96 Speers, C., Zhao, S., Liu, M., Bartelink, H., Pierce, L.J., and Feng, F.Y. (2015). Development and validation of a novel radiosensitivity signature in human breast cancer. *Clinical Cancer Research: An Official Journal of the American Association for Cancer Research* Aug 15 21 (16): 3667–3677.

97 Chang-Claude, J., Ambrosone, C.B., Lilla, C. et al. (2009). Genetic polymorphisms in DNA repair and damage response genes and late normal tissue complications of radiotherapy for breast cancer. *British Journal of Cancer* May 19 100 (10): 1680–1686.

98 Hall, W.A., Bergom, C., Thompson, R.F., et al. Precision Oncology and Genomically Guided Radiation Therapy: A Report From the American Society for Radiation Oncology/ American Association of Physicists in Medicine/National Cancer Institute Precision Medicine Conference. *International journal of radiation oncology, biology, physics.* Jun 1 2018;101(2):274–284.

99 Carabe, A., Moteabbed, M., Depauw, N., Schuemann, J., and Paganetti, H. (2012). Range uncertainty in proton therapy due to variable biological effectiveness. *Physics in Medicine and Biology* Mar 7 57 (5): 1159–1172.

100 Peeler, C.R., Mirkovic, D., Titt, U. et al. (2016). Clinical evidence of variable proton biological effectiveness in pediatric patients treated for ependymoma. *Radiotherapy and Oncology: Journal of the European Society for Therapeutic Radiology and Oncology* Dec 121 (3): 395–401.

101 Underwood, T. and Paganetti, H. (2016). Variable proton relative biological effectiveness: how do we move forward? *International Journal of Radiation Oncology, Biology, Physics* May 1 95 (1): 56–58.

102 Paganetti, H., Blakely, E., Carabe-Fernandez, A. et al. (2019). Report of the AAPM TG-256 on the relative biological effectiveness of proton beams in radiation therapy. *Medical Physics* Mar 46 (3): e53–e78.

103 Liu, C., Zheng, D., Bradley, J.A., et al. (2020) Incorporation of the LETd-weighted biological dose in the evaluation of breast intensity-modulated proton therapy plans. *Acta Oncologica (Stockholm, Sweden)*. In press.

104 Underwood, T.S.A., Grassberger, C., Bass, R. et al. (2018). Asymptomatic Late-phase Radiographic Changes Among Chest-Wall Patients Are Associated With a Proton RBE Exceeding 1.1. *International Journal of Radiation Oncology, Biology, Physics* Jul 15 101 (4): 809–819.

105 Paganetti, H. (2014). Relative biological effectiveness (RBE) values for proton beam therapy. Variations as a function of biological endpoint, dose, and linear energy transfer. *Physics in Medicine and Biology* Nov 21 59 (22): R419–472.

106 Rorvik, E., Fjaera, L.F., Dahle, T.J. et al. (). Exploration and application of phenomenological RBE models for proton therapy. *Physics in Medicine and Biology* Sep 13 63 (18): 185013.

107 Giovannini, G., Bohlen, T., Cabal, G. et al. (2016). Variable RBE in proton therapy: Comparison of different model predictions and their influence on clinical-like scenarios. *Radiation Oncology (London, England)* May 17 11: 68.

108 Verhoeven, K., Weltens, C., Remouchamps, V. et al. (2015). Vessel based delineation guidelines for the elective lymph node regions in breast cancer radiation therapy - PROCAB guidelines. *Radiotherapy and Oncology: Journal of the European Society for Therapeutic Radiology and Oncology* Jan 114 (1): 11–16.

109 Kirk, M., Freedman, G., Ostrander, T., and Dong, L. (2017). Field-specific intensity-modulated proton therapy optimization technique for breast cancer patients with tissue expanders containing metal ports. *Cureus* Sep 18 9 (9): e1698.

110 Berg, M., Lorenzen, E.L., Jensen, I. et al. (2018). The potential benefits from respiratory gating for breast cancer patients regarding target coverage and dose to organs at risk when applying strict dose limits to the heart: Results from the DBCG HYPO trial. *Acta Oncologica (Stockholm, Sweden)* Jan 57 (1): 113–119.

111 Ahmed, K.A., Liveringhouse, C.L., Mills, M.N. et al. (2019). Utilizing the genomically adjusted radiation dose (GARD) to personalize adjuvant radiotherapy in triple negative breast cancer management. *EBioMedicine* Sep 47: 163–169.

112 Chen, F., Jen, Y.M., He, K., Yin, Z., and Shi, J. (2020). Heart-sparing effect of postmastectomy radiotherapy for breast cancer patients: A dosimetric study of cardiac substructures. *Medical Dosimetry: Official Journal of the American Association of Medical Dosimetrists. Autumn* 45 (3): 246–251.

21

Prostate Cancer

Cameron S. Thorpe, MD, Ronik S. Bhangoo, MD, Justin D. Anderson, MD, Jiajian (Jason) Shen, PhD, and Carlos E. Vargas, MD

Department of Radiation Oncology, Mayo Clinic, Phoenix, Arizona
Corresponding A retrospective cohort consisting of 1,327 uthor: Carlos E. Vargas, MD, 5881 East Mayo Boulevard, Phoenix, Arizona 85054

21.1   Introduction

Prostate cancer is the second most common cancer diagnosis in men, trailing only skin cancer. In 2020, an estimated 190,000 men were diagnosed with prostate cancer with more than 33,000 predicted deaths from the disease [1]. Numerous treatment options exist for localized prostate cancer including radical prostatectomy, radiation therapy, and active surveillance. Radical prostatectomy is the most common treatment utilized for prostate cancer while radiation therapy is more common for patients over the age of 65 [2]. Prostate cancer is a very curable disease, especially for low and intermediate risk prostate cancers; even patients with high-risk prostate cancer can often expect to live for many years with their disease. Despite high cure rates, most treatments are associated with significant and sometimes life-altering side effects. Prostatectomy negatively affects urinary continence and sexual function while radiation therapy negatively affects bowel function, urinary voiding, and nocturia [3]. Given the long survival of prostate cancer patients and the risk for significant toxicity, it is important to investigate new ways to improve both disease control and toxicity outcomes for this patient population. Heavy particle therapy such as proton beam therapy is a promising treatment approach to maintain high cure rates and reduce toxicity through the unique properties of particle therapy.

Proton beam therapy is the most common heavy particle therapy utilized in the United States. There are over 30 treatment centers with more being announced or under construction each year [4]. Proton beam therapy has a number of potential benefits for prostate cancer over conventional photon techniques. Most hypothesized benefits of proton beam therapy come from the reduced dose to normal tissues. This is due to the finite distance traveled by protons in the body and lack of exit dose of radiation beyond the treatment target. For example, several investigators have demonstrated significant dose reductions to nearby organs at risk such as the rectum and bladder when comparing proton beam therapy to conventional radiation therapy for prostate cancer patients [5,6]. Nichols et al. reported no decrease in testosterone levels from proton beam therapy for prostate cancer while photon radiation has been shown to decrease testosterone levels by as much as 27% [7,8]. As a result, sexual function may be less disrupted by proton beam therapy due to minimal impact on testosterone production and improved sparing of the penile bulb. Proton beam therapy also has the potential to decrease the risk of secondary cancers due to radiotherapy by reducing the integral dose of excess radiation [9]. Newer techniques of proton beam therapy, such as intensity modulated proton therapy (IMPT), show added promise to deliver more conformal treatment and greater sparing of organs at risk.

Since it was first used to treat prostate cancer in 1979, proton beam therapy has become a very unique and specialized treatment modality [10]. New and innovative techniques have been developed to assist with treatment planning and treatment delivery. Conventionally fractionated and hypofractionated protocols have been investigated and implemented with proton beam therapy for prostate cancer treatment. Data exist for its use in the definitive, adjuvant, and salvage setting. While retrospective and nonrandomized data are frequently reported, no randomized control trials exist that directly compare proton beam therapy and photon radiation for prostate cancer. This lack of randomized data makes it difficult to evaluate the clinical benefits of proton beam therapy over photon radiation in prostate cancer. Most reports suggest that proton beam therapy is well tolerated and severe toxicity from treatment is rare. The benefits of proton beam therapy may provide more benefit when pelvic nodes are treated in addition to the prostate or prostate bed.

The potential benefits of proton beam therapy have also led to an increased interest in other heavy ions for treatment of cancer. Carbon-ion therapy has been used in a few centers around the world to treat prostate cancer. With promising early results and additional potential benefits, the development and implementation of carbon-ion therapy may increasingly influence how we think about treatment for prostate cancer.

As more particle treatment centers are built, new opportunities to conduct clinical trials and identify patients that will benefit the most from particle therapy will arise. There are still many questions about how to optimize treatment for patients with prostate cancer but particle therapy is an exciting development that may continue to improve patient outcomes.

21.2 Proton Beam Therapy

The first report of proton beam therapy in prostate cancer was in 1979 [10]. Here, protons were given as a perineal boost following a course of photons. This approach, with a proton beam boost, comprised many of the earliest experiences with proton beam therapy in prostate cancer [11–13]. Subsequently, there have been numerous studies reporting on proton beam

therapy in various settings including in combination with photons [13,14], conventional fractionation [15–20], hypofractionation [21–29], and in the adjuvant or salvage setting (Table 21.1) [30,31].

21.2.1 Conventional Fractionation

Conventional fractionation is defined as radiation given in fractions of 180–200 cGy and has the longest data supporting its use [32,33]. Likewise, some of the largest proton series with the longest follow-up are patients treated with conventional fractionation. Takagi et al. reported a retrospective cohort from a single institution of patients treated with proton beam therapy [20]. Patients received either 74 Gy relative biological effectiveness (RBE) or 78 Gy RBE in 2 Gy per fraction. Treatment was well tolerated and yielded 5-year freedom from biochemical relapse rates of 99%, 91%, and 83% for low, intermediate, and high-risk patients, respectively. Iwata et al. reported a large multi-institutional retrospective review of prostate cancer patients treated with proton beam therapy at seven centers in Japan [16]. Patients were treated to 70–80 Gy RBE in 35–40 fractions and reported 5-year biochemical progression-free survival rates of 97%, 91.1%, and 83.1% for low, intermediate, and high risk, respectively.

Bryant et al. also reported on a large retrospective cohort consisting of 1,327 patients with prostate cancer treated mostly with 78 Gy RBE (range, 74–82 Gy RBE in 37–41 fractions) [15]. Five-year biochemical progression-free survival was 99%, 94%, and 74% for low, intermediate, and high-risk groups, respectively. Predictors of biochemical failure on MVA included Gleason score (4–7 vs. 8 vs. ≥9–10, $p = 0.2$), prostate-specific antigen (PSA) (0–<10 vs. 10–<20 vs. ≥20, $p = 0.2$), perineural invasion (yes vs. no, $p = 0.02$), and percentage of positive zones on biopsies (<50% vs. ≥50%, $p = 0.02$). These results are comparable to conventionally fractionated photon trials with 5-year freedom from biochemical failure rates of >90%, 60–85%, and 50–70% for low, intermediate, and high-risk groups, respectively [33].

21.2.2 Hypofractionation

In recent years, several large moderate hypofractionation trials with photons have been reported that show non-inferior disease outcomes compared to standard fractionation [34–39]. Taken together, these trials have shown acceptable toxicity rates and comparable disease outcomes compared to conventional fractionation. As a result, hypofractionation is becoming more prevalent and is now included in guidelines as first-line options [32,40–43]. Several studies have reported on hypofractionation with proton beam therapy [21,24–27,44]. Grewal et al. reported disease outcomes in a cohort of mostly

Table 21.1 Selected proton beam therapy studies in prostate cancer.

| Author | n | Risk Category (%) | | | ADT (%) | Dose (Gy RBE) | Median follow-up (month) | Biochemical Control (%) | | | | | Overall Survival | | | | | Toxicity - GI | | Toxicity - GU | |
		Low	Int.	High				Year	Low	Int.	High	Overall	Year	Low	Int.	High	Overall	Acute	Late	Acute	Late
Conventional Fractionation																					
Takagi (2017)	1375	18	44	38	57	74 in 37 fractions or 78 Gy in 39 fractions	70	5	99	91	83		5	98	96	High 96 Very High 90			Grade 2: 3.8 Grade 3: 0.1		Grade 2: 1.9 Grade 3 0.1
Iwata (2018)	1291	17	40	43	59.5	70-80 Gy in 35-40 fractions, 63-66 Gy in 21-22 fractions	69	5	97	91.1	83.1		5	98.4	96.8	95.2			Grade ≥2: 4.1		Grade ≥2: 4
Mendenhall (2014)	211	42	39	19	26	78-82 Gy in 39-41 fractions	62.4	5	99	99	76								Grade ≥3: 0.5		Grade 3≥: 1
Bryant (2016)	1327	41	42	17	18	74-82 Gy in 37 to 41 fractions	63.6	5	99	94	74								Grade ≥3: 0.6		Grade 3≥: 2.9
Lee (2018)	192	19.8	54.2	26	37	75.6-81 Gy in 42-44 fractions (not sure on # of fractions 1.8-2 Gy/fraction)	20.4												Grade ≥2: 21.3		Grade ≥2: 26.4
Pugh (2013)	291	41.2	58.4	0.3	36.8	76 Gy in 38 fractions	NR (minimum 24 months)												Grade ≥2: 9.6		Grade ≥2: 13.4
Hypofractionation																					
Kubes (2019)	200	46.5	53.5		14.5	36.25 Gy in 5 fractions	36	At follow-up	99	93.4		98.5						Grade 2: 3.5 Grade 3: 0	Grade 2: 5.5 Grade 3: 0	Grade 2: 19 Grade 3: 0	Grade 2: 4 Grade 3: 0
Grewal (2019)	184	10	90 (Fav. 42, Unfav. 48)		25.5	70 Gy in 28 fractions	49.2	4	94.4	Fav. 92.5 Unfav. 93.8		95.8		95.8			95.8	Grade ≥2: 3.8 Grade 3: 0.5	Grade ≥2: 13.6 Grade 3: 0.5	Grade ≥2: 12.5 Grade 3: 0	Grade ≥2: 7.6 Grade 3: 0

(Continued)

Table 21.1 (Continued)

Author	n	Risk Category (%)			ADT (%)	Dose (Gy RBE)	Median follow-up (month)	Biochemical Control (%)					Overall Survival					Toxicity - GI		Toxicity - GU	
		Low	Int.	High				Year	Low	Int.	High	Overall	Year	Low	Int.	High	Overall	Acute	Late	Acute	Late
Slater (2019)	146	100				60 Gy in 20 fractions	42	3	99.3									Grade ≥2: 1.7	Grade 2: 5.1 Grade 3:0	Grade ≥2: 16	Grade 2: 9.5 Grade 3: 0.7
Nakajima (2018)	526	17.1	42	40.9	82.1	74-78 Gy in 37-39 fractions (conventional) or 60-63 Gy in 20-21 fractions (HF)	NR											Grade 2: Conventional or HF 0		Grade 2: Conventional 15, HF 5.9 Grade 3: 0 in either arm	
Henderson (2017)	215	56	44		55	70-72.5 Gy in 28-29 fractions	62.4	5	98.3	92.7			5	96	96.4			Grade 3: 0	Grade ≥3: 0.5	Grade 3: 0	Grade ≥3: 1.7
Combined Photon and Proton																					
Johansson (2019)	531	18.7	31.3	50	55	50 Gy in 25 fractions photons + 20 Gy in 4 fractions proton boost	113	5	100	94	High 82 Very High 72								Grade 3: 0		Grade 3: 2
After Cryosurgery or High-Intensity Focused Ultrasound																					
Holtzman (2015)	21	NR			38	74-82 Gy in 37-41 fractions	37	3				77									Grade 3: 17%
Adjuvant/ Salvage/ Recurrent																					
Deville (2020)	100				34	66.6 - 75.6 in 37-42 fractions*	55	5				56	5				99				

*31 patients had combined IMRT+Proton

Abbreviations: ADT, androgen deprivation therapy; Fav, favorable; GI, gastrointestinal; GU, genitourinary; Gy, gray; HF, hypofractionation; Int, intermediate; NR, not reported; Unfav, unfavorable; RBE, relative biological effectiveness intermediate risk patients treated with moderate hypofraction-ation (70 Gy RBE in 28 fractions). Four-year biochemical pro-gression-free survival was 94.4%, 92.5%, and 93.8% in low-, favorable intermediate-, and unfavorable intermediate-risk patients, respectively. Treatment was well tolerated with acute grade ≥ 2 genitourinary (GU) toxicity of 12.5% and 4-year grade ≥ 2 GU toxicity of 7.6%. Kubes et al. reported on cohort of low- and intermediate-risk patients treated with extreme or ultra-hypofractionation [25]. All patients received 36.25 Gy RBE in 5 fractions. Treatment was well tolerated with no acute grade 3 gastrointestinal (GI) or GU toxicity and 19% acute grade 2 GU toxicity. With a median follow-up of 36 months, they reported biochemical control of 99% for low-risk and 93.4% for interme-diate-risk patients.

There is very little proton beam-specific data comparing hypofractionation to conventional fractionation. Nakajima et al. reported on over 500 patients with about half treated with conventional fractionation (74–78 Gy RBE in 37–39 fractions) and the other half receiving hypofractionation (60–63 Gy RBE in 20–21 fractions) [26]. They showed less grade 2 GU toxicity in the hypofractionation arm (15% vs. 5.9%, $p < 0.001$). However, disease outcomes were not reported.

There are numerous benefits to hypofractionation over con-ventional fractionation including reduced treatment time and cost. This has led to its adoption as a standard of care and its utilization will likely increase over the coming years. Although there are currently limited data on hypofractionation with pro-ton beam therapy, it is likely equally as safe and effective as photon hypofractionation and its utilization will also likely increase over time.

21.2.3 Adjuvant and Salvage Radiation

Indications for adjuvant and salvage radiation after prostatec-tomy are well established [43,45,46]. Adjuvant radiation is gen-erally recommended after prostatectomy for adverse pathology including positive surgical margin, seminal vesicle invasion, or extraprostatic extension [45,46]. Three randomized clinical tri-als (ARO 96-02, EORTC 22911, and SWOG 8794) investigated adjuvant radiation versus observation [47–50]. All three showed improved biochemical control with adjuvant radiation, but only SWOG 8794 showed improved survival on long-term analysis (hazard ratio [HR] 0.72, 95% CI: 0.55–0.96; $p = 0.023$) [49].

Salvage radiation is recommended with PSA or local recur-rence with two of the previous studies suggesting a benefit in subgroup analyses [45,46,48,49]. Androgen deprivation ther-apy (ADT) is also recommended in this setting based off of three randomized trials (GETUG-AFU 16, RTOG 0534, and RTOG 9601) that showed a benefit [51–54]. RTOG 0534 also investigated the addition of whole pelvis radiation and reported their findings in abstract form. With over 5 years of follow-up,

they showed improved freedom from failure and freedom from metastases with the addition of whole pelvis radiation [54]. However, there was no difference in 5-year freedom from dis-tant metastasis between prostate bed radiation with short-term ADT and prostate bed radiation with whole pelvis radiation and short-term ADT (94.4% and 95.2%, respectively, $p = 0.28$). Proton beam therapy may be able to offer additional advan-tages in patients requiring pelvic lymph node radiation with reduced doses to organs at risk [55].

Several randomized trials have investigated whether adju-vant or salvage radiation is optimal. Recently, a preplanned meta-analysis, ARTISTIC, combining three randomized trials (RADICALS, GETUG-AFU 17, and RAVES) investigating adju-vant radiation versus early salvage radiation was presented at European Society for Medical Oncology (ESMO) [56]. Although only in abstract, adjuvant radiation did not improve event-free survival compared to early salvage radiation. Furthermore, the updated ESMO Clinical Practice Guidelines for prostate cancer now recommends against routine adjuvant radiation and instead advocates for early salvage radiation when is PSA <0.5 ng/mL [43]. Regardless of timing, radiation is often used after prostatectomy. However, there is very limited literature on PBT in this setting.

Santos et al. reported on a case-matched cohort of 307 patients in the postoperative setting with 237 receiving inten-sity-modulated radiation therapy (IMRT) and 70 receiving pro-ton beam therapy [31]. Patients were treated in either the adjuvant or salvage setting. Median follow-up was 48.6 months for IMRT and 46.1 months for PBT. A dosimetric analysis showed that proton beam therapy was superior to IMRT at minimizing low doses (V10–V40) to the bladder and rectum and high dose (V50–V65) to the anterior rectal wall. However, proton beam therapy resulted in higher V50–V70 to the rectum and mean femoral head dose. Despite these findings, there was no significant difference between modality in acute or late GI or GU toxicity. Acute grade ≥ 1 GI toxicity was 39.6% with IMRT and 27.1% with proton beam therapy ($p = 0.082$). Late grade ≥ 1 GI toxicity was 25.9% with IMRT and 24.3% with proton beam therapy ($p = 0.874$). Acute grade ≥ 2 GU toxicity was 21.8% with IMRT and 17.1% with proton beam therapy ($p = 0.492$). Late grade ≥ 2 GU toxicity was 38.6% with IMRT and 30% with pro-ton beam therapy ($p = 0.247$). On univariate analysis, no blad-der DVH parameters were associated with acute or late grade ≥ 2 GU toxicity. Also, no rectal DVH parameters were associ-ated with acute or late grade ≥ 1 GI toxicity. The authors noted that this study may have been underpowered to detect a differ-ence between modalities and called for prospective data.

Disease outcomes have also been reported in a retrospective analysis of 100 patients by Deville et al. with a median follow-up of 55 months [30]. Thirty-one patients required combined IMRT and proton beam plans due to either not being able to achieve target coverage or organs at risk dose constraints.

Furthermore, 34% received concurrent ADT and 20% were treated to the whole pelvis. Biochemical failure-free survival at 5 years was 56% with a median time to failure of 23 months. These results compare favorably to a multi-institutional study of salvage radiation where 5-year freedom from biochemical progression was 56% [57]. Furthermore, Deville et al. reported 5-year biochemical failure-free survival of 79% in the patients who received whole pelvic radiation compared to 50% for patients who received prostate only radiation. These findings mirror the preliminary findings from RTOG 0534 that suggest improved freedom from progression with whole pelvis radiation with reported 5-year rates of 89% in the whole pelvis radiation plus ADT arm [54]. Additionally, Deville et al. reported 5-year distant metastasis-free survival and overall survival were 93% and 99%, respectively.

21.2.4 Toxicity

Many studies have reported on quality of life and toxicity of proton beam therapy in prostate cancer. Some have found associations of various clinical and treatment parameters with higher toxicity, but these findings are not consistent. For example, Bryant et al. reported that grade ≥3 GU toxicity on multivariate analysis (MVA) was associated with pretreatment transurethral resection of the prostate (TURP) ($p < 0.0001$), prostate volume ≥60 cm [3] ($p < 0.0001$), pretreatment α-blockers ($p = 0.0002$), and various bladder dose–volume histogram (DVH) parameters. Patients with 0, 1, 2, or 3 or more risk factors had 1.9%, 3.6%, 11.3%, and 17.8% of grade ≥3 toxicity at 5 years, respectively [15]. However, others have found that prostate gland size is not associated with toxicity [21,58,59].

Although there are limited data comparing proton beam therapy directly with other radiation modalities, comparable toxicity rates and quality-of-life changes have been reported with proton beam therapy [60,61]. Gray et al. reported on quality of life of prostate cancer patients treated with 3D conformal radiation therapy (3DCRT), IMRT, or proton beam therapy [62]. Patients treated with 3DCRT or IMRT reported worse bowel quality of life immediately after treatment. All three cohorts reported clinically meaningful decrements in bowel quality of life at 12 and 24 months. Similarly, IMRT patients reported worse urinary quality of life immediately following treatment while the proton beam cohorts were the only ones to report worse urinary quality of life at 12 months. However, at 24 months, all three cohorts reported no clinically meaningful urinary quality-of-life changes. Although the patterns were different, the overall effect on quality of life was similar across the three modalities. Yu et al. reported on a matched cohort of Medicare prostate cancer patients treated with IMRT or proton beam therapy [63]. They also showed that IMRT had worse GU toxicity at 6 months (5.9% proton beam therapy vs. 9.5% IMRT, $p = 0.03$), but there was no difference at 12 months (18.8% proton beam therapy vs. 17.5% IMRT, $p = 0.66$). Additionally, there was no difference of GI toxicity. Sheets et al. performed a SEER-based study of prostate cancer patients and found that there was no difference in GU toxicity or hip fractures between IMRT and proton beam [64]. However, proton beam patients had more GI toxicity (12.2 vs. 17.8 per 100 person-years; RR, 0.66; 95% CI: 0.55–0.79).

More recently, a systematic review investigating toxicities after primary radiotherapy found high-grade toxicities are uncommon regardless of treatment modality and toxicities are similar with proton beam therapy or photons [61]. In keeping with this finding, Dutz et al. recently reported quality of life and toxicities in a matched analysis of proton beam therapy versus IMRT [65]. There was no difference in acute grade 2 or 3 GU toxicity with 41% and 3% with IMRT and 24% and 3% with proton beam, respectively ($p = 0.45$). There was also no difference in late grade 2 or 3 GU toxicity with 27% and 5% with IMRT and 23% and 0% with proton beam, respectively ($p = 0.53$). Likewise, acute grade 2 or 3 GI toxicity was 17% and 0% with IMRT and 14% and 3% with proton beam therapy, respectively ($p = 0.6$). Late grade 2 or 3 GI toxicity was 9% and 0% with IMRT and 9% and 5% with proton beam, respectively ($p = 0.35$). The only difference noted was in late grade 1 urinary urgency with 25% with IMRT and 0% with proton beam therapy ($p = 0.047$). They also found that late grade 2 urinary obstruction was associated with anterior bladder wall receiving 70 Gy and the entire bladder V60Gy. Quality of life was similar for most items between IMRT and proton beam therapy.

Sexual side effects are an important consideration among prostate cancer patients [66]. Although erectile function has many factors, including patient age, body mass index, diabetes, and other comorbidities, some studies, including those with proton beam therapy, have found dose to the penile bulb is associated with erectile dysfunction [67–69]. Furthermore, one study utilizing hydrogel spacer showed a decrease in penile bulb dose with spacer and a subsequent improvement in erections adequate for intercourse at 3 years (66.7% vs. 37.5%, $p = 0.046$) [70]. Proton beam therapy offers potential advantages in this regard and has been shown to decrease penile bulb dose compared to photon-based treatments [44,71,72]. Holtzman et al. reported a 2-year potency rate of 68% in a cohort treated with proton beam therapy and found their rates compared favorably to the PROSTQA study where 2-year potency rates were 40%, 58%, and 63% for surgery, external beam radiotherapy, and brachytherapy, respectively [73,74]. Ho et al. reported 1-year potency of 72% that only declined to 67% at 5 years after proton beam therapy [75].

Proton beam therapy has been used to treat the whole pelvis with prostate cancer [30,44,55,76]. Compared to IMRT, whole pelvis radiation with proton beam results in less dose to the rectum, small and large bowel, and bladder largely due to the reduction of the low-dose wash that occurs with IMRT [55]. Using a prospective registry, Chuong et al. reviewed prostate cancer patients who received whole pelvis radiation with proton beam therapy. They identified 85 patients who met their criteria and reported acute grade 2 or 3 GI toxicity rates of 2.4% and 0%, respectively. Acute grade 2 or 3 GU toxicity was 34.1% and 0%, respectively. They noted the acute GI toxicity seen in their study was less compared to historical controls with IMRT [77–82].

Hip fractures are another known complication following prostate radiation [61,83]. Elliott et al. found that men who were treated with 3DCRT were at increased risk of hip fractures compared to surgical patients (HR, 1.76; 95% CI: 1.38–2.40) [84]. Furthermore, Sheets et al. showed that IMRT has a lower risk compared to 3DCRT likely due IMRT being able to better limit dose to the femoral heads [64]. Proton beam therapy plans, on the other hand, have a higher mean femoral head dose due to generally being planned with lateral beams [55,85,86]. Despite the higher dose, Sheets et al. showed no difference in hip fracture rates between proton beam and IMRT [64]. Valery et al. also showed no increased risk of hip fracture compared to expected rates based on World Health Organization Fracture Risk Assessment Tool (FRAX) in a cohort of prostate cancer patients treated with proton beam therapy with a median follow-up of 4 years [87].

A few studies have reported on toxicity between pencil beam scanning and passive scatter [17,19,88]. Pugh et al. reported no significant differences between passive scatter and pencil beam scanning [19]. Contrary to this, Nakajima et al. reported worse acute GU toxicity with spot scanning [26]. However, only 6.1% of patients in this trial were treated with spot scanning and thus a small sample size could have contributed to this finding. Mishra et al. compared prospectively collected patient-reported outcomes utilizing Expanded Prostate Cancer Index Composite (EPIC) between pencil beam scanning and passive scatter in a multicenter registry [88]. Both changes in mean EPIC score and percentage of men experiencing a minimally important difference (MID) were analyzed. MID was defined as declines of 5 points for bowel, 6 points for urinary, and 11 points for sexual or as a half-standard deviation difference from the mean baseline domain score. The average scores and proportion of men experienced 1 MID did not differ between groups at 12 months. However, the proportion of mean reporting 2 MID decline in urinary quality of life at 12 months was greater for mean in the pencil beam scanning cohort (26.9% vs. 13.2%, $p = 0.01$). Additional studies are needed to investigate the difference in technologies.

Another complication of radiation treatment is secondary malignancies. Secondary malignancies after radiation treatment are uncommon, but the lower integral dose with proton beam therapy compared to photons is a potential advantage. Although prostate cancer patients are older, this concern applies to these patients as men treated with radiation for prostate cancer have a higher incidence of secondary malignancy with most common secondary cancers being bladder, colon, and rectal [89]. Fortunately, there is some emerging evidence that proton beam therapy can decrease these risks [90]. A National Cancer Database study including over 450,000 patients reported on risks of a second cancer diagnosis after primary treatment with radiation [91]. Though this study included more than just prostate cancer patients, prostate cancer represented 40% of all IMRT and 61% of all proton beam patients included. They found that the incidence of second cancer diagnosis was less with PBT compared to IMRT (adjusted OR, 0.31; 95% CI: 0.26–0.36; $p < 0.0001$) [91]. The benefit of PBT appeared to be greatest in prostate cancer patients (adjusted OR, 0.18; 95% CI: 0.14–0.24; $p < 0.0001$). Mohamad et al. performed a similar retrospective study with patients treated with carbon ion radiation at the National Institute of Radiological Sciences (NIRS) in Japan [92]. They also found that carbon ion radiation had a lower risk of second cancer diagnosis compared to photon radiation with a HR of 0.81 ([95% CI: 0.66–0.99]; $p = 0.038$). However, others have not found differences in secondary malignancies between IMRT and proton beam therapy [64]. Future studies with long follow-up are needed to identify to true benefit of particle therapy in its ability to decrease secondary malignancies.

21.3 Carbon-ion Therapy

Carbon-ion therapy may be advantageous in the treatment of prostate cancer given its physical and biologic characteristics. Carbon ions are heavy particles that allow for more conformal dose distributions when treating deeper tumors [93]. Additionally, carbon ions have an estimated RBE of 2–5 which may result in more effective treatment with respect to tumor control [94].

Clinical experiences with the use of carbon-ion therapy for prostate cancer have been reported since the early 2000s with the majority of published data coming from Japanese centers (Table 21.2). The NIRS (Chiba, Japan) reported their early experience of prostate cancer patients treated with carbon-ion therapy in 2004 [95]. Ninety-six patients with prostate cancer of all risk categories were treated with carbon-ion therapy on phase I/II dose escalation trials. Doses ranged from 54 to 72 Gy RBE in 20 fractions. A patient-specific compensation bolus was used to better conform the dose to the target and an RBE

Table 12.2 Selected carbon ion therapy studies in prostate cancer.

| Author | n | Risk Category (%) | | | ADT (%) | Dose (Gy RBE) | Median follow-up (months) | Biochemical Control (%) | | | | | Overall Survival | | | | | Toxicity - GI | | Toxicity - GU | |
		Low	Int.	High				Year	Low	Int.	High	Overall	Year	Low	Int.	High	Overall	Acute	Late	Acute	Late
Akakura (2004)	96	NR	NR	NR	79.2	54-72 Gy in 20 fractions	47	5				82.6	5				87.7	Grade 3: 0	Grade 3 GI or GU: 6.3	Grade 3: 0	Grade 3 GI or GU: 6.3
Ishikawa (2015)	76	4	38	53	91	57.6 Gy in 16 fractions	51	4				94.6	4				97.4	Grade 2: 0Grade 3: 0	Grade 2: 1Grade 3: 0	Grade 2: 9Grade 3: 0	Grade 2: 7Grade 3: 0
Kasuya (2017)	608			100	100	57.6 Gy in 16 fractions or 63-66 Gy in 20 fractions	88.4	At follow-up			84		5				95		Grade 2: 1.7		Grade ≥2: 11.7
Katoh (2014)	213	NR	NR	NR	81.2	66 Gy in 20 fractions	NR	3				91.4	3				93.4		Grade 2: 2.3Grade 3: 0		Grade 2: 6.1Grade 3: 0
Kawamura (2020)	304	5	47	48	78	57.6 Gy in 16 fractions	60	5	91.7	93.4	92	92.7	5				96.6	Grade 2: 0 Grade 3: 0	Grade 2: 0.3 Grade 3 0	Grade 2: 4 Grade 3: 0	Grade 2: 9Grade 3: 0.3
Maruyama (2017)	417	19	21	60	81	63-66 Gy in 20 fractions	60												Grade 2: 2.9Grade 3: 0		Grade 2: 7Grade 3: 0.2
Nomiya (2014)	46	26	20	54	98	51.6 Gy in 12 fractions	32.3	At follow-up				100						Grade 2: 0	Grade ≥2: 0	Grade 2: 4	Grade ≥2: 0
Nomiya (2016)	2157	12	31	56	81.3	51.6 - 66 Gy in 12 - 20 fractions	29	5	92	89	92		5	100	99	96		Grade 2: 0Grade 3: 0	Grade 2: 0.4Grade 3: 0	Grade 2: 5.5Grade 3: 0	Grade 2: 4.6Grade 3: 0
Okada (2012)	740	18.1	24.2	57.7	81.9	57.6 Gy in 16 fractions or 63-66 Gy in 20 fractions	59.3	5				89.7	5				95.2	Grade 2: 0Grade 3: 0	Grade 2: 2.4Grade 3: 0		Grade 2: 7.8Grade 3: 0.2

Study						Dose		At follow-up								
Shimazaki (2012)	728	17	26	57	NR	54-72 Gy in 20 fractions or 57.6 Gy in 16 fractions	87		88	94	85	87.6	Grade 2: 0	Grade 2: 1.2	Grade 2: 4.7	Grade 2: 6.7
Takakusagi (2020)	253	3.2	34.8	62.1	96.4	51.6 Gy in 12 fractions	35.3	3	87.5	88	97.5		Grade 2: 0 Grade 3: 0	Grade 2: 0 Grade 3: 0		
Zhang (2019)	64	4.7	37.5	57.8	95.3	59.2-60.8 Gy in 16 fractions or 66 Gy in 24 fractions	19						Grade 2: 0 Grade 3: 0	Grade 2: 0 Grade 3: 0	Grade 2: 10.9 Grade 3: 0	Grade 2: 1.6Grade 3: 0
Combined Modality																
Nikoghosyan (2011)	14		64.3	35.7	85.7	60 Gy in 30 fractions IMRT + 18 Gy in 6 fractions Carbon Ion boost	28	3	86	100			Grade ≥3: 0	Grade ≥3: 0		

Abbreviations: ADT, androgen deprivation therapy; GI, gastrointestinal; GU, genitourinary; Gy, gray; Int, intermediate; NR, not reported; RBE, relative biological effectiveness value of 3.0 was assumed for the carbon ion treatment. With a median follow-up of 47 months, the 5-year biochemical recurrence-free survival was 83% with a clinical recurrence-free survival of 90%. Acute toxicity was limited to grade ≤2 or lower whereas late grade ≥3 toxicity was seen in six patients—five of which were treated to 72 Gy RBE. Due to these late toxicities, the total dose was decreased to 66 Gy RBE. This early report of the NIRS experience helped set the stage for future carbon ion studies in the setting of prostate cancer.

Since that publication, multiple reports on the use of carbon-ion therapy to treat prostate cancer have been published. Most series included a majority of high-risk prostate cancer patients (approximately 50–60%) compared to low–intermediate risk prostate cancer patients. Clinical outcomes have been excellent with 5-year biochemical recurrence-free survival rates of approximately 90%. Carbon-ion therapy has been generally very well tolerated with several series not reporting any grade ≥3 GU or GI toxicity—acute or late. Grade 2 toxicities have also been low (generally ≤10% for both GU and GI). The NIRS group reported no late grade ≥3 rectal toxicity in their phase II trial and found that a rectal V50 Gy >50% was significantly associated with late grade ≤2 GI toxicity on MVA [96]. The use of anticoagulation was also significantly associated with late grade ≤2 GI toxicity in the same analysis.

The dose fractionation employed with carbon-ion therapy has primarily been hypofractioantion (between 10 and 20 fractions). Common dose fractionations have included 51.6 Gy RBE in 12 fractions, 57.6 Gy RBE in 16 fractions, and 66 Gy RBE in 20 fractions [97–99]. As discussed above, these dose fractionations have resulted in low-grade toxicities and have been safely employed in clinical practice. Selection of dose fractionation is particularly important with heavy ion therapy given the increased RBE and concerns of LET at the end of range.

In addition to clinical outcomes and toxicities, quality-of-life data after carbon ion treatment for prostate cancer have also been reported. For patients enrolled on their phase II clinical trial, the NIRS group assessed quality of life using the Functional Assessment of Cancer Therapy for Prostate Cancer Patients (FACT-P) [100]. Their results revealed no significant changes in FACT-P for patients who underwent carbon ion treatment alone, whereas patients who also received hormone therapy had a significant decline in scores at 12 months post-treatment compared to pretreatment. Additionally, there was no difference in urinary, bowel, and sexual function at 12 months for patients who had carbon ion treatment alone. On 5-year follow-up, both groups (ADT and no ADT) developed significantly lower FACT-P and FACT-General (FACT-G) scores but the absolute decline from baseline was only noted to be about 2 points [101]. This decline in scores at 5 years was attributed to the Social/Family Well-being score which remained significantly lower than baseline at both 1 year and 5 years. In one of the few carbon ion for prostate cancer reports from outside Japan, the Shangai Proton and Heavy Ion Center published their quality-of-life data with 2-year follow-up [102]. They assessed patient's quality of life using EPIC. Their results demonstrated stable urinary continence, bowel, and sexual quality of life at both end of treatment and at 2 years. While urinary irritation/obstruction scores significantly declined immediately after treatment, these scores had recovered by 2 years post-treatment.

Thus, the literature supports carbon-ion therapy as an effective treatment for prostate cancer. The above data suggest that carbon-ion therapy may benefit prostate cancer patients in terms of decreased toxicity and improved quality of life. Further randomized comparisons are needed to discover the value of carbon-ion therapy for prostate cancer compared to the more commonly utilized proton and photon therapy.

21.4 Randomized Clinical Trials

Although randomized controlled trials are the gold standard for evidence to determine clinical practice, only four randomized clinical trials of proton beam therapy or carbon-ion therapy in prostate cancer have published results and in one trial proton beam therapy was used only as a boost (Table 21.3) [13,22,23,28,29,103–105]. Vargas et al. randomized low-risk prostate cancer patients to standard fractionation (79.2 Gy RBE in 44 fractions) versus hypofractionation (38 Gy RBE in 5 fractions) in a phase III trial [28,29,103]. The primary endpoint of the trial is 2-year non-inferior freedom from failure in the hypofractionation arm. The interim analysis reported on adverse events and quality of life and included 75 patients; 46 patients in the hypofractionation arm and 29 patients in the standard fractionation arm. All patients underwent a treatment planning MRI, daily kV imaging matching to gold fiducials, and daily rectal balloon placement. The clinical target volume (CTV) was the prostate only in either arm. With a median follow-up of 36 months, no grade 3 GI or GU adverse events were reported in either arm. There were significantly more grade 2 GU adverse events at 6 months in the hypofractionation arm (20% in the hypofractionation arm vs. 0% in the standard arm, $p = 0.01$). However, there was no significant difference at 12 months. Furthermore, the overall cumulative rates were 34% with standard fractionation and 30.4% with hypofractionation ($p = 0.8$). There was no difference in cumulative grade 2 GI events at any point. There was an early, small, non-clinically significant difference in urinary quality of life and AUASI scores favoring the standard fractionation arm that disappeared after 18 months. Freedom from failure rates has not been reported.

Ha et al. performed a single institution phase II where they randomized low (34%), intermediate (45%), or high-risk (21%)

Table 21.3 Published results from randomized clinical trials in prostate cancer utilizing proton beam therapy or carbon ion therapy.

Author	n	Arms* (Gy RBE)	Risk Category (%)			ADT (%)	Median follow-up	Biochemical Control (%)				Overall Survival	Toxicity - GI		Toxicity - GU	
			Low	Int.	High			Year	Low	Int.	High		Acute	Late	Acute	Late
Ha (2019)	82	EHF 35 Gy in 5 fractions in 2.5 weeks 35 Gy in 5 fractions in 4 weeks MHF 47 Gy in 10 fractions 54 Gy in 15 fractions 60 Gy in 20 fractions	34	45	21	90	7	7	MHF 90.5 EHF 57.1	MHF 83.5 EHF 42.9	MHF 41.7 EHF 40	All Arms: 97.5	Grade 2: 0 MHF, 0 EHF	Grade 2: MHF 15, EHF 13 Grade 3: MHF 4, EHF 0	Grade 2: MHF 4, EHF 7 Grade 3: 0 MHF and EHF	Grade 2: MHF 12, EHF 7 Grade 3: 0 MHF and EHF
Vargas (2018 - Adv in Radiation Oncology)	75	79.2 Gy in 44 fractions 38 Gy in 5 fractions	100				36							Grade 2: 79.2 Gy 17.2, 38 Gy 19.6, Grade 3: 79.2 Gy 0, 38 Gy 0		Grade 2: 79.2 Gy 30.4, 38 Gy 34.5 Grade 3: 79.2 Gy 0, 38 Gy 0
Habl (2016)	91	Proton 66 Gy in 20 fractions Carbon 66 Gy in 20 fractions	23	59	17	23	22.3						Grade 3: Proton 4.3, Carbon 0		Grade 2: Proton 21.7, Carbon 13.3	
Combined Photon and Proton																
Zietman (2010)	393	70.2 Gy in 39 fractions (19.8 Gy in 11 fractions proton boost) 79.2 Gy in 44 fractions (28.8 Gy in 16 fractions with proton boost)	57.8	36.6	4.3		106.8	10	70.2 Gy: 71.8 79.2 Gy: 92.9	70.2 Gy: 57.9 79.2 Gy: 69.6		70.2 Gy: 78.4 79.2 Gy: 83.4		Grade 3: 70.2 Gy: 1 79.2 Gy: 0		Grade 3: 70.2 Gy: 2 79.2 Gy: 2

*Proton unless otherwise stated

Abbreviations: ADT, androgen deprivation therapy; EHF, extreme hypofractionation; GI, gastrointestinal; GU, genitourinary; Int, intermediate; MHF moderate hypofractionation patients to one of five different hypofractionation schedules [22,104]. According to the authors, moderate hypofractionation schedules included 60 Gy RBE in 20 fractions, 54 Gy RBE in 15 fractions, or 47 Gy RBE in 10 fractions. Extreme hypofractionation schedules were treated to 35 Gy RBE in five fractions either over 2.5 weeks or 4 weeks. A treatment planning MRI, gold fiducials, and a rectal balloon for each treatment were required. The CTV was the prostate and proximal 1 cm of the seminal vesicle or whole seminal vesicles if involved. The primary end point was acute toxicity and 82 patients were randomized. Median follow-up was 90 months. Slightly worse acute grade 2 GU toxicity was seen in the extreme hypofractionation arm with 7% compared to 4% with moderate hypofractionation ($p = 0.009$). No acute grade 3 GU toxicity was seen. Late grade 2 GU toxicity was similar with 12% with moderate hypofractionation and 7% with extreme hypofractionation ($p = 0.835$). Acute and late grade 2 GI toxicity were similar with 11% and 15% with moderate hypofractionation and 20% and 13% with extreme hypofractionation, respectively. Late grade 3 GI toxicity was seen in 4% of moderate hypofractionation and 0% of extreme hypofractionation ($p = 0.891$). The 7-year biochemical failure-free survival with moderate hypofractionation and extreme hypofractionation were 90.5% and 57.1% in low-risk ($p = 0.154$), 83.5% and 42.9% in intermediate risk ($p = 0.018$), and 41.7% and 40% in high-risk group ($p = 0.786$), respectively. The seemingly worse disease outcomes in the extreme hypofractionation arms led the authors to conclude that extreme hypofractionation is potentially inferior to moderate hypofractionation. However, they also acknowledged that this was an exploratory analysis and was not the primary end point of the study. Additionally, the authors noted that the worse results could be attributed to their α/β ratio assumption of 1.5 Gy for prostate cancer, overall treatment time in the extreme hypofractionation arms, and/or small sample size. As discussed previously, the results from Kubes et al. are superior with ultra-hypofractionation and protons but are retrospective. It should also be noted that Widmark et al. showed non-inferior failure-free survival in a photon-only trial with extreme or ultra-hypofractionation compared to conventional fractionation [106]. In this trial, patients were randomized to 42.7 Gy in 7 fractions versus 78 Gy in 39 fractions. Most patients were intermediate risk (89%). With a median follow-up of 5 years, they reported 5-year failure-free survival of 84% in both treatment groups ($p = 0.99$). Thus, it is unlikely that the results from Ha et al. are representative of the effectiveness of hypofractionation with proton beam therapy.

Lastly, Habl et al. reported on a phase II trial of low (23%), intermediate (59%), or high-risk (17%) patients randomized to 66 Gy RBE in 20 fractions with proton beam therapy or carbon-ion therapy [23,105]. Ninety-two patients were randomized and a hydrogel spacer was used for each patient. Median follow-up was 22.3 months. No significant difference

in acute GI or GU toxicities was observed. However, two patients (4.3%) treated with proton beam therapy developed a rectal fistula. Quality of life was assessed with the European Organization for Research and Treatment of Cancer (EORTC) questionnaire and showed worse quality of life at the end of treatment for urinary symptoms, fatigue, and pain. Urinary symptoms and pain improved and were not different than baseline scores 6 months after treatment. Differences were seen between proton beam therapy and carbon-ion therapy in urinary and bowel subdomains with carbon-ion therapy being slightly better (urinary $p = 0.026$, bowel $p = 0.046$). However, the authors note that the study was not powered for this analysis. The authors concluded that hypofractionation with either proton beam therapy or carbon-ion therapy is feasible and resulted in similar acute toxicities and quality of life. Disease outcomes have not been reported.

21.5 Proton Prostate Treatment Planning

Our treatment planning approach at Mayo Clinic Arizona is described in detail in this section.

21.5.1 Fiducial and Spacer Placements

Our preference is to place four carbon fiducial markers (size: 1 mm × 3 mm) into the prostate gland using a transperineal approach: one each at the left and right base and one each at the left and right apex. The benefit of carbon fiducials, as compared to higher density fiducials such as gold viscoil, is negligible artifacts in a computed tomography (CT) scan. Figure 21.1 shows that carbon fiducials can be seen clearly in kV X-rays (Figure 21.1a) and do not cause artifacts in CT (Figure 21.1b). Additionally, when placing fiducial markers, qualified patients may get hydrogel (SpaceOAR) placed in between rectum and prostate. The SpaceOAR provides a physical gap between the prostate and anterior rectal wall and remains in place for 3 months [107,108]. SpaceOAR is not recommended for patients with high-risk prostate cancer. An example of hydrogel placement is shown in Figure 21.2.

21.5.2 CT and MRI Simulations

In regards to simulation, patients are instructed to have a full bladder. The patient is simulated similar to photon patients—that is, the patient is supine using a leg immobilizer indexed at a fixed position on the couch (Figure 21.3). A water-filled endoretal balloon (100 cm^3) is used for prostate immobilization and reproducibility. The endoretal balloon can significantly reduce intrafraction motion of prostate to within 2–3 mm [109,110].

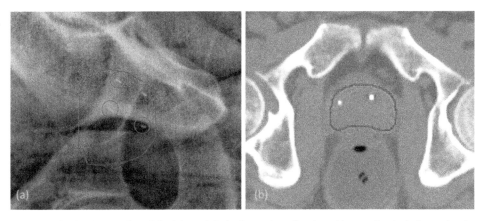

Figure 21.1 (a) Four carbon fiducials and their dimensions (enclosed by purple circles) are clearly seen in kV X-rays; and (b) carbon fiducial in a CT slice shows no artifacts caused by fiducial. Red structures are CTV.

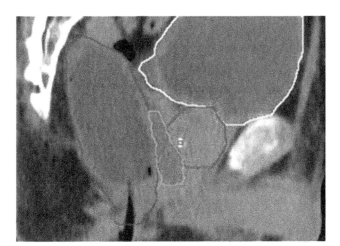

Figure 21.2 A CT sagittal view that shows hydrogel placement (orange contour) between prostate and anterior rectum wall.

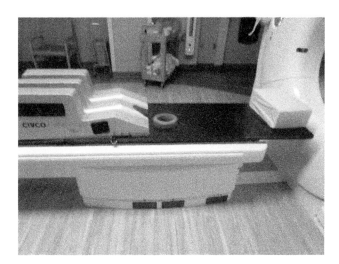

Figure 21.3 Patient immobilization devices (left to right): dual leg immobilizer, O-ring for hand rest, and square pillow.

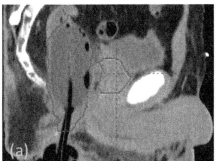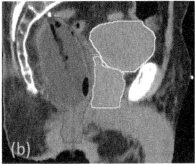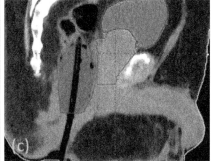

Figure 21.4 Example of endorectal balloon in rectum: (a) good depth, (b) too deep, and (c) too shallow.

The patient is then scanned with 2 mm slice thickness. The rectal balloon needs to be checked to make sure it is properly placed. Some common issues include air between the endorectal balloon and the prostate, depth of insertion that best immobilizes the prostate (Figure 21.4 shows an endorectal balloons at an appropriate depth, and two depths that are either too deep or too shallow), no significant stool in the rectum that affects balloon position, and an insufficiently full bladder (e.g., 200–250 cm^3). Care should be taken to make sure the bladder is not too full because a very large bladder volume can be difficult to reproduce for treatment each day.

The same immobilization devices used at the CT simulation are also used for the magnetic resonance imaging (MRI) in treatment planning position. "AX T2 Cube" and "water LAVA" MRI sequences are acquired for fusion with CT and target delineation.

21.5.3 Fiducial and Target Contours

The carbon fiducial marker is contoured first. To assist with this, the window and level of the CT images are changed to show only the high-density structure within the treatment planning system (TPS). The center of the carbon fiducials is located in two CT slices and a circle with a 4-mm diameter is contoured in each of the two CT slices, with center of the circle aligned to the center of the carbon markers. The contour does not need to fit the exact shape of the fiducial markers since this contour is used to ensure proper alignment for image-guided radiation therapy (IGRT). It is critical to have an accurate center location of the fiducials to allow for proper alignment during IGRT. An example of a fiducial contour is shown in Figure 21.5.

The MRI is used to precisely delineate the CTV that encompasses the prostate gland or prostate bed and seminal vesicles. The quality of the CT and MRI fusion will affect the target accuracy on the planning CT. As shown in Figure 21.6, fiducials are easily distinguishable in the "water LAVA" sequence, but not in the "AX T2 Cube" sequence. Thus, the "water LAVA" sequence is used for initial registration. The first step is to auto-match the CT and the "water LAVA" MRI images to bony anatomy. Next, the carbon fiducials are aligned to the fiducial contours in the CT. The prostate gland is well defined in the "AX T2 Cube" images, which is used to contour the prostate. Hence, the final step is to fine tune the fiducials in the "AX T2 Cube" sequence to align with fiducial contours in the CT. The prostate gland and optional target volumes depending on stage and involvement, such as the proximal seminal vesicles, full seminal vesicles, and/or pelvic lymph nodes, are then contoured.

Our typical target volumes and doses for the definitive and adjuvant/salvage setting are in Table 21.4. In the definitive setting, we typically deliver 20 or 5 fractions, although other dose and fractionation schedules are acceptable. In the adjuvant/

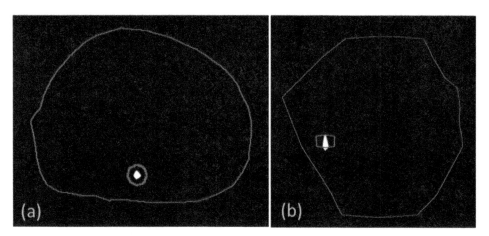

Figure 21.5 Example of fiducial marker contour in planning CT at axial view (a) and sagittal view (b). Window and level of CT images were set to only show the high-density structures.

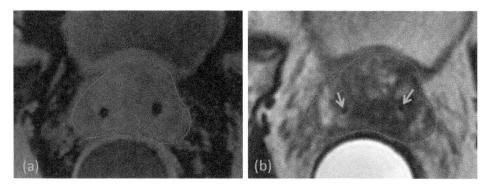

Figure 21.6 Example of fiducial images in MRI sequences (a) "water LAVA" that shows fiducials clearly, and (b) "T2 Cube" shows that fiducials (green arrow) are more difficult to identify.

Table 21.4 Recommended target volumes and radiation doses for treatment of prostate cancer.

		Volume	Dose/Constraint
Definitive - Moderate hypofractionation (20 fractions)			
	CTV	Prostate ± Seminal Vesicles	60 Gy RBE
Organs at risk			
	Bladder		V90% ≤ 10%
	Bladder		D0.03cc <103-105%
	Rectum		V90% ≤ 10%
Definitive - Ultra hypofractionation (5 fractions)			
	CTV	Prostate ± Seminal Vesicles	35 Gy RBE
Organs at risk			
	Bladder		V90% ≤ 10%
	Bladder		D0.03cc <103-105%
	Rectum		V90% ≤ 10%
Adjuvant/Salvage (33-35 fractions)			
	CTV	Prostate bed	66-70 Gy RBE
Organs at risk			
	Bladder		V61 Gy RBE ≤ 8-11%
	Rectum		V61 Gy RBE ≤ 9-12%

Abbreviations: CTV, clinical target volume; RBE, relative biological effectiveness

salvage setting, we generally deliver 66–70 Gy RBE in standard fractionation (i.e., 2 Gy RBE per fraction). However, hypofractionation is being investigated in the adjuvant/salvage setting and we recently completed a clinical trial utilizing hypofractionation (five fractions) in this setting. Figure 21.7 shows an example of a target contour (prostate gland + proximal seminal vesicles) in CT and MRI images.

21.5.4 Volume Expansion and Plan Optimization

The optimization target volume (OTV) is expanded from the CTV with 3 mm margins in all directions, except 5 mm in lateral directions. The OTV includes a 3-mm setup uncertainty and 3% of range uncertainty along the beam direction. The scanning target volume (STV) is expanded from the OTV with 7 mm margins universally. The STV defines the area where the proton pencil beam spots can be placed. Figure 21.8 shows the OTV and the STV structures expanded from the CTV. The artifacts caused by the carbon fiducials and BB need to be contoured and the Hounsfield unit (HU) overridden to "0." Additionally, the gas in the rectum and air inside the rectum balloon need to be contoured and the HU overridden to "0."

Typically, we employ two parallelly opposed lateral beams because lateral beams are robust and can spare the rectum and bladder. Figure 21.9 shows the high linear energy transfer (LET) (>6 keV/μm) distribution of right lateral beam. It is clear that this beam selection places the high LET only in the muscle and far away from rectum and bladder.

The plan is optimized by single field uniform dose (SFUD), that is, each lateral field is optimized individually to uniformly cover the target. After optimization, the dose is renormalized to the OTV (D95 = 100%). A typical DVH is shown in Figure 21.10. It is clear that proton pencil beam scanning generates very conformal plans, for example, the min and max doses for CTV are 100.4% and 102.1%, respectively. Setting appropriate optimization parameters in plan optimization are essential to get a conformal plan. Figure 21.11 shows a DVH comparison of two plans generated for the same patient. The only difference for the two plans is that the OTV upper dose limits in optimization were set to 102% (triangle) and 105% (square), respectively. Both the DVH and the axial dose show that the plan with the higher upper dose limit for optimization (square) is less conformal than plan with the lower upper dose limit for optimization (triangle). Another thing for plan optimization is

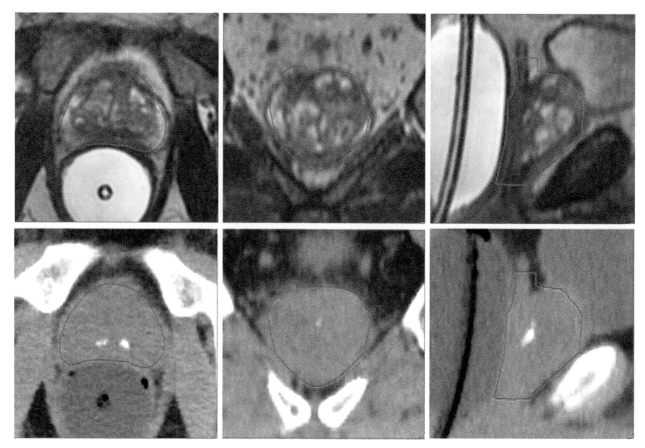

Figure 21.7 Example of target contour (prostate + proximal seminal vesicles) in MRI (top row) and CT (bottom row). From left to the right are axial, coronal and sagittal views, respectively.

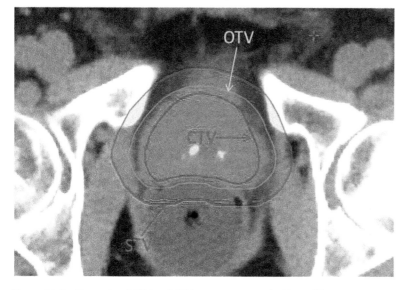

Figure 21.8 Example of OTV and STV structure expanded from CTV.

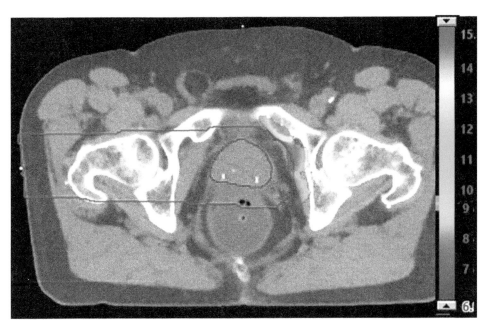

Figure 21.9   High LET (>6 keV/μm) distribution of the right lateral beam. The magenta curve shows the 50% isodose line.

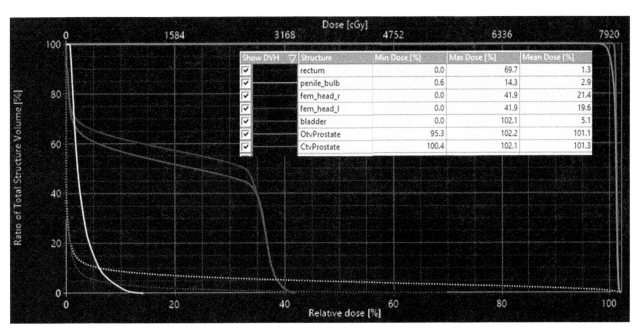

Show DVH	Structure	Min Dose [%]	Max Dose [%]	Mean Dose [%]
✓	rectum	0.0	69.7	1.3
✓	penile_bulb	0.6	14.3	2.9
✓	fem_head_r	0.0	41.9	21.4
✓	fem_head_l	0.0	41.9	19.6
✓	bladder	0.0	102.1	5.1
✓	OtvProstate	95.3	102.2	101.1
✓	CtvProstate	100.4	102.1	101.3

Figure 21.10   Typical DVH histogram for prostate shows that the plan generated by proton pencil beam scanning technique is highly conformal.

to avoid any hot spots in the rectum and bladder. Figure 21.12 shows an example of conformal dose distribution to the over-lap area between OTV and rectum where enough dose (>95%) is delivered for coverage and plan robustness, but dose to the rectum is kept to less than prescription dose.

TPS provides plan robustness evaluation. We apply a 3-mm setup uncertainty and 3% range uncertainty to the CTV. This creates a set of 12 uncertainty dose scenarios, as shown in

Figure 21.13. Alternatively, we can evaluate CTV robustness using the OTV, since the OTV covers our setup errors and range uncertainty. If the OTV D95 = 100%, we know that the CTV will be robust and will always be better than D95 = 100%. Our minimum dose to the OTV is 90%.

Hip prostheses require a different approach than the one outlined above. Due to the limitations of beam arrangement (i.e., lateral beams), proton beam therapy is not used for

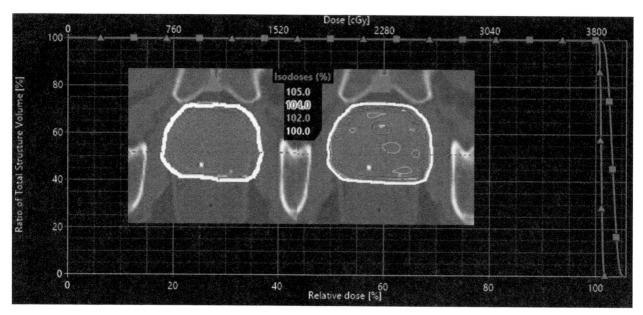

Figure 21.11 Example of an ideal plan (triangle) and not-ideal plan (square) by using different upper dose limits for OTV (102% vs. 105%) during plan optimization.

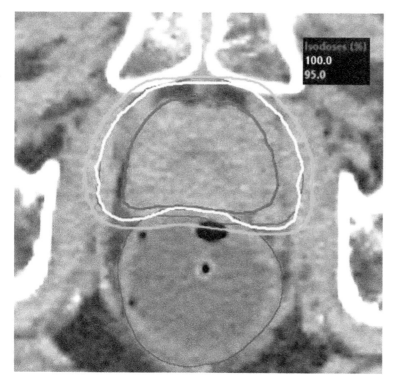

Figure 21.12 Example of conformal dose distribution that gives full dose to the CTV (red curve), more than 95% dose to the OTV (magenta), but not more than the prescription dose to the rectum.

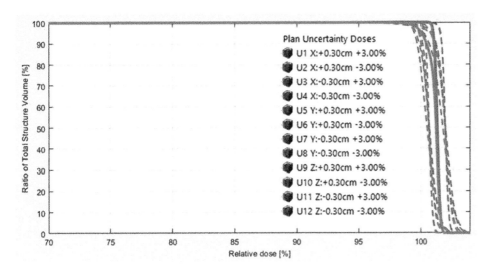

Figure 21.13 Example of 12 scenarios of uncertainty doses with 3-mm setup and 3% range uncertainties to evaluate plan robustness for the CTV (red dashed lines). The pink line is the OTV.

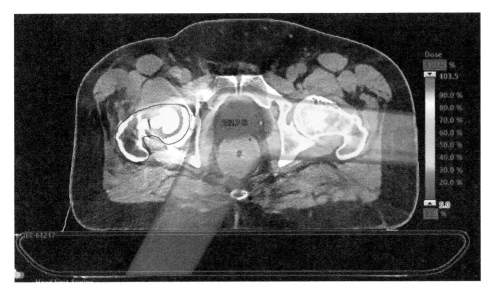

Figure 21.14 Posterior oblique beam is used for patient with a hip prosthesis. For this case, the posterior oblique beam is weighted slightly less than the lateral beam (45% vs. 55%) to spare more of the rectum.

patients with bilateral hip prophesies. For patients with unilateral hip prosthesis, a posterior oblique beam on the ipsilateral side as the prosthesis is used. A typical lateral beam is used on the contralateral side. The beam path of the posterior beam should completely avoid the hip prosthesis, as shown in Figure 21.14. The couch structure should be included in the beam path for dose calculation. If an endorectal balloon is not used, a posterior beam may not be a good choice because the extra range uncertainty caused by day-to-day variations of rectum filling. Anterior oblique beam(s) is an alternative, but high

LET ending in the rectum is a concern [111]. Artifact reduction algorithm in CT reconstruction should always be applied, which can significantly reduce the CT image streak artifacts caused by high-density prosthesis (as shown in Figure 21.14). In certain situations, whole pelvic nodal radiation in addition to prostate radiation may be indicated. We use lateral beams and the volume expansions to the prostate are the same as outlined above. The OTV for the pelvic node volume has a 7-mm expansion in all directions. Separate STVs are assigned for each field in order to spare the midline of the pelvis. IMPT with robust optimization is used in plan optimization. Figure 21.15 shows an example of the separate STVs for both fields and the low dose to the midline of the pelvis. The STV structures for left and right lateral fields are turquoise color (Figure 21.15a) and purple color (Figure 21.15b), respectively. The STV of the left lateral field does not include the nodes on the right side and vice versa for the STV of the right lateral field. This approach allows proton spots to be placed only on the proximal side for each lateral field. As shown in Figure 21.15c and d, the midline of the pelvis has very low dose because no beam passes through the midline.

21.5.5 Treatment Delivery, IGRT, and Troubleshooting

For treatment, the patient will have the same bladder preparation and immobilization as in CT simulation. The patient is setup with orthogonal kV images and is first aligned to bony structures with 6 degrees of freedom. The patient is then aligned to fiducials in kV images to the fiducial contours from the planning CT with 3 degrees of freedom (i.e., only translational shifts). We use the following criteria for IGRT: (a) bony deviation should be less than 10 mm for regular prostate alignment in order to avoid potential large radiological path length change, (b) bony deviation should be within 7 mm for cases including pelvic nodes because pelvis nodes move with bones and this 7 mm is required to make sure that pelvic node targets are still in the radiation field, and (c) all fiducials from kV X-rays should be aligned to inside or at least touching the fiducial contours from the planning CT. We treat both fields per day, although a single field delivery on alternative days is feasible [112]. IGRT is applied for each treatment field, which can correct potential prostate intrafraction motion between fields.

In cases where the fiducials cannot be aligned well, verification CT would be helpful for troubleshooting. In Figure 21.16a, the fiducials in kV X-rays are closer to each other than the contours from the planning CT (blue). The new contours of fiducials (green) from verification CT confirmed that prostate

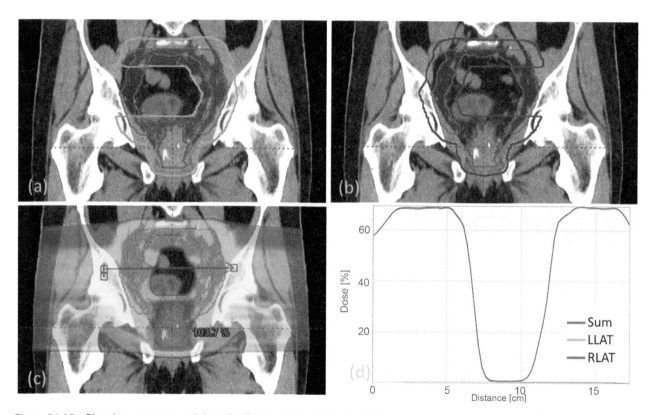

Figure 21.15 Planning structures and dose distributions for prostate cancer including pelvic nodes. Separate STV structures for the left lateral (turquoise) and the right lateral (purple) are shown in (a) and (b), respectively. (c) The dose distribution in color wash shows low dose to the midline of the pelvis. (d) Green, red, and blue curves are dose profiles of the line drawn in (c) for the left lateral, the right lateral field, and the sum of both fields, respectively.

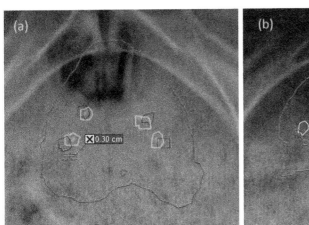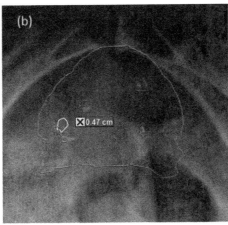

Figure 21.16 Two examples of drifted fiducials: (a) fiducials had systematic drifts due to tumor shrink during treatment. The blue and green structures are fiducial contours in planning CT and verification CT. The red curve is the CTV structure, and the background is the kV image taken in the treatment room. (b) Three fiducials (blue) were aligned well, but one (yellow) may have drifted.

gland contracted, which is probably due to the effect of radiation. In Figure 21.16b, three fiducials (blue) can be aligned well, but the yellow one is suspected to have drifted from its original position at planning CT. A verification CT can be requested to verify that. In cases where there are consistent large bony deviations from the planning CT, a verification CT would be requested to investigate its effect to the dose distribution and a replan would be needed when the dose degradation is not acceptable.

21.6 Conclusions and Future Direction

Prostate cancer is a very common indication for proton beam therapy and is often the most common type of cancer treated at a proton beam facility [113,114]. However, many aspects of prostate cancer treatment have yet to be answered concerning proton beam therapy. In particular, prospective randomized trials need to address disease outcomes and toxicity advantages, if any, that proton beam therapy offers over other forms of radiation. Consequently, there are many open clinical trials investigating proton beam therapy in prostate cancer (Table 21.5).

The PARTIQoL study (NCT01617161) is enrolling low- or intermediate-risk prostate cancer patients and randomizing them to IMRT or proton beam therapy [115]. The primary outcome is mean EPIC bowel scores. This trial will help to answer if the dosimetric advantages seen with proton beam therapy result in less toxicity. Another important study is the Prostate

Cancer Patients Treated with Alternative Radiation Oncology Strategies (PAROS) (NCT04083937) [116]. This multicenter study is randomizing postoperative patients to conventional fractionation with photons versus hypofractionation with photons or protons. The goal is to show improved quality of life with protons with biochemical progression-free survival as a secondary outcome. These studies will provide randomized evidence directly comparing protons to photons. Other studies, such as the Phase III Study of Image Guided Radiation Therapy with or without Androgen Suppression for Intermediate Risk Adenocarcinoma of the Prostate (NCT01492972), will help advance prostate cancer treatment by answering if ADT is needed with modern dose escalation delivered with the latest technology [117].

In recent years, we have seen a proliferation of proton beam facilities and will likely continue to see this as costs come down and technical challenges are overcome [118,119]. There will certainly be other heavy ion facilities built in the years to come. These changes will continue to provide prostate cancer patients with additional treatment options to consider when deciding on treatment. Because prostate cancer can be effectively treated with surgery, external beam radiation, brachytherapy, proton beam therapy, or carbon-ion therapy, it will remain important for patients to consider the quality-of-life impact of the various treatment options. Future prospective randomized studies utilizing the latest technology including particle therapy need to be performed to help ensure the best outcomes for our patients.

Table 21.5 Ongoing clinical trials in prostate cancer uttilizing proton beam therapy.

ClinicalTrials.gov Identifier	Phase	Official Name	Country
Definitive			
NCT01617161	III	Prostate Advanced Radiation Technologies Investigating Quality of Life (PARTIQoL): A Phase III Randomized Clinical Trial of Proton Therapy vs IMRT for Low or Intermediate Risk Prostate	USA
NCT03561220	NA	A Prospective Comparative Study of Outcomes With Proton and Photon Radiation in Prostate Cancer (COMPPARE)	USA
NCT01230866	III	A Phase III Prospective Randomized Trial of Standard-fractionation vs. Hypo-fractionation With Proton Radiation Therapy for Low Risk Adenocarcinoma of the Prostate	USA
NCT01492972	III	Phase III Study of Image Guided Radiation Therapy With or Without Androgen Suppression for Intermediate Risk Adenocarcinoma of the Prostate	USA
NCT01950351	II	Phase II Trial of Hypofractionated Proton Beam Therapy in Men With Localized Prostate Adenocarcinoma	USA
NCT03285815	II	A Phase II Randomized Trial of Hypofractionated Proton Therapy in Patients With a Localized Prostate Adenocarcinoma	South Korea
NCT03624660	II	A Phase II Study of Dose-Escalated Proton-Based Radiation Therapy Delivered With a Simultaneous Integrated Boost (SIB) to Intraprostatic Tumors (IPT) Visible on Pretreatment Magnetic Resonance Image	USA
NCT02040610	II	A Phase II Study of Hypofractionated Image Guided Proton Therapy for Low and Intermediate Risk Prostate Cancer	USA
NCT02766686	NA	Preference-based Comparative Study on Definitive Radiotherapy of Prostate Cancer With Protons in Standard Fractionation and Standard Dosage (ProtoChoice-P)	Germany
NCT03740191	NA	Spot-Scanning Based Hypofractionated Proton Therapy for Low and Intermediate Risk Prostate Cancer	Austria
UMIN000025453		A multi-institutional clinical trial of proton beam therapy for localized intermediate-risk prostate cancer	Japan
Adjuvant/Salvage			
NCT04083937	III	Prostate Cancer Patients Treated With Alternative Radiation Oncology Strategies (PAROS)	Germany
NCT00969111	NA	Postoperative or Salvage Radiotherapy for Node Negative Prostate Cancer Following Radical Prostatectomy	USA
Recurrent			
NCT04190446	II	A Randomized, Parallel Phase II Trial of Hypofractionated Proton Beam Therapy or IMRT for Recurrent, Oligometastatic Prostate Cancer Involving Only Pelvic and/or Para-Aortic Lymph Nodes Following Primary Localized Treatment	USA

Abbreviations: NA, Not applicable

Bibliography

1 Siegel, R.L., Miller, K.D., and Jemal, A. (2020). Cancer statistics. *CA: A Cancer Journal for Clinicians* 70: 7–30.

2 Burt, L.M., Shrieve, D.C., and Tward, J.D. (2018). Factors influencing prostate cancer patterns of care: An analysis of treatment variation using the SEER database. *Advances in Radiation Oncology* 3: 170–180.

3 Donovan, J.L., Hamdy, F.C., Lane, J.A. et al. (2016). Patient-reported outcomes after monitoring, surgery, or radiotherapy for prostate cancer. *The New England Journal of Medicine* 375(15):1425–1437. doi: 10.1056/NEJMoa1606221. Epub 2016 Sep 14. PMID: 27626365; PMCID: PMC5134995.

4 Particle therapy facilities in clinical operation (2020). (Accessed July 30, at https://www.ptcog.ch/index.php/facilities-in-operation.)

5 Trofimov, A., Nguyen, P.L., Coen, J.J. et al. (2007). Radiotherapy treatment of early-stage prostate cancer with IMRT and protons: A treatment planning comparison. *International Journal of Radiation Oncology, Biology, Physics* 69: 444–453.

6 Vargas, C., Fryer, A., Mahajan, C. et al. (2008). Dose-volume comparison of proton therapy and intensity-modulated radiotherapy for prostate cancer. *International Journal of Radiation Oncology, Biology, Physics* 70: 744–751.

7 Daniell, H.W., Clark, J.C., Pereira, S.E. et al. (2001). Hypogonadism following prostate-bed radiation therapy for prostate carcinoma. *Cancer* 91: 1889–1895.

8 Nichols, R.C., Jr., Morris, C.G., Hoppe, B.S. et al. (2012). Proton radiotherapy for prostate cancer is not associated with post-treatment testosterone suppression. *International Journal of Radiation Oncology, Biology, Physics* 82: 1222–1226.

9 Bryant, C., Henderson, R.H., Hoppe, B.S. et al. (2016). Controversies in proton therapy for prostate cancer. *The Chinese Clinical Oncology* 5: 55.

10 Shipley, W.U., Tepper, J.E., Prout, G.R., Jr. et al. (1979). Proton radiation as boost therapy for localized prostatic carcinoma. *Jama* 241: 1912–1915.

11 Shipley, W.U., Verhey, L.J., Munzenrider, J.E. et al. (1995). Advanced prostate cancer: The results of a randomized comparative trial of high dose irradiation boosting with conformal protons compared with conventional dose irradiation using photons alone. *International Journal of Radiation Oncology, Biology, Physics* 32: 3–12.

12 Slater, J.D., Rossi, C.J., Jr., Yonemoto, L.T. et al. (2004). Proton therapy for prostate cancer: The initial Loma Linda University experience. *International Journal of Radiation Oncology, Biology, Physics* 59: 348–352.

13 Zietman, A.L., Bae, K., Slater, J.D. et al. (2010). Randomized trial comparing conventional-dose with high-dose conformal radiation therapy in early-stage adenocarcinoma of the prostate: Long-term results from Proton Radiation Oncology Group/American College of Radiology 95-09. *Journal of Clinical Oncology: Official Journal of the American Society of Clinical Oncology* 28: 1106–1111.

14 Johansson, S., Isacsson, U., Sandin, F., and Turesson, I. (2019). High efficacy of hypofractionated proton therapy with 4 fractions of 5Gy as a boost to 50Gy photon therapy for localized prostate cancer. *Radiotherapy and Oncology: Journal of the European Society for Therapeutic Radiology and Oncology* 141: 164–173.

15 Bryant, C., Smith, T.L., Henderson, R.H. et al. (2016). Five-year biochemical results, toxicity, and patient-reported quality of life after delivery of dose-escalated image guided proton therapy for prostate cancer. *International Journal of Radiation Oncology, Biology, Physics* 95: 422–434.

16 Iwata, H., Ishikawa, H., Takagi, M. et al. (2018). Long-term outcomes of proton therapy for prostate cancer in Japan: A multi-institutional survey of the Japanese Radiation Oncology Study Group. *Cancer Medicine* 7: 677–689.

17 Lee, H.J., Jr., Macomber, M.W., Spraker, M.B. et al. (2018). Early toxicity and patient reported quality-of-life in patients receiving proton therapy for localized prostate cancer: A single institutional review of prospectively recorded outcomes. *Radiation Oncology* 13: 179.

18 Mendenhall, N.P., Hoppe, B.S., Nichols, R.C. et al. (2014). Five-year outcomes from 3 prospective trials of image-guided proton therapy for prostate cancer. *International Journal of Radiation Oncology, Biology, Physics* 88: 596–602.

19 Pugh, T.J., Munsell, M.F., Choi, S. et al. (2013). Quality of life and toxicity from passively scattered and spot-scanning proton beam therapy for localized prostate cancer. *International Journal of Radiation Oncology, Biology, Physics* 87: 946–953.

20 Takagi, M., Demizu, Y., Terashima, K. et al. (2017). Long-term outcomes in patients treated with proton therapy for localized prostate cancer. *Cancer Medicine* 6: 2234–2243.

21 Grewal, A.S., Schonewolf, C., Min, E.J. et al. (2019). Four-year outcomes from a prospective phase II clinical trial of moderately hypofractionated proton therapy for localized prostate cancer. *International Journal of Radiation Oncology, Biology, Physics* 105: 713–722.

22 Ha, B., Cho, K.H., Lee, K.H. et al. (2019). Long-term results of a phase II study of hypofractionated proton therapy for prostate cancer: Moderate versus extreme hypofractionation. *Radiation Oncology* 14: 4.

23 Habl, G., Uhl, M., Katayama, S. et al. (2016). Acute toxicity and quality of life in patients with prostate cancer treated with protons or carbon ions in a prospective randomized phase II study–the IPI trial. *International Journal of Radiation Oncology, Biology, Physics* 95: 435–443.

24 Henderson, R.H., Bryant, C., Hoppe, B.S. et al. (2017). Five-year outcomes from a prospective trial of image-guided accelerated hypofractionated proton therapy for prostate cancer. *Acta Oncologica* 56: 963–970.

25 Kubes, J., Vondracek, V., Andrlik, M. et al. (2019). Extreme hypofractionated proton radiotherapy for prostate cancer using pencil beam scanning: Dosimetry, acute toxicity and preliminary results. *Journal of Medical Imaging and Radiation Oncology* 63: 829–835.

26 Nakajima, K., Iwata, H., Ogino, H. et al. (2018). Acute toxicity of image-guided hypofractionated proton therapy for localized prostate cancer. *International Journal of Clinical Oncology* 23: 353–360.

27 Slater, J.M., Slater, J.D., Kang, J.I. et al. (2019). Hypofractionated proton therapy in early prostate cancer: Results of a phase I/II trial at Loma Linda University. *International Journal of Particle Therapy Impact Factor* 6: 1–9.

28 Vargas, C.E., Hartsell, W.F., Dunn, M. et al. (2018). Hypofractionated versus standard fractionated proton-beam therapy for low-risk prostate cancer: Interim results of a randomized trial PCG GU 002. *American Journal of Clinical Oncology* 41: 115–120.

29 Vargas, C.E., Schmidt, M.Q., Niska, J.R. et al. (2018). Initial toxicity, quality-of-life outcomes, and dosimetric impact in a randomized phase 3 trial of hypofractionated versus standard fractionated proton therapy for low-risk prostate cancer. *Advances in Radiation Oncology* 3: 322–330.

30 Deville, C., Jr., Hwang, W.T., Barsky, A.R. et al. (2020, Oct). Initial clinical outcomes for prostate cancer patients undergoing adjuvant or salvage proton therapy after radical prostatectomy. *Acta Oncologica* 59(10): 1235–1239 doi: 10.1080/0284186X.2020.1766698. Epub 2020 May 18. PMID: 32421456.

31 Santos, P.M.G., Barsky, A.R., Hwang, W.T. et al. (2019). Comparative toxicity outcomes of proton-beam therapy versus intensity-modulated radiotherapy for prostate cancer in the postoperative setting. *Cancer* 125: 4278–4293.

32 Morgan, S.C., Hoffman, K., Loblaw, D.A. et al. (2019). Hypofractionated radiation therapy for localized prostate cancer: Executive summary of an ASTRO, ASCO and AUA evidence-based guideline. *The Journal of Urology* 201: 528–534.

33 Zaorsky, N.G., Shaikh, T., Murphy, C.T. et al. (2016). Comparison of outcomes and toxicities among radiation therapy treatment options for prostate cancer. *Cancer Treatment Reviews* 48: 50–60.

34 Aluwini, S., Pos, F., Schimmel, E. et al. (2016). Hypofractionated versus conventionally fractionated radiotherapy for patients with prostate cancer (HYPRO): Late toxicity results from a randomised, non-inferiority, phase 3 trial. *The Lancet Oncology* 17: 464–474.

35 Aluwini, S., Pos, F., Schimmel, E. et al. (2015). Hypofractionated versus conventionally fractionated radiotherapy for patients with prostate cancer (HYPRO): Acute toxicity results from a randomised non-inferiority phase 3 trial. *The Lancet Oncology* 16: 274–283.

36 Incrocci, L., Wortel, R.C., Alemayehu, W.G. et al. (2016). Hypofractionated versus conventionally fractionated radiotherapy for patients with localised prostate cancer (HYPRO): Final efficacy results from a randomised, multicentre, open-label, phase 3 trial. *The Lancet Oncology* 17: 1061–1069.

37 Dearnaley, D., Syndikus, I., Mossop, H. et al. (2016). Conventional versus hypofractionated high-dose intensity-modulated radiotherapy for prostate cancer: 5-year outcomes of the randomised, non-inferiority, phase 3 CHHiP trial. *The Lancet Oncology* 17: 1047–1060.

38 Lee, W.R., Dignam, J.J., Amin, M.B. et al. (2016). Randomized phase III noninferiority study comparing two radiotherapy fractionation schedules in patients with low-risk prostate cancer. *Journal of Clinical Oncology: Official Journal of the American Society of Clinical Oncology* 34: 2325–2332.

39 Catton, C.N., Lukka, H., Gu, C.S. et al. (2017). Randomized trial of a hypofractionated radiation regimen for the treatment of localized prostate cancer. *Journal of Clinical Oncology: Official Journal of the American Society of Clinical Oncology* 35: 1884–1890.

40 Mahase, S.S., D'Angelo, D., Kang, J., Hu, J.C., Barbieri, C.E., and Nagar, H. (2020). Trends in the use of stereotactic body radiotherapy for treatment of prostate cancer in the united states. *JAMA Network Open* 3: e1920471.

41 McClelland, S., III, Sandler, K.A., Degnin, C., Chen, Y., Hung, A.Y., and Mitin, T.E. (2019). Is moderate hypofractionation accepted as a new standard of care in North America for prostate cancer patients treated with external beam radiotherapy? Survey of genitourinary expert radiation oncologists. *International Braz J Urol: Official Journal of the Brazilian Society of Urology* 45: 273–287.

42 Prostate Cancer (Version 2.2020) (2020). (Accessed July 7, 2020, at https://www.nccn.org/professionals/physician_gls/pdf/prostate.pdf.)

43 Parker, C., Castro, E., Fizazi, K. et al. (2020, Sep). Prostate cancer: ESMO clinical practice guidelines for diagnosis, treatment and follow-up. *Annals Of Oncology: Official Journal Of The European Society For Medical Oncology / ESMO* 31(9):1119–1134. doi: 10.1016/j.annonc.2020.06.011. Epub 2020 Jun 25. PMID: 32593798.

44 Widesott, L., Pierelli, A., Fiorino, C. et al. (2011). Helical tomotherapy vs. intensity-modulated proton therapy for whole pelvis irradiation in high-risk prostate cancer patients: Dosimetric, normal tissue complication probability, and generalized equivalent uniform dose analysis. *International Journal of Radiation Oncology, Biology, Physics* 80: 1589–1600.

45 Thompson, I.M., Valicenti, R.K., Albertsen, P. et al. (2013). Adjuvant and salvage radiotherapy after prostatectomy: AUA/ASTRO guideline. *The Journal of Urology* 190: 441–449.

46 Pisansky, T.M., Thompson, I.M., Valicenti, R.K., D'Amico, A.V., and Adjuvant, S.S. (2019). Salvage radiotherapy after prostatectomy: ASTRO/AUA guideline amendment 2018-2019. *The Journal of Urology* 202: 533–538.

47 Wiegel, T., Bartkowiak, D., Bottke, D. et al. (2014). Adjuvant radiotherapy versus wait-and-see after radical prostatectomy: 10-year follow-up of the ARO 96-02/AUO AP 09/95 trial. *European Urology* 66: 243–250.

48 Bolla, M., Van Poppel, H., Tombal, B. et al. (2012). Postoperative radiotherapy after radical prostatectomy for high-risk prostate cancer: Long-term results of a randomised controlled trial (EORTC trial 22911). *Lancet* 380: 2018–2027.

49 Thompson, I.M., Tangen, C.M., Paradelo, J. et al. (2009). Adjuvant radiotherapy for pathological T3N0M0 prostate cancer significantly reduces risk of metastases and improves survival: Long-term followup of a randomized clinical trial. *The Journal of Urology* 181: 956–962.

50 Swanson, G.P., Hussey, M.A., Tangen, C.M. et al. (2007). Predominant treatment failure in postprostatectomy patients is local: Analysis of patterns of treatment failure in SWOG 8794. *Journal of Clinical Oncology: Official Journal of the American Society of Clinical Oncology* 25: 2225–2229.

51 Carrie, C., Magne, N., Burban-Provost, P. et al. (2019). Interest of short hormonotherapy (HT) associated with radiotherapy (RT) as salvage treatment for metastatic free survival (MFS) after radical prostatectomy (RP): Update at 9 years of the GETUG-AFU 16 phase III randomized trial (NCT00423475). *Journal of Clinical Oncology* 37: 5001-.

52 Shipley, W.U., Seiferheld, W., Lukka, H.R. et al. (2017). Radiation with or without antiandrogen therapy in recurrent prostate cancer. *The New England Journal of Medicine* 376: 417–428.

53 Carrie, C., Hasbini, A., De Laroche, G. et al. (2016). Salvage radiotherapy with or without short-term hormone therapy for rising prostate-specific antigen concentration after radical prostatectomy (GETUG-AFU 16): A randomised, multicentre, open-label phase 3 trial. *The Lancet Oncology* 17: 747–756.

54 Pollack, A., Karrison, T.G., Balogh, A.G. et al. (2018). Short term androgen deprivation therapy without or with pelvic lymph node treatment added to prostate bed only salvage radiotherapy: The NRG oncology/RTOG 0534 SPPORT Trial. *International Journal of Radiation Oncology, Biology, Physics* 102: 1605-.

55 Whitaker, T.J., Routman, D.M., Schultz, H. et al. (2019). IMPT versus VMAT for pelvic nodal irradiation in prostate cancer: A dosimetric comparison. *International Journal of Particle Therapy Impact Factor* 5: 11–23.

56 Vale, C.L., Brihoum, M., Chabaud, S. et al. (2019). Adjuvant or salvage radiotherapy for the treatment of

localised prostate cancer? A prospectively planned aggregate data meta-analysis. *Annals of Oncology* 30: 883-.

57 Tendulkar, R.D., Agrawal, S., Gao, T. et al. (2016). Contemporary update of a multi-institutional predictive nomogram for salvage radiotherapy after radical prostatectomy. *Journal of Clinical Oncology: Official Journal of the American Society of Clinical Oncology* 34: 3648–3654.

58 Goenka, A., Newman, N.B., Fontanilla, H. et al. (2017). Patient-reported quality of life after proton beam therapy for prostate cancer: The effect of prostate size. *Clinical Genitourinary Cancer* 15: 704–710.

59 McGee, L., Mendenhall, N.P., Henderson, R.H. et al. (2013). Outcomes in men with large prostates (>/= 60 cm(3)) treated with definitive proton therapy for prostate cancer. *Acta Oncologica* 52: 470–476.

60 Fang, P., Mick, R., Deville, C. et al. (2015). A case-matched study of toxicity outcomes after proton therapy and intensity-modulated radiation therapy for prostate cancer. *Cancer* 121: 1118–1127.

61 Matta, R., Chapple, C.R., Fisch, M. et al. (2019). Pelvic complications after prostate cancer radiation therapy and their management: An international collaborative narrative review. *European Urology* 75: 464–476.

62 Gray, P.J., Paly, J.J., Yeap, B.Y. et al. (2013). Patient-reported outcomes after 3-dimensional conformal, intensity-modulated, or proton beam radiotherapy for localized prostate cancer. *Cancer* 119: 1729–1735.

63 Yu, J.B., Soulos, P.R., Herrin, J. et al. (2013). Proton versus intensity-modulated radiotherapy for prostate cancer: Patterns of care and early toxicity. *Journal of the National Cancer Institute* 105: 25–32.

64 Sheets, N.C., Goldin, G.H., Meyer, A.M. et al. (2012). Intensity-modulated radiation therapy, proton therapy, or conformal radiation therapy and morbidity and disease control in localized prostate cancer. *Jama* 307: 1611–1620.

65 Dutz, A., Agolli, L., Baumann, M. et al. (2019). Early and late side effects, dosimetric parameters and quality of life after proton beam therapy and IMRT for prostate cancer: A matched-pair analysis. *Acta Oncologica* 58: 916–925.

66 Sidana, A., Hernandez, D.J., Feng, Z. et al. (2012). Treatment decision-making for localized prostate cancer: What younger men choose and why. *Prostate* 72: 58–64.

67 Nukala, V., Incrocci, L., Hunt, A.A., Ballas, L., and Koontz, B.F. (2020). Challenges in reporting the effect of radiotherapy on erectile function. *The Journal of Sexual Medicine* 17: 1053–1059.

68 Roach, M., 3rd, Nam, J., Gagliardi, G., El Naqa, I., Deasy, J.O., and Marks, L.B. (2010). Radiation dose-volume effects and the penile bulb. *International Journal of Radiation Oncology, Biology, Physics* 76: S130–4.

69 Hoppe, B.S., Nichols, R.C., Henderson, R.H. et al. (2012). Erectile function, incontinence, and other quality of life outcomes following proton therapy for prostate cancer in men 60 years old and younger. *Cancer* 118: 4619–4626.

70 Hamstra, D.A., Mariados, N., Sylvester, J. et al. (2018). Sexual quality of life following prostate intensity modulated radiation therapy (IMRT) with a rectal/prostate spacer: Secondary analysis of a phase 3 trial. *Practical Radiation Oncology* 8: e7–e15.

71 Schwarz, M., Pierelli, A., Fiorino, C. et al. (2011). Helical tomotherapy and intensity modulated proton therapy in the treatment of early stage prostate cancer: A treatment planning comparison. *Radiotherapy and Oncology: Journal of the European Society for Therapeutic Radiology and Oncology* 98: 74–80.

72 Kole, T.P., Nichols, R.C., Lei, S. et al. (2015). A dosimetric comparison of ultra-hypofractionated passively scattered proton radiotherapy and stereotactic body radiotherapy (SBRT) in the definitive treatment of localized prostate cancer. *Acta Oncologica* 54: 825–831.

73 Alemozaffar, M., Regan, M.M., Cooperberg, M.R. et al. (2011). Prediction of erectile function following treatment for prostate cancer. *Jama* 306: 1205–1214.

74 Holtzman, A.L., Bryant, C.M., Mendenhall, N.P. et al. (2019). Patient-reported sexual survivorship following high-dose image-guided proton therapy for prostate cancer. *Radiotherapy and Oncology: Journal of the European Society for Therapeutic Radiology and Oncology* 134: 204–210.

75 Ho, C.K., Bryant, C.M., Mendenhall, N.P. et al. (2018). Long-term outcomes following proton therapy for prostate cancer in young men with a focus on sexual health. *Acta Oncologica* 57: 582–588.

76 Chuong, M.D., Hartsell, W., Larson, G. et al. (2018). Minimal toxicity after proton beam therapy for prostate and pelvic nodal irradiation: Results from the proton collaborative group REG001-09 trial. *Acta Oncologica* 57: 368–374.

77 Ishii, K., Ogino, R., Hosokawa, Y. et al. (2016). Comparison of dosimetric parameters and acute toxicity after whole-pelvic vs prostate-only volumetric-modulated arc therapy with daily image guidance for prostate cancer. *The British Journal of Radiology* 89: 20150930.

78 Deville, C., Both, S., Hwang, W.T., Tochner, Z., and Vapiwala, N. (2010). Clinical toxicities and dosimetric parameters after whole-pelvis versus prostate-only intensity-modulated radiation therapy for prostate cancer. *International Journal of Radiation Oncology, Biology, Physics* 78: 763–772.

79 Bayley, A., Rosewall, T., Craig, T. et al. (2010). Clinical application of high-dose, image-guided intensity-modulated radiotherapy in high-risk prostate cancer.

80 Pervez, N., Small, C., MacKenzie, M. et al. (2010). Acute toxicity in high-risk prostate cancer patients treated with androgen suppression and hypofractionated intensity-modulated radiotherapy. *International Journal of Radiation Oncology, Biology, Physics* 76: 57–64.

81 Sanguineti, G., Endres, E.J., Parker, B.C. et al. (2008). Acute toxicity of whole-pelvis IMRT in 87 patients with localized prostate cancer. *Acta Oncologica* 47: 301–310.

82 Muren, L.P., Wasbø, E., Helle, S.I. et al. (2008). Intensity-modulated radiotherapy of pelvic lymph nodes in locally advanced prostate cancer: Planning procedures and early experiences. *International Journal of Radiation Oncology, Biology, Physics* 71: 1034–1041.

83 Melton, L.J., 3rd, Lieber, M.M., Atkinson, E.J. et al. (2011). Fracture risk in men with prostate cancer: A population-based study. *Journal of Bone and Mineral Research: The Official Journal of the American Society for Bone and Mineral Research* 26: 1808–1815.

84 Elliott, S.P., Jarosek, S.L., Alanee, S.R., Konety, B.R., Dusenbery, K.E., and Virnig, B.A. (2011). Three-dimensional external beam radiotherapy for prostate cancer increases the risk of hip fracture. *Cancer* 117: 4557–4565.

85 Tran, A., Zhang, J., Woods, K. et al. (2017). Treatment planning comparison of IMPT, VMAT and 4π radiotherapy for prostate cases. *Radiation Oncology* 12: 10.

86 Rana, S., Cheng, C., Zheng, Y. et al. (2014). Dosimetric study of uniform scanning proton therapy planning for prostate cancer patients with a metal hip prosthesis, and comparison with volumetric-modulated arc therapy. *Journal Of Applied Clinical Medical Physics / American College of Medical Physics* 15: 4611.

87 Valery, R., Mendenhall, N.P., Nichols, R.C., Jr. et al. (2013). Hip fractures and pain following proton therapy for management of prostate cancer. *Acta Oncologica* 52: 486–491.

88 Mishra, M.V., Khairnar, R., Bentzen, S.M. et al. (2020). Patient reported outcomes following proton pencil beam scanning vs. passive scatter/uniform scanning for localized prostate cancer: Secondary analysis of PCG 001-09. *Clinical and Translational Radiation Oncology* 22: 50–54.

89 Wallis, C.J., Mahar, A.L., Choo, R. et al. (2016). Second malignancies after radiotherapy for prostate cancer: Systematic review and meta-analysis. *Bmj* 352: i851.

90 Eaton, B.R., MacDonald, S.M., Yock, T.I., and Tarbell, N.J. (2015). Secondary malignancy risk following proton radiation therapy. *Frontiers in Oncology* 5: 261.

91 Xiang, M., Chang, D.T., and Pollom, E.L. (2020). Second cancer risk after primary cancer treatment with three-dimensional conformal, intensity-modulated, or proton beam radiation therapy. *Cancer* 126: 3560–3568.

92 Mohamad, O., Tabuchi, T., Nitta, Y. et al. (2019). Risk of subsequent primary cancers after carbon ion radiotherapy, photon radiotherapy, or surgery for localised prostate cancer: A propensity score-weighted, retrospective, cohort study. *The Lancet Oncology* 20: 674–685.

93 Nikoghosyan, A., Schulz-Ertner, D., Didinger, B. et al. (2004). Evaluation of therapeutic potential of heavy ion therapy for patients with locally advanced prostate cancer. *International Journal of Radiation Oncology, Biology, Physics* 58: 89–97.

94 Choi, J. and Kang, J.O. (2012). Basics of particle therapy II: Relative biological effectiveness. *Radiation Oncology Journal* 30: 1–13.

95 Akakura, K., Tsujii, H., Morita, S. et al. (2004). Phase I/II clinical trials of carbon ion therapy for prostate cancer. *Prostate* 58: 252–258.

96 Ishikawa, H., Tsuji, H., Kamada, T. et al. (2006). Risk factors of late rectal bleeding after carbon ion therapy for prostate cancer. *International Journal of Radiation Oncology, Biology, Physics* 66: 1084–1091.

97 Ishikawa, H., Tsuji, H., Kamada, T. et al. (2006). Carbon ion radiation therapy for prostate cancer: Results of a prospective phase II study. *Radiotherapy and Oncology: Journal of the European Society for Therapeutic Radiology and Oncology* 81: 57–64.

98 Kawamura, H., Kubo, N., Sato, H. et al. (2020). Moderately hypofractionated carbon ion radiotherapy for prostate cancer; A prospective observational study "GUNMA0702". *BMC Cancer* 20: 75.

99 Takakusagi, Y., Katoh, H., Kano, K. et al. (2020). Preliminary result of carbon-ion radiotherapy using the spot scanning method for prostate cancer. *Radiation Oncology* 15: 127.

100 Wakatsuki, M., Tsuji, H., Ishikawa, H. et al. (2008). Quality of life in men treated with carbon ion therapy for prostate cancer. *International Journal of Radiation Oncology, Biology, Physics* 72: 1010–1015.

101 Maruyama, K., Tsuji, H., Nomiya, T. et al. (2017). Five-year quality of life assessment after carbon ion radiotherapy for prostate cancer. *Journal of Radiation Research* 58: 260–266.

102 Zhang, Y., Li, P., Yu, Q. et al. (2019). Preliminary exploration of clinical factors affecting acute toxicity and quality of life after carbon ion therapy for prostate cancer. *Radiation Oncology* 14: 94.

103 Vargas, C.E., Hartsell, W.F., Dunn, M. et al. (2016). Image-guided hypofractionated proton beam therapy for low-risk prostate cancer: Analysis of quality of life and toxicity, PCG GU 002. *Reports of Practical Oncology and Radiotherapy* 21: 207–212.

104 Kim, Y.J., Cho, K.H., Pyo, H.R. et al. (2013). A phase II study of hypofractionated proton therapy for prostate cancer. *Acta Oncologica* 52: 477–485.

105 Habl, G., Hatiboglu, G., Edler, L. et al. (2014). Ion Prostate Irradiation (IPI) – A pilot study to establish the safety and feasibility of primary hypofractionated irradiation of the prostate with protons and carbon ions in a raster scan technique. *BMC Cancer* 14: 202.

106 Widmark, A., Gunnlaugsson, A., Beckman, L. et al. (2019, Aug 3). Ultra-hypofractionated versus conventionally fractionated radiotherapy for prostate cancer: 5-year outcomes of the HYPO-RT-PC randomised, non-inferiority, phase 3 trial. *Lancet* 394(10196):385–395. doi: 10.1016/S0140-6736(19)31131-6. Epub.

107 Hamstra, D.A., Mariados, N., Sylvester, J. et al. (2017). Continued benefit to rectal separation for prostate radiation therapy: Final results of a phase III trial. *International Journal of Radiation Oncology, Biology, Physics* 97: 976–985.

108 Navaratnam, A., Cumsky, J., Abdul-Muhsin, H. et al. (2020). Assessment of polyethylene glycol hydrogel spacer and its effect on rectal radiation dose in prostate cancer patients receiving proton beam radiation therapy. *Advances in Radiation Oncology* 5: 92–100.

109 Wang, K.K., Vapiwala, N., Deville, C. et al. (2012). A study to quantify the effectiveness of daily endorectal balloon for prostate intrafraction motion management. *International Journal of Radiation Oncology, Biology, Physics* 83: 1055–1063.

110 Both, S., Wang, K.K., Plastaras, J.P. et al. (2011). Real-time study of prostate intrafraction motion during external beam radiotherapy with daily endorectal balloon. *International Journal of Radiation Oncology, Biology, Physics* 81: 1302–1309.

111 Tang, S., Both, S., Bentefour, H. et al. (2012). Improvement of prostate treatment by anterior proton fields. *International Journal of Radiation Oncology, Biology, Physics* 83: 408–418.

112 Kirk, M.L., Tang, S., Zhai, H. et al. (2015). Comparison of prostate proton treatment planning technique, interfraction robustness, and analysis of single-field treatment feasibility. *Practical Radiation Oncology* 5: 99–105.

113 Forsthoefel, M.K., Ballew, E., Unger, K.R. et al. (2020). Early experience of the first single-room gantry mounted active scanning proton therapy system at an integrated cancer center. *Frontiers in Oncology* 10: 861.

114 Parikh-Patel, A., Morris, C.R., Maguire, F.B., Daly, M.E., and Kizer, K.W. (2020). A population-based assessment of proton beam therapy utilization in California. *The American Journal of Managed Care* 26: e28–e35.

115 (2020). Identifier: NCT01617161 – Proton therapy vs. IMRT for low or intermediate risk prostate cancer (PARTIQoL). (Accessed July, 14, at https://www.clinicaltrials.gov/ct2/show/NCT01617161.)

116 Clinicaltrials.gov. Identifier: NCT04083937 – Prostate cancer patients treated with alternative radiation oncology strategies access July 14, 2021.

117 Clinicaltrials.gov. Identifier: NCT01492972 – Phase III study of image guided radiation therapy with or without androgen suppression for intermediate risk adenocarcinoma of the prostate.

118 Farr, J.B., Flanz, J.B., Gerbershagen, A., and Moyers, M.F. (2018). New horizons in particle therapy systems. *Medical Physics* 45: e953–e83.

119 Kamran, S.C., Light, J.O., and Efstathiou, J.A. (2019). Proton versus photon-based radiation therapy for prostate cancer: Emerging evidence and considerations in the era of value-based cancer care. *Prostate Cancer and Prostatic Diseases* 22: 509–521.

22

Non-prostate Genitourinary Cancers

Justin Cohen, MD, Gregory Alexander, MD, and Mark V. Mishra, MD

Department of Radiation Oncology, University of Maryland, Baltimore, MD
Corresponding Author: Mark V. Mishra, MD, Associate Professor, Department of Radiation Oncology, University of Maryland, UMMC GGK19 655 W. Baltimore Street, Baltimore, MD 21201

22.1 Introduction

Particle therapy, particularly proton therapy, serves as a promising treatment modality for the treatment of non-prostate genitourinary malignancies. Given its characteristic Bragg peak and potential to decrease integral dose and total irradiated volume, proton therapy has the ability to reduce dose to organs at risk, potentially decreasing the rate and severity of acute and late toxicity in appropriately selected cases. In this chapter, we review the available evidence to support the safety and efficacy of particle therapy to treat testicular tumors, bladder cancer, and tumors of renal pelvis.

22.2 Seminoma

22.2.1 Background

Testicular cancer is predicted to account for only 0.5% of all new cancer cases in 2020, but it remains the most common solid malignancy in young adult males (https://seer.cancer.gov/statfacts/html/testis.html). Risk factors include family history of testicular cancer, undescended testis, and Klinefelter syndrome. Ninety to ninety-five percent of testicular tumors are germ cell tumors (GCT) with seminomas accounting for 40% of the germ cell histology (Sarici, Telli, and Eroğlu, 2013). Patients most often present with a painless mass but can present with a dull ache or less commonly acute pain (Gilligan et al., 2019).

22.2.2 Seminoma

The initial management of a suspected testicular malignancy involves radical inguinal orchiectomy with high ligation of the spermatic cord. This approach is preferred over a transcrotal approach as there is a concern for seeding of the scrotal skin and spread to the lymphatic drainage (Khan et al., 2007). Up-front radical orchiectomy serves as definitive treatment and allows for the establishment of a histopathologic diagnosis. If life-threatening metastatic disease is present with elevated tumor markers, patients can be treated with upfront chemotherapy with delay of orchiectomy (Gilligan et al., 2019).

Historically, the standard of care for post-orchiectomy radiotherapy for seminoma was elective treatment of the inguinal, iliac, para-aortic, mediastinal, and supraclavicular lymph nodes (Maier et al., 1968). Over the past 40 years, the treatment paradigm for adjuvant radiation therapy has seen an evolution from large volume higher dose radiotherapy to smaller volumes and lower dose. This evolution has been largely fueled by several retrospective studies demonstrating increased cardiac toxicity and secondary malignancies (Hay, Duncan, and Kerr, 1984; Sherman et al., 1990; Steinfeldet al., 1990; Mccormick, Abramson, and Ellsworth, 1994; Zagars et al., 2015). Perhaps most notably, MD Anderson published their experience of 453 early stage patients, all having received adjuvant radiation, who were cured of their cancer. Beyond 15 years from the completion of radiation treatment, overall mortality was 1.85 times than what was predicted based on expected survival curves. Secondary cancer and cardiac mortality were 2.02 and 1.95 times that expected, respectively. This paradigm shift to reduced field and dose radiotherapy was also fueled by the incidence of acute and late gastrointestinal toxicity associated with abdominal radiation (Dieckmann et al., 1996). The German testicular cancer group published a single arm prospective study of 675 patients with stage I testicular seminoma treated with a para-aortic field without inclusion of the ipsilateral pelvic lymph nodes to 26 Gy. Disease-free and disease-specific survivals were 95.8% and 99.6% at 5 years, respectively, and 94.9% and 99.6% at 8 years, respectively. These results were similar to published reports of patients treated with inclusion of the ipsilateral pelvic lymph nodes (Bamberg et al., 1999). Reduced dose was evaluated in a randomized study in which patients with stage I seminoma were randomized to 30 Gy vs. 20 Gy. The authors found that patients receiving 30 Gy experienced significantly more moderate-to-severe lethargy (20% vs. 5%) and an inability to perform their normal work (46% vs. 28%) within the first 12 weeks from therapy, with similar rate of relapse between the arms (Jones et al., 2005).

Chemotherapy with single agent carboplatin in stage I disease has emerged as an alternative adjuvant therapy. Oliver et al. published their results of a large randomized trial including 1,477 patients, comparing adjuvant radiation to one injection of adjuvant carboplatin. Relapse-free survival rates were similar for radiation and chemotherapy (96.7 % vs. 97.7% at 2 years and 95.9% vs. 94.8% at 3 years, respectively). Rates of lethargy and time off of work were lower in the chemotherapy arm (Oliver et al., 2005).

Given the excellent cure rates and the concerns regarding acute and late morbidity associated with radiation, surveillance has emerged as an alternative to adjuvant therapy. Perhaps the most comprehensive published study on this approach is a systematic review of testis cancer surveillance literature which demonstrated a cause-specific survival of 99.7% in seminoma patients who proceed with surveillance (Groll, Warde, and Jewett, 2007). Critics of the observation approach point to the 17% relapse rate and thus the potential for salvage therapy, which may be more toxic, the need for longer follow-up, and the potential for greater psychological stress (Krege et al., 2008). Nonetheless, in stage I patients, given the high cure rate of salvage therapy, surveillance is the preferred approach as per NCCN, though radiotherapy or carboplatin remains acceptable alternatives. In stage IIA disease, patients should be treated with adjuvant radiation or multi-agent chemotherapy, and in stage IIB disease, the preferred adjuvant therapy is multi-agent chemotherapy with radiation being an acceptable alternative in select non-bulky disease (Sarma, Mclaughlin, and Schottenfeld, 2009). In patients who decline or are not good candidates for chemotherapy in stage I and II disease and who are hesitant to proceed with surveillance or are deemed to be noncompliant with follow-up in stage I disease, adjuvant radiation is the recommended approach. The current standard of care following orchiectomy for patients with stage I disease is 20–25.5 Gy to the para-aortic chain. For patients with stage II disease, treatment is to the para-aortic and ipsilateral iliac lymph nodes (modified "dogleg") with a boost to the gross nodes to a total dose of 30 Gy (Sarma, Mclaughlin, and Schottenfeld, 2009).

22.2.3 Intensity Modulated Radiotherapy

Intensity modulated radiotherapy (IMRT) is an advanced form of radiotherapy that employs nonuniform intensity of radiation beams and computerized inverse planning, allowing for the delivery of highly conformal radiation dose to targets with irregular shapes. This treatment modality allows for dose escalation with better sparing of neighboring organs at risk from high-dose radiation (Taylor and Powell, 2004). While IMRT has demonstrated dosimetric and clinical superiority in the treatment of various disease sites, it can increase the integral dose and total irradiated volume, thereby potentially increasing the risk of secondary malignancies (Hall et al., 2003). Given the young age and high cure rate of patients with seminoma, the risk of secondary cancers is higher when compared to most malignancies, thus IMRT is not the recommended radiation treatment modality.

22.2.4 Proton-beam Therapy

Given its characteristic Bragg peak, proton-beam therapy has the potential to deliver a highly conformal dose distribution (similar to IMRT), while also minimizing integral dose to the healthy tissues. The use of protons compared to photon-based radiotherapy can minimize radiation dose to neighboring stomach, pancreas, small bowel, large bowel, kidneys, liver, rectum, and bladder, potentially reducing the risk of acute and late toxicity.

A dosimetric advantage in stage I seminoma was demonstrated by Simone et al. in which the authors compared protons to photons in 10 consecutive patients. They demonstrated a statistically significant decrease in dose to the stomach, pancreas, large bowel, and liver (most dramatic difference was mean dose to the stomach). In patients who had a life expectancy of at least 40 years, they predicted a reduction of one secondary malignancy per 50 patients treated with protons vs. photons (Simone et al., 2012). Hoppe et al. published a dosimetric analysis in which they planned two representative patients with seminomas for stage I and II seminoma with 3D CRT, IMRT, and protons. Proton therapy demonstrated a reduction in mean dose to stomach, ipsilateral kidney, pancreas, bowel space, small bowel, and colon in stage I seminoma. For stage II disease, they were able to reduce dose to the aforementioned in addition to bladder and rectum (Hoppe et al., 2013). Efstathiou et al. similarly published a dosimetric analysis in which they analyzed 10 stage I patients treated with 3D CRT to 25.5 Gy and generated comparative proton plans. The authors demonstrated a decreased equivalent uniform dose by 46% for stomach and 64% to large bowel. The volume of whole body normal tissue spared 0.1 Gy was 9 L for PA and 7.8 L for AP/PA. Based on this difference, it was predicted that proton therapy would decrease the risk of secondary malignancies by 612 per 10,000 patients treated (Efstathiou et al., 2012).

A clinical difference has been demonstrated at least retrospectively in a SEER database analysis in which the investigators evaluated 559 patients treated with protons, matched to 558 SEER patients treated with photons. At a median follow-up of 6.7 years, they found a 5.2% rate of second malignancies in patients treated with proton, 7.5% in patients treated with photon. Once adjusted for sex, age at treatment, primary site, and year of diagnosis, proton therapy was not associated with a risk of developing a secondary malignancy.

Taken together, given the young age of most patients with a seminoma and risk of acute-, subacute-, and long-term treatment morbidities, proton-beam therapy should be strongly considered for treatment of patients with classic seminoma if the clinical scenario warrants adjuvant RT as compared to chemotherapy or surveillance.

22.2.5 Simulation and Treatment Planning

A planning noncontrast CT scan is acquired with the patient in the supine position. In contrast to simulation for photon therapy, testicular shielding should not be used as scattering neutrons are produced when protons hit a heavy-metal target. The para-aortic CTV volume is generated by creating a 1.2–1.9-cm expansion from the aorta and inferior vena cava which is modified around natural barriers. The superior border should extend to the T10/T11 interspace and the inferior border should extend to the L5/S1 interspace (Table 22.2). When including the pelvic lymph nodes, a 7-mm expansion from iliac vessels is generated. Loops of bowel must be contoured so that density override is possible during proton planning, though bowel bags may be used for constraints when clinically appropriate.

In stage I patients, an SFO (single field optimization) plan should be generated, typically utilizing two posterior obliques for treatment of the para-aortic nodes. For stage II patients who are treated with a modified dogleg, a MFO (multi-field optimization) plan should be generated, utilizing two lateral or anterior oblique beams, a posterior beam (without rectal block, but blocking inguinals), and an anterior beam with a range shifter if treating the inguinal nodes (to help increase superficial coverage of the inguinals) (Figure 22.1; Table 22.1).

Table 22.1   Comparison of doses given to organs at risk for proton vs 3D plans.

Anatomic region of interest	PROTON planDVH value		3D planDVH value	
Left kidney D15 < 20 Gy	D15	13.2 Gy	D15	21 Gy
Right kidney D50 < 8 Gy	D50	0.3 Gy	D50	19.7 Gy
Total kidney mean	4.4 Gy		15.2 Gy	
Liver mean dose	2.3 Gy		13.6 Gy	
Bowel max dose	37 Gy		37.9 Gy	
Spinal cord max dose	21.9 Gy		24.3 Gy	
Stomach mean dose	15.2 Gy		25.6 Gy	
Duodenum mean dose	2.7 Gy		18.0 Gy	

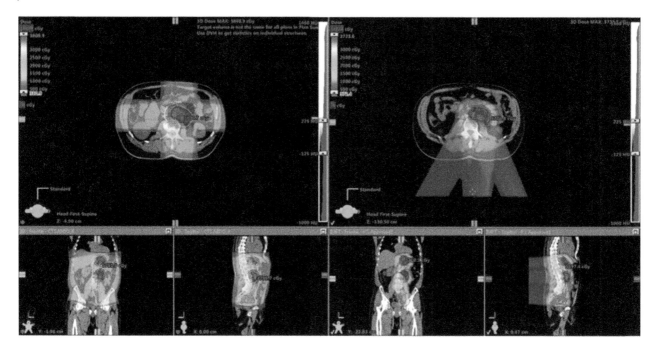

Figure 22.1 Figure of intensity modulated proton therapy with pencil beam scanning versus 3D CRT photon comparative plan (photon on left, proton on right). The above patient was a 65-year-old with Stage IIB T2N2M0S0 pure seminoma of the left testicle). Underwent orchiectomy but declined chemotherapy. The patient underwent proton therapy which he tolerated well with mild fatigue and acute nausea managed with anti-emetics. He had no late toxicity. He was prescribed 20 Gy to the elective para-aortic and ipsilateral pelvic lymph nodes (modified "dog-leg") with a 16-Gy small-field boost to the gross nodes. This was a three field MFO plan with one posterior and two posterior-oblique beams. The proton plan was able to significantly reduce dose to the bilateral kidneys, liver, stomach, and duodenum.

Table 22.2 Recommended target volumes for seminoma.

Stage	Volume	Definitive	Postoperative	Dose
IA, IB	CTV	Para-aortic chain	–	20–25.5 Gy (RBE) in 10–17 fractions
IIA	GTV	Gross lymph node as delineated on CT imaging + 5 mm CTV expansion		Cone down to gross node to a total dose of 30 Gy RBE
	CTV	Modified dog leg		20–25.5 Gy (RBE) in 10–17 fractions
IIB	GTV	Gross lymph node as delineated on CT imaging 5 mm CTV expansion		Cone down to gross node to a total dose of 36 Gy RBE
	CTV	Modified dog leg		20–25.5 Gy (RBE) in 10–17 fractions

CTV = Clinical target volume; GTV = gross tumor volume.

22.3 Bladder Cancer

22.3.1 Background

Bladder cancer is the 9th most common cancer worldwide and 13th most common cause of death from cancer (Antoni et al., 2017; Cumberbatch et al., 2018). Risk factors include cigarette smoking, exposure to aromatic amines, polycyclic aromatic hydrocarbons, hair dyes, schistosomiasis, history of UTIs, drinking tap-water with chlorination by-products or arsenic, cyclophosphamide, heavy use of phenacetin-containing anal-

gesics, and prior exposure to radiation (Pelucchi et al., 2006). Greater than 90% of bladder cancers are urothelial carcinoma and patients most commonly present with hematuria (Chalasani, Chin, and Izawa, 2009).

Bladder cancer can be classified as either muscle invasive bladder cancer (MIBC) or non-MIBC. MIBC (T2–T4) was classically treated with cystectomy, though radiotherapy ± concurrent chemotherapy preceded by maximal transurethral resection of bladder tumor (TURBT) has emerged as the bladder preservation treatment paradigm and is often utilized in patients who are not surgical candidates due to medical comorbidity, advanced age or in those who do not want to undergo cystectomy. In patients who undergo definitive radiotherapy, cystectomy can then be reserved as a salvage option. Neoadjuvant radiotherapy is often utilized to downstage patients prior to cystectomy. Additionally, as per NCCN adjuvant radiotherapy following cystectomy is a category 2B recommendation for positive margins, positive nodes, or pT3/T4 disease (Morgan et al., 2010).

22.3.2 Proton Therapy

The rationale for proton therapy includes the potential for dose escalation which may improve rates of local control, as well as the ability to spare critical organs at risk such as the small and large bowel, the rectum, bone marrow, and uninvolved bladder wall. This may be of more significance in cases of re-irradiation when normal tissue dose constraints cannot be met with photon therapy, or in the postoperative setting given tissue hypoxia and postsurgical scarring, both contributing to the potential risk of late radiation toxicity.

The University of Tsukuba (Japan) published a retrospective review on the role of proton therapy as part of tri-modality bladder preservation therapy. Patients with cT2-3N0M0 bladder cancer were treated with TURBT followed by small pelvic external beam radiotherapy to 41.4 Gy in 23 fractions and concurrent intra-arterial chemotherapy with methotrexate and CDDP followed by proton therapy to the primary site to 36.3 GyE in 11 fractions. One-hundred and thirty-five patients were treated with the induction regimen of TURBT, small pelvis radiation with concurrent chemotherapy. Only those patients who demonstrated a complete response received a small field boost to the primary site with proton therapy. Those who had an incomplete response underwent a radical cystectomy. Tumor response was established with rebiopsy of the primary site, urine cytology, and imaging. One-hundred and fifteen patients (85.1%) experienced a complete response. Seventy of those underwent proton therapy, the rest chose either a photon boost, cystectomy, or declined further treatment. Patients underwent tumor reevaluation 3–4 weeks after induction therapy, which included a biopsy of the primary site, urine cytology, and diagnostic imaging. At a median follow-up of 3.4 years, 3-year overall survival, progression-free survival, and time to progression rates were 90%, 80%, and 82%, respectively, for patients treated with protons. Eighteen percent demonstrated acute grade 3–4 acute hematologic toxicity and 3% had late grade GU toxicity. No patients discontinued therapy due to acute toxicity (Takaoka et al., 2017). Though retrospective, the above-described trimodality bladder preservation therapy with proton therapy as a small field boost demonstrated that dose escalation with protons is feasible, with a high local control rate and an acceptable rate of grade ≥3 toxicities.

Meeting normal tissue dose constraints, particularly for the small bowel, can often be challenging when treating bladder cancer with radiotherapy. This challenge is only compounded in the setting of re-irradiation. Though there may exist scenarios where clinically appropriate, treating with protons as opposed to photons introduces a set of challenges. This is due to end-rage uncertainties secondary to organ motion, setup reproducibility, dose calculation approximations, and variations of relative biological effectiveness (RBE) across the spread out Bragg peak (SOBP) with data suggesting a significant increase in RBE at the distal edge and distal fall-off (Paganetti, 2012; Lühr et al., 2018). These present themselves as even more of a challenge in bladder cancer as achieving reproducible bladder volumes from the time of simulation through the duration of treatment can be difficult to achieve, particularly as acute radiation cystitis sets in over the course of treatment. Proton therapy thus serves as a more attractive treatment modality in the post-cystectomy scenario (in cases where post-cystectomy radiotherapy is indicated) where bladder position is not an issue. Photon therapy does not have as steep of a dose fall-off as proton therapy, and thus less of a risk of missing the target volume with motion compared to proton therapy. Thus, if treating with protons, a full and empty bladder internal target volume (ITV) should be created to ensure target coverage. But that technique itself will likely just increase the volume exposed to the high-dose isodose lines, thus increasing dose to organs at risk. Additionally, though we recognize there is variation from practitioner to practitioner, at our institution we generally use a 1-cm CTV margin extension from the bladder. As the small bowel may not overlap to a significant degree with the CTV target created from the CT simulation, the small bowel is a mobile organ and may very well fall into the field periodically throughout treatment, thus receiving more radiation dose than what was predicted. While this is an inherent challenge regardless of treatment modality, given the increased RBE at the distal range of the proton beam, this "end-ranging" effect can result in the overdose of an organ at risk, possibly resulting in significant morbidity. Thus, proton therapy can be considered if unable to meet normal organ constraints, in cases of re-irradiation, or if there's a history of prior abdominal/pelvic surgeries, inflammatory bowel disease or other significant gastrointestinal pathology, or if patients have cytopenias or become cytopenic when undergoing chemotherapy. However, we recommend generating a comparative IMRT/volumetric modulated arc therapy (VMAT) plan for all patients undergoing proton planning. These should be created and evaluated with careful attention to meeting normal organ dose constraints while not significantly sacrificing target coverage and ensuring the proton plan is robustly optimized.

22.3.3 Neutron Therapy

Though not as widely used as protons, neutrons have been investigated at various centers as a radiation treatment modality for bladder cancer. Neutrons have high linear energy transfer (LET) properties in comparison to photons and possess a RBE that is three times that of photons (Russell et al., 1989). This difference in RBE has prompted investigators to evaluate the effectiveness of neutron therapy for the treatment of bladder cancer, given the relative radioresistance of this malignancy. A review of the literature reveals mixed results with some studies demonstrating a high percentage of severe complications (Laramore et al., 1984; Duncan et al., 1985; Pointon, Read, and Greene, 1985; Batterman et al, 1986). However, a criticism of these older studies is they utilized now-outdated equipment which had poor dose penetration. It is possible as centers begin to use next-generation cyclotrons that have more desirable dose penetration; neutron therapy may emerge as an effective treatment, though randomized clinical trials comparing it to the standard of care are needed to change practice.

22.3.4 Simulation and Treatment Planning for Proton Therapy

A planning noncontrast CT scan is acquired with the patient in the supine position. An empty and full bladder scan should be obtained. The bladder should be emptied 10–15 min before simulation and treatment. Patients should be asked to empty their rectum. Oral contrast can be used if small bowel will be within the radiation field based on review of prior diagnostic imaging. In contrast to simulation for photon therapy, testicular shielding should not be used as scattering neutrons are produced when protons hit a heavy-metal target. If planning partial bladder boost, patients should be resimulated with a comfortably full bladder. This limits the volume of uninvolved bladder receiving boost dose, though it is very likely the patient may not be able to hold a full bladder due to acute urinary symptoms secondary to radiation. Fiducials should ideally be placed at the time of TURBT to help with target delineation and to assist in alignment with image-guidance.

For an intact bladder, an initial CTV volume is generated which includes the whole bladder plus a 0.6-cm margin if no extravesicular changes and 1 cm if extravesicular changes are present. This is prescribed 41.4–50.4 Gy in 1.8 Gy per fraction. The boost volume consists of the gross disease plus a 1-cm margin and is prescribed to a total dose of 61.2–64.8 Gy per fraction. If treating the whole bladder, then prescribe the aforementioned boost dose to the whole bladder (Table 22.3).

For image guidance, when treating with photons we perform radiographs every fraction and cone-beam computed tomography (CBCT) first three fractions and then weekly. However, when treating with protons, we recommend daily CBCT to ensure bladder position reproducibility and confirm that a significant amount of bowel has not fallen within the radiation field. We recommend weekly QA-CT.

Our beam arrangement consists of a three-field approach with a posterior beam and two posterior oblique beams to best spare small bowel and bone marrows (Figure 22.2). Similar to other pelvic disease sites, if hip prostheses are present, care should be taken use beam angles which avoid the prostheses.

22.4 Kidney and Renal Pelvis

Cancers of the kidney and the renal pelvis result in approximately 73,000 new cancer diagnoses a year with approximately 14,830 deaths in the United States (Siegel, Miller, and Jemal, 2020). They occur more frequently in men with associated risk factors being cigarette smoking, obesity, and hypertension along with familial cancer syndromes such as Von Hippel–Lindau Syndrome and hereditary papillary renal cell carcinoma (Chow, Dong, and Devesa, 2010).

The general treatment paradigm for cancers of the renal pelvis includes surgery, with the role of radiation therapy to the primary mass historically relegated to symptom palliation (Tselis and Chatzikonstantinou, 2019). While adjuvant radiotherapy may be considered for select cases of urethral cancers of the renal pelvis or in the setting of renal cell carcinoma with positive margins or lymph node involvement, it is generally not recommended (Tselis and Chatzikonstantinou,

Table 22.3 Recommended target volumes for bladder cancer.

Volume	Definitive	Postoperative (category 2B for patients with pT3pT4 disease following radical cystectomy with ileal conduit)	Dose
Initial CTV	–	Area at risk for having residual microscopic disease (may include cystectomy bed and pelvic lymph nodes)	45–50.4 Gy (RBE) in 25–28 fractions
Boost CTV	–	Involved margins and areas of ECE	Cone down to a total dose of 54–60 Gy in 1.8 Gy per fraction if normal tissue constraints allow

CTV = Clinical target volume.

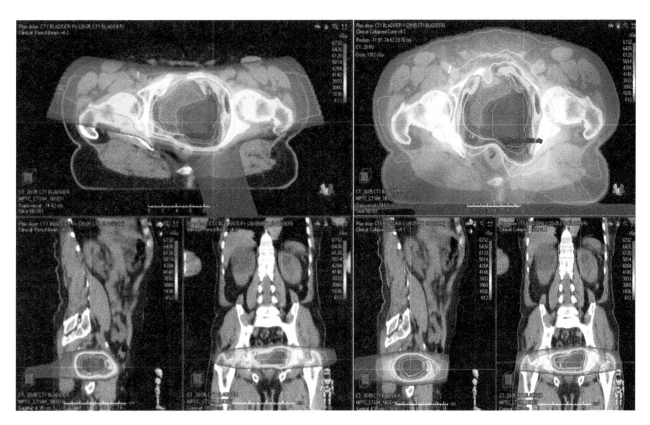

Figure 22.2 Figure of intensity modulated proton therapy with pencil beam scanning versus VMAT photon comparative plan (proton on left, photon on right). The above patient was an 85-year-old male with a history of prostate cancer treated 20 years ago with external beam radiotherapy followed by radioactive seed implants, who presented to us with stage IIIA (T3bN0M0) high-grade muscle invasive urothelial carcinoma involving the left bladder and extending into the trigone with perivesicular involvement. Given his prior history of radiation, he was referred to us for proton therapy. Besides the inherent challenge of treating bladder cancer with protons due to bladder position uncertainty, this particular case made protons less than ideal due to the presence of radioactive seeds. Though we can usually treat through metal by performing a density override, radioactive seeds are small and numerous and there will be day-to-day variability in their position, making it impossible to do a density override. Additionally, there was small bowel that was abutting the superior and right lateral bladder wall. Two opposed lateral beams would have been the beam arrangement of choice to minimize a large volume of bowel falling within the beams path, but such an arrangement would have resulted in significant "end-ranging" on that loop of small bowel abutting the bladder. To meet are small bowel constraints and minimize the degree of "end-ranging" on the small bowel, we would have had to significantly undercover the boost volume with a non-robust plan. A comparative VMAT plan was generated which demonstrated superior target coverage which met our small bowel constraints. Thus, we proceeded with the VMAT plan.

2019). Historic randomized trials demonstrated clinical detriment with high rates of severe complication associated with adjuvant therapy including several grade 5 toxicities (Finney, 1973; Kjaer, Iversen, and Hvidt et al., 1987). While these trials utilized older radiotherapy techniques, given the rarity of local recurrences (approximately ~2%), there is unlikely to be a clinically meaningful benefit to adjuvant treatment standardly even if the toxicity profile is reduced with advanced techniques such as VMAT or particle therapy. Unsurprisingly, retrospective studies with more modern techniques reported disappointing results with adjuvant radiotherapy being associated with increased toxicity and lack of survival improvement (Gez et al., 2002; Ulutin et al., 2006).

While surgery will remain the standard for localized disease, SBRT is an emerging treatment option in special circumstances where surgery is contraindicated such as medically inoperable patients or unique clinical situations (i.e., unilateral kidney or bilateral disease). So far reports of patients treated with SBRT with photon-based techniques have demonstrated local control rates of varying between 60% and 90% with acceptable rates of toxicity (Ponsky, Lo, and Zhang et al., 2015).

Historically, there was also a defined role for surgery with cytoreductive nephrectomy in patients with metastatic renal cell carcinoma. Non-randomized retrospective analyses suggested higher rates of response to systemic therapy following nephrectomy which prompted further investigation. A randomized trial comparing radical nephrectomy followed by interferon alfa-2b versus interferon alfa-2b therapy alone with improved median survival in the nephrectomy group (Flanigan, Salmon, and Blumenstein et al., 2001; Choueiri and Motzer, 2017). However, since this trial has been reported, systemic options for patients with metastatic renal cell carcinoma have expanded to include VEGF-targeted therapies and immune checkpoint inhibitors which have drastically increased efficacy compared to interferon based treatment (Choueiri and Motzer, 2017). In the era of improved systemic therapy, more recent randomized trials in patients with metastatic renal cell carcinoma found sunitinib alone to be noninferior to nephrectomy and sunitinib (Méjean, Ravaud, and Thezenas et al., 2018; Bex, Mulders, and Jewett et al., 2019). Following the results of these trials, cytoreductive nephrectomy is now mainly be offered in specific, well-selected patients to avoid unnecessary morbidity (Culp, 2015; Bhindi, Abel, and Albiges et al., 2019; Larcher, Wallis, and Bex et al., 2019).

While local therapy with surgery is falling out of favor in most patients with metastatic renal cell carcinoma, there is an emerging interest in combining radiotherapy with immune checkpoint blockade to potentially achieve a synergistic immunostimulatory interaction in a multitude of disease sites (Wang, Deng, and Li et al., 2018). Clinical trials combining SBRT to primary or metastatic sites of disease with immune checkpoint blockade are ongoing areas of research and could potentially expand the role of radiotherapy in renal cell carcinoma (Hammers, Vonmerveldt, and Ahn et al., 2020; Lalani, Swaminath, and Pond et al., 2020).

As the role of radiotherapy has the potential to expand in the coming years for medically inoperable patients with local disease and possibly patients with metastatic renal cell carcinoma, the advantages of particle therapy in this disease site must be explored. In challenging clinical scenarios such as when there is abutment of the clinical target volume by small or large bowel, particle therapy may be of particular benefit. There is also potential reduction in radiation doses to other critical OARs, such as the contralateral kidney and potentially the uninvolved ipsilateral kidney. With improved OAR sparing, particle therapy may allow for dose escalate with possibly improved local control. Given the radioresistance of renal cell carcinoma, dose escalation may be especially important.

Dosimetric studies comparing Gamma Knife SBRT, VMAT, and proton therapy have shown equivalent to improved coverage of the clinical target volume with improved OAR sparing with proton therapy (Baydoun, Vapiwala, and Ponsky et al., 2018). Clinical outcomes of patients treated with particle therapy are an emerging body of research that will continue to mature as particle therapy becomes more widely accessible and the role of radiotherapy in renal cell carcinoma continues to evolve.

The short-term results of proton SBRT have been reported on a patient with bilateral renal cell carcinoma. The patient had only a marginal decrease in glomerular filtration rate when compared to baseline at 1-year follow-up (Frick et al., n.d.).

So far, small series of patients being treated with carbon ion therapy have been reported with encouraging results. One prospective clinical trial demonstrated 100% local control and no grade 3 or higher treatment toxicities in eight patients with a median follow-up of 43.1 months (Kasuya, Tsuji, and Nomiya et al., 2019). Another retrospective analysis of 19 patients who underwent carbon-ion radiotherapy demonstrated excellent local control and acceptable rates of renal function preservation. There were no non-urologic grade 3 toxicities and progression to advanced chronic kidney disease occurred only in a minority of patients with pre-existing renal comorbidities such as solitary kidney, diabetic nephropathy, or sclerotic kidney (Kasuya, Tsuji, and Nomiya et al., 2018).

22.4.1   Simulation and Treatment Planning

Patients should be simulated supine with an empty bladder. An immobilization device such as a vac lock or an alpha cradle should also be employed to limit patient motion. Noncontrast CT images should be for treatment planning. For motion management, a 4D CT should be obtained for the generation of an ITV target to account for any motion. If there is significant motion during 4D CT, then SDX or other breath hold technology could be employed to reduce motion. Three scans with SDX should be obtained and an ITV should be generated from these scans to account for slight differences between breath

Table 22.4   Recommended target volumes for renal cell carcinoma proton SBRT.

Volume	Definitive	Postoperative	Dose
GTV	Gross tumor as delineated on CT imaging; MRI fusion may be helpful to define tumor extent	–	40–50 Gy (RBE) in 5 fractions per tolerance of surrounding structures
ITV	GTV should be contoured in all respiratory phases to generate an ITV	–	40–50 Gy (RBE) in 5 fractions per tolerance of surrounding structures

holds. OARs such as spinal cord, liver, small bowel, large bowel, ipsilateral, and contralateral kidneys should be contoured for treatment planning purposes. To evaluate dose to the uninvolved ipsilateral kidney, a kidney minus GTV structure should be generated.

In general, posterior oblique beams should be utilized to minimize setup differences that may occur from bladder filling, pannus, and other patient-specific factors. When possible, the plan should attempt to be SFO (Figures 22.3 and 22.4 and Tables 22.4 and 22.5). When delivering radiotherapy with SBRT dosing, we recommended the utilizing of dose repainting to minimize the interplay effect. Additionally, daily IGRT with kV and CBCT should be performed in accordance with institutional practices.

22.4.2 Future Directions

Taken together, the evident dosimetric benefits associated with particle therapy for treatment of non-prostate genitourinary malignancies requiring radiation therapy support the need for robust clinical trials. Given the continued of expansion of proton centers nationally and internationally, it is our hope that these trials will be performed, and we will see published prospective data in the not-too-distant future. Outside of a clinical trial, patients with known risk factors for developing radiation toxicity should be considered for particle therapy, as should patients in whom established dose constraints cannot be achieved when using photon therapy.

Table 22.5 Recommended target volumes for adjuvant radiotherapy for carcinomas of the renal pelvis and bladder.

Volume	Definitive	Postoperative	Dose
Postoperative bed (CTV54)	–	Postoperative bed contoured per clinician judgment incorporating preoperative imaging, surgical records, and consultation with performing surgeon	54 Gy (RBE) with standard fractionation; if OAR constraints cannot be met, may reduce dose or consider SIB approach
Interval target volume (ITV54)	–	If there is significant motion of target, CTV54 should be contoured in all respiratory phases to generate an ITV	54 Gy (RBE) with standard fractionation; if OAR constraints cannot be met, may reduce dose or consider SIB approach

CTV = Clinical target volume; ITV = internal target motion.

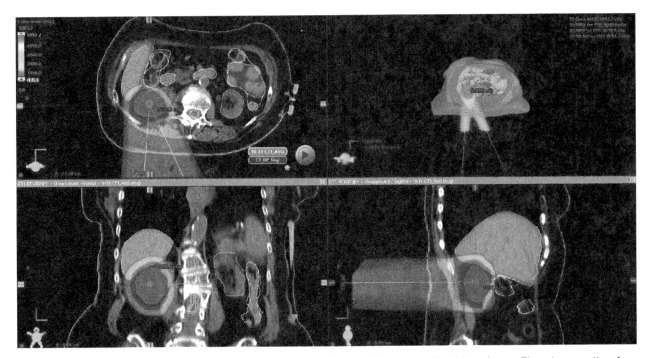

Figure 22.3 An example of a proton SBRT plan for renal cell carcinoma with two posterior oblique beams. These images allow for visualization of the advantages of the steep dose fall-off with protons particularly in sparing of the adjacent small bowel and liver.

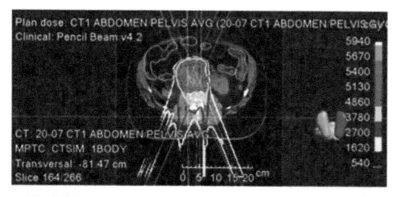

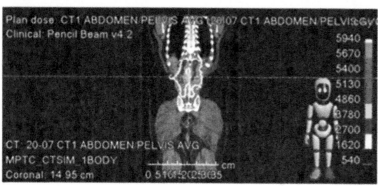

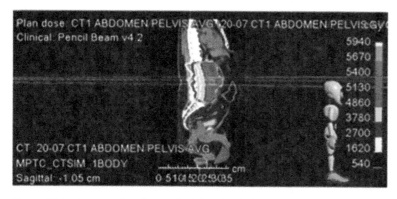

Figure 22.4 An example of a standard fractionated EBRT plan utilizing proton therapy as adjuvant therapy for a T3N1 high-grade papillary urothelial carcinoma of the right renal pelvis and bladder.

References

Antoni, S., Ferlay, J., Soerjomataram, I., Znaor, A., Jemal, A., and Bray, F. (2017). Bladder Cancer Incidence and Mortality: A global overview and recent trends. *European Urology* 71 (1): 96–108. https://doi.org/10.1016/j.eururo.2016.06.010.

Bamberg, M., Schmidberger, H., Meisner, C., Classen, J., Souchon, R., Weinknecht, S., Schorcht, J., Walter, F., Engenhart-Cabillic, R., Schulz, U., Born, H., and Flink, M. (1999). Radiotherapy for stages I and IIA/B testicular seminoma. *International Journal of Cancer* 83 (6): 823–827. https://onlinelibrary.wiley.com/doi/full/10.1002/(SICI)1097-0215(19991210)83:6<823::AID-IJC22>3.0.CO;2-V.

Batterman, J.J. and Mijnheer, B.J. (1986). The Amsterdam Fast Neutron Therapy Project: A final report. *International Journal of Radiation Oncology*Biology*Physics* 12 (12): 2093–2099. https://doi.org/10.1016/0360-3016(86)90007-6.

Baydoun, A., Vapiwala, N., Ponsky, L.E. et al. (2018). Comparative analysis for renal stereotactic body radiotherapy using Cyberknife, VMAT and proton therapy based treatment planning. *Journal of Applied Clinical Medical Physics* Published online March 14 10.1002/acm2.12308.

Bex, A., Mulders, P., Jewett, M. et al. (2019). Comparison of Immediate vs Deferred Cytoreductive Nephrectomy in patients with synchronous Metastatic Renal Cell Carcinoma Receiving Sunitinib: The SURTIME randomized clinical trial. *JAMA Oncology* 5 (2): 164–170. doi:10.1001/jamaoncol.2018.5543.

Bhindi, B., Abel, E.J., Albiges, L. et al. (2019). Systematic review of the role of Cytoreductive Nephrectomy in the Targeted

Therapy Era and Beyond: An individualized approach to metastatic Renal Cell Carcinoma. *European Urology* 75 (1): 111–128. doi:10.1016/j.eururo.2018.09.016.

Chalasani, V., Chin, J.L., and Izawa, J.I. (2009). Histologic variants of urothelial bladder cancer and nonurothelial histology in bladder cancer. *Journal of the Canadian Urological Association* 3 (6 SUPPL. 4): 193–198. https://doi.org/10.5489/cuaj.1195.

Choueiri, T.K. and Motzer, R.J. (2017). Systemic therapy for Metastatic Renal-Cell Carcinoma. *The New England Journal of Medicine* 376 (4): 354–366. 10.1056/NEJMra1601333.

Chow, W.-H., Dong, L.M., and Devesa, S.S. (2010). Epidemiology and risk factors for kidney cancer. *Nature Reviews Urology* 7 (5): 245–257. doi:10.1038/nrurol.2010.46.

Culp, S.H. (2015). Cytoreductive nephrectomy and its role in the present-day period of targeted therapy. *Therapeutic Advances in Urology* 7 (5): 275–285. doi:10.1177/1756287215585501.

Cumberbatch, M.G.K., Jubber, I., Black, P.C., Esperto, F., Figueroa, J.D., Kamat, A.M., Kiemeney, L., Lotan, Y., Pang, K., Silverman, D.T., Znaor, A., and Catto, J.W.F. (2018). Epidemiology of bladder cancer: A systematic review and contemporary update of risk factors in 2018. *European Urology* 74 (6): 784–795. https://doi.org/10.1016/j.eururo.2018.09.001.

Dieckmann, K.P., Krain, J., Küster, J., and Brüggeboes, B. (1996). Adjuvant carboplatin treatment for seminoma clinical stage I. *Journal of Cancer Research and Clinical Oncology* 122 (1): 63–66. https://doi.org/10.1007/BF01203075.

Duncan, W., Arnott, S.J., Jack, W.J.L., Macdougall, R.H., Quilty, P.M., Rodger, A., Kerr, G.R., and Williams, J.R. (1985). A report of a randomized trial of d(15)+Be neutrons compared with megavoltage X ray therapy of bladder cancer. *International Journal of Radiation Oncology, Biology, Physics* 11 (12): 2043–2049. https://doi.org/10.1016/0360-3016(85)90082-3.

Efstathiou, J.A., Paly, J.J., Lu, H.M., Athar, B.S., Moteabbed, M., Niemierko, A., Adams, J.A., Bekelman, J.E., Shipley, W.U., Zietman, A.L., and Paganetti, H. (2012). Adjuvant radiation therapy for early stage seminoma: Proton versus photon planning comparison and modeling of second cancer risk. *Radiotherapy and Oncology* 103 (1): 12–17. https://doi.org/10.1016/j.radonc.2012.01.012.

Finney, R. (1973). The value of radiotherapy in the treatment of hypernephroma: a clinical trial. *Br Journal of Urology* 45 (3): 258–269. doi:10.1111/j.1464-410X.1973.tb12152.x.

Flanigan, R.C., Salmon, S.E., Blumenstein, B.A. et al. (2001). Nephrectomy followed by interferon alfa-2b compared with interferon alfa-2b alone for metastatic renal-cell cancer. *The New England Journal of Medicine* 345 (23): 1655–1659. doi:10.1056/NEJMoa003013.

Frick, M.A., Chhabra, A.M., Lin, L., and Simone, C.B. n.d. first ever use of proton stereotactic body radiation therapy delivered with curative intent to bilateral synchronous primary Renal Cell Carcinomas. *Cureus* 9 (10): doi:10.7759/cureus.1799.

Gez, E., Libes, M., Bar-Deroma, R., Rubinov, R., Stein, M., and Kuten, A. (2002). Postoperative irradiation in localized renal cell carcinoma: The Rambam Medical Center experience. *Tumori* 88 (6): 500–502.

Gilligan, T., Lin, D.W., Aggarwal, R., Chism, D., Cost, N., Derweesh, I.H., Emamekhoo, H., Feldman, D.R., Geynisman, D.M., Hancock, S.L., LaGrange, C., Levine, E.G., Longo, T., Lowrance, W., McGregor, B., Monk, P., Picus, J., Pierorazio, P., Rais-Bahrami, S., and Pluchino, L.A. (2019). Testicular cancer, version 2.2020. *JNCCN Journal of the National Comprehensive Cancer Network* 17 (12): 1529–1554. https://doi.org/10.6004/jnccn.2019.0058.

Groll, R.J., Warde, P., and Jewett, M.A.S. (2007). A comprehensive systematic review of testicular germ cell tumor surveillance. *Critical Reviews in Oncology/Hematology* 64 (3): 182–197. https://doi.org/10.1016/j.critrevonc.2007.04.014.

Hall, E.J. and Wuu, C.S. (2003). Radiation-induced second cancers: The impact of 3D-CRT and IMRT. *International Journal of Radiation Oncology Biology Physics* 56 (1): 83–88. https://doi.org/10.1016/S0360-3016(03)00073-7.

Hammers, H.J., Vonmerveldt, D., Ahn, C. et al. (2020). Combination of dual immune checkpoint inhibition (ICI) with stereotactic radiation (SBRT) in metastatic renal cell carcinoma (mRCC) (RADVAX RCC). *Journal of Clinical Oncology* 38 (6_suppl): 614-614. doi:10.1200/JCO.2020.38.6_suppl.614.

Hay, J.H., Duncan, W., and Kerr, G.R. (1984). Subsequent malignancies in patients irradiated for testicular tumours. *British Journal of Radiology* 57 (679): 597–602. https://doi.org/10.1259/0007-1285-57-679-597.

Hoppe, B.S., Mamalui-Hunter, M., Mendenhall, N.P., Li, Z., and Indelicato, D.J. (2013). Improving the therapeutic ratio by using proton therapy in patients with stage I or II seminoma. *American Journal of Clinical Oncology: Cancer Clinical Trials* 36 (1): 31–37. https://doi.org/10.1097/COC.0b013e3182354b9e.

Jones, W.G., Fossa, S.D., Mead, G.M., Roberts, J.T., Sokal, M., Horwich, A., and Stenning, S.P. (2005). Randomized trial of 30 versus 20 Gy in the adjuvant treatment of stage I testicular seminoma: A report on Medical Research Council Trial TE18, European Organisation for the Research and Treatment of Cancer Trial 30942 (ISRCTN18525328). *Journal of Clinical Oncology* 23 (6): 1200–1208. https://doi.org/10.1200/JCO.2005.08.003.

Kasuya, G., Tsuji, H., Nomiya, T. et al. (2018). Updated long-term outcomes after carbon-ion radiotherapy for primary renal cell carcinoma. *Cancer Science* 109 (9): 2873–2880. doi:10.1111/cas.13727.

Kasuya, G., Tsuji, H., Nomiya, T. et al. (2019). Prospective clinical trial of 12-fraction carbon-ion radiotherapy for primary renal cell carcinoma. *Oncotarget* 10 (1): 76–81. doi:10.18632/oncotarget.26539.

Khan, O. and Protheroe, A. (2007). Testis cancer. *Postgraduate Medical Journal* 83 (984): 624–632. https://doi.org/10.1136/pgmj.2007.057992.

Kjaer, M., Iversen, P., Hvidt, V. et al. (1987). A Randomized Trial of Postoperative Radiotherapy Versus Observation in Stage II and III Renal Adenocarcinoma: A study by the Copenhagen Renal Cancer Study Group. *Scandinavian Journal of Urology and Nephrology* 21 (4): 285–289. doi:10.3109/00365598709180784.

Krege, S., Beyer, J., Souchon, R., Albers, P., Albrecht, W., Algaba, F., Bamberg, M., Bodrogi, I., Bokemeyer, C., Cavallin-Ståhl, E., Classen, J., Clemm, C., Cohn-Cedermark, G., Culine, S., Daugaard, G., de Mulder, P.H.M., de Santis, M., de Wit, M., de Wit, R., and von der Maase, H. (2008). European Consensus Conference on Diagnosis and Treatment of Germ Cell Cancer: A Report of the Second Meeting of the European Germ Cell Cancer Consensus group (EGCCCG): Part I. *European Urology* 53 (3): 478–496. https://doi.org/10.1016/j.eururo.2007.12.024.

Lalani, A.-K.A., Swaminath, A., Pond, G.R. et al. (2020). Phase II trial of cytoreductive stereotactic hypofractionated radiotherapy with combination ipilimumab/nivolumab for metastatic kidney cancer (CYTOSHRINK). *Journal Clinical Oncology* 38 (6_suppl): TPS761–TPS761. doi:10.1200/JCO.2020.38.6_suppl.TPS761.

Laramore, G.E., Davis, R.B., Hussey, D.H., Griffin, T.W., Maor, M.H., Hendrickson, F.R., Davis, L.W., and Dupre, E. (1984). Radiation therapy oncology group phase I–II study on fast neutron teletherapy for carcinoma of the bladder. *Cancer* 54 (3): 432–439. https://pubmed.ncbi.nlm.nih.gov/6375854.

Larcher, A., Wallis, C.J.D., Bex, A. et al. (2019). Individualised Indications for Cytoreductive Nephrectomy: Which Criteria define the Optimal Candidates? *European Urology Oncology* 2 (4): 365–378. doi:10.1016/j.euo.2019.04.007.

Lühr, A., Von Neubeck, C., Krause, M., and Troost, E.G.C. (2018). Relative biological effectiveness in proton beam therapy – Current knowledge and future challenges. *Clinical and Translational Radiation Oncology* 9: 35–41. https://doi.org/10.1016/j.ctro.2018.01.006.

Maier G.J., Sulak H.M., and Mittemeyer T.B. (1968). Seminoma of the testis: analysis of treatment success and failure. *American Journal of Roentgenology* 102 (3): 596–602.

Mccormick, B., Abramson, D.H., and Ellsworth, R.M. (1994). 0 clinical original contribution. *Science* 29 (4): 729–733.

Méjean, A., Ravaud, A., Thezenas, S. et al. (2018). Sunitinib Alone or after Nephrectomy in Metastatic Renal-Cell Carcinoma. *The New England Journal of Medicine* 379 (5): 417–427. doi:10.1056/NEJMoa1803675.

Morgan, T.M. and Clark, P.E. (2010). Bladder cancer. *Current Opinion in Oncology* 22 (3): 242–249. https://doi.org/10.1097/CCO.0b013e3283378c6b.

Oliver, R.T.D., Mason, M.D., Mead, G.M., von der Maase, H., Rustin, G.J.S., Joffe, J.K., de Wit, R., Aass, N., Graham, J.D., Coleman, R., Kirk, S.J., and Stenning, S.P. (2005). Radiotherapy versus single-dose carboplatin in adjuvant treatment of stage I seminoma: A randomised trial. *Lancet* 366 (9482): 293–300. https://doi.org/10.1016/S0140-6736(05)66984-X.

Paganetti, H. (2012). Range uncertainties in proton therapy and the role of Monte Carlo simulations. *Physics in Medicine and Biology* 57: 11. https://iopscience.iop.org/article/10.1088/0031-9155/57/11/R99.

Pelucchi, C., Bosetti, C., Negri, E., Malvezzi, M., and la Vecchia, C. (2006). Mechanisms of disease: The epidemiology of bladder cancer. *Nature Clinical Practice Urology* 3 (6): 327–340. https://doi.org/10.1038/ncpuro0510.

Pointon, R.S., Read, G., and Greene, D. (1985). A randomised comparison of photons and 15 MeV neutrons for the treatment of carcinoma of the bladder. *British Journal of Radiology* 58 (687): 219–224. https://doi.org/10.1259/0007-1285-58-687-219.

Ponsky, L., Lo, S.S., Zhang, Y. et al. (2015). Phase I dose-escalation study of stereotactic body radiotherapy (SBRT) for poor surgical candidates with localized renal cell carcinoma. *Radiother Oncology* 117 (1): 183–187. doi:10.1016/j.radonc.2015.08.030.

Russell, K.J., M.D., Laramore, G.E., Ph.D., M.D., Griffin, T.W., M.D., Parker, R.G., M.D., Davis, L.W., M.D., and Krall, J.W., Ph.D. (1989) Fast Neutron Radiotherapy for the treatment of Carcinoma of the Urinary Bladder. *American Journal of Clinical Oncology* August 12 (4): 301–306.

Sarici, H., Telli, O., and Eroğlu, M. (2013). Bilateral testiküler germ hücreli tümörler. *Turk Uroloji Dergisi* 39 (4): 249–252. https://doi.org/10.5152/tud.2013.062.

Sarma, A., Mclaughlin, J.C., and Schottenfeld, D. (2009). Testicular Cancer. *Cancer Epidemiology and Prevention* https://doi.org/10.1093/acprof:oso/9780195149616.003.0060.

Sherman, N.E., Romsdahl, M., Evans, H., Zagars, G., and Oswald, M.J. (1990 July). Desmoid tumors: a 20-year radiotherapy experience. International Journal of Radiation Oncology Biology Physics *Original Contribution Experience* 19 (1): 37–40. doi: 10.1016/0360-3016(90)90131-3. PMID: 2380093.

Siegel, R.L., Miller, K.D., and Jemal, A. Cancer statistics. (2020). *CA Cancer Journal of Clinicians* 2020 70 (1): 7–30. doi:10.3322/caac.21590.

Simone, C.B., Kramer, K., O'Meara, W.P., Bekelman, J.E., Belard, A., McDonough, J., and O'Connell, J. (2012). Predicted rates of secondary malignancies from proton versus photon radiation therapy for stage I seminoma. *International Journal of*

Radiation Oncology Biology Physics 82 (1): 242–249. https://doi.org/10.1016/j.ijrobp.2010.11.021.

Steinfeld, A.D. and Shore, R.E. (1990). Second malignancies following radiotherapy for testicular seminoma. *Clinical Oncology* 2 (5): 273–276. https://doi.org/10.1016/S0936-6555(05)80954-9.

Takaoka, E.I., Miyazaki, J., Ishikawa, H., Kawai, K., Kimura, T., Ishitsuka, R., Kojima, T., Kanuma, R., Takizawa, D., Okumura, T., Sakurai, H., and Nishiyama, H. (2017). Long-term single-institute experience with trimodal bladder-preserving therapy with proton beam therapy for muscle-invasive bladder cancer. *Japanese Journal of Clinical Oncology* 47 (1): 67–73. https://doi.org/10.1093/jjco/hyw151.

Taylor, A. and Powell, M.E.B. (2004). Intensity-modulated radiotherapy - What is it? *Cancer Imaging* 4 (2): 68–73. https://doi.org/10.1102/1470-7330.2004.0003.

Tselis, N. and Chatzikonstantinou, G. (2019). Treating the Chameleon: Radiotherapy in the management of Renal Cell Cancer. *Clinical and Translation Radiation Oncology* 16: 7–14. doi:10.1016/j.ctro.2019.01.007.

Ulutin, H.C., Aksu, G., Fayda, M., Kuzhan, O., Tahmaz, L., and Beyzadeoglu, M. (2006). The value of postoperative radiotherapy in renal cell carcinoma: A single-institution experience. *Tumori* 92 (3): 202–206.

Wang, Y., Deng, W., Li, N. et al. (2018). Combining immunotherapy and radiotherapy for cancer treatment: Current challenges and future directions. *Frontiers in Pharmacology* 9. doi:10.3389/fphar.2018.00185.

Zagars, G.K., Ballo, M.T., Lee, A.K., and Strom, S.S. (2015). *Journal of Clinical Oncology Mortality after Cure OF Testicular Seminoma* 22 (4): https://doi.org/10.1200/JCO.2004.05.205.

23

Gynecologic Cancers

Ariel E. Pollock, MD[1], Jill S. Remick MD[2], and Pranshu Mohindra MD, MBBS[1]

[1]*Department of Radiation Oncology, University of Maryland School of Medicine and Maryland Proton Treatment Center, Baltimore, MD*
[2]*Department of Radiation Oncology, Winship Cancer Institute, Emory University Hospital, Atlanta GA*

Corresponding Author: *Pranshu Mohindra MD, MBBS, Associate Professor, Department of Radiation Oncology, University of Maryland School of Medicine, Maryland Proton Treatment Center, 22 S. Greene St., Rm GGJ35 Baltimore, MD 21201 Phone: (410) 328-9155 Fax: (410) 328-5279*

TABLE OF CONTENTS

23.1 Introduction

Gynecologic malignancies represent 12% of cancers diagnosed in woman, with endometrial cancer being the most common [1]. In contrast to other common cancers in which outcomes are improving, the survival rate for patients diagnosed with cervix and endometrial cancer has remained stable or slightly declined [2,3]. These trends have largely been attributed to lack of good salvage treatment options [4,5] and an increasing prevalence of more aggressive histology such as cervical adenocarcinoma and other uterine histologies [3,6,7].

Radiation therapy plays a key role in the treatment of gynecologic malignancies and is often combined with chemotherapy. The toxicity associated with multi-modality therapy can be debilitating for patients, particularly when radiation and chemotherapy are given concurrently [8–13]. For example, in a randomized trial for patients with advanced endometrial cancer, 60% of patients treated with adjuvant concurrent chemoradiation experienced a severe side effect (defined as grade 3 or higher) during treatment compared to 12% of patients treated with radiation alone [14]. Likewise, in a randomized trial investigating post-hysterectomy radiation with or without chemotherapy in cervical cancer, 17% of patients treated with adjuvant chemoradiation experienced grade 4 toxicity compared to 3% of patients treated with adjuvant radiation alone [8]. The most prevalent acute severe side effects include gastrointestinal and hematologic which occur in 13–26% and 21–45% of patients, respectively [13–15]. This often prevents patients from completing a full course of therapy, which has been postulated to negatively impact outcomes [13]. Chronic side effects from radiation can include irritable bowel symptoms, rectal proctitis, hematochezia, hematuria, dysuria, fistulas, ulcers, and vaginal stenosis. Among patients that receive definitive pelvic radiation, late grade 2 or higher gastrointestinal and genitourinary toxicity has been reported in up to 15–33% and 9–19% of patients, respectively [11,16]. Pelvic insufficiency fracture is a common and often debilitating late consequence of definitive pelvic radiation which has been reported to occur in 14–19% of patients [17,18].

Several dosimetric parameters associated with pelvic radiation have been correlated with acute and chronic toxicity. The volume of bone marrow receiving a dose of 40 Gy was correlated with an increased risk of developing hematologic toxicity with a cutoff of 37% found to be most prognostic [19]. Studies involving radiation for rectal cancer have demonstrated a strong relationship between the volume of small bowel receiving a certain dose and the development of severe acute gastrointestinal (GI) toxicity [20,21]. Late GI toxicity in the adjuvant setting for cervical cancer has been correlated with the V15 Gy (volume of bowel receiving 15 Gy) which was less than 5% when V15 Gy was limited to <275 and <250 cm^3 for the small and large bowel, respectively [22]. The incidence of grade 3 or higher late GI toxicity was less than 5% when the V15 Gy was limited to <275 and <250 cm^3 for the small and large bowel, respectively. Furthermore, the risk of developing a pelvic insufficiency fracture has been correlated with maximum dose [17,23].

Despite technical advances in both external and internal radiation delivery techniques [24–26], reducing dose to the anterior pelvic organs and bone structures remains a challenge, particularly when treating the para-aortic lymph nodes and in the re-irradiation setting. Proton therapy provides the unique advantage of a steep dose fall-off at the distal end of the beam path resulting in lack of exit dose. In passive scatter proton therapy (PSPT), a single beam is spread out by a beam-scattering material. The beam is shaped laterally and distally by an aperture and range compensator, respectively. Pencil beam scanning (PBS) is a more modern proton delivery technique that utilizes a scanning magnet to move the narrow pencil beam throughout the tumor target layer by layer while the proton energy is adjusted [27]. PBS has allowed for intensity-modulated proton therapy (IMPT) in which the dose delivered by each beam can be uniquely modulated to fit the tumor shape and avoid nearby organs [28]. Unlike PSPT, IMPT can

conform the dose at both the distal and proximal ends of the tumor target which may improve the therapeutic window for dose escalation.

The unique physical properties of proton therapy provide several potential advantages in radiation therapy for gynecologic malignancies. The significant reduction in low-to-moderate dose to the bowel and bone marrow may reduce acute treatment-limiting toxicities. This may improve therapy-completion rates and also enable dose escalation or treatment intensification in appropriately selected patients. Furthermore, the decreased amount of low-dose spillage may improve the safety and efficacy of re-irradiation in the setting of recurrent disease. Other potential benefits include minimizing dose to critical organs such as the external genitalia and ovaries. While proton therapy for gynecologic malignancies is very promising, there are several unique challenges associated with proton therapy that need to be considered. This includes careful consideration of patient positioning, selecting beam arrangements to maximize robustness, and accounting for daily setup variation and internal organ motion. The purpose of this review is to discuss the dosimetric and clinical data that are currently available for proton therapy in gynecologic cancers, present our institutional planning techniques and considerations when treating gynecologic cancers with proton therapy, and discuss some of the challenges and future directions of proton therapy in gynecologic malignancies.

23.2 General Treatment Paradigms

Radiation therapy is an integral component in the management cancers of the endometrium, cervix, vagina, and vulva with possible role in patients with locally recurrent ovarian cancers. Adjuvant radiation therapy is recommended in the setting of one or more adverse pathologic features depending on disease subsite as follows. Indications for adjuvant external beam radiation therapy in endometrial cancer include tumor grade, presence of deep myometrial invasion, and lymph-vascular space invasion (LVSI) [29–31]. Definitive chemoradiation is standard for locally advanced cervical cancer; however, adjuvant indications for radiation therapy in cervical cancer include tumor size >4 cm, presence of middle or deep stromal invasion, and lymphovascular invasion [32]. In vulvar cancer, adjuvant radiation therapy should be considered for patients with margins <8 mm, LVSI, and lymph node involvement [33,34]. Definitive chemoradiation is the standard of care for locally advanced cervical and vulvovaginal cancers with radiotherapy (external beam and/or brachytherapy) for medically inoperable patients with endometrial cancer [15,35–38]. Definitive or neoadjuvant chemoradiation has also emerged as a promising treatment approach for patients with locally advanced or unresectable vulvar cancer [39,40].

External beam radiation typically involve radiation to the elective nodes to 45–50.4 Gy, with boost to gross nodes to a total dose of 55–65 Gy, respectively. Intracavitary and/or interstitial (IS) brachytherapy is often used for to boost the primary tumor or in the adjuvant setting if there are high-risk pathologic features. When treating definitively, the combined total dose goal in 2 Gy equivalents (EQD2) is generally aimed at 85–90 Gy and 70–75 Gy for cervical and distal vaginal tumors, respectively.

23.3 Proton Dosimetric Data

23.3.1 Whole Pelvis Irradiation

As there is a dosimetric benefit with IMRT for treatment of the whole pelvis for gynecologic malignancies, various institutions have investigated the role of proton beam therapy (PBT) for treatment of the whole pelvis.

A dosimetric study from Italy included 20 patients treated with cervical cancer and compared IMRT, volumetric-arc therapy (VMAT), helical tomotherapy (HT), and IMPT plans [41]. Ten patients received EBRT to the whole pelvis and were prescribed 50.4 Gy to the elective lymph node volume with a simultaneous integrated boost to 59.36 Gy to the high-risk volume (parametrium and surrounding lymphatic tissue). To treat the pelvis, three proton beams were used including two anterior obliques and one posterior beam, with various gantry angles for the oblique beams depending on the individual patient and bowel anatomy. They achieved more homogeneous dose distribution for treatment of their simultaneous integrated boost (SIB) volumes with the IMPT plans versus photon-based plans; however, differences were small. The authors reported significantly lower bowel V10–V30 and mean bladder doses with IMPT when compared to HT, IMRT, and VMAT. For example, mean bowel dose was 18.6 ± 5.9 for IMPT versus 27.6 ± 5.6, 30.2 ± 4.0, and 34.1 ± 7.0 for HT, IMRT, and VMAT, respectively. Bowel V50 was significantly lower with IMPT compared to IMRT and VMAT, but not HT.

Another dosimetric study from the Netherlands further evaluated the dosimetric advantages to IMPT for the treatment of cervical and endometrial cancer [42]. Patients were divided into three groups based on target volume: pelvic only ($n = 10$), pelvic and para-aortic ($n = 6$), and para-aortic nodes only ($n = 5$), all prescribed 48.6 Gy with an SIB to 58.05 Gy. The dosimetric methods and findings for the para-aortic groups are reported in the following section. For treatment of the pelvis only, two lateral beams were used. IMPT led to a reduction in dose to all organs at risk (OARs) when compared with IMRT, with the largest benefit seen in the lower dose region rather than the higher dose region, which is often characteristic of proton plans. The bowel bag V15 Gy was 383 cm^3 with IMPT

and 535 cm^3 with IMRT, while the V45 Gy was similar. Mean rectal dose was 38.2 Gy with IMPT versus 42.1 Gy with IMRT and mean bladder dose was 34.5 Gy with IMPT and 40.6 Gy with IMRT.

23.3.2 Extended Field Radiation and Small Bowel Dose

The para-aortic lymph node chains are generally included in the radiation field if they are positive for metastatic disease or electively treated in the presence of considerable pelvic nodal burden. Microscopic disease can extend as high as the renal vessels and even to the retrocrural lymph nodes in the presence of gross paraortic nodes [43]. An extended field technique results in a larger volume of the abdominal organs exposed to radiation which leads to increased toxicity to the bowel and bone marrow with possible impact on kidney, liver, and other abdominal viscera. It also makes it more difficult to deliver a definitive dose to gross nodes while respecting normal tissue (i.e., small bowel) constraints.

Single-institution series have demonstrated excellent local control associated with extended-field IMRT to the para-aortic lymph node chain with a simultaneous integrated boost technique to gross nodes to a total median dose of 55–63.8 Gy [44–46]; however, the incidence of severe toxicity is variable. For example, the MD Anderson Cancer Center reported duodenal toxicity occurred in nine patients (11.7%) in which two patients experienced grade 3 toxicity, 4 patients experienced grade 4 and 2 patients experienced grade 5 [45]. The volume of the small bowel receiving 55 Gy was found to significantly correlate with duodenal toxicity [45]. Other series using a similar approach reported only 4% grade 3 GI/duodenal toxicity and no grade 4 or higher toxicity [46,47].

Several institutions have investigated the potential role of PBT in extended-field radiation for gynecologic malignancies to reduce dose to the anterior abdominal organs. A summary of dosimetric comparison studies are shown in Table 23.1. A study from Austria compared 3D CRT, IMRT, PSPT, and IMPT plans for five patients who had advanced cervical cancer with radiographic lymph node involvement who received radiation to the pelvic and para-aortic lymph nodes [48]. Beam arrangements included a four-field box for 3D CRT plans, seven coplanar beams for IMRT and a split field (upper and lower) with anterior–posterior (AP)/posterior–anterior (PA) beams for both of the proton plans. The volume of the small bowel receiving 30 Gy (V30) and V45 were both lower with both PSPT (14.6% and 6.6%) and IMPT (19% and 2.7%) compared to 3D CRT (38.2% and 9.5%) and IMRT (41% and 13.1%), respectively. Mean dose to small bowel was 26 ± 6.8 with 3D CRT, 27.2 ± 5.5 with IMRT, 13.5 ± 4.5 with passive scatter, and 13.4 ± 5.1 with IMPT. Mean doses to various normal organs were lower with

Table 23.1 Dosimetric comparison studies of normal tissue dose-volume metrics between photons and protons.

tabPelvic RT

Study	Dose/Technique		Photons		Protons
Dinges et al. (U Iowa, 2015)	45 Gy/1.8 IMRT IMPT (3 beams: AI, 2 PO)	–	Small bowel: D_{mean} (Gy): 23 Gy V40: 20% Large bowel/Rectum: D_{mean} (Gy): 40 Gy V30: 80% Bladder: D_{mean} (Gy): 42 Gy V45: 44% Bone marrow: V5: 78% V10: 72% V15: 70% V20: 60% V35: 46% V40: 37%	–	Small bowel: D_{mean} (Gy): 14 Gy V40: 18% Large bowel/Rectum: D_{mean} (Gy): 34 Gy V30: 62% Bladder: D_{mean} (Gy): 37 Gy V45: 31% Bone marrow: V5: 50% V10: 39% V15: 32% V20: 27% V35: 15% V40: 12%
De Boer et al. (Netherlands, 2018)	46 Gy/2 VMAT IMPT (4 beams: 2 laterals, 2 PO)	–	Small bowel: D_{mean} (Gy): 12 Gy V15: 899 cm³ V30: 501 cm³ V45: 268 cm³ Rectum: D_{mean} (Gy): 43 Gy V30: 99% Sigmoid: D_{mean} (Gy): 39 Gy V15: 96% V30: 81% V45: 55% Bladder: D_{mean} (Gy): 37 Gy V15: 95% V30: 74%	–	Small bowel: D_{mean} (Gy): 20 Gy V15: 559 cm³ V30: 382 cm³ V45: 227 cm³ Rectum: D_{mean} (Gy): 39 Gy V30: 84% Sigmoid: D_{mean} (Gy): 34 Gy V15: 83% V30: 71% V45: 44% Bladder: D_{mean} (Gy): 33 Gy V15: 86% V30: 62%
Vyfhius et al. (UMaryland, 2019)	45 Gy/1.8 VMAT IMPT (3 beams: PA, R, and L lateral)	–	Small bowel: V10: 72% V20: 6% Bladder: V10: 100% V20: 93% Bone marrow: V10: 94% V20: 76% Ovary: D_{mean} (Gy): 15.3 Gy V7.5: 98%	–	Small bowel: V10: 43% V20: 28% Bladder: V10: 93% V20: 81% Bone marrow: V10: 79% V20: 52% Ovary: D_{mean} (Gy): 14 Gy V7.5: 86%

Pelvic and PA RT

Study	Dose/Technique	Photons	Photons	Protons	Protons
Georg et al. (Austria, 2008)	50.4 Gy/1.8 IMRT PSPT (2 beams: AP/PA) IMPT (2 beams: AP/PA)	Small bowel: D_{mean} (Gy): 26.0 V30: 38.2% V45: 9.5% Large bowel/Rectum: D_{mean} (Gy): 17.2 Gy Femoral Head (R): D_{mean} (Gy): 20.5 Gy Kidney (R): D_{mean} (Gy): 11.4 Gy	Small bowel: D_{mean} (Gy): 27.2 Gy V30: 41% V45: 13.1% Large bowel/Rectum: D_{mean} (Gy): 18.3 Gy Femoral head: D_{mean} (Gy): 15.3 Gy Kidney (R): D_{mean} (Gy): 16.9 Gy	Small bowel: D_{mean} (Gy): 13.5 Gy V30: 14.6% V45: 6.6% Large bowel/Rectum: D_{mean} (Gy): 5.2 Gy Femoral head: D_{mean} (Gy): 1.1 Gy Kidney (R): D_{mean} (Gy): 2.0 Gy	Small bowel: D_{mean} (Gy): 13.4 Gy V30: 19% V45: 2.7% Large bowel/Rectum: D_{mean} (Gy): 3.2 Gy Femoral head: D_{mean} (Gy): 0.7 Gy Kidney (R): D_{mean} (Gy): 1.4 Gy

(Continued)

Table 23.1 (Continued)

tabPelvic RT

Milby et al. (UPenn, 2011)	50.4 Gy/1.8 IMRT IMRT/PSPT[a] (1 beam: PA) IMRT/IMPT[a] (1 beam: PA)	–	Small bowel: D_{mean} (Gy): 39.8 Gy Large bowel/Rectum: D_{mean} (Gy): 28.4 Gy R pelvis bone marrow: D_{mean} (Gy): 11.3 Gy	Small bowel: D_{mean} (Gy): 27.3 Gy Large bowel/Rectum: D_{mean} (Gy): 12.6 Gy R pelvis bone marrow: D_{mean} (Gy): 10.8 Gy	Small bowel: D_{mean} (Gy): 29 Gy Large bowel/Rectum: D_{mean} (Gy): 13.5 Gy R pelvis bone marrow: D_{mean} (Gy): 10.9 Gy
Marnitz et al. (Italy, 2015)	50.4 Gy/1.8 59.36 Gy/2.12 (parametrium and surrounding lymphatics) IMRT HT VMAT IMPT (3 beams: 2 AO, 1 PA)	–	Small bowel (IMRT): D_{mean} (Gy): 26 Gy V10: 91% V20: 61% V30: 34% V50: 9% Rectum: D_{mean} (Gy): 48 Gy Bladder: D_{mean} (Gy): 49 Gy Small bowel (VMAT): D_{mean} (Gy): 25 Gy V10: 94% V20: 60% V30: 33% V50: 8% Rectum: D_{mean} (Gy): 48 Gy Bladder: D_{mean} (Gy): 49 Gy	–	Small bowel: D_{mean} (Gy): 14 Gy V10: 40% V20: 28% V30: 18% V50: 3% Rectum: D_{mean} (Gy): 41 Gy Bladder: D_{mean} (Gy): 41 Gy
Van de Sande (Netherlands, 2016)	48.6 Gy/1.8 IMRT IMPT (variable)	–	Small bowel: V15: 1,915 cm^3 V45: 355 cm^3 Rectum: D_{mean} (Gy): 46 Gy Sigmoid: D_{mean} (Gy): 46 Gy Bladder: D_{mean} (Gy): 48 Gy Femoral heads: D_{mean} (Gy): 27 Gy Pelvic bone marrow: D_{mean} (Gy): 34 Gy R kidney: D_{mean} (Gy): 12 Gy Spinal cord: D_{mean} (Gy): 28 Gy	–	Small bowel: V15: 684 cm^3 V45: 234 cm^3 Rectum: D_{mean} (Gy): 38 Gy Sigmoid: D_{mean} (Gy): 39 Gy Bladder: D_{mean} (Gy): 37 Gy Femoral heads: D_{mean} (Gy): 11 Gy Pelvic bone marrow: D_{mean} (Gy): 20 Gy R kidney: D_{mean} (Gy): 2 Gy Spinal cord: D_{mean} (Gy): 14 Gy

[a]Pelvic nodes treated with IMRT, PA nodes treated with protons. 3D CRT = 3D conformal radiation therapy; IMRT = intensity modulated radiation therapy; VMAT = volumetric arc therapy; HT = helical therapy; AI = anterior inferior; AO = anterior oblique; PO = posterior oblique; PA = posterior–anterior; AP = anterior–posterior; V10 = volume of "x" receiving 10 Gy; D_{mean} (Gy) = mean dose.

proton modality than photon modalities including colon (17.2 ± 4.0 and 18.3 ± 5.4 with 3D CRT and IMRT, respectively, versus 5.2 ± 2.4 and 3.2 ± 2.8 with passive scatter and IMPT, respectively), right kidney (11.4 ± 4.0 and 16.9 ± 4.8 with 3D CRT and IMRT versus 2.0 ± 2.5 and 1.4 ± 1.8 with passive scatter and IMPT, respectively), left kidney (9.0 ± 3.7 and 17.3 ± 7.1 with 3D CRT and IMRT versus 2.7 ± 3.7 and 2.2 ± 3.6 with passive scatter and IMPT, respectively), right femur (20.5 ± 3.2 and 15.3 ± 3.7 with 3D CRT and IMRT, respectively, versus 1.1 ± 1.4 and 0.7 ± 0.6 with passive scatter and IMPT, respectively), and left femur (20.8 ± 3.4 and 15.9 ± 3.5 with 3D CRT and IMRT, respectively, versus 1.0 ± 0.9 and 0.6 ± 0.4 with passive scatter and IMPT, respectively).

The University of Pennsylvania performed a dosimetric comparison of IMRT, PSPT, and IMPT for the treatment of pelvic and para-aortic lymph nodes in 10 patients with locally advanced gynecologic malignancies [49]. The pelvic IMRT portion utilized seven coplanar beams with one beam used to treat the para-aortic nodes. For all proton plans, a single PA proton beam (either PSPT or IMPT) was used to treat the para-aortic field and IMRT was used to treat the pelvic nodes due to concern for field matching and range uncertainty with protons. All plans demonstrated similar, adequate planning target volume (PTV) coverage. The integral mean dose to the large bowel, small bowel, left kidney, and pelvic bones were significantly lower with both proton modalities compared to IMRT. Dose–volume comparison for the small bowel revealed a significant reduction in V20, V30, V35, and V40 by 40%, 27%, 18%, and 11% associated with PSPT compared to IMRT. For IMPT plans, only V20 was significantly reduced compared to IMRT (56% vs. 82.5%).

As mentioned earlier, a dosimetric study from Italy that included twenty patients treated with cervical cancer, compared IMPT to photon modalities including HT, IMRT, and VMAT [41]. Half of the patients received extended-field radiation therapy to the para-aortic lymph nodes. The dosimetric results for the whole pelvis was reported earlier in the chapter. For treatment of the para-aortic lymph nodes, their same whole pelvis field three-field arrangement (two anterior obliques and one posterior beam) was used with an additional anterior–posterior fields for the para-aortic lymph nodes. There was a significant reduction in the volume of small bowel receiving 10–50 Gy when using IMPT compared to the other three modalities and notably, this difference was more pronounced when the para-aortic lymph nodes were treated. For example, the bowel V30 was 47.1%, 44.8%, 45.6%, and 28.4% with HT, VMAT, IMRT, and IMPT, respectively, when just treating the pelvic lymph nodes, and 36%, 32.7%, 34.2%, and 18.2%, respectively, when treating the para-aortic nodes. Additionally, there was a significantly lower mean bowel dose with IMPT (13.8 Gy; compared to 25.3 Gy with VMAT) as well as a 57% reduction in the volume of bowel receiving 10 Gy (40.3% vs. 94%).

A previously mentioned study from the Netherlands included a total of 11 patients that received treatment to the para-aortic lymph nodes, 6 of whom had treatment to the pelvis and para-aortic lymph nodes [42]. For treatment of the pelvis and para-aortic nodes, a four-field box was used, and for the treatment of para-aortic nodes alone, an AP/PA beam arrangement was used. When using standard PTV margins (0.7–1.5 cm), they observed IMPT provided the greatest dosimetric advantage when treating the para-aortic lymph nodes. For patients receiving para-aortic radiation, IMPT reduced V15 Gy and V45 Gy to the bowel bag by 64–75% and 26–34%, respectively. Mean dose to rectum was 38.3 Gy with IMPT versus 45.9 Gy with IMRT and mean dose to bladder was 37.5 Gy with IMPT and 48.5 Gy with IMRT. Furthermore, IMPT reduced the dose to the right and left kidneys were reduced by 86–89% and 80–91%, respectively.

Based on these simulation studies, IMPT demonstrates the greatest dosimetric advantage when treating the para-aortic lymph nodes; however, dose reductions to the small bowel, bladder, and rectum have also been observed when treating the whole pelvis alone. Given the strong correlation of small bowel dose–volume metrics and acute bowel toxicity, it is likely these reductions in small bowel dose will minimize acute toxicity for patients undergoing definitive chemoradiation, with possible extension of benefit to chronic bowel symptoms.

23.3.3 Bone Marrow

Hematologic toxicity is the most common acute severe toxicity observed with concurrent chemoradiation to the pelvis and often limits the number of chemotherapy cycles a patient can receive [13–15]. The number of chemotherapy cycles a patient receives has been shown to correlate with disease outcomes, including a decrease in progression-free and overall survival [50]. The volume of the bone marrow receiving 40 Gy (V40) has been shown to significantly correlate with the risk of grade 2 or higher hematologic toxicity [19]. Other studies suggest the volume of bone marrow receiving low dose, in the range of 10–20 Gy, is a strong predictor for hematologic toxicity [51,52].

By reducing integral dose, proton therapy has the potential to minimize dose to the bone marrow. A dosimetric comparison study of IMPT versus IMRT for the treatment of stage I–II cervical cancer patients at the University of Iowa utilized a three-beam approach including one anterior inferior beam with a couch kick to avoid bowel, and two posterior oblique beams angled at 150° and 210° [53]. The posterior oblique beams were chosen to maximize bone marrow sparing and avoid passing through bowel. They evaluated and compared dose to functional bone marrow as defined by and SUV threshold of >4 on an ^{18}F-flourothymidine (FLT)-positron emission tomography scan [53]. They reported a significant reduction in the volume of functional bone marrow receiving 5–40 Gy with relative reductions of 32% (V5 Gy), 47% (V10 Gy), 51% (V15 Gy), 54% (V20 Gy), 60% (V35 Gy), and 57% (V40 Gy). These metrics remained significantly lower with IMPT after performing robust optimization to account for proton range uncertainty (±3 mm) and errors in stopping power calculations (±3%). Target coverage was similar between the two modalities.

Similarly, a dosimetric study from Austria that utilized an AP/PA proton beam arrangement to treat the pelvis and para-aortic lymph nodes demonstrated a significant reduction in the mean femoral head dose from 15 Gy (IMRT) to approximately 1 Gy (PSPT) and <1 Gy (IMPT) while also maintaining a significantly lower mean small bowel dose with both proton modalities compared to IMRT [48]. Using a single PA proton beam to treat the para-aortic lymph node chain, the University of Pennsylvania reported a small but significant reduction in mean dose to the pelvic bones of 3% and 4% for IMPT and PSPT, respectively [49]. The University of Maryland demonstrated a significant reduction in volume of the bone marrow receiving 10–20 Gy using a single PA and two opposed lateral beams compared to VMAT; however, V40 was similar between the two modalities [54].

These dosimetric simulation data suggest that proton therapy may minimize hematologic toxicity by reducing the amount of bone marrow exposed to low-to-moderate doses of radiation. Clinically, if these dosimetric observations translate into a reduced risk of treatment-limiting toxicity, then IMPT has the potential to improve completion rates of chemoradiotherapy and thus disease outcomes.

23.3.4 Other Organs

Ovarian preservation is an important consideration for premenopausal patients undergoing pelvic radiation. Options that are available to preserve fertility and ovarian endocrine function, including ovarian transposition and cryopreservation, are not always successful and can delay initiation of treatment. A dosimetric feasibility study performed at the University of Maryland explored the ability of IMPT and VMAT to spare dose to a single ovary as an alternative approach to ovarian endocrine preservation. The ovarian dose goal of mean <15 Gy was considered a conservative estimate based on data from prior studies of ovarian radio-ablation in breast cancer. In this study of 10 patients treated with definitive chemoradiation, all IMPT plans were able to meet the ovary constraint of mean <15 Gy without compromising target coverage whereas only four of the VMAT plans were able to achieve this. The authors concluded that sparing of a single ovary when treating whole pelvis radiation is feasible with IMPT without compromising target coverage. Figure 23.1 shows an example of an IMPT plan for the treatment of locally advanced cervical cancer for a premenopausal patient where an ovarian sparing technique was used.

23.3.5 Boost Treatment

Definitive chemoradiation followed by an intracavitary or IS brachytherapy is standard of care for locally advanced cervical cancer. Brachytherapy offers a highly conformal radiation delivery technique with sharp dose fall-off making it the optimal delivery method for a cervical boost. The total dose in EQD2 to the high-risk target volume has been shown to significantly correlate with local control [55]. To adequately encompass areas of subclinical and gross residual disease, IS needles are often used to improve target coverage which generally requires ultrasound-guidance and/or MRI adaptive planning. While this is a resource- and labor-intensive approach requiring multidisciplinary care coordination across different specialties, it results in a superior dose distribution compared to any other external beam technique. Indeed, prior efforts using EBRT as an alternative to a brachytherapy boost revealed unacceptably high rates of in-field recurrences [56]. This was attributed to inadequate tumor dose to achieve durable local control. However, the unique physical properties of proton therapy may allow for a higher target dose escalation without exceeding constraints to normal tissue.

Several institutions have explored using proton therapy to simulate a brachytherapy boost for patients with advanced cervical cancers. A dosimetric comparison study comparing VMAT, IMRT, and IMPT as a boost demonstrated adequate PTV coverage for all modalities, with the IMPT plans having a more homogenous dose distribution [57]. The dose to 2 cm^3 of the rectum and bladder was not significantly different across the plans. Another dosimetric study evaluated 11 patients with locally advanced cervical cancer treated with definitive chemoradiation followed by an IMPT boost as an alternative to brachytherapy [58]. IMPT target coverage and dose to OARs were compared to reference VMAT plans. Both treatment modalities were able to achieve an EQD2 of 89.6 Gy with acceptable target coverage. IMPT resulted in a significantly lower D2 cm^3, D5 cm^3, and mean dose to the rectum by 34%, 71%, and 47%, respectively, and to the sigmoid by 37%, 74%, and 56%, respectively, compared to VMAT. When combined with the EBRT dose, the IMPT boost plans were able to achieve a mean EQD2 to 2 cm^3 of the rectum, sigmoid and bladder of 62, 57.8, and 80.6 Gy, respectively, all of which were within the recommended dose limits based on American Society for Radiation Oncology (ASTRO) consensus recommendations [59]; in comparison, the EQD2 with VMAT plans was 75, 66.9, and 89 Gy, respectively, with only the mean 2 cm^3 of the sigmoid falling within the recommended dose limits.

A key difference in IMPT dose distribution from brachytherapy is the lack of the high doses in the center of target volume that are otherwise achieved with an intracavitary brachytherapy. Further, day-to-day uncertainties in uterocervical

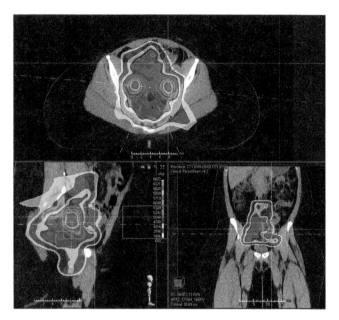

Figure 23.1 Ovarian avoidance. A 35-year-old patient with locally advanced cervical cancer who received 50.4 Gy to the whole pelvis, para-aortics and gross disease as well as an SIB to 60.2 Gy to the gross nodal volume. Ovary contoured in red with ovarian avoidance structure contoured in brown. In order to block the ovary, this was a multi-field optimization plan with two laterals and two posterior oblique beams.

positioning from variations in bladder and rectal filling can have significant impact on actual dose distribution from IMPT. As such, brachytherapy remains the standard of care after chemoradiation in the definitive management cervical cancer. Use of IMPT in this setting remains investigational and should not be clinically implemented outside of a clinical trial or be considered only in settings where brachytherapy may not be feasible due to medical or technical reasons. In such settings, IMPT may have the advantage over VMAT to reach an adequate EQD2 while limiting dose to critical structures.

23.4 Clinical Data

Clinical data on outcomes from proton RT in the management of gynecological cancers is limited. The reported literature describes early institutional experiences.

23.4.1 Reported Outcomes and Toxicity

University of Tsukuba, Japan, reported on their experience treating patients with external proton therapy as an alternative to intracavitary radiation for cervical cancer [60]. Patients were treated with photon RT to the pelvis and passive scatter proton RT to the primary tumor and adjacent tissue. Median combined dose to tumor was 86 Gy. At 10 years, overall sur-

vival was 59% and cause-specific survival was 65%. Five-year local control rates for all patients, Stage IIB, and IIIB/IVA were 75%, 100%, and 61%, respectively. BED was associated with better overall survival, and clinical stage was associated with local control. Fifty percent of patients had late bowel complications, mostly with rectal bleeding as symptom and 20% of patients had late complications in the bladder. These were predominantly grade 1 and grade 2 toxicities; however, 1 patient did develop grade 4 GI toxicity.

University of Pennsylvania prospectively enrolled 11 posthysterectomy patients in their image-guided PBS proton therapy study. They additionally reported dosimetric comparison between PBS proton and IMRT plans. Patients with endometrial, cervical, and vaginal cancer received 45–50.4 Gy to the pelvis with or without a brachytherapy boost; para-aortic lymph nodes were not treated. Treatment technique evolved with time, involving use of laterally opposed beams when using fixed beam room to posterior obliques once PBS on gantry was available. Robustness was achieved by accounting for 3.5% range uncertainty, with additional 1 mm margin for beam calibration uncertainty and ±5 mm for positional uncertainty. Pelvic bone marrow was divided into three subsites for contouring (lower pelvis, ilium, and lumbosacral spine). Very limited hematological toxicity was seen. One patient (11%) developed grade 3 leukopenia and three (33%) developed grade 2 leukopenia. One patient developed grade 3 GI toxicity, while no patients had grade 3 GU toxicity. On dosimetric comparison within the treated patients, the small bowel V0–V32 was lower with PBS than with IMRT; however, this was not statistically different at doses greater than 32 Gy. The V0–V29 for bone marrow was lower with PBS; however, IMRT was lower in the high-dose region. Bone marrow V10 was 64% with PBS and 88% with IMRT and V20 was 57% versus 74% ($p < 0.05$). They further looked at the individual bone marrow components and found that ilium V10 and V20 were lower with PBS; however, the lumbosacral spine was higher with PBS than with IMRT. V10 and V20 for the lower pelvis were lower with PBS than IMRT. The authors suggested that IMRT is possibly better at sparing total bone marrow dose in the high-dose region because the posteriorly situated proton beams pass through the sacrum.

Preliminary data from the University of Maryland-affiliated Maryland Proton Treatment Center evaluated 28 consecutive patients with uterine (86%) or cervical (14%) cancers treated with PBS-IMPT to a dose was 55.4 Gy (relative biologic effectiveness [RBE]) (range, 45–66) in 28 once-daily fractions [61]. Target volume involved pelvis alone (57%) and/or peri-aortic fields (43%). Using robustness analysis performed for setup (3–5 mm) and range uncertainty (3.5%) and 78.5% plans using multi-field optimization, a median of 3 beams (range, 2–5) were used in treatment delivery. Typical beam set involved a combination of posterior and lateral beams (including obliques). Quality assurance CT (QACT) scans were performed through the treatment course resulted in replans in a little less than one-third of the patients. Causes for replan included changes in setup or surface anatomy (66%), and tumor swelling or shrinkage in 1 patient each. Despite pre-IMPT or concurrent chemotherapy use in 75% patients, treatment was very well tolerated with only 10% of patients developing grade 2 GI toxicity and no patients developing ≥grade 3 GI or GU toxicities.

A report of clinical practice patterns for proton therapy in gynecological cancers from the Proton Collaborative Group (PCG) identified 83 patients enrolled in a prospective registry from 2012 to 2019 [62]. Spread of disease sites included uterine (68.7%) followed by vulvovaginal (16.9%), ovarian (8.4%), and cervical (6%). Median PT dose was 50.4 Gy (RBE) (range, 16–72.17) with a median fraction size of 1.8 Gy (RBE) (range, 1.1–7) targeting pelvis alone (69.8%), abdomen alone (16.8%), both abdomen-pelvis (3.6%). Grade 3–4 adverse events were noted in seven patients.

23.4.2 Carbon Ions

Carbon ions share many similar properties with protons with some important differences. Similar to PBT, carbon ions demonstrate the characteristic energy-dependent dose-fall off at depth known as the "Bragg peak" [63]. In contrast to protons where the dose beyond this point is essentially zero, with carbon ions, there is a low-dose trail as a result of nuclear fragmentation. However, the lateral dose penumbra is steeper with carbon ions and increases with depth. Importantly, carbon ions are high light-energy transfer radiations resulting in more effective DNA damage and thus a higher RBE. The RBE of carbon ions decreases with higher dose per fraction and this effect appears to be more pronounced in normal tissues compared to tumor cells [64,65]. These unique properties of carbon ions may provide the opportunity for greater dose escalation to the target and sparing of dose to OARs.

The first center to treat with carbon ions, The National Institute of Radiological Sciences (NIRS), has provided the majority of clinical data for the use of carbon ions in gynecologic cancer. The NIRS performed a phase I/II clinical trial (9902) investigating the safety and effectiveness of carbon-ion radiation therapy alone for bulky cervical cancer [66]. They treated 22 patients to the whole pelvis to 39 GyE in 13 fractions with a two-step cone down to boost the gross disease to 64–72 Gy in 20 fractions. They reported a 5-year overall survival and local control rate of 50% and 68%, respectively. No patients developed grade 2 or higher acute toxicity; however seven patients (32%) developed late GI complications (grade 1 and grade 2 toxicity) including bleeding.

NIRS subsequently evaluated the safety and efficacy of carbon-ion radiation therapy with concurrent chemotherapy in a phase I/II clinical trial [67]. Similarly to their earlier study, patients were treated to 72 Gy in 20 fractions, but with the addition of weekly cisplatin 40 mg/m [2]. Two of 22 patients developed grade 3 GI toxicity. Two-year local control and overall survival were superior for patients with tumors less than 7.1 cm versus greater than 7.1 cm (92% vs. 33% and 100% vs. 60%, respectively).

Carbon-ion radiation therapy has also been demonstrated to be safe with extended-field and prior to brachytherapy [68,69]. NIRS has treated patients with inoperable endometrial cancers with carbon-ion radiotherapy to 62.4–74.4 Gy. In this series, vaginal packing and Foley catheters were used in order to minimize target motion. Of the 14 patients, 5 developed grade 2 late toxicity with no patients developing grade 3 or higher toxicity. With a median follow-up of 50 months, 5-year local control was 86%, progression-free survival 64%, and overall survival 68%.

23.4.3 Re-irradiation

Historically, there have been limitations in the tolerability of re-irradiation with external beam therapy for gynecological malignancies due to risk of excessive toxicities such as radiation proctitis, cystitis, small bowel obstruction, fistula, and aseptic necrosis of the femoral neck [70]. Brachytherapy and stereotactic body radiotherapy therefore emerged as primary modalities for re-irradiation for gynecologic malignancies, given the ability to treat small volumes in a conformal manner [71,72]. Several small studies have demonstrated the ability to treat lateral sidewall disease or nodal recurrences with SBRT, with local control ranging between 50% and 90% at 2 years [73–75]. Brachytherapy and SBRT, however, are not suited for treatment for larger targets or recurrences. Proton therapy has been used for re-irradiation in many disease sites in the abdomen and pelvis, as the physical properties allow for treatment of a larger target with acceptable cumulative dose to organs-at-risk [76,77]. At this time, there is paucity of data regarding re-irradiation for gynecologic malignancies with proton therapy. A case report from the University of Pennsylvania demonstrated the feasibility of re-irradiation with protons for a vaginal recurrence of cervical cancer, initially treated with definitive radiation alone 27 years prior [78]. In the PCG registry experience described above, one-quarter of the patients underwent re-irradiation with protons. Of the seven patients with grade 3–4 adverse events, four underwent re-irradiation.

In our experience, patients with large recurrences are likely most suitable candidates for re-irradiation with proton therapy over conformal photon techniques with SBRT employed for small volume recurrences and brachytherapy for lesions accessible to intracavitary/IS brachytherapy. Figures 23.2 and 23.3 represent two patients who received re-irradiation for recurrent cervical and ovarian cancer, not amenable to SBRT.

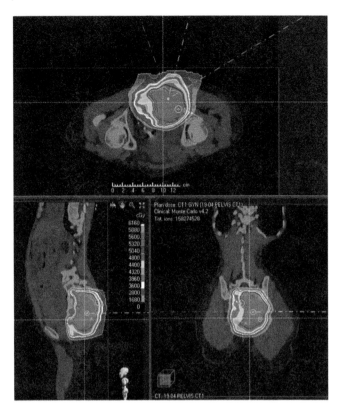

Figure 23.2 Re-irradiation for recurrent cervical cancer of a 55-year-old female who had prior definitive chemoradiation (45 Gy to pelvis with 9 Gy SFB to gross lymph node (LN) and parametrial disease) and intracavitary brachytherapy for locally advanced cervical cancer 2 years prior. Proton re-irradiation was offered for presacral recurrence targeting gross disease to 56 Gy with simultaneous integrated boost while treating microscopic margin to 44 Gy. Patient was treated in the prone position with three posterior beams with multi-field optimization and a 3-cm range shifter.

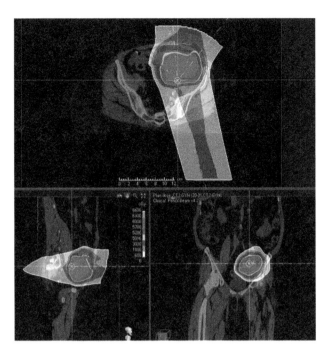

Figure 23.3 Re-irradiation for recurrent ovarian cancer of a 41-year-old female who had previously received 54 Gy to a left ovarian mass that was chemo-refractory. Proton re-irradiation was offered 2.5 years later, prescribing 60 Gy in 48 twice-daily fractions to the recurrent ovarian mass. Patient was treated supine with two anterior and one posterior beam with multi-field optimization.

23.5 Ongoing Studies

Aside from the prospective study from University of Pennsylvania mentioned earlier, there are currently no published prospective trials evaluating the use of proton therapy in gynecologic malignancies. A group of researchers in Germany are conducting a phase II prospective study (APROVE trial, NCT03184350) of 25 participants to assess the ability of proton therapy to decrease radiation dose to the pelvic organs and to evaluate whether this clinically translates into a meaningful reduction in toxicity. This single-armed study is enrolling patients requiring adjuvant radiation therapy for histologically confirmed cervical or endometrial cancer. Patients will be treated with PBS proton radiation to a total dose of 45–50.4 Gy in 1.8 Gy per fraction followed by a high-dose rate vaginal brachytherapy boost. The primary end point of this study is absence of severe toxicity as defined by no grade 3 or high adverse events based on CTCAE version 4. Secondary end points to be evaluated include all toxicities, quality of life metrics including patient-reported outcomes and progression-free survival. The Massachusetts General Hospital is also conducting a prospective pilot study of 30 patients with cervical or endometrial cancer with histologically confirmed metastasis to regional lymph nodes treated with adjuvant PBS proton therapy (NCT01600040). This study will primarily assess normal tissue dose reductions and treatment-related toxicity. At the University of Maryland-affiliated Maryland Proton Treatment Center, a phase 2 study for up to 21 patients has been initiated with the primary objective of testing treatment compliance of Upfront Intensity Modulated Proton Beam Therapy (IMPT) and Concurrent Chemotherapy (UPPROACH) for Post-operative Treatment in Loco-regionally Advanced Endometrial Cancer (NCT04527900).

23.6 Proton Therapy Planning Techniques

23.6.1 Considerations and Contraindications

While dosimetric studies and early clinical outcomes with proton therapy suggest a potential for benefitting many patients by reducing bowel, hematological and bladder toxicity, there are some patients and clinical situations in which proton therapy may be associated with unique challenges. Patients with metallic implants, such as bilateral hip replacements, is one such group who pose great challenges for proton planning when treating pelvic target volume. The stopping power of high-*Z* materials make it such that the proton beam should not traverse the metal. If a patient has a unilateral hip prosthesis, then a possible solution includes replacement of a lateral beam with an alternative beam angle such as posterior oblique (Figure 23.4). If a patient has bilateral hip prostheses, neither right nor left lateral beam angles can be utilized limiting beam angles to posterior obliques. It should be noted that these patients are also a challenge for IMRT/VMAT planning often requiring partial arcs or beam angles restricted to the anterior and posterior direction with resultant increase in bowel and bladder dose.

Body habitus is another consideration when selecting patients for proton therapy. There is greater tissue dependent dose inhomogeneity as well as subsequent range uncertainty with protons as compared to photons and therefore setup reproducibility is crucial. Patients with a large body habitus, notably with a large pannus or multiple skin folds, make setup reproducibility challenging. This should be considered at time of CT simulation in an effort to minimize skin folds, as well as during treatment planning in order to optimize beam angles from surfaces that are likely to be reproducible during day-to-day setups. Figure 23.5 compares an IMPT and VMAT plan for

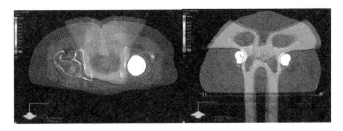

Figure 23.4 Unilateral or bilateral hip prosthesis. Choice of beam angles are adjusted to prevent direct entry through the prosthesis. This can pose challenges especially with bilateral prosthesis leaving limited choice of posterior and oblique beam angles.

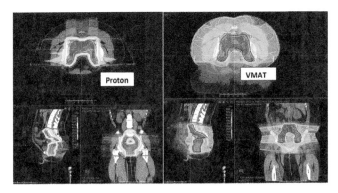

Figure 23.5 IMPT and VMAT comparative plans for locally advanced postoperative endometrial cancer of a 35-year-old female who received 50.4 Gy to the pelvis. Pictured above are the comparison IMPT plan (left) and VMAT plan (right). Patient had a large pannus, which due to setup uncertainty could have made the IMPT plan less robust. However, prone positioning and posterolateral beams were used to minimize uncertainty. Comparative analysis of IMPT versus VMAT plan for this patient is shown below.

the treatment of locally advanced endometrial cancer in the adjuvant setting.

Proton (IMPT)		IMRT	
% PTV receiving 95% of Rx dose	N/A	% PTV receiving 95% of Rx dose	98%
% CTV receiving 100% of Rx dose	98%	% CTV receiving 100% of Rx dose	99%
% Max point dose	108%	% Max point dose	105%

Anatomic region of interest	PROTON plan DVH value		IMRT plan DVH value	
	Goal	**Actual**	**Goal**	**Actual**
Small bowel loops	V15 < 120 cm^3	156.84 cm^3	V15 < 120 cm^3	395.76 cm^3
Bladder	V40 < 40%	42.89%	V40 < 40%	57.56%
	V45 < 15%	39.52%	V45 < 15%	49.56%
Bone marrow	V40 < 37%	23.81%	V40 < 37%	23.61%
	V20 < 80%	58.13%	V20 < 80%	79.23%

Finally, patients may develop greater acute skin reaction with proton therapy, which is to be considered especially when treating inguinal nodes or when treating vulvovaginal cancers. While the incidence of acute skin toxicity with proton therapy has not been studied in gynecologic malignancies, it has been demonstrated in breast cancer patients. In a University of Maryland experience of 86 patients undergoing adjuvant breast radiation therapy, a higher rate of grade ≥2 radiation dermatitis (69.2% vs. 29.8%, $p = 0.002$) was observed with proton RT [79].

23.6.2 Simulation (for All Gynecologic Disease Sites with Special Considerations per Disease Site)

Both supine and prone positioning are feasible and should be considered as clinically appropriate for bowel and marrow sparing, based on patient's tolerability. However since prone positioning is less reproducible, the impact on the radiation plan is more pronounced with proton therapy, which needs to be accounted for in the decision process. Generally, frail patients or those with a high BMI have more difficulty with prone position. When treating inguinal nodes or vulvar site, frog-leg positioning may limit possible beam angles due to length limitation from beam accessories that come close to the patient (apertures/compensators with passive scattering machines and range-shifters with PBS), which needs to be balanced against the benefit of reducing skin folds.

Immobilization devices are similar to those used with photon therapy and (for supine positioning) include vacuum bag immobilization device bag under upper thigh, with the addition of an upper bag if treating para-aortics. Prone belly board without an anterior insert allows for maximal bulging of anterior abdominal wall and subsequent bowel dose optimization. Immobilization devices should be indexed to the simulation table.

Skin folds should be minimized as much as possible, especially along interfaces of anticipated or possible beam entry, as this can increase range uncertainty. Skin folds should also be minimized especially around inguinal region for treatment of lymph nodes, to minimize skin toxicity. It is very important to include the dosimetry team in the simulation process supplemented by clear communication of target volume by the physician team.

Treatment planning and dose calculations are performed on a noncontrast CT scan. Oral and IV contrast are useful for better bowel and vessel delineation, and if being administered, should be done after a noncontrast CT scan is obtained.

When targeting an intact uterus/vaginal cuff, patients should be scanned with both a full and empty bladder in order to create an ITV. Typically, if patient is able to tolerate, the full bladder scan will be used for both planning and treatment. Both the full and empty bladder scans should be done noncontrast as well with the final contrast scan done with the bladder filling anticipated to be used for daily treatments.

Since proton planning is significantly impacted by tissue heterogeneity variations, it is important for patients to establish a good bowel routine prior to planning simulation. At the time of simulation, images should be assessed for any gaseous distention in the region of target volume and if needed, simulation to be repeated after instructing patients to empty rectum or reschedule on a different day after using stool softeners/laxatives. It is important for this conversation to start during the consultation step itself.

If any special markers are used for simulation, this should be performed on the contrast-enhanced scan, as these markers may create artifact and can interfere with dose calculation on the noncontrast scan. For the treatment of cervical cancer and endometrial cancer, a radiopaque marker may be placed at the vaginal introitus and a cotton swab/Q-tip may be placed in the vagina to help determine vaginal length. For treatment of vulvar cancer, radiopaque markers may be placed at the vaginal introitus, anus, urethra, and clitoris, or marking the surgical bed, to aid in target delineation. Gross disease and surgical scars if visible should be wired.

23.6.3 Treatment Planning

23.6.3.1 Target Definitions and Margins

The planning target for proton therapy is the CTV, consistent with standard practice. Available contouring atlases and consensus guidelines from experts should be followed [80–82]. See Tables 23.2 and 23.3 for summary of target volumes and prescription doses for cervical and endometrial cancer. Setup and range uncertainties are accounted for using robust optimization, described below.

23.6.3.2 Robustness

Robust optimization is used to ensure adequate coverage in 13 scenarios (1 nominal plan, 6 cardinal directions, ±3.5% range uncertainty). Goal robustness should be to have 97% of the volume covered by 97% of the prescribed dose for each dose level, at minimum 95%/95%, in the "worst case scenario" of robust evaluation. For all pelvic plans where beam entry and passage through bowel is anticipated, two special density-override (DO) scans could be derived to account for uncertainty in bowel filling. In one, loops of bowel are considered to have the density of air, and in the other, the density of muscle. Robust optimization is then performed on these two DO scans in addition to the nominal scan.

Table 23.2 Recommended target volumes and radiation doses for treatment of cervical cancer.

Volume	Definitive	Adjuvant	Dose
GTVp	Primary tumor including parametria	N/A	45–50.4 Gy (RBE) Brachytherapy boost to attain an EQD2 ≥ 85 Gy
GTVn	LNs >1 cm or PET-positive lymph nodes	LNs >1 cm or PET-positive lymph nodes	>54–56 Gy to gross nodes using SIB technique or sequential boost depending on size and proximity to bowel
CTVp	GTV, entire cervix, uterus, parametria, ovaries, and vaginal tissue (treatment length depends on extent of involvement)	Vagina (treatment length depends on extent of involvement) and paravaginal soft tissue	45–50.4 Gy (RBE)
Primary ITV	Contour CTV on full and empty bladder scans. there is considerable stool/gas	Extend ITV 1–1.5 cm into rectum if	45–50.4 Gy (RBE)
CTVn	Superior border 7 mm below L4–L5 interspace or the level of bifurcation of aorta into common iliac arteries. Include a 7-mm margin around the common iliac, internal, and external iliac vessels, obturator nodes and anterior 1–2 cm presacral soft tissues to the level of S3. If treating para-aortics consider extending treatment field to level of renal vessels. If lower 1/3 vaginal involvement, include inguinal lymph nodes		45–50.4 Gy (RBE)

GTVp = Primary gross tumor volume; GTVn = nodal gross tumor volume; CTVp = primary clinical tumor volume; ITV = internal target volume; CTVn = nodal clinical tumor volume.

Table 23.3 Recommended target volumes and radiation doses for treatment of endometrial cancer.

Volume	Definitive	Adjuvant	Dose
GTVp	Primary tumor	N/A	45–50.4 Gy (RBE)
GTVn	LNs >1 cm or PET-positive lymph nodes	LNs >1 cm or PET-positive lymph nodes	>54–56 Gy to gross nodes using SIB technique or sequential boost depending on size and proximity to bowel
CTVp	GTV, entire uterus, paravaginal/parametrial tissues, proximal vagina	Vaginal cuff, paravaginal/parametrial tissues, proximal vagina	45–50.4 Gy (RBE)
Primary ITV	Contour CTV on full and empty bladder scans. Extend ITV 1–1.5 cm into rectum if there is considerable stool/gas		45–50.4 Gy (RBE)
CTVn	Superior border 7 mm below L4–L5 interspace or the level of bifurcation of aorta into common iliac arteries. Include a 7-mm margin around the common iliac, internal and external iliac vessels, obturator nodes and anterior 1–2 cm presacral soft tissues to the level of S3. If treating para-aortics consider extending treatment field to level of renal vessels. If lower 1/3 vaginal involvement, include inguinal lymph nodes		45–50.4 Gy (RBE)

23.6.3.3 Range Shifter/Skin Considerations for PBS Planning

When a target is near the skin surface, for example, with treatment of inguinal nodes, a range shifter should be used. Spot size does increase with range shifters, so it is preferable to use ≤3 cm range shifter.

23.6.3.4 Beam Arrangements

Beam arrangement may vary for different disease sites and treatment volumes as below. It is generally advisable for the target to be covered by at least two beams so as to minimize end-ranging on a critical structure and beam-specific hot spots.

For treatment of a pelvic primary + pelvic lymph nodes with supine positioning, a commonly used beam arrangement with multi-field optimization includes two laterals, each with a midline block to allow treating the uterus/cervix or vaginal cuff and ipsilateral nodal volume, as well as a PA field with a rectal block to treat the pelvic nodal volumes. Another approach is using two posterior obliques with single-field optimization treating the entire volume though this is more dependent on the variability in rectal distention. For prone treatment positioning, a four-field technique with opposed laterals and paired posterior obliques may be used.

When treating para-aortic lymph nodes, two posterior obliques should be used superiorly for coverage of para-aortic lymph nodes. This component of the plan is single-field optimization. While a single posterior beam may be sufficient for target coverage, this may increase toxicity due to the end-range effect and should not be used. Figure 23.6 shows a single posterior beam for the treatment of the para-aortic lymph nodes for a patient with locally advanced endometrial cancer in the adjuvant setting. This patient unfortunately developed enteritis during her course of radiation therapy. On the other hand, Figure 23.7 demonstrates an alternative beam arrangement with two posterior obliques for coverage of the para-aortic lymph nodes.

When treating inguinal nodes, a common multi-field optimization beam arrangement includes two laterals with midline block (or two anterior obliques), PA beam with anterior inguinal node block, and an AP beam with all targets except for inguinal nodes blocked and up to a 3-cm range shifter. Figure 23.8 compares an IMPT plan to a VMAT plan for the adjuvant treatment of a locally advanced vulvar cancer with positive lymph nodes and positive margin.

Proton (IMPT)		IMRT	
% CTV receiving 100% of Rx dose	100%	% CTV receiving 100% of Rx dose	100%
% Max point dose	105.2%	% Max point dose	104.3%

Anatomic region of interest	PROTON plan DVH value		IMRT plan DVH value	
	Goal	Actual	Goal	Actual
Small bowel	V15 < 120 cm^3	43.8 cm^3	V15 < 120 cm^3	108.5 cm^3
Bladder	V50 < 0.5 cm^3	2.99 cm^3	V50 < 0.5 cm^3	2.25 cm^3
Bone marrow	V40 < 37%	12.24%	V40 < 37%	19.42%

23.6.4   Dose Constraints

Proton-specific organ at risk dose constraints has not been established. It is feasible for proton plans to meet tighter dose constraints and therefore this should be attempted by dosimetrists.

23.6.5   Plan Evaluation

Evaluation of a proton radiation plan includes the standard aspects of photon evaluation with a few additions. Total nominal dose (0 mm, 0%) should be evaluated first as well as target coverage and dose to OARs, as with photon plans. With IMPT,

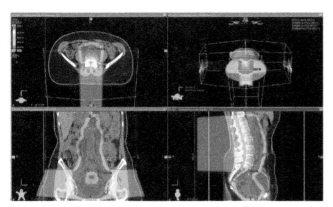

Figure 23.6   Single posterior beam for para-aortic nodes. Patient was prescribed 45 Gy to the pelvis and para-aortic nodes with a sequential boost to a gross para-aortic node to an additional 10.8 Gy. This was a multi-field optimization plan with two laterals and a posterior beam, each with a 2-cm range shifter. The para-aortic nodal chain was covered by only the posterior beam.

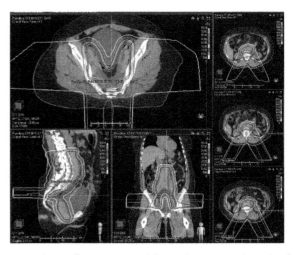

Figure 23.7   Two posterior obliques for para-aortic nodes. Patient was prescribed 50.4 Gy to the pelvis and para-aortic nodes. This was a multi-field optimization plan with two laterals and a posterior beam for the pelvis and two posterior obliques for coverage of the para-aortic nodes.

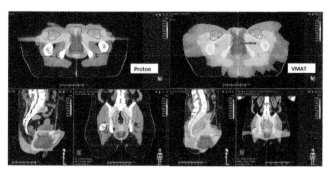

Figure 23.8 IMPT and VMAT comparative plans for locally advanced vulvar cancer. Patient received 45 Gy to the whole pelvis with a small-field boost to 66.6 Gy to the postoperative bed. Proton plan was multi-field optimization with four fields, AP/PA, two laterals. VMAT plan used three full arcs with bolus for adequate coverage of the inguinal nodes and vulva. Comparative analysis of IMPT versus VMAT plan for this patient is shown below.

additional evaluation steps include the looking at the beam specific dose for multi-field optimization plans, maximum monitor units, as well as spot size. Physicians often request less than 110% hot spot per beam as well as less than 50–70% dose contribution per beam. While there is no data correlating maximum MU with toxicity, it is advisable to limit the maximum MU per spot in IMPT, as there is concern about the distal range effect of proton beams. Physicians should evaluate where each beam is end-ranging so as to avoid end-ranging in

critical structures such as spinal cord/cauda equina or bowel. The final step in proton plan evaluation is the robust optimization as mentioned earlier.

23.6.6 QACT

A QACT at some point during treatment course is required. For gynecologic malignancies, this may be performed every other week but is ultimately up to the discretion of treating physician.

Dose is recalculated on the QACT using a rigid registration with the planning CT by dosimetry, and subsequently evaluated by the treating physician. Deformable registration may be utilized to adapt OARs and targets to the QACT position, with subsequent modification performed by the physician, if required. The physician should always evaluate the dose based on visualization of the dose distribution on the patient's anatomy rather than DVH review alone. Recognizing that creating a new proton plan takes considerable extra effort, QACTs are best avoided to close to the end of treatment to allow sufficient time for replanning should it be indicated. Our initial experience with using QACTs for gynecological cancers has been described above.

See Figure 23.9 for an additional comparison between a proton and photon plan with the corresponding dosimetric analysis in the table.

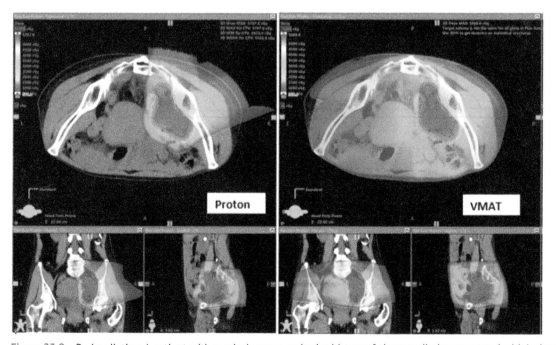

Figure 23.9 Re-irradiation. A patient with cervical cancer and prior history of chemoradiation presented with isolated nodal recurrence. IMPT allowed restriction of dose to the target volume while limiting dose to other pelvic visceral. Comparative analysis of IMPT versus VMAT plan for this patient is shown below.

Proton (IMPT)		IMRT	
% CTV receiving 100% of Rx dose	100%	% CTV receiving 100% of Rx dose	99.9%
% GTV receiving 95% of Rx dose	97.3%	% GTV receiving 95% of Rx dose	99.5%
% Max point dose	104.8%	% Max point dose	103.1%

Anatomic region of interest	PROTON plan DVH value		IMRT plan DVH value	
	Goal	Actual	Goal	Actual
Small bowel	$V15 < 120$ cm^3	65.1 cm^3	$V15 < 120$ cm^3	240.8 cm^3
	$V50 < 2$ cm^3	0.3 cm^3	$V50 < 2$ cm^3	6.1 cm^3
Bladder	$V48 < 2$ cm^3	2.4 cm^3	$V48 < 2$ cm^3	4.0 cm^3
Rt femoral head	Max < 50 Gy	41.5 Gy	Max < 50 Gy	30.0 Gy

23.7 Conclusions

Radiation therapy is indicated for most gynecologic malignancies in the definitive, adjuvant, and palliative setting. This treatment is associated with gastrointestinal, genitourinary, and hematologic toxicity, all of which can be exacerbated when given concurrently with chemotherapy or after a patient has been pretreated with chemotherapy. Given the associated toxicities with radiation therapy, technological advancements have been made in an attempt to reduce these while still maintaining appropriate tumor control and oncologic outcomes. Proton therapy, both in the form of passive scatter and PBS, has dosimetric advantages over photon modalities given the dose deposition profile with protons. Many dosimetric studies have been published which demonstrate the reduction in bowel, bladder, rectum, kidney, and bone marrow dose with both passive scatter and PBS proton therapy. These dosimetric benefits have been established for both treatment of the whole pelvis only as well as treatment of the whole pelvis and para-aortic lymph nodes. There have also been dosimetric studies demonstrating the ability to reduce dose to the ovary and to dose-escalate in patients potentially unable to receive brachytherapy boost. While there is sufficient dosimetric data to demonstrate a dosimetric benefit, there is not as much clinical data on the role of proton therapy for gynecologic malignancies. The published studies have, however, demonstrated the feasibility of proton therapy for treatment of the whole pelvis with low rate of grade 2+ toxicities. Like with other disease sites, re-irradiation may be the primary indication in these initial stages with consideration of use in patients with gross nodal disease or need to treat para-aortic chain. Ongoing clinical experiences will help further refine the planning and optimization process along with establishing clinical guidelines for OAR constraints when using proton therapy. Learning from research comparing 3D CRT with IMRT, patient reported outcomes will be key in establishing the true clinical benefit of proton therapy over IMRT/VMAT. There are ongoing clinical trials investigating whether there is a reduction in toxicity with proton therapy for the adjuvant treatment of endometrial or cervical cancer. More studies are needed to explore the role of proton therapy in gynecologic malignancies.

References

1 Siegel, R.L., Miller, K.D., and Jemal, A. (2020). Cancer statistics, 2020. *CA: A Cancer Journal for Clinicians* 70: 7–30. doi: 10.3322/caac.21590.

2 Jemal, A., Ward, E.M., Johnson, C.J., et al. (2017). Annual report to the nation on the status of cancer, 1975-2014, featuring survival. *Journal of the National Cancer Institute* 1–22. doi: 10.1093/jnci/djx030.

3 Henley, S.J., Miller, J.W., Dowling, N.F., Benard, V.B., and Richardson, L.C. (2018). Uterine cancer incidence and mortality — United States, 1999–2016. *MMWR. Morbidity and Mortality Weekly Report*. doi: 10.15585/mmwr. mm6748a1.

4 Boussios, S., Seraj, E., Zarkavelis, G., et al. (2016). Management of patients with recurrent/advanced cervical cancer beyond first line platinum regimens: Where do we stand? A literature review. *Critical Reviews in Oncology/hematology* 164–174. doi: 10.1016/j.critrevonc.2016.11.006.

5 McAlpine, J.N., Temkin, S.M., and Mackay, H.J. (2016:2787-2798). Endometrial cancer: Not your grandmother's cancer. *Cancer*. doi: 10.1002/cncr.30094.

6 Smith, H.O., Tiffany, M.F., Qualls, C.R., and Key, C.R. (2000). The rising incidence of adenocarcinoma relative to squamous cell carcinoma of the uterine cervix in the United States - A 24-year population-based study. *Gynecologic Oncology* 78 (2): 97–105. doi: 10.1006/gyno.2000.5826.

7 Wang, S.S., Sherman, M.E., Hildesheim, A., Lacey, J.V., and Devesa, S. (2004). Cervical Adenocarcinoma and Squamous Cell Carcinoma Incidence Trends among White Women and Black Women in the United States for 1976-2000. *Cancer* 100 (5): 1035–1044. doi: 10.1002/cncr.20064.

8 Peters, W.A., Liu, P.Y., Barrett, R.J., et al. (2000). Concurrent chemotherapy and pelvic radiation therapy compared with pelvic radiation therapy alone as adjuvant therapy after radical surgery in high-risk early-stage cancer of the cervix. *Journal of Clinical Oncology: Official Journal of the American Society of Clinical Oncology*. doi: 10.1200/JCO.2000.18.8.1606.

9 Stehman, F.B., Ali, S., Keys, H.M., et al. (2007). Radiation therapy with or without weekly cisplatin for bulky stage 1B cervical carcinoma: Follow-up of a Gynecologic Oncology Group trial. *American Journal of Obstetrics and Gynecology* 197 (5): 503.e1–503.e6. doi: 10.1016/j.ajog.2007.08.003.

10 Nout, R.A., Van De Poll-Franse, L.V., Lybeert, M.L.M., et al. (2011). Long-term outcome and quality of life of patients with endometrial carcinoma treated with or without pelvic radiotherapy in the post operative radiation therapy in endometrial carcinoma 1 (PORTEC-1) trial. *Journal of Clinical Oncology: Official Journal of the American Society of Clinical Oncology* 29: 1692–1700. doi: 10.1200/JCO.2010.32.4590.

11 Lei, C., Ma, S., Huang, M., et al. (2019). Long-term survival and late toxicity associated with pelvic intensity modulated radiation therapy (IMRT) for cervical cancer involving CT-based positive lymph nodes. *Frontiers in Oncology* 9: 520. doi: 10.3389/fonc.2019.00520.

12 De Boer, S.M., Powell, M.E., Mileshkin, L., et al. (2019). Adjuvant chemoradiotherapy versus radiotherapy alone in women with high-risk endometrial cancer (PORTEC-3): Patterns of recurrence and post-hoc survival analysis of a randomised phase 3 trial. *The Lancet Oncology* 20: 1273–1285. doi: 10.1016/S1470-2045(19)30395-X.

13 Matei, D., Filiaci, V., Randall, M.E., et al. (2019). Adjuvant chemotherapy plus radiation for locally advanced endometrial cancer. *The New England Journal of Medicine* 380 (24): 2317–2326. doi: 10.1056/NEJMoa1813181.

14 De Boer, S.M., Powell, M.E., Mileshkin, L., et al. (2018). Adjuvant chemoradiotherapy versus radiotherapy alone for women with high-risk endometrial cancer (PORTEC-3): Final results of an international, open-label, multicentre, randomised, phase 3 trial. *The Lancet Oncology* 19: 295–309. doi: 10.1016/S1470-2045(18)30079-2.

15 Keys, H.M., Bundy, B.N., Stehman, F.B., et al. (1999). Cisplatin, radiation, and adjuvant hysterectomy compared with radiation and adjuvant hysterectomy for bulky stage IB cervical carcinoma. *The New England Journal of Medicine*. doi: 10.1056/NEJM199904153401503.

16 Sung, U.L., Young, A.K., Young-Ho, Y., et al. (2017). General health status of long-term cervical cancer survivors after radiotherapy. *Strahlentherapie Und Onkologie* 193: 543–551. doi: 10.1007/s00066-017-1143-8.

17 Oh, D., Huh, S.J., Nam, H., et al. (2008). Pelvic insufficiency fracture after pelvic radiotherapy for cervical cancer: Analysis of risk factors. *International Journal of Radiation Oncology, Biology, Physics* 70 (4): 1183–1188. doi: 10.1016/j.ijrobp.2007.08.005.

18 Sapienza, L.G., Salcedo, M.P., Ning, M.S., et al. (2020). Pelvic insufficiency fractures after external beam radiation therapy for gynecologic cancers: A meta-analysis and meta-regression of 3929 patients. *International Journal of Radiation Oncology, Biology, Physics*. doi: 10.1016/j.ijrobp.2019.09.012.

19 Klopp, A.H., Moughan, J., Portelance, L., et al. (2013). Hematologic toxicity in RTOG 0418: A phase 2 study of postoperative IMRT for gynecologic cancer. *International Journal of Radiation Oncology, Biology, Physics* 86 (1): 83–90. doi: 10.1016/j.ijrobp.2013.01.017.

20 Robertson, J.M., Lockman, D., Yan, D., and Wallace, M. (2008). The dose-volume relationship of small bowel irradiation and acute grade 3 diarrhea during chemoradiotherapy for rectal cancer. *International Journal of Radiation Oncology, Biology, Physics* 70: 413–418. doi: 10.1016/j.ijrobp.2007.06.066.

21 Baglan, K.L., Frazier, R.C., Yan, D., Huang, R.R., Martinez, A.A., and Robertson, J.M. (2002). The dose-volume relationship of acute small bowel toxicity from concurrent 5-FU-based chemotherapy and radiation therapy for rectal cancer. *International Journal of Radiation Oncology, Biology, Physics* 52: 176–183. doi: 10.1016/S0360-3016(01)01820-X.

22 Chopra, S., Dora, T., Chinnachamy, A.N., et al. (2014). Predictors of grade 3 or higher late bowel toxicity in patients undergoing pelvic radiation for cervical cancer: Results from a prospective study. *International Journal of Radiation Oncology, Biology, Physics* 88: 630–635. doi: 10.1016/j.ijrobp.2013.11.214.

23 Bazire, L., Xu, H., Foy, J.P., et al. (2017). Pelvic insufficiency fracture (PIF) incidence in patients treated with intensity-modulated radiation therapy (IMRT) for gynaecological or anal cancer: Single-institution experience and review of the literature. *The British Journal of Radiology* 90: 20160885. doi: 10.1259/bjr.20160885.

24 Klopp, A.H., Yeung, A.R., Deshmukh, S., et al. (2018). Patient-reported toxicity during pelvic intensity-modulated radiation therapy: NRG oncology-RTOG 1203. *Journal of Clinical Oncology: Official Journal of the American Society of Clinical Oncology* 36 (24): 2538–2544. doi: 10.1200/JCO.2017.77.4273.

25 Tanderup, K., Fokdal, L.U., Sturdza, A., et al. (2016). Effect of tumor dose, volume and overall treatment time on local control after radiochemotherapy including MRI guided brachytherapy of locally advanced cervical cancer. *Radiotherapy and Oncology: Journal of the European Society for Therapeutic Radiology and Oncology* 120: 441–446. doi: 10.1016/j.radonc.2016.05.014.

26 Sturdza, A., Pötter, R., Fokdal, L.U., et al. (2016). Image guided brachytherapy in locally advanced cervical cancer: Improved pelvic control and survival in RetroEMBRACE, a multicenter cohort study. *Radiotherapy and Oncology: Journal of the European Society for Therapeutic Radiology and Oncology* 120 (3): 428–433. doi: 10.1016/j.radonc.2016.03.011.

27 Liu, H. and Chang, J.Y. (2011 May). Proton therapy in clinical practice. *Chinese Journal of Cancer* 30(5) 315–326. doi: 10.5732/cjc.010.10529. PMID: 21527064; PMCID: PMC4013396.

28 Lomax, A. (1999). Intensity modulation methods for proton radiotherapy. *Physics in Medicine and Biology*. doi: 10.1088/0031-9155/44/1/014.

29 Keys, H.M., Roberts, J.A., Brunetto, V.L., et al. (2004). A phase III trial of surgery with or without adjunctive external pelvic radiation therapy in intermediate risk endometrial adenocarcinoma: A Gynecologic Oncology Group study. *Gynecologic Oncology*. doi: 10.1016/j.ygyno.2003.11.048.

30 Wortman, B.G., Creutzberg, C.L., Putter, H., et al. (2018). Ten-year results of the PORTEC-2 trial for high-intermediate risk endometrial carcinoma: Improving patient selection for adjuvant therapy. *British Journal of Cancer*. doi: 10.1038/s41416-018-0310-8.

31 Bosse, T., Peters, E.E.M., Creutzberg, C.L., et al. (2015). Substantial lymph-vascular space invasion (LVSI) is a significant risk factor for recurrence in endometrial cancer - A pooled analysis of PORTEC 1 and 2 trials. *European Journal of Cancer (Oxford, England: 1990)*. doi: 10.1016/j.ejca.2015.05.015.

32 Rotman, M., Sedlis, A., Piedmonte, M.R., et al. (2006). A phase III randomized trial of postoperative pelvic irradiation in Stage IB cervical carcinoma with poor prognostic features: Follow-up of a gynecologic oncology group study. *International Journal of Radiation Oncology, Biology, Physics*. doi: 10.1016/j.ijrobp.2005.10.019.

33 Heaps, J.M., Fu, Y.S., Montz, F.J., Hacker, N.F., and Berek, J.S. (1990). Surgical-pathologic variables predictive of local recurrence in squamous cell carcinoma of the vulva. *Gynecologic Oncology*. doi: 10.1016/0090-8258(90)90064-R.

34 Kunos, C., Simpkins, F., Gibbons, H., Tian, C., and Homesley, H. (2009). Radiation therapy compared with pelvic node resection for node-positive vulvar cancer: A randomized controlled trial. *Obstetrics and Gynecology*. doi: 10.1097/AOG.0b013e3181b12f99.

35 Rao, Y.J., Chin, R.I., Hui, C., et al. (2017). Improved survival with definitive chemoradiation compared to definitive radiation alone in squamous cell carcinoma of the vulva: A review of the National Cancer Database. *Gynecologic Oncology*. doi: 10.1016/j.ygyno.2017.06.022.

36 Rajagopalan, M.S., Xu, K.M., Lin, J.F., Sukumvanich, P., Krivak, T.C., and Beriwal, S. (2014). Adoption and impact of concurrent chemoradiation therapy for vaginal cancer: A National Cancer Data Base (NCDB) study. *Gynecologic Oncology*. doi: 10.1016/j.ygyno.2014.09.018.

37 Van Der Steen-banasik, E., Christiaens, M., Shash, E., et al. (2016). Systemic review: Radiation therapy alone in medical non-operable endometrial carcinoma. *European Journal of Cancer (Oxford, England: 1990)*. doi: 10.1016/j.ejca.2016.07.005.

38 Schwarz, J.K., Beriwal, S., Esthappan, J., et al. (2015). Consensus statement for brachytherapy for the treatment of medically inoperable endometrial cancer. *Brachytherapy* 14 (5): 587–599. doi: 10.1016/j.brachy.2015.06.002.

39 Moore, D.H., Ali, S., Koh, W.J., et al. (2012). A phase II trial of radiation therapy and weekly cisplatin chemotherapy for the treatment of locally-advanced squamous cell carcinoma of the vulva: A gynecologic oncology group study. *Gynecologic Oncology*. doi: 10.1016/j.ygyno.2011.11.003.

40 Montana, G.S., Thomas, G.M., Moore, D.H., et al. (2000). Preoperative chemo-radiation for carcinoma of the vulva with N2/N3 nodes: A gynecologic oncology group study. *International Journal of Radiation Oncology, Biology, Physics*. doi: 10.1016/S0360-3016(00)00762-8.

41 Marnitz, S., Wlodarczyk, W., Neumann, O., et al. (2015). Which technique for radiation is most beneficial for patients with locally advanced cervical cancer? Intensity modulated proton therapy versus intensity modulated photon treatment, helical tomotherapy and volumetric arc therapy for primary radiation - an. *Radiation Oncology* 10 (1): 91. doi: 10.1186/s13014-015-0402-z.

42 Mae, V.D.S., Creutzberg, C.L., Van De Water, S., Sharfo, A.W., and Hoogeman, M.S. (2016). Which cervical and endometrial cancer patients will benefit most from intensity-modulated proton therapy? *Radiotherapy and Oncology: Journal of the European Society for Therapeutic Radiology and Oncology* 120 (3): 397–403. doi: 10.1016/j.radonc.2016.06.016.

43 Kabolizadeh, P., Fulay, S., and Beriwal, S. (2013). Are radiation therapy oncology group para-aortic contouring guidelines for pancreatic neoplasm applicable to other malignancies - Assessment of nodal distribution in gynecological malignancies. *International Journal of Radiation Oncology, Biology, Physics* 87 (1): 106–110. doi: 10.1016/j.ijrobp.2013.05.034.

44 Vargo, J.A., Kim, H., Choi, S., et al. (2014). Extended field intensity modulated radiation therapy with concomitant boost for lymph node-positive cervical cancer: Analysis of regional control and recurrence patterns in the positron emission tomography/computed tomography era. *International Journal of Radiation Oncology, Biology, Physics* 90: 1091–1098. doi: 10.1016/j.ijrobp.2014.08.013.

45 Verma, J., Sulman, E.P., Jhingran, A., et al. (2014). Dosimetric predictors of duodenal toxicity after intensity modulated radiation therapy for treatment of the para-aortic nodes in gynecologic cancer. *International Journal of Radiation Oncology, Biology, Physics* 88 (2): 357–362. doi: 10.1016/j.ijrobp.2013.09.053.

46 Townamchai, K., Poorvu, P.D., Damato, A.L., et al. (2014). Radiation dose escalation using intensity modulated radiation therapy for gross unresected node-positive endometrial cancer. *Practical Radiation Oncology* 4: 90–98. doi: 10.1016/j.prro.2013.07.002.

47 Xu, K.M., Rajagopalan, M.S., Kim, H., and Beriwal, S. (2015). Extended field intensity modulated radiation therapy for gynecologic cancers: Is the risk of duodenal toxicity high? *Practical Radiation Oncology* 5: E291–E297. doi: 10.1016/j.prro.2014.10.013.

48 Georg, D., Georg, P., Hillbrand, M., Pötter, R., and Mock, U. (2008). Assessment of improved organ at risk sparing for advanced cervix carcinoma utilizing precision radiotherapy techniques. *Strahlentherapie Und Onkologie* 184 (11): 586–591. doi: 10.1007/s00066-008-1872-9.

49 Milby, A.B., Both, S., Ingram, M., and Lin, L.L. (2012). Dosimetric comparison of combined intensity-modulated radiotherapy (IMRT) and proton therapy versus IMRT alone for pelvic and para-aortic radiotherapy in gynecologic malignancies. *International Journal of Radiation Oncology, Biology, Physics* 82 (3): e477–84. doi: 10.1016/j.ijrobp.2011.07.012.

50 Nugent, E.K., Case, A.S., Hoff, J.T., et al. (2010). Chemoradiation in locally advanced cervical carcinoma: An analysis of cisplatin dosing and other clinical prognostic factors. *Gynecologic Oncology* 116 (3): 438–441. doi: 10.1016/j.ygyno.2009.09.045.

51 Mell, L.K., Schomas, D.A., Salama, J.K., et al. (2008). Association between bone marrow dosimetric parameters and acute hematologic toxicity in anal cancer patients treated with concurrent chemotherapy and intensity-modulated radiotherapy. *International Journal of Radiation Oncology, Biology, Physics* 70: 1431–1437. doi: 10.1016/j.ijrobp.2007.08.074.

52 Albuquerque, K., Giangreco, D., Morrison, C., et al. (2011). Radiation-related predictors of hematologic toxicity after concurrent chemoradiation for cervical cancer and implications for bone marrow-sparing pelvic IMRT. *International Journal of Radiation Oncology, Biology, Physics* 79: 1043–1047. doi: 10.1016/j.ijrobp.2009.12.025.

53 Dinges, E., Felderman, N., McGuire, S., et al. (2015). Bone marrow sparing in intensity modulated proton therapy for cervical cancer: Efficacy and robustness under range and setup uncertainties. *Radiotherapy and Oncology: Journal of the European Society for Therapeutic Radiology and Oncology* 115 (3): 373–378. doi: 10.1016/j.radonc.2015.05.005.

54 Vyfhuis, M.A.L., Fellows, Z., McGovern, N., et al. (2019). Preserving endocrine function in premenopausal women undergoing whole pelvis radiation for cervical cancer. *International Journal of Particle Therapy* 6 (1): 10–17. doi: 10.14338/IJPT-D-19-00061.1.

55 Dimopoulos, J.C.A., Pötter, R., Lang, S., et al. (2009). Dose-effect relationship for local control of cervical cancer by magnetic resonance image-guided brachytherapy. *Radiotherapy and Oncology: Journal of the European Society for Therapeutic Radiology and Oncology* 93: 311–315. doi: 10.1016/j.radonc.2009.07.001.

56 Barraclough, L.H., Swindell, R., Livsey, J.E., Hunter, R.D., and Davidson, S.E. (2008). External beam boost for cancer of the cervix uteri when intracavitary therapy cannot be performed. *International Journal of Radiation Oncology, Biology, Physics* 71: 772–778. doi: 10.1016/j.ijrobp.2007.10.066.

57 Sharma, M.K., Hug, E.B., Bhushan, M., et al. (2017). Dosimetric comparison of pencil-beam scanning and photon-based radiation therapy as a boost in carcinoma of cervix. *International Journal of Particle Therapy* 4 (2): 1–10. doi: 10.14338/ijpt-17-00009.

58 Clivio, A., Kluge, A., Cozzi, L., et al. (2013). Intensity modulated proton beam radiation for brachytherapy in patients with cervical carcinoma. *International Journal of Radiation Oncology, Biology, Physics* 87 (5): 897–903. doi: 10.1016/j.ijrobp.2013.08.027.

59 Chino, J., Annunziata, C.M., Beriwal, S., et al. (2020). Radiation therapy for cervical cancer: Executive summary of an ASTRO clinical practice guideline. *Practical Radiation Oncology*. doi: 10.1016/j.prro.2020.04.002.

60 Kagei, K., Tokuuye, K., Okumura, T., et al. (2003). Long-term results of proton beam therapy for carcinoma of the uterine cervix. *International Journal of Radiation Oncology, Biology, Physics* 55 (5): 1265–1271. doi: 10.1016/S0360-3016(02)04075-0.

61 Mohindra, P., Pollock, A., Patel, A., Roque, D., Rao, G., and Nichols, E. (2020). First clinical experience of quality assurance CT scan adapted intensity modulated proton therapy for utero-cervical cancers. In: *ASTRO Annual Meeting.* Virtual.

62 Mohindra, P., Nichols, E.M., and Kesslering, C.M. Clinical practice patterns for proton therapy in gynecological cancers: Report from a prospective multi-institutional registry. In: *2020 ASTRO Annual Meeting.* 108, 3, e498–e499

63 Rackwitz, T. and Debus, J. (2019). Clinical applications of proton and carbon ion therapy. *Seminars in Oncology*. doi: 10.1053/j.seminoncol.2019.07.005.

64 Karger, C.P., Peschke, P., Sanchez-Brandelik, R., Scholz, M., and Debus, J. (2006). Radiation tolerance of the rat spinal cord after 6 and 18 fractions of photons and carbon ions: Experimental results and clinical implications. *International Journal of Radiation Oncology, Biology, Physics*. doi: 10.1016/j.ijrobp.2006.08.045.

65 Hopewell, J.W., Barnes, D.W.H., Robbins, M.E.C., et al. (1990 Oct). The relative biological effectiveness of fractionated doses of fast neutrons (42 MeV(d→Be)) for normal tissues in the pig. II. Late effects on cutaneous and subcutaneous tissues. *The British Journal of Radiology*. 63(754):760–770. doi: 10.1259/0007-1285-63-754-760. PMID: 2242473.

66 Wakatsuki, M., Kato, S., Ohno, T., et al. (2014). Dose-escalation study of carbon ion radiotherapy for locally advanced squamous cell carcinoma of the uterine cervix (9902). *Gynecologic Oncology*. doi: 10.1016/j.ygyno 2013.10.021.

67 Okonogi, N., Wakatsuki, M., Kato, S., et al. (2019). A phase 1/2 study of carbon ion radiation therapy with concurrent chemotherapy for locally advanced uterine cervical squamous cell carcinoma (Protocol 1302). *International Journal of Radiation Oncology, Biology, Physics*. doi: 10.1016/j.ijrobp.2019.02.042.

68 Wakatsuki, M., Kato, S., Kiyohara, H., et al. (2015). Clinical trial of prophylactic extended-field carbon-ion radiotherapy for locally advanced uterine cervical cancer (Protocol 0508). *PLoS One*. doi: 10.1371/journal.pone.0127587.

69 Ohno, T., Noda, S.E., Murata, K., et al. (2018). Phase I study of carbon ion radiotherapy and image-guided brachytherapy for locally advanced cervical cancer. *Cancers (Basel)*. doi: 10.3390/cancers10090338.

70 Russell, A.H., Koh, W.J., Markette, K., et al. (1987). Radical reirradiation for recurrent or second primary carcinoma of the female reproductive tract. *Gynecologic Oncology* 27 (2): 226–232. doi: 10.1016/0090-8258(87)90297-6.

71 Llewelyn, M. and Taylor, A. (2017). Re-irradiation of cervical and endometrial cancer. *Current Opinion in Oncology* 29 (5): 343–350. doi: 10.1097/CCO.0000000000000392.

72 Sadozye, A.H. (2018). Re-irradiation in Gynaecological Malignancies: A Review. *Clinical Oncology*. doi: 10.1016/j.clon.2017.11.013.

73 Dewas, S., Bibault, J.E., Mirabel, X., et al. (2011). Robotic image-guided reirradiation of lateral pelvic recurrences: Preliminary results. *Radiation Oncology* 6 (1): 77. doi: 10.1186/1748-717X-6-77.

74 Park, H.J., Chang, A.R., Seo, Y., et al. (2015). Stereotactic body radiotherapy for recurrent or oligometastatic uterine cervix cancer: A cooperative study of the Korean radiation oncology group (KROG 14-11). *Anticancer Research* 35 (9): 5103–5110.

75 Abusaris, H., Hoogeman, M., and Nuyttens, J.J. (2012). Re-irradiation: Outcome, cumulative dose and toxicity in patients retreated with stereotactic radiotherapy in the abdominal or pelvic region. *Technology in Cancer Research & Treatment* 11 (6): 591–597. doi: 10.7785/tcrt.2012.500261.

76 Barsky, A.R., Reddy, V.K., Plastaras, J.P., Ben-Josef, E., Metz, J.M., and Wojcieszynski, A.P. (2020). Proton beam re-irradiation for gastrointestinal malignancies: A systematic review. *Journal of Gastrointestinal Oncology* 11 (1): 187–202. doi: 10.21037/jgo.2019.09.03.

77 DeCesaris, C.M., McCarroll, R., Mishra, M.V., et al. (2020). Assessing outcomes of patients treated with re-irradiation utilizing proton pencil-beam scanning for primary or recurrent malignancies of the esophagus and gastroesophageal junction. *Journal of Thoracic Oncology: Official Publication of the International Association for the Study of Lung Cancer* 15 (6): 1054–1064. doi: 10.1016/j.jtho.2020.01.024.

78 Li, Y.R., Kirk, M., and Lin, L. (2016). Proton therapy for vaginal reirradiation. *International Journal of Particle Therapy* 3 (2): 320–326. doi: 10.14338/ijpt-16-00013.1.

79 DeCesaris, C.M., Rice, S.R., Bentzen, S.M., Jatczak, J., Mishra, M.V., and Nichols, E.M. (2019). Quantification of acute skin toxicities in patients with breast cancer undergoing adjuvant proton versus photon radiation therapy: A single institutional experience. *International Journal of Radiation Oncology, Biology, Physics*. doi: 10.1016/j.ijrobp.2019.04.015.

80 Small, W., Mell, L.K., Anderson, P., et al. (2008). Consensus guidelines for delineation of clinical target volume for intensity-modulated pelvic radiotherapy in postoperative treatment of endometrial and cervical cancer. *International Journal of Radiation Oncology, Biology, Physics* 71 (2): 428–434. doi: 10.1016/j.ijrobp.2007.09.042.

81 Lim, K., Small, W., Portelance, L., et al. (2011). Consensus guidelines for delineation of clinical target volume for intensity-modulated pelvic radiotherapy for the definitive treatment of cervix cancer. *International Journal of Radiation Oncology, Biology, Physics* 79 (2): 348–355. doi: 10.1016/j.ijrobp.2009.10.075.

82 Gaffney, D.K., King, B., Viswanathan, A.N., et al. (2016). Consensus recommendations for radiation therapy contouring and treatment of vulvar carcinoma. *International Journal of Radiation Oncology, Biology, Physics* 95: 1191–1200. doi: 10.1016/j.ijrobp.2016.02.043.

24

Lymphoma and Leukemia

Chirayu G. Patel and Yolanda D. Tseng

Department of Radiation Oncology, Massachusetts General Hospital, 55 Fruit St, Boston, MA, 02114
Department of Radiation Oncology, University of Washington, 1959 NE Pacific St. Box 356043, Seattle, WA, 98195

24.1   Introduction

As the first curative treatment for Hodgkin lymphoma (HL), the role and delivery of radiation monotherapy for lymphoma have evolved since its initial descriptions in the 1960s [1,2] based on lessons learned from survivors of HL and integration of multi-agent chemotherapy. Late toxicity observed among survivors of HL (see Section 23.2) demonstrated the radiosensitivity of thoracic and abdominal normal structures including the heart, lung, and breast tissue. With chemotherapy, radiation fields and dose could be safely reduced while maintaining and even improving rates of cure. Technological advancements in radiation therapy image-guidance and delivery permitted smaller margins for setup error (i.e., planning target volume [PTV]) and higher dose conformality, respectively. All together, these advancements have allowed improved sparing of critical organs at risk from radiation dose with the goal of maintaining high rates of cure but decreasing late treatment-related toxicity.

24.2 The Rationale for Proton Therapy

24.2.1 Late Toxicities Learned from Hodgkin Lymphoma Survivors

As one of the most curable cancers, HL is a prototype for striking a balance between curative treatments and the treatment-associated toxicities that patients may live long enough to develop. Though radiotherapy was the first curative treatment for early stage HL, the price of cure was noted two decades later when the causes of death from secondary cancers and cardiovascular disease (CVD) outnumbered that from HL recurrence [3]. In addition to death from late toxicity, radiotherapy has also been associated with late morbidity from cardiac disease, pulmonary toxicity, and endocrine dysfunction.

24.2.2 Secondary Malignancies

Secondary cancers represent the most common cause of death among survivors of HL [3,4], with cancers of the breast, lung, and gastrointestinal tract representing the most common solid tumors [5]. Dose–response relationships have been implicated in deaths from secondary breast [6], esophageal [7], and lung cancer [8]. Relatively low-dose thresholds (≥4 Gy for breast cancer, ≥5 Gy for lung cancer) are significantly associated with increased relative risk of secondary cancer.

24.2.3 Breast Cancer

The breast tissue in young females is radiosensitive. Female HL survivors treated in the second and third decade of life have the highest cumulative incidence of secondary breast cancer, with a 10–15-year latency between treatment and secondary cancer [9]. The cumulative incidence in HL female survivors that were treated before age 21 years was as high as 26%, 30 years after treatment [9]. Several studies have established a dose–response relationship with increased risk observed with higher radiation dose to the breast (e.g., >20–40 Gy) [10,11]. With more granular estimates of breast dose and location of secondary breast cancer reconstructed through simulation films and mammography reports, a Dutch-nested

case-control study demonstrated a linear, radiation dose–response relationship between the adjusted excess odds ratio and estimated dose to the breast tissue, 6.1% per Gy [12].

Besides radiation dose, length of gonadal hormone exposure and radiation fields can modify the risk of breast cancer. Patients with longer intact ovarian function (e.g., younger patients) have higher risk of secondary breast cancer [9,11]. Premature ovarian suppression through pelvic radiation and/or receipt of alkylating chemotherapy can be protective with a lower, though still nonzero, risk of secondary breast cancer [9,11]. In like manner, smaller thoracic radiation fields may lower the risk of secondary breast cancer through reduction of breast volume irradiated. In a series from the British Columbia Cancer Agency (BCCA), the 20-year cumulative incidence of secondary breast cancer was 7.5% among HL patients treated with mantle field versus 3.1% with smaller radiation fields (involved field radiation therapy, involved site radiation therapy [ISRT], or involved node radiation therapy [INRT]) [13]. Similarly, female HL patients treated in the Netherlands with mantle field irradiation experienced a nearly threefold increased risk for breast cancer compared with those treated with mediastinal radiation alone (hazard ratio [HR] 2.8, 95% confidence interval [CI] 1.1–7.2) [9]. Together, these findings support the premise that techniques that reduce the volume of breast tissue irradiated may reduce breast cancer risk.

24.2.4 Lung Cancer

The risk of secondary lung cancer in survivors of HL is influenced by radiation dose to the lung, receipt of alkylating chemotherapy, and other comorbidities such as smoking. While the risk of lung cancer from alkylating agents is increased within the first 10 years from treatment, risk from radiotherapy does not occur until 5–9 years after radiation and persists for more than 20 years [8]. In a nested case-control study conducted within population-based cancer registries, a dose response was observed with elevated lung cancer risks observed with ≥5 Gy and with increasing dose to the lung [8]. Older age at HL diagnosis, male sex, increasing cycles with alkylating chemotherapy, and history of smoking were also associated with higher relative risk of lung cancer. There appeared to be a synergistic effect between radiation ≥5 Gy, smoking, and alkylating agents. Among patients receiving ≥5 Gy radiation and no alkylating agents, relative risk (RR) of secondary lung cancer was 7.2 among non- or light smokers and 20.2 among moderate–heavy smokers. However, in patients that received both RT and alkylating agents and were a moderate–heavy smoker, RR for secondary lung cancer was 49.1 [8]. Given the poor outcomes in treating secondary lung cancer [14], reduction of lung dose and consequent lung cancer risk are expected to be beneficial.

24.2.5 Gastrointestinal Cancers

Irradiated HL survivors are at risk of radiation-associated cancers of the esophagus [7], stomach [15], and pancreas [16], with risk being dose-dependent. Significantly increased incidence of cancers of the colon and rectum also have been observed compared to the general population [17]. Median time from HL treatment to secondary GI cancers is 15–20 years; prognosis is generally poor after diagnosis of the secondary cancer. Irradiation of the esophagus ≥30 Gy is associated with a 4.3-fold higher (95% CI 1.5–15.3) esophageal cancer risk compared to <30 Gy or no radiotherapy, with suggestion of linearity (excess odds ratio [EOR]/Gy 0.38; 95% CI 0.04–8.17; $p_{trend} < 0.001$) [7]. Risk of pancreatic cancer among HL survivors is also related to dose, with increasing odds ratio (OR) with increasing radiation dose: OR 0.5 (0.5–5 Gy), OR 1.8 (10–40 Gy), and OR 9.1 (≥40 Gy) [16]. In addition, there is a greater than additive risk of pancreatic cancer with radiation and number of cycles of alkylating agents. Risk of secondary gastric cancer among HL survivors is also dose-dependent, with increasing dose to the stomach associated with increasing risk of stomach cancer (EOR/Gy 0.09; 95% CI 0.04–0.21; $p_{trend} < 0.001$) [15]. Alkylating agents influence the risk of gastric cancer and may interact with radiation dose. Receipt of procarbazine ≥5,600 mg/m^2 and ≥25 Gy radiation to the stomach was associated with a 77.5-fold increased risk (95% CI 14.7–1,452), but risk was not elevated with ≥5,600 mg/m^2 procarbazine if dose to stomach was <25 Gy. Despite these relative risks, the absolute excess risks of secondary GI cancers are relatively low and typically below five per 10,000 per years of follow-up [17].

24.2.6 Cardiovascular Disease after Mediastinal Radiation

Among long-term HL survivors, CVD death is the most common, nonmalignant cause of death. HL survivors have a 2.5- to 6.5-fold higher incidence of CVD death compared to the general population [3,18,19]. Risk of CVD death remains elevated even >20 years from treatment [19] and is dose dependent: radiation dose of >30 Gy to the heart is associated with a 3.5 times relative risk (95% CI 2.7–4.3) of death compared to <30 Gy [19]. Though males and females have similar RR of death from CVD and myocardial infarction (MI), given the higher CVD mortality rate of men in the general population, the absolute excess risk (AER) of CVD death among male HL survivors is higher [3,19]. Age at irradiation also appears to impact risk of cardiovascular death. In a series from Stanford, younger patients at treatment (<19 years) had the highest RR for death from MI (RR 44.1; 95% CI 17.8–91.8), with RR decreasing with increasing age. However, given that the incidence of death from MI increases with increasing age, the AER of MI deaths increases with increasing age despite decline in RR [19]. These observations highlight that while it is important to minimize dose to young mediastinal lymphoma patients, given the higher absolute risk of CVD and associated death among older patients, cardiac sparing should be considered for all patients, regardless of age.

Besides cardiac mortality, HL survivors are at risk of chronic cardiac conditions including coronary artery disease (CAD), valvular dysfunction, pericardial disease, cardiomyopathy, and conduction defects [20]. CAD is the most predominant clinical manifestation of radiation-related heart disease [21]. Incidence of CVD is 3–6-fold higher than the general population [22,23]. In a Dutch cohort of HL survivors, the 40-year cumulative incidence of CVD was 50% (95% CI 47–52) [22].

Over the last decade, the dose–response relationship between heart dose and risk of CVD has been better characterized (Table 24.1), though 3D treatment planning data is still needed to better identify the relative radiosensitivity of various cardiac substructures. These findings, which demonstrate a linear, no threshold relationship between mean heart dose

Table 24.1 Summary of dose–response relationship of radiation dose to heart or cardiac substructures and risk of cardiovascular toxicity.

End point	Cohort	Shape of dose–response relationship
Symptomatic CVD (MI, angina pectoris)	5-year HL survivors treated in Netherlands, 1965–1995	Linear with mean heart dose: ERR 7.4%/Gy (95% CI 3.3–14.8) [71]
CVD	HL patients treated on 9 EORTC-LYSA trials	Linear with mean heart dose: HR 1.015 (95% CI 1.006–1.024) per 1 Gy [73]
Valvular heart disease	5-year HL survivors treated in Netherlands, 1965–1995	Nonlinear with dose to heart valve: ≤30, 31–35, 36–40, and >40 Gy associated with RR 2.5%, 6.5%, 11.2%, and 24.3% per 1 Gy, respectively [72]
Symptomatic heart failure or cardiomyopathy	5-year HL survivors treated in Netherlands, 1965–1995	Nonlinear with mean heart dose: ≤25, 26–30, and >30 Gy associated with RR 1.00, 2.43, and 3.67, respectively Linear with mean dose to left ventricle: ERR 9.0%/Gy [92]

CI = Confidence interval; CVD = cardiovascular disease; ERR = excess relative risk; HL = Hodgkin lymphoma; HR = hazard ratio; MI = myocardial infarction.

and risk of CVD highlight that even low doses of the heart may increase the relative risk of CVD for patients with mediastinal lymphoma and the importance of reducing heart dose to the extent possible.

HL survivors are also at risk of CVD from anthracycline-based chemotherapy, which most commonly manifests as valvular heart disease and heart failure [22]. A linear dose–response relationship is observed between dose of anthracyclines per 50 mg/m^2 increase in dose and risk of CVD events (HR 1.077, 95% CI 1.021–1.137) [22], highlighting the importance of cardiac radiation dose sparing in those patients who are heavily pretreated and/or who have received higher cumulative anthracycline exposure given their already elevated risk of CVD.

24.2.7 Stroke

HL patients irradiated to the mediastinum and/or neck have an increased risk of cerebrovascular disease, which can be 2–3-fold higher compared to the general population with the median time to event being over 15 years after treatment [24]. Among HL survivors treated in the Netherlands, most ischemic events were from large artery atherosclerosis or cardioembolism [24], presumably due to neck irradiation and and/or valvular disease from mediastinal radiation.

24.2.8 Pulmonary Toxicity

Treatment-associated pulmonary toxicity in patients with mediastinal lymphoma include radiation pneumonitis (RP) and bleomycin toxicity [25], which occur in the acute and subacute settings. RP risk is related to radiation dose to the lungs, with mean lung dose >13.5 Gy, V5 >55%, and V20 >30–33.5% predictive of risk among patients treated with 3D-conformal and IMRT photon techniques [26,27]. Among patients treated with 3D-conformal radiation, risk of RP also increased if mediastinal radiation was given in the relapsed/refractory (r/r) versus upfront setting (35% vs. 10%) and if peri-transplant radiation was given before versus after transplant (grade 3 RP, 57% vs. 0%; $p = 0.015$) [26]. Rates of reduced diffusing capacity for carbon monoxide (diffusing capacity of lung for carbon monoxide [DLCO]) are observed 6 months after treatment of HL, which are higher among patients treated with combined modality treatment versus chemotherapy alone (52% vs. 20%; $p = 0.03$) and patients with larger volume of lung irradiated to higher dose [28]. Besides the potential direct impact in terms of diminished lung function, pulmonary dysfunction has also been associated with fatigue in HL survivors [29].

24.2.9 Endocrine Dysfunction

Approximately 50–60% of patients with lymphoma irradiated to the neck will develop hypothyroidism [30,31]. Smaller thyroid gland volume in addition to volume of thyroid irradiated are predictive of risk [31,32]. Childhood cancer survivors and adult HL survivors irradiated to the abdomen are at increased risk of diabetes [33,34], which is dose- and location-dependent. The tail of the pancreas, in contrast to the pancreatic body or head, appears especially radiosensitive and corresponds to where the islets of Langerhans are concentrated. Children who received >10 Gy to the pancreatic tail had a 11.5-fold increased RR of diabetes (95% CI 3.9–34), which increased with increasing radiation dose [33]. Among adult HL survivors, risk of diabetes was also increased with increasing mean dose to the pancreatic tail (HR 1.017 per Gy) [34].

24.2.10 Summary

The late toxicities learned from HL survivors have established the radiosensitivity of critical structures within the head and neck, thoracic, and upper abdominal regions, with risk often being dose-dependent. In efforts to reduce risk of late toxicity, radiotherapeutic management of lymphoma has focused on the three-prong approach of (1) reducing field size (i.e., ISRT, INRT), (2) reducing radiation dose, and pertinent to this chapter, and (3) improving radiation delivery. Proton therapy represents one avenue to improve the conformality of radiation dose to the head and neck, mediastinum, abdomen/pelvis, and cranial spinal axis.

24.3 Proton Therapy for Head and Neck Lymphomas

The head and neck regions can be divided into nodal, extranodal, and brain sites. Irradiation of the brain (i.e., primary or secondary CNS lymphomas) will not be discussed here as standard therapy involves whole brain radiation therapy with or without a boost. Extranodal sites include the orbit, sinuses, parotids, thyroid, cavernous sinus, and nasal cavity, which lie in proximity to organs at risk, including the temporal lobes, optic nerves/chiasm, pituitary gland, and salivary glands. Nodal sites include the Waldeyer's ring, cervical, retropharyngeal, and facial nodal tissue. Though doses used for definitive or adjuvant treatment (24–36 Gy) of indolent and aggressive non-HLs generally are within tolerance of many critical structures, for a subset of patients (e.g., extranodal NK/T-cell lymphoma), higher doses (≥50 Gy) are required for local control.

24.3.1 Dosimetric Comparisons

Two dosimetric studies have compared proton therapy to modern photon techniques including 3D conformal and volumetric modulated arc therapy (VMAT) in HL patients with cervical nodal involvement [35,36]. The greatest reduction in dose to critical structures such as the common carotid artery, thyroid, larynx, pharynx, and salivary glands was achieved not through radiation technique but instead by reduction in field size (i.e., mantle field to INRT) [35,36].

Though little information is provided on type of proton technique used, both 3D conformal and proton therapy had low dose (e.g., <20 Gy) to the thyroid, larynx, and pharynx compared to VMAT. However, at higher doses (e.g., ≥20 Gy), the dose volume histograms (DVH) overlapped with that of VMAT. For the parotid gland, 3D conformal and proton therapy had lower low dose (<5 Gy) compared to VMAT, but the DVH curve was similar to VMAT by 5–10 Gy, both for ipsilateral and contralateral glands [36]. Proton therapy appeared to have better sparing of the ipsilateral submandibular gland for low and moderate doses compared to 3D conformal and better sparing of low dose compared to VMAT. Dose >10 Gy was equally spared to the contralateral submandibular gland with all three techniques, with proton therapy and 3D conformal having the lowest low dose (<10 Gy) [36]. Though the number of studies is small, these findings mirror the anecdotal experience of the authors: proton therapy appears to spare low radiation dose to contralateral paired structures. However, for ipsilateral structures adjacent to the target (e.g., parotid gland organ at risk adjacent to level II cervical lymph node target), high dose conformality may be equivalent or better with VMAT/IMRT compared to proton therapy, at least for non-intensity modulated proton therapy techniques.

For radioresistant tumors, proton therapy may permit dose escalation through better OAR sparing [37] in attempts to improve local control. However, as adequate local control can be achieved for most lymphoma histologies with doses lower than typically required for primary head and neck tumors, the role of proton therapy for head and neck lymphoma is less well defined. Additionally, one must be mindful of the sharp dose gradients of proton therapy to avoid marginal recurrence [37].

24.3.2 Outcomes

Outcome studies of proton radiotherapy focusing on head and neck lymphoma are limited given the long latency to late effects and relatively few patients available for study [38]. University of Florida investigators published a case series of 11 non-HL patients who were treated with proton therapy. This included seven patients with the following sites and his-

tologies: four orbit (two MALT, two follicular), one base of skull/paranasal sinuses (plasmablastic), one oropharynx/hypopharynx/hard palate (NK/T cell), and one orbit/infratemporal fossa/cavernous sinus (NK/T cell) [39]. Proton therapy was well tolerated, with no grade 3 or higher acute toxicity. Local control rate was 91%, with a single patient with NK/T-cell lymphoma recurring within the RT field [39].

Recent population-based data from the National Cancer Database found that proton therapy was associated with reduced risk of secondary cancer among lymphoma and primary head/neck patients compared to IMRT [40], presumably due to lower integral dose to normal tissues. The overall adjusted odds ratio for second malignancy in comparing proton therapy to IMRT for all histologies was 0.31 (95% CI 0.26–0.36) [40]. These early findings suggest that proton therapy is important to consider for younger patients with excellent prognoses, who may live long enough to develop a secondary cancer from treatment (Figure 24.1).

24.3.3 Simulation

Patients are simulated in the supine position with a thermoplastic mask for immobilization. For nodal radiation, neck extension is required if anterior fields may be used. For certain sites, such as the sinonasal region, a bite block may be considered to help spare dose to the oral cavity. Intravenous contrast is recommended for cases requiring treatment of neck lymph nodes.

24.3.4 Treatment Planning

The fusion of PET/CTs (including pre- and post-chemotherapy, if relevant) will help to delineate volumes as per ISRT approach [41,42], or if PET/CT and CT simulation are obtained in the same position, involve node radiation therapy (INRT) can be done [43]. For sinonasal and nasopharyngeal sites, an MRI is recommended. Ideally, both pre-chemotherapy and post-chemotherapy MRIs would be available for treatment planning, especially in cases of uncertain metabolic response to chemotherapy based on PET/CT. Finally, direct evaluation by flexible nasopharyngolaryngoscopy and review of any operative reports may further guide volume delineation.

Several proton techniques can be considered for irradiation of the head and neck region. The most advanced proton therapy, intensity-modulated proton therapy (IMPT), uses pencil beam scanning (PBS), which can help with skin-sparing and achieve excellent target conformality [44]. IMPT can be planned with single-field optimization (SFO) or multi-field optimization (MFO) [44]. With SFO, each beam covers the entire target volume, which improves the plan robustness to

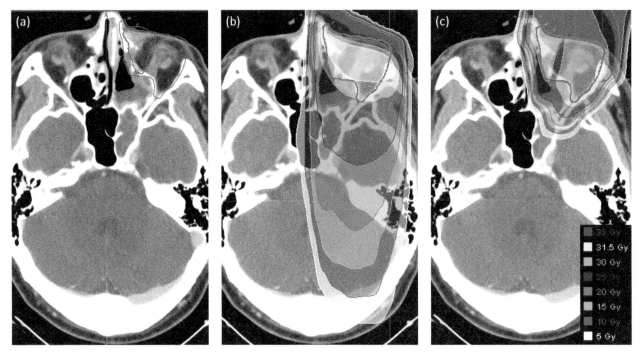

Figure 24.1 Passive scatter proton therapy plan for a 32-year-old patient with grade 3A follicular lymphoma of the medial orbital adnexa, including a small focus of invasion into the nasal cavity. He received combined modality therapy, with a post-chemotherapy PET/CT indicative of a complete metabolic response followed by involved site radiotherapy of the whole orbit to 30 Gy (RBE). Proton therapy was utilized to help minimize integral dose to surrounding structures and reduce his long-term risk of second malignancy. (a) Pre-chemotherapy GTV in red, CTV in pink. (b) Radiation dose distribution with standard-of-care 3D-conformal radiation therapy with superior/inferior wedged pair to avoid contralateral orbit. (c) Radiation dose distribution using passive scatter proton technique with a single LAO field.

changes in patient setup, anatomy, and less likely, motion during treatment. In contrast, with MFO, different beams may be treating different portions of the target. A simple example would be treating the bilateral neck, in which left and right anterior oblique beams would only be treating the left and right neck, respectively, instead of both neck targets. However, when viewed together, the entire target is covered to the prescription dose. While more conformal, MFO can be more sensitive to changes in tumor volume as treatment progresses, potentially reducing its robustness relative to SFO or passive scattering [44]. SFO is particularly well suited for unilateral tumors due to high conformality and robustness that can be achieved relative to complex, bilateral tumors [44]. Traversing surgical or dental hardware is not recommended as CT artifact may affect the treatment plan accuracy and be associated with dose shadowing distal to the hardware [44].

For irradiation of the sinonasal region, in which radiation-associated irritation of the sinuses may cause thickening of the mucosa and/or blockage, consideration should be given to performing quality assurance (QA) CT scans during treatment to confirm no changes along the proton beam path(s), which may influence the proton dose distribution. The same is true for patients in whom at the time of radiation treatment planning has blockage or thickening of the nasal sinuses, which may open during treatment.

24.3.5 Acute Toxicities

Mucositis, xerostomia, dysgeusia, and dry eye are commonly encountered acute toxicities of radiotherapy in the head and neck region, though acute toxicity requiring treatment break is rare. Acute toxicities with regard to proton radiotherapy in head and neck lymphomas have not been systematically studied. Many comparative studies examining proton versus photon radiation therapy in the head and neck region, but not involving lymphoma, have shown comparable or modest improvements in acute toxicities, in addition to select toxicities being potentially worse with protons (dermatitis, neurologic toxicity, temporal lobe necrosis) [44]. However, due to the differences in prescription dose used for lymphoma and other solid tumors, it is difficult to extrapolate these clinical toxicity outcomes to lymphoma patients that are treated to lower doses.

24.4 Proton Therapy for Mediastinal Lymphomas

The mediastinum is a commonly involved site in lymphoma. Given the adjacent normal tissues at risk—breast, lung, and heart—mediastinal lymphoma patients are at risk of long-term cardiotoxicity and second malignancy, as discussed earlier. Besides the location of the target volume and patient anatomy (see Section 24.4.1), patient, and prior treatment factors may also modulate the relative benefit of proton therapy. These include sex, age, r/r disease, presence of cardiac comorbidities, receipt of cardiotoxic systemic therapy, and prior mediastinal radiation therapy. Identification of patients who may benefit from mediastinal proton therapy has nicely been summarized by consensus guidelines from the International Lymphoma Radiation Oncology Group (ILROG). These include (1) patients with mediastinal disease below the origin of left main stem coronary artery (i.e., lower mediastinal involvement), (2) young female patients in whom dose to the breast tissue should be minimized, and (3) heavily pretreated patients (i.e., r/r) who may benefit from sparing of lung, heart, and bone marrow given higher risk of pneumonitis and exposure to anthracyclines [45]. As patient-specific anatomy and mediastinal disease distribution greatly influence the relative benefit of proton therapy over IMRT, case-by-case comparative planning is advised for personalized selection of the optimal radiation technique [45].

24.4.1 Dosimetric Comparisons

A number of dosimetric comparisons of proton therapy to photons with 3D CRT and/or IMRT have been published [46–59], with an emphasis on comparing dose to normal surrounding tissues that bear the burden of morbidity and mortality. Excellent target coverage is possible with any of the radiation modalities. A systematic review of dosimetric studies performed by the Particle Therapy Co-Operative Group lymphoma subcommittee showed reduced dose to the heart, lungs, breasts, esophagus, and thyroid, as well as integral dose, with proton therapy compared with IMRT or 3D-conformal techniques [60]. DIBH has been selectively implemented in patients being treated with proton therapy [51,53,54,57–59].

Cardiac sparing is one of the major reasons to consider proton therapy, given that for certain cardiac endpoints (e.g., CVD), there is no threshold below which the risk of toxicity is zero. Furthermore, risk is linearly and positively associated with cardiac dose (Table 24.1). By reducing low dose to the heart and improving conformality, proton therapy can be asso-

ciated with lower mean heart dose. Disease extent may help select which patients may derive the greatest benefit with proton over photon therapy. Greater cardiac sparing, at least based on mean heart dose, was seen for proton therapy over 3D conformal or IMRT/VMAT among patients with lower (vs. upper) mediastinal involvement [51]. Of note, the definition of "lower mediastinal involvement" varies by study or guideline, but generally reflects disease that spans inferiorly to the level of the heart (Table 24.2). Currently, little is known whether cardiac substructures have differential radiosensitivity, and hence, whether radiation dose should be differentially distributed across the heart. Future attention should be paid to radiation dose of cardiac substructures [45].

Proton therapy is also associated with significant reduction in mean lung dose, with larger benefits noted with IMRT (mean difference, 3.28 Gy [relative biological effectiveness (RBE)]) compared to 3D conformal (mean difference, 2.81 Gy [RBE]) [60]. High-dose conformality within the lung (i.e., V20) is generally similar between proton therapy and IMRT [53,57,58]. Not surprisingly for low lung dose (i.e., V5), proton therapy is associated with greater reduction of V5 compared to IMRT [53,57,58] and 3D-conformal techniques as well [49,53]. However, attention should be paid to the type of proton techniques used in comparative dosimetric studies, which have included passive scatter and PBS techniques. As PBS may have higher dose conformality compared to uniform scanning and passive scattering, lung dose may be further reduced with use of this technique [49].

In attempts to further improve cardiac and lung dosimetry, DIBH has been widely utilized with 3D CRT and IMRT photon techniques. Several studies have now examined DIBH in protons [51,53,54,57–59]. By increasing the lung volume with DIBH, a smaller percentage of the entire lung is irradiated, leading to improvement in lung metrics [61]. By elongating the mediastinum downward, DIBH also has the potential to reduce radiation exposure to the heart. However, this benefit is primarily seen in those patients whose disease is located superior to the heart [62]. For lower mediastinal disease (Table 24.2), the additional cardiac sparing by incorporating DIBH with proton therapy may be modest at best, as there will continue to be disease adjacent to the heart even with DIBH [57,59,61].

Table 24.2 Definition of lower mediastinal involvement used across various studies and/or guidelines.

ILROG [45]	Mediastinal disease spans below the origin of the left main stem coronary artery
Institut Gustav Roussy [62]	Mediastinal disease whose lower border extends >3 cm below the carina
Oxford Cancer Centre [51]	Mediastinal disease whose inferior border of CTV is inferior to the 7th thoracic level (T7)
Authors' definition	Mediastinal disease that spans below the left pulmonary artery (i.e., superior aspect of the heart as defined by the heart contouring atlas [70])

Breast dose is another metric of interest in comparative dosimetry studies given the young age of mediastinal lymphoma patients being considered for radiotherapy. Posterior beam angle(s) can lower breast dose, but potentially at the cost of higher lung and heart dose [63]. Even when exclusively posterior beams are not used, proton therapy has been associated with reduced mean breast dose, again with greater benefits noted when compared with IMRT/VMAT (average difference, 2.45 Gy [RBE]) versus 3D-conformal techniques (average difference, 1.47 Gy [RBE]) [60]. Patients with axillary involvement may derive greater benefit with proton therapy compared to photon techniques. In one study, proton therapy was associated with significantly lower mean breast dose compared to 3D conformal (2.7 Gy reduction, $p < 0.01$) or VMAT with three partial arcs (3.3 Gy reduction, $p < 0.01$) in patients with axillary involvement, but not in patients without axillary involvement (0.6 Gy reduction, $p = 0.06$; 0.4 Gy reduction, $p = 0.09$, respectively) [51].

Proton therapy may help with thyroid sparing [60]. The impact of DIBH on thyroid dose due to changes in positioning has not been well-studied, but data to date does not show a significant difference in thyroid dose with DIBH versus free breathing [64]. In a dosimetric study of esophageal dose and estimated risk of complications including esophagitis, esophageal stricture, and esophageal cancer, proton therapy did better on all measures, except esophageal stricture risk, which was similar to 3D CRT. Protons, IMRT, and 3D CRT all had substantially improved mean esophageal dose relative to mantle field techniques of the past [65].

Based on these reviewed dosimetric comparison studies, we favor use of proton therapy for patient with lower mediastinal and/or axillary involvement. DIBH, which is expected to improve lung dosimetry, may be incorporated if the proton clinic is able to confirm daily reproducibility of breath hold (e.g., volumetric IGRT). For patients with exclusively upper mediastinal involvement, prior dosimetric studies and our anecdotal experience suggest that DIBH and photons can yield plans with very good cardiac and lung sparing, although integral dose will be improved with protons as compared to photons and is of increasing relevance with younger patient age due to concerns of secondary malignancies over time.

24.4.2 Outcomes

Mediastinal proton radiation therapy is well tolerated. Among 138 HL patients (30% favorable early stage, 28% unfavorable early stage, 42% advanced stage) who underwent consolidative mediastinal proton radiation therapy, no grade 3 toxicities were observed during a median 32-month follow-up [66]. The three-year relapse-free survival (RFS) was 92%, which was lower for pediatric patients (87%) compared to adults (96%). Among the 10 recurrences observed, 6 were in-field, 1 in- and

out-of-field, and 3 out-of-field in immediately adjacent nodal ranges. Most recurrences with an in-field component (six out of seven) were observed in pediatric patients treated <30 Gy (RBE). Notably, no marginal recurrences were seen at the edge of the proton field. These data suggest that despite the conformal dose distribution with proton therapy, that rates of cure and RFS are not compromised.

Given the latency between radiation treatment and onset of cardiac toxicity and secondary cancers, which generally require >10–20 years, little, if any clinical data, is currently available on late toxicity among patients treated with proton therapy. Recent data from the National Cancer Database evaluated rates of secondary cancer by histology and radiation technique (proton therapy vs. IMRT). Though not statistically significant, the adjusted odds ratio for risk of secondary cancer favored proton therapy among lymphoma patients. Across all tumor types, proton therapy was associated with significantly lower risk of secondary cancer compared to IMRT (adjust OR 0.31; 95% CI 0.26–0.36; $p < 0.0001$) [40]. This highlights the importance of following patients treated with proton therapy to ensure future data to assess the clinical value of proton therapy.

Models have been created to estimate risk of late effects based on dosimetric differences observed between photons and proton therapy. Based on dosimetric data of IMRT versus proton therapy and free breathing versus DIBH techniques for 22 early stage HL patients, Rechner et al. estimated life years lost (LYL) secondary to late effects from radiotherapy by techniques [58]. LYL was calculated accounting for age at radiotherapy, sex, and potential risk of various cardiac toxicities and secondary lung and breast cancers. Valvular heart disease and lung cancer were found to dominate LYL. Proton therapy with DIBH had the least LYL, but LYL with proton therapy with free breathing was comparable to IMRT with DIBH. IMRT with free breathing had greatest LYL. Limitations of this study include the uncertainties in the risk models, lack of 4D imaging for simulation, generous PTV margins, lack of an integral dose measure, no description about disease extent (which could influence relative benefit of proton therapy), and a focus limited to mortality that would miss morbidity-related improvement of proton therapy. In a separate modeling study, Toltz et al. found no excess risk of cardiac mortality at 15 years after radiation for IMPT or helical TomoTherapy compared to 3D-conformal therapy for 20 HL patients. This was attributed in part to lower radiation doses now prescribed for consolidation (20–30 Gy). However, subsets of patients had more pronounced differences in estimated cardiac mortality among the three studied techniques, including those with disease anterior to the heart and lungs and those with higher prescribed radiation dose. Risks of lung cancer and breast cancer were predicted to be reduced for all patients with IMPT as compared to 3D-conformal and helical TomoTherapy [67].

24.4.3 Simulation

Patients are simulated in the supine position with the use of custom body immobilization. Arm and neck positioning may be chosen in attempts to reproduce the pre-chemotherapy PET/CT scan position, which may facilitate fusion of PET/CT to CT simulation scan for target delineation. For young female patients, we favor treating with arms down or akimbo given this brings less breast tissue medially [68] and into the proton beam path. A 10°–15° incline board may also help reduce breast dose [69]. For patients with concurrent neck disease, a thermoplastic head and neck mask is incorporated for immobilization. With mid-neck involvement, having mild neck extension may help with minimizing dose to the chin with a straight anterior beam. However, with high neck involvement (e.g., high level II), alternate beam angles may be preferred (e.g., anterior oblique or posterior beam) over a straight anterior beam. As such, neck extension is less beneficial and complicates fusion with the pre-chemotherapy PET/CT scan, which is generally taken with the neck in a neutral or a mildly flexed position.

Motion management strategies include a 4D CT scan if free breathing or DIBH, if available within the proton clinic. DIBH may be more challenging to implement given the longer treatment times required and that confirmation of a reproducible breath hold (i.e., volumetric image guided radiotherapy) may not be readily available at all proton clinics. A surrogate or surface monitoring system could otherwise be considered but should be validated to accurately predict the mediastinal target volume location. For DIBH, we recommend three separate CT scans in DIBH to assess reproducibility of the breath hold. Regardless of motion management strategy, IV contrast is recommended.

24.4.4 Treatment Planning

ISRT [41] is recommended by ILROG when there are differences in body position between PET/CT and CT simulation; otherwise, if immobilization and position are exactly the same, INRT can be used [42,43]. The following OARs are recommended to be contoured: thyroid, esophagus, lungs, breasts, heart, and cardiac substructures (atria, ventricles, valves, common carotid, left anterior descending artery, right circumflex) [45]. The use of a cardiac contouring atlas is recommended to facilitate contouring of cardiac substructures [70]. ILROG recommends the following recommended mediastinal dose constraints based on applicable literature [45]: heart/left ventricle/coronary arteries/valves (mean < 5 Gy; 5–15 Gy allowable; avoid >30 Gy) [71–73], breast (age dependent; mean < 4 Gy; 4–15 allowable; avoid >30 Gy), lung V5 (<55%; 55–60% allowable, avoid >60%), lung V20 (<30%), lung mean (<10 Gy; 10–13.5 Gy allowable; avoid >13.5 Gy) [27], and thy-

roid V25 (<62.5%) [32]. We note that modern proton therapy may allow for even lower doses to OARs than these ideal constraints, depending on the target volume and patient anatomy. As such, these constraints should be used help guide clinical judgment but should be modified to be more stringent whenever feasible. Of note, with more conformal techniques, the mean heart dose may have less relevance than dose to specific cardiac substructures, which may vary greatly even if mean heart dose is similar between two plans [74].

Recent work has shown substantial motion of cardiac substructures, mainly in the craniocaudal direction [75], though further work is needed first to identify which cardiac substructures are radiosensitive and then how to account for these substructures' movement during treatment. The Mayo Clinic has published early work on electrocardiogram-gated CT with coronary angiography to assist in cardiac substructure identification and creation of an organ-at-risk structure that is incorporated as part of the radiation plan optimization. While the first study patients were treated with VMAT with DIBH, the investigators are now enrolling patients that will be treated with proton therapy [76].

Beam angle selection is dependent on the target volume (i.e., anterior vs. posterior mediastinal involvement, treatment of the neck) and patient anatomy. Anterior or anterior oblique beams are generally chosen, especially if disease resides in the anterior mediastinum. With posterior mediastinal involvement, posterior beams may be included as these targets may drape behind the heart. Especially with PBS, the CTV or ITV target may be split with different beams treating different regions of the target (Figure 24.2). A gradient junction approach can be used to transition between beams from one region to another within a target.

Proton therapy has unique treatment planning considerations that need to be considered, especially when irradiating a mediastinal target volume. The first, most basic aspect is accounting for range calculation uncertainties that arise from inaccuracies in converting Hounsfield units to proton stopping power and variation in setup. In efforts to improve robustness to these range uncertainties, one of two strategies is typically employed. A margin can be added along the beam path both distally and proximally to the target volume; or, planning occurs with a larger volume than the ITV or CTV.

A second consideration is accounting for various tissue densities that a proton beam may traverse to the target volume: soft tissue, bone, and air. Historically, pencil beam analytical (PBA) algorithms have been used to calculate proton dose. However, in thoracic targets, PBA may not calculate proton dose accurately given the heterogeneous tissue densities [77], leading to undercoverage of mediastinal target volumes [59]. As such, Monte Carlo dose algorithms, which are now commercially available, are preferred for treatment planning to ensure appropriate coverage of the target volume and accurate

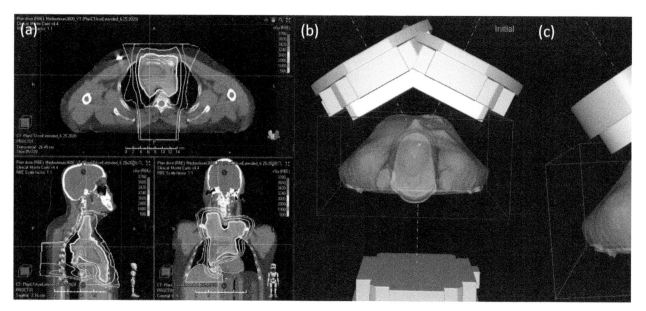

Figure 24.2 A 53-year-old man with stage IIA unfavorable classical Hodgkin lymphoma of the right neck, bilateral supraclavicular region, mediastinum, internal mammary lymph nodes, and cardiophrenic lymph nodes. He was treated with two cycles of ABVD with a Deauville 4 on interim PET. As such, his treatment was escalated to BEACOPP for four cycles. (a) In the setting of persistent disease (Deauville 4), he underwent consolidation radiotherapy with PBS to his initial extent of disease (30 Gy) followed by a boost to his area of partial response (6 Gy). (b) The target volume was split into four regions, each with different beam angles. The right neck disease was treated with two beams: a right anterior oblique (RAO) and PA beam. The left neck disease was treated with two beams: a left anterior oblique (LAO) and PA beam. In the mediastinum, the anterior mediastinal and internal mammary targets were treated with two beams (LAO and RAO), whereas the posterior mediastinal and cardiophrenic lymph nodes (see sagittal images) were treated with only a PA beam using volumetric repainting. A gradient junction was used to transition between these three regions. (c) As his residual disease was only in the anterior mediastinum, the sequential boost volume was treated with LAO and RAO beams.

estimates of physical dose to organs at risk. However, Monte Carlo is more time-intensive for computation and can lengthen the treatment planning process. Furthermore, it is important to note that dose levels were set through historical data based on PBA calculations and patient outcomes, emphasizing the importance of following the outcomes of patients planned with Monte Carlo dose algorithms.

A third consideration, especially if patients are treated free breathing, is generating a plan robust to respiratory and cardiac motion to minimize the risk of missing a moving target (i.e., interplay effect). This is handled both through motion management strategies (4D CT scans, DIBH, beam gating) and selection of proton technique and beams. Whereas passive scattering technique is the most robust given that the dose for a field is delivered instantaneously, many proton clinics have adopted PBS given improved conformality. With uniform scanning and PBS, dose is delivered on a layer-by-layer basis through changes in proton beam energy. While uniform scanning delivers all dose to a single layer nearly instantaneously, PBS uses a magnet to steer the beam in a raster-like pattern along the x- and y-axis of a single layer. Hence, PBS is most prone to the interplay effect given that the proton delivery and target volume are both moving over time. Strategies to minimize risk of interplay with PBS include use of volumetric

repainting and using a larger spot size [49,78–80]. Fractionated treatment can also provide effective rescanning.

A final consideration is being mindful of potential changes in target volume during treatment. This refers specifically to cases in which gross disease is being treated (i.e., salvage therapy). Given the radioresponsive nature of lymphoma, the target volume may change during treatment, potentially leading to under- or overranging of the proton beam to adjacent organs at risk. In these circumstances, QA CT scans during treatment may be helpful.

Discussion thus far has focused on the physical dose distribution of proton therapy. Accurately estimating biological dose is also an active area of research, in particular developing models to estimate variability in the RBE at the end of the Bragg peak. This may be of concern when the distal edge of an anterior field is adjacent to coronary vessels, though as the coronary artery moves with cardiac and respiratory motion, a point maximum dose may be less pronounced. With the availability of Monte Carlo treatment planning algorithms, future dose calculations may be able to incorporate spatial variations in proton RBE, although there is no one accepted variable RBE model to estimate biological dose currently. Preliminary data using a published model for DNA double-strand break induction found that the putative increase in RBE at the end of range did not decrease the dosimetric advantages of proton therapy in cardiac substructures compared to advanced photon techniques [59].

24.4.5 Acute Toxicities

Acute toxicities with mediastinal proton therapy include dermatitis and esophagitis, most frequently grade 1–2 based on RTOG grading for dermatitis and CTCAEv5 for esophagitis. Esophagitis is well managed with diet modification and use of over-the-counter analgesics and/or mouthwash containing viscous lidocaine (e.g., Magic or Miracle Mouthwash). Pneumonitis is a subacute toxicity, with mean lung dose and lung V20 predictive of CTCAEv4 grade 2 or higher pneumonitis [81]. Though numbers are small ($n = 59$), rates of pneumonitis after proton therapy in a series from University of Florida were 1.7% (grade 2) [82], with 81% of the cohort being treated after initial chemotherapy versus the r/r setting. Rates of symptomatic pneumonitis among r/r mediastinal lymphoma patients treated with proton therapy are 12.8% (CTCAEv4 grade 2) [81], which is consistent or slightly lower than historical rates observed among patients treated with photons [26]. Pulmonary function remained relatively unchanged compared to baseline at 12 months after proton therapy in a small case series of HL patients who completed mediastinal proton therapy [83].

24.5 Proton Therapy for Infradiaphragmatic Lymphoma

Among early stage HL patients, infradiaphragmatic involvement is less common (10–15%) but can be seen as part of advanced stage disease. Patients with aggressive non-HL, most commonly diffuse large B-cell lymphoma, may also have abdominal and/or pelvic involvement as part of localized or advanced disease. Proton therapy for infradiaphragmatic lymphoma may lower dose to the stomach, bowel, kidneys, and liver in the upper abdomen or bone marrow and bowel in the pelvis. Though the dose used for consolidation (20–30 Gy) is generally lower than the tolerance of the abdominal and pelvic OARs, in some cases, such as r/r disease, dose escalation (40–55 Gy) is required and may be facilitated through use of proton therapy.

24.5.1 Dosimetric Comparisons

To date, few dosimetric comparison studies have compared proton therapy with photon techniques for abdominal and pelvic targets in patients with lymphoma. Twelve consecutive HL patients from University of Florida with subdiaphragmatic

targets had 3D conformal, IMRT, and proton therapy (primarily passive scattering technique) plans generated on 4D CT simulation scans [84]. Beam-specific margins were incorporated for range uncertainty. The most common targets were the para-aortic lymph nodes ($n = 7$) and spleen ($n = 6$). Compared to 3D conformal, the greatest benefit of IMRT was seen with gastric sparing (median 5 Gy difference; $p = 0.0022$), though dose to the right kidney was higher with IMRT (median 1 Gy difference; $p = 0.0077$). Compared with IMRT, proton therapy had significantly lower dose to all OARs, with the greatest median difference observed for stomach (median 8 Gy difference; $p = 0.0022$), liver (6 Gy; $p = 0.0022$), pancreas (4 Gy; $p = 0.0058$), and bowel (4 Gy; $p = 0.0051$). The relative benefit in terms of left kidney sparing, especially given half the targets were left sided, was modest (median 1 Gy difference, $p = 0.0382$) [84].

24.5.2 Simulation

Upper abdominal targets may move with respiration and/or gastrointestinal filling and peristalsis. Therefore, motion management strategies should be considered, such as 4D CT and/or consideration of patients being treated in the fasting state. Not all upper abdominal targets are amenable to proton therapy. For example, given that a gastric target moves with respiration, may change volume between treatments (despite patients fasting prior to treatment), and may not be visualized during daily treatment (i.e., lack of volumetric IGRT), proton therapy may risk underdosing the target and overdosing adjacent OARs given the potential for interplay, changes in density along the beam path with respiratory movement, and proton therapy's conformal dose distribution.

Targets in the pelvis generally do not require motion management strategies. CT simulation scans are acquired with and without IV contrast for purposes of contouring and treatment planning, respectively. As doses used for treatment of lymphoma are below the small and large bowel dose constraints, oral contrast is generally not required to help delineate between the two, unless this would help define the target volume.

24.5.3 Treatment Planning

Given potential inter- and intra-fractional movement and/or changes in bowel content, proton beam angles are chosen to avoid treating through these unstable structures. The proton beam path length is sensitive to the density of material it traverses. Changes in density along the beam path during and between beam delivery, for example, the presence of gas during treatment when the bowel was simulated without gaseous contents, may lead to under or overshooting of the target volume by the spread-out Bragg peak. In the upper abdomen, when treating the porta-caval and/or para-aortic lymph nodes, posterior beams are preferred. In situations with large motion (>0.5–1 cm), a volumetric repainting approach may be considered to minimize the risk of interplay. If a beam must traverse bowel, preferably more than one beam angle is chosen to mitigate uncertainty with changes in the beam path. QA CT scan(s) during treatment or volumetric IGRT, if available, should be considered to confirm reproducibility of bowel loops that may be in the beam path (Figure 24.3).

24.5.4 Acute Toxicities

Treatment is well tolerated with potential of fatigue and dermatitis. Risk of nausea is less common and if needed, daily pretreatment with an anti-nausea medication such as ondansetron can be considered. Doses used for consolidation of lymphoma (20–30 Gy) generally are not associated with loose or increased bowel movements, but when dose is increased, for example, given the need to treat gross and/or r/r disease, patients should be counseled about the potential for bowel irritation, especially if bowel is within the radiation field.

24.6 Proton Therapy for Cranial Spinal Irradiation

Irradiation of the whole brain and spine axis may be considered in patients with CNS leukemia as part of cytoreduction or consolidation after allogeneic stem-cell transplant, consolidation after salvage chemotherapy, or salvage for r/r disease. Though whole brain can be considered, given that the CSF space is involved, treating the entire cranial spinal axis is more

comprehensive with one retrospective series suggesting a trend to improved progression-free survival among patients radiated prior to transplant with cranial spinal irradiation (CSI) compared to a cranial boost (HR 3.23; $p = 0.14$) [85].

24.6.1 Dosimetric Comparisons

For both photons and proton therapy, the spine fields for CSI use posterior beams. Here, the physical dose distribution of protons is most clearly evident given the lack of exit radiation dose to anterior OARs of the neck (thyroid), thorax (lungs, heart, esophagus), and abdomen/pelvis (bowel, kidneys, stomach, liver, ovaries). This is confirmed by several dosimetric studies comparing photons with proton therapy in patients with CNS malignancies, generally primitive neuroectodermal tumors such as medulloblastoma in which irradiation of the cranial spinal axis is indicated. Compared to photon treatment with either 3D conformal or advanced techniques such as TomoTherapy, proton therapy passive scattering technique was associated with lower dose to esophagus, heart, breast, stomach, liver, lung, pancreas, and kidney [86,87]. Dose to the ovaries was also lowest with proton passive scattering technique compared to 3D conformal or IMRT photon techniques [88]. Not surprisingly, given the greater distance between the spinal canal and thoracic, abdominal, and pelvic OARs compared to those of the head and neck region (e.g., thyroid), greater sparing was seen in OARs of these regions.

24.6.2 Outcomes

Given the dosimetric benefits seen in comparative studies, it is not surprising that proton CSI is better tolerated compared

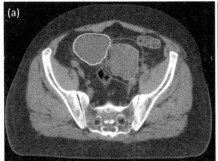 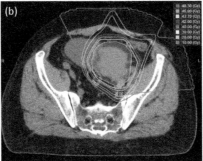 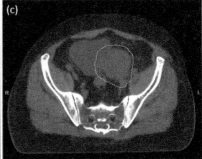

Figure 24.3 A 57-year-old man with chemorefractory diffuse large B-cell lymphoma with persistent, bulky pelvic lymph node involvement after multiple lines of systemic therapy, including CAR-T cells. His only site of disease in the left pelvis was irradiated to 46 Gy (RBE) in 23 fractions with plans for him to proceed to an allogeneic stem-cell transplant. To limit dose to the pelvic bone and bowels, especially in light of his upcoming stem-cell transplant, proton therapy was used. (a) Axial image of treatment planning scan with contours: CTV in pink, PTV in purple, sigmoid colon in brown, bladder in yellow, and large bowel in teal. (b) Radiation dose distribution using uniform scanning proton technique with three beams: a 30° left anterior oblique, 30° right anterior oblique, and left lateral beam. Two of the three beams treated through a portion of the large bowel. The volume of pelvic bone receiving 10 Gy or higher was <8%. (c) Because a portion of the large bowel was present within the proton beam paths, a QA CT scan was done during treatment. The loop of large bowel was not present at this scan, but given minimal differences in dose distribution, no replanning was performed.

to photon CSI. Among adults with medulloblastoma (median CSI dose 30.6 Gy), patients treated with proton CSI had lower >5% weight loss (16% vs. 64%; $p = 0.004$), grade 2 nausea and vomiting (26% vs. 71%; $p = 0.004$), and medical management of esophagitis (5% vs. 57%; $p < 0.001$) compared to patients treated with photon CSI [89]. Lower doses to the anterior vertebral bodies were observed among proton CSI patients (median, 69% of CSI dose vs. 100%; $p < 0.0001$), which was associated with smaller reduction in white blood cells, hemoglobin, and platelets (i.e., less myelosuppression) [89]. Similar findings were seen among patients with hematologic malignancies receiving CSI with either photon or proton techniques for consolidation or salvage treatment prior to stem-cell transplant. Though the median dose used to treat this cohort was lower (24 Gy photons CSI, 21.8 Gy proton CSI), significant differences in acute toxicity were still observed with proton versus photon CSI, including lower risk of grade 1–3 mucositis (7% vs. 44%; $p = 0.03$) [90]. No difference in risk of CNS relapse or toxicity during stem-cell transplant was observed among patients treated with photon versus proton CSI.

24.6.3 Simulation

Patients are typically simulated in the supine position with a thermoplastic mask for immobilization. In contrast to photons, where a neck extension is preferred to avoid exit radiation dose through the oral cavity, the neck is simulated in the neutral position. CT scans are taken from vertex to mid-femur.

24.6.4 Treatment Planning

The CTV includes the whole brain, cribriform plate, most inferior portion of the temporal lobes, pituitary fossa, and skull base foramina through which the cranial nerves pass. Though no consensus exists, the full length of the optic nerves should also be considered for inclusion given that the CSF tracks around the optic nerve and reaches to the back of the globe [91]. In the spine, the entire subarachnoid space including nerve roots laterally should be drawn as part of the CTV. Consensus guidelines on craniospinal target volume have been published by the European Society for Paediatric Oncology (SIOPE) cooperative group [91]. In adults, the anterior vertebral bodies are spared to minimize myelosuppression. Site-specific treatment planning recommendations are discussed in Table 24.3.

Treatment planning differs by proton technique. For passive scattering or uniform scanning, the whole brain is treated with two slight posterior oblique beams (15° off lateral) to have non-diverging dose to the upper spine. Two posterior beams are used to treat the spine in adult patients (upper and lower). Junctions of 1 cm are created between the whole brain, upper spine, and lower spine fields. Because three match lines are typically used, this effectively requires three different CSI plans and patient-specific hardware to be created. Treatment alternates between the three plans to feather out the junctions.

With PBS, treatment planning and delivery is greatly simplified with the use of a gradient junction (Figure 24.4). All beams, including the brain field, are treated with a single posterior field. In contrast to planning with passive scattering or

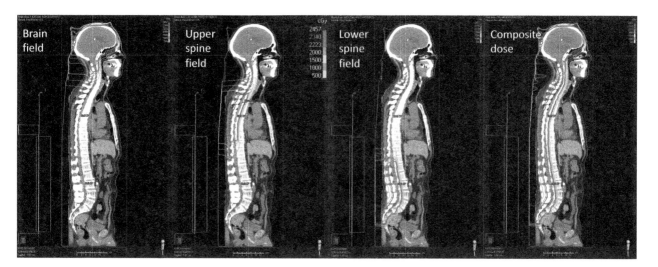

Figure 24.4 Proton CSI treatment using a gradient junction technique. Three posterior fields are used for the brain, upper spine, and lower spine. In this patient with relapsed acute myelogenous leukemia with CNS involvement, a prescription dose of 23.4 Gy (RBE) was given (blue). A junction of several centimeters is used, in which dose from the inferior brain field slowly decreases from the prescription dose to 0 cGy over the same region that dose from the upper spine field is increasing from 0 cGy to the prescription dose. The resulting composite dose has no hot or cold spots.

Table 24.3   Site-specific simulation, contouring, and treatment planning considerations.

Site	Treatment planning considerations	
Head and neck	Simulation	• Supine, thermoplastic mask, IV contrast • If using anterior beams: neck extension • Sinonasal site: bite block
	Contouring	• ISRT approach [41,42]*: anatomically confined CTV should cover at least the pre-chemotherapy extent of disease, with margins for uncertainty based on clinical judgment ○ Consider an expanded CTV for patients undergoing definitive RT alone following nodal regions of spread • Fusions: PET/CT, MRI (for sinonasal/NPX sites) • Incorporate findings from flexible endoscopy and relevant operative reports
	Planning	• Avoid hardware • Consider SFO for unilateral cases to improve robustness • Sinonasal: consider QA CT scans during treatment
Mediastinal	Simulation	• Supine with custom body immobilization, IV contrastConsider positioning similar to PET/CT ○ Concurrent neck disease: mild neck extension if low neck involvement, thermoplastic mask • Young female patients: arms down or akimbo, 10°–15° incline board [69] • Motion management: 4D scan if free breathing, or DIBH with 3 separate scans
	Contouring	• ISRT approach [41,42]* • Fusion of all relevant PET/CTs • OARs: thyroid, esophagus, lungs, breasts, heart, and cardiac substructures (atria, ventricles, valves, common carotid, left anterior descending artery, right circumflex)—see ILROG Proton Therapy for Adults with Mediastinal Lymphoma Guidelines [45]
	Planning	• Beam angle selection depends on target volume ○ Anterior disease: anterior or anterior oblique ○ Posterior disease: posterior beams • Gradient junction approach may be used if target volume requires splitting between different beams • Robustness analysis is important due to motion • PBS more conformal than PS but can be less robust—larger spot size, volumetric repainting can improve robustness if required • QA CT scan(s) recommended if there is concern for changing lymphoma size during RT (i.e., if treating gross disease)
Infradiaphragmatic	Simulation	• GI sites: Overnight fasting with early morning appointments, or at ≥4 h fasting prior to simulation and all treatments • 4D CT scan if motion may be a concern (gastric, duodenal, renal, splenic lymphomas) • Small volume (<50 cm3) oral contrast for gastric or duodenal sites to help define treatment volume
	Contouring	• ISRT approach [41,42]* • ITV generated using 4D for upper GI sites
	Planning	• Portacaval or para-aortic lymph nodes: posterior beams preferred to avoid bowels • Volumetric repainting when ≥0.5–1 cm motion • QA CT scan(s) during treatment or volumetric IGRT to confirm reproducibility of bowel loops that may be in the beam path
Cranial and spinal	Simulation	• Supine, neck neutral, thermoplastic mask • Scan from vertex to mid-femur
	Contouring	• CTV includes the whole brain, cribriform plate, most inferior portion of the temporal lobes, pituitary fossa, and skull base foramina, consider treating full length of optic nerves • Adults: anterior vertebral bodies can be spared to minimize myelosuppression
	Planning	• PS/US: whole brain is treated with two slight posterior oblique beams (15° off lateral) to have non-diverging dose to the upper spine. Two posterior beams are used to treat the spine in adult patients (upper and lower). Use 1-cm junctions with feathering between the whole brain, upper spine, and lower spine fields • PBS: gradient junction with all beams, including brain field, treated with single posterior field

DIBH = Deep inspiration breath hold; ISRT = involved-site radiotherapy; NPX = nasopharyngeal; PBS = pencil beam scanning; PS = passive scattering; QA = quality assurance; SFO = single-field optimization; US = uniform scanning; *Note: involved node radiotherapy (INRT) [43] can be done instead of ISRT [41,42] if PET/CT and CT simulation is done in exactly the same position.

uniform scanning, the whole brain, upper and lower spine fields with PBS overlap, and the same fields are delivered on all days of treatment. Both fields contribute dose in the region of overlap (i.e., junction), which may be several centimeters long. Over the junction, the dose from one field gradually increases from 0% to 100% while the dose from the other overlapping field gradually decreases from 100% to 0%. Use of a PBS gradient junction technique improves plan robustness to patient setup errors, shortens treatment planning time as no patient-specific hardware needs to be created, and shortens time for patient delivery as apertures and compensators do not need to be changed for each field.

24.6.5 Acute Toxicities

CSI with proton therapy is very well tolerated. Given the risk of myelosuppression with treatment, weekly complete blood counts with differential are obtained. Patients may note fatigue, dermatitis, hair loss (depending on prescription dose) and less likely headaches, nausea, or esophagitis. Patients treated with the single posterior beam to the whole brain (i.e.,

with PBS gradient junction technique) may note dermatitis of the forehead, which is not always seen with lateral or lateral oblique fields.

24.7 Summary

Proton therapy may contribute toward the three-prong approach to lower acute and late toxicity in patients with lymphoma or leukemia. Appropriate patient selection and technical considerations need to be incorporated into clinical decision making given that proton therapy remains a more time intensive and expensive resource with unique treatment planning considerations. The role of proton therapy for mediastinal lymphoma and cranial spinal radiation has been established through dosimetric comparison studies and early clinical data. Future directions include better defining the role of proton therapy for other sites, evaluating the radiosensitivity of cardiac substructures in the era of conformal radiotherapy, and working toward incorporating spatial variations in proton RBE into treatment planning.

References

1 Easson, E.C. and Russell, M.H. (1963). The cure of Hodgkin's disease. *British Medical Journal* 1 (5347): 1704–1707. doi:10.1136/bmj.1.5347.1704.

2 Kaplan, H.S. (1962). The radical radiotherapy of regionally localized Hodgkin's disease. *Radiology* 78: 553–561. doi:10.1148/78.4.553.

3 Aleman, B.M.P., Van Den Belt-dusebout, A.W., Klokman, W.J., Van't Veer, M.B., Bartelink, H., and Van Leeuwen, F.E. (2003). Long-term cause-specific mortality of patients treated for Hodgkin's disease. *Journal of Clinical Oncology: Official Journal of the American Society of Clinical Oncology* 21 (18): 3431–3439. doi:10.1200/JCO.2003.07.131.

4 Ng, B.A.K., Bernardo, M.P., Weller, E., et al. (2002). Long-term survival and competing causes of death in patients with early-stage Hodgkin's disease treated at age 50 or younger conclusion: Patients. *Journal of Clinical Oncology: Official Journal of the American Society of Clinical Oncology* 20 (8): 2101–2108.

5 Hodgson, D.C., Gilbert, E.S., Dores, G.M., et al. (2007). Long-term solid cancer risk among 5-year survivors of Hodgkin's lymphoma. *Journal of Clinical Oncology: Official Journal of the American Society of Clinical Oncology* 25 (12): 1489–1497. doi:10.1200/JCO.2006.09.0936.

6 Travis, L.B., Hill, D.A., Gospodarowicz, M., et al. (2003). Breast cancer following radiotherapy and chemotherapy among young women with Hodgkin disease. *JAMA* 290 (4): 465–476.

7 Morton, L.M., Gilbert, E.S., Stovall, M., et al. (2014). Risk of esophageal cancer following radiotherapy for Hodgkin lymphoma. *Haematologica* 99 (10): e193–e196. doi:10.3324/haematol.2014.108258.

8 Travis, L.B., Gospodarowicz, M., Curtis, R.E., et al. (2002). Lung cancer following chemotherapy and radiotherapy for Hodgkin's disease. *Journal of the National Cancer Institute* 94 (3): 182–192. http://www.ncbi.nlm.nih.gov/pubmed/11830608. Accessed March 19, 2015.

9 De Bruin, M.L., Sparidans, J., Van't Veer, M.B., et al. (2009). Breast cancer risk in female survivors of Hodgkin's lymphoma: Lower risk after smaller radiation volumes. *Journal of Clinical Oncology: Official Journal of the American Society of Clinical Oncology* 27 (26): 4239–4246. doi:10.1200/JCO.2008.19.9174.

10 Van Leeuwen, F.E., Klokman, W.J., and Stovall, M., et al. *Roles of radiation dose, chemotherapy, and hormonal factors in breast cancer following Hodgkin's disease.* https://academic.oup.com/jnci/article-abstract/95/13/971/2520315. Accessed June 11, 2020

11 Travis, L.B., Hill, D., Dores, G.M., et al. (2005). Cumulative absolute breast cancer risk for young women treated for Hodgkin lymphoma. *Journal of the National Cancer Institute* 97 (19): 1428–1437. doi:10.1093/jnci/dji290.

12 Krul, I.M., Awj, O.W., Aleman, B.M.P., et al. (2017). Clinical investigation breast cancer risk after radiation therapy for Hodgkin lymphoma: Influence of Gonadal Hormone Exposure Radiation Oncology. *International Journal of Radiation Oncology, Biology, Physics* 99 (4): 843–853. doi:10.1016/j.ijrobp.2017.07.016.

13 Conway, J.L., Connors, J.M., Tyldesley, S., et al. (2017). Clinical investigation secondary breast cancer risk by Radiation Volume in Women With Hodgkin Lymphoma Radiation Oncology. *International Journal of Radiation Oncology, Biology, Physics* 97 (1): 35–41. doi:10.1016/j.ijrobp.2016.10.004.

14 Milano, M.T., Li, H., Constine, L.S., and Travis, L.B. (2011). Survival after second primary lung cancer: A population-based study of 187 Hodgkin lymphoma patients. *Cancer* 117 (24): 5538–5547. doi:10.1002/cncr.26257.

15 Morton, L.M., Dores, G.M., Curtis, R.E., et al. (2013). Stomach cancer risk after treatment for Hodgkin lymphoma. *Journal of Clinical Oncology: Official Journal of the American Society of Clinical Oncology* 31 (27): 3369–3377. doi:10.1200/JCO.2013.50.6832.

16 Dores, G.M., Curtis, R.E., Van Leeuwen, F.E., et al. (2014). Pancreatic cancer risk after treatment of Hodgkin lymphoma. *Annals of Oncology: Official Journal of the European Society for Medical Oncology / ESMO* 25: 2073–2079. doi:10.1093/annonc/mdu287.

17 Schaapveld, M., Aleman, B.M.P., Van Eggermond, A.M., et al. (2015). Second cancer risk up to 40 years after treatment for Hodgkin's lymphoma. *The New England Journal of Medicine* 373 (26): 2499–2511. doi:10.1056/NEJMoa1505949.

18 Swerdlow, A.J., Higgins, C.D., Smith, P., et al. (2007). Myocardial infarction mortality risk after treatment for Hodgkin disease: A collaborative British cohort study. *Journal of the National Cancer Institute* 99 (3): 206–214. doi:10.1093/jnci/djk029.

19 Hancock, S.L., Hoppe, R.T., and Tucker, M.A. (1993). Factors affecting late mortality from heart disease after treatment of Hodgkin's disease. *JAMA: The Journal of the American Medical Association* 270 (16): 1949–1955. doi:10.1001/jama.1993.03510160067031.

20 Aleman, B.M.P., Van Den Belt-dusebout, A.W., De Bruin, M.L., et al. (2007). Late cardiotoxicity after treatment for Hodgkin lymphoma. *Blood* 109 (5): 1878–1886. doi:10.1182/blood-2006-07-034405.

21 Darby, S.C., Cutter, D.J., Boerma, M., et al. (2010). Radiation-related heart disease: Current knowledge and future prospects. *International Journal of Radiation Oncology, Biology, Physics* 76 (3): 656–665. doi:10.1016/j.ijrobp.2009.09.064.

22 Van Nimwegen, F.A., Schaapveld, M., Janus, C.P.M., et al. (2015). Cardiovascular disease after Hodgkin lymphoma treatment: 40-year disease risk. *JAMA Internal Medicine* 175 (6): 1007–1017. doi:10.1001/jamainternmed.2015.1180.

23 Galper, S.L., Yu, J.B., Mauch, P.M., et al. (2011). Clinically significant cardiac disease in patients with Hodgkin lymphoma treated with mediastinal irradiation. *Blood* 117 (2): 412–418. doi:10.1182/blood-2010-06-291328.

24 De Bruin, M.L., Dorresteijn, L.D.A., Van't Veer, M.B., et al. (2009). Increased risk of stroke and transient ischemic attack in 5-year survivors of Hodgkin lymphoma. *Journal of the National Cancer Institute* 101 (13): 928–937. doi:10.1093/jnci/djp147.

25 Hirsch, A., Vander Els, N., Straus, D.J., et al. (1996). Effect of ABVD chemotherapy with and without mantle or mediastinal irradiation on pulmonary function and symptoms in early-stage Hodgkin's disease. *Journal of Clinical Oncology: Official Journal of the American Society of Clinical Oncology* 14 (4): 1297–1305. doi:10.1200/JCO.1996.14.4.1297.

26 Fox, A.M., Dosoretz, A.P., Mauch, P.M., et al. (2012). Predictive factors for radiation pneumonitis in Hodgkin lymphoma patients receiving combined-modality therapy. *International Journal of Radiation Oncology, Biology, Physics* 83 (1): 277–283. doi:10.1016/j.ijrobp.2011.05.078.

27 Pinnix, C.C., Smith, G.L., Milgrom, S., et al. (2015). Predictors of radiation pneumonitis in patients receiving intensity modulated radiation therapy for Hodgkin and non-Hodgkin lymphoma. *International Journal of Radiation Oncology, Biology, Physics* 92 (1): 175–182. doi:10.1016/j.ijrobp.2015.02.010.

28 Ng, A.K., Li, S., Neuberg, D., et al. (2008). A prospective study of pulmonary function in Hodgkin's lymphoma patients. *Annals of Oncology: Official Journal of the European Society for Medical Oncology / ESMO* 19 (10): 1754–1758. doi:10.1093/annonc/mdn284.

29 Knobel, H., Loge, J.H., Lund, M.B., Forfang, K., Nome, O., and Kaasa, S. (2001). Late medical complications and fatigue in Hodgkin's disease survivors. *Journal of Clinical Oncology: Official Journal of the American Society of Clinical Oncology* 19 (13): 3226–3233. doi:10.1200/JCO.2001.19.13.3226.

30 Hancock, S.L., Cox, R.S., and McDougall, I.R. (1991). Thyroid diseases after treatment of Hodgkin's disease. *The New England Journal of Medicine* 325 (9): 599–605. doi:10.1056/NEJM199108293250902.

31 Cella, L., Conson, M., Caterino, M., et al. (2012). Thyroid V30 predicts radiation-induced hypothyroidism in patients treated with sequential chemo-radiotherapy for Hodgkin's lymphoma. *International Journal of Radiation Oncology, Biology, Physics* 82 (5): 1802–1808. doi:10.1016/j.ijrobp.2010.09.054.

32 Pinnix, C.C., Cella, L., Andraos, T.Y., et al. (2018). Predictors of Hypothyroidism in Hodgkin lymphoma survivors after intensity modulated versus 3-dimensional radiation therapy. *International Journal of Radiation Oncology, Biology, Physics* 101 (3): 530–540. doi:10.1016/j.ijrobp.2018.03.003.

33 De Vathaire, F., El-Fayech, C., Ben Ayed, F.F., et al. (2012). Radiation dose to the pancreas and risk of diabetes mellitus in childhood cancer survivors: A retrospective cohort study. *The Lancet Oncology* 13 (10): 1002–1010. doi:10.1016/S1470-2045(12)70323-6.

34 Van Nimwegen, F.A., Schaapveld, M., Janus, C.P.M., et al. (2014). Risk of diabetes mellitus in long-term survivors of

Hodgkin lymphoma. *Journal of Clinical Oncology: Official Journal of the American Society of Clinical Oncology* 32 (29): 3257–3263. doi:10.1200/JCO.2013.54.4379.

35 Maraldo, M.V., Brodin, P., Aznar, M.C., et al. (2013). Doses to carotid arteries after modern radiation therapy for Hodgkin lymphoma: Is stroke still a late effect of treatment? *International Journal of Radiation Oncology, Biology, Physics* 87 (2): 297–303. doi:10.1016/j.ijrobp.2013.06.004.

36 Maraldo, M.V., Brodin, N.P., Aznar, M.C., et al. (2014). Hodgkin lymphoma Doses to head and neck normal tissues for early stage Hodgkin lymphoma after involved node radiotherapy. *Radiotherapy and Oncology: Journal of the European Society for Therapeutic Radiology and Oncology* 110: 441–447. doi:10.1016/j.radonc.2013.09.027.

37 Dagan, R., Bryant, C., Li, Z., et al. (2016). Outcomes of sinonasal cancer treated with proton therapy. *International Journal of Radiation Oncology, Biology, Physics* 95 (1): 377–385. doi:10.1016/j.ijrobp.2016.02.019.

38 Ho, C.K., Flampouri, S., and Hoppe, B.S. (2014). Proton therapy in the management of lymphoma. *Cancer Journal (United States)* 20 (6): 387–392. doi:10.1097/PPO.0000000000000076.

39 Sachsman, S., Flampouri, S., Li, Z., Lynch, J., Mendenhall, N.P., and Hoppe, B.S. (2015). Proton therapy in the management of non-Hodgkin lymphoma. *Leukemia & Lymphoma* 56 (9): 2608–2612. doi:10.3109/10428194.2015.1014364.

40 Xiang, M., Chang, D.T., and Pollom, E.L. (2020). Second cancer risk after primary cancer treatment with three-dimensional conformal, intensity-modulated, or proton beam radiation therapy. *Cancer* 1–9. doi:10.1002/cncr.32938.

41 Specht, L., Yahalom, J., Illidge, T., et al. (2014). Modern radiation therapy for Hodgkin lymphoma: Field and dose guidelines from the international lymphoma radiation oncology group (ILROG). *International Journal of Radiation Oncology, Biology, Physics* 89 (4): 854–862. doi:10.1016/j.ijrobp.2013.05.005.

42 Wirth, A., Mikhaeel, N.G., Pauline Aleman, B.M., et al. (2020). Involved site radiation therapy in adult lymphomas: An overview of International Lymphoma Radiation Oncology Group guidelines. *International Journal of Radiation Oncology*. doi:10.1016/j.ijrobp.2020.03.019.

43 Girinsky, T., Van Der Maazen, R., Specht, L., et al. Involved-node radiotherapy (INRT) in patients with early Hodgkin lymphoma: Concepts and guidelines. doi:10.1016/j.radonc.2006.05.015

44 Leeman, J.E., Romesser, P.B., Zhou, Y., et al. (2017). Proton therapy for head and neck cancer: Expanding the therapeutic window. *The Lancet Oncology* 18 (5): e254–e265. doi:10.1016/S1470-2045(17)30179-1.

45 Dabaja, B.S., Hoppe, B.S., Plastaras, J.P., et al. (2018). Proton therapy for adults with mediastinal lymphomas: The international lymphoma radiation oncology group

guidelines. *Blood* 132 (16): 1635–1646. doi:10.1182/blood-2018-03-837633.

46 Chera, B.S., Rodriguez, C., Morris, C.G., et al. (2009). Dosimetric comparison of three different involved nodal irradiation techniques for stage II Hodgkin's lymphoma patients: Conventional radiotherapy, intensity-modulated radiotherapy, and three-dimensional proton radiotherapy. *International Journal of Radiation Oncology, Biology, Physics* 75 (4): 1173–1180. doi:10.1016/j.ijrobp.2008.12.048.

47 Lautenschlaeger, S., Iancu, G., Flatten, V., et al. (2019). Advantage of proton-radiotherapy for pediatric patients and adolescents with Hodgkin's disease. *Radiation Oncology* 14: 157. doi:10.1186/s13014-019-1360-7.

48 Maraldo, M.V., Brodin, N.P., Aznar, M.C., et al. (2013). Estimated risk of cardiovascular disease and secondary cancers with modern highly conformal radiotherapy for early-stage mediastinal Hodgkin lymphoma. *Annals of Oncology: Official Journal of the European Society for Medical Oncology / ESMO* 24 (8): 2113–2118. doi:10.1093/annonc/mdt156.

49 Zeng, C., Plastaras, J.P., James, P., et al. (2016). Proton pencil beam scanning for mediastinal lymphoma: Treatment planning and robustness assessment. *Acta Oncologica (Madr)* 55 (9-10): 1132–1138. doi:10.1080/0284186X.2016.1191665.

50 Knäusl, B., Lütgendorf-Caucig, C., Hopfgartner, J., et al. (2013). Can treatment of pediatric Hodgkin's lymphoma be improved by PET imaging and proton therapy? *Strahlentherapie und Onkologie: Organ der Deutschen Rontgengesellschaft. [et al]* 189: 54–61. doi:10.1007/s00066-012-0235-8.

51 Ntentas, G., Dedeckova, K., Andrlik, M., et al. (2019). Clinical intensity modulated proton therapy for Hodgkin lymphoma: Which patients benefit the most? *Practical Radiation Oncology* 9 (3): 179–187. doi:10.1016/j.prro.2019.01.006.

52 König, L., Bougatf, N., Hörner-Rieber, J., et al. (2019). Consolidative mediastinal irradiation of malignant lymphoma using active scanning proton beams: Clinical outcome and dosimetric comparison. *Strahlentherapie und Onkologie* 195 (7): 677–687. doi:10.1007/s00066-019-01460-7.

53 Edvardsson, A., Kügele, M., Alkner, S., et al. (2019). Comparative treatment planning study for mediastinal Hodgkin's lymphoma: Impact on normal tissue dose using deep inspiration breath hold proton and photon therapy. *Acta Oncologica (Madr)* 58 (1): 95–104. doi:10.1080/0284186X.2018.1512153.

54 Baues, C., Marnitz, S., Engert, A., et al. (2018). Proton versus photon deep inspiration breath hold technique in patients with Hodgkin lymphoma and mediastinal radiation. *Radiation Oncology* 13 (1): 1–11. doi:10.1186/s13014-018-1066-2.

55 Li, J., Dabaja, B., Reed, V., et al. (2011). Rationale for and preliminary results of proton beam therapy for mediastinal lymphoma. *International Journal of Radiation Oncology,*

Biology, Physics 81 (1): 167–174. doi:10.1016/j.
ijrobp.2010.05.007.

56 Hoppe, B.S., Flampouri, S., Zaiden, R., et al. (2014). Involved-node proton therapy in combined modality therapy for Hodgkin lymphoma: Results of a phase 2 study. *International Journal of Radiation Oncology, Biology, Physics* 89 (5): 1053–1059. doi:10.1016/j.ijrobp.2014.04.029.

57 Everett, A.S., Hoppe, B.S., Louis, D., et al. (2019). Comparison of techniques for involved-site radiation therapy in patients with lower mediastinal lymphoma. *Practical Radiation Oncology* 9 (6): 426–434. doi:10.1016/j.prro.2019.05.009.

58 Rechner, L.A., Maraldo, M.V., Vogelius, I.R., et al. (2017). Life years lost attributable to late effects after radiotherapy for early stage Hodgkin lymphoma: The impact of proton therapy and/or deep inspiration breath hold. *Radiotherapy and Oncology: Journal of the European Society for Therapeutic Radiology and Oncology* 125 (1): 41–47. doi:10.1016/j.radonc.2017.07.033.

59 Tseng, Y.D., Maes, S.M., Kicska, G., et al. (2019). Comparative photon and proton dosimetry for patients with mediastinal lymphoma in the era of Monte Carlo treatment planning and variable relative biological effectiveness. *Radiation Oncology* 14 (1): 1–13. doi:10.1186/s13014-019-1432-8.

60 Tseng, Y.D., Cutter, D.J., Plastaras, J.P., et al. (2017). Critical review evidence-based review on the use of proton therapy in lymphoma from the Particle Therapy Cooperative Group (PTCOG) lymphoma subcommittee radiation oncology. *International Journal of Radiation Oncology, Biology, Physics* 99 (4): 825–842. doi:10.1016/j.ijrobp.2017.05.004.

61 Petersen, P.M., Aznar, M.C., Berthelsen, A.K., et al. (2015). Prospective phase II trial of image-guided radiotherapy in Hodgkin lymphoma: Benefit of deep inspiration breath-hold. *Acta Oncologica (Madr)* 54 (1): 60–66. doi:10.3109/02841 86X.2014.932435.

62 Paumier, A., Ghalibafian, M., Gilmore, J., et al. (2012). Dosimetric benefits of intensity-modulated radiotherapy combined with the deep-inspiration breath-hold technique in patients with mediastinal Hodgkin's lymphoma. *International Journal of Radiation Oncology, Biology, Physics* 82 (4): 1522–1527. doi:10.1016/j.ijrobp.2011.05.015.

63 Andolino, D.L., Hoene, T., Xiao, L., Buchsbaum, J., and Chang, A.L. (2011). Dosimetric comparison of involved-field three-dimensional conformal photon radiotherapy and breast-sparing proton therapy for the treatment of Hodgkin's lymphoma in female pediatric patients. *International Journal of Radiation Oncology, Biology, Physics* 81: 4. doi:10.1016/j.ijrobp.2011.01.061.

64 Aznar, M.C., Maraldo, M.V., Schut, D.A., et al. (2015). Minimizing late effects for patients with mediastinal Hodgkin lymphoma: Deep inspiration breath-hold, IMRT, or both? *International Journal of Radiation Oncology, Biology, Physics* 92 (1): 169–174. doi:10.1016/j.ijrobp.2015.01.013.

65 Jorgensen, A.Y.S., Maraldo, M.V., Brodin, N.P., et al. (2013). The effect on esophagus after different radiotherapy techniques for early stage Hodgkin's lymphoma. *Acta Oncologica (Madr)* 52 (7): 1559–1565. doi:10.3109/02841 86X.2013.813636.

66 Hoppe, B.S., Hill-Kayser, C.E., Tseng, Y.D., et al. (2017). Consolidative proton therapy after chemotherapy for patients with Hodgkin lymphoma. *Annals of Oncology: Official Journal of the European Society for Medical Oncology / ESMO* 28 (9): 2179–2184. doi:10.1093/annonc/mdx287.

67 Toltz, A., Shin, N., Mitrou, E., et al. (2015). Late radiation toxicity in Hodgkin lymphoma patients: Proton therapy's potential. *Journal Of Applied Clinical Medical Physics / American College of Medical Physics* 16 (5): 167–178. doi:10.1120/jacmp.v16i5.5386.

68 Denniston, K.A., Verma, V., Bhirud, A.R., Bennion, N.R., and Lin, C. (2016). Effect of Akimbo versus raised arm positioning on breast and cardiopulmonary dosimetry in pediatric Hodgkin lymphoma. *Frontiers in Oncology* 6 (JUL): 176. doi:10.3389/fonc.2016.00176.

69 Dabaja, B.S., Rebueno, N.C.S., Mazloom, A., et al. (2011). Radiation for Hodgkin's lymphoma in young female patients: A new technique to avoid the breasts and decrease the dose to the heart. *International Journal of Radiation Oncology, Biology, Physics* 79 (2): 503–507. doi:10.1016/j.ijrobp.2009.11.013.

70 Feng, M., Moran, J.M., Koelling, T., et al. (2011). Development and validation of a heart atlas to study cardiac exposure to radiation following treatment for breast cancer. *International Journal of Radiation Oncology, Biology, Physics* 79 (1): 10–18. doi:10.1016/j.ijrobp.2009.10.058.

71 Van Nimwegen, F.A., Schaapveld, M., Cutter, D.J., et al. (2016). Radiation dose-response relationship for risk of coronary heart disease in survivors of Hodgkin lymphoma. *Journal of Clinical Oncology: Official Journal of the American Society of Clinical Oncology* 34 (3): 235–243. doi:10.1200/JCO.2015.63.4444.

72 Cutter, D.J., Schaapveld, M., Darby, S.C., et al. (2015). Risk of valvular heart disease after treatment for Hodgkin lymphoma. *Journal of the National Cancer Institute* 107: 4. doi:10.1093/jnci/djv008.

73 Maraldo, M.V., Giusti, F., Vogelius, I.R., et al. (2015). Cardiovascular disease after treatment for Hodgkin's lymphoma: An analysis of nine collaborative EORTC-LYSA trials. *Lancet Haematology* 2 (11): e492–502. doi:10.1016/S2352-3026(15)00153-2.

74 Hoppe, B.S., Bates, J.E., Mendenhall, N.P., et al. (2020). The meaningless meaning of mean heart dose in Mediastinal lymphoma in the modern radiation therapy era. *Practical Radiation Oncology* 10 (3): e147–e154. doi:10.1016/j.prro.2019.09.015.

75 Guzhva, L., Flampouri, S., Mendenhall, N.P., Morris, C.G., and Hoppe, B.S. (2019). Intrafractional displacement of cardiac substructures among patients with mediastinal lymphoma or lung cancer. *Advances in Radiation Oncology* 4 (3): 500–506. doi:10.1016/j.adro.2019.03.008.

76 Lester, S.C., Taparra, K., Petersen, M.M., et al. (2020). Electrocardiogram-gated computed tomography with coronary angiography for cardiac substructure delineation and sparing in patients with mediastinal lymphomas treated with radiation therapy. *Practical Radiation Oncology* 10 (2): 104–111. doi:10.1016/j.prro.2019.10.016.

77 Taylor, P.A., Kry, S.F., and Followill, D.S. (2017). Pencil beam algorithms are unsuitable for proton dose calculations in lung. *International Journal of Radiation Oncology, Biology, Physics* 99 (3): 750–756. doi:10.1016/j.ijrobp.2017.06.003.

78 Dowdell, S., Grassberger, C., Sharp, G.C., Paganetti, H., and Org, S. (2013). Interplay effects in proton scanning for lung: A 4D Monte Carlo study assessing the impact of tumor and beam delivery parameters. *Physics in Medicine and Biology* 58 (12): 4137–4156. doi:10.1088/0031-9155/58/12/4137.

79 Grassberger, C., Dowdell, S., Sharp, G., and Paganetti, H. (2015). Motion mitigation for lung cancer patients treated with active scanning proton therapy. *Medical Physics* 42 (5): 2462–2469. doi:10.1118/1.4916662.

80 Chang, J.Y., Zhang, X., Knopf, A., et al. (2017). Consensus guidelines for implementing pencil-beam scanning proton therapy for thoracic malignancies on behalf of the PTCOG thoracic and lymphoma subcommittee. *International Journal of Radiation Oncology, Biology, Physics* 99 (1): 41–50. doi:10.1016/j.ijrobp.2017.05.014.

81 Tseng, Y.D., Hoppe, B.S., Miller, D., Maity, A., Nanda, R., Mendenhall, N.P., Flampouri, M.P., Hartsell, W.F., and Vargas, C.E.P.J. (2017). Rates of toxicity and outcomes after mediastinal proton therapy for relapsed/Refractory lymphoma. In: *ASTRO Annual Meeting* 99, 2, S62–S63 Oral Presentation.

82 Nanda, R., Flampouri, S., Mendenhall, N.P., et al. (2017). Pulmonary toxicity following proton therapy for Thoracic lymphoma. *International Journal of Radiation Oncology, Biology, Physics* 99 (2): 494–497. doi:10.1016/j.ijrobp.2017.04.001.

83 O'Steen, L., Bellardini, J., Cury, J., et al. (2019). Pulmonary function after proton therapy for Hodgkin lymphoma. *International Journal of Particle Therapy* 5 (3): 1–4. doi:10.14338/IJPT-18-00040.1.

84 Sachsman, S., Hoppe, B.S., Mendenhall, N.P., et al. (2015). Proton therapy to the subdiaphragmatic region in the management of patients with Hodgkin lymphoma.

Leukemia & Lymphoma 56 (7): 2019–2024. doi:10.3109/10428194.2014.975802.

85 Hiniker, S.M., Agarwal, R., Modlin, L.A., et al. (2014). Survival and neurocognitive outcomes after cranial or craniospinal irradiation plus total-body irradiation before stem cell transplantation in pediatric leukemia patients with central nervous system involvement. *International Journal of Radiation Oncology, Biology, Physics* 89 (1): 67–74. doi:10.1016/j.ijrobp.2014.01.056.

86 Zhang, R., Howell, R.M., Taddei, P.J., Giebeler, A., Mahajan, A., and Newhauser, W.D. (2014). A comparative study on the risks of radiogenic second cancers and cardiac mortality in a set of pediatric medulloblastoma patients treated with photon or proton craniospinal irradiation. *Radiotherapy and Oncology: Journal of the European Society for Therapeutic Radiology and Oncology* 113 (1): 84–88. doi:10.1016/j.radonc.2014.07.003.

87 Yoon, M., Shin, D.H., Kim, J., et al. (2011). Craniospinal irradiation techniques: A dosimetric comparison of proton beams with standard and advanced photon radiotherapy. *International Journal of Radiation Oncology, Biology, Physics* 81 (3): 637–646. doi:10.1016/j.ijrobp.2010.06.039.

88 Pérez-Andújar, A., Newhauser, W.D., Taddei, P.J., Mahajan, A., and Howell, R.M. (2013). The predicted relative risk of premature ovarian failure for three radiotherapy modalities in a girl receiving craniospinal irradiation. *Physics in Medicine and Biology* 58 (10): 3107–3123. doi:10.1088/0031-9155/58/10/3107.

89 Brown, A.P., Barney, C.L., Grosshans, D.R., et al. (2013). Proton beam craniospinal irradiation reduces acute toxicity for adults with medulloblastoma. *International Journal of Radiation Oncology, Biology, Physics* 86 (2): 277–284. doi:10.1016/j.ijrobp.2013.01.014.

90 Gunther, J.R., Rahman, A.R., Dong, W., et al. (2017). Craniospinal irradiation prior to stem cell transplant for hematologic malignancies with CNS involvement: Effectiveness and toxicity after photon or proton treatment. *Practical Radiation Oncology* 7 (6): e401–e408. doi:10.1016/j.prro.2017.05.002.

91 Ajithkumar, T., Horan, G., Padovani, L., et al. (2018). SIOPE – Brain tumor group consensus guideline on craniospinal target volume delineation for high-precision radiotherapy. *Radiotherapy and Oncology: Journal of the European Society for Therapeutic Radiology and Oncology* 128 (2): 192–197. doi:10.1016/j.radonc.2018.04.016.

92 Van Nimwegen, F.A., Ntentas, G., Darby, S.C., et al. (2017). Risk of heart failure in survivors of Hodgkin lymphoma: Effects of cardiac exposure to radiation and anthracyclines. *Blood* 129 (16): 2257–2265. doi:10.1182/blood-2016-09-740332.

25

Sarcomas and Soft Tissue Malignancies

Jonathan B. Ashman, MD, PhD

Assistant Professor, Department of Radiation Oncology, Mayo Clinic, 5881 E. Mayo Blvd. Phoenix, AZ 85254

25.1   Introduction

Sarcomas are a heterogeneous group of malignancies with more than 80 subtypes [1]. They are typically classified by site of origination either as soft tissue sarcomas (STSs) or bone sarcomas (BSs). Sarcomas can occur throughout the body, but the most common sites for STS are the extremities and retroperitoneum. In contrast to carcinomas that arise from epithelial cells, sarcomas originate from mesenchymal stem cells. As a whole, they are less common cancers with an estimated incidence of 13,130 cases of STS and 3,600 cases of BS in 2020 in the United States [2]. Surgery is the primary treatment, but complete resection can be challenging while also preserving function and quality of life. Therefore, radiation therapy is routinely used either preoperatively or postoperatively as an adjuvant to surgery to improve local control (LC) [3,4]. However, these tumors have been considered "radioresistant" and often require high doses of radiation to achieve substantial cell kill or cure. Particle therapy may provide a meaningful advantage over photon irradiation, especially in the setting of unresectable STS or BS.

25.2   Biology of Sarcoma

From a genetic perspective, sarcomas are classified as having either a single driver mutation or a complex genomic profile [5]. There are multiple genetic pathways associated with sarcoma genesis. Gene translocations result in classical fusion transcripts that drive several sarcoma types. The most common genetic alteration in Ewing sarcoma is the t[11;22] translocation of EWSR1 gene to the FLI1 genes, which is associated with activation of the insulin growth factor (IGF) pathway. Another alteration associated with activating the IGF pathway is found in alveolar rhabdomyosarcoma with either the PAX3 or PAX7 translocation to FKHR (t[2;13] or t[1;13], respectively). For malignant peripheral nerve sheath tumors (MPNST), loss of the tumor suppressor gene NF1 is a characteristic finding. In liposarcomas, amplification of the MDM2 gene leads to inactivation of the other major tumor suppressor gene p53. Mutations in either KIT or PGDFRA account for most cases of gastrointestinal stroma tumor (GIST) and result in receptor tyrosine kinase activation. Currently, approximately 20% of STS have driver mutations that could be therapeutic targets.

Compared to these examples of relatively straightforward genetic alterations, undifferentiated STSs are characterized by complex genomics [6]. Nevertheless, common genetic pathway alterations still have been identified in many of these tumors as well. For example, 43–65% of undifferentiated pleomorphic sarcoma (UPS) and myxofibrosarcoma cases harbor p53 mutations [7]. Other common mutations involve the CDK2NA and RB1 genes. The heterogeneity of undifferentiated sarcomas is related to aberrations in ploidy and copy number alterations. Osteosarcoma also represents a disease with high genetic complexity [8]. In children, the development of osteosarcoma may be associated with inherited syndromes such as Li–Fraumeni (p53) or Hereditary Retinoblastoma (RB1). Prior to advanced genomic sequencing technology, osteosarcoma was characterized by aneuploidy and genetic instability. However, modern genetic analytics have suggested multiple gene candidates where mutations could be driving osteosarcoma development.

Sarcomas have been regarded as radioresistant. Early analyses of pathologic specimens that had been treated with preoperative radiation suggested that a response to radiation could be observed in a substantial portion of sarcoma but that a complete or even partial clinical response was difficult to achieve [9,10]. Clinical experiences reported that doses greater than 66–70 Gy were required to provide adequate tumor control [11,12]. However, histologic subtype is a factor for radiation response. For example, major responses to radiation were observed in approximately 50% of liposarcomas, fibrosarcoma, and leiomyosarcoma cases but less than that in UPS, synovial sarcoma, or neurogenic sarcoma [13]. In particular, myxoid liposarcoma is notable for being radiosensitive. A statistically significantly greater volume reduction after radiotherapy was demonstrated in myxoid liposarcomas compared to malignant fibrous histiocytoma (MFH), which is now classified as UPS [14]. Nevertheless, the relative radioresistance of sarcoma has led to significant interest in particle therapy.

25.3 Preclinical Data

There are limited preclinical data investigating the radiobiology of particle therapy specifically for sarcoma. The relative biologic effectiveness (RBE) of carbon ions was tested in a murine model of fibrosarcoma [15]. The calculated α/β ratio varied with increasing linear energy transfer (LET) and ranged from 129 ± 10 Gy for Cs-137 gamma rays up to 475 ± 168 Gy for 74 keV/μM. The RBE also varied with LET and with the number of fractions for the higher LET energies. The calculated RBE range was 1.4 with 14 keV/μM beams up to 3.0 for 74 keV/μM beam energies using four fractions.

Brownstein et al. conducted a more recent study comparing carbon-ion radiotherapy (CIRT) to photon radiotherapy in a primary sarcoma mouse tumor model [16]. The RBE was three times higher for CIRT than for photons. Interestingly, differences in growth kinetics were observed after isoeffective doses of 10 GyE CIRT compared to 30 Gy X-rays. After CIRT, there was initially less tumor cell division compared to cells treated with photons. However, at the time of tumor regrowth, there was accelerated proliferation in the carbon-treated cells that eventually outpaced photon-treated cells. A larger T-cell infiltrate also was observed in the tumor stroma after CIRT compared to after photon treatment.

25.4 Clinical Outcomes

25.4.1 Particle Therapy for Unresectable Sarcoma

Most of the interest in using particle therapy for sarcoma has focused on treating patients with unresectable disease. In this setting with a need for dose escalation, the superior dose distribution and increased biologic potency were hypothesized to improve the therapeutic window compared to photons. The modern era for using particle therapy for unresectable sarcoma started initially in the 1970s and 1980s with heavy particle therapy and then shifted in more recent decades to CIRT and proton-beam therapy (PBT). Due to the relative rarity of patients, most of the studies described were by necessity generated from single institutions and included a heterogeneous mix of tumor histologies and disease sites. This group of studies is subdivided the next several sections by type of particle beam and summarized in Table 25.1.

25.4.1.1 Helium, Neon, Pions
An early phase I–II trial from the University of California Lawrence Berkeley Laboratory (UCLBL) used mainly helium and neon ions [17]. Between 1978 and 1985, 41 patients were treated with curative intent doses of 50–78.5 GyE. The largest individual cohorts of patients were

Table 25.1 Particle therapy for unresectable sarcoma

Ref.	Year	Patients (no.)	Particle	Dose (GyE; median; range)	LC (%; 5 years)	OS (%; 5 years)	Late Gr. 3 + toxicity (%)
[17]	1986	41	He/Ne	50–78.5	75[a]	60[a]	15
[18]	1989	27	Pion	30–36	61	52	7
[19]	1989	94	Neutron	16.8	56	26	28
[22]	1999	61	Neutron	14.1 (5.01–18.37)	51.8	47.5	11
[20]	2001	42	Neutron	18.3 (4.8–22)	68[b]	60[b]	15
[23]	2002	57	Carbon	52.8–73.6	73[c]	46[c]	10
[24]	2010	128	Carbon	70.4 (64–73.6)	65	46	3
[28]	2005	112	Proton	64 (25–87.5)	45	35	14
[29]	2007	13	Proton	69.4 (50.4–76)	74.1[b]	82.5[b]	15
[26]	2017	91	Carbon/Proton	70.4	92	83	25

Ref.: Reference; no.: number; He: helium; Ne: neon; GyE: Gray equivalent; LC: local control; OS: overall survival; Gr.: grade;

[a]2 years; [b]4 years; [c]3 years.

paraspinal chondrosarcoma ($n = 11$) and osteosarcoma ($n = 9$). The remaining 21 patients were a mix of STS histologies, and LC was achieved in 14 of these patients. Only seven patients were treated for microscopic residual disease after gross total resection, and LC was achieved in six of these patients. The remaining patients were treated either after resection with gross residual ($n = 22$) or unresectable disease ($n = 12$), and LC was achieved in 16 and 6 cases, respectively. At 2 years, actuarial LC and overall survival (OS) for the entire treatment group was 75% and 60%, respectively. Late severe complications occurred in six patients, including fatal brain necrosis ($n = 1$), spinal cord injury ($n = 2$), cauda equina injury ($n = 1$), bone necrosis ($n = 1$), and bowel injury ($n = 1$).

The Paul Scherrer Institute (PSI) in Switzerland published their initial experience treating unresectable STS with negative Pi-Mesons (pions) on a prospective phase I–II trial [18]. Between 1981 and 1987, 27 patients were treated with "high dose" therapy to 30–36 GyE. The most common histologies were liposarcoma ($n = 6$), MFH/undifferentiated sarcoma ($n = 5$), and leiomyosarcoma ($n = 3$). LC and OS at 5 years were 64% and 52%, respectively. Significant acute toxicity was limited to three patients with grade 3 dermatitis. Two cases of severe late toxicities were attributable to radiation, including one patient with chronic diffuse bowel obstruction and a second patient with disturbed liver function.

25.4.1.2 Neutrons

The largest study of particle therapy for the treatment of STS was reported from Essen, Germany using neutrons [19]. At total of 221 patients were treated between 1978 and 1983 for either unresectable or gross residual disease ($n = 94$) or after gross total resection ($n = 127$). Patients treated for gross dis-

ease received the entire dose with neutrons, but patients treated after gross total resection received a neutron boost after initial treatment with photons or electrons. The tumor histologies included liposarcoma ($n = 54$), fibrosarcoma ($n = 34$), synovial sarcoma ($n = 27$), MFH ($n = 21$), neurofibrosarcoma ($n = 17$), leiomyosarcoma ($n = 16$), and spindle cell sarcoma ($n = 12$). LC was 87% after R0 resection, 78% after R1 resection, and 56% for gross disease. Among the patients treated for gross disease, tumor size was a prognostic factor for LC. LC was achieved in 76% of patients with tumors 5–10 cm in size but in only 42% of patients with tumors larger than 10 cm. Severe late grade 3–4 toxicities occurred in 28% of patients treated only with neutrons and in 7% of patients treated with neutrons as a boost.

The University of Washington reported results for 42 patients treated between 1984 and 1996 with neutrons for curative intent [20,21]. The tumor sites were extremity ($n = 15$), torso ($n = 15$), head and neck ($n = 8$), retroperitoneum ($n = 2$), and viscera ($n = 2$). Liposarcoma ($n = 11$), leiomyosarcoma ($n = 6$), and spindle cell sarcoma ($n = 5$) were the most common STS histology, and eight patients had chondrosarcoma. Most patients were treated after resection ($n = 35$), and the remaining patients were unresectable ($n = 7$). Treatment was for primary disease in 33 patients and for recurrent disease in nine patients. Local relapse-free survival (RFS) was 68% at 4 years. The only factor predictive for worse LC was recurrent disease compared to primary disease (35.7% vs. 78.7%; $p = 0.045$). Serious late toxicity was observed in 15% of patients.

The results of neutron or photon therapies for STS were retrospectively compared by the group from the University of Munster, Germany [22]. A cohort of 61 patients treated with neutrons was compared to 100 patients treated with photons.

Of the neutron group, most ($n = 46$) were treated only with neutrons and the remaining 15 patients were treated with a combination of neutrons and photons. The groups were similar in their distribution of tumor site (lower extremity: 37% vs. 45%). However, there were fewer grade 3 tumors (9.7% vs. 32%) and a higher percentage of patients with gross disease (52% vs. 11%) in the neutron cohort. Moreover, the most common tumor histologies among patients treated with neutrons were MFH ($n = 15$), liposarcoma ($n = 11$), and neurogenic sarcoma ($n = 10$), but there were more cases of fibrosarcoma ($n = 26$), synovial sarcoma ($n = 19$), and rhabdomyosarcoma ($n = 14$) among the photon-treated patients. For patients who were treated only with neutron therapy, the average dose was 14.1 GyE (range 5.01–18.37 GyE) delivered three fractions per week. In the combined modality group, the average dose was 8.5 GyE (range 3.34–10.02) neutrons plus 36.5 Gy (36.5–60 Gy) photons. Patients who received only photons were treated between 45 and 66 Gy. The 5-year local RFS was similar for neutrons compared to for photons (51.8% vs. 44.8%, respectively). Median (27 vs. 35 months) and 5-year OS (42.5% vs. 43.1%) were also equivalent between neutrons and photons, respectively. Severe grade 3–4 side effects were moderately more common in the patients after neutron therapy compared to photon therapy (11% vs. 4%).

25.4.1.3 Carbon Ions

The National Institute of Radiological Sciences (NIRS) in Japan initially conducted a prospective phase I–II trial between 1996 and 1999 of CIRT for unresectable sarcoma [23]. The total accrual was 57 patients with 64 lesions. The majority of patients ($n = 41$) had primary BS, including osteosarcoma ($n = 15$) and chordoma/chondrosarcoma ($n = 17$). The remaining patients ($n = 16$) were classified as STS, including MPNST ($n = 6$) and liposarcomas ($n = 3$). Tumors mostly were located in the pelvis ($n = 36$) or spine/paraspinal ($n = 21$) locations, and only seven patients had extremity sarcomas. The initial dose level was 52.8 GyE for pelvic and spine tumors and 57.6 GyE for extremity tumors. Keeping the number of fractions fixed at 16, a dose escalation strategy increased the dose to a maximum of 73.6 GyE. The primary end point of the study was safety, and the only cases of grade 3 or 4 toxicity that were observed involved the skin and soft tissue. Almost all of these toxicities occurred at the highest dose level of 73.6 GyE (seven of eight acute cases; four of six late cases). Other than skin and soft tissue side effects, only seven cases were recorded of late grade 2 peripheral neuropathy. Tumor outcomes were also encouraging with a 3-year LC rate of 73%. Moreover, a dose response was observed with a superior LC at 3 years for doses of at least 64 GyE (84% vs. 53%; $p = 0.035$). Median and 3-year OS were 31 months and 46%, respectively. The authors concluded that CIRT delivered in this dose range with 16 fractions was safe and produced encouraging tumor control outcomes.

This trial also established the institutional standard dose of 73.6 GyE in 16 fractions, except for a dose reduction to 70.4 GyE or less for tumors with a subcutaneous component.

A recent report from NIRS updated their subsequent experience by focusing on CIRT for unresectable axial (non-extremity, non-spine) STS [24]. A retrospective review was reported of 128 patients treated between 2000 and 2015. Most of the tumors were in the retroperitoneum, pelvis, abdominal wall or chest wall ($n = 123$). The major tumor histologies were UPS ($n = 29$), MPNST ($n = 15$), liposarcoma ($n = 15$), synovial sarcoma ($n = 14$), and leiomyosarcoma ($n = 10$). The most common dose was 70.4 GyE in 16 fractions ($n = 115$), and a minority of patients were treated to 64 GyE ($n = 8$) or 73.6 GyE ($n = 5$). LC at 5 years was very good at 65%, but no factors could be identified as prognostic. Similar to the earlier phase I–II study, median and 5-year OS were 42 months and 46%, respectively. On multivariate analysis, LC and tumor size larger than 500 cm^3 were both independent prognostic factors for OS. Toxicities were low. One patient experienced a grade 4 colon injury resulting in a colostomy. Three other grade 3 toxicities were observed including spinal cord injury, peripheral neuropathy, and skin injury. However, it was noted that the spinal cord injury occurred in a patient who received two courses of CIRT due to local disease recurrence.

A small report from Heidelberg, Germany, focused on CIRT for patients with MPNST who were either unresectable or had gross residual disease [25]. This study retrospectively identified 11 consecutive patients treated between 2010 and 2013. Tumors were located in the pelvis/sacrum ($n = 5$), sinonasal/orbit ($n = 5$), or cervical neck ($n = 1$). Only three patients had associated neurofibromatosis type 1. Tumors were primary in six patients and recurrent in five patients; three of these patients had received prior radiation. Treatment was delivered only with CIRT ($n = 7$) or as a boost after initial photon intensity-modulated radiation therapy (IMRT; $n = 4$). For patients receiving CIRT only, dose was 60–66 GyE in 20–22 fractions and reduced to 54–60 GyE in 18–20 fractions for re-irradiation cases. For patients receiving mixed modality therapy, the initial IMRT course was 50 Gy in 25 fractions followed by a CIRT boost of 24 GyE in 8 fractions. At a median follow-up of 17 months, 2-year LC was 65%. Of the three patients with local progression, one case was in-field and two cases were marginal. Acute toxicities were minimal with only one case of grade 2 dermatitis and no grade 3 or higher toxicities. Two patients experienced severe late toxicities including one patient who developed trismus and one patient who developed delayed wound healing after carbon ion re-irradiation.

The use of particle therapy for the treatment of unresectable or incompletely resected pelvis sarcoma also was studied at the Hyogo Ion Beam Medical Center in Japan. This center has the capability to deliver both PBT and CIRT. A retrospective study reported on 91 nonmetastatic patients treated between 2005 and 2014 [26]. Most of these patients had either chordoma ($n = 53$) or chondrosarcoma ($n = 14$). The remaining patients had osteosarcoma ($n = 10$), UPS ($n = 5$), MPNST ($n = 3$), or other ($n = 6$). Proton therapy was used for 52 patients. A uniform dose of 70.4 GyE was used for all patients, which was delivered either in 16 fractions ($n = 36$) based on the NIRS experience or in 32 fractions ($n = 55$) if tumors were adjacent to organs at risk. A surgical spacer to displace adjacent bowel was used in 38 patients. With a median follow-up of 32 months, the 3-year LC and OS were 92% and 83%, respectively. No significant differences were observed in the outcomes after treatment with either PBT or CIRT for patients with chordoma, chondrosarcoma, or osteosarcoma. Toxicities were observed more frequently in this study. Both grade 3 ($n = 20$) and grade 4 ($n = 2$) acute dermatitis were observed, but all patients completed treated and recovered completely. One quarter of the patients ($n = 23$) developed late grade ≥3 toxicities, and eight patients experienced more than one severe late toxicity. The only late grade 4 toxicities involved the skin in nine patients. Late grade 3 effects included pain ($n = 5$) or injury to peripheral nerves ($n = 6$), bone ($n = 2$), genitourinary system ($n = 2$), skin ($n = 2$), muscle ($n = 2$), and vascular system ($n = 1$). Significantly more late severe toxicities occurred in patients after the 16 fraction regimen than the 32 fraction regimen (50% vs. 9%; $p < 0.001$). After excluding skin events, the significant difference persisted in favor of the 32 fraction regimen persisted (28% vs. 9%; $p = 0.024$). Specifically for the patients who developed late peripheral neuropathy, five of the six patients were treated with the 16 fraction regimen. The authors concluded that the 32 fraction regimen appeared to be favored as achieving equivalent oncologic outcome with less toxicity.

Given the known risk of late skin toxicities after CIRT, an analysis was performed at NIRS to identify dosimetric factors associated with grade ≥3 skin toxicities [27]. The study cohort included 35 patients with bone and STS mostly located in the pelvis ($n = 21$) and spine ($n = 10$). The strongest independent prognostic factor to be identified was when the surface area receiving at least 60 GyE exceeded 20 square centimeters (HR 5.107; 95% CI: 1.068–24.20; $p = 0.041$).

25.4.1.4 Proton Therapy

An early experience using PBT to treat patients with unresectable sarcoma was reported by the Massachusetts General Hospital (MGH) [28]. Between 1970 and 2001, 112 patients were treated for gross disease located in the lower extremity ($n = 32$), upper extremity ($n = 17$), head and neck ($n = 26$), chest and abdominal wall ($n = 8$), and retroperitoneum ($n = 29$). The most common histologies included MFH ($n = 22$), liposarcomas ($n = 21$), MPNST ($n = 16$), angiosarcoma ($n = 13$), fibrosarcoma ($n = 12$), and unclassified sarcoma ($n = 10$). Median radiation dose was 64 GyE (range 25–87.5 GyE) and 22 patients received doses of 70 GyE or higher. Median follow-up was 29 months. At 5 years, LC and OS were 45% and 35%, respectively. Tumor size was predictive of LC with a 5-year rate of 51% and 45% for tumors <5 cm and 5–10 cm, respectively, compared to only 9% for tumors >10 cm ($p < 0.001$). Dose was another significant predictor of LC with a 5-year rate of 60% for patients treated to at least 63 GyE compared to only 22% for patients treated to less than 63 GyE. Dose remained a significant independent prognostic factor for LC on multivariate analysis ($p = 0.02$). Major complications occurred in 16 patients (14%), which mostly were related to serious wound healing damage, skin necrosis, or soft tissue necrosis ($n = 10$). There were only two cases of neuropathy and one case of bowel injury.

The initial experience of treating unresectable STS with spot scanning PBT was published by Weber and colleagues at the PSI [29]. Thirteen patients were treated between 1998 and 2005. Tumor histologies included liposarcoma ($n = 3$), MPNST ($n = 3$), leiomyosarcoma ($n = 2$), desmoid tumor ($n = 2$), angiosarcoma ($n = 1$), spindle cell sarcoma ($n = 1$), and malignant hemangiopericytoma ($n = 1$). The most common tumor location was paraspinal ($n = 6$). Patients were treated after gross total resection with positive microscopic margins ($n = 7$), subtotal resection ($n = 4$), or only biopsy ($n = 2$). The median dose was 69.4 GyE (range 50.4–76 GyE), and seven patients were treated with a combination of photons and protons. Median follow-up was 48.1 months for surviving patients. Local failure was observed in three patients, although two of these patients had desmoid or hemangiopericytoma, which are known to have higher risk of local recurrence. The third case of local failure was a patient with MPNST. At 4 years, the rates of LC and OS were 74.1% and 82.5%. No late toxicities were observed in the patients treated for paraspinal tumors. The only two late adverse events (cataract and symptomatic brain necrosis) occurred after treatment of head and neck sarcomas.

25.4.1.5 Case 1

A 70-year-old woman presented with left hip pain, leg weakness, and left foot drop. Imaging demonstrated a $15.1 \times 12.5 \times 11$-cm destructive mass of the left ilium without metastasis (Figure 25.1a,c). Based on the imaging, the differential diagnosis favored primary BS over STS or other malignancy. A CT-guided biopsy was reviewed by subspecialty pathologists at two tertiary care institutions with findings consistent for a high-grade pleomorphic sarcoma with numerous intermixed multinucleated giant cells. A focus of matrix raised the suspicion of a giant cell osteosarcoma, but it could not definitively be determined to represent osteoid. Ultimately, while osteosarcoma could not be completely excluded, the final diagnosis was a high-grade UPS.

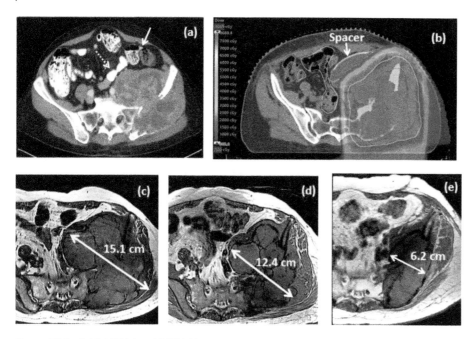

Figure 25.1 Initial CT (a) and MRI (c) imaging demonstrating a large, destructive pleomorphic sarcoma centered in the left ilium in close proximity to small bowel (dotted arrow) and large bowel (solid arrow). A favorable response to neoadjuvant chemotherapy resulted in modest reduction in the tumor size (d). After chemotherapy, the patient received definitive proton beam therapy to a prescription dose of 74 GyE (b). The doses represented by the colorwash are indicated on the left and range from 500–8,000 cGyE. A spacer was positioned to displace the bowel from the gross tumor volume (red line) and clinical target volume (pink line). MRI 1 year after completion of proton beam (e) demonstrated significant additional tumor response, which has subsequently remained stable.

An initial multidisciplinary tumor board recommended against radical surgery, and the patient also did not want surgery. Neoadjuvant doxorubicin, ifosfamide, and mesna were delivered for three cycles and achieved a partial clinical tumor response with no metastatic progression (Figure 25.1d). Definitive PBT was recommended, but bowel immediately abutting the tumor was dose-limiting. Therefore, surgical oncology placed a 10 × 12-cm tissue expander with 250 mL of saline in the retroperitoneal space. The first report of facilitating PBT by surgically creating space between the target and the surrounding bowel used multiple layers of biomaterial [30]. Interesting preclinical and phase I studies are underway in the development of a biodegradable spacer [31,32]. Our technique of using a tissue expander was similar to a recent report by Chan et al. [33].

Simulation was performed supine, with arms across her chest, and in a thermoplastic mask fabricated over her lower abdomen and pelvis. A dose of 74 GyE in 37 fractions was prescribed using a three-field plan with pencil-beam scanning (PBS) and single-field optimization (SFO) technique (Figure 25.1b). The dose to 1 cm^3 of large and small bowel was 45.22 GyE and 11.70 GyE, respectively. Acute toxicity included only grade 1 dermatitis. The spacer was removed without incident at the 3-month follow-up appointment.

Imaging with MRI at 1-year post-treatment demonstrated further favorable tumor response compared to the post-chem-

otherapy imaging (Figure 25.1e), which subsequently remained stable. The patient reported an increase in mild, aching pain in the left hip 2 years and 4 months after treatment. A MRI demonstrated a small fracture in the acetabulum and anterior femoral head. The patient began using a cane more regularly but did not require opioid analgesics or surgical intervention. This was classified as a grade 2 late toxicity. The patient remained ambulatory 4 years status post-completion of radiotherapy with no evidence of local or distant disease progression.

25.4.2 Anatomic Subsites

As described, much of the literature on particle therapy for sarcoma includes a variety of anatomic subsites in each analysis. However, several studies have focused on common sites where particle therapy may prove to be of particular benefit such as spinal/paraspinal sarcoma, retroperitoneal sarcoma (RPS), and extremity STS. In addition, case reports have described the use of PBT for the rare occurrences of primary cardiac sarcoma.

25.4.2.1 Spine

Particle therapy has been most established in the setting of chordoma and chondrosarcoma of the base of skull and spine. However, other sarcomas may also occur in this location. An initial experience using helium and neon ions to treat paraspinal tumors was reported from the UCLBL [34]. A total of 52 patients were treated between 1976 and 1987. Although approximately one-half of the patients in this study were treated for chordoma and chondrosarcoma, the results were reported separately for a group of 14 patients with osteosarcoma ($n = 5$), neurofibrosarcoma ($n = 4$), MFH ($n = 2$), fibrosarcoma ($n = 1$), synovial sarcoma ($n = 1$), and undifferentiated sarcoma ($n = 1$). All of these 14 patients were treated for gross residual disease after incomplete resection with a median follow-up of 28 months. The median dose was 66 GyE (range 50–76 GyE) using a RBE of 1.3 and 2.5 for non-CNS tissue and 1.6 and 4.5 for CNS tissue for late effects after helium and neon, respectively. Local tumor control was achieved in seven patients with a median time to local failure of 7 months. At 4 years, actuarial LC and OS was 56% and 77%, respectively.

Matsumoto et al. described the NIRS experience using CIRT to treat non-sacral, unresectable spine sarcoma [35]. A retrospective review of patients enrolled on their phase I and II trials included 47 patients treated between 1996 and 2001. Osteosarcoma ($n = 13$), chondrosarcoma ($n = 13$), and chordoma ($n = 13$) were the most common histologies, but patients were also included with MFH ($n = 7$), Ewing sarcoma ($n = 2$), and other STSs ($n = 4$). The median dose was 64.0 GyE (range 52.8–70.4 GyE) delivered in 16 fractions. The median follow-up was 25 months. LC at 5 years was 79%. Both tumor volume and dose were prognostic factors for LC. The 5-year LC was 100% in tumors ≤ 100 cm^3 but only 67% in larger tumors ($p = 0.0194$). Patients treated with at least 64 GyE had fewer local recurrences compared to patients treated with a lower dose ($p = 0.0252$). Although not statistically significant, the 5-year LC rate was 75% for tumors located within 5 mm of the spinal cord compared to 100% for tumors at least 5 mm away. No differences in LC were identified by histology. The 5-year OS was 52%. Late toxicities included one patient each with a grade 3 skin reaction, a grade 4 skin ulcer, and a grade 3 spinal cord myelopathy. Vertebral body compression occurred in seven patients, and all of these cases went on to surgical fixation at a median of 35 months (range 4–47 months) post-radiotherapy.

Hug et al. reported the initial experience from the Harvard Cyclotron Laboratory using a combination of photons and protons [36]. A total of 47 patients were treated between 1980 and 1982. Patients were grouped by histology: chordoma and chondrosarcoma ($n = 20$); osteosarcoma ($n = 15$); giant cell tumors, osteoblastoma, and chondroblastoma ($n = 12$). For the osteosarcoma group, the median dose was 69.8 GyE (range 61.1–80.0 GyE). LC was achieved in 11 of the 15 patients for a 5-year actuarial LC rate of 59%. In further analysis of the osteosarcoma group, it was noted that LC was achieved in 10 of 12 patients (83%) presenting with primary disease but in only one

of three patients (33%) presenting with recurrent disease. All four patients (100%) treated with a combination of pre- and postoperative radiation achieved LC compared to only six of eight patients (75%) treated with surgery plus only postoperative radiation and only one of three patients (33%) treated with radiation after only a biopsy.

This early experience was extended with a prospective phase II trial [37,38]. Chordoma and chondrosarcoma were the predominant histologies (43 of 50 patients), but the remaining patients included one case each of osteosarcoma, Ewing sarcoma, giant cell tumor, MPNST, liposarcoma, angiosarcoma, and spindle/round cell sarcoma. The median dose was 76.6 GyE (range 59.4–77.41 GyE). LC at 8 years was excellent at 74% for the entire group and 85% for the patients with primary tumor presentation. However, these outcomes were not further broken out for the minority subgroup of patients with STS. The only toxicities noted for the non-chordoma/chondrosarcoma patients included a grade 4 radiation-associated sarcoma and a grade 1 scoliosis identified 8.4 and 9.5 years after protocol radiation, respectively.

To explore using more modern PBS proton techniques, Weber et al. performed a treatment planning study to compare IMRT and intensity-modulated protons (IMPT) [39]. Five patients with tumors (STS, $n = 4$; chondrosarcoma, $n = 1$) of the thoracic or lumbar spine were planned using both techniques to a definitive dose of 77.4 GyE. Proton therapy plans were more homogeneous and delivered significant dose reductions to normal organs at risk. Based on their institutional normal tissue tolerance, it was modeled that a 20% dose escalation to over 90 GyE could be achieved with IMPT for each of the five test patients regardless of tumor size or location.

25.4.2.2 Retroperitoneum

The PSI group initially used pion therapy for 21 patients with RPS [40]. Local recurrence occurred in three patients (one, in-field; two, marginal) for an actuarial rate of LC at 3 and 5 years of 90% and 60%, respectively. The OS rate at 5 years was 33%. Radiation was thought to contribute to late toxicities in three patients, including liver dysfunction, leg edema, and skin necrosis.

The CIRT experience from NIRS focused on their experience treating 24 patients with unresectable RPS [41]. The dose ranged 52.8–73.6 GyE in 16 fractions. LC and OS were excellent at 69% and 50% at 5 years, respectively. No grade 3 or higher toxicities were observed. One caveat to the interpretation of these results was the atypical distribution of tumor histology for this anatomic site. Only three patients had liposarcoma and six patients had MFH/UPS, and the remainder either had MPNST ($n = 3$), Ewing sarcoma ($n = 2$), or "miscellaneous" tumors ($n = 10$).

A treatment planning study compared the use of 3D-conformal photons (3DCRT), IMRT, or 3D conformal protons for preoperative treatment of RPS [42]. While all of the techniques provided adequate target coverage, treatment plans were more conformal and homogeneous with both IMRT and PBT compared to 3DCRT. However, PBT significantly decreased the dose to the bowel compared to photons. The small bowel volume receiving 15 Gy (V15) was 16.4% for proton beam, 52.2% for IMRT, and 66.1% for 3DCRT. Even more significantly in this disease where surgery often requires ipsilateral nephrectomy, the median volume of the contralateral kidney receiving 5 GyE (V5) was 0% for protons compared to 49.9% for IMRT and 99.7% for 3DCRT.

Yoon et al. reported the initial experience from MGH with PBT for sarcomas of the retroperitoneum or pelvis [43]. Twenty patients with primary tumors and eight patients with recurrent tumors were treated between 2003 and 2007. Radiotherapy was performed preoperatively for 20 patients, and proton beam was incorporated into the treatment for 18 patients. Compared to IMRT plans, the authors noted that PBT significantly reduced the dose exposure to the spinal cord, contralateral kidney, kidney, liver, and small bowel. Surgical complications were observed in eight patients (28.6%) and radiotherapy complications in four patients (14%), although only one case of postoperative bleeding appeared to be related

to PBT specifically. Oncologic outcomes were excellent with 3-year LC of 90% for patients with primary tumors.

This initial experience with proton therapy was then extended into a prospective phase I trial [44]. The study recruited 11 patients with primary RPS. The high-risk margin was treated to escalated doses of 60.2, 61.6, and 63 GyE using a simultaneous integrated boost technique while treating the entire tumor volume to a standard dose of 50.4 GyE in 28 fractions. The treatment was well tolerated with no dose-limiting toxicities up to the maximum dose and no grade 3 acute toxicities. One patient had delayed ureteral stenosis after receiving 57.5 GyE; the ureteral dose was limited to 50.4 GyE in the subsequently treated patients without any further complications. With a median follow-up of 18 months, no local recurrences were observed among the nine patients who underwent resection. A phase II study is underway at the highest dose level of 63 GyE.

25.4.2.3 Case 2

A 73-year-old woman presented to the emergency department with severe reflux and nausea. On questioning, she acknowledged that symptoms of anorexia and early satiety have been presented for approximately 1 year. A CT scan demonstrated a

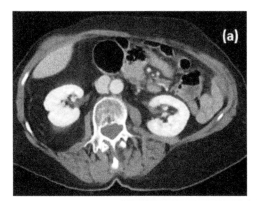
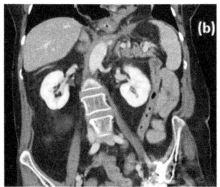
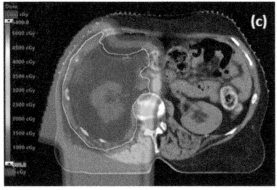

Figure 25.2 Axial (a) and coronal (b) CT images demonstrating a well-differentiated liposarcoma of the right retroperitoneum. Treatment was delivered preoperatively to a prescription dose of 50 GyE with proton beam (c). The doses represented by the colorwash are indicated on the left and range from 500–5,400 cGyE. Highlighted structures include the gross tumor volume (red line), the clinical target volume (pink line), and the contralateral left kidney (blue).

15 × 10 × 7-cm right retroperitoneal mass primarily of fat density, surrounding the right kidney, and causing displacement of the bowel to the left (Figure 25.2a,b). A biopsy was performed and pathology was consistent with a MDM2-amplified, well-differentiated liposarcoma. Our institutional practice has been to treat RPS with preoperative radiation followed by surgery combined with intraoperative electron radiation therapy (IOERT) [45,46]. The phase III randomized EORTC STRASS trial was recently reported in abstract form [47]. In this multinational trial, 266 patients were randomized between 2012 and 2017 either to preoperative radiation (3DCRT or IMRT) to a dose of 50.4 Gy followed by surgery or to surgery alone. As would be expected for a study of patients with RPS, liposarcoma (74%) represented the most common histology. For the overall study group, there was no difference in the 3-year rate of abdominal recurrence between study arms. However, on sensitivity analysis, for the liposarcoma subgroup, the 3-year abdominal-free recurrence rate was borderline significant in favor of the preoperative radiation arm (71.6% vs. 60.4%; HR 0.64; 95% CI: 0.40–1.01; $p = 0.049$).

Therefore, the patient was taken for simulation and placed supine with her arms over her head and immobilized in a thermoplastic body mask. A 4D CT scan was performed to assess for organ and target motion. Target volumes were contoured per consensus guidelines [48]. A PBT plan using PBS with two fields and a SFO technique was designed to deliver 50 GyE in 25 fractions (Figure 25.2 c). Target coverage was achieved with 99.3% of the clinical target volume (CTV) receiving 100% of the prescription dose while also limiting the maximum cord dose to 30.5 GyE and a mean liver dose of 17.7 GyE. The maximum small bowel dose was 50.75 GyE, and only 2.3 cm^3 exceeded 45 Gy. In a patient where ipsilateral nephrectomy is planned, the Quantitative Analyses of Normal Tissue Effects in the Clinic (QUANTEC) report recommends limiting the volume of contralateral kidney receiving at least 6 Gy to less than 30% [49]. In the current patient's plan, the maximum dose to the left kidney was 4.5 GyE and only 1% received 1 Gy. Surgery with IOERT will be planned 4 weeks after the completion of radiotherapy.

25.4.2.4 Extremity

There are limited data specifically focusing on particle therapy for sarcoma of the extremity. In the previously described study by Schmitt et al., a large subgroup of 143 patients with extremity STS treated with neutrons were broken out for analysis [19]. There were 49 local failures (34%), and 20 of these patients required amputation resulting in an overall limb preservation rate of 86%. Functional outcome was reported as good in 70% of patients.

The experience at NIRS treating sarcomas of the extremity with CIRT was reported by Sugahara et al. [50]. A prospective analysis was performed for 17 patients treated between 2000 and 2010. Patients were treated for both primary ($n = 9$) and recurrent ($n = 8$) tumors. Most of the tumors were located in the lower extremity ($n = 13$), most were soft tissue tumors ($n = 13$), and most were at least 10 cm ($n = 13$). There were four cases of primary tumors of the bone (osteosarcoma, $n = 3$; chondrosarcoma, $n = 1$). All of the patients were treated in 16 fractions, 4 days per week, and over 4 weeks. The most common dose was 70.4 GyE ($n = 13$). Median follow-up was 37 months. At both 3 and 5 years, LC was 76%. All of the cases of local failure ($n = 4$) were treated with the highest prescription dose level of 70.4 GyE. Severe late grade 3 toxicity only occurred in one patient with a femoral fracture, and four patients developed late grade 2 neuropathy.

There are no case series exclusively addressing PBT for the treatment of extremity STS. Fogliata et al. performed a planning study comparing photon IMRT with volumetric-modulated arc therapy to IMPT [51]. Treatment plans were generated for 10 patients with STS of the leg with a prescription dose of 66.5 Gy in 25 fractions and a normal tissue constraint of 50 Gy to the adjacent bone. Acceptable plans were achieved with both techniques, but plan homogeneity and the sparing of normal tissue from low and medium doses were superior in the proton plans.

A case report from the University of Maryland described a patient treated with preoperative PBT for a 7.5-cm UPS of the thigh adjacent to the femoral head and shaft [52]. A PBS proton plan delivered 50.4 GyE in 28 fractions to the target while limiting the mean dose to the left femoral head to 24.4 GyE. During treatment, the patient experienced increased pain associated with a significant increase in tumor size and cystic change that required a replan after 41.4 GyE. Due to these symptoms, the patient was taken to the operating room only 12 days after radiation. A gross total resection with negative margins was achieved, and consistent with a favorable treatment effect, the pathology revealed approximately 80% tumor necrosis. The patient developed a wound complication requiring intravenous antibiotics and debridement two weeks after surgery, but good healing was achieved by 1 month after this intervention.

Two institutions have suggested the combination of PBT with hyperthermia for extremity STS. The hypothesis is that hyperthermia may act to kills cells in a manner similar to high LET radiation such as heavy particles and that combining hyperthermia with the superior dose distribution of PBT may produce an effect similar to CIRT [53]. The PSI reported an initial two patients with lower extremity STS who required definitive PBT after refusing amputation [54]. Both patients were treated to 70–72 GyE in 2.0 GyE fractions combined with hyperthermia delivered weekly during radiotherapy. Acute toxicity was limited to grade 1–2 dermatitis with no observed late toxicities. Both patients achieved an apparent complete response and LC at last follow up at 5 and 14 months, respectively. A third case was reported from the University of Tsukuba also describing a patient who refused amputation for a high-grade STS of the leg [55]. He was treated with an accelerated course of PBT to a dose of 72 GyE in 18 fractions of 4.0 GyE each combined with twice weekly hyperthermia sessions. Acute toxicity was limited to grade 2 dermatitis. Late toxicities included grade 1 edema, telangiectasia, hyperpigmentation, and contracture. The patient was followed for 7 years and remained ambulatory and free of disease progression. The HYPROSAR trial was designed as a prospective phase I–II trial combining proton beam with hyperthermia (NCT01904565) with a goal to accrue 26 patients. The primary end point was safety, and the secondary end point was local tumor response [53].

25.4.2.5 Case 3

A 70-year-old woman presented with a painless mass in the right thigh above the knee that had rapidly increased in size over approximately 3 months. A MRI demonstrated a 3.7 × 14.4 × 4.8-cm, heterogeneously enhancing mass associated with the vastus intermedius and medialis possibly contiguous with the suprapatellar region (Figure 25.3a,b). A core biopsy yielded a diagnosis of intermediate grade myxofibrosarcoma. After multidisciplinary discussion between orthopedic oncology, radiation oncology, and medical oncology, the decision was made to proceed with preoperative radiation therapy. The patient was simulated in the supine, feet-first position with her hands on her chest, with IV contrast, and immobilized in a vacuum cradle. A two-field PBS proton plan with SFO technique was generated to deliver a prescription dose of 50 GyE (Figure 25.3c). The mean dose to the femur was 11.90 GyE, and the volume of femur receiving 50 GyE was 3.9%. Acute toxicity was limited to grade 2 dermatitis. One month after radiation, a preoperative MRI demonstrated a significant decrease in tumor size and contrast enhancement (Figure 25.3d). A gross total resection was performed with negative margins. Pathology demonstrated extensive treat-

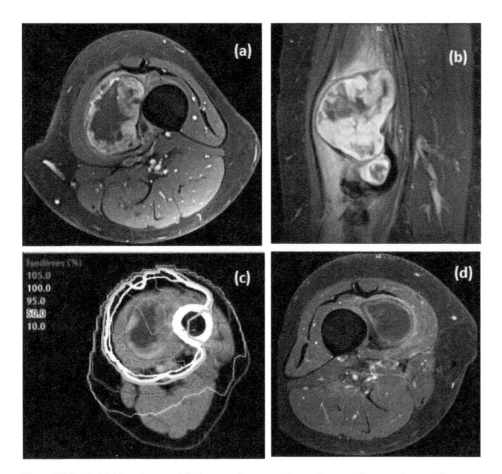

Figure 25.3 Axial (a) and coronal (b) images demonstrating an intermediate grade myxofibrosarcoma of the right leg adjacent to the femur. Treatment was delivered preoperatively to a prescription dose of 50 GyE with proton beam (c). The isodose lines representing 105% (pink), 100% (yellow), 95% (green), 50% (blue), and 10% (cyan) of the prescription dose are shown in relation to the gross tumor volume (red) and clinical target volume (white) and the adjacent femur. Favorable treatment response based on decrease tumor size and enhancement was observed on a MRI one month post-radiotherapy (d).

ment effect with 90% necrosis and only focal residual sarcoma. The patient remains disease free 1 year after surgery with no apparent late toxicities and good function.

25.4.2.6 Head and Neck

Although tumors of the head and neck were included in several of the previously discussed studies, two centers have published results focused on the use of particle therapy for this anatomic subsite. Mizoe et al. reported the results from NIRS of a phase II trial of CIRT for head and neck cancers [56]. Between 1997 and 2006, a total of 236 patients were treated on the protocol to a dose of either 57.6 or 64.0 GyE in 16 fractions. The patient cohort was a mixture of tumor histologies; the majority of patients had mucosal melanoma ($n = 85$) and adenoid cystic carcinoma ($n = 69$), but 14 patients with sarcoma were also included in the treatment cohort. The 5-year LC rate for the entire group was 68%. However, outcomes were poor for the patients treated for sarcoma (5-year LC, 24%) compared to mucosal melanoma, adenoid cystic carcinoma, and adenocarcinoma (5-year LC 75%, 73%, and 73%, respectively). The 5-year OS rate for the sarcoma patients was 36%.

Given the poor results observed among the sarcoma patients, a second study was initiated to study dose escalation with CIRT in this subgroup of head and neck patients [57]. A total of 27 patients with unresectable but nonmetastatic disease were enrolled between 2001 and 2008. Patients with both STS ($n = 16$) and primary BS (osteosarcoma, $n = 9$; chondrosarcoma, $n = 2$) were enrolled in the study. The dose was 70.4 GyE in 16 fractions. Median follow-up was 37 months (range 4.1–37.0 months). At 5 years, LC and OS were 80.4% and 57.8%, respectively. Late toxicities included one patient with grade 4 loss of vision after treatment of a tumor involving the optic nerve and four patients with grade 3 bone pain. Based on a cross-study comparison, the authors concluded that dose escalation was safe and produced statistically significant improvements in oncologic outcomes compared to patients treated on the earlier lower dose protocol.

A recent report from the Shanghai Proton and Heavy Ion Center described their initial experience treating 51 patients with head and neck sarcoma between 2014 and 2018 [58]. Patients were mostly unresectable, including 47 patients treated after incomplete resection or biopsy only. Approximately half of the patients were primary BS (chondrosarcoma, $n = 20$; osteosarcoma, $n = 4$). Consistent with a young patient population with a median age of 36 (range 14–68), another 10 patients had rhabdomyosarcoma. Although 22 patients were treated for recurrent disease, only 12 patients had received prior radiation. Patient were treated either with CIRT ($n = 41$), PBT ($n = 2$), or a combination of both modalities ($n = 8$). A wide range of dose and fractionation schedules were used depending on the modality. Among the patients treated with CIRT only, the most common prescriptions were 60–63 GyE in 18–21 fractions ($n = 28$), and PBT was delivered with standard fractionation. Median follow-up was relatively short at 15.7 months (range 2.8–56.7 months). At 2 years, local RFS was 78.9% and OS was 90%. On multivariate analysis, only re-irradiation was prognostic for worse LC. Acute toxicities were limited to one patient with a grade 4 hemorrhage and one patient with grade 3 mucositis. The patient who suffered from the acute hemorrhage suffered a recurrent grade 5 hemorrhage 3.4 months after completion of CIRT, which was the only late toxicity more severe than grade 2.

25.4.2.7 Cardiac

Primary cardiac tumors are rare and mostly benign. However, sarcomas are the most common histology when these tumors are malignant. One of the few studies to report specifically on cardiac sarcoma was from the Cleveland Clinic [59]. The retrospective series included 42 patients treated between 1998 and 2013. The most common histologies were angiosarcoma ($n = 9$), synovial sarcoma ($n = 7$), and MFH ($n = 5$). Treatment involved a variety of combinations of surgery, chemotherapy, and radiation therapy. Surgery was performed for most patients ($n = 30$), and photon radiation was included in the treatment for 15 patients. Median survival for the whole group was 25 months but was significantly better for the eight patients who received all three modalities at 82.7 months ($p = 0.007$).

Given the high doses of radiation required to treat sarcoma and the need to spare as much normal cardiac volume as possible, it would be expected that particle therapy could be beneficial in this setting. Two case reports described PBT for primary cardiac sarcoma. Aoka et al. reported a case from NIRS of a 33-year-old female diagnosed with a rapidly growing angiosarcoma [60]. After a biopsy, the patient was treated to a dose of 64 GyE in 16 fractions with definitive intent CIRT. Post-treatment imaging demonstrated a favorable response with a calculated volume reduction of 86% and resolution of uptake on PET/CT. Lung metastases developed 4 months after CIRT, and the patient subsequently was treated with interleukin 2. The patient remained alive without evidence for local recurrence for more than 1.5 years. A second case was described by Abe et al. [61]. A 41-year-old male underwent primary surgical resection for a cardiac UPS without adjuvant therapy. Local recurrence was identified five months after surgery, and then he was treated with PBT to a total dose of 75 GyE. Post-radiotherapy imaging demonstrated significant tumor decrease in tumor size, and the patient was alive more than 1 year after treatment without progression of disease.

25.4.2.8 Case 4

A 37-year-old male presented with progressive dyspnea. Echocardiography and MRI demonstrated a mass in the left atrium spanning the atrial septum. Surgery was performed to

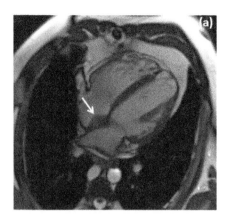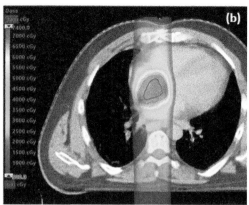

Figure 25.4 Primary cardiac high-grade pleomorphic sarcoma residual after surgery (arrow) demonstrated on MRI (a). Treatment was delivered with definitive intent to the gross disease to a dose of 68 GyE in 34 fractions with proton beam (b). The doses represented by the colorwash are indicated on the left and range from 500 to 7,400 cGyE. Highlighted structures include the gross tumor volume (thick red line) and the clinical target volume (thin pink line).

decompress the cardiac flow, and a subtotal resection was achieved. Pathology was confirmed as an UPS. After recovery, systemic therapy was initiated with doxorubicin and ifosfamide. Treatment was discontinued after three cycles due to pancytopenia. Restaging showed no evidence for metastatic disease and stable residual intracardiac primary tumor (Figure 25.4a). Definitive intent radiation therapy was recommended with PBT. He was simulated supine, arms up, with a thermoplastic mask, and without and with intravenous contrast. A 4D CT was performed to assess the impact of diaphragm motion on the heart. Sequences from a cardiac MRI and cardiac CT angiogram were fused with the simulation CT to facilitate contouring of the GTV. An iGTV was constructed based on the motion of the tumor and heart estimated from the 4DCT and cine MRI images. The iGTV was uniformly expanded by 0.5 cm to create the CTV. The treatment plan prescribed a dose of 64 GyE in 34 fractions using PBS with SFO technique (Figure 25.4b). The mean heart dose was 10.92 GyE and the heart volume receiving 40 GyE was 11.2%. The maximum and mean dose to the right coronary artery was 25.62 and 12.74 GyE, respectively. The left main, the left anterior descending, and the circumflex coronary arteries each received less than 1 GyE. Acute toxicity was limited to grade 1 fatigue. No definite late toxicity was noted, but imaging at three months was concerning for new adrenal metastases. Systemic therapy was restarted, but metastatic disease continued to progress. The patient expired from disease progression 2 years after initial diagnosis and 1 year after completion of radiotherapy.

25.4.3 Re-irradiation

Re-irradiation is a common indication for particle therapy. Although multiple series described in the previous sections also included recurrent and re-irradiation patients, specific outcomes in this patient population can difficult to discern from heterogeneous studies. Recently, early results were published from a prospective trial from the University of Pennsylvania using PBT for re-irradiation of patients with sarcoma [62]. A total of 23 patients were enrolled between 2010 and 2016. The most common histology was liposarcoma ($n = 6$), UPS ($n = 5$), and spindle cell sarcoma ($n = 4$). As only two cases were chordoma and chondrosarcoma, this trial was predominantly STS. Tumor locations included the lower extremity ($n = 9$), pelvis ($n = 4$), thorax ($n = 4$), retroperitoneum ($n = 3$), head and neck ($n = 2$), and upper extremity ($n = 1$). Proton re-irradiation was performed to a dose of 50 GyE in preoperative cases ($n = 8$), 64.8 GyE in postoperative cases ($n = 7$), and 74.7 GyE in definitive cases ($n = 8$). The only acute grade 3 or higher toxicity observed was dysphagia in a recurrent head and neck sarcoma. Two patients experienced late wound complications. There were four cases of late grade 2 musculoskeletal complications including fracture ($n = 1$), lymphedema ($n = 2$), and fibrosis ($n = 1$). At a median follow-up of 10 months, 12 patients experienced a local failure. The cumulative incidence of local failure at 36 months was 41%. The 3-year PFS and OS were 43% and 64%, respectively. The authors concluded that proton re-irradiation was well tolerated, and given the high-risk patient population, that oncologic outcomes were encouraging.

25.4.4 Osteosarcoma

Several series previously discussed have included osteosarcoma patients in the study cohort. However, there are additional studies that have focused exclusively on these patients (Table 25.2). Laramore et al. summarized the early experience using neutrons in 73 patients from 7 institutions with a 55%

Table 25.2 Particle therapy for osteosarcoma

Ref.	Year	Patients (no.)	Particle	Dose (GyE; median; range)	LC (%; 5 years)	OS (%; 5 years)	Late Gr. 3 + toxicity (%)
[21]	1989	73	Neutron	N/R	55[a]	N/R	N/R
		73	Photons	55–80	21[a]	N/R	N/R
[63]	1992	17	He/Ne	64 (52–76)	48	41	24
[64]	2012	79	Carbon	70.4 (52.8–73.6)	62	33	15
[65]	2018	24	Carbon	70.4 (52.8–73.6)	62.9	41.7	24
[66]	2011	55	Proton	68.4	72	67	31

Ref.: Reference; no.: number; He: helium; Ne: neon; GyE: Gray equivalent; LC: local control; OS: overall survival; Gr.: grade; N/R: not reported; [a]crude incidence.

crude LC rate compared to only 21% LC rate from contemporaneous studies of 73 patients from 3 institutions treated with photons [21]. Uhl et al. also utilized heavy particles in a report of the early experience at UCLBL specifically with unresectable BS [63]. Between 1979 and 1989, 17 patients were treated with helium or neon to a median dose of 64 GyE (range 52–76 GyE). The majority of patients had osteosarcoma ($n = 13$). With a mean follow-up of 40 months (range 7–118 months), the crude LC was 53% for an actuarial 5-year rate of 48%. When the analysis was limited to the osteosarcoma cases, the 5-year LC rate was 53% with no local failures after 24 months. Four patients experienced serious late complications including one patient with partial cauda equina injury. Two patients who developed osteoradionecrosis had been treated in a prior radiation field for presumed radiation-induced osteosarcoma. A fourth patient developed presumed heavy particle-induced angiosarcoma at the site of treatment for an osteosarcoma which was itself radiation-induced 20 years after treatment for retinoblastoma as a child.

Two studies described the carbon ion experience at NIRS treated on their institutional prospective clinical trials. Matsunobu et al. described 78 patients with unresectable osteosarcoma of the pelvis ($n = 61$), spine or paraspinal ($n = 15$), or other trunk site ($n = 2$) [64]. The median age was 41 years (range 11–83). Most were primary tumors ($n = 74$) and treated without prior surgery ($n = 67$). The most common dose delivered was 70.4 GyE in 16 fractions ($n = 57$). Median follow-up was 42 months (range 14–166). At 5 years, LC and OS were 62% and 33%, respectively. Tumor volume ≥ 500 cm^3 was predictive for significantly worse LC (88% vs. 31%; $p < 0.003$). Grade 3 and 4 soft tissue late toxicities occurred in six patients. Severe neurologic deficits were attributed to radiation in four patients, and two patients developed fractures requiring surgery.

More recently, Mohamad et al. reported the NIRS experience treating unresectable osteosarcoma in 26 patients between the ages of 11 and 20 years [65]. Most of the tumors were located in the pelvis ($n = 24$). The common dose was 70.4 GyE in 16 fractions for 18 patients. Median follow-up was 32.7 months (range 1.2–248 months). LC at 5 years was 62.9%, and there were two cases of late local failure beyond 5 years. OS at 5 years was 41.7%. The only significant factor for LC was tumor size. At 5 years, LC for tumors ≤ 9.5 cm compared to > 9.5 cm was 75% versus 45%, respectively ($p = 0.03$). Grade 3–4 late toxicities included two cases of skin toxicity and two cases of neurologic dysfunction. One patient experienced a grade 4 sacral fracture requiring fixation. No growth defects or cases of second malignancy were attributable to CIRT.

Ciernik et al. reported the MGH experience using protons for incompletely resected or unresectable osteosarcoma [66]. A retrospective review identified 55 patients treated between 1983 and 2009 with a median age of 29 (range 2–76) years. Tumors were primarily located in the skull ($n = 22$), mobile spine ($n = 17$), or pelvis and sacrum ($n = 13$). Treatment was delivered without surgery ($n = 12$), after partial resection ($n = 19$), or after gross total resection with positive margins ($n = 24$). Prescription doses were between 60 and 70 GyE for 22 patients and at least 70 GyE for 28 patients; only 3 patients were treated to a dose less than 60 GyE. LC at 3 and 5 years were 82% and 72%, respectively. No local recurrences were observed in the 12 patients treated for grade 1 disease. There was a trend toward increased risk for local failure in patients treated for skull tumors compared to other anatomic sites. The benefit of combining surgery and radiation on LC was apparent with radiation doses less than 70 GyE, but this benefit of surgery could not be appreciated for patients treated with over 70 GyE. OS was 67% at 5 years. Grade 3 or 4 toxicities were observed in 17 patients, including 6 patients with loss of vision and 2 patients with severely impaired gait.

25.4.5 Ongoing Clinical Trials

Several notable clinical trials are ongoing in the United States, Europe, and Japan. Building on the MGH experience using proton beam for preoperative treatment for RPS, a phase I–II trial is using either intensity modulated PBT or photon IMRT to boost the high-risk retroperitoneal margin with a simultaneously integrated boost technique (NCT01659203). The trial is now in phase II with the primary outcome being LC rate after protocol therapy and surgery. The trial is open to recruit 80 patients at several centers in the United States.

The center in Heidelberg, Germany, also is exploring the use of particle therapy in the neoadjuvant treatment of RPS (NCT04219202). A phase II study is randomizing patients 1:1 to either PBT or CIRT with both arms receiving an accelerated, hypofractionation course of 39 GyE in 13 fractions with 6 fractions delivered per week. The primary objective is safety with oncologic outcomes and quality of life as secondary end points.

The ETOILE trial is a transnational European study based in France comparing CIRT with either PBRT or photon therapy for radioresistant tumors (NCT02838602). Patients with sarcoma at any site (except base of skull chondrosarcoma), chordoma (except base of skull site), and adenoid cystic carcinoma are eligible if no surgery or chemotherapy is planned during the clinical trial period. If the patients are randomized to the experimental arm, they will be treated at one of the European carbon ion facilities. If they are randomized to PBT or photons, they will be treated at the nearest participating facility in France. The accrual goal is 250 patients with a primary end point to detect a 20% difference in 5-year progression-free survival.

Loma Linda University is conducting a single institution phase II trial of proton therapy in the neoadjuvant treatment of extremity and body wall STS (NCT01819831). The dose is a standard preoperative regimen of 50.4 GyE in 28 fractions followed by surgery with a planned accrual of 51 patients. The primary end point is late toxicities 2 years after treatment including grade >2 lymphedema, subcutaneous fibrosis, and joint stiffness.

Two additional trials in Japan are studying CIRT for unresectable sarcoma. The HIMAT1341 protocol is a phase II trial through the SAGA HIMAT foundation (UMIN000012373). The primary objective is 2-year LC rate with secondary end points including OS, progression-free survival, and toxicities. The second trial is running in parallel at Gunma University Heavy-ion Medical Center with a similar patient population and end points (UMIN000009720).

Tips and Advice

Site	Sim technique	Contouring	Treatment planning considerations
Head and Neck	Head/shoulders mask IV contrast Proton compatible headframe	CTV = Tumor or postop bed + 1.5–2.0 cm	More often postop treatment Typically two fields but may benefit from IFSO technique if larger target volume [67]
Retroperitoneal	Supine Arms up 4D CT IV contrast No oral contrast	Per consensus guidelines [48] iGTV based on GTV + motion CTV = iGTV + 1.5 cm edited at interfaces	Lateral and posterior beams Avoid single beam design to spread out protons ranging out into bowel Interfraction variability in bowel filling requires caution with anterior beams
Extremity	Neutral position favored for stability but variable based on tumor location Consider using mask for hand or foot to improve reproducibility of positioning	Per consensus guidelines [68] 3 cm longitudinal and 1.5 cm radial for preoperative treatment of high-grade lesions	Two beams preferred over single beam to limit skin dose Angles vary based on tumor location and limb position Avoiding dose to the circumferential limb typically easier with particle beam than photons
Spine	Supine Arms at side body mask MRI in treatment position and/or CT myelogram	GTV + 1–1.5 cm for extraosseous tumor extension and grossly involved vertebral body plus 1 above and below [37] Postop boost to preop GTV Postop final boost to gross residual disease, if any Contour cord-surface and cord-core	2–3 posterior oblique beams arranged either superior/inferior or right/left laterals Max of 1 beam with end of range into cord Cord dose constraints D2% of 54 GyE for core and 64 GyE for surface [69]

References

1 Fletcher C.D.M., Bridge J.A., Hogendoorn P.C.W.,Mertens F., eds. (2013). *WHO Classification of Tumors of Tissue and Bone.* 4th ed. Lyon: IARC Press.

2 Siegel, R.L., Miller, K.D., and Jemal, A. (2020). Cancer statistics. *CA: A Cancer Journal for Clinicians* 70 (1): 7–30.

3 Yang, J.C., Chang, A.E., Baker, A.R., Sindelar, W.F., Danforth, D.N., Topalian, S.L. et al. (1998). Randomized prospective study of the benefit of adjuvant radiation therapy in the

treatment of soft tissue sarcomas of the extremity. *Journal of Clinical Oncology* 16 (1): 197–203.

4 O'Sullivan, B., Davis, A.M., Turcotte, R., Bell, R., Catton, C., Chabot, P. et al. (2002). Preoperative versus postoperative radiotherapy in soft-tissue sarcoma of the limbs: A randomised trial. *Lancet* 359 (9325): 2235–2241.

5 Dufresne, A., Brahmi, M., Karanian, M., and Blay, J.Y. (2018). Using biology to guide the treatment of sarcomas and aggressive connective-tissue tumours. *Nature Reviews. Clinical Oncology* 15 (7): 443–458.

6 Steele, C.D. and Pillay, N. (2020). The genomics of undifferentiated sarcoma of soft tissue: Progress, challenges and opportunities. *Seminars in Cancer Biology* 61: 42–55.

7 Cancer Genome Atlas Research Network. (2017). Electronic address edsc, Cancer Genome Atlas Research N. Comprehensive and Integrated Genomic Characterization of Adult Soft Tissue Sarcomas. *Cell* 171 (4): 950–965. e28.

8 Rickel, K., Fang, F., and Tao, J. (2017). Molecular genetics of osteosarcoma. *Bone* 102: 69–79.

9 Willett, C.G., Schiller, A.L., Suit, H.D., Mankin, H.J., and Rosenberg, A. (1987). The histologic response of soft tissue sarcoma to radiation therapy. *Cancer* 60 (7): 1500–1504.

10 Hew, L., Kandel, R., Davis, A., O'Sullivan, B., Catton, C., and Bell, R. (1994). Histological necrosis in soft tissue sarcoma following preoperative irradiation. *Journal of Surgical Oncology* 57 (2): 111–114.

11 Gilbert, H.A., Kagan, A.R., and Winkley, J. (1975). Soft tissue sarcomas of the extremities: Their natural history, treatment, and radiation sensitivity. *Journal of Surgical Oncology* 7 (4): 303–317.

12 Tepper, J.E. and Suit, H.D. (1985). Radiation therapy alone for sarcoma of soft tissue. *Cancer* 56 (3): 475–479.

13 Rhomberg, W. (2006). The radiation response of sarcomas by histologic subtypes: A review with special emphasis given to results achieved with razoxane. *Sarcoma* 2006 (1): 87367.

14 Pitson, G., Robinson, P., Wilke, D., Kandel, R.A., White, L., Griffin, A.M. et al. (2004). Radiation response: An additional unique signature of myxoid liposarcoma. *International Journal of Radiation Oncology, Biology, Physics* 60 (2): 522–526.

15 Koike, S., Ando, K., Oohira, C., Fukawa, T., Lee, R., Takai, N. et al. (2002). Relative biological effectiveness of 290 MeV/u carbon ions for the growth delay of a radioresistant murine fibrosarcoma. *Journal of Radiation Research* 43 (3): 247–255.

16 Brownstein, J.M., Wisdom, A.J., Castle, K.D., Mowery, Y.M., Guida, P., Lee, C.L. et al. (2018). Characterizing the potency and impact of carbon ion therapy in a primary mouse model of soft tissue Sarcoma. *Molecular Cancer Therapeutics* 17 (4): 858–868.

17 Reimers, M., Castro, J.R., Linstadt, D., Collier, J.M., Henderson, S., Hannigan, J. et al. (1986). Heavy charged particle therapy of bone and soft tissue sarcoma. A Phase I-II Trial of the University of California Lawrence Berkeley Laboratory and the Northern California Oncology Group. *American Journal of Clinical Oncology* 9 (6): 488–493.

18 Greiner, R.H., Blattmann, H.J., Thum, P., Coray, A., Crawford, J.F., Kann, R.H. et al. (1989). Dynamic pion irradiation of unresectable soft tissue sarcomas. *International Journal of Radiation Oncology, Biology, Physics* 17 (5): 1077–1083.

19 Schmitt, G., Mills, E.E., Levin, V., Pape, H., Smit, B.J., and Zamboglou, N. (1989). The role of neutrons in the treatment of soft tissue sarcomas. *Cancer* 64 (10): 2064–2068.

20 Schwartz, D.L., Einck, J., Bellon, J., and Laramore, G.E. (2001). Fast neutron radiotherapy for soft tissue and cartilaginous sarcomas at high risk for local recurrence. *International Journal of Radiation Oncology, Biology, Physics* 50 (2): 449–456.

21 Laramore, G.E., Griffith, J.T., Boespflug, M., Pelton, J.G., Griffin, T., Griffin, B.R. et al. (1989). Fast neutron radiotherapy for sarcomas of soft tissue, bone, and cartilage. *American Journal of Clinical Oncology* 12 (4): 320–326.

22 Schonekaes, K.G., Prott, F.J., Micke, O., Willich, N., and Wagner, W. (1999). Radiotherapy on adult patients with soft tissue sarcoma with fast neutrons or photons. *Anticancer Research* 19 (3B): 2355–2359.

23 Kamada, T., Tsujii, H., Tsuji, H., Yanagi, T., Mizoe, J.E., Miyamoto, T. et al. (2002). Efficacy and safety of carbon ion radiotherapy in bone and soft tissue sarcomas. *Journal of Clinical Oncology* 20 (22): 4466–4471.

24 Imai, R., Kamada, T., and Araki, N. (2018). Working Group for Carbon Ion Radiotherapy for B, Soft Tissue S. Carbon ion radiotherapy for unresectable localized axial soft tissue sarcoma. *Cancer Medicine* 7 (9): 4308–4314.

25 Jensen, A.D., Uhl, M., Chaudhri, N., Herfarth, K.K., Debus, J., and Roeder, F. (2015). Carbon Ion irradiation in the treatment of grossly incomplete or unresectable malignant peripheral nerve sheaths tumors: Acute toxicity and preliminary outcome. *Radiation Oncology* 10: 109.

26 Demizu, Y., Jin, D., Sulaiman, N.S., Nagano, F., Terashima, K., Tokumaru, S. et al. (2017). Particle therapy using protons or carbon ions for unresectable or incompletely resected bone and soft tissue sarcomas of the pelvis. *International Journal of Radiation Oncology, Biology, Physics* 98 (2): 367–374.

27 Yanagi, T., Kamada, T., Tsuji, H., Imai, R., Serizawa, I., and Tsujii, H. (2010). Dose-volume histogram and dose-surface histogram analysis for skin reactions to carbon ion radiotherapy for bone and soft tissue sarcoma. *Radiotherapy and Oncology* 95 (1): 60–65.

28 Kepka, L., DeLaney, T.F., Suit, H.D., and Goldberg, S.I. (2005). Results of radiation therapy for unresected soft-tissue sarcomas. *International Journal of Radiation Oncology, Biology, Physics* 63 (3): 852–859.

29 Weber, D.C., Rutz, H.P., Bolsi, A., Pedroni, E., Coray, A., Jermann, M. et al. (2007). Spot scanning proton therapy in the curative treatment of adult patients with sarcoma: The Paul Scherrer institute experience. *International Journal of Radiation Oncology, Biology, Physics* 69 (3): 865–871.

30 Fukumoto, T., Komatsu, S., Hori, Y., Murakami, M., Hishikawa, Y., and Ku, Y. (2010). Particle beam radiotherapy with a surgical spacer placement for advanced abdominal leiomyosarcoma results in a significant clinical benefit. *Journal of Surgical Oncology* 101 (1): 97–99.

31 Akasaka, H., Sasaki, R., Miyawaki, D., Mukumoto, N., Sulaiman, N.S., Nagata, M. et al. (2014). Preclinical evaluation of bioabsorbable polyglycolic acid spacer for particle therapy. *International Journal of Radiation Oncology, Biology, Physics* 90 (5): 1177–1185.

32 Sasaki, R., Demizu, Y., Yamashita, T., Komatsu, S., Akasaka, H., Miyawaki, D. et al. (2019). First-In-Human Phase 1 Study of a Nonwoven Fabric Bioabsorbable Spacer for Particle Therapy: Space-Making Particle Therapy (SMPT). *Advances in Radiation Oncology* 4 (4): 729–737.

33 Chan, D.K.H., Cheo, T., and Cheong, W.K. (2019). Successful use of tissue expander and pelvic sling to exclude small bowel for high-dose pelvic irradiation. *International Journal of Colorectal Disease* 34 (6): 1043–1046.

34 Nowakowski, V.A., Castro, J.R., Petti, P.L., Collier, J.M., Daftari, I., Ahn, D. et al. (1992). Charged particle radiotherapy of paraspinal tumors. *International Journal of Radiation Oncology, Biology, Physics* 22 (2): 295–303.

35 Matsumoto, K., Imai, R., Kamada, T., Maruyama, K., Tsuji, H., Tsujii, H. et al. (2013). Impact of carbon ion radiotherapy for primary spinal sarcoma. *Cancer* 119 (19): 3496–3503.

36 Hug, E.B., Fitzek, M.M., Liebsch, N.J., and Munzenrider, J.E. (1995). Locally challenging osteo- and chondrogenic tumors of the axial skeleton: Results of combined proton and photon radiation therapy using three-dimensional treatment planning. *International Journal of Radiation Oncology, Biology, Physics* 31 (3): 467–476.

37 DeLaney, T.F., Liebsch, N.J., Pedlow, F.X., Adams, J., Dean, S., Yeap, B.Y. et al. (2009). Phase II study of high-dose photon/proton radiotherapy in the management of spine sarcomas. *International Journal of Radiation Oncology, Biology, Physics* 74 (3): 732–739.

38 DeLaney, T.F., Liebsch, N.J., Pedlow, F.X., Adams, J., Weyman, E.A., Yeap, B.Y. et al. (2014). Long-term results of Phase II study of high dose photon/proton radiotherapy in the management of spine chordomas, chondrosarcomas, and other sarcomas. *Journal of Surgical Oncology* 110 (2): 115–122.

39 Weber, D.C., Trofimov, A.V., Delaney, T.F., and Bortfeld, T. (2004). A treatment planning comparison of intensity modulated photon and proton therapy for paraspinal sarcomas. *International Journal of Radiation Oncology, Biology, Physics* 58 (5): 1596–1606.

40 Greiner, R.H., Munkel, G., Blattmann, H., Coray, A., Kann, R., Pedroni, E. et al. (1992). Conformal radiotherapy for unresectable retroperitoneal soft tissue sarcoma. *International Journal of Radiation Oncology, Biology, Physics* 22 (2): 333–341.

41 Serizawa, I., Kagei, K., Kamada, T., Imai, R., Sugahara, S., Okada, T. et al. (2009). Carbon ion radiotherapy for unresectable retroperitoneal sarcomas. *International Journal of Radiation Oncology, Biology, Physics* 75 (4): 1105–1110.

42 Swanson, E.L., Indelicato, D.J., Louis, D., Flampouri, S., Li, Z., Morris, C.G. et al. (2012). Comparison of three-dimensional (3D) conformal proton radiotherapy (RT), 3D conformal photon RT, and intensity-modulated RT for retroperitoneal and intra-abdominal sarcomas. *International Journal of Radiation Oncology, Biology, Physics* 83 (5): 1549–1557.

43 Yoon, S.S., Chen, Y.L., Kirsch, D.G., Maduekwe, U.N., Rosenberg, A.E., Nielsen, G.P. et al. (2010). Proton-beam, intensity-modulated, and/or intraoperative electron radiation therapy combined with aggressive anterior surgical resection for retroperitoneal sarcomas. *Annals of Surgical Oncology* 17 (6): 1515–1529.

44 DeLaney, T.F., Chen, Y.L., Baldini, E.H., Wang, D., Adams, J., Hickey, S.B. et al. (2017). Phase 1 trial of preoperative image guided intensity modulated proton radiation therapy with simultaneously integrated boost to the high risk margin for retroperitoneal sarcomas. *Advances in Radiation Oncology* 2 (1): 85–93.

45 Petersen, I.A., Haddock, M.G., Donohue, J.H., Nagorney, D.M., Grill, J.P., Sargent, D.J. et al. (2002). Use of intraoperative electron beam radiotherapy in the management of retroperitoneal soft tissue sarcomas. *International Journal of Radiation Oncology, Biology, Physics* 52 (2): 469–475.

46 Stucky, C.C., Wasif, N., Ashman, J.B., Pockaj, B.A., Gunderson, L.L., and Gray, R.J. (2014). Excellent local control with preoperative radiation therapy, surgical resection, and intra-operative electron radiation therapy for retroperitoneal sarcoma. *Journal of Surgical Oncology* 109 (8): 798–803.

47 Bonvalot, S., Gronchi, A., Le Pechoux, C., Swallow, C.J., Strauss, D.C., Meeus, P. et al. (2019). STRASS (EORTC 62092): A phase III randomized study of preoperative radiotherapy plus surgery versus surgery alone for patients with retroperitoneal sarcoma. *Journal of Clinical Oncology* 37, no. 15_suppl (May 20, 2019) 11001–11001. DOI: 10.1200/JCO.2019.37.15_suppl.11001

48 Baldini, E.H., Wang, D., Haas, R.L., Catton, C.N., Indelicato, D.J., Kirsch, D.G. et al. (2015). Treatment guidelines for preoperative radiation therapy for retroperitoneal Sarcoma: Preliminary consensus of an international expert panel.

International Journal of Radiation Oncology, Biology, Physics 92 (3): 602–612.

49 Dawson, L.A., Kavanagh, B.D., Paulino, A.C., Das, S.K., Miften, M., Li, X.A. et al. (2010). Radiation-associated kidney injury. *International Journal of Radiation Oncology, Biology, Physics* 76 (3 Suppl): S108–S115.

50 Sugahara, S., Kamada, T., Imai, R., Tsuji, H., Kameda, N., Okada, T. et al. (2012). Carbon ion radiotherapy for localized primary sarcoma of the extremities: Results of a phase I/II trial. *Radiotherapy and Oncology* 105 (2): 226–231.

51 Fogliata, A., Scorsetti, M., Navarria, P., Catalano, M., Clivio, A., Cozzi, L. et al. (2013). Dosimetric comparison between VMAT with different dose calculation algorithms and protons for soft-tissue sarcoma radiotherapy. *Acta Oncology* 52 (3): 545–552.

52 Remick, J., Regine, W., Malyapa, R., Ng, V., Vyfhuis, M., Diwanji, T. et al. (2017). Excellent pathologic response and atypical clinical course of high-grade extremity Sarcoma to Neoadjuvant pencil beam scanning proton therapy. *Cureus* 9 (9): e1687.

53 Datta, N.R., Puric, E., Schneider, R., Weber, D.C., Rogers, S., and Bodis, S. (2014). Could hyperthermia with proton therapy mimic carbon ion therapy? Exploring a thermo-radiobiological rationale. *International Journal of Hyperthermia* 30 (7): 524–530.

54 Datta, N.R., Schneider, R., Puric, E., Ahlhelm, F.J., Marder, D., Bodis, S. et al. (2016). Proton Irradiation with Hyperthermia in Unresectable Soft Tissue Sarcoma. *International Journal of Particle Theory* 3 (2): 327–336.

55 Iizumi, T., Shimizu, S., Numajiri, H., Takei, H., Yamada, N., Mizumoto, M. et al. (2019). Large malignant fibrous histiocytoma treated with hypofractionated proton beam therapy and local Hyperthermia. *International Journal of Particle Theory* 6 (1): 35–41.

56 Mizoe, J.E., Hasegawa, A., Jingu, K., Takagi, R., Bessyo, H., Morikawa, T. et al. (2012). Results of carbon ion radiotherapy for head and neck cancer. *Radiotherapy and Oncology* 103 (1): 32–37.

57 Jingu, K., Tsujii, H., Mizoe, J.E., Hasegawa, A., Bessho, H., Takagi, R. et al. (2012). Carbon ion radiation therapy improves the prognosis of unresectable adult bone and soft-tissue sarcoma of the head and neck. *International Journal of Radiation Oncology, Biology, Physics* 82 (5): 2125–2131.

58 Yang, J., Gao, J., Qiu, X., Hu, J., Hu, W., Wu, X. et al. (2019). Intensity-modulated proton and carbon-ion radiation therapy in the management of head and neck sarcomas. *Cancer Medicine* 8 (10): 4574–4586.

59 Randhawa, J.S., Budd, G.T., Randhawa, M., Ahluwalia, M., Jia, X., Daw, H. et al. (2016). Primary Cardiac Sarcoma: 25-year Cleveland Clinic experience. *American Journal of Clinical Oncology* 39 (6): 593–599.

60 Aoka, Y., Kamada, T., Kawana, M., Yamada, Y., Nishikawa, T., Kasanuki, H. et al. (2004). Primary cardiac angiosarcoma treated with carbon-ion radiotherapy. *The Lancet Oncology* 5 (10): 636–638.

61 Abe, D., Sato, A., Takeyasu, N., Tokunaga, C., Akishima, S., Iijima, T. et al. (2014). Life-threatening acute heart failure due to primary cardiac undifferentiated pleomorphic sarcoma. *Internal Medicine* 53 (16): 1775–1777.

62 Guttmann, D.M., Frick, M.A., Carmona, R., Deville, C., Jr., Levin, W.P., Berman, A.T. et al. (2017). A prospective study of proton reirradiation for recurrent and secondary soft tissue sarcoma. *Radiotherapy and Oncology* 124 (2): 271–276.

63 Uhl, V., Castro, J.R., Knopf, K., Phillips, T.L., Collier, J.M., Petti, P.L. et al. (1992). Preliminary results in heavy charged particle irradiation of bone sarcoma. *International Journal of Radiation Oncology, Biology, Physics* 24 (4): 755–759.

64 Matsunobu, A., Imai, R., Kamada, T., Imaizumi, T., Tsuji, H., Tsujii, H. et al. (2012). Impact of carbon ion radiotherapy for unresectable osteosarcoma of the trunk. *Cancer* 118 (18): 4555–4563.

65 Mohamad, O., Imai, R., Kamada, T., Nitta, Y., Araki, N. Working Group for B. et al. (2018). Carbon ion radiotherapy for inoperable pediatric osteosarcoma. *Oncotarget* 9 (33): 22976–22985.

66 Ciernik, I.F., Niemierko, A., Harmon, D.C., Kobayashi, W., Chen, Y.L., Yock, T.I. et al. (2011). Proton-based radiotherapy for unresectable or incompletely resected osteosarcoma. *Cancer* 117 (19): 4522–4530.

67 Anand, A., Bues, M., Gamez, M.E., Stefan, C., and Patel, S.H. (2019). Individual Field Simultaneous Optimization (IFSO) in spot scanning proton therapy of head and neck cancers. *Medical Dosimetry* 44 (4): 375–378.

68 Wang, D., Bosch, W., Roberge, D., Finkelstein, S.E., Petersen, I., Haddock, M. et al. (2011). RTOG sarcoma radiation oncologists reach consensus on gross tumor volume and clinical target volume on computed tomographic images for preoperative radiotherapy of primary soft tissue sarcoma of extremity in Radiation Therapy Oncology Group studies. *International Journal of Radiation Oncology, Biology, Physics* 81 (4): e525–e528.

69 Stieb, S., Snider, J.W., 3rd, Placidi, L., Kliebsch, U., Lomax, A.J., Schneider, R.A. et al. (2018). Long-term clinical safety of high-dose proton radiation therapy delivered with pencil beam scanning technique for extracranial chordomas and chondrosarcomas in adult patients: clinical evidence of spinal cord tolerance. *International Journal of Radiation Oncology, Biology, Physics* 100 (1): 218–225.

26

Pediatric Central Nervous System Tumors

Danielle A. Cunningham and Anita Mahajan

Department of Radiation Oncology, Mayo Clinic 200 1ˢᵗ St. SW Rochester, MN, 55905
cunningham.daniell@mayo.edu; mahajan.anita@mayo.edu

TABLE OF CONTENTS

26.1   Introduction

Over 890 pediatric central nervous system tumors are treated with particle therapy internationally each year (Journy et al., 2019). The goal of particle therapy for pediatric central nervous system tumors is to spare adjacent critical structures including hypothalamus, optic apparatus, hippocampus, and uninvolved brain in order to avoid neurocognitive sequelae, hearing loss, neuroendocrine abnormalities, vascular disease, and secondary malignancy. Particle therapy also provides a mechanism to control radiation dose to adjacent nontarget structures such as the vertebral bodies in children requiring craniospinal irradiation (CSI). Additionally, particle therapy has been shown to reduce the incidence of secondary malignancies by reducing the integral dose delivered to the patient.

26.2   Considerations for Specific Tumor Types

26.2.1   Medulloblastoma

Approximately 400 cases of medulloblastoma are diagnosed each year in the United States. Standard-risk medulloblastoma includes children 3 years of age and older with less than 1.5 cm² residual tumor and M0 disease. High-risk medulloblastoma includes children with larger volume residual tumor and M+ disease. Patients with medulloblastoma are treated with maximal safe resection, as presence of more than 1.5 cm² residual tumor is associated with worse survival outcomes (Zeltzer et al., 1999). Following surgery, 8–25% of patients experience posterior fossa syndrome, seen as transient mutism, ataxia, hypotonia, swallowing dysfunction, and irritability with onset 1–2 days postoperatively (Doxey et al., 1999). Posterior fossa syndrome should not delay the start of radiation.

All patients, 3 years of age or older with medulloblastoma, should receive CSI, 23.4 Gy for standard risk and 36–39.6 Gy for high-risk disease, followed by boost(s) to a dose of 54 Gy. While historically the boost targeted the entire posterior fossa, we now advocate for a conformal boost to the tumor bed and residual disease with a 1–1.5-cm clinical target volume (CTV) expansion based on ACNS0331 (Michalski et al., 2016). Spinal metastases are treated with a 45-Gy boost if above the conus medullaris and 50.4 Gy if below. Diffuse gross disease of the spinal cord can be treated with a 39.6-Gy boost.

Proton therapy has been shown to reduce long-term cardiac, pulmonary, and gastrointestinal toxicities for medulloblastoma patients by 25–50% relative to photon treatment. In a study of 59 patients enrolled on a phase 2 trial, no cardiac, pulmonary, or gastrointestinal late effects were described after proton CSI (Yock et al., 2016).

The role of chemotherapy in medulloblastoma is to allow for reduced radiation dose in standard risk children and to improve overall survival in high risk children. For some very young patients, chemotherapy can serve as a bridge between surgery and radiation to delay the onset of CSI. Currently, weekly vincristine during radiotherapy is included in many regimens. Otherwise, all children receive 6–8 cycles of maintenance chemotherapy after completion of radiation. The specific chemotherapy agents vary but generally include a combination of the following: cyclophosphamide, cisplatinum, vincristine, lomustine, or carboplatin.

The future of medulloblastoma lies in molecular guided therapy, with current protocols investigating deescalation for Wnt-pathway tumors and more intensive treatment for Group 3 and 4 subtypes.

26.2.2 Ependymoma

There are approximately 200 cases of ependymoma per year in the United States, with 40% of patients under the age of three (Merchant, 2009a). Approximately 90% of pediatric ependymomas are intracranial, with the most common location being the ependymal lining of the fourth ventricle (Smyth et al., 2000). Spread beyond the site of the primary tumor occurs in 10–15% of patients at diagnosis but is more common with relapsed disease (Smyth et al., 2000; Dhall et al., 2008). Ependymomas are generally treated with maximal surgical resection followed by radiation to the primary site (van Veelen-vincent et al., 2002; Merchant and Fouladi, 2005). It is critically important to obtain a gross total resection, as extent of resection is the single most important prognostic factor in ependymoma. Historically, chemotherapy was used as a bridge between surgery and radiation for infants with

ependymoma; however, this approach has been abandoned since COG ACNS 0121 confirmed the safety and feasibility of radiotherapy in infants as young as 18 months immediately after surgery. Now two cycles of chemotherapy are considered after a subtotal resection to facilitate an attempt at a complete resection prior to adjuvant radiotherapy. Otherwise, adjuvant chemotherapy is being evaluated for anaplastic ependymoma in a prospective randomized trial (ACNS 0831).

Local control following gross total resection followed by adjuvant proton therapy is 75–80%, which is similar to outcomes after adjuvant photon therapy (MacDonald et al., 2008; Merchant, 2009a and 2009b). We typically treat patients with 54 Gy, though 52.2 Gy is now allowed on COG protocols due to concerns of brainstem injury. The standard tumor bed CTV expansion is 1 cm; however, ACNS0831 is investigating a 5-mm CTV to 54 Gy without a CTV expansion on the 59.4-Gy volume (Chan et al., 2012). As most ependymomas occur in the fourth ventricle, and tend to extend to the cerebellopontine angle through the foramina of Luschka or Magendie, the tumor is often in close proximity to the brainstem, cranial nerves, cochlea, and temporal lobes. Proton therapy offers superior sparing of the optic chiasm, cochlea, hypothalamus, pituitary gland, and pharynx relative to intensity-modulated radiation therapy (IMRT) (MacDonald et al., 2008).

26.2.3 Low-grade Glioma

Twenty-five percent of primary brain tumors in patients 0–19 years old are low-grade gliomas, and 17% of all pediatric CNS tumors are pilocytic astrocytomas (Ostrom et al., 2013). Maximal safe resection is a critical component of glioma management, with extent of resection being the most important factor in progression-free survival (Youland et al., 2013). While adjuvant radiation demonstrates a local control benefit in pediatric low-grade glioma, utilization is decreasing due to desire to avoid long-term toxicity. Ongoing protocols aim to identify if hippocampal sparing results in improvements in neurocognitive outcomes in these patients over time. Systemic therapy is increasingly playing a role in pediatric low-grade glioma, particularly in children 10 years old and younger to avoid immediate adjuvant radiotherapy.

Radiation in low-grade glioma is typically used for residual disease, progression, or recurrence. For Grade 1 tumors, we utilize a 5-mm CTV expansion on the resection cavity and residual disease, while we utilize a 1–1.5cm expansion for Grade 2 tumors. We prescribe 50.4–54 Gy at 1.8 Gy per fraction. Particle therapy is extremely relevant for patients with pediatric low-grade glioma as survival is measured in decades. Pediatric patients treated with proton therapy to the brain experience stable IQ, while patients treated with photon treatment experienced a 1.57-point annual IQ decline, based on a study of 54 patients (Kahalley et al., 2016). Patients age 5 or younger at the time of radiation experience worse neurocognitive outcomes, making the reduced brain integral dose seen with particle therapy even more important.

26.2.4 High-grade Glioma

High-grade gliomas represent 7–11% of pediatric brain tumors, with the most common being anaplastic astrocytoma and glioblastoma (Ostrom et al., 2013). Maximal safe resection is an important mainstay of treatment, and greater extent of resection is associated with significant improvements in progression-free survival. Systemic therapy such as temozolomide is routinely used for patients with high-grade glioma during and after radiation, though the data to support the use of temozolomide for pediatric high-grade glioma are not as strong as it is for adults with high-grade glioma. Particle therapy can be considered for select Grade 3 tumors, particularly tumors with better prognosis. We typically prescribe 54–60 Gy in 1.8–2 Gy fractions to the tumor bed and residual disease, with a 1.5–2-cm CTV expansion.

26.2.5 Brainstem Glioma

Brainstem gliomas represent approximately 10% of childhood brain tumors, with the most common being H3K27 mutation positive tumors (formerly known as diffuse intrinsic pontine glioma). We do not routinely advocate for proton therapy in children with diffuse midline glioma (H3K27 mutation positive) due to the poor overall prognosis. Those patients with the following better prognosis gliomas that involve the brainstem (focal pontine, dorsal exophytic, cervicomedullary, or tectal plate gliomas) should be classified as low-grade gliomas and could be considered for proton therapy.

26.2.6 Atypical Teratoid Rhabdoid Tumor

Atypical teratoid rhabdoid tumor (ATRT) is a rare, embryonal CNS tumor comprising 1–2% of pediatric brain tumors that tends to affect infants and children under age 3 with a median age of diagnosis at age 1 (Rickert and Paulus, 2001; Lafay-Cousin et al., 2012). ATRT is an aggressive tumor with a historical poor median survival of 6–11 months (Burger et al., 1998; Weiss et al., 1998). A recent COG protocol (ACNS0333), however, has reported 4-year event-free and overall survival rates of 37% and 43%, respectively, with an aggressive trimodality regimen of surgery, high-dose chemotherapy with stem-cell rescue, and radiotherapy for patients older than 6 months (Reddy et al., 2020).

Due to the very young age of patients with ATRT, radiation oncologists are understandably reluctant to use radiation, though particle therapy may offer a more acceptable alternative (Packer et al., 2002; Squire, Chan, and Marcus, 2007) due to the substantial reduction in integral brain dose (De Amorim Bernstein et al., 2013). In historical series, older patients are more likely to have been treated with CSI, and outcomes appear to be superior in these patients.

We treat patients postoperatively with focal irradiation as per the COG protocol; however, if the patient has metastatic disease, then CSI with appropriate boosts would be considered. When less intense chemotherapy protocols are considered, especially in older children, CSI may be warranted even in nonmetastatic situations.

26.2.7 Craniopharyngioma

Craniopharyngioma is the third most common brain tumor in children, with approximately 350 cases per year in the United States, with a peak incidence between ages 5 and 14 years. Histologically, adamantinomatous craniopharyngiomas are more commonly seen in pediatric patients while papillary-squamous histology is more commonly seen in adults (Louis et al., 2016).

While craniopharyngiomas are technically benign, patients tend to have substantial neurocognitive and psychological morbidity after tumor-directed therapies due to the close proximity of the optic pathway, pituitary, hypothalamus, temporal lobes, brainstem, and major intracerebral blood vessels (Bradley et al., 2014). Previously, patients were standardly treated with aggressive surgery with a goal of gross total resection; however, treatment has transitioned to subtotal resection with adjuvant radiation or radiation at the time of recurrence. Patients who receive subtotal resection followed by postoperative radiation therapy appear to have similar control rates to gross total resection, with disease relapse occurring in 0–12% of patients (Bishop et al., 2014). A select subset of tumors, generally small and separate from the hypothalamus and optic pathway, can be treated with surgery alone.

Patients with craniopharyngioma have an estimated 10-year survival of 80–91% (Bishop et al., 2014) and benefit from the normal structure sparing offered by particle therapy. Radiation doses for craniopharyngioma range from 50.4 to 54 Gy delivered at 1.8 Gy per fraction. The gross tumor volume (GTV) is delineated by fusion between the treatment planning CT and the MRI. Both cystic and solid areas are included in the GTV, as tumor cells may be present in cyst walls. Unlike gliomas, craniopharyngiomas are not inherently infiltrative, thus we do not utilize CTV expansions in our practice. Radiation oncologists should carefully review preoperative imaging, the operative report, and communicate with the surgeon to ensure coverage of areas of adhesion or remaining cyst walls noted intraoperatively. Weekly CT or MRI brain verifications are standard during radiation for craniopharyngioma to monitor the cystic component and adapt the treatment plan as needed

(Beltran, Naik, and Merchant, 2010). Cyst volume fluctuation can cause the GTV to change an average 28.5% through the course of treatment (range of –20.7% to 82%) when monitoring with weekly MRIs (Beltran, Naik, and Merchant, 2010). In an analysis of surveillance MR imaging during radiation, 17 patients with craniopharyngioma during proton therapy, significant cyst growth occurred in 6 patients, requiring 4 proton replans to account for cyst enlargement and prevent underdosing the tumor (Winkfield et al., 2009).

26.2.8 Germ-cell Tumor

Approximately 200 germ-cell tumors are diagnosed in the United States each year, with approximately 75% occurring in children and young adults (Ostrom et al., 2017). Germ-cell tumors are classified into two groups: pure germinoma and non-germinomatous germ-cell tumors (NGGCT). Treatment paradigms have developed for each of these tumor groups.

Pure germinomas most commonly arise in suprasellar or pineal regions and are present in both regions 5–10% of the time—known as bifocal germinoma (Jellinger, 1973). Pure germinomas can be treated with radiation alone, or a combination of radiation and chemotherapy (Huh et al., 1996). Localized germinomas can be treated with 21–24 Gy whole ventricle RT, with a tumor bed boost to 45–50 Gy. Patients with disseminated pure germinoma still have excellent prognosis and can be treated with 30 Gy CSI with a 45-Gy boost(s) to gross disease. The goal of induction chemotherapy in germinoma, such as 2–4 cycles of platinum-based chemotherapy, allows for radiation dose reduction, such as 18–21 Gy whole ventricular dose with a tumor bed boost to 30–36 Gy for non-metastatic disease, and 24 Gy CSI with a boost to 36–40 Gy for patient with metastatic disease for patients who have a good response to chemotherapy.

In contrast, radiotherapy alone has yielded poor outcomes, with local control ranging between 20% and 40% for patients with NGGCT. Currently, the standard of care is 6 cycles of alternating carboplatin/etoposide with ifosfomide/etoposide followed by RT with or without surgery (Robertson, DaRosso, and Allen, 1997; Kim et al., 2012). Following, patients with a complete response are treated with 36 Gy CSI with a 54-Gy primary tumor boost. Patients without a complete response can be considered for second look surgery to rule out a growing teratoma. If patients have persistent disease, high-dose chemotherapy with stem-cell rescue has been considered, followed by radiation as noted above.

Patients with CNS germ-cell tumors tend to have an excellent prognosis and are likely to be cured of their disease, making normal tissue sparing a high priority for long-term neurocognitive outcomes and prevention of late effects. Proton therapy in germ-cell tumors offers significant advantage given the large fields to be irradiated with whole ventric-ular radiation or CSI. For example, whole ventricle RT with proton therapy allows for significant sparing of normal, non-targeted brain tissue when compared to IMRT plans. Specifically, doses to whole brain, temporal lobes, and optic nerve, retinal, and lacrimal doses demonstrate significant sparing (MacDonald et al., 2011).

26.2.9 Chordoma

Chordomas are rare tumors with 0.1 case per year per 1,000,000 population, with 5% of chordomas arising in the pediatric population (Rombi, 2013). Approximately 50–66% arise in the sacrococcygeal region while approximately 35% arise in the skull base (Dahlin et al., 1986). Chordomas are generally treated with surgical resection followed by adjuvant high-dose radiation, preferentially with particle therapy. It is currently unclear whether radiation should be delivered immediately after gross total resection for young children, or whether close observation should be pursued. For children with large tumors, we recommend maximal safe debulking for symptom control and optimal radiation planning.

It is critical that pediatric skull-base tumors are managed by a highly specialized team due to age-related anatomic issues. Good communication with the surgical team is necessary for patient management and radiotherapy planning. If possible, hardware placement should be discussed in advance of the surgery. Placement of metal spine stabilization hardware in the beam path can impact the ability to deliver a robust particle therapy plan. Strategic resections to create "space" next to critical structures such as the brainstem and optic chiasm can lead to better dose delivery to the target. Operative findings and review of the postoperative imaging with the skull-base surgery team is valuable to understand what was seen and done at the time of surgery. For example, whether or not dural penetration was noted will impact CTV extension into the brain parenchyma.

We prescribe 70 Gy for small residual disease targets and 75 Gy for large volume disease. In patients who have achieved a gross total resection, high-risk areas can be treated to 66–68 Gy. Particle therapy via carbon or proton treatment is ideal for treatment of chordomas due to their excellent conformality of the high doses needed for these tumors, while substantially reducing integral dose. A study of 17 pediatric patients with skull-base or low-grade chondrosarcoma treated with carbon ion radiotherapy demonstrated that treatment was well tolerated with 94% local control (Combs et al., 2009).

26.3.1 Anesthesia

Approximately two-third of pediatric patients being referred to proton centers are under the age of 10 and approximately 1/2 overall will require anesthesia to tolerate treatment.

Though we do not utilize prespecified age cutoffs to determine whether anesthesia will be used, nearly all children 5 years old and younger will require anesthesia, and others depending on their specific needs. For maximal optimization of the patient experience to avoid sedation, we use child life specialists, play therapy, and portable screens containing videos and games. When anesthesia is needed, we utilize total intravenous anesthesia (TIVA) with propofol without airway manipulation by intubation or laryngeal mask airway, which has led to excellent safety outcomes while enhancing patient comfort (Owusu-Agyemang et al., 2014). It is critical that anesthesiologists have input on the design of proton therapy centers in order to maximize patient safety as particle therapy treatment is generally delivered in a free-standing center. In designing a facility, anesthesia induction, patient setup, and recovery should be thoughtfully considered. In many centers, induction and recovery occur outside of the treatment room, and treatment positioning takes place in the gantry room or in a separate setup room.

26.3.2 Immobilization

Setup rooms can be used to improve efficiency of the process for patients with complex setups such as CSI (Figures 26.1a and 26.1b). This allows the treating gantry to be utilized for other patients while complex setups are maximized, and then patients are transferred via the docking functionality of the robotic couch. Most patients require a thermoplastic mask to immobilize the head and shoulders to reduce setup uncertainty. It is important that immobilization devices are evaluated by a physicist to ensure they will not interfere with treatment planning or delivery. For older children, a bite block is integrated into the mask to improve immobilization. If needed for patient comfort or to allow for anesthesia, holes can be cut out of the mask around the eyes or nose.

26.3.3 Volume Delineation

For most cases, an MRI in treatment position and selected preoperative imaging should be fused to images acquired during CT simulation, with a goal of keeping treatment volumes as small as possible while covering all residual tumor and at-risk tissue, such as the surgical bed. MRI is also helpful in normal tissue delineation, but it is critical that all structures are verified on the CT. Adjacent extracranial structures must be contoured and protected, with special attention to the lacrimal glands, parotids, cochlea, lens, and retina (Figure 26.3).

26.3.4 Image-Guided Radiation Therapy

For children treated with particle therapy, the most common method of image guided radiation is with daily X-rays. In a pediatric population, minimizing radiation exposure from the treatment and treatment-associated imaging is particularly important. We recommend selecting the scan range and imaging technique that minimizes radiation dose as much as pos-

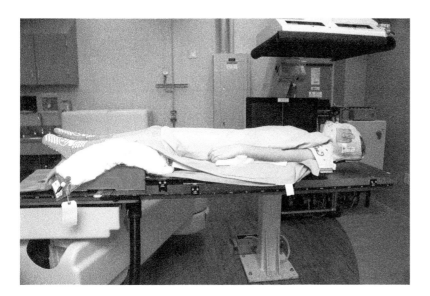

Figure 26.1a and 26.1b Example of our institutional craniospinal irradiation setup. Patients are initially immobilized in our setup rooms (Figure 26.1a) and then transferred into the treatment room (Figure 26.1b) using the docking functionality of our robotic couch. Patients are treated supine in mask with a bite-block to immobilize the head and shoulder, with a lower vacuum mold immobilization device. Child-life specialists assist the patients in decorating their masks and are present for daily treatments to maximize the patient experience. Photos obtained with written permission from the patient and family.

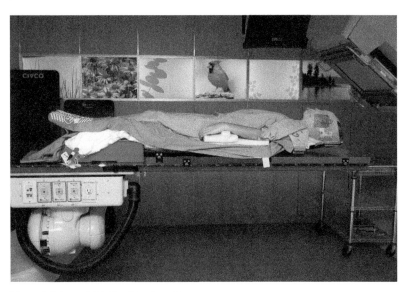

Figure 26.1a and 26.1b (Continued)

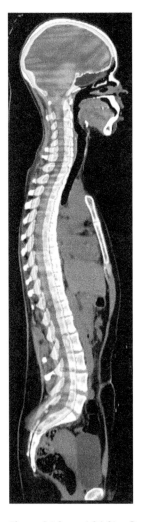

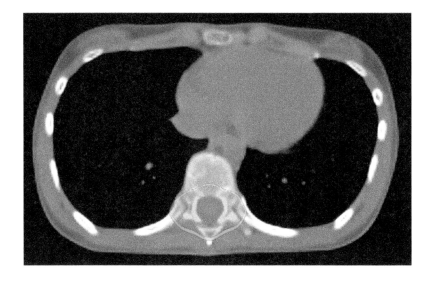

Figure 26.2a and 26.2b   Proton plan of age-adjusted craniospinal irradiation, with sagittal (Figure 26.2a) and axial (Figure 26.2b) views of a 17-year-old female with medulloblastoma, who had attained skeletal maturity by bone age assessment.

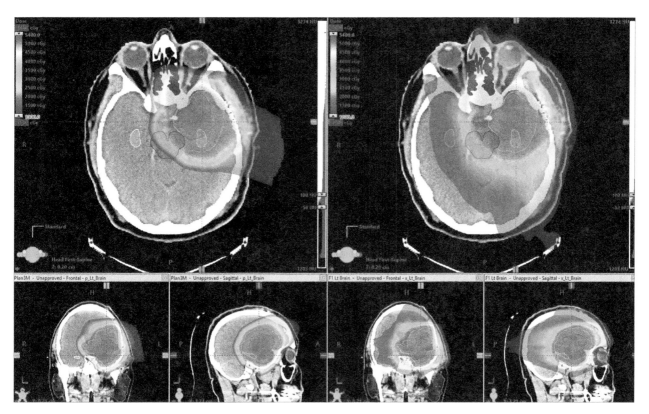

Figure 26.3   Left temporal low-grade glioma, with proton plan (left) demonstrating superior sparing of optic structures, brainstem, and normal brain compared to IMRT plan (right).

sible while maintaining visibility of anatomic structures required for localization. Isocentric cone beam CT scan technology is becoming increasingly available and may be used if available. CT-on-rails is another in-room technology and may be helpful for verification scans due to positioning uncertainty, or to detect changes in tumor or normal tissue. A future direction for image-guided particle therapy for pediatric patients may be MR-guided treatment, as MR imaging does not utilize ionizing radiation.

Surface imaging and tracking can be useful for some sites for particle therapy alignment and verification; however, in general, it is not as helpful for pediatric populations since body contours are less variable than in adult patients.

Monitoring patients with weekly imaging verifications via CT or MRI is more commonly needed with particle therapy compared to photons. Even small changes in tissue thickness can impact the dose to target volumes and organs at risk; careful verification scans allow for close monitoring of radiation dose, with replanning employed as needed.

26.3.5   Craniospinal Irradiation

CSI is recommended for patients where there is a risk or presence of tumor spread in the cerebrospinal fluid or leptome-

ninges. Proton therapy for the cranial target volume has limited advantage over X-ray-based modalities, though there is potential dose reduction to the salivary glands and orbital structures including the lacrimal glands. The greater benefit of proton CSI is the dose reduction afforded by the spinal and boost volumes, including sparing of the heart, lungs, liver, and thyroid (Howell et al., 2012). Future directions that improve target and normal tissue delineation by functional imaging, advanced MRI imaging, or PET imaging may facilitate additional benefits for proton CSI.

Historically, patients were treated with CSI in the prone position to allow for direct visualization of match lines, but we now prefer to treat patients in supine position to improve patient comfort, reduce setup uncertainty, and optimize airway access for anesthesia providers. We utilize a head and shoulders mask. After investigating multiple immobilization devices and setup procedures, including vacuum bag immobilization, and input from physicists and radiation therapists, we find it optimal for patients to lay supine on a 2-cm thick foam pad to decrease skin wrinkling at the couch surface, improve inter and intra-fraction uncertainty, and ease of daily set up.

The spine is treated with PA fields, and the head can be treated with 2–3 fields depending on the technique used. IMPT is able to modulate between fields using pencil beam scanning, with a goal of having smooth interfaces without hot or cold spots at overlapping edges. The specific technique is well described by Stoker et al. (2014) (Figures 26.3 and 26.4).

Young children treated with CSI should have dose to the entire vertebral body to prevent asymmetric growth that can result from radiation stopping mid-vertebral body. For these patients, care should be taken to avoid end of range effect into esophagus and pharynx, as severe mucositis can result. Exit dose to the thyroid gland should be monitored to lower the risk of subsequent malignancies. Patients with skeletal maturity can have a targeted CSI surrounding the spinal canal, while avoiding the majority of the anterior vertebral body to spare bone marrow and reduce the overall irradiated volume. Proton CSI reduces acute toxicities of nausea and vomiting, cytopenias, and medical interventions for esophagitis and weight loss compared to patients treated with photons (Brown et al., 2013). Of note, in our experience, approximately 40% of our patients experience nausea with proton CSI, presumably due to dose to the area postrema in the floor of the fourth ventricle.

26.3.6 Toxicities

As the overall survival for pediatric brain tumors has increased, identification and management of treatment-related side effects have grown in importance. The most worrisome complications of radiation therapy for pediatric brain tumors are necrosis, neuropsychological changes, and secondary brain tumors. Children are also at risk for vasculopathy, endocrinopathies, reduction in vision and hearing, and are monitored accordingly in survivorship.

Radiation necrosis is thought to arise from radiation induced microvascular damage and most often occurs 1–12 months after treatment. The most common presentation is asymptomatic changes on imaging, such as T2 prolongation and parenchymal enhancement on MRI, though some cases can be severely symptomatic or even fatal. Proton therapy may increase the risk of necrosis as a result of the higher radiobiologic equivalent dose, especially at the distal beam edge Bragg peak phenomena. A study of 166 pediatric patients with brain tumors treated with proton therapy demonstrated a 0.7% rate of symptomatic brainstem necrosis with a median follow-up of 19.6 months (Vogel et al., 2019). Symptomatic brainstem necrosis following proton therapy for pediatric CNS tumors is rare, with a 0.7% incidence at 19.6 months, while asymptomatic imaging changes are more common and reported in up to 31% of patients (Kralik et al., 2015; Vogel et al., 2019). Treating tumors of the posterior fossa requires special consideration to reduce the risk of brainstem injury. We recommend review of the paper by Haas-Kogan et al. describing practical considerations to reduce the risk of proton therapy induced brainstem injury (Haas-Kogan et al., 2018).

The developing cerebrovascular system is sensitive to the effects of radiation which can lead to ischemic stroke, Moyamoya, aneurysm, cavernoma, hemorrhage, necrosis, and complex migraines. It appears that radiation may accelerate the aging process of blood vessels, with irradiated vessels displaying smaller arterial lumens, increased thickness of the tunica media, stiffness, and plaque (Vatanen, 2015). Moyamoya translates to "puff of smoke" in Japanese and is seen as collateral blood vessel development as a result of narrowing of large arteries. It can be seen in children with radiation to the circle of Willis, particularly doses over 45 Gy (Morris et al., 2009). Specifically contouring and avoiding dose to vascular structures via particle therapy may reduce the incidence of these complications over time.

Secondary malignancy following treatment for pediatric CNS tumors is estimated to be 4.7–17.4 times higher than the general population (Cardous-Ubbink et al., 2007). This risk is impacted by genetic, tumor, radiation, and chemotherapy-related factors. The most common secondary malignancies after treatment for pediatric CNS tumors are meningiomas and gliomas, with a mean latency time of 15.5 years (Taylor et al., 2010). The most important radiation factors that appear to modulate the risk of secondary malignancy are overall radiation dose, and the volume irradiated including integral dose spillage. Particle therapy has the potential to reduce the incidence of secondary malignancies by reducing the volume of irradiated tissue. A retrospective cohort study with a median follow-up of 6.7 years demonstrated a rate of second malignancy of 5.2% for patients treated with proton therapy compared to 7.5% with photon therapy (hazard ratio 0.52; 95% CI: 0.32–0.85; $p = 0.009$) (Chung et al., 2013). Additionally in a National Cancer Database study of 450,373 patients treated with radiation, proton therapy demonstrated a reduction in secondary malignancies compared to 3D conformal radiation and IMRT (Xiang et al., 2020). Due to a reduction in integral dose with particle therapy, proton therapy is suspected to offer a 2–15-fold decreased rate of secondary malignancy compared to that of photon treatment (Miralbell et al., 2002). In a study of 1,580 patients with prostate cancer treated with carbon radiotherapy, a propensity score-weighted analysis demonstrated a reduction in secondary malignancy for carbon treatment compared to photon therapy (Mohamad et al., 2019). Imaging surveillance is needed after treatment for pediatric CNS tumors, and we favor MRI, as diagnostic scans using ionizing radiation can further increase the risk of secondary malignancy.

Neuropsychological changes are a common morbidity experienced by pediatric brain tumor survivors and impact cognitive, academic, socioemotional, and behavioral domains. These changes are multifactorial and can be impacted by radiation, surgery, chemotherapy, and tumor-related factors. Craniospinal and whole brain radiotherapy carries the greatest risk, and it is known that higher radiation dose carries greater deficits. In patients with medulloblastoma, reduced dose CSI has been associated with less intellectual decline over time (Moxon-Emre et al., 2014). Particle therapy is an important way to reduce the neurocognitive burden of treatment over time. A study by Kahalley et al. of 54 patients treated with proton therapy for brain tumors demonstrated stable IQ, while patients treated with photon treatment experienced an IQ decline of 1.57 points per year (Kahalley et al., 2016). Future directions to reduce the impact of treatment on neurocognition may include molecularly tailored radiation dose and volume reduction, avoidance of functional structures such as the hippocampi, and neuroprotectants such as memantine.

Radiation for pediatric CNS tumors can lead to endocrinopathies, and particle therapy aims to decrease the incidence by decreasing dose to endocrine structures. The two areas at greatest risk are the anterior pituitary and the thyroid gland. As mentioned above, dose to the thyroid gland should be monitored when planning CSI. For all patients, dose to the pituitary gland and hypothalamus should be minimized. Endocrine

dysfunction can impact height, metabolism, pubertal development, and fertility. Patients should be followed closely by an endocrinologist after treatment for early identification and intervention of endocrine abnormalities.

Dose reduction to optic structures at risk via particle therapy aims to preserve visual function. Identification and protection of the lacrimal glands reduce the incidence of dry eye which can improve patient comfort and visual outcomes. Children are monitored with visual acuity and visual field testing prior to treatment and over time.

Patients with pediatric CNS tumors are at high risk for hearing loss, as many children receive platinum containing chemotherapy, and dose to the cochlea. Particle therapy is often able to attain reduced dose to the cochlea for hearing preservation, and we try to keep cochlear doses <30 Gy if possible (Grewal et al., 2010). Children are evaluated by an audiologist prior to radiation and over time. Assistive listening devices, hearing aids, or cochlear implants can be utilized if needed.

References

1 Beltran, C., Naik, M., and Merchant, T.E. (2010). Dosimetric effect of target expansion and setup uncertainty during radiation therapy in pediatric craniopharyngioma. *Radiotherapy and Oncology : Journal of the European Society for Therapeutic Radiology and Oncology* 97: 399–403.

2 Bishop, A.J. et al. (2014). Proton beam therapy versus conformal photon radiation therapy for childhood craniopharyngioma: Multi-institutional analysis of outcomes, cyst dynamics, and toxicity. *International Journal of Radiation Oncology, Biology, Physics* 90(2): 354–361.

3 Bradley, J.A. et al. (2014). Craniopharyngioma and proton therapy. *International Journal of Particle Therapy* 1(2): 386–398.

4 Brown, A.P. et al. (2013). Proton beam craniospinal irradiation reduces acute toxicity for adults with medulloblasoma. *IJROBP* 86(2): 277–284.

5 Burger, P.C. et al. (1998). Atypical teratoid/rhabdoid tumor of the central nervous system: A highly malignant tumor of infancy and childhood frequently mistaken for medulloblastoma: A pediatric oncology group study. *The American Journal of Surgical Pathology* 22(9): 1083–1092.

6 Cardous-Ubbink, M.C. et al. (2007). Risk of second malignancies in long term survivors of childhood cancer. *European Journal of Cancer (Oxford, England : 1990)* 43(2): 351–362.

7 Chan, M.D. et al. (2012). Multidisciplinary management of intracranial ependymoma. *Current Problems in Cancer* 36(1): 6–19.

8 Chung, C.S., Yock, T.I., Nelson, K., Xu, Y., Keating, N.L., and Tarbell, N.J. (2013). Incidence of second malignancies among patients treated with proton versus photon radiation. *International Journal of Radiation Oncology, Biology, Physics* 87: 46–52.

9 Combs, S.E. et al. (2009). Carbon ion radiotherapy for pediatric patients and young adults treated for tumors of the skull base. *Cancer* 115(6): 1348–1355.

10 Dahlin, D.C. et al. (1986). *Bone Tumors: General Aspects and Data on 8542 Cases, Ed 4*. 119–140. Springfield III: Charles C Thomas. P.

11 De Amorim Bernstein, K. et al. (2013). Early clinical outcomes using proton radiation for children with central nervous system atypical teratoid rhabdoid tumors. *International Journal of Radiation Oncology, Biology, Physics* 86(1): 114–120.

12 Dhall, G. et al. (2008). Outcome of children less than three years old at diagnosis with non-metastatic medulloblastoma treated with chemotherapy on the "Head Start" I and II protocols. *Pediatric Blood & Cancer* 50(6): 1169–1175.

13 Doxey, D. et al. (1999). Posterior fossa syndrome: Identifiable risk factors and irreversible complications. *Pediatric Neurosurgery* 31(3): 131–136.

14 Grewal, S. et al. (2010). Auditory late effects of childhood cancer therapy: A report from the children's oncology group. *Pediatrics* 125(4): e938–950.

15 Haas-Kogan, et al. (2018). National cancer institute workshop on proton therapy for children: Considerations regarding brainstem injury. *International Journal of Radiation Oncology, Biology, Physics* 101(1): 152–168.

16 Howell, R.M. et al. (2012). Comparison of therapeutic dosimetric data from passively scattered proton and photon craniospinal irradiations for medulloblastoma. *Radiation Oncology* 7: 116.

17 Huh, S.J. et al. (1996). Radiotherapy of intracranial germinomas. *Radiotherapy and Oncology : Journal of the European Society for Therapeutic Radiology and Oncology* 38(1): 19–23.

18 Jellinger, K. (1973). Primary intracranial germ cell tumours. *Acta Neuropathologica* 25(4): 291–306.

19 Journy, N. et al. (2019, Mar). Patterns of proton therapy use in pediatric cancer management in 2016: An international survey. *Radiotherapy and Oncology : Journal of the European Society for Therapeutic Radiology and Oncology* 132: 155–161.

20 Kahalley, L.S. et al. (2016). Comparing intelligence quotient change after treatment with proton versus photon radiation therapy for pediatric brain tumors. *Journal of Clinical Oncology : Official Journal of the American Society of Clinical Oncology* 34(10): 1043–1049.

21 Kim, J.W. et al. (2012). A multimodal approach including craniospinal irradiation improves the treatment outcome of high-risk intracranial nongerminomatous germ cell tumors. *International Journal of Radiation Oncology, Biology, Physics* 84(3): 625–631.

22 Kralik, S.F. et al. (2015). Radiation Necrosis in pediatric patients with brain tumors treated with proton radiotherapy. *AJNR* 36(8): 1572–1578.

23 Lafay-Cousin, L. et al. (2012). Central nervous system atypical teratoid rhabdoid tumours: The Canadian Paediatric Brain Tumour Consortium experience. *European Journal of Cancer (Oxford, England : 1990)* 48: 353–359.

24 Louis, D. et al. (2016). *WHO Classification of Tumours of the Central Nervous System*, 4th ed. Lyon: IARC.

25 MacDonald, S.M. et al. (2008). Proton radiotherapy for childhood ependymoma: Initial clinical outcomes and dose comparisons. *International Journal of Radiation Oncology, Biology, Physics* 71(4): 979–986.

26 MacDonald, S.M. et al. (2011). Proton radiotherapy for pediatric central nervous system germ cell tumors: Early clinical outcomes. *International Journal of Radiation Oncology, Biology, Physics* 79(1): 121–129.

27 Merchant, T.E. et al. (2009a). Conformal radiotherapy after surgery for paediatric ependymoma: A prospective study. *The Lancet Oncology* 10(3): 258–266.

28 Merchant, T.E. (2009b). Three-dimensional conformal radiation therapy for ependymoma. *Child's Nervous System : ChNS : Official Journal of the International Society for Pediatric Neurosurgery* 25(10): 1261–1268.

29 Merchant, T.E. and Fouladi, M. (2005). Ependymoma: New therapeutic approaches including radiation and chemotherapy. *Journal of Neuro-oncology* 75(3): 287–299.

30 Michalski, J.M. et al. (2016). Results of COG ACNS0331: A Phase III Trial of Involved-Field Radiotherapy (IFRT) and Low Dose Craniospinal Irradiation (LD-CSI) with chemotherapy in average-risk medulloblastoma: A report from the children's oncology group. *International Journal of Radiation Oncology, Biology, Physics* 96: 937–938.

31 Miralbell, R., Lomax, A., Cella, L., and Schneider, U. (2002). Potential reduction of the incidence of radiation-induced second cancers by using proton beams in the treatment of pediatric tumors. *International Journal of Radiation Oncology, Biology, Physics* 54: 824–829.

32 Mohamad, O. et al. (2019). Risk of subsequent primary cancers after carbon ion radiotherapy, photon radiotherapy, or surgery for localized prostate cancer: A propensity score-weighted, retrospective, cohort study. *The Lancet Oncology* 20: 674–685.

33 Morris, B. et al. (2009). Cerebrovascular disease in childhood cancer survivors: A childrens oncology group report. *Neurology* 73(22): 1906–1913.

34 Moxon-Emre, et al. (2014). Impact of craniospinal dose. *Boost Volume, and Neurologic Complications on Intellectual Outcome in Patients with Medulloblastoma. J Clin Oncol* 32(17): 1760–1768.

35 Ostrom, Q.T. et al. (2013). CBTRUS statistical report: Primary brain and central nervous system tumors diagnosed in the United States in 2006-2010. *Neuro-Oncology* 15(2): ii1–i56.

36 Ostrom, Q.T. et al. (2017). CBTRUS statistical report: Primary brain and other central nervous system tumors diagnosed in the United States in 2010-2014. *Neuro-Oncology* 19(suppl_5): v1–v88.

37 Owusu-Agyemang, P. et al. (2014, Apr). Non-invasive anesthesia for children undergoing proton radiation therapy. *Radiotherapy and Oncology: Journal of the European Society for Therapeutic Radiology and Oncology* 111(1): 30–34.

38 Packer, R.J. et al. (2002). Atypical teratoid/rhabdoid tumor of the central nervous system: Report on workshop. *Journal of Pediatric Hematology/oncology* 24(5): 337–342.

39 Reddy, A.T. et al. (2020, Apr 10). Efficacy of high-dose chemotherapy and three-dimensional conformal radiation for atypical teratoid/rhabdoid tumor: A report from the children's oncology group trial ACNS0333. *Journal of Clinical Oncology : Official Journal of the American Society of Clinical Oncology* 38(11): 1175–1185.

40 Rickert, C.H. and Paulus, W. (2001). Epidemiology of central nervous system tumors in childhood and adolescence based on the new WHO classification. *Child's Nervous System : ChNS : Official Journal of the International Society for Pediatric Neurosurgery* 17(9): 503–511.

41 Robertson, P.L., DaRosso, R.C., and Allen, J.C. (1997). Improved prognosis of intracranial non-germinoma germ cell tumors with multimodality therapy. *Journal of Neuro-oncology* 32(1): 71–80.

42 Rombi, B. (2013). Spot Scanning proton radiation therapy for pediatric chordoma and chondrosarcoma: Clinical outcome of 26 patients treated at Paul Scherrer Institute. *IJROBP* 28(3): 578–584.

43 Smyth, M.D. et al. (2000). Intracranial ependymomas of childhood: Current management strategies. *Pediatric Neurosurgery* 33(3): 138–150.

44 Squire, S.E., Chan, M.D., and Marcus, K.J. (2007). Atypical teratoid/rhabdoid tumor: The controversy behind radiation therapy. *Journal of Neuro-oncology* 81(1): 97–111.

45 Stoker, J.B. et al. (2014). Intensity modulated proton therapy for craniospinal irradiation: Organ at risk exposure and a low gradient junctioning technique. *International Journal of Radiation Oncology, Biology, Physics* 90(3): 637–644.

46 Taylor, A.J. et al. (2010). Survival after second primary neoplasms of the brain or spinal cord in survivors of childhood cancer: Results from the British childhood cancer survivor study. *JCO* 27(34): 5781–5787.

47 Van Veelen-vincent, M.L. et al. (2002). Ependymoma in childhood: Prognostic factors, extent of surgery, and adjuvant therapy. *Journal of Neurosurgery* 97(4): 827–835.

48 Vatanen, A., Sarkola, T., Ojala, T.H., Turanlahti, M., Jahnukainen, T., Saarinen-Pihkala, U.M., and Jahnukainen, K. (2015). Radiotherapy-related arterial intima thickening and plaque formation in childhood cancer survivors detected with veryhigh resolution ultrasound during young adulthood. *Pediatric Blood Cancer*, 62: 2000–2006.

https://doi.org/10.1002/pbc.25616 https://onlinelibrary.wiley.com/doi/full/10.1002/pbc.25616.

49 Vogel, J. et al. (2019). Risk of brainstem necrosis in pediatric patients with central nervous system malignancies after pencil beam scanning proton therapy. *Acta Oncologica* 58(12): 1752–1756.

50 Weiss, E. et al. (1998). Treatment of primary malignant rhabdoid tumor of the brain: Report of three cases and review of the literature. *International Journal of Radiation Oncology, Biology, Physics* 41(5): 1013–1019.

51 Winkfield, K.M., Linsenmeier, C., Yock, T.I., Grant, P.E., Yeap, B.Y., Butler, W.E., and Tarbell, N.J. (2009). Surveillance of craniopharyngioma cyst growth in children treated with proton radiotherapy. *International Journal of Radiation Oncology, Biology, Physics* 73: 716–721.

52 Xiang, M. et al. (2020). Second cancer risk after primary cancer treatment with three-dimensional conformal, intensity modulated, or proton beam radiation therapy. *Cancer* 126: 3560–3568.

53 Yock, T.I. et al. (2016). Long-term toxic effects of proton radiotherapy for paediatric medulloblastoma: A phase 2 single-arm study. *The Lancet Oncology* 17(3): 287–298.

54 Youland, R.S. et al. (2013). Prognostic factors and survival patterns in pediatric low grade gliomas over 4 decades. *Journal of Pediatric Hematology/oncology* 35(3): 197–205.

55 Zeltzer, P.M. et al. (1999). Metastasis stage, adjuvant treatment, and residual tumor are prognostic factors for medulloblastoma in children: Conclusions from the children's cancer group 921 randomized phase III study. *Journal of Clinical Oncology : Official Journal of the American Society of Clinical Oncology* 17(3): 832–845.

27

Particle Therapy for Non-CNS Pediatric Malignancies

Fantine Giap MD, Daniel J Indelicato MD, and Raymond Mailhot Vega MD, MPH

Department of Radiation Oncology, University of Florida College of Medicine

Corresponding author: Raymond Mailhot Vega, MD, MPHDepartment of Radiation Oncology, University of Florida College of Medicine2015 N Jefferson St, Jacksonville, FL 32206

TABLE OF CONTENTS

27.1   Ewing Sarcoma

27.1.1   Epidemiology

In the United States, about 1% of all childhood cancers are Ewing tumors with about 200 children and teens diagnosed with Ewing tumors each year [1]. Ewing sarcoma is primarily a disease seen in pediatric patients with a median age of diagnosis of 15 years; however, 30% of all Ewing sarcoma family of tumors (ESFT) are diagnosed in adults above the age of 20. Slightly more males than females develop Ewing tumors.

27.1.2   Clinical Evaluation

Ewing sarcoma is a type of small round blue cell tumor with relatively undifferentiated cells. The 2020 WHO classification system introduced a new system for distinguishing Ewing sarcoma and the three main categories of undifferentiated small round cell tumors by cytogenetics. Ewing sarcoma is characterized by gene fusions involving a gene of the FET family of genes (typically *EWSR1*) and a gene of the ETC family of transcription factors, most commonly *EWSR1-FL11* (85%) and *EWSR1-ERG* (10%) [2–4]. The other three categories include round cell sarcomas with *EWSR1* and non-ETS fusions, sarcomas with *CIC*-rearrangements, and sarcomas with *BCOR* genetic alterations [2–4]. These tumors most often arise in the pelvic and extremities (femur, tibia, fibula, and humerus). The spine, hands, and feet are less often sites of disease.

Clinical presentation is typically characterized by localized pain and/or swelling over a period of a few weeks or months and may be associated with fever, fatigue, weight loss, or anemia. Diagnostic evaluation initially usually includes a radiograph which demonstrates a destructive lesion with poorly defined margins, often with an associated soft tissue mass. MRI is then typically obtained to delineate intra- and extraosseous extent, as well as evaluate the potential involvement of adjacent nerves, vessels, and organs. The MRI should include T1 and T2-weighted sequences and should cover the entire involved bone as well as 4–10 cm on either side of each joint. A CT-guided core needle biopsy of the tumor is then obtained. Labs include a complete blood count, complete metabolic panel, erythrocyte sedimentation rate (ESR), and lactate dehydrogenase (LDH). Additional evaluation for metastatic spread of disease includes CT chest, PET, and often

at least a unilateral bone marrow biopsy. Of note, while bone marrow biopsy has been considered gold standard for detection of bone marrow metastasis in pediatric Ewing sarcoma, a recent systematic review has suggested that bone marrow biopsy/aspirate may be omitted in patients with localized disease after staging imaging, as PET imaging has high sensitivity and specificity for detection of bone marrow metastasis [5].

Poor prognostic factors include age greater than 15 years, pelvic and or axial site of disease, tumor size greater than 8 cm, and poor response to chemotherapy (i.e., greater than 10% viable tumor).

There is no specific staging system for Ewing sarcoma, though there is a TNM staging system that exists for primary tumors of bone and soft tissue advocated by the Musculoskeletal Tumor Society and American Joint Committee on Cancer. In regards to management, Ewing's Family of Tumors (EFST) are often categorized as local and metastatic.

27.1.3   Clinical Management

Treatment paradigm typically follows the standard arm of the Children's Oncology Group (COG) AEWS 1031 protocol, which includes chemotherapy, followed by local therapy, and then chemotherapy. The chemotherapy regimen in North America includes vincristine, adriamycin, cyclophosphamide, ifosfamide, and etoposide every 2 weeks. Typically, induction chemotherapy occurs on weeks 1–12 (6 cycles). Then, during weeks 13 and 14 local therapy options including surgery, concurrent chemoradiation, and surgery followed by postoperative chemoradiation. After local therapy, consolidative chemotherapy is delivered in the remaining 11 cycles over 22 weeks. As noted above, local therapy occurs at approximately week 13. The decision for radiotherapy versus surgery versus a combination of the two relates to the morbidity and feasibility of resection. Obviously, a benefit of surgery alone would be obviating risks of radiotherapy for a pediatric patient. The decision for local therapy is a multidisciplinary one and should be made at a multidisciplinary conference.

In 2012, Rombi et al. reported their initial clinical experience treating Ewing sarcoma with proton therapy (Rombi, 2012) (Table 27.1). All 30 patients were younger than 22 years old (median 10 years) and had tumors in the pelvis, trunk, head and neck region, and base of skull. The median dose was 54 GyRBE, range 45–59.4 GyRBE. For patients with vertebral body tumors (*n* = 14), typically a decompressive laminectomy

Table 27.1 Clinical experiences utilizing particle therapy for Ewing sarcoma.

Publication	Number of patients	Median RT dose GyRBE (range)	Disease site	Outcomes
Rombi et al. [10]	30	54 (45–59.4)	Pelvis, trunk, head and neck, base of skull	3-year EFS 60% 3-year LC 86% 3-year DSS 68% 3year OS 89%
Nakao et al. [7]	15	55.8 (45–55.8)	Pelvis, trunk, head and neck, base of skull	4year EFS 84.8% 4-year OS 94.6%
Kharod et al. [8]	25	50.4 GTR 54 STR 55.8 unresectable	Cranium and skull base	4-year LC 96% 4-year DFS 86% 4-year OS 92%
Uezono et al. [9]	35	As noted above	Pelvis	3-year LC 92% 3-year PFS 64% 3-year OS 83%
Vogel et al. [6]	10	55.8 (55.2–65.6)	Head and neck	1-year FFLR 86% 1-year FFRR 100% 1-year FFDR 86% 1-year OS 83%

was completed followed by proton therapy, with prescribed dose 45–57.6 GyRBE with a limiting dose constraint to the spinal cord of 45 GyRBE. With a median follow-up of 38.4 months, their 3-year actuarial rate of local control was 86% and of overall survival was 89% (Rombi, 2012). Seventeen percent of patients were alive with disease (2 patients with local failure, 1 patient with distant failure, 2 patients with combined local and distant failures). Thirteen percent of patients died (3 of 4 with disease progression); 13% patients developed secondary malignancies (none of which were secondary solid tumors).

In 2018, Vogel et al. reported their clinical experience treating pediatric head and neck malignancies. Ten patients of the 69 had Ewing sarcoma and were treated to a median dose of 55.8 GyRBE with double scatter proton therapy, pencil beam scanning proton therapy, or mixed intensity-modulated radiation therapy/proton beam therapy (IMRT/PBT) [6]. Nine of these 10 patients had stage I Ewing sarcoma and only 2 of the 10 patients underwent resection. These tumors were located in the ethmoid sinus, mandible, mastoid, maxillary sinus, and orbit. There was one reported patient death of the patients with Ewing sarcoma. One-year overall survival was 83% [6].

Also, in 2018, Nakao et al. reported their clinical experience treating Ewing sarcoma with proton therapy, involving patient transfer during chemotherapy to a different institution for radiation treatment [7]. All 15 patients were younger than 21 years old (median 4 years) with disease sites including base of skull, head and neck, trunk, spine, and pelvis. The median dose was 55.8 GyRBE range 45–55.8 GyRBE. The protocol utilized out-

lined 45–50.4 GyRBE for microscopic residual tumor and 54–55.8 GyRBE for gross residual tumor in 1.8 GyRBE daily fractions to the preoperative and pre-chemotherapy disease (10–15 mm margin), with CTV reduction after 41.4–45 GyRBE. At the initiation of proton radiotherapy, 13 of 15 patients had partial response (PR) to induction therapy and 2 patients had complete response. With a median follow-up of 52 months, 66.7% of patients achieved complete response. Four of the 15 patients were alive with disease (1 patient with in-field secondary osteosarcoma, 3 patients with residual tumor without progression). One patient died of combined local and distant recurrence.

The year 2020 saw the publication of two-site specific publications for Ewing sarcoma for patients enrolled on prospective outcome studies from the University of Florida. Kharod et al. reported disease control and toxicity for patients with nonmetastatic Ewing sarcoma of the cranium and skull base [8]. With 25 patients included and median follow-up of 3.7 years, 25 patients were identified. Median patient age was 5.89 years with a range of 1–21.7 years. The authors' volume description was described as follows: CTV1 was defined as the GTV with a 1-cm anatomically constrained margin and encompasses any tissue infiltrated with gross disease at the time of diagnosis. CTV2 was defined as the GTV. The dose prescribed to PTV1 was 45 GyRBE, and the dose prescribed to PTV2 was 50.4 GyRBE for patients who undergo gross total resection, 54 GyRBE for patients who undergo subtotal resection, or 55.8 GyRBE if the tumor was unresectable. The 4-year local control, disease-free survival, and overall survival rates were 96%, 86%, and 92%, respectively. Two patients experienced in-field recurrences, and two experienced distant progression. There were no marginal recurrences.

The second publication by Uezono et al. reported children treated for Ewing sarcoma of the pelvis [9]. Thirty-five patients were included with median age 14 years with nonmetastatic Ewing sarcoma. Most patients received definitive radiation ($n = 26$; median dose 55.8 GyRBE; range, 54.0–64.8), seven received preoperative radiation (50.4 GyRBE), and two received postoperative radiation (45 GyRBE and 54 GyRBE). CTV expansion was completed as in the experience by Kharod above. However, based on intent, doses were prescribed as follows: PTV1 received 45 GyRBE. Patients treated in the preoperative or postoperative setting received 50.4 GyRBE or 54 GyRBE to PTV2, respectively. Patients with an unresectable tumor <8 cm at diagnosis received 55.8 GyRBE. For patients with an unresectable tumor measuring ≥8 cm at diagnosis, the dose was escalated to a maximum of 64.8 GyRBE since 2017. For those aged <5 years and with a tumor ≥8 cm at diagnosis, dose escalation was not employed if the postinduction tumor measured <8 cm. Most (74%) received definitive radiation with the remaining receiving preoperative or postoperative radiotherapy. The median primary tumor size was 10.5 cm. With a median follow-up of 3 years (range, 0.3–9.0 years), the 3-year overall survival, progression-free survival, and local control rates were 83% (95% confidence interval [CI], 65–93%), 64% (95% CI, 45–79%), and 92% (95% CI, 74–98%), respectively. Of the five patients with tumors ≥8 cm, none experienced tumor recurrence. Current studies investigating the use of particle therapy for the treatment of Ewing Sarcoma are summarized in Table 27.2.

27.1.3.1 Toxicities

The Massachusetts General Hospital experience reported that all patients endured acute skin toxicity: grade 1 ($n = 16$), grade 2 ($n = 9$), grade 3 ($n = 5$) [10]. Many patients reported fatigue: grade 1 ($n = 18$), grade 2 ($n = 2$), grade 3 ($n = 1$) [10]. Grade 1–2 anorexia was reported in 14 patients, 9 patients of which had grade 2 anorexia. One patient with an orbital primary lesion developed grade 2 kerato-conjunctivitis; one patient with a base of tongue primary was hospitalized due to in field mucositis. In regards to late adverse events, scolioses/kyphoses developed in five patients who all had vertebral body primary tumors. One patient with a pelvic primary tumor had a limb length discrepancy requiring no intervention. Other late effects reported included alopecia, telangiectasias, and hyperpigmentation. Two patients developed endo-

crine deficiencies and one patient developed unilateral hearing loss after base of skull primary tumors and two patients with orbital primaries developed late effects involving the orbital adnexa (lid paralytic lagophthalmos, corneal ulcer). Four patients developed secondary malignancies: acute myelogenous leukemia ($n = 3$) and myelodysplastic syndrome ($n = 1$).

The Japanese retrospective review noted 18 non-hematological acute adverse events of grade 3 but no grade 4 non-hematological acute adverse events during proton therapy [7]. Febrile neutropenia (10%), mucositis (6.8%), and dermatitis (5.1%) were the most common grade 3 acute adverse events; other adverse events included bacteremia, cellulitis, in field pharyngeal abscess, and transaminitis [7]. Late adverse events included growth hormone deficiency ($n = 2$), alopecia ($n = 2$), spinal atrophy ($n = 1$), eyelid function disorder ($n = 1$), corneal opacity ($n = 1$), and adhesive ileus ($n = 1$).

The experience of Kharod et al. with patients with Ewing sarcoma of the cranium or skull base noted three patients who experienced grade 3 acute toxicity—two with grade 3 radiation dermatitis and one with grade 3 oral mucositis [8]. Regarding late toxicity, the authors note one case of Moya moya disease approximately 3 years after radiotherapy with silent infarction of the right caudate nucleus; one case of bilateral conductive hearing loss requiring bilateral hearing aids; three cases of epiphora (with maximum doses to lacrimal ducts of 48–54 GyRBE); one case of sinusitis requiring surgical repair in a patient with Ewing sarcoma of the maxillary sinus; one case of right frontal lobe hemorrhage for a case with primary of the paranasal sinuses. Six patients required hormone replacement for neuroendocrine deficits.

Regarding the cohort of children with pelvic Ewing sarcoma described by Uezono et al., five patients experienced grade ≥2 late toxicity [9]. These events included unequal limb length ($n = 1$), pelvic pain ($n = 1$), premature ovarian deficiency ($n = 1$), wound infection ($n = 1$), hip dislocation ($n = 1$), and bladder perforation ($n = 1$).

27.1.3.2 Active Clinical Trials

27.1.4 Treatment Planning

Setup and selection of beam angles for treatment of patients with Ewing sarcoma is heterogeneous, given the fact that the

Table 27.2 Active clinical trials utilizing particle therapy for Ewing sarcoma.

Title	Sponsor	Status	Clinical trial identifier
Proton Radiation for the Treatment of Pediatric Bone and Non-Rhabdomyosarcoma Soft Tissue Sarcomas	Massachusetts General Hospital	Active, study completion date September 2021	NCT00592293
Phase I Trial of Safety of Carbon-ion Radiotherapy for Primary Malignant Bone and Soft Tissue Tumor in the Childhood	Gunma University	Active	GUNMA1102
Combination Chemotherapy in Treating Patients with Non-Metastatic Extracranial Ewing Sarcoma (AEWS1031)	Children's Oncology Group	Active, not recruiting	NCT01231906
Combination Chemotherapy with or without Ganitumab in Treating Patients with Newly Diagnosed Metastatic Ewing Sarcoma (AEWS1221)	National Cancer Institute	Active, not recruiting	NCT02306161

primary site will be different child to child. However, there are a few clinical scenarios worth describing.

As Ewing sarcoma represents a malignancy for which metastatic disease may be approached with curative intent, there are some clinical cases where treatment may involve a hybrid photon–proton approach. The normal treatment paradigm recommends whole lung consolidation at the end of chemotherapy; however, for children with primary sites that approximate metastatic sites (like the chest wall and pulmonary metastases), metastatic treatment is delivered at the time that the primary is treated. In such instances where hemithorax or whole lung treatment happens concomitantly with radiotherapy directed to the primary, a dose-painted photon plan is used for the duration of the hemithorax or whole lung treatment and treatment to the primary is completed with a proton therapy plan. Dose-painting is employed as fractionation for whole lung and hemithorax typically at 1.5 Gy/fraction whereas radiotherapy directed to the primary is delivered in 1.8 Gy/fraction. Given the location of a chest wall primary, 4D simulation is recommended for creation of an internal target volume (ITV) to capture the motion of the target.

Another location which merits comment is pelvic primaries. For young male patients with primaries such as the ischium, testicular dose can be reduced not only through particle therapy but also by repositioning the penis and testes at simulation. Beam angle selection for pelvic primaries may also be influenced by the bladder and bowels for which their size and location may vary. As such, we typically avoid angles crossing either structure in order to reach their target.

27.1.4.1 Volume Construction
The University of Florida approach to treatment and planning is described in Table 27.3:

27.1.5 Case

Below we present a case of a 17-year-old child treated for an unresectable pelvic Ewing sarcoma. After fusing pertinent MRI and imaging to the simulation imaging, we proceeded with identifying the contour of the pre-chemotherapy tumor volume (blue).

A GTV was identified from his most recent MRI imaging just prior to simulation (red).

CTV expansion was conducted as noted above, respecting barriers to tumor extension (CTV1 = yellow).

Table 27.3 Recommended target volumes and radiation doses for Ewing sarcoma.

Volume	Definitive	Postoperative	Dose (GyRBE)	
GTV1	Visible gross tumor consisting of the *pre-chemotherapy* bone involvement and *pre-chemotherapy* soft tissue mass defined by MR (T1, T2, FLAIR, etc.)	Visible gross tumor consisting of the *pre-chemotherapy* bone involvement and residual *pre-chemotherapy* soft tissue mass defined by MR (T1, T2, FLAIR, etc.) AND Include the operative bed (not including the scar or operative tract, unless felt to be at risk)	–	
GTV2	The pretreatment abnormalities in bone but the residual *post-chemotherapy* soft tissue mass defined by MR (T1, T2, FLAIR, etc.)	The pretreatment abnormalities in bone but the residual *post-chemotherapy* soft tissue mass defined by MR (T1, T2, FLAIR, etc.)		
CTV1	1. Clinical margin of 1 cm around the GTV, respecting anatomic barriers that limit tumor spread AND 2. Tissue that harbored gross disease that now has no visible gross disease (specifically bone or other "infiltrated" tissues)	1. Clinical margin of 1 cm around the GTV, respecting anatomic barriers that limit tumor spread AND 2. Tissue that harbored gross disease that now has no visible gross disease (specifically bone or other "infiltrated" tissues)	45	
CTV2	GTV2 + 1 cm as above	GTV2 + 1 cm as above	*Resected with positive margin* 50.4*	*Definitive or gross residual* 55.8

Note: PTV expansions are isotropic and based on factors of immobilization and daily image guidance (3 mm for CNS, skull base, and head and neck; 5 mm for remainder of disease sites). [a]Dose modifications are made for the following scenarios: for spinal primaries above the spinal cord, the dose is 50.4 GyRBE. *Per AEWS1031 and 1221, for tumors with microscopic positive margins, the volume to which is treated to 50.4 is noted by the amount of necrosis in the pathologic specimen. For those tumors with >90% necrosis, the volume treated is PTV2. For those with <90% necrosis, the volume treated is PTV1.

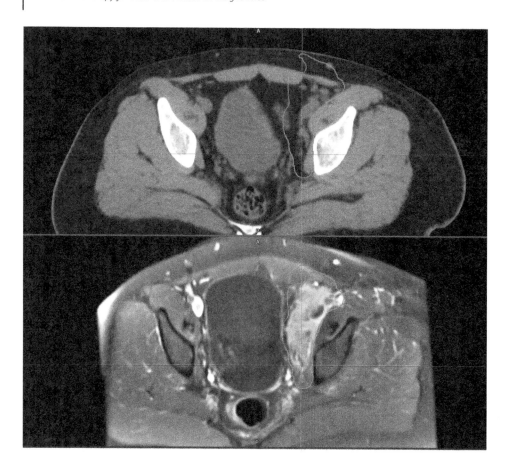

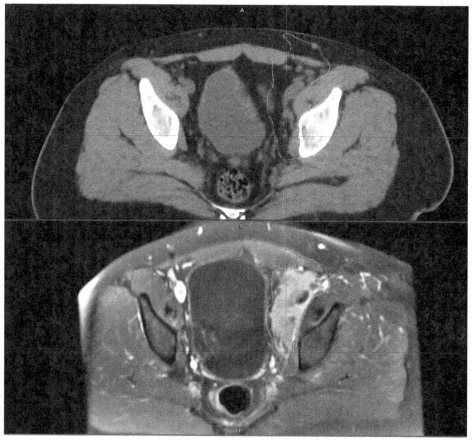

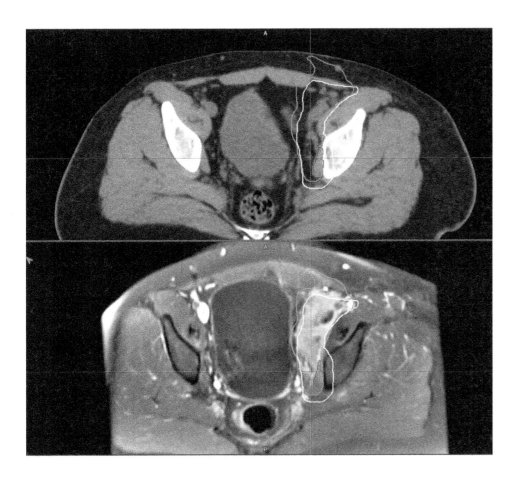

27.2 Hodgkin Lymphoma

27.2.1 Epidemiology

Hodgkin lymphoma is a hematologic cancer occurring in both children and adults with a bimodal distribution. While it is most common in young adults with an average age at diagnosis of 39 [1], it is one of the most common cancers diagnosed in teens between the ages of 15–19 [1]. It is very rare in children under the age of 14 years.

Although there are several subtypes of Hodgkin lymphoma, they can primarily be divided into two categories: classical (typically CD15+/CD30+/CD20−/CD45−) and nodular lymphocyte predominant (CD15−/CD30−/CD20+/CD45+). Risk factors for Hodgkin lymphoma include HIV infection, EBV infection, and family history (American Cancer Society). Overall survival of pediatric Hodgkin lymphoma is excellent, leading to additional research in how to minimize late effects of oncologic interventions.

27.2.2 Clinical Evaluation

Evaluation is initiated by a thorough history and physical documenting B symptoms, which includes recurrent fevers >38°C, drenching night sweats, and or weight loss greater than 10% of body weight within 6 months. Diagnosis is made by initial excisional biopsy with immunohistochemistry evaluation. Classical Hodgkin lymphoma typically stains positive for CD15 and CD30, negative for CD20 and CD45. While classical Hodgkin lymphoma has four histological subtypes, the most common in children are mixed cellularity and nodular sclerosing variants, with mixed cellularity having improved prognosis. Complete workup includes labs (complete blood count with differential, ESR and or CRP, comprehensive metabolic panel with serum albumin, pregnancy test in post-pubescent females), echocardiogram and pulmonary function tests (for purposes of chemotherapy management), and imaging. Additional labs such as HIV and hepatitis B and C testing are encouraged but not mandatory. Pretreatment diagnostic imaging is critical for radiation treatment planning, which can include CT neck, chest, abdomen, and pelvis with contrast or CT chest with MRI neck, abdomen, and pelvis (pediatric Hodgkin lymphoma, NCCN, Version 2.2021). Of note, pretreatment PET/CT imaging is preferred if radiotherapy is anticipated in the treatment course and should be performed with the patient in the treatment planning position if possible.

27.2.3 Clinical Management

In general, Hodgkin lymphoma management is dominated by systemic therapies with more recent PET adaptive strategies. Radiation oncologists should pursue radiotherapy strategy as per the chemotherapy following a multidisciplinary pediatric oncology discussion, as different strategies have utilized different radiotherapy recommendations. Risk stratification of classic Hodgkin lymphoma has been developed by clinical protocols, namely, EuroNet-PHL-C1, AHOD0031, AHOD0431, AHOD0831, and AHOD01331. As defined by COG protocols AHOD0031, 0431, and 0831, low-risk cHL includes stages IA and IIA without bulky disease or B symptoms. Intermediate-risk cHL includes stages I and II with any risk factor, including bulky disease, B symptoms, and extranodal disease. Notably, the definition of intermediate and high-risk cHL has evolved over the last decade. By AHOD0831, high risk was defined as stages IIIB and IVB. For the most recent COG trial AHOD1331, high-risk cHL evolved to represent IIB with bulk, IIIB, IVA, and IVB.

For low-risk cHL, the EuroNet-PHL-C1 chemotherapy regimen is preferred if the patient is not on a clinical trial, though ABVD or the AHOD0431 regimen could be used (pediatric Hodgkin lymphoma, NCCN, Version 2.2021). Response assessment with PET and contrast enhanced CT or MRI then determines if involved site radiotherapy (ISRT) is recommended for inadequate response to primary chemotherapy.

For intermediate risk cHL, the AHOD0031 regimen of ABVE-PC × 2 cycles is preferred if not on clinical trial, though OEPA × 2 cycles per the EUroNet-PHL-C1 regimen or ABVD could be utilized (pediatric Hodgkin lymphoma, NCCN, Version 2.2021). If there is an inadequate response, then additional chemotherapy is indicated followed by ISRT. Notably, AHOD0031 defined slow responding lesions using anatomic CT criteria, predating Deauville score decision-making (whereas Deauville 4+ is generally considered positive for lymphoma management). If adequate response, only additional chemotherapy is generally indicated. However, analyses of the results of AHOD0031 denoted that children with anemia and bulk at presentation have a higher risk of relapse. For those children, we recommend consideration of radiotherapy consolidation.

For high-risk cHL, the AHOD1331 regimen of ABVE-PE × 2 cycles is commonly used for those not on clinical trial, though OEPA × 2 cycles per the EUroNet-PHL-C1 regimen or ABVD or BEACOPP could be utilized (pediatric Hodgkin lymphoma, NCCN, Version 2.2021). Regardless of treatment response, oftentimes ISRT is indicated after additional chemotherapy for inadequate response with either ABVE-PC × 3 cycles or COPDAC × 4 cycles. Notably, AHOD1331 employs adaptive radiotherapy such that sites of mediastinal bulk are consolidated as well as sites of inadequate response after PET-2. The Euronet-C2 protocol however recommends radiotherapy consolidation to all sites of disease for those children with inadequate response.

Additionally, nodular lymphocyte predominant HL generally presents as early stage (stages I and II). If the patient has a single lymph node involved, surgery alone with subsequent close surveillance may be acceptable and is under investigation by COG. If the patient has stage IA or IIA disease, their management is often similar to that of low-risk classical HL.

In regards to the use of proton therapy for pediatric Hodgkin lymphoma, there has been one phase II trial led by Hoppe et al. that evaluated involved node proton therapy technique for patients with stage I–IIIB disease and mediastinal involvement, for which five pediatric patients were enrolled [11] (Table 27.4). The 3-year recurrence-free survival was 93% overall for the entire cohort. The other published experiences were also led by the University of Florida, for which INRT to a total of 21 GyRBE

Table 27.4 Clinical experiences utilizing particle therapy for Hodgkin lymphoma.

Publication	Number of patients	Median RT dose GyRBE (range)	Disease site	Outcomes
Hoppe et al.[13]	10	21 ISRT + 9 boost	Mediastinal	Dosimetric outcomes study. Escalated residual target dose by 42% but reduced OAR dose by 25–46%
Hoppe et al.[12]	138 (42% of patients were pediatric)	21 (20–45)	–	3-year RFS 87% (for pediatric patients)
Wray et al.[14]	22	21 (15–36)	Cervical/supraclavicular, infraclavicular, lung hilum, para-aortic, mesenteric, splenic, pelvic/inguinal, extranodal	2-year OS 94% \ 3-year OS 94% \ Recurrences ($n = 3$): in-field and out of field
Hoppe et al.[11]	15 ($n = 5$ pediatric patients)	15–25.5 INPT	Mediastinal	3-year RFS 93% \ 3-year EFS 87% (overall)

Table 27.5 Active clinical trials utilizing particle therapy for Hodgkin lymphoma.

Title	Sponsor	Status	Clinical trial identifier
UFPTI 1431–HL02: Investigating Early Markers of Radiation-Induced Cardiac Injury in Hodgkin Lymphoma Survivors Treated With Either Photon or Proton Radiation	University of Florida	Active, not recruiting	NCT02404818
A Prospective Observational Study with Longitudinal Cardiopulmonary Surveillance in Lymphoma Patients Undergoing Mediastinal Radiotherapy in the Era of Modern Chemoradiation	Chang Gung Memorial Hospital	Recruiting Note: inclusion includes patients with age greater than 15 years old	NCT03969693
Immunotherapy Plus Combination Chemotherapy in Treating Patients with Newly Diagnosed Stage II–IV Classic Hodgkin Lymphoma (S1826)	National Cancer Institute (NCI)	Recruiting	NCT03907488

was delivered [12–14]. Survival outcomes were comparable to published photon radiotherapy, with the decrease noted in organs at risk dose [13]. Potential improvement of late effects from ISRT would necessitate longer follow-up. Current clinical trials investigating particle therapy in the treatment of Hodgkin Lymphoma are summarized in Table 27.5.

27.2.3.1 Toxicities

In the University of Florida experience, no grade 3 acute or late toxicities occurred. In the phase II INPT study, while pediatric patient-specific toxicities were not specified, there were in total three grade 2 esophagitis and one grade 2 skin toxicity; there were no other acute grade 2 toxicities and no late grade 2 toxicities [11]. None of the other series report proton therapy related grade 3 or higher toxicities [11–14].

27.2.3.2 Active Clinical Trials

27.2.4 Treatment Planning

As above, the decision for radiotherapy is very much influenced and supported by the chemotherapy regimen per which our pediatric patients are treated. As a tertiary center, we have the privilege of seeing children treated with many different regimens. For adolescents (18 and above) who received ABVD, please refer to the adult section of this book.

27.2.4.1 Intermediate Risk Classical Hodgkin Lymphoma

For those children treated as per AHOD0031, it is important to note that radiotherapy was prescribed to all sites of involvement for those children with an inadequate response. As such, we recommend 21 GyRBE to all sites. Relapses were higher than expected, and for children with Deauville 3 + PET-CT at end of therapy or with gross residual >2.5 cm on CT, we recommend a 9-GyRBE boost to those residual foci. We employ involved-site radiotherapy as described by the International Lymphoma Radiation Oncology Group (ILROG) [15]. As

noted above, we also discuss radiotherapy for children treated as per AHOD0031 who had bulk and anemia at diagnosis.

For children treated with an OEPA-COPDAC backbone, institutional series have been published from the United States. However, phase III data from EURONET C1 and C2 are pending. Notably, the EURONETC2 strategy also dictates radiotherapy delivery to all sites, whereas institutional series from the United States have individualized consolidation to the sites of inadequate response. As such, we contextualize radiotherapy volumes (all sites versus those sites of inadequate response) based on the anatomic sites of involvement and the subsequent elevation in OAR dose by being more comprehensive. As above, we recommend a dose of 21 GyRBE (as per EURONET) with a boost to 30 GyRBE for residual disease/partial PET response.

27.2.4.2 High-risk Classical Hodgkin Lymphoma

For those children treated as per AHOD1331, it is important to note that radiotherapy was recommended for large mediastinal adenopathy (LMA) as well as sites of PR at interim PET after two cycles. This contrasts AHOD0031 for which all sites were consolidated. We similarly utilize a dose of 21 GyRBE utilizing ISRT techniques to the LMA and PR sites reserving a 9-GyRBE boost for residual disease (Deauville 3+ as above).

For those children treated with OEPA-COPDAC, our decision-making is the same as noted above under Intermediate risk classical Hodgkin lymphoma.

27.2.4.3 Positioning and Image Verification

Simulation for patients is guided by anatomic site of involvement. For Hodgkin lymphoma, the most common sites are cervical and mediastinal. For the common simulation that involves both sites, we utilize an Aquaplast mask to affix the head and neck in an extended position with a base of skull frame and shoulder pulls for upper extremity stabilization. We obtain a 3D CT with contrast in addition to a 4D CT (particularly for spleen and mediastinum) for ITV creation. For splenic treatment, patients are both simulated and treated while NPO.

The treatment of young women with mediastinal targets can be challenging. With much evidence demonstrating that breast tissue needs to be included as an OAR, it is imperative to have reproducible setup for which breast soft tissue image verification is necessary. We do not typically employ a breast board (as noted in our description above) as the positioning raises breast tissue superiorly. As such, we also include the nipple and other breast marks as leveling marks at simulation such that placement of BBs in those same positions in treatment with kV imaging can identify alignment before confirming with CBCT. This allows reduction of the times CBCT needs to be utilized. For those centers with capability, optical surface imaging would be recommended to similarly achieve this.

Given the variability in setup, we also repeat a verification scan the first week of treatment to ensure reproducibility and calculated dose delivery.

27.2.4.4 Volume Construction

The University of Florida approach to treatment and planning is described in Table 27.6:

As per the aforementioned ILROG guidelines, a GTV is created informed by the sites of involvement from both the PET and CT information provided at diagnosis. Notably, this may not reflect a "true" GTV as this disease may have resolved at time of therapy. However, any residual disease present at time of treatment (typically from diagnostic imaging that may accompany) will be included in the GTV. The CTV though will incorporate the GTV from diagnosis with modifications to reflect changes in treatment response (such that if mediastinal disease earlier entered what is now healthy lung tissue or bone) is reflected by cropping it from non-invaded structures. The GTV from the end of therapy imaging will be included in the CTV without modification. At our center, we

employ ISRT, and as such, an expansion to account for uncertainty between diagnostic imaging and simulation is utilized. Unfortunately, there is no set value for this expansion but an approximation of 5 mm in the superior–inferior direction is useful. Similarly, evaluating the change in setup helps inform as neck flexion can vary quite a bit. Also, given the displacement of mediastinal anatomy, it is useful to reflect on the relation of disease to cardiac structures, great vessels, and ribs to better localize what surfaces may be at risk of harboring microscopic disease. For splenic treatment, the whole spleen is treated.

PTV expansion is institutionally specific as always. At our center, we utilize a 3-mm expansion for head and neck locations with 5 mm for other sites.

27.2.5 Case

Below we present a case of a 17-year-old female treated for Stage IIA bulky classical HL with chemotherapy as per AHOD0031. Interval PET noted slow early response by anatomic criteria with less than 60% reduction in size in addition to Deauville 4 persistence in the mediastinum and left neck. Consolidative radiotherapy to 21 GyRBE was prescribed to all sites with 9 GyRBE to residual disease. A 4D simulation scan and a 3D scan with contrast were obtained.

In the panels below, represented are PET-CT and PET from diagnosis (top-right and top-left). Below are the 4D scan (left) and contrasted 3D scan (right). In pink is the pre-chemotherapy disease used to inform the CTV (orange). ITV is represented in yellow.

The same patient is shown with coronal sections for the same imaging studies as above with the ITV redemonstrated in yellow.

The dose of the plan is shown on the simulation slices below with 50% and 95% dose shown in color wash with green and

Table 27.6 Recommended target volumes and radiation doses for Hodgkin lymphoma.

Volume	Definitive	Postoperative	Dose (GyRBE)
$GTV_{pre-chemo}$	Sites of involvement from both the PET and CT information provided *at diagnosis*	–	–
$GTV_{post-chemo}$	Any residual disease present *at time of treatment*	–	–
CTV	$GTV_{pre-chemo} + GTV_{post-chemo}$	–	21
	+ clinically informed expansion to reflect uncertainty as a reflection of ISRT		Consider 9 GyRBE boost to residual disease, considering HL risk group and treatment protocol as defined above
	− edited off uninvolved tissue for $GTV_{pre-chemo}$		
	If there is target motion:		
	ITV = CTV + 1.5–2 cm if there is no 4DCT (or as visualized by 4DCT)		

Note: PTV expansions are isotropic (3 mm for CNS, skull base, and head and neck; 5 mm for remainder of disease sites).

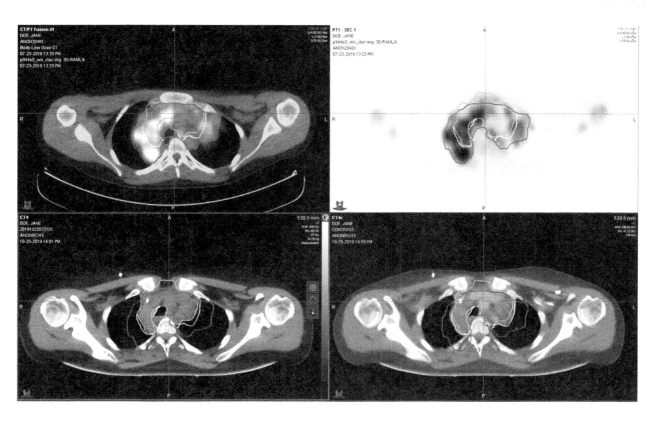

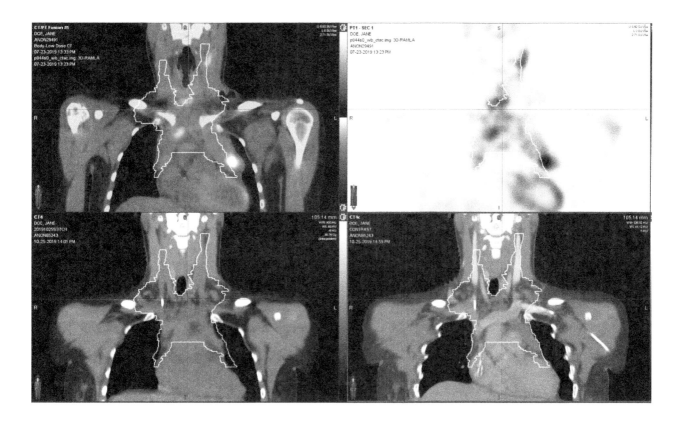

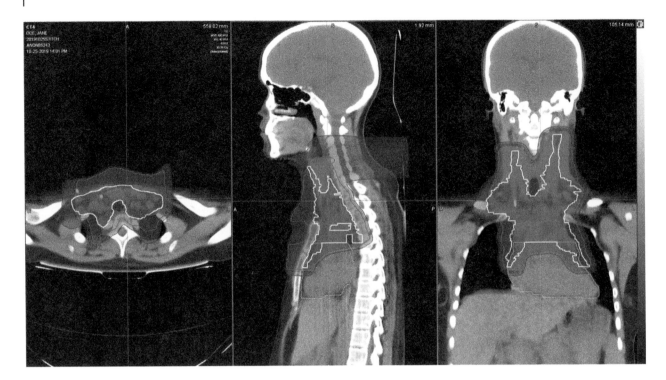

magenta, respectively. The ITV and heart contours are shown in yellow and orange, respectively.

27.3 Neuroblastoma

27.3.1 Epidemiology

In the United States, there are about 800 new cases of neuroblastoma yearly, accounting for 6% of all childhood cancers [1]. It is the most common cancer in children less than 1 year old, and most cases are diagnosed by age 5. It rarely occurs in patients over 10 years of age. There are no known environmental risk factors for neuroblastoma. However, about 1–2% of neuroblastoma cases are familial, and these patients tend to be younger than patients who have the sporadic form of neuroblastoma. There is also a positive association between children born with birth defects and development of neuroblastoma [1].

27.3.2 Clinical Evaluation

A careful history and physical may reveal clinical findings unique to neuroblastoma. On physical exam, periorbital ecchymosis, opsoclonus, and the "blueberry muffin sign" of skin metastases may indicate this diagnosis. Paraneoplastic syndromes such as the "pepper syndrome" of the liver may lead to respiratory compromise, Hutchinson syndrome may present as pain and refusal to walk, and bone marrow involve-

ment leading to pancytopenia may present as pallor and infection. Evaluation includes lab work; notably diagnosis is made from elevated urine or serum catecholamines (VMA, HMA) and core needle biopsy. If a core needle biopsy is not obtained, then a bone marrow biopsy of bilateral sites must be obtained to confirm diagnosis, unless the patient is less than 6 months of age. Imaging includes abdominal CT or MRI, as well as MIBG (if MIBG negative, then bone scan to confirm).

Negative prognostic factors include: N-myc/MYCN gene amplification, DNA ploidy (triploid less aggressive), LOH at 1p 11q, age greater than 1.5 years of age, and poorly differentiated.

27.3.3 Clinical Management

The International Neuroblastoma Staging System (INSS) was used to classify surgical treatment outcomes, which the COG has combined with molecular prognostic factors and age to determine risk groups. There are three risk groups: low, intermediate, and high risk.

- Low-risk group patients generally undergo primary surgery followed by chemotherapy or radiotherapy only for persistent or recurrent disease.
- Intermediate-risk group patients underwent surgery followed by chemotherapy with cyclophosphamide, doxorubicin, and etoposide × 4 cycles if favorable histology (×8 cycles if not). Radiotherapy was reserved for persistent or recurrent disease.

- High-risk group patients undergo neoadjuvant chemotherapy × 6 cycles, followed by surgery, adjuvant chemotherapy and stem-cell transplant, then radiotherapy and subsequent systemic therapy.
- Patients with Stage 4S by the INSS received palliative treatment for acute respiratory or abdominal compartment syndrome from massive hepatomegaly.

Of note, the International Neuroblastoma Risk Group Staging System (INRGSS) is a newer system used for treatment management prior to surgery. It considers not only pretreatment imaging tests but also patient age, tumor histology, presence of MYCN gene amplification, chromosome 11q aberration, and DNA ploidy. The INRGSS has four stages:

- L1: tumor has not spread or grown into vital organs and is confined to one area of the body
- L2: tumor has not spread far from origin, but has at least one image-defined risk factor
- M: tumor that has metastasized
- MS: metastatic disease in patients <18 months (with metastatic disease limited to skin, liver, and or bone marrow with ≤10% marrow involvement). MIBG scan with no evidence of bone involvement.

Radiotherapy in neuroblastoma is used for patients with high-risk disease after neoadjuvant chemotherapy, surgery, and transplant. High-risk disease most commonly refers to those children positive for n-myc amplification or with metastatic disease and above 18 months of age. Also, metastatic sites, in addition to the primary, may be treated depending upon response to neoadjuvant systemic treatment. There is limited experience reported as well of using radiotherapy as a form of local control in the relapse setting [16]. Additionally, radiotherapy can be used for palliation due to hepatomegaly or spinal cord compression.

Consolidative radiotherapy may be used neuroblastoma for treatment of metastatic sites. If children have ≤5 metastatic sites that are still MIBG positive after induction chemotherapy, ANBL0532 and ANBL1531 note consolidative radiotherapy to the primary and those sites. For those children who may have >5 sites, an MIBG scan is recommended post-transplant with consolidation to those sites still positive after stem cell transplant. If >5 sites are still positive at that time, discussion in a multidisciplinary setting is recommended.

Recent strides with the publication of an analysis of ANBL0532 also have refined the idea of boosting residual disease for children with neuroblastoma after publication by Liu et al. noted that boost radiotherapy to gross residual tumor present at end of induction did not improve 5-year cumulative incidence of local progression [17].

Proton therapy has been studied in multiple retrospective series over the past decade for treatment of the primary site status post-maximum safe resection as well as for metastatic MIBG-avid sites (Table 27.7). Efficacy in terms of local control at up to 5 years is acceptable [18–21].

27.3.3.1 Toxicities

Of the retrospective series published in the past 5 years, in the Hosaka et al. experience, most of the reported grade 3–4 events were neutropenia, though there was one acute grade 3 pericardial effusion and hypertension in a patient who received RT to the mediastinum and one acute grade 3 renal dysfunction in a patient who received RT to the abdomen [18]. In total, there were 2 events of late grade 3–4 toxicity, both involving chronic kidney disease in patients who received abdominal RT [18]. In the Lim et al. experience, there were two events of acute grade 3–4 toxicity, which were hematological and in patients ($n = 2$) with preexisting low counts prior to RT [19]. In the Bagley et al. experience, no acute grade 3 toxicities were reported [20]. Similarly, in the Hill-Kayser et al. experience, there was only

Table 27.7 Clinical experiences utilizing particle therapy for neuroblastoma..

Publication	Number of patients	Median RT dose GyRBE (range)	Disease site	Outcomes
Hosaka et al. [18]	18	Primary: 19.8 (residual tumor boost, total dose 30.6) Metastatic sites: 19.8	Primary site, MIBG-avid metastatic sites	3-year LC 100% 3-year EFS 44% 3-year OS 71%
Lim et al. [19]	19	Primary: 21 (residual disease boost, $n = 1$, total dose 36)	Primary site	No LR at 14.9-month median follow-up 2-year OS 94% 2-year PFS 76%
Bagley et al. [20]	18	Primary: 21–24 (residual tumor boost in $n = 2$, total dose 36) Entire vertebra: 15–18	Primary site and up to 3 MIBG-avid metastatic sites	2-year LC 94% 5-year LC 87% No failures at distant met sites 5-year PFS 64% 5-year OS 94%

(Continued)

Table 27.7 (Continued)

Publication	Number of patients	Median RT dose GyRBE (range)	Disease site	Outcomes
Hill-Kayser et al. [21]	45	Primary: 21.6 (residual tumor boost, total 36) Metastatic sites: 21.6	Primary site, MIBG-avid metastatic sites	3-year LC 97% 4-year LC 97% 5-year LC 97% 3-year DFS 77% 4-year DFS 70% 5-year DFS 70% 3-year OS 89% 4-year OS 80% 5-year OS 80%
Hishiki et al. [22] JNBSG Phase II trial (JN-H-07)	50	Primary: 19.8 (residual tumor boost, total dose 30.6)	Primary site, MIBG-avid bone metastases	3-year PFS 36.5% 3-year OS 69.5%
Oshiro et al. [23]	14	19.8–45.5 *Some patients underwent IORT and some underwent combination PBT and photon RT	Primary site, MIBG-avid metastatic sites	$N = 7$ with NED $N = 1$ with disease progression $N = 6$ died due to tumor 3-year LRC 82%
Hill-Kayser et al. [24]	13	Primary: 21.6 (residual tumor boost, total dose 36) Metastatic sites: 21.6	Primary site, MIBG-avid metastatic sites	For patients with lateralized disease, proton therapy demonstrated better sparing of the contralateral kidney but did not reduce ipsilateral kidney dose compared to IMRT
Hattangadi et al. [25]	9	Primary: 21.6–23.4 (residual tumor boost in $n = 4$, total dose 36) Metastatic sites: 21.6 (bone mets)	Primary site, MIBG-avid metastatic sites	No local failures at median follow-up 38 months Distant failure in $n = 4$, of which $n = 2$ death due to disease

one acute grade 3 toxicity (anorexia) and there were notably no late grade 3 or 4 renal or hepatic toxicities [21]. The Oshiro et al. experience reports one patient who developed aortic narrowing and vertebral growth retardation, found 28 years after radiotherapy to the abdomen due to premature birth of her baby [23].

27.3.3.2 Active Clinical Trials

Current clinical trials utilizing particle therapy for neuroblastoma are described in Table 27.8.

27.3.4 Treatment Planning

27.3.4.1 Positioning and Image Verification

For simulation, we typically obtain a 4D CT and a 3D CT with contrast. Many of these tumors may be large at the time of surgery and susceptible to respiratory motion in the abdomen or in the mediastinum. Given the age of diagnosis for many of these tumors, we include the vertebral bodies in the PTV with

Table 27.8 Active clinical trials utilizing particle therapy for neuroblastoma.

Title	Sponsor	Status	Clinical trial identifier
Phase II Study of Proton Radiation Therapy for Neuroblastoma	Massachusetts General Hospital	Recruiting	NCT02112617
Neuroblastoma Protocol 2012: Therapy for Children with Advanced Stage High-risk Neuroblastoma	St. Jude Children's Research Hospital	Active, not recruiting	NCT01857934
Local Control with Reduced-dose Radiotherapy for High-risk Neuroblastoma	Memorial Sloan Kettering Cancer Center	Recruiting	NCT02245997
A Phase 3 Study of ^{131}I-Metaiodobenzylguanidine (^{131}I-MIBG) or Crizotinib Added to Intensive Therapy for Children with Newly Diagnosed High-risk Neuroblastoma (NBL) (ANBL1531)	Children's Oncology Group	Active, not recruiting	NCT03126916

a goal to treat them to 18 GyRBE. With utilization of PBS, we achieve this in a dose-painting fashion.

27.3.4.2 Logistic Considerations

As noted above, indications exist for both treating the primary after resection as well as metastatic sites. At our institution, we similarly follow COG guidelines with treatment to the primary and up to five metastatic sites—those sites that are still active on MIBG at end of induction. If greater than five sites were still positive as by MIBG (or PET), then we repeat MIBG and treat those metastatic sites that are positive after stem cell transplant.

As recovery from stem-cell transplant can be arduous, special care should be taken with how a child is recovering after transplant. In prior COG protocols, RT was recommended to start by day 42 although for the currently enrolling ANBL1531 the span is increased to day 120. In balancing treatment start delay concerns with recovery, our goal has been to have ANC >500 and platelet count >40,000 although with multidisciplinary discussion treatment start may be warranted with the expectation of transfusion support throughout radiotherapy.

27.3.4.3 Volume Construction

The University of Florida approach to treatment and planning is described in Table 27.9:

For the primary, the GTV is informed by the extent of disease present at the time of induction chemotherapy just before surgery (as opposed to extent at diagnosis). This informs the superior–inferior extent of GTV. GTV includes any residual volume or disease after surgery as well as the volume of postinduction presurgery space (reflecting the postoperative bed) after accounting for mass effect changes. Pathology reports should be included in informing GTV. Elective nodal irradiation is not performed.

The CTV is a 1-cm expansion on the GTV, accounting for barriers of spread to disease (e.g., past diaphragm superiorly into the lung; invasion into bone). However, if clear invasion is identified, then trimming for that adjacent organ should not be performed to reflect residual disease.

PTV expansions would be isometric and informed by institutional guidelines. As noted previously, we utilize a 3-mm expansion for head and neck sites and 5 mm elsewhere. As noted with recent evidence, we treat to a dose of 21.6 GyRBE without any boost for residual disease.

27.3.5 Case

Below are representative slices used to inform the treatment planning of a 4-year-old girl with stage IV N-myc-negative, ALK-negative, high-risk neuroblastoma treated per ANBL12P1 with a paraspinal primary. She underwent resection of the left primary paraspinal tumor and was referred for proton consolidative radiotherapy.

The panels demonstrate MRI sequences from the time of surgery postinduction (top panels), MIBG-SPECT at postinduction presurgery shown axially (middle), and the average 4D scan from simulation (bottom). The pre-op volume is shown in blue.

The preop tumor volume was then used to inform the GTV, CTV, and ITV. Pre-op tumor, GTV, and ITV are shown in blue, yellow, and magenta, respectively.

Given its extent into the spinal canal, care was ensured to allow expansion of the CTV for any microscopic disease as emphasized in the panels below.

27.4 Osteosarcoma

27.4.1 Epidemiology

Osteosarcoma is the most common primary bone tumor arising in pediatric and young adult patients, accounting for 2% of childhood cancers and about half of all bone cancers in pediatric patients [1]. There are about 800–900 new cases diagnosed in the United States each year. Of note, the incidence of osteosarcoma has a bimodal age distribution, with the pediatric peak incidence occurring between 13 and 16 years of age.

Table 27.9 Recommended target volumes and radiation doses for neuroblastoma.

Volume	Definitive	Postoperative	Dose (GyRBE)
GTV	Extent of disease present at the time of induction chemotherapy just before surgery (as opposed to extent at diagnosis). This informs the sup-inf extent	Any residual volume or disease after surgery as well as the volume of postinduction presurgery space (reflecting the postoperative bed) after accounting for mass effect changes	–
CTV	GTV+ 1 cm edited for barriers to tumor spread	GTV+ 1 cm edited for barriers to tumor spread (but including known invasion into adjacent organs if applicable)	21.6

Note: PTV expansions are isotropic (3 mm for CNS, skull base, and head and neck; 5 mm for remainder of disease sites). [a]No boost for residual disease. Elective nodal irradiation is not performed.

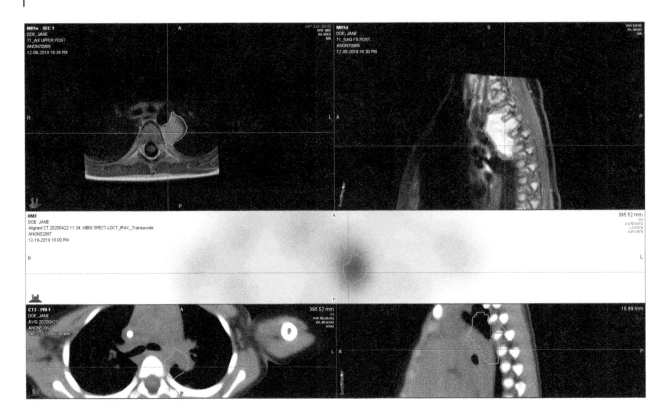

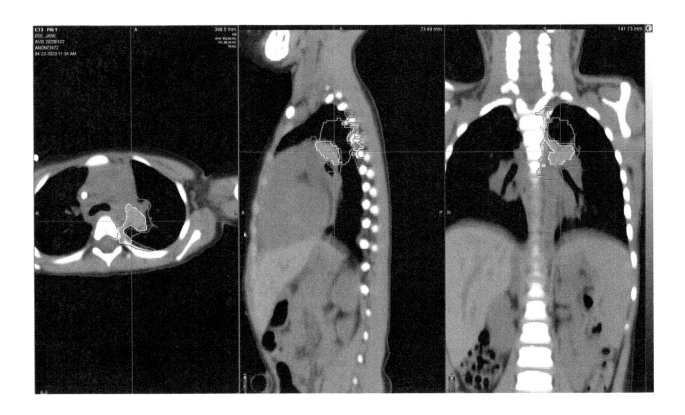

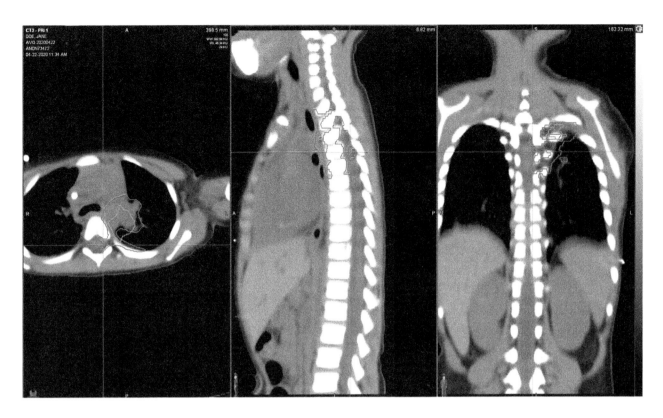

Common sites of osteosarcomas include the metaphysis of long bones such as the femur, tibia, and humerus.

27.4.2 Clinical Evaluation

Osteosarcomas arise from mesenchymal stem cells, which can differentiate into bone, cartilage, or fibrous tissue. Histologic diagnosis is based on the presence of malignant sarcomatous stroma characterized by woven bone matrix. Intramedullary, high-grade osteosarcomas account for about 90% of osteosarcomas and are subclassified by its predominant cellular component: osteoblastic, fibroblastic, and chondroblastic osteosarcoma. There are several variants from the conventional osteosarcomas and these include small cell, telangiectatic, multifocal, malignant fibrous histiocytoma; these were thought to have a worse prognosis, but with modern management appear to respond similarly to conventional osteosarcoma. Surface osteosarcomas, namely, the low grade (parosteal) and intermediate grade (periosteal) subcategories, appear to be more indolent in nature and are often curative with surgery alone [26].

Clinical presentation is characterized by localized pain over several months that may wax and wane without associated symptoms. Exam is typically significant for a tender palpable soft tissue mass, most commonly involving the distal femur, proximal tibia, and proximal humerus.

Initial evaluation involves a plain radiograph, which would characteristically show cortical destruction and periosteal new bone formation with indistinct margins (Codman triangle), surrounded by mixture of radiodense and radiolucent bone; surrounding soft tissue may demonstrate a "sunburst" pattern due to variable ossification. About 12% of patients may have a pathologic fracture at diagnosis [27]. If radiograph findings are subtle, an MRI of the entire length of affected bone may be obtained if suspicion remains high for a bone tumor and is indicated for surgical planning. Biopsy is recommended and can either be an open biopsy completed by an orthopedic surgeon or a core needle biopsy completed by interventional radiology with a biopsy tract confirmed by the surgeon. To complete staging, a CT chest is required due to prevalence of pulmonary metastasis. A radionuclide bone scan with technetium is preferred for evaluation of synchronous lesions, though a PET/CT may be obtained instead and is useful for evaluating response to chemotherapy (NCCN, ESMO, COG Bone Tumor Committee).

The Musculoskeletal Tumor Society created a surgical staging system that classifies primary tumor by grade, local anatomical extent, and presence of metastasis. In brief, metastatic osteosarcoma, regardless of tumor grade or extent, is stage III. High-grade (G2) localized osteosarcoma is stage II. Low-grade (G1) localized osteosarcoma is stage I. For stage I and II osteosarcoma, further classification is designated for intracompartmental (T1) or extracompartmental (T2). This commonly used staging system is summarized below:

Grade	Tumor	Metastasis	Stage
G1	T1	M0	IA
G1	T2	M0	IB
G2	T1	M0	IIA
G2	T2	M0	IIB
G1 or G2	T1 or T2	M1	III

27.4.3 Clinical Management

Function and limb-preserving surgery is the goal for osteosarcoma, usually preceded by neoadjuvant chemotherapy. Notably, optimal timing for chemotherapy, which has greatly improved survival outcomes for patients with osteosarcoma, has not been established. As defined by the POG-8651 study evaluating preoperative versus postoperative chemotherapy for pediatric osteosarcoma, the 44-week chemotherapy regimen used included: doxorubicin, cisplatin, bleomycin, cyclophosphamide, dactinomycin, and high-dose methotrexate with leucovorin [28]. This trial demonstrated similar incidence of limb salvage and event-free survival at 5 years for both arms. Of note, recommended chemotherapy for osteosarcoma typically follows the protocol defined by the control arm of the COG AOST-0331 (EURAMOS-1) clinical trial: doxorubicin, cisplatin, and methotrexate for induction chemotherapy in weeks 1–10, surgery in week 11, followed by postoperative chemotherapy with this three-drug regimen in weeks 12–29 [27].

For osteosarcoma involving the limb, limb sparing surgery is preferred over amputation and has been shown to be as effective. Conventional osteosarcomas are more radioresistant than Ewing sarcoma, thus surgery remains the mainstay local therapy. In patients who undergo surgery for primary management of their osteosarcoma, radiation therapy is only indicated postoperatively when there are positive margins or close margin with poor histologic response to neoadjuvant chemotherapy. It may also be indicated for cases with presentation of a pathologic fracture or status post-intramedullary rod placement through the tumor prior to diagnosis of osteosarcoma.

For patients with non-appendicular sites of disease such as the sacrum or base of skull or if the patient's comorbidities preclude a safe resection, definitive radiation therapy may be indicated for local control. Of note, one such retrospective series from Massachusetts General Hospital [29] describes a single institution experience with utilizing proton therapy for unresectable or incompletely resected osteosarcoma. While not all patients in this series were children, this remains the largest published series describing proton therapy technique and outcomes for osteosarcoma. Initial treatment fields covered preoperative clinical tumor using CT-based 3D planning. Most patients were treated using a daily fractionation scheme, except four patients treated with hyperfractionated RT. In regards to the total dose used, 50.1% of patients received at least 70 GyRBE and 40% of patients received between 60 and 70 GyRBE. The patients who received less than 60 GyRBE typically had disease of the spine, though one patient had osteosarcoma of the maxilla and one patient had an incompletely resected distal femur osteosarcoma. Only 20% of patients received protons only, but most of these patients had head and neck osteosarcomas. In this series, 13% of patients received some preoperative RT (typically to a dose of 19.8 GyRBE). Median gross tumor volume of disease receiving maximum dose was 82 cm^3. Results are summarized in Table 27.10.

27.4.3.1 Toxicities

From the Massachusetts General Hospital experience [29], significant grade 3 or 4 toxicity occurred in 17 of 55 patients. Grade 3 toxicity included pain requiring morphine ($n = 3$), cranial nerve damage with diplopia ($n = 1$), and limb immobility ($n = 2$), headaches ($n = 1$), and bowel dysfunction secondary to denervation ($n = 1$). Grade 4 toxicity included enucleation ($n = 4$), severe immobility and handicap ($n = 2$), maxillary bone prosthesis ($n = 1$), and acute lymphocytic leukemia less than 2 years after successful RT for osteosarcoma

Table 27.10 Clinical experiences utilizing particle therapy for osteosarcoma.

Publication	Number of patients	Mean RT dose GyRBE (range)	Disease site	Outcomes
Ciernik et al.[29]	55 Note: patient age range 2–74 (median age 29)	68.4 (SD 5.4)	Spine, sacrum, pelvis, femur	2-year OS: 84% 5-year OS: 67% 2-year DFS: 68% 5-year DFS: 65% 5-year LCR: 72%

and subsequent death ($n = 1$), and secondary squamous cell carcinoma of the maxilla 16 years after successful RT for osteosarcoma and subsequent death ($n = 1$).

27.4.3.2 Active Clinical Trials

Clinical trials utilizing particle therapy for osteosarcoma are described in Table 27.11.

27.4.4 Treatment Planning

As surgery is the standard of care, unresectable disease sites or locations where patients may not desire surgical resection (such as a hemipelvectomy) make sites such as base of skull or pelvis more common locations a radiation oncologist may manage primarily. For pelvic sites of disease, careful attention to beam selection, typically avoiding crossing the bowel and bladder to reach the target, is similar to techniques described previously for Ewing sarcoma. Given the high dose, particular care must be given for meeting bowel constraints for pelvic primaries, and similar care needs to be given for base of skull primaries given the myriad of sensitive OARs in that location. For these reasons and high dose, daily image guidance is recommended.

27.4.4.1 Volume Construction

The University of Florida approach to treatment and planning is described in Table 27.12:

27.4.5 Case

A representative case is shared. The patient is a 21-year-old male with osteosarcoma of the right ilium (cT2N0M0, grade 2, stage IIB) treated with MAP chemotherapy.

Displayed are CT sim slices on the top panels with T2 MRI sequences shown below. GTV is shown in red, CTV1 in teal, and CTV2 in yellow.

27.5 Rhabdomyosarcoma (Non-CNS)

27.5.1 Epidemiology

Rhabdomyosarcoma (RMS) is the most common soft tissue tumor diagnosed in children, accounting for about one half of all pediatric sarcomas. Overall, they represent 3% of pediatric cancers, with about 400–500 new cases diagnosed in the United States each year [1]. More than half of RMS are diagnosed in children younger than 10 years old. It occurs more commonly in boys than in girls. Most cases of RMS are sporadic, though 7–8% of cases are associated with inherited syndromes, including neurofibromatosis, Li–Fraumeni syndrome, Beckwith–Wiedemann syndrome, DICER1 syndrome, and Costello syndrome.

27.5.2 Clinical Evaluation

In regards to histology, RMS is notable for immunohistological stains positive for polyclonal desmin (99%), muscle-specific actin (95%), myogenin (95%), and myoglobin (78%). There are four major histologic subtypes of rhabdomyosarcoma, which have differing prognosis and thus treatment paradigms. Classic embryonal RMS is the most common (59%), with variants including botryoid (6%), spindle cell (3%), and sclerosing. Alveolar RMS (21%) has generally poorer prognosis and is often distinguished by FOXO1 rearrangement by FISH or RT-PCR.

Table 27.11 Active clinical trials utilizing particle therapy for osteosarcoma.

Title	Sponsor	Status	Clinical trial identifier
Proton Radiation for the Treatment of Pediatric Bone and Non-Rhabdomyosarcoma Soft Tissue Sarcomas	Massachusetts General Hospital	Active, not recruiting	NCT00592293

Table 27.12 Recommended target volumes and radiation doses for osteosarcoma.

Volume	Definitive	Postoperative	Dose (GyRBE)
GTV	Residual tumor at the time of radiation	Residual tumor at the time of radiation	–
CTV1	GTV + 1.5 cm	GTV + 1.5 cm	50.4
CTV2	GTV + 0.5 cm	GTV + 0.5 cm	70.2 (68.4 if microscopic residual)

Note: PTV expansions are isotropic (3 mm for skull base and head and neck; 5 mm for remainder of disease sites).

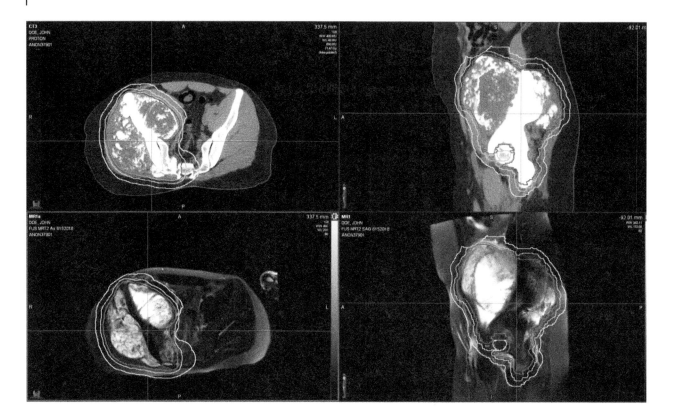

Patients' risk stratification is determined primarily by the COG risk classification system. This classification system involves both the pretreatment TNM staging system and a surgical clinical grouping system, which was established by the Intergroup Rhabdomyosarcoma Study Group (IRSG) and is highly prognostic. Additionally, patient age at diagnosis and tumor histology are also prognostic.

The pretreatment TNM staging is notably dependent on tumor location anatomically and accounts for tumor size and extent of invasion. Tumors of any site with metastasis are considered stage 4. Tumors of the bladder/prostate, extremity, parameningeal, or other (including trunk, retroperitoneum, etc.) are at least stage 2 if N0 but are considered stage 3 if N1 (any regional nodes) or classified as T1b or T2b (tumors >5 cm in diameter). Tumors of the orbit, head, and neck (non-parameningeal), GU (excluding bladder/prostate), and biliary tract are considered stage 1 regardless of tumor extent, size, or nodal involvement, unless metastasis is present.

In general, the IRSG grouping system is based on the extent of residual disease after surgery and includes regional lymph node involvement. Group I is defined by localized disease that is completely resected. Group II is defined by a total gross resection with evidence of regional spread, subcategorized into three groups: A (grossly resected tumor with microscopic

residual disease), B (involved regional nodes completely resected with no microscopic residual disease), and C (involved regional nodes completely resected with microscopic residual disease). Group III is defined by biopsy only or incomplete resection with gross residual disease. Group IV includes distant metastatic disease (excluding regional nodes and invasion of adjacent organs).

Thus, the current COG-STS risk stratification accounts for the stage, group, and histology and reflects a rapidly decreasing failure-free survival at 5 years from 90% with the low-risk (subset 1) disease to less than 30% with the high-risk disease (Table 27.13) [30].

27.5.3 Clinical Management

Multimodality therapy is most often indicated for rhabdomyosarcoma. In regards to chemotherapy regimen, treatment protocols including COG ARST 0331, COG ARST 0431, COG ARST 0531, and EpSSG 2005 have been utilized with regimens that vary based on risk stratification [30, 31]. Chemotherapy precedes localized therapy and typically includes vincristine, actinomycin, and cyclophosphamide or ifosfamide. As the site of disease often presents challenges for safe resection in RMS, radiotherapy often is the primary local therapy for low-risk

Table 27.13   COG-STS risk stratification.

Risk	Stage	Group	Histology
Low (subset 1)	1, 2	I, II	Embryonal
	1	III orbit	
Low (subset 2)	1	III non-orbit	Embryonal
	3	I, II	
Intermediate	2,3	III	Embryonal
	1,2,3	I, II, III	alveolar
High	4	IV	Embryonal, alveolar

and intermediate-risk RMS. However, in the case of planned surgical resection, radiotherapy could be used pre- or postoperatively. Surgical planning varies widely with the location of the primary disease.

In regards to radiotherapy, proton therapy has been studied mainly in retrospective series at single institutions since 2007 table 27.14. As reflected in the table below, the median dose to the primary site varies by disease site. Highlighting the single phase II trial from Massachusetts General Hospital, which started accrual in 2004 from MGH and in 2010 from MD Anderson Cancer Center, patients with low- and intermediate-risk RMS from a variety of sites underwent neoadjuvant chemotherapy followed by local therapy (proton therapy, with or without gross total surgical resection) (Table 27.14) [32].

Table 27.14   Clinical experiences utilizing particle therapy for rhabdomyosarcoma.

Publication	Number of patients	Median RT dose GyRBE (range)	Disease site (non-CNS)	Outcomes
Timmermann et al. [33]	16	50 (46–61.2)	Head and neck, parameningeal, paraspinal, pelvic	LC in 12 patients at 1.5 years median follow-up All 4 patients with failure of LC died of tumor recurrence
Cotter et al. [34]	7	36–50.4	Pelvic (bladder/prostate)	LC in 5 patients at 27-month median follow-up
Childs et al. [35]	17	50.4 (50.4–56.0)	Parameningeal	5-year FFS 59% 5-year OS 64%
Ladra et al. [32] Phase II trial	57	50.4 (36–50.4)	Head and neck, perineal, biliary, bladder/prostate, extremities, chest/abdomen, perianal	5-year EFS 69% 5-year LC 78% 5-year OS 81%
Fukushima et al. [36]	5	47.7 (41.4–50.4)	Genitourinary/Pelvic	100% OS at median 36-month follow-up
Mizumoto et al. [37]	55	50.4 (36–60)	Head and neck, parameningeal, prostate, other	1-year OS 91.1% 2-year OS 84.8% Grade 3+ radiation induced toxicities 16%
Vogel et al. [6]	35	50.4 (36.0–59.4)	Head and neck	1-year FFLR 84% 1-year FFRR 85% 1-year FFDR 95% 1-year OS 96%
Buszek et al. [38]	19	50.4 (36.0–50.51)	Bladder/Prostate	5-year OS 76% 5-year PFS 76% 5-year LC 76%
Indelicato et al. [39]	31	50.4	Pelvic	5-year LC 83% 5-year PFS 80% 5-year OS 84%

(Continued)

Table 27.14 (Continued)

Publication	Number of patients	Median RT dose GyRBE (range)	Disease site (non-CNS)	Outcomes
Ludmir et al. [31]	46	50.4 (36–50.8)	Head and neck	5-year OS 76% 5-year PFS 57% 5-year LC 84%
Bradley et al. (2020) [40]	24	50.4 (41.4–59.4)	Parameningeal alveolar	3-year LC 66% 3-year RC 94% 3-year DFS 40% 3-year OS 58%
Buszek et al.[41]	94	50.4 (36.0–50.8)	Orbit, head and neck, GU including bladder and prostate, biliary, parameningeal, trunk, extremity	4-year LC 85% 4-year PFS 63% 4-year OS 71%

27.5.3.1 Toxicities

In the phase II trial evaluating proton therapy, there were no acute or late grade 4 toxicities [32]. There were acute grade 3 odynophagia in 10% of patients treated for parameningeal and or head and neck sites attributable to radiotherapy, as well as 9% of patients overall who experienced grade 3 radiation dermatitis. There was one patient with acute grade 3 mucositis. These all resolved without prolonged weight loss or infectious complications. Seven percent of patients developed late grade 3 toxicity including unilateral cataract, chronic otitis, and retinopathy ($n = 3$ patients had either an orbital or parameningeal disease site) [32]. There was an incidence of about 28% late grade 2 toxicities, including endocrine dysfunction, facial hypoplasia, dry eye, and unilateral hearing loss not requiring intervention. One patient who underwent limb sparing surgery and RT had grade 2 muscular atrophy. There were no secondary malignancies reported.

The retrospective series otherwise did not report any radiation attributable acute or late grade 4 toxicities [6,31,34–39, Bradley, 2020].

A notable finding in children with pelvic masses (such as prostate location or abutting the bladder) from the publication by Indelicato et al. was that exploratory surgery to address persistent mass or thickened bladder wall after radiotherapy was the most common source of serious toxicity [39]. For this reason, urologic exploration for such findings par-ticularly after definitive treatment benefits from multidisciplinary discussion as exploration may be associated with toxicity.

27.5.3.2 Active Clinical Trials

Current clinical trials for rhabdomyosarcoma are described in Table 27.15.

27.5.4 Treatment Planning

27.5.4.1 Volume Construction

The University of Florida approach to treatment and planning is described in Table 27.16:

27.5.5 Case

The following clinical case is a 22-month-old boy with intermediate-risk pelvic RMS, stage III (T2bN0M0), Group 3 as biopsy only, treated by VAC chemotherapy per D9803. Given the timing of the patient's diagnosis and chemotherapy initiation, MR imaging was not performed before the start of chemotherapy; hence, a CT was used to determine pre-chemotherapy extent of disease. The panels above show the CT at time of diagnosis with simulation images below.

Table 27.15 Active clinical trials utilizing particle therapy for rhabdomyosarcoma.

Title	Sponsor	Status	Clinical trial identifier
A Phase II Trial of Proton RT for the Treatment of Pediatric Rhabdomyosarcoma	Massachusetts General Hospital	Active, recruiting	NCT00592592
Combination Chemotherapy with or Without Temsirolimus in Treating Patients with Intermediate Risk Rhabdomyosarcoma (ARST1431)	National Cancer Institute	Recruiting	NCT02567435

Table 27.16   Recommended target volumes and radiation doses for rhabdomyosarcoma.

Volume	Definitive	Postoperative	Dose (GyRBE)
GTV1	Visible gross tumor consisting of the *pre-chemotherapy* and *presurgical* mass defined by MR (T1, T2, FLAIR, etc.) and other imaging	Visible gross tumor consisting of the *pre-chemotherapy* and *presurgical* mass defined by MR (T1, T2, FLAIR, etc.) and other imaging	
CTV1	1. GTV1+ 1 cm respecting anatomic barriers that limit tumor spread (*exception*: For embryonal orbital tumors: GTV + 5 mm) AND 2. Tissue that harbored gross disease that now has no visible gross disease (specifically bone or other "infiltrated" tissues) AND 3. Any lymph nodes that were clinically or pathologically involved with tumor	1. GTV1+ 1 cm respecting anatomic barriers that limit tumor spread AND 2. Tissue that harbored gross disease that now has no visible gross disease and postoperative bed (not including the scar or operative tract, unless felt to be at risk) AND 3. Any lymph nodes that were clinically or pathologically involved with tumor	36

For patients if the total dose will exceed 36 Gy

Volume	Definitive	Postoperative	Dose (GyRBE)		
GTV2	Visible gross tumor in the lymphatics consisting of the residual post-chemotherapy mass defined by MR (T1, T2, FLAIR, etc.), CT, and PET	Visible gross tumor in the lymphatics consisting of the residual post-chemotherapy mass defined by MR (T1, T2, FLAIR, etc.), CT, and PET			
CTV2	1. GTV2+ 1 cm respecting anatomic barriers that limit tumor spread	1. GTV-L+ 5 mm respecting anatomic barriers that limit tumor spread	**Total doses are dependent on group and risk**		
				Fusion negative	**Fusion positive**
			Group I	No RT	36 Gy
			Group II	36 Gy	36 Gy
			Group III	50.4 Gy	50.4 Gy

Note: PTV expansions are isotropic (3 mm for CNS, skull base, and head and neck; 5 mm for remainder of disease sites). *Resected lymph nodes receive a dose of 41.4 Gy, while unresected nodes receive a dose of 50.4 Gy.

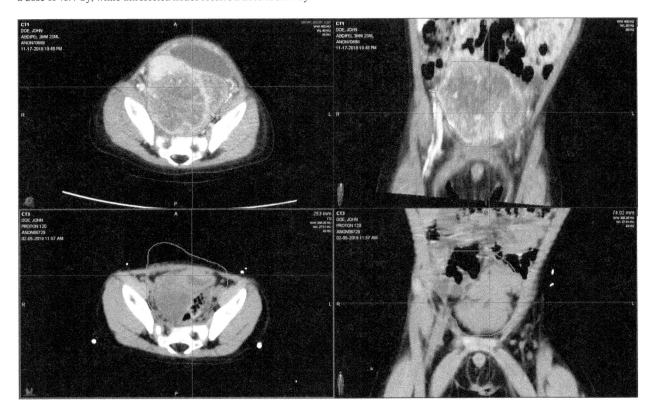

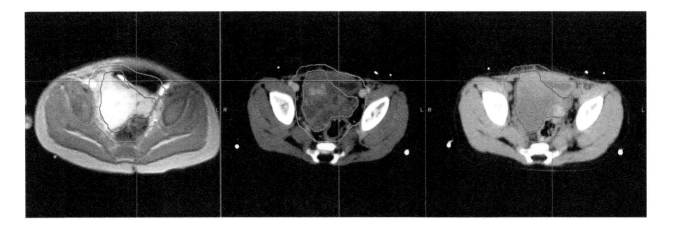

Representative axial slices from MR at time of simulation, CT with contrast, and CT simulation (left to right) are shown below. GTV is delineated in red and CTV1 in pink. For these sites, bladder reproducibility should be assessed. Ultrasound or CBCT represent ways to confirm setup, and establishing a protocol for bladder volume with anesthesia is a useful setup maneuver to assure reproducibility.

References

1 Siegel, R.L., Miller, K.D., and Jemal, A. (2020). Cancer statistics, 2020 CA. *A Cancer Journal for Clinicians* 70 (1): 7–30.

2 De Álava, E., Lessnick, S.L., and Stamenkovic, I. (2020). Ewing sarcoma. In: *The WHO Classification of Tumours Editorial Board*, 5th e (ed. WHO Classification of Tumours Soft Tissue and Bone Tumours), 323–325. Lyon: IARC Press.

3 Choi, J.H. and Ro, J.Y. (2021). *The 2020 WHO Classification of Tumors of Bone*. Publish Ahead of Print.

4 Sbaraglia, M., Righi, A., Gambarotti, M., and Dei Tos, A.P. (2019). Ewing sarcoma and Ewing-like tumors. *Virchows Archiv : An International Journal of Pathology* 476 (1): 109–119.

5 Campbell, K.M., Shulman, D.S., Grier, H.E., and DuBois, S.G. (2020). Role of bone marrow biopsy for staging new patients with Ewing sarcoma: A systematic review. *Pediatric Blood & Cancer* 68: 2.

6 Vogel, J., Both, S., Kirk, M., et al. (2018). Proton therapy for pediatric head and neck malignancies. *Pediatric Blood & Cancer* 65 (2): e26858-.

7 Nakao, T., Fukushima, H., Fukushima, T., et al. (2018). Interinstitutional patient transfers between rapid chemotherapy cycles were feasible to utilize proton beam therapy for pediatric Ewing sarcoma family of tumors. *Reports of Practical Oncology & Radiotherapy* 23 (5): 442–450.

8 Kharod, S.M., Indelicato, D.J., Rotondo, R.L., et al. (2019). Outcomes following proton therapy for Ewing sarcoma of the cranium and skull base. *Pediatric Blood & Cancer* 67: 2.

9 Uezono, H., Indelicato, D.J., Rotondo, R.L., et al. (2020). Treatment outcomes after proton therapy for Ewing sarcoma of the pelvis. *International Journal of Radiation Oncology*Biology*Physics* 107 (5): 974–981.

10 Rombi, B., DeLaney, T.F., MacDonald, S.M., et al. (2012). Proton radiotherapy for pediatric Ewing's sarcoma: Initial clinical outcomes. *International Journal of Radiation Oncology*Biology*Physics* 82 (3): 1142–1148.

11 Hoppe, B.S., Flampouri, S., Zaiden, R., et al. (2014). Involved-node proton therapy in combined modality therapy for Hodgkin lymphoma: Results of a phase 2 study. *International Journal of Radiation Oncology*Biology*Physics* 89 (5): 1053–1059.

12 Hoppe, B., Hill-Kayser, C., Tseng, Y., et al. (2017). Consolidative proton therapy after chemotherapy for patients with Hodgkin lymphoma. *Annals of Oncology* 28 (9): 2179–2184.

13 Hoppe, B.S., Vega, R.B.M., Mendenhall, N.P., et al. (2020). Irradiating residual disease to 30 Gy with proton therapy in pediatric mediastinal Hodgkin lymphoma. *International Journal of Particle Therapy* 6 (4): 11–16.

14 Wray, J., Flampouri, S., Slayton, W., et al. (2016). Proton therapy for pediatric Hodgkin lymphoma. *Pediatric Blood & Cancer* 63 (9): 1522–1526.

15 Specht, L., Yahalom, J., Illidge, T., et al. (2014). Modern radiation therapy for Hodgkin lymphoma: Field and dose

guidelines from the International Lymphoma Radiation Oncology Group (ILROG). *International Journal of Radiation Oncology*Biology*Physics* 89 (4): 854–862.

16 Dove, A.P., Manole, B., Wakefield, D.V., et al. (2018). Managing local-regional failure in children with high-risk neuroblastoma: A single institution experience. *Pediatric Blood & Cancer* 65 (12): e27408-.

17 Liu, K.X., Naranjo, A., Zhang, F.F., et al. (2020). Prospective evaluation of radiation dose escalation in patients with high-risk neuroblastoma and gross residual disease after surgery: A report from the Children's Oncology Group ANBL0532 study. *JCO* 38 (24): 2741–2752.

18 Hosaka, S., Fukushima, H., Nakao, T., et al. (2020). Patient transfer to receive proton beam therapy during intensive multimodal therapy is safe and feasible for patients with newly diagnosed high-risk neuroblastoma. *Journal of Pediatric Hematology/Oncology* 42 (1): e18–e24.

19 Lim, P., Pica, A., Hrbacek, J., et al. (2020). Pencil beam scanning proton therapy for paediatric neuroblastoma with motion mitigation strategy for moving target volumes. *Clinical Oncology* 32 (7): 467–476.

20 Bagley, A.F., Grosshans, D.R., Philip, N.V., et al. (2019). Efficacy of proton therapy in children with high-risk and locally recurrent neuroblastoma. *Pediatric Blood & Cancer* 66 (8).

21 Hill-Kayser, C.E., Tochner, Z., Li, Y., et al. (2019). Outcomes after proton therapy for treatment of pediatric high-risk neuroblastoma. *International Journal of Radiation Oncology*Biology*Physics* 104 (2): 401–408.

22 Hishiki, T., Matsumoto, K., Ohira, M., et al. (2018). Results of a phase II trial for high-risk neuroblastoma treatment protocol JN-H-07: A report from the Japan Childhood Cancer Group Neuroblastoma Committee (JNBSG). *International Journal of Clinical Oncology* 23 (5): 965–973.

23 Oshiro, Y., Mizumoto, M., Okumura, T., et al. (2013). Clinical results of proton beam therapy for advanced neuroblastoma. *Radiation Oncology* 8 (1): 142-.

24 Hill-Kayser, C., Tochner, Z., Both, S., et al. (2013). Proton versus photon radiation therapy for patients with high-risk neuroblastoma: The need for a customized approach. *Pediatric Blood & Cancer* 60 (10): 1606–1611.

25 Hattangadi, J.A., Rombi, B., Yock, T.I., et al. (2012). Proton radiotherapy for high-risk pediatric neuroblastoma: Early outcomes and dose comparison. *International Journal of Radiation Oncology*Biology*Physics* 83 (3): 1015–1022.

26 Kaste, S.C., Fuller, C.E., Saharia, A., Neel, M.D., Rao, B.N., and Daw, N.C. (2006). Pediatric surface osteosarcoma: Clinical, pathologic, and radiologic features Pediatr. *Blood Cancer* 47 (2): 152–162.

27 Smeland, S., Bielack, S.S., Whelan, J., et al. (2019). Survival and prognosis with osteosarcoma: Outcomes in more than 2000 patients in the EURAMOS-1 (European and American Osteosarcoma Study) cohort. *European Journal of Cancer* 109: 36–50.

28 Goorin, A.M., Schwartzentruber, D.J., Devidas, M., et al. (2003). Presurgical chemotherapy compared with immediate surgery and adjuvant chemotherapy for nonmetastatic osteosarcoma: Pediatric Oncology Group study POG-8651. *JCO* 21 (8): 1574–1580.

29 Ciernik, I.F., Niemierko, A., Harmon, D.C., et al. (2011). Proton-based radiotherapy for unresectable or incompletely resected osteosarcoma. *Cancer* 117 (19): 4522–4530.

30 Malempati, S. and Hawkins, D.S. (2012). Rhabdomyosarcoma: Review of the Children's Oncology Group (COG) soft-tissue Sarcoma committee experience and rationale for current COG studies. *Pediatric Blood & Cancer* 59 (1): 5–10.

31 Ludmir, E.B., Grosshans, D.R., McAleer, M.F., et al. (2019). Patterns of failure following proton beam therapy for head and neck rhabdomyosarcoma. *Radiotherapy and Oncology* 134: 143–150.

32 Ladra, M.M., Szymonifka, J.D., Mahajan, A., et al. (2014). Preliminary results of a phase II trial of proton radiotherapy for pediatric rhabdomyosarcoma. *JCO* 32 (33): 3762–3770.

33 Timmermann, B., Schuck, A., Niggli, F., et al. (2007). Spot-scanning proton therapy for malignant soft tissue tumors in childhood: First experiences at the Paul Scherrer Institute. *International Journal of Radiation Oncology*Biology*Physics* 67 (2): 497–504.

34 Cotter, S.E., Herrup, D.A., Friedmann, A., et al. (2011). Proton radiotherapy for pediatric bladder/prostate rhabdomyosarcoma: Clinical outcomes and dosimetry compared to intensity-modulated radiation therapy. *International Journal of Radiation Oncology*Biology*Physics* 81 (5): 1367–1373.

35 Childs, S.K., Kozak, K.R., Friedmann, A.M., et al. (2012). Proton radiotherapy for parameningeal rhabdomyosarcoma: Clinical outcomes and late effects. *International Journal of Radiation Oncology*Biology*Physics* 82 (2): 635–642.

36 Fukushima, H., Fukushima, T., Sakai, A., et al. (2015). Tailor-made treatment combined with proton beam therapy for children with genitourinary/pelvic rhabdomyosarcoma. *Reports of Practical Oncology & Radiotherapy* 20 (3): 217–222.

37 Mizumoto, M., Murayama, S., Akimoto, T., et al. (2018). Preliminary results of proton radiotherapy for pediatric rhabdomyosarcoma: A multi-institutional study in Japan. *Cancer Medicine* 7 (5): 1870–1874.

38 Buszek, S.M., Ludmir, E.B., Grosshans, D.R., et al. (2019). Patterns of failure and toxicity profile following proton beam therapy for pediatric bladder and prostate rhabdomyosarcoma. *Pediatric Blood & Cancer* 66 (11).

39 Indelicato, D.J., Rotondo, R.L., Krasin, M.J., et al. (2020). Outcomes following proton therapy for group III pelvic rhabdomyosarcoma. *International Journal of Radiation Oncology*Biology*Physics* 106 (5): 968–976.

40 Bradley, J.A., Indelicato, D.J., Uezono, H., et al. (2020). Patterns of Failure in Parameningeal Alveolar Rhabdomyosarcoma. *International Journal of Radiation Oncology Biology Physics* 107(2): 325-333. doi: 10.1016/j. ijrobp.2020.01.035. Epub 2020 Feb 7. PMID: 32044412.

41 Buszek, S.M., Ludmir, E.B., Grosshans, D.R., et al. (2021). Disease control and patterns of failure after proton beam therapy for rhabdomyosarcoma. *International Journal of Radiation Oncology*Biology*Physics* 109 (3): 718–725.

Index

Note: Page numbers are followed by *f* indicates figure and *t* indicates table respectively.

Principles and Practice of Particle Therapy, First Edition. Edited by Timothy D. Malouff and Daniel M. Trifiletti.
© 2022 John Wiley & Sons Ltd. Published 2022 by John Wiley & Sons Ltd.